# Faust's
# Anesthesiology Review

# Faust's Anesthesiology Review

## *Sixth Edition*

EDITED BY:

**Terrence L. Trentman, MD**
Professor and Chair Emeritus
Department of Anesthesiology and
Perioperative Medicine
Mayo Clinic
Phoenix, Arizona

ASSOCIATE EDITORS:
**Brantley D. Gaitan, MD**
Assistant Professor of Anesthesiology
Department of Anesthesiology and
Perioperative Medicine
Mayo Clinic
Phoenix, Arizona

**Bhargavi Gali, MD**
Associate Professor
Department of Anesthesiology and
Perioperative Medicine
Mayo Clinic
Rochester, Minnesota

**Rebecca L. Johnson, MD**
Professor of Anesthesiology
Department of Anesthesiology and
Perioperative Medicine
Mayo Clinic
Rochester, Minnesota

**J. Ross Renew, MD**
Associate Professor
of Anesthesiology
Department of Anesthesiology and
Perioperative Medicine
Mayo Clinic
Jacksonville, Florida

**Jeffrey T. Mueller, MD**
Assistant Professor of Anesthesiology
Department of Anesthesiology and
Perioperative Medicine
Mayo Clinic
Phoenix, Arizona

**Toby N. Weingarten, MD**
Professor of Anesthesiology
Department of Anesthesiology and
Perioperative Medicine
Mayo Clinic
Rochester, Minnesota

ELSEVIER

Elsevier
1600 John F. Kennedy Blvd.
Ste 1800
Philadelphia, PA 19103-2899

FAUST'S ANESTHESIOLOGY REVIEW, SIXTH EDITION

ISBN: 978-0-323-87916-3

---

**Notice**

Practitioners and researchers must always rely on their own experience and knowledge in evaluating and using any information, methods, compounds, or experiments described herein. Because of rapid advances in the medical sciences, in particular, independent verification of diagnoses and drug dosages should be made. To the fullest extent of the law, no responsibility is assumed by Elsevier, authors, editors, or contributors for any injury and/or damage to persons or property as a matter of product liability, negligence or otherwise, or from any use or operation of any methods, products, instructions, or ideas contained in the material herein.

---

*Content Strategist:* Kayla Wolfe
*Content Development Specialist:* Kristen Helm
*Publishing Services Manager:* Shereen Jameel
*Project Manager:* Beula Christopher
*Design Direction:* Bridget Hoette

Printed in India

Last digit is the print number:  9  8  7  6  5  4  3  2  1

*To the memory of my mother, Wynefred Trentman,*
*whose unwavering love and support made*
*so many good things possible.*

# CONTRIBUTORS

**Arnoley S. Abcejo, MD**
Assistant Professor of Anesthesiology
Department of Anesthesiology and Perioperative Medicine
Mayo Clinic
Rochester, Minnesota

**Devon Aganga, MD**
Assistant Professor
Departments of Anesthesiology and Pediatrics
Mayo Clinic
Rochester, Minnesota

**Chelsea Camba Alfafara, MD**
Anesthesiologist
Department of Anesthesiology and Perioperative Medicine
Mayo Clinic
Phoenix, Arizona

**Wesley L. Allen, MD**
Assistant Professor of Anesthesiology
Department of Anesthesiology
Mayo Clinic Florida
Jacksonville, Florida

**Adam W. Amundson, MD**
Assistant Professor of Anesthesiology and Perioperative
   Medicine
Department of Anesthesiology
Mayo Clinic
Rochester, Minnesota

**Alexandra L. Anderson, MD**
Assistant Professor
Department of Anesthesiology and Perioperative Medicine
Mayo Clinic Rochester
Rochester, Minnesota

**Alberto E. Ardon, MD, MPH**
Anesthesiologist
Department of Anesthesiology and Perioperative Medicine
Mayo Clinic Florida
Jacksonville, Florida

**Sarah K. Armour, MD**
Assistant Professor
Department of Anesthesiology
Mayo Clinic
Rochester, Minnesota

**Trygve K. Armour, MD**
Resident
Department of Anesthesiology and Perioperative Medicine
Mayo Clinic Rochester
Rochester, Minnesota

**Christopher Bailey, MD**
Interventional Pain Physician
Pain Institute of Southern Arizona
Tucson, Arizona

**Lindsay Barendrick, MD**
Resident Anesthesiologist
Department of Anesthesiology
Mayo Clinic Arizona
Phoenix, Arizona

**Ross Barman, DO**
Resident Physician
Department of Anesthesiology
Mayo Clinic
Rochester, Minnesota

**William Brian Beam, MD**
Assistant Professor
Department of Anesthesiology and Perioperative Medicine
Mayo Clinic
Rochester, Minnesota

**Markus A. Bendel, MD**
Consultant
Department of Anesthesiology
Mayo Clinic
Rochester, Minnesota

**Layne M. Bettini, MD, JD**
Instructor
Department of Anesthesiology and Perioperative Medicine
Mayo Clinic
Phoenix, Arizona

**Megan Hamre Blackburne, MD**
Anesthesiologist
Department of Anesthesiology
Comprehensive Anesthesia Care, PC
Chesterfield, Missouri

**Patrick B. Bolton, MD**
Assistant Professor
Department of Anesthesiology
Mayo Clinic
Phoenix, Arizona

**Sherri A. Braksick, MD**
Assistant Professor of Neurology
Department of Neurology
Mayo Clinic
Rochester, Minnesota

**Kaitlyn Brennan, DO, MPH**
Assistant Professor
Department of Anesthesiology Critical Care Medicine
Vanderbilt University
Nashville, Tennessee

**Marcus Bruce, MD**
Anesthesiology Resident
Department of Anesthesiology
Mayo Clinic Arizona
Phoenix, Arizona

**Sorin J. Brull, MD, FCARCSI (Hon)**
Professor Emeritus, Consultant
Department of Anesthesiology and Perioperative Medicine
Mayo Clinic Florida
Jacksonville, Florida

**Jason M. Buehler, MD**
Assistant Professor
Department of Anesthesiology
University of Tennessee, Knoxville
Knoxville, Tennessee

**David M. Buric, MD**
Instructor of Anesthesiology
Department of Anesthesiology and Perioperative Medicine
Mayo Clinic Florida
Jacksonville, Florida

**Nicholas Canzanello, DO**
Division of Pain Medicine
Mayo Clinic
Rochester, Minnesota

**Paul E. Carns, MD**
Anesthesiologist
Department of Anesthesiology
Mayo Clinic
Rochester, Minnesota

**Ryan Chadha, MD**
Assistant Professor
Department of Anesthesiology and Perioperative Medicine
Mayo Clinic Florida
Jacksonville, Florida

**Andrew N. Chalupka, MD, MBA**
Assistant Professor of Anesthesiology
Department of Anesthesiology and Perioperative Medicine
Mayo Clinic
Rochester, Minnesota

**Jonathan E. Charnin, MD**
Consultant
Department of Anesthesiology
Mayo Clinic
Assistant Professor of Anesthesiology
Mayo Clinic College of Medicine
Rochester, Minnesota

**Thomas J. Christianson, MD**
Assistant Professor
Department of Anesthesiology
University of Tennessee Medical Center
Knoxville, Tennessee

**Frances Chung, MBBS, MD, FRCPC**
Professor
Department of Anesthesiology
University of Toronto
Toronto, Ontario, Canada

**Kathryn Clark, MB, BCh, BAO**
Physician
Department of Anesthesiology and Perioperative Medicine
Mayo Clinic
Rochester, Minnesota

**Steven R. Clendenen, MD**
Professor of Anesthesiology
Department of Anesthesiology
Mayo Clinic
Jacksonville, Florida

**Daniel J. Cole, MD**
Professor of Clinical Anesthesiology
Department of Anesthesiology
Ronald Reagan UCLA Medical Center
Los Angeles, California

**Rachel Corbitt, MD**
Anesthesiologist Resident
Department of Anesthesiology and Perioperative Medicine
Mayo Clinic
Rochester, Minnesota

**Stephen Covington, DO**
Consultant
Department of Anesthesiology
Mayo Clinic Arizona
Phoenix, Arizona

**Robert M. Craft, MD**
Professor of Anesthesiology
Department of Anesthesiology
The University of Tennessee Graduate School of Medicine
Knoxville, Tennessee

**Ryan C. Craner, MD**
Assistant Professor of Anesthesiology
Division of Cardiovascular and Thoracic Anesthesiology
Department of Anesthesiology and Perioperative Medicine
Mayo Clinic
Phoenix, Arizona

**Ryan S. D'Souza, MD**
Interventional Pain Physician, Director of Neuromodulation
Department of Anesthesiology and Pain Medicine
Mayo Clinic Hospital
Rochester, Minnesota

**Benjamin T. Daxon, MD**
Assistant Professor of Anesthesiology
Department of Anesthesiology and Perioperative Medicine
Mayo Clinic
Rochester, Minnesota

**Martin L. De Ruyter, MD, MS, FASA**
Professor
Department of Anesthesiology
Kansas University Medical Center
Kansas City, Kansas

**Onur Demirci, MD**
Assistant Professor of Anesthesiology
Department of Anesthesiology and Perioperative Medicine
Mayo Clinic
Rochester, Minnesota

**Peter A. DeSocio, DO, MBA, CPE, FASA**
Director
UH East Anesthsia Services
Department of Anesthesiology
The Ohio State University Wexner Medical Center
Columbus, Ohio

**John A. Dilger, MD**
Associate Professor of Anesthesiology and Perioperative
   Medicine
Department of Anesthesiology and Perioperative Medicine
Mayo Clinic
Rochester, Minnesota

**Sarah E. Dodd, MD**
Assistant Professor
Department of Anesthesiology and Perioperative Medicine
Mayo Clinic
Rochester, Minnesota

**Gifty A. Dominah-Agyemang, MD**
Department of Anesthesia and Critical Care Medicine
The Johns Hopkins University
Baltimore, Maryland

**Karen B. Domino, MD, MPH**
Professor and Vice Chair for Clinical Research
Department of Anesthesiology and Pain Medicine
University of Washington
Seattle, Washington

**Brian S. Donahue, MD, PhD**
Professor of Anesthesiology and Pediatrics
Department of Anesthesiology
Monroe Carell Jr Children's Hospital at Vanderbilt
Nashville, Tennessee

**Catalina Dumitrascu, MS, MD**
Assistant Professor
Department of Anesthesiology
Mayo Clinic
Phoenix, Arizona

**Tyler Dunn, MD**
Anesthesiologist
Department of Anesthesiology and Perioperative Medicine
Mayo Clinic
Phoenix, Arizona

**Holly B. Ende, MD, MS**
Associate Professor
Department of Anesthesiology
Vanderbilt University Medical Center
Nashville, Tennessee

**Kirstin M. Erickson, MD**
Assistant Professor of Anesthesiology
Department of Anesthesiology and Perioperative Medicine
Mayo Clinic College of Medicine
Rochester, Minnesota

**Jennifer L. Fang, MD, MS**
Associate Professor of Pediatrics
Department of Pediatric and Adolescent Medicine
Division of Neonatal Medicine
Mayo Clinic
Rochester, Minnesota

**Amanda R. Fields, MD**
Physician
Department of Anesthesiology
Mayo Clinic
Rochester, Minnesota

**James Y. Findlay, MB, ChB**
Consultant
Department of Anesthesiology and Perioperative Medicine
Mayo Clinic
Rochester, Minnesota

**Roseanne M. Fischoff, MPP**
Center for Perioperative Medicine
Executive Director
American Society of Anesthesiologists
Schaumburg, Illinois

**Randall Paul Flick, MD, MPH**
Professor
Departments of Anesthesiology and Pediatrics
Mayo Clinic
Rochester, Minnesota

**Tarrah Folley, MD**
Anesthesiologist
Department of Anesthesia
Mayo Clinic Phoenix
Phoenix, Arizona

**Robert J. Friedhoff, MD**
Assistant Professor of Anesthesiology
Department of Anesthesiology and Perioperative Medicine
Mayo Clinic
Rochester, Minnesota

**Ashley V. Fritz, DO**
Assistant Professor of Anesthesiology
Department of Anesthesiology and Perioperative Medicine
Mayo Clinic
Jacksonville, Florida

**Brantley D. Gaitan, MD**
Assistant Professor of Anesthesiology
Department of Anesthesiology and Perioperative Medicine
Mayo Clinic
Phoenix, Arizona

**Jonathan Gal, MD, MBA, MS, FASA**
Assistant Professor, Anesthesiology
Department of Anesthesiology, Perioperative, and Pain Medicine
Icahn School of Medicine at Mount Sinai
**System Medical Director,** Facility Revenue Integrity and
    Optimization
**System Medical Director,** Offsite Ambulatory Surgery Centers
    Anesthesia
Mount Sinai Health System
New York, New York

**Rosemarie E. Garcia Getting, MD**
Associate Member
Department of Anesthesiology
H. Lee Moffitt Cancer Center and Research Institute
Associate Professor
Department of Oncologic Sciences
University of South Florida
Tampa, Florida

**Halena M. Gazelka, MD**
Professor of Anesthesiology and Perioperative Medicine
Division of Pain Medicine
Mayo Clinic
Rochester, Minnesota

**Adrian W. Gelb, MBChB, FRCPC**
Professor
Department of Anesthesia and Perioperative Care
University of California, San Francisco
San Francisco, California

**James A. Giacalone, PhD, MS, BS**
Lecturer
Department of Biology
Humboldt State University
Arcata, California

**Nigel Gillespie, MD**
Anesthesiologist
Department of Anesthesiology and Perioperative Medicine
Mayo Clinic Florida
Jacksonville, Florida

**Michael D. Godbold, MD**
Assistant Professor
Department of Anesthesiology
University of Tennessee
Knoxville, Tennessee

**Andrew Gorlin, MD**
Anesthesiologist
Department of Anesthesiology
Mayo Clinic Arizona
Phoenix, Arizona

**Mark Grant, MD, PhD**
Senior Methodologist
Department of Analytics and Research Services
American Society of Anesthesiologists
Schaumburg, Illinois
Adjunct Assistant Professor
Division of Epidemiology and Biostatistics
University of Illinois at Chicago School of Public Health
Chicago, Illinois

**Roy A. Greengrass, MD, FRCP**
Professor of Anesthesiology
Department of Anesthesiology and Perioperative Medicine
Mayo Clinic College of Medicine
Jacksonville, Florida

**Benjamin Fredrick Gruenbaum, MD, PhD**
Assistant Professor
Department of Anesthesiology and Perioperative Medicine
Mayo Clinic
Jacksonville, Florida

**Shaun Evan Gruenbaum, MD, PhD**
Associate Professor
Department of Anesthesiology and Perioperative Medicine
Mayo Clinic
Jacksonville, Florida

**Lindsay Royce Hunter Guevara, MD**
Assistant Professor of Anesthesiology
Department of Anesthesiology and Perioperative Medicine
Mayo Clinic
Rochester, Minnesota

**Patrick J. Guffey, MD, MHA**
Associate Professor
Department of Anesthesiology
University of Colorado
Denver, Colorado
Chief Medical Information Officer
Children's Hospital Colorado
Aurora, Colorado

**Carmelina Gurrieri, MD**
Assistant Professor of Anesthesiology
Department of Anesthesia
Mayo Clinic Health System
Eau Claire, Wisconsin

**Dawit T. Haile, MD**
Assistant Professor of Anesthesiology
Department of Anesthesiology
Mayo Clinic
Rochester, Minnesota

**Brian A. Hall, MD**
Assistant Professor
Mayo Clinic Department of Anesthesiology
Mayo Clinic
Rochester, Minnesota

**Kathryn S. Handlogten, MD**
Assistant Professor of Anesthesiology
Department of Anesthesiology and Perioperative Medicine
Mayo Clinic
Rochester, Minnesota

**James D. Hannon, MD**
Assistant Professor of Anesthesiology, Central Division
    Chair
Department of Anesthesiology and Perioperative Medicine
Mayo Clinic
Rochester, Minnesota

**Daniel A. Hansen, MD**
Anesthesiologist
Reno, Nevada

**Barry A. Harrison, MBBS, FRACP, FANZCA**
Assistant Professor
Department of Anesthesiology and Perioperative Medicine
Mayo Clinic Florida
Jacksonville, Florida

**Molly M.H. Herr, MD**
Instructor
Department of Anesthesiology and Perioperative Medicine
Mayo Clinic
Rochester, Minnesota

**Denzil R. Hill, MD**
Instructor of Anesthesiology
Department of Anesthesiology and Perioperative Medicine
Mayo Clinic
Rochester, Minnesota

**Ryan E. Hofer, MD**
Assistant Professor of Anesthesiology
Department of Anesthesiology and Perioperative Medicine
Mayo Clinic
Rochester, Minnesota

**Terese Toddie Horlocker, MD**
Professor of Anesthesiology and Orthopaedics
Department of Anesthesiology and Perioperative Medicine
Mayo Clinic
Rochester, Minnesota

**Frances Hu, MD**
Consultant
Department of Anesthesiology and Perioperative Medicine
Mayo Clinic
Phoenix, Arizona

**Christine L. Hunt, DO, MS**
Assistant Professor
Department of Pain Medicine
Mayo Clinic
Jacksonville, Florida

**Timothy J. Ingall, MB BS, PhD**
Co-Director
Clinical Ethics Program
Mayo Clinic Arizona
Phoenix, Arizona

**Michael G. Ivancic, MD**
Anesthesiologist
Department of Anesthesiology
St. Luke's East Anesthesia Services
Lee's Summit, Missouri

**Malinporn Jampong, MD**
Department of Medicine
Golden Jubilee Medical Center
Faculty of Medicine Siriraj Hospital
Mahidol University, Phutthamonthon
Nakhon Pathom, Thailand

**Michael E. Johnson, MD, PhD**
Assistant Professor
Department of Anesthesiology and Perioperative Medicine
Mayo Clinic College of Medicine
Rochester, Minnesota

**Rebecca L. Johnson, MD**
Professor of Anesthesiology
Department of Anesthesiology and Perioperative Medicine
Mayo Clinic
Rochester, Minnesota

**Matthew Johnston, MD**
Resident Physician
Department of Anesthesiology and Perioperative Medicine
Mayo Clinic
Rochester, Minnesota

**Nycole K. Joseph, MD**
Vascular Neurology Fellow
Department of Neurology
Mayo Clinic
Jacksonville, Florida

**Marissa L. Kauss, MD**
Assistant Professor
Department of Anesthesiology
Mayo Clinic
Rochester, Minnesota

**Melissa Kenevan, MD**
Physician
Department of Pain Medicine
Mayo Clinic Health System
Eau Claire, Wisconsin

**Mitchell Kerfeld, MD**
Assistant Professor of Anesthesiology
Department of Anesthesiology and Perioperative Medicine
Mayo Clinic
Rochester, Minnesota

**Narjeet Khurmi, MD**
Anesthesiologist
Department of Anesthesiology and Perioperative Medicine
Medical Director
Perioperative and Surgical Services
Mayo Clinic Arizona
Phoenix, Arizona

**Michelle A. Ochs Kinney, MD**
Assistant Professor of Anesthesiology and Perioperative
    Medicine
Department of Anesthesiology and Perioperative Medicine
Mayo Clinic
Rochester, Minnesota

**Allan M. Klompas, MB, BCh, BAO**
Assistant Professor
Department of Anesthesiology and Laboratory Medicine and
    Pathology
Mayo Clinic
Rochester, Minnesota

**Helga Komen, MD**
Assistant Professor of Anesthesiology
Department of Anesthesiology
Washington University in St. Louis School of Medicine
St Louis, Missouri

**Suneerat Kongsayreepong, MD**
Professor in Anesthesiology
Department of Anesthesiology
Siriraj Hospital, Mahidol University
Bangkok, Thailand

**Sandra L. Kopp, MD**
Professor
Department of Anesthesiology
Mayo Clinic
Rochester, Minnesota

**Benjamin T. Kor, MD**
Consultant
Department of Anesthesiology and Perioperative Medicine
Mayo Clinic
Rochester, Minnesota

**Todd M. Kor, MD**
Consultant
Department of Anesthesiology and Perioperative Medicine
Mayo Clinic
Rochester, Minnesota

**Sarang S. Koushik, MD**
Assistant Professor, Pain Clinic Director
Department of Anesthesiology
Valleywise Health Medical Center
Creighton University School of Medicine
Phoenix, Arizona

**Molly B. Kraus, MD**
Associate Professor
Department of Anesthesiology
Mayo Clinic Hospital
Phoenix, Arizona

**Beth L. Ladlie, MD, MPH**
Assistant Professor
Department of Anesthesiology and Perioperative Medicine
Mayo Clinic Florida
Jacksonville, Florida

**Tim J. Lamer, MD**
Professor of Anesthesiology
Department of Anesthesiology and Perioperative Medicine
Mayo Clinic
Rochester, Minnesota

**Brendan J. Langford, MD**
Resident Physician
Department of Anesthesiology
Mayo Clinic
Rochester, Minnesota

**Micah T. Long, MD**
Assistant Professor
Department of Anesthesiology
University of Wisconsin School of Medicine and Public Health
Madison, Wisconsin

**Timothy R. Long, MD**
Professor of Anesthesiology
Department of Anesthesia and Perioperative Medicine
Mayo Clinic
Rochester, Minnesota

**Christopher V. Maani, MD**
Vice Chair of Quality
Department of Anesthesiology
San Antonio Military Medical Center (SAMMC)
Fort Sam Houston, Texas
Vice Chair of Safety
Department of Anesthesiology
San Antonio Uniformed Services Health Education
    Consortium (SAUSHEC)
San Antonio, Texas
Associate Professor
Department of Anesthesiology
Uniformed Services University of Health Sciences
Bethesda, Texas
Associate Professor
Department of Anesthesiology
University of Texas Health Science Center San Antonio
San Antonio, Texas

**Shawn Malan, MD**
Resident Physician
Department of Anesthesiology and Perioperative Medicine
Mayo Clinic
Phoenix, Arizona

**Jillian Maloney, MD**
Assistant Professor, Consultant
Department of Anesthesiology
Mayo Clinic
Phoenix, Arizona

**Megan N. Manento, MD**
Assistant Professor of Anesthesiology
Department of Anesthesiology
Division of Critical Care Medicine
Mayo Clinic
Rochester, Minnesota

**Carlos B. Mantilla, MD, PhD**
Professor and Chair
Department of Anesthesiology and Perioperative Medicine
Professor
Department of Physiology and Biomedical Engineering
Mayo Clinic
Rochester, Minnesota

**Archer Kilbourne Martin, MD**
Chair
Division of Cardiovascular and Thoracic Anesthesiology
Mayo Clinic
Associate Professor of Anesthesiology
Mayo Clinic College of Medicine and Science
Jacksonville, Florida

**David P. Martin, MD, PhD**
Professor of Anesthesiology
Department of Anesthesiology and Perioperative Medicine
Mayo Clinic
Rochester, Minnesota

**Yvette N. Martin McGrew, MD, PhD**
Assistant Professor
Department of Anesthesiology
Mayo Clinic
Rochester, Minnesota

**Stephanie C. Mavis, MD**
Assistant Professor of Pediatrics
Department of Pediatric and Adolescent Medicine
Mayo Clinic
Rochester, Minnesota

**Robert L. McClain, MD**
Assistant Professor of Anesthesiology
Department of Anesthesiology and Perioperative Medicine
Mayo Clinic
Jacksonville, Florida

**Patrick O. McConville, MD, FASA**
Associate Professor
Chair
Department of Anesthesiology
The University of Tennessee Graduate School of Medicine
Knoxville, Tennessee

**Patrick J. McCormick, MD, MEng**
Associate Attending
Department of Anesthesiology and Critical Care Medicine
Memorial Sloan Kettering Cancer Center
Associate Professor of Clinical Anesthesiology
Department of Anesthesiology
Weill Cornell Medical College
New York, New York

**K.A. Kelly McQueen, MD, MPH, FASA**
Chair and Professor
Department of Anesthesiology
University of Wisconsin–Madison
Madison, Wisconsin
Professor
Department of Anesthesiology and Surgery
Vanderbilt University Medical Center
Nashville, Tennessee

**Ellen C. Meltzer, MD, MSc**
Medical Director
Office of Experience,
Co-Director
Clinical Ethics Program
Mayo Clinic Arizona
Phoenix, Arizona
Director of Performance Improvement
Office of Clinical Ethics
Mayo Clinic Rochestor
Rochester, Minnesota
Consultant
General Internal Medicine
Mayo Clinic Arizona
Scottsdale, Arizona

**Sharon K. Merrick, MS, CCS-P**
Past Director of Payment and Practice Management
American Society of Anesthesiologists
Washington, District of Columbia

**Gregory James Mickus, MD**
Cardiothoracic Anesthesiologist
Baptist Medical Center
Jacksonville, Florida

**Adam J. Milam, MD, PhD**
Associate Professor of Anesthesiology
Department of Anesthesiology and Perioperative Medicine
Mayo Clinic
Phoenix, Arizona

**Lopa Misra, DO**
Assistant Professor
Department of Anesthesiology and Perioperative Medicine
**Vice Chair of Admissions**
Mayo Clinic Alix School of Medicine
Mayo Clinic
Phoenix, Arizona

**Susan Moeschler, MD**
**Professor of Anesthesiology and Perioperative Medicine**
Mayo Clinic
Rochester, Minnesota

**Rajat N. Moman, MD, MA**
Pain and Spine Centers of Florida
Leesburg, Florida

**Monica Myers Mordecai, MD**
Assistant Professor
Department of Anesthesiology
Mayo Clinic Florida
Jacksonville, Florida

**Steven T. Morozowich, DO, FASE, FASA**
Assistant Professor
Division of Cardiovascular and Thoracic Anesthesiology
Mayo Clinic
Phoenix, Arizona

**Jeffrey T. Mueller, MD**
**Assistant Professor of Anesthesiology**
Department of Anesthesiology and Perioperative Medicine
Mayo Clinic
Phoenix, Arizona

**David R. Mumme, MD**
Anesthesiologist
Indiana University Health
Indianapolis, Indiana

**Andrew Murray, MBChB**
Consultant
Department of Anesthesiology and Perioperative Medicine
Mayo Clinic Arizona
Phoenix, Arizona

**Julian Naranjo, DO**
**Assistant Professor of Anesthesiology**
Department of Anesthesiology and Perioperative Medicine
Mayo Clinic
Rochester, Minnesota

**Michael E. Nemergut, MD, PhD**
Assistant Professor
Departments of Anesthesiology and Pediatrics
Mayo Clinic
Rochester, Minnesota

**Reka Nemes, MD, PhD**
**Consultant in Anesthesiology and Intensive Care**
Department of Anesthesiology and Intensive Care
University of Debrecen
Debrecen, Hungary

**Wayne T. Nicholson, MD, PharmD**
Consultant
Department of Anesthesiology and Perioperative Medicine
Mayo Clinic
Rochester, Minnesota

**Adam D. Niesen, MD**
Assistant Professor
Department of Anesthesiology and Perioperative Medicine
Mayo Clinic
Rochester, Minnesota

**Sindhuja R. Nimma, MD**
**Instructor of Anesthesiology**
Department of Anesthesiology and Perioperative Medicine
Mayo Clinic
Jacksonville, Florida

**Catherine Wanjiru Njathi-Ori, MD**
Assistant Professor
Department of Anesthesiology and Perioperative Medicine
Mayo Clinic
Rochester, Minnesota

**Oludare O. Olatoye, MD**
**Interventional Pain Physician**
Director of Inpatient Pain Service
Department of Anesthesiology and Pain Medicine
Rochester, Minnesota

**David Olsen, MD**
**Assistant Professor of Anesthesiology**
Department of Anesthesiology and Perioperative Medicine
Mayo Clinic
Rochester, Minnesota

**Sher-Lu Pai, MD**
**Director, Preoperative Evaluation Clinic**
Department of Anesthesiology and Perioperative Medicine
Mayo Clinic
Jacksonville, Florida

**Jason K. Panchamia, DO**
**Director**
Preoperative Evaluation Clinic
Department of Anesthesiology and Perioperative Medicine
Mayo Clinic
Rochester, Minnesota

**Jeffrey J. Pasternak, MS, MD**
**Professor of Anesthesiology**
Department of Anesthesiology and Perioperative Medicine
Mayo Clinic
Rochester, Minnesota

**Richard K. Patch III, MD**
**Assistant Professor of Anesthesiology and Medicine**
Department of Anesthesiology
Division of Critical Care Medicine
Mayo Clinic
Rochester, Minnesota

**Perene V. Patel, MD**
**Assistant Professor of Anesthesiology**
Department of Anesthesiology and Perioperative Medicine
Mayo Clinic
Phoenix, Arizona

**Roxann Barnes Pike, MD**
**Assistant Professor**
Department of Anesthesiology and Perioperative Medicine
Mayo Clinic College of Medicine
Rochester, Minnesota

**Jordan S. Pogu, MD**
**Resident Physician**
Department of Anesthesiology and Perioperative Medicine
Mayo Clinic
Rochester, Minnesota

**Rochelle J. Pompeian, MD**
**Assistant Professor of Anesthesiology**
Department of Anesthesiology and Perioperative Medicine
Mayo Clinic
Rochester, Minnesota

**Matthew Thomas Popovich, PhD**
**Quality and Regulatory Affairs Executive**
Department of Quality and Regulatory Affairs
American Society of Anesthesiologists
Washington, District of Columbia

**Steven B. Porter, MD**
**Assistant Professor**
Department of Anesthesiology and Perioperative Medicine
Mayo Clinic
Jacksonville, Florida

**Karl A. Poterack, MD**
**Associate Professor**
Department of Anesthesiology and Perioperative Medicine
Mayo Clinic College of Medicine
Phoenix, Arizona

**Bridget P. Pulos, MD**
**Assistant Professor**
Department of Anesthesiology and Perioperative Medicine
Mayo Clinic
Rochester, Minnesota

**Misty A. Radosevich, MD**
**Assistant Professor**
Department of Anesthesiology and Critical Care
Mayo Clinic
Rochester, Minnesota

**Harish Ramakrishna, MD, FACC, FESC, FASE**
**Professor**
Department of Anesthesiology
Mayo Clinic College of Medicine
Rochester, Minnesota

**Manoch Rattanasompattikul, MD, FASN**
Department of Medicine
Golden Jubilee Medical Center
Faculty of Medicine Siriraj Hospital
Mahidol University, Phutthamonthon
Nakhon Pathom, Thailand

**Gwendolyn Raynor, MD**
**Senior Associate Consultant**
Department of Anesthesiology and Perioperative Medicine
Mayo Clinic Arizona
Phoenix, Arizona

**Kent H. Rehfeldt, MD, FACC, FASE**
**Associate Professor of Anesthesiology**
Department of Anesthesiology
Mayo Clinic
Rochester, Minnesota

**J. Ross Renew, MD**
**Associate Professor of Anesthesiology**
Department of Anesthesiology and Perioperative Medicine
Mayo Clinic
Jacksonville, Florida

**Mariana Restrepo-Holguin, MD**
**Anesthesiology Resident**
Department of Anesthesiology and Perioperative Medicine
Mayo Clinic
Rochester, Minnesota

**Edwin H. Rho, MD**
**Consultant**
Department of Anesthesiology
Mayo Clinic
Rochester, Minnesota

**Juan G. Ripoll, MD**
**Mayo Clinic Scholar**
Department of Anesthesiology and Perioperative Medicine
Mayo Clinic
Rochester, Minnesota

**Kevin T. Riutort, MD, MS**
**Assistant Professor**
Department of Anesthesiology and Perioperative Medicine
Mayo Clinic Florida
Jacksonville, Florida

**Sara B. Robertson, MD**
**Associate Professor**
Department of Anesthesiology
Division of Pediatric Anesthesiology
University of Mississippi Medical Center
Jackson, Mississippi

**Kip D. Robinson, MD**
**Assistant Professor**
Department of Anesthesia
University of Tennessee
Knoxville, Tennessee

**Eduardo S. Rodrigues, MD**
Assistant Professor
Department of Anesthesiology
Mayo Clinic
Jacksonville, Florida

**Adam Paul Roth, MD**
Assistant Professor
Department of Anesthesiology
The University of Tennessee Graduate School of Medicine
Knoxville, Tennessee

**Vanessa Salcedo, MPH**
Associate Director of Payment and Practice Policy
American Society of Anesthesiologists
Schaumberg, Illinois

**Rebecca A. Sanders, MD**
Physician
Institute of Pain Management
Freeman Health System
Joplin, Missouri

**Troy G. Seelhammer, MD**
Assistant Professor of Anesthesiology
Department of Anesthesiology and Perioperative Medicine
Mayo Clinic
Rochester, Minnesota

**Leal G. Segura, MD**
Assistant Professor
Department of Anesthesiology
Mayo Clinic Rochester
Rochester, Minnesota

**Anna Bovill Shapiro, MD**
Senior Associate Consultant
Department of Anesthesiology and Perioperative Medicine
Mayo Clinic Florida
Jacksonville, Florida

**Emily E. Sharpe, MD**
Assistant Professor of Anesthesiology
Department of Anesthesiology and Perioperative Medicine
Mayo Clinic
Rochester, Minnesota

**Yu Shi, MD, MPH**
Assistant Professor in Anesthesiology
Department of Anesthesiology and Perioperative Medicine
Mayo Clinic
Rochester, Minnesota

**Eric R. Simon, MD**
Assistant Professor
Department of Anesthesiology
University of Wisconsin School of Medicine and Public Health
Madison, Wisconsin

**Mandeep Singh, MBBS, MD, MSc, FRCPC**
Associate Professor
Department of Anesthesia and Pain Management
University of Toronto
Toronto, Ontario, Canada

**Nathan J. Smischney, MD, MSc**
Associate Professor
Department of Anesthesiology
Mayo Clinic
Rochester, Minnesota

**Bradford B. Smith, MD**
Assistant Professor of Anesthesiology
Department of Anesthesiology and Perioperative Medicine
Mayo Clinic
Phoenix, Arizona

**J. Robert Sonne, JD, BA**
Legal Counsel
Legal Department
Mayo Clinic
Scottsdale, Arizona

**Wolf H. Stapelfeldt, MD**
Chief of Anesthesiology Services
Department of Anesthesiology
Richard L. Roudebush VA Medical Center
Professor of Anesthesia
Department of Anesthesia
Indiana University School of Medicine
Indianapolis, Indiana

**Chris Steel, MD**
Inpatient Chief Medical Officer
Department of Administration
White River Health System
Chief Medical Consultant
E1 Precision Consulting
Batesville, Arkansas
Director of Anesthesia Services
Department of Anesthesiology
Jefferson Regional Medical Center
Pine Bluff, Arkansas

**Thomas M. Stewart, MD**
Assistant Professor of Anesthesiology
Department of Anesthesiology and Perioperative Medicine
Mayo Clinic
Rochester, Minnesota

**Hans P. Sviggum, MD**
Associate Professor of Anesthesiology
Department of Anesthesiology
Mayo Clinic
Rochester, Minnesota

**Heidi A. Tavel, MD, FASA**
Physician Anesthesiologist
Old Pueblo Anesthesia
Tucson, Arizona

**Brian J. Thomas, JD**
**Vice President, Risk Management**
Preferred Physicians Medical
Overland Park, Kansas

**Daniel Thum, MD**
**Clinical Assistant Professor**
Department of Surgery
University of South Dakota, Sanford School of Medicine
Sioux Falls, South Dakota

**Christopher A. Thunberg, MD**
**Assistant Professor of Anesthesiology**
Department of Anesthesiology and Perioperative Medicine
Mayo Clinic
Phoenix, Arizona

**Klaus D. Torp, MD**
**Assistant Professor**
Department of Anesthesiology
Mayo Clinic Florida
Jacksonville, Florida

**Ali Akber Turabi, MD**
Department of Pain
Medstar Good Samaritan
Baltimore, Maryland

**Kristen Vanderhoef, MD**
**Assistant Professor**
Department of Anesthesiology
University of Florida Jacksonville
Saint Johns, Florida

**Michael Vega, MD**
**Associate Professor**
Department of Anesthesiology and Perioperative Medicine
Oregon Health and Science University
Portland, Oregon

**Ricardo Verdiner, MD**
**Assistant Professor**
Mayo Clinic
Phoenix, Arizona

**Amy G. Voet, DO, MS, BS**
**Department of Anesthesiology**
St. Joseph Eureka
Eureka, California

**Elizabeth R. Vogel, MD, PhD**
**Anesthesiologist**
Department of Anesthesiology and Perioperative Medicine
Mayo Clinic
Rochester, Minnesota

**Matthew N. Vogt, MD**
**Assistant Professor**
Department of Anesthesiology and Perioperative Medicine
Mayo Clinic
Rochester, Minnesota

**Robalee L. Wanderman, MD**
Rochester, Minnesota

**R. Doris Wang, MD**
**Consultant**
Department of Anesthesiology and Perioperative Medicine
Mayo Clinic Florida
Jacksonville, Florida

**Lindsay Warner, MD**
**Anesthesiologist**
Department of Anesthesiology
Mayo Clinic
Rochester, Minnesota

**Matthew A. Warner, MD**
**Associate Professor of Anesthesiology**
Department of Anesthesiology and Perioperative Medicine
Mayo Clinic
Rochester, Minnesota

**Paul A. Warner, MD**
**Assistant Professor**
Department of Anesthesiology
Mayo Clinic
Rochester, Minnesota

**Edward J. Washington, MD**
**Instructor in Anesthesiology**
Department of Anesthesiology and Perioperative Medicine
Mayo Clinic Arizona
Phoenix, Arizona

**Kelli C. Watson, MD, MPH**
**Anesthesiology Resident**
Department of Anesthesiology and Perioperative Medicine
Mayo Clinic
Rochester, Minnesota

**Toby N. Weingarten, MD**
**Professor of Anesthesiology**
Department of Anesthesiology and Perioperative Medicine
Mayo Clinic
Rochester, Minnesota

**Ricardo Weis, MD**
**Assistant Professor of Anesthesiology**
Division of Cardiovascular and Thoracic Anesthesiology
Department of Anesthesiology and Perioperative Medicine
Mayo Clinic
Phoenix, Arizona

**Tasha L. Welch, MD**
**Assistant Professor**
Department of Anesthesiology and Perioperative Medicine
Mayo Clinic
Rochester, Minnesota

**Carson C. Welker, MD**
Assistant Professor of Anesthesiology
Department of Anesthesiology and Perioperative Medicine,
    Division of Critical Care
Mayo Clinic
Rochester, Minnesota

**Christopher Wie, MD**
Consultant
Department of Anesthesiology
Mayo Clinic Arizona
Phoenix, Arizona

**Erica D. Wittwer, MD, PhD**
Associate Professor of Anesthesiology
Department of Anesthesiology and Perioperative Medicine
Mayo Clinic
Rochester, Minnesota

**Katherine Wochos, MPPA, CAE (past)**
AQI Director of Operations
Anesthesia Quality Institute
American Society of Anesthesiologists
Schaumburg, Illinois

**Risa L. Wolk, MD**
Assistant Professor
Department of Anesthesiology and Pain Medicine
University of Washington
Seattle, Washington

**Ashley V. Wong Grossman, MD**
Pediatric Anesthesia Fellow
Department of Anesthesiology and Perioperative Medicine
Mayo Clinic
Rochester, Minnesota

**Jason M. Woodbury, MD**
Assistant Professor of Anesthesiology
Department of Anesthesiology and Perioperative Medicine
Mayo Clinic
Rochester, Minnesota

**Suraj M. Yalamuri, MD**
Assistant Professor of Anesthesiology
Department of Anesthesiology
Mayo Clinic
Rochester, Minnesota

**Tonia M. Young-Fadok, MD, MS, FACS, FASCRS**
Professor of Surgery
Mayo Clinic College of Medicine
Chair
Division of Colon and Rectal Surgery
Mayo Clinic
Phoenix, Arizona

**Soojie Yu, MD**
Assistant Professor, Senior Associate Consultant
Department of Anesthesiology
Mayo Clinic
Phoenix, Arizona

**Kaiying Zhang, MD**
Assistant Professor
Department of Anesthesiology
University of Utah
Salt Lake City, Utah

# PREFACE

As of this writing (Fall '23), it has been 32 years since I began my career in anesthesia. As it happens, my first anesthesiology attending was Dr. Ronald Faust. At the time, Dr. Faust was the Program Director of the Mayo Clinic Rochester Anesthesiology residency, and in addition, that same year he published the 1st edition of Anesthesiology Review. Dr. Faust's textbook was designed to be a rapid review for anesthesia providers, and the chapter topics were based on the "key words" from the annual in-training exam for anesthesiology residents.

After my first month of anesthesia training, my second attending was Dr. Leslie Milde, one of the Associate Editors of the 1st edition of Faust. She succeeded Dr. Faust as the Program Director in Rochester and later became Chair of the Anesthesiology Department at Mayo Clinic Arizona, where she kindly recruited me to the staff a few years later. I mention these historical notes only to point out how frequently we are influenced by mentors, and how often we are indebted to them.

I know I speak for our current associate editors when I say it is a great pleasure to present the 6th edition of *Faust's Anesthesiology Review*. This book represents the efforts of hundreds of authors, many of whom are current or former anesthesiology trainees and staff at the Mayo Clinic. Without their dedication and the hard work of our associate editors and the team at Elsevier, this book would not be possible.

Since the last edition, much has changed in anesthesia and the world. The Covid pandemic has ended yet subvariants persist, and a land war continues to rage in Europe. Further, each day brings more news of the impact of climate change on our planet. Simultaneously, medical knowledge accumulates faster than ever, and computer learning / AI become more common. Now more than ever we need well-informed anesthesia providers to address these challenges and opportunities.

In addition to updating topics that have always been important to the field of anesthesiology, this edition includes information on the current pandemic and guidance on how to prepare for the next one. We've added thoughts on sustainability and invite every anesthesia provider to consider what they can do to stem the tide of global warming.

It is with gratitude that I look back on teachers and mentors like Drs. Faust and Milde, and it is with confidence that I look forward to our future as both a medical specialty and as a human family that can face and overcome the challenges that are so prominent today.

I, along with the associate editors, thank you for investing your time and resources in this textbook. We are confident it will make you a more knowledgeable and prepared provider, ultimately bringing about the best possible outcomes for our patients. Finally, as always, we look for opportunities to improve our work. Please feel free to contact me directly with comments or suggestions at the email address below.

Terrence L. Trentman, MD
Editor-in-Chief
*Faust's Anesthesiology Review*
trentman.terrence@mayo.edu

# CONTENTS

## SECTION XIII
## Risk Management   715

## SECTION XIV
## Practice Management   749

# SECTION I

# Operating Room, Equipment, and Monitoring

# 1

# Medical Gas Supply

MARTIN L. DE RUYTER, MD, MS, FASA

Medical gases most common to anesthesia include oxygen ($O_2$), nitrous oxide ($N_2O$), and air. Less frequently used medical gases include helium (He), nitrogen ($N_2$), and carbon dioxide ($CO_2$), but there has been a recent surge in the use of $CO_2$ secondary to the advancement of laparoscopic and robotic procedures. Several governing bodies regulate medical gases, but the containment and delivery of these gases via a medical gas cylinder system are controlled via standards set by the U.S. Department of Transportation. Medical gas cylinders are the foundation for central pipeline supply of gases to the operating room (OR) and hospital. Additionally, a cylinder system (typically the smaller E cylinders) exists in the OR as a backup for unanticipated failure of the central pipeline supply.

Medical gas cylinders store compressed gas. Cylinder sizes and thus capacity vary and traditionally have been designated by letters, with "A" being the smallest and "H" being the largest (most commonly). The new naming system begins with the letter "M" to signify "medical" gas, and the number that follows is the capacity of the cylinder expressed as cubic feet (Table 1.1). Most clinicians remain familiar with older nomenclature, and that will be used in this chapter. H cylinders are large-capacity storage containers that typically provide the central pipeline supply of medical gas that is piped into the OR. E cylinders are smaller, portable, and are the most commonly encountered cylinders in the OR. A typical anesthesia machine will have an attachment for two ($O_2$ and $N_2O$) or three (two $O_2$ and one $N_2O$) E cylinders. E cylinders are also commonly used to supply $O_2$ to patients during transport. Cylinders are color coded according to the gas they contain. Unfortunately, there is no global agreement, and the colors in the United States are not the same as those accepted internationally. Table 1.2 lists the common medical gases, the cylinder capacity, the color of the cylinders, and the state (liquid/gas) under which medical gases are stored.

Based on their physical properties, at ambient temperature when gases are compressed and stored in cylinders, they will either liquefy or remain in a gas state. When stored at ambient temperature in medical cylinders, compressed $O_2$, He, and air remain in a gas state. In contrast, $N_2O$ stored in the same conditions becomes a liquid. Knowledge of the state of gases in these cylinders as either liquid or nonliquid allows one to estimate the amount of gas that remains in a cylinder as it is being consumed. Pressure gauges on cylinders will decrease in a linear proportion as the vaporized gas is consumed. For example, an E cylinder filled with $O_2$ contains approximately 660 L of nonliquid $O_2$ gas at a pressure of approximately 2000 pounds per square inch gauge (psig). When the gauge reads 1000 psig, approximately 330 L of $O_2$ remain. One can, therefore, estimate how long before an oxygen cylinder will empty when delivering gas at a certain flow rate. An equation to estimate the time remaining is as follows:

$$\text{Approximate remaining time (h)} = \frac{O_2 \text{ cylinder pressure (psi)}}{200 \times O_2 \text{ flow rate (L/min)}}$$

The volume remaining in a cylinder of liquid gases, such as $N_2O$, cannot be estimated in the same manner. The pressure gauge of the $N_2O$ cylinder reads the pressure of the small amount of vapor above the liquid. As gas is consumed, more gas moves from the liquid phase to the vapor phase, maintaining the vapor pressure, and the reading of the pressure gauge does not change. Only when nearly all of the liquid $N_2O$ is vaporized does the pressure start to fall. For example, a full E cylinder of $N_2O$ contains 1590 L and reads 745 psig; this pressure will remain constant until nearly all of the $N_2O$ is vaporized, at which point the pressure starts to drop. At this point, approximately 400 L of $N_2O$ remain in the cylinder. The only reliable way to estimate the volume of $N_2O$ remaining in a cylinder is to weigh the cylinder. Each cylinder is stamped with a tare weight (empty weight), and the difference between the measured weight and tare weight represents the amount of liquid gas present.

E cylinders attach directly to the anesthesia machine via a hanger-yoke assembly. This assembly orients and supports the cylinder, provides a gas-tight seal, and ensures unidirectional flow of gases into the machine. In addition, a pin index safety system has been developed as a safety measure to prevent inadvertently connecting the wrong gas cylinder to the wrong machine inlet (and thus potentially delivering a hypoxic mixture). Each gas cylinder has two holes in its cylinder valve that interface with corresponding pins in the yoke of the anesthesia machine. The positioning of the holes on the cylinder valve and the pins on the yoke are unique for each gas, and only when they align correctly will the hanger-yoke assembly properly engage (Figs. 1.1 and 1.2). This safety mechanism can be breached if the yoke pins are broken, missing, or intentionally instrumented.

Today's ORs commonly have a pipeline supply of medical gases. Large-capacity tanks, such as liquid $O_2$ storage tanks or H cylinders connected in series by a manifold, use pipes to deliver $O_2$ throughout the hospital. In the OR, these pipes connect to one of three common systems: gas columns, hose drops, or articulating arms. Color-coded hoses from the anesthesia machines with a quick-coupling mechanism and a diameter index safety system (DISS) connect to these systems. The color and DISS are specific for each gas and represent a safety mechanism to ensure proper connection and hence delivery of the desired gas (Fig. 1.3).

| TABLE 1.1 | Medical Gas Cylinders | | | | |
|---|---|---|---|---|---|
| | CYLINDER | | CAPACITY | | VALVE TYPE |
| Previous Nomenclature | New Nomenclature | ft³ | L | |
| A | M4 | 4.0 | 113 | Pin index |
| B | M6 | 7.4 | 164–210 | Pin index |
| D | M15 | 15 | 400–425 | Pin index |
| E | M24 | 24.9 | 680–704 | Pin index |
| H | M250 | 250 | 6900–7986 | Bullnose |

Medical gas is ubiquitous in health care, and safe delivery to patients is paramount. Portable devices and pipeline systems have been developed with patient safety in mind, and pin index systems and DISS serve to achieve this purpose. However, these safety measures are not flawless. Best practice would suggest that prior to exposing patients, providers should confirm that they are delivering the proper gas. In the OR, this confirmation is reaffirmed with monitors such as $O_2$ analyzers, pulse oximetry, and gas analyzers.

| TABLE 1.2 | Commonly Encountered Operating Room Medical Gases | | | | | |
|---|---|---|---|---|---|---|
| | CYLINDER CAPACITY (L) | | | TANK COLOR | | |
| Gas | E | H | Pressure (psig) at 20°C | U.S. | International | State |
| $O_2$ | 625–700 | 6000–8000 | 1800–2200 | Green | White | Gas |
| Air | 625–700 | 6000–8000 | 1800–2200 | Yellow | Black and white | Gas |
| $N_2O$ | 1590 | 15,900 | 745 | Light blue | Light blue | Liquid |
| He | 500 | 6000 | 1600 | Brown | Brown | Gas |
| $CO_2$ | 1800 | | 830 | Gray | Gray | liquid |

*psig,* Pounds per square inch gauge.

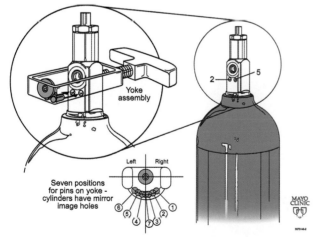

**Fig. 1.1** The pin index safety system is one of several features of medical gas cylinders that is in place to ensure that the correct cylinder is attached to the correct gas inlet in the back of the anesthesia machine. Cylinders are color coded; each cylinder has a label identifying which gas it contains, and the cylinders attach to the back of the anesthesia machine using the pin index safety system. Two pins incorporated into the yoke of the machine, just below the gas inlet, and line up with two holes on the gas cylinder, allowing only the correct cylinder to be connected to the correct inlet. (From Mayo Foundation for Medical Education and Research. All rights reserved.)

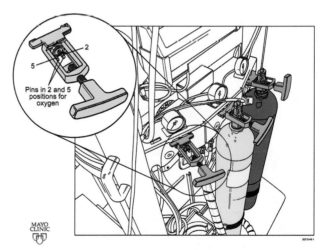

**Fig. 1.2** A close-up view of the yoke assembly in the back of the anesthesia machine. The two pins that are immediately below the gas inlet on the anesthesia machine occupy one of seven possible standardized positions. For $O_2$, the pins are in the 2 and 5 position and line up with the corresponding inlet on the $O_2$ cylinder. As the clamp on the yoke assembly is tightened, the cylinder is secured up against the gas inlet for $O_2$. If the pins line up correctly, when the valve on the cylinder is open, the correct gas will flow into the correct inlet. If the pins are *not* lined up correctly, the cylinder cannot be tightened into the yoke; no contact will be made between the gas inlet and the cylinder, and gas will not flow into the inlet. (From Mayo Foundation for Medical Education and Research. All rights reserved.)

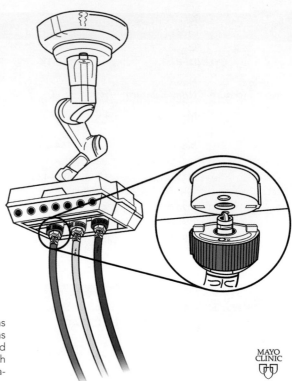

**Fig. 1.3**   Hoses, color coded for each gas, can be connected to the appropriate gas outlet with an adapter that has a diameter index safety system (DISS) unique to the gas for that outlet. The system comprises a central tube, through which the gas flows, and two small metal rectangles placed on the surface of the adapter that are unique to each gas, such that an $O_2$ hose can only be connected to an $O_2$ outlet. (From Mayo Foundation for Medical Education and Research. All rights reserved.)

MAYO
CLINIC

## SUGGESTED READINGS

Dorsch, J. A., & Dorsch, S. E. (2007). Medical gas cylinders and containers. In J. A. Dorsch, & S. E. Dorsch (Eds.), *Understanding anesthesia equipment* (5th ed., pp. 1–24). Philadelphia: Wolters Kluwer/Lippincott Williams & Wilkins.

Dorsch, J. A., & Dorsch, S. E. (2007). Medical gas pipeline systems. In J. A. Dorsch, & S. E. Dorsch (Eds.), *Understanding anesthesia equipment* (5th ed., pp. 25–50). Philadelphia: Wolters Kluwer/Lippincott Williams & Wilkins.

Ishimura, T., Ikuta, Y., & Yamamoto, T. (2016). Failure of a "foolproof" pin-index medical pipeline system. *JA Clinical Reports, 2*, 20.

Malayaman, S. N., Mychaskiw, G., II., & Ehrenwerth, J. (2013). Medical gases: Storage and supply. In J. Ehrenwerth, J. B. Eisenkraft, & J. M. Berry (Eds.), *Anesthesia equipment: Principles and applications* (2nd ed., pp. 3–24). Philadelphia: Saunders/Elsevier Inc.

# 2

# Electricity in the Operating Room

BRIAN A. HALL, MD

## Electrical Supply

Benjamin Franklin is credited with the discovery of electricity in 1752. Commercial electricity came to New York City in 1882 and subsequently became ubiquitous in the modern world. After 140 years, however, the same major hazards still exist: fire, shock, and electrocution. In the operating room (OR), all three of these must be recognized and guarded against.

All sources of electrical energy have two poles (e.g., the positive and negative ends of a dry cell battery, the terminals of a car battery, the blades of an outlet). When nothing conductive bridges the poles, the circuit is said to be "open," and electrical current does not flow through the circuit. When a conductive load is inserted between them, like a light bulb, the circuit is "closed," and electrical current flows. If a metallic conductor with little to no impedance closes the circuit, the circuit becomes "shorted," and current flows relatively unimpeded.

In health care facilities there are two types of power systems: a grounded power system (GPS) and an isolated power system (IPS). A GPS consists of a live (hot, positive) wire carrying alternating current at 120 V, a neutral (cold, negative) wire that completes the circuit by transmitting the current back to the power-generating station, and a ground (earth) wire. If a person is grounded (e.g., standing in water) and comes in contact with the hot limb, an electric shock will be delivered. Ground-fault circuit interrupters (GFCIs) are safety devices in GPS systems that "trip" (interrupt electrical flow through the circuit) if a current greater than 4 to 6 mA begins to flow between the live wire and any pathway other than the neutral wire. A GFCI reduces the chance for "macroshock" (discussed later) in a GPS, but it also causes all electrical devices sharing power from that circuit to lose power. The National Electrical Code (NEC 210.8) requires that all bathrooms, kitchens, garages, and other wet locations use GFCIs. ORs (IPS electrical systems) have similar electrical shock potential as other wet locations (residential and commercial), thus special protective provisions are mandated. In such cases, the line isolation monitor (LIM) sounds, and it is incumbent on the OR personnel to manually cut off electrical flow to the offending branch circuit because a current leak (ground fault) is detected. This is a different approach to the same hazard used in homes and businesses (the difference being a manual response vs. automatic using a GFCI). Both residential dwellings and ORs use overcurrent devices (circuit breakers or fuses) to protect against excessive current passing through a metallic conductor (cord, cable, wire) if that current exceeds the current rating of the circuit breaker (based on wire thickness or gauge).

Electricity in an IPS is supplied by a transformer that is separate from the power station electrical supply. In an IPS, both wires are "hot," and the voltage between either of the lines and the ground is zero, making the system isolated from the earth ground. Thus a person could stand in a pool of water while holding either of the wires of the circuit without receiving a shock. However, touching both wires simultaneously would deliver a shock. To reduce the likelihood of injury, the chassis of all devices should be checked by a biomedical engineer every 3 months, and current leakage cannot be greater than 300 µA.

The possibility of electric shock in the OR becomes more likely when a ground fault has occurred. This means that one side of the circuit has become grounded. This may occur, for example, when the steel collar of an electric cord has worn through to one of the electrical conductors. Because the collar is part of the steel electrical plug, which is intentionally grounded when plugged in, a ground fault will occur under these conditions. Even with a ground fault, no shock will occur unless a second fault exists.

When grounding occurs in the OR, the LIM (Fig. 2.1) will sound, alerting the OR personnel to the fact that a fault exists, so that it can be corrected. Appropriate reaction to this alarm would be to disconnect the last item connected, then the next to last, and then successively backward until the alarm stops. The threshold for activation of the LIM is about 3 to 5 mA. For this reason, the LIM offers no protection against microshock (discussed later), which can occur if the current is as low as 0.05 to 0.1 mA (50–100 µA).

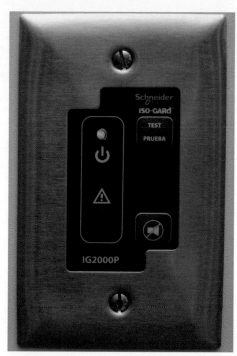

**Fig. 2.1** Example of a line isolation monitor, the ISO-GardTM IG2000 Line Isolation Monitor, Schneider Electric (Rueil-Malmaison, France). (Courtesy Brian A. Hall, Mayo Clinic.)

## Electrical Injuries

Sometimes the patient is deliberately introduced into an electrical circuit such as with a pacemaker or electrocautery. These devices are designed to limit current and to function with minimal risk to the patient when used properly; however, it is important to be familiar with the types of electrical injury that can still occur.

With electrocautery, a *thermal injury* hazard exists. Electrocautery relies on electrical current to heat a small probe that then destroys tissue in a controlled fashion. The electricity flows through the patient and exists in a large dispersive electrode (grounding pad). This dispersive electrode provides a large surface area for electrical energy returning from the patient to return to the electrical circuit without damaging tissues at the exit site. However, if the dispersive electrode pad is not firmly placed against the patient or if the conductive medium becomes dried out, the electrical current will become concentrated and may burn the skin because of the high current density ($mA/cm^2$).

*Macroshock* is what most people envision when discussing electrical shock. Macroshock is the passage of electricity through the body via external pathways. Most people have experienced a static electrical shock or a 120 volt AC shock through a frayed electrical cord. The passage of as little as 100 mA directly through the myocardium can produce ventricular fibrillation. There is also the possibility of thermal injury from high voltage even without passage through the heart.

*Microshock* can only occur when there is an electrical conductor in or on the heart, like a pacemaker lead. Because the skin, fat, bones, and other tissues (which offer significant impedance to current) are bypassed in this scenario, the current threshold for ventricular fibrillation (50–100 µA) is considerably less than with macroshock. The National Electrical Manufacturers Association has set the maximum acceptable current leakage for any device implanted on or in the heart at 10 µA.

## SUGGESTED READINGS

Barker, S. J., & Doyle, D. J. (2010). Electrical safety in the operating room: Dry versus wet. *Anesthesia and Analgesia, 110*(6), 1517–1518.

Ehrenwerth, J., Eisenkraft, J., & Berry, J. (2020). Electrical and fire safety. *Anesthesia equipment* (3rd ed., pp. 526–558). Philadelphia: Saunders.

Fish, R. M., & Geddes, L. A. (2009). Conduction of electrical current to and through the human body: A review. *Eplasty, 9,* e44.

Gropper, M. (2020). *Miller's anesthesia* (9th ed., p. 1880). Philadelphia: Elsevier.

Hemmings, H., & Egan, T. *Pharmacology and physiology for anesthesia* (2nd ed., pp. 145–173). Philadelphia: Elsevier.

Hull, C. J. (1978). Electrocution hazards in the operating theatre. *British Journal of Anaesthesia, 50,* 647–657.

Leeming, M. N. (1973). Protection of the "electrically susceptible patient": A discussion of systems and methods. *Anesthesiology, 38,* 370–383.

# 3

# Operating Room Fires

ROSEMARIE E. GARCIA GETTING, MD

With the movement away from the use of flammable anesthetic gases, the incidence of fires in the operating room (OR) has decreased. However, closed claims data analysis revealed a dramatic increase in OR fires from 1985 to 2009; most commonly, these were electrosurgery-induced fires that occurred during monitored anesthesia care with open delivery of oxygen for cases involving the upper chest, head, and neck. Several OR fire safety initiatives were launched to raise awareness of the risks of this rare, catastrophic, and largely preventable event. These fire safety education efforts may have facilitated the 44% decrease in OR fires reported in Pennsylvania from 2011 to 2018. Although the precise incidence of OR fires nationwide is difficult to determine because of a lack of mandatory reporting in all states, it is estimated that 100 OR fires continue to occur annually in the United States resulting in 1 to 2 patient deaths per year.

## Fire Triangle

For a fire to occur, three elements must come together: (1) an oxidizer, (2) fuel, and (3) an ignition source. These three elements are commonly called the "fire triad" and can be represented as a "fire triangle" (Fig. 3.1). An OR fire can be prevented by removing any one element of the triangle.

The two oxidizing agents that are most prevalent in the OR are oxygen ($O_2$) and nitrous oxide ($N_2O$). In the OR, many potential fuel sources are present (Box 3.1). The most common ignition source is electrosurgery (e.g., electrocautery); other ignition sources are listed in Box 3.1.

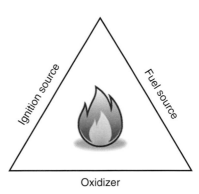

**Fig. 3.1**  The fire triangle.

## Prevention

General OR fire prevention strategies, summarized in Box 3.2, should be used in all cases and involve minimizing or avoiding oxidizer-enriched atmospheres near the surgical site and safely managing fuels and ignition sources. A useful strategy for prevention of an OR fire is identification of a high-risk procedure (e.g., a procedure in which an ignition source will be used in proximity to an oxidizer-enriched environment). The presence of an oxidizer ($O_2$ and $N_2O$) lowers the combustion threshold, decreases time to ignition, and increases the intensity of a fire. This oxidizer-enriched atmosphere exists in (and around) the patient's airway, and the risk of fire is increased in these areas (e.g., head, neck,

---

**BOX 3.1   COMPONENTS OF THE FIRE TRIANGLE**

**OXIDIZERS**

Oxygen ($O_2$)
Nitrous oxide ($N_2O$)

**FUEL**

Drapes and gowns
Alcohol-containing solutions
Tracheal tubes
Nasal cannulas
Face masks
Ventilator circuits
Patient
Intestinal gases
Blankets
Sponges and gauze
Dressings
Ointment

**IGNITION SOURCES**

Electrosurgical devices
Electrocautery devices
Lasers
Fiber-optic light sources
Defibrillators
Drills and burrs
Heated probes
Static electricity
Malfunctioning electrical devices

---

**BOX 3.2   GENERAL OPERATING ROOM FIRE PREVENTION STRATEGIES**

- Avoid or minimize an oxidizer-enriched environment close to the surgical site.
- Allow sufficient drying time of flammable skin-prepping solution, and remove any presoaked towels prior to draping.
- Configure surgical drapes to avoid trapping oxidizer-enriched gases.
- Moisten sponges and gauze that are placed near an $O_2$-enriched environment.
- Protect heat sources when not in use (e.g., laser or fiber-optic source on standby; active electrosurgical unit electrode tip in holster).

---

**BOX 3.3   TECHNIQUES TO MINIMIZE THE RISK OF FIRE IN THE OPERATING ROOM DURING HIGH-RISK PROCEDURES**

- Communicate a team plan, with assignment of individual team member roles and tasks for fire prevention and management before surgery.
- Communicate the presence of, and increases in, the oxidizer-enriched environment.
- Communicate the intent to use an ignition source before activating it.
- Before activation of an ignition source, decrease the inspired oxygen concentration as low as physiologically acceptable, as guided by pulse oximetry, and discontinue the use of nitrous oxide. Wait a period of time after discontinuation for oxidizers to dissipate from the surgical site; in closed oxygen delivery, wait until the fractions of inspired and expired oxygen are reduced to safe levels before activating the heat source. A cuffed tracheal tube (TT) should be used for airway procedures. For laser procedures, select a TT that is resistant to the type of laser being used, and ensure that the cuffs are filled with colored saline to allow detection of a perforation.
- In lieu of open oxygen delivery (i.e., via nasal cannula, face mask, high-flow nasal oxygen), consider securing the airway with a laryngeal mask airway or TT for procedures of the head, neck, and upper chest with monitored anesthesia care requiring moderate to deep sedation and/or for patients who are oxygen dependent.
- If open oxygen delivery is required, avoid using a 100% oxygen source (instead use a common gas outlet, blender, or adapter in standard breathing circuit) and keep $Fio_2 \le 0.3$.

---

and upper chest). Fire risk assessment should occur before surgery, allowing identification of high-risk procedures (i.e., tracheostomy, craniotomy under monitored anesthesia care). A number of techniques can be used to reduce fire risk during these high-risk procedures (Box 3.3).

## Preparation

The development of a multidisciplinary fire prevention and management plan is an important strategy that can minimize the risk and severity of an OR fire. It involves communication among all personnel and should begin with a team meeting before surgery (i.e., during the preoperative time-out). The meeting should focus on (1) determining whether the procedure has a high risk of fire and (2) assigning specific roles in fire prevention and specific tasks in fire management if a fire should occur. Inadequate communication is frequently cited in root cause analyses of OR fires and other serious preventable surgical events. Although communication is important at all times, it is critical in high-risk situations to minimize the risk of OR fires. In addition to daily preparation and communication, all OR patient care team members should participate in recurring (e.g., yearly) education and practice via dedicated OR fire prevention and management in-services and drills.

## Management of an Operating Room Fire

An overall strategy for management of an OR fire has been developed by the American Society of Anesthesiologists (Fig. 3.2). Once a fire is suspected, the surgical procedure should be immediately halted to allow further evaluation and, if present, all OR personnel should simultaneously execute the necessary fire management tasks depending on the location of the fire (e.g., airway vs. nonairway).

If the fire involves an airway device, ventilation and gas flows should be stopped and the airway device or any burning material should be removed immediately. Saline or water should be used to extinguish the fire. Once the fire is extinguished, a patent airway should be reestablished and ventilation resumed. Reassessment of the patient and situation should occur. Retained intraluminal fragments should be removed by bronchoscopy.

For a nonairway fire, ventilation and gas flows should be stopped. Patient drapes and all burning material should be immediately removed from the patient, and saline or other means (e.g., water or smothering) should be used to extinguish the fire. Once all burning material has been extinguished, ventilation should be resumed and reassessment of the patient and situation should occur.

If fire is not extinguished on the first attempt, a $CO_2$ fire extinguisher is recommended on second attempt. If that fails, initiate the RACE fire protocol (Rescue/evacuate patient; activate fire Alarm; Confine/close OR door; Extinguish with $CO_2$ extinguisher as you retreat and turn off gas supply to the room).

After any fire, the involved personnel should be debriefed appropriately. A review of procedural techniques, including the fire response, should also be conducted.

**OPERATING ROOM FIRES ALGORITHM**

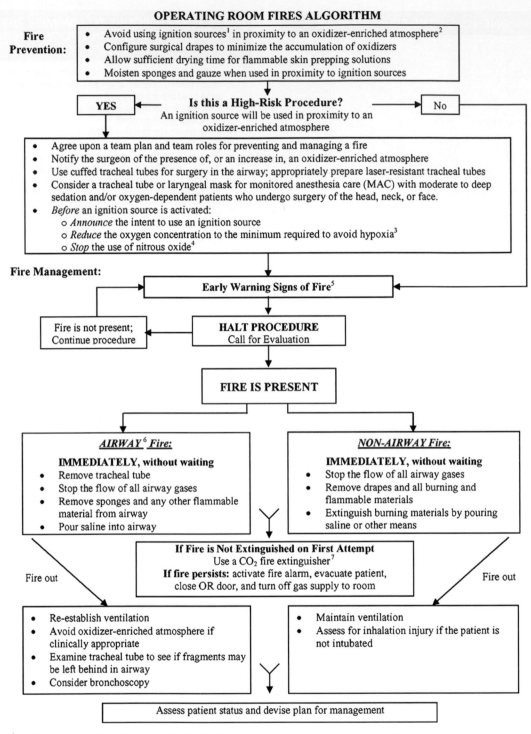

**Fire Prevention:**

- Avoid using ignition sources[1] in proximity to an oxidizer-enriched atmosphere[2]
- Configure surgical drapes to minimize the accumulation of oxidizers
- Allow sufficient drying time for flammable skin prepping solutions
- Moisten sponges and gauze when used in proximity to ignition sources

**Is this a High-Risk Procedure?**
An ignition source will be used in proximity to an oxidizer-enriched atmosphere

YES        No

- Agree upon a team plan and team roles for preventing and managing a fire
- Notify the surgeon of the presence of, or an increase in, an oxidizer-enriched atmosphere
- Use cuffed tracheal tubes for surgery in the airway; appropriately prepare laser-resistant tracheal tubes
- Consider a tracheal tube or laryngeal mask for monitored anesthesia care (MAC) with moderate to deep sedation and/or oxygen-dependent patients who undergo surgery of the head, neck, or face.
- *Before* an ignition source is activated:
  - *Announce* the intent to use an ignition source
  - *Reduce* the oxygen concentration to the minimum required to avoid hypoxia[3]
  - *Stop* the use of nitrous oxide[4]

**Fire Management:**

**Early Warning Signs of Fire[5]**

Fire is not present;
Continue procedure

**HALT PROCEDURE**
Call for Evaluation

**FIRE IS PRESENT**

*AIRWAY[6] Fire:*

**IMMEDIATELY, without waiting**
- Remove tracheal tube
- Stop the flow of all airway gases
- Remove sponges and any other flammable material from airway
- Pour saline into airway

Fire out

*NON-AIRWAY Fire:*

**IMMEDIATELY, without waiting**
- Stop the flow of all airway gases
- Remove drapes and all burning and flammable materials
- Extinguish burning materials by pouring saline or other means

Fire out

**If Fire is Not Extinguished on First Attempt**
Use a CO₂ fire extinguisher[7]
**If fire persists:** activate fire alarm, evacuate patient, close OR door, and turn off gas supply to room

- Re-establish ventilation
- Avoid oxidizer-enriched atmosphere if clinically appropriate
- Examine tracheal tube to see if fragments may be left behind in airway
- Consider bronchoscopy

- Maintain ventilation
- Assess for inhalation injury if the patient is not intubated

Assess patient status and devise plan for management

[1] Ignition sources include but are not limited to electrosurgery or electrocautery units and lasers.
[2] An oxidizer-enriched atmosphere occurs when there is any increase in oxygen concentration above room air level, and/or the presence of any concentration of nitrous oxide.
[3] After minimizing delivered oxygen, wait a period of time (*e.g.,* 1-3 min) before using an ignition source.   For oxygen dependent patients, *reduce* supplemental oxygen delivery to the minimum required to avoid hypoxia.  Monitor oxygenation with pulse oximetry, and if feasible, inspired, exhaled, and/or delivered oxygen concentration.
[4] After stopping the delivery of nitrous oxide, wait a period of time (*e.g.,* 1-3 min) before using an ignition source.
[5] Unexpected flash, flame, smoke or heat, unusual sounds (*e.g.,* a "pop," snap or "foomp") or odors, unexpected movement of drapes, discoloration of drapes or breathing circuit, unexpected patient movement or complaint.
[6] In this algorithm, airway fire refers to a fire in the airway or breathing circuit.
[7] A CO₂ fire extinguisher may be used on the patient if necessary.

**Fig. 3.2** American Society of Anesthesiologists operating room fire algorithm. (Copyright 2013, American Society of Anesthesiologists, Inc. Lippincott Williams & Wilkins. *Anesthesiology* 2013;118:271-290.)

## SUGGESTED READINGS

Anesthesia Patient Safety Foundation. (2010). *Prevention and management of operation room fires video.* Retrieved from http://www.apsf.org/safetynet/apsf-safety-videos/or-fire-safety-video/. Accessed November, 2021.

Apfelbaum, J. L., Caplan, R. A., Barker, S. J., Connis, R. T., Cowles, C., Ehrenwerth, J., et al. (2013). Practice advisory for the prevention and management of operating room fires. *Anesthesiology, 118,* 271–290.

Cowles, C., Lake, C., & Ehrenwerth, J. (2020). Surgical fire prevention: A review. *APSF Newsletter, 35,* 82–84. Retrieved from https://www.apsf.org/article/surgical-fire-prevention-a-review/. Accessed November 6, 2021.

Feldman, J., & Stoelting, R. (2010). *OR fire safety video commentary for the anesthesia professional.* Retrieved from https://www.apsf.org/videos/or-fire-safety-video/or-fire-safety-video-commentary-for-the-anesthesia-professional/. Accessed November, 2021.

Jones, T. S., Black, I. H., Robinson, T. N., & Jones, E. L. (2019). Operating room fires. *Anesthesiology, 130,* 492–501.

Mehta, S. P., Bhananker, S. M., Posner, K. L., & Domino, K. B. (2013). Operating room fires: A closed claims analysis. *Anesthesiology, 118,* 1133–1139.

Wahr, J. A. (2021). *Fire safety in the operating room.* Retrieved from https://www.uptodate.com/contents/fire-safety-in-the-operating-room. Accessed November, 2021.

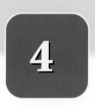

# 4

# Vaporizers

KEVIN T. RIUTORT, MD, MS  |  BARRY A. HARRISON, MBBS, FRACP, FANZCA

When a volatile anesthetic in the liquid state is added to a closed container at room temperature, it begins to evaporate into a gas (a *vapor*). As the liquid anesthetic continues to evaporate, the pressure in the container continues to increase until the liquid and vapor phases of the anesthetic reach a state of equilibrium. At this point, the vapor is said to be *saturated*, and the pressure in the container is called the *saturated vapor pressure* (SVP). If the temperature were to increase or decrease, the anesthetic would reach a new equilibrium point and the SVP would change; thus SVP is dependent on temperature but independent of ambient pressure.

At normal temperature and pressure (defined as 20°C, 1 atmosphere), volatile anesthetic agents such as halothane, isoflurane, sevoflurane, and desflurane exist as liquids (Table 4.1). However, these agents have much higher SVPs than the partial pressure needed to produce anesthesia. Thus a vaporizer is necessary to deliver clinical and safe concentrations to the patient. To illustrate this point, sevoflurane inhaled without a vaporizer delivers about *10 times* the required minimum alveolar concentration (MAC).

Although the vaporizer's output is the partial pressure of the anesthetic gas, it is expressed as a concentration (volume %).

$$\text{Volume \%} = \left( \frac{\text{Partial Pressure of Vapor}}{\text{Total Ambient Pressure}} \right) \times 100$$

## Concentrated-Calibrated Variable Bypass Vaporizers

The American Society for Testing and Materials International standard requires that all vaporizers must be placed between the

| TABLE 4.1 | Saturated Vapor Pressure, Boiling Point, and Minimum Alveolar Concentration of Inhaled Anesthetic Agents | | |
|---|---|---|---|
| Anesthetic Agent | SVP at 20°C and 1 atm | BP at 1 atm (°C) | MAC Adult (vol %) |
| Isoflurane | 238 | 48.5 | 1.15 |
| Sevoflurane | 160 | 58.5 | 1.7 |
| Desflurane | 669 | 22.8 | 6.0- 7.25 |

*BP,* boiling point; *MAC,* minimum alveolar concentration; *SVP,* saturated vapor pressure.

flowmeters and the gas outlet on the anesthesia machine, and the control dial must turn counterclockwise to increase anesthetic concentration. Modern vaporizers are (1) concentration calibrated, (2) flow-over, (3) temperature compensated, and (4) agent specific. Examples of this type of vaporizer delivering isoflurane and sevoflurane include GE Datex-Ohmeda Tec 4, Tec 5, and Tec 7; and Drager Vapor 19n, 2000, and 3000 series.

## CONCENTRATION CALIBRATED

The fresh gas flow (FGF) originates from the common gas inlet. A proportion of the FGF enters the vaporizer which contains the liquid anesthetic and exits as the carrier gas. The FGF that does not enter the vaporizer continues as the bypass gas. The ratio of the FGF entering the vaporizer to the FGF bypassing the vaporizer is called the *splitting ratio* and depends on the resistance in the two pathways (Fig. 4.1). This splitting ratio is determined by the vaporizer concentration dial.

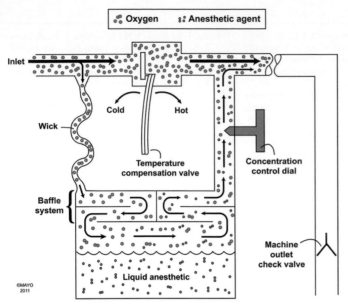

**Fig. 4.1** A schematic of a variable-bypass vaporizer. Oxygen, air, or both flow into the inlet, and a small amount is diverted into the vaporizing chamber. The concentration valve and a temperature compensation valve control the amount that is diverted. As the gas flowing through the vaporizing chamber absorbs the inhalation agent, the temperature of the liquid drops. To maintain a constant output of the inhalation agent, the temperature compensation valve diverts more gas into the vaporizing chamber. Conversely, if the room temperature were to rise (and therefore the temperature of the entire vaporizer), the valve would move to the left and less gas would be diverted into the vaporizing chamber.

## FLOW-OVER

In flow-over vaporizers the gas flow entering the vaporizer passes over the anesthetic liquid. Increasing the surface area of the carrier gas liquid interface increases the efficiency of vaporization. Baffles, spiral tracks to lengthen the gas pathway, and capillary wicks are techniques used to increase efficiency of vaporization.

## TEMPERATURE COMPENSATED

As the anesthesia liquid is vaporized, heat energy is lost. A decrease in the anesthesia liquid temperature decreases the vapor pressure and thus the partial pressure. Most concentration-calibrated vaporizers will compensate for changes in vapor pressure by using temperature-sensitive valves that increase the flow of the carrier gas through the vaporizer. In a mechanical vaporizer, a thermostatic element increases the resistance to the bypass gas flow, allowing more carrier gas through the vaporizer chamber. Other temperature-compensation techniques are computer-controlled injected and "electronic heat supply."

## AGENT SPECIFIC

The physiochemical properties of liquid anesthetics vary, thus agent-specific vaporizers are constructed and calibrated for different liquid anesthetics. For each liquid anesthetic, the vaporizer is labeled and color coded. Also, the filling of vaporizers is now anesthetic agent specific. This is achieved by using agent-specific connections between the anesthetic liquid container and the vaporizer. These connections are also usually color coded. Provided there has not been contamination of the anesthetic liquid within the container, only anesthetic that is agent specific to that vaporizer can be filled from the respective container.

## FACTORS AFFECTING VAPOR CONCENTRATION

Fresh gas flow rate and composition: Vaporizers are calibrated through a wide range of FGFs, from 250 mL/min to 15 L/min. Vaporizers are usually calibrated using 100% oxygen as the carrier gas. Substituting air for oxygen causes little change in concentration. However, adding nitrous oxide to the carrier gas usually decreases the vapor concentration, at least temporarily. Depending on the vaporizer, longer-term effects may either be increased or decreased vapor concentration.

Decreased barometric pressure (high altitude): Vaporizers are calibrated to sea level. As SVP is independent of ambient pressure, the partial pressure of the anesthetic in the carrier gas will remain the same. However, because gas density decreases with increasing altitude, the splitting ratio will change, causing a minor increase in gas concentration, but this effect on the partial pressure (and thus the clinical effect) is minimal.

Increased barometric pressure (hyperbaric chambers): In a hyperbaric chamber, or increased depth, the partial pressure of the anesthetic gas will remain the same. With an increase in depth the density will decrease, leading to a decrease in concentration; however, the partial pressure and clinical effects remain relatively unchanged. The effects of increased barometric pressure on the vaporizer function have not been extensively studied, and the results of the limited studies are possibly contradictory.

# Desflurane Vaporizer and Electronic Temperature-Regulated, Pressure-Controlled Vaporizer

Desflurane liquid anesthetic has a high SVP that is close to atmospheric pressure at room temperature. Thus a mechanical concentration-calibrated vaporizer is unsuitable; instead, an electronic temperature-regulated, pressure-controlled vaporizer is required (essentially a gas blender). The TEC 6 Plus (GE Healthcare, USA) heats the desflurane in a sealed sump to 39°C to a SVP of 1500 mm Hg. There is no carrier gas in the sump. This saturated gas is then blended into the bypass gas flow and continuously adjusted via a pressure transducer sited in the rotary valve. The concentration dial and rotary valve control the blending process, thus the gas exiting the vaporizer is the dialed-in or set concentration of desflurane. The TEC 6 Plus is calibrated using 100% oxygen. Unlike the concentration-calibrated vaporizer, the TEC 6 Plus vaporizer accurately delivers the set concentration (vol %) at different altitudes. At higher altitudes with a set concentration and a decrease in atmospheric pressure, there will be decrease in partial pressure and thus clinical effect. An increase in the set concentration is indicated. At higher ambient pressure, the opposite is correct, and a lower set concentration is indicated.

## Problems With Vaporizers

### VAPORIZER FILLING

Tipping/Overfilling: If the vaporizer is tipped onto its side, usually during positioning or if overfilled, excess anesthesia liquid may contaminate the gas bypass pathway. With subsequent use of the vaporizer, an increase concentration of anesthesia vapor may be administered to a patient. Modern vaporizers are designed to prevent overfilling.

Misfilling: Agent-specific filling connections prevent misfilling a vaporizer. However, a deliberate action may result in misfilling. If a vaporizer designed for a higher potency agent is filled with a less potent agent, it will deliver a lower anesthetic dose. Conversely, if a vaporizer designed for a lower potency agent is filled with a more potent agent, it will deliver a higher anesthetic dose.

Mislabeled: An example is an isoflurane vaporizer that is labeled "sevoflurane."

### VAPORIZER IN USE

Use of two vaporizers simultaneously: If two vaporizers are in use simultaneously, their side effects may be additive, potentially leading to hemodynamic instability. The use of interlocking devices on the anesthesia back bar prevents simultaneous use.

Vaporizer leaks: Before each case the level of liquid anesthetic in the vaporizer must be checked. There is no alarm in a regular vaporizer when a volatile anesthetic approaches empty (except the desflurane vaporizer, which has a low-level alarm).

Vaporizer not turned off: At the end of a case the vaporizer must be turned to the "off" position. This prevents inadvertent administration of the anesthetic agent to the subsequent patient.

Pumping: In older anesthesia machines the downstream ventilator or oxygen flush control caused a "pumping" effect in the anesthesia system that changed the gas flow distribution potential resulting in increased anesthesia concentration. Anesthesia machines now have one-way valves to prevent the pumping effect; the valves limits but do not eliminate this effect. The latest anesthesia machines do not have check valves but use other techniques to eliminate this problem.

## Miscellany

The American Society of Anesthesiologist guideline "Determining Anesthesia Obsolescence" (posted 2004) stated that measured flow (flowmeter-controlled) vaporizers such as the Verni-Trol ("vernitrol") and Copper Kettle had unacceptable features that made them obsolete. These included lack of serviceability, anesthesia provider knowledge, and safety features.

Nitrous oxide, cyclopropane, and xenon are examples of anesthetic gases (i.e., they are in the gaseous state at room temperature and do not require a vaporizer).

### SUGGESTED READINGS

Dorsch, J. A., & Dorsch, S. E. (2011). Vaporizers. In J. A. Dorsch, & S. E. Dorsch (Eds.), *A practical approach to anesthesia equipment* (pp. 78–107). Philadelphia: Wolters Kluwer Health / Lippincott Williams & Wilkins.

Eisenkraft, J. B. (2021). Vaporizers. In J. Ehrenwerth, J. B. Eisenkraft, & J. M. Berry (Eds.), *Anesthesia equipment: Principles and application* (pp. 66–99). St Louis, Missouri: Elsevier.

Riutort, K. T., & Eisenkraft, J. B. (2017). The anesthesia workstation and delivery systems for inhaled anesthetics. In P. G., Cullen, B. F., Stoelting, R. K., Cahalan, M. K., Stock, M. C., Ortega, R., & Holt, N. F. (Eds.), *Clinical anesthesia* (8th ed., pp. 1618–1738). Philadelphia: Wolters Kluwer.

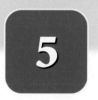

# 5

# Carbon Dioxide Absorption

PERENE V. PATEL, MD

## Carbon Dioxide Absorbers

Carbon dioxide absorbers remove carbon dioxide ($CO_2$) from circle breathing systems to avoid $CO_2$ rebreathing and hypercapnia. It allows for the use of lower fresh gas flows (FGFs) and use of less inhalation agent, thus minimizing waste. Characteristics of an ideal $CO_2$ absorbent would include a lack of reactivity with common anesthetics, absence of toxicity, low resistance to airflow, high-efficiency $CO_2$ absorption, low cost, ease of handing, and minimal dust production. The absorber canister should be easy to remove and replace, maintain breathing circuit integrity if quickly replaced during use, and have minimal risk of causing breathing system leaks or obstruction.

$CO_2$ absorber canisters should be visible and transparent to monitor for absorbent color. Modern workstations use single-canister absorbers, which are disposable and readily replaceable while maintaining circuit integrity (bypass feature). As a result, it is important to routinely inspect the absorber, as the machine may pass a leak test without the absorber attached. Changing an absorbent canister during a procedure also bypasses the leak test, and there are reports of leaks being introduced due to a damaged canister.

## Absorbent Chemistry

Most modern $CO_2$ absorbents contain calcium hydroxide [$Ca(OH)_2$], which reacts with $CO_2$ to yield calcium carbonate and water. Because $CO_2$ does not react quickly with $Ca(OH)_2$, water and small amounts of stronger base catalysts are required to speed up the reaction. Strong bases, such as sodium hydroxide (NaOH), potassium hydroxide (KOH), and barium hydroxide, are used to enhance the speed of the reaction and the capacity to absorb $CO_2$. An example of the chemical reaction is as follows:

1. $CO_2 + H_2O \leftrightharpoons H_2CO_3$
2. $H_2CO_3 + NaOH \leftrightharpoons NaHCO_3 + H_2O$
3. $NaHCO_3 + Ca(OH)_2 \leftrightharpoons CaCO_3 + H_2O + NaOH + Heat$

Absorbents with $Ca(OH)_2$ contain varying contents of water, metal hydroxide catalysts, and humectants (to prevent drying, i.e., calcium chloride). Newer absorbents have only trace amounts of NaOH or KOH because these bases are associated with anesthetic degradation. Absorbents differ in their absorptive capacity and their propensity to react with volatile anesthetics, and they produce degradation products such as carbon monoxide (CO) and compound A.

Lithium hydroxide is an alternative to $Ca(OH)_2$; it does not interact with anesthetic agents to produce either compound A or CO, and it provides an even better absorbent capacity. It does not require an additional catalyst to react with $CO_2$ and generates less heat in circle breathing circuits. Unfortunately, the cost of lithium has prohibited its widespread use.

## Interactions With Inhaled Anesthetic Agents and Formation of Degradation Products

Volatile anesthetics interact with the strong bases present in $Ca(OH)_2$-based absorbents, such as KOH and NaOH, to produce degradation products. Sevoflurane interaction with absorbents can produce compound A, which is nephrotoxic in rats. However, the data does not show an adverse effect on renal function in humans, and studies demonstrate safety at lower flow rates. The type and ratio of strong bases within the $CO_2$ absorbent affects the degree of sevoflurane degradation. KOH seems to cause more breakdown than NaOH. Newer $Ca(OH)_2$-based absorbents that are nearly free of KOH and NaOH (<2% concentration) generate negligible amounts of compound A. The sevoflurane package insert states that patient exposure should not exceed 2 minimum alveolar concentration (MAC)-hours at flow rates between 1 and 2 L/min to minimize risk from compound A. Based on the safe track record of sevoflurane and improvements in $CO_2$ absorbents, compound A poses minimal risk to patients during routine clinical practice.

Desiccated (dry) strong-base absorbents can degrade inhaled anesthetics to CO. This reaction can produce high caryhemoglobin concentrations reaching 35% or more. Patient exposure to a high level of CO typically would occur during the first case on Monday morning if continuous high gas flows were left on throughout the weekend and caused absorbent desiccation. Machines in remote locations are at higher risk of absorbent desiccation. Desiccation of absorbent is unlikely to occur during anesthesia delivery because $CO_2$ absorption produces water and patients exhale humidified gas.

Factors that increase CO production include inhaled anesthetic used (desflurane ≥ enflurane > isoflurane >> halothane = sevoflurane), degree of absorbent dessication, type of absorbent, higher temperature, higher concentration of anesthetic, low FGF rates, and smaller patient size. To reduce CO exposure risk, turn off the anesthesia machine at the end of the day and change the $CO_2$ absorber if gas is found flowing in the machine. Measurement of arterial blood-gas concentrations with a co-oximeter will document the concentration of caryhemoglobin. Most types of granules contain more calcium hydroxide with lesser amounts of the stronger bases because of the risk of compound A and carbon monoxide accumulation. Thus Baralyme (now withdrawn from the market) and to a lesser extent soda lime were more likely to produce CO.

## Thermal Injury

Fires within the breathing system are an extremely rare complication related to the interaction of desiccated strong-base absorbents and sevoflurane. Several case reports have documented patient injuries related to this problem (specifically with Baralyme). Sevoflurane and Baralyme can produce temperatures of more than 200°C with associated smoldering, melting of plastic, explosion, and fire. As a result of reported dangerous reactions, Baralyme was withdrawn from the market in 2004. Newer $CO_2$ absorbents (Amsorb Plus, LoFloSorb, and Dragersorb) do not contain NaOH or KOH. These absorbents are composed of $Ca(OH)_2$ with small amounts of calcium chloride and calcium sulfate and are not known to react with volatile anesthetic agents or produce compound A or CO. The Anesthesia Patient Safety Foundation consensus statement recommends the use of a $CO_2$ absorbent that does not significantly degrade volatile anesthetics when absorbent desiccation occurs, or if conventional $CO_2$ absorbents are used, specific policies be instituted to prevent their desiccation.

## Carbon Dioxide Removal Capacity

The size and shape of the absorptive granules are designed with the goal of maximizing absorptive surface and flow through the canister while minimizing the resistance to airflow. The absorptive capacity increases as the surface area for $CO_2$ absorption increases. However, as granule size decreases (and total surface area increases), resistance to airflow through the canister increases. The granular size of some common absorbents is between 4 and 8 mesh, a size at which absorptive surface area and resistance to flow are optimized.

*Channeling* refers to the preferential passage of exhaled gases through the canister via the pathway of least resistance. Excessive channeling will bypass much of the granule bulk and decrease the efficiency of $CO_2$ absorption.

## Indication of Absorbent Exhaustion

Absorbents contain an indicator dye, ethyl violet, to visually assess for absorbent depletion. Ethyl violet changes from colorless to violet when the pH of the absorbent drops below 10.3 as a result of $CO_2$ absorption. The color change signals that the absorptive capacity of the material has been consumed. Of note, prolonged exposure to fluorescent lights can deactivate ethyl violet so that the absorbent appears white, although its absorptive capacity is exhausted. Many newer-generation absorbent indicators are more resistant to color reversion, and some produce permanent color change. An alternative to using the indicator dye is to monitor inspired $CO_2$ and change the absorbent when the inspired $CO_2$ level reaches approximately 5 mm Hg or 0.05%. Although exhausted $CO_2$ absorbent is the most common cause of a horizontal elevation of the capnogram indicating inspired $CO_2$, incompetent valves will also cause elevation of inspired $CO_2$. In both situations, increasing FGF above minute ventilation will return inspired $CO_2$ to baseline. Absorbent desiccation cannot be detected via visual inspection; therefore some newer generation $Ca(OH)_2$ absorbents also include desiccation indicators.

## SUGGESTED READINGS

Bokoch, M. P., & Weston, S. D. (2020). Inhaled anesthetics delivery systems. In R. D. Miller (Ed.), *Millers anesthesia*. Philadelphia: Elsevier.

Feldman, J. M. (2012). Managing fresh gas flow to reduce environmental contamination. *Anesthesia and Analgesia, 114,* 1093–1101.

Feldman, J. M., Hendrickx, J., & Kennedy, R. R. (2021). Carbon dioxide absorption during inhalation anesthesia: A modern practice. *Anesthesia and Analgesia, 132,* 993–1002.

Feldman, J. M., Lo, C., & Hendrickx, J. (2020). Estimating the impact of carbon dioxide absorbent performance differences on absorbent cost during low-flow anesthesia. *Anesthesia and Analgesia, 130,* 374–381.

Jiang, Y., Bashraheel, M. K., Liu, H., Poelaert, J., Van de Velde, M., Vandenbroucke, G., et al. (2019). In vitro efficiency of 16 different Ca(OH)2 based CO2 absorbent brands. *Journal of Clinical Monitoring and Computing, 33,* 1081–1087.

Kennedy, R. R., Hendrickx, J. F., & Feldman, J. M. (2019). There are no dragons: Low-flow anaesthesia with sevoflurane is safe. *Anaesthesia and Intensive Care, 47,* 223–225.

Kuruma, Y., Kita, Y., & Fujii, S. (2013). Exchanging the CLIC absorber in the middle of surgery. *APSF Newsletter, 27,* 64–65.

Levy, R. J. (2016). Anesthesia-related carbon monoxide exposure: Toxicity and potential therapy. *Anesthesia and Analgesia, 123*(3), 670–681.

Olympio, M. A. (2005). Carbon dioxide absorbent desiccation safety conference convened by APSF. *APSF Newsletter, 20,* 25–29.

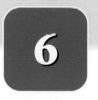

# 6

# Carbon Dioxide Retention and Capnography

MICHAEL G. IVANCIC, MD

Monitoring of carbon dioxide ($CO_2$) is a noninvasive process that has no contraindications and has been deemed a standard of practice by the American Society of Anesthesiologists (ASA). The ASA's updated 2020 Standards for Basic Anesthetic Monitoring now include the monitoring of $CO_2$ for all anesthetics with any level of sedation. Besides general anesthesia, this now encompasses moderate, deep, and regional with sedation. $CO_2$ is a by-product of aerobic cellular metabolism, and it is the most abundant gas produced by the human body. Using capnography during an anesthetic provides not only information on patient metabolism but also perfusion and ventilation status. In addition, it gives valuable information on possible mechanical complications related to the anesthetic equipment.

Perhaps no other monitor routinely used in anesthesia provides such a broad outlook on patient care.

## Terminology

Retention of $CO_2$ is synonymous with hypercarbia/hypercapnia and suggests elevated levels of $CO_2$ in the blood. $PETCO_2$ refers to the pressure of end-tidal $CO_2$ just before inspiration. $Paco_2$ is the partial pressure of $CO_2$ in the arterial blood. Capnometry is the measurement and numeric display of the partial pressure or gas concentration of $CO_2$. A capnometer is the device that measures and numerically displays the concentration of $CO_2$, typically in millimeters of mercury. Capnography is the graphic record of $CO_2$ concentration, the capnograph is the device that generates the waveform, and the capnogram is the actual graphic waveform.

## Retention of Carbon Dioxide

The rebreathing of $CO_2$ is undesirable during mechanical ventilation except during the rare occasion when it can be helpful to maintain normocarbia in patients who are being hyperventilated (i.e., when large tidal volumes may be desirable for other reasons).

Although short-term $CO_2$ retention likely is not deleterious, it can suggest a more concerning process requiring the clinician's attention. A leak or obstruction in the anesthesia machine circuit, common gas outlet, or fresh gas supply line may also cause an increase in $CO_2$ concentration.

Retention of $CO_2$ in the anesthesia circle system may be found anytime the mechanical or physiologic dead space is increased, such as the use of a heat and moisture exchanger or pulmonary hypoperfusion, respectively. These effects are more pronounced in smaller patients. In the closed-circle systems of modern anesthesia machines, minimal rebreathing and $CO_2$ retention, if any, should occur. However, malfunction of either of the unidirectional valves may lead to $CO_2$ rebreathing. If an inspiratory valve is held open, rebreathing can occur because, during expiration, alveolar gases can backfill the inspiratory limb of the circuit, so as the next delivered breath ensues, $CO_2$ will be present. A malfunctioning expiratory valve can lead to $CO_2$ rebreathing as well, and both will produce changes on the capnogram.

Other causes of inadvertent $CO_2$ rebreathing typically involve the $CO_2$ absorber. If the absorbent color indicator malfunctions and therefore does not reflect the true level of $CO_2$ in the system, rebreathing can occur without the anesthesia provider being aware of the problem. In some older anesthesia machines, the $CO_2$ absorber could be bypassed. Older absorbent canisters had a rebreathing valve that, if engaged, would lead to $CO_2$ rebreathing. Today's machines are still susceptible to channeling of gas through the canister without contacting any active absorbent, leading to rebreathing of $CO_2$. Independent of the cause, $CO_2$ rebreathing is best corrected immediately by increasing fresh gas flows and troubleshooting the underlying cause, because absorbent problems typically improve with increased flows but unidirectional valve issues do not. Malfunctions of circle systems are summarized in Box 6.1.

---

**BOX 6.1  REBREATHING OF $CO_2$ IN A CLOSED-CIRCLE ANESTHESIA SYSTEM**

**ABSORBENT-RELATED PROBLEMS**

Channeling of gas through the canister without contacting any active absorbent
Exhausted absorbent (soda lime or Amsorb)
Malfunction of the color indicator
Unintentional engagement of the rebreathing valve[a]
Intentional or unintentional bypass of the absorber[a]

**UNIDIRECTIONAL VALVE MALFUNCTION DURING SPONTANEOUS OR MECHANICAL VENTILATION**

Inspiratory valve
Expiratory valve

[a]Older machine.

---

When Mapleson systems are used, inadequate fresh gas flow is the primary culprit of an increase in $CO_2$, because these systems do not contain unidirectional valves or absorbent canisters. Specifically, systems with concentric inner tubes, such as the Mapleson D (Bain circuit), can cause rebreathing if there is any dysfunction (kink) in that tube. Of note, the Mapleson D circuit is the most efficient for controlled ventilation with regard to fresh gas flow; the Mapleson A circuit is most suitable for patients who are breathing spontaneously. Specific minimum fresh gas flow rates for the various Mapleson apparatuses are recommended for spontaneous and controlled ventilation (see Chapter 191, Pediatric Breathing Circuits).

During the induction and emergence phases of anesthesia, rebreathing of $CO_2$ will lengthen each process because of alterations in alveolar tensions associated with rebreathing of exhaled alveolar anesthetic gases. Capnography can help alert the clinician to rebreathing, regardless of the cause, so that appropriate steps can be taken to correct the problem.

## Capnography

Assessment of $CO_2$ can be done in a variety of ways. The devices used vary greatly in complexity and scope, but they all evaluate $P_{CO_2}$ in the expired gas noninvasively. Infrared spectroscopy is the most commonly used method to measure $CO_2$ concentration. Other methods include mass spectrometry, Raman scattering, and chemical colorimetric analysis.

### SIDESTREAM VERSUS MAINSTREAM SAMPLING

The $CO_2$ may be measured from a mainstream or sidestream device. Mainstream sampling uses a device that is placed close to the tracheal tube, with all of the inhaled and exhaled gas flowing through this measuring system. A benefit of mainstream sampling is that the response time is faster, so there is no uncertainty about the rate of gas sampling. Drawbacks include the bulkiness of the device and the need for it to be heated to $40°C$, increasing the risk of patient burns.

Sidestream sampling is most commonly used today. This method draws a continuous sample of gas from the breathing circuit into the measuring cell. Sampling flow rate is an important aspect of this system and is usually 150 to 250 mL/min. Lower sampling flows may be advantageous for patients with smaller tidal volumes, such as neonates, and also may have a lower occlusion rate. A higher sampling flow rate has the benefit of less time delay but is more likely to be inaccurate in patients with low tidal volumes because of the possibility of contamination of the sample with fresh gas. Various water trap systems have been devised but may fail and lead to erroneous $CO_2$ readings and waveforms. Purging the $CO_2$ sampling tubing with an air-filled syringe or replacing it will alleviate some moisture-caused sampling errors; however, filter replacement may be required.

### MEASUREMENT METHODS

Infrared spectroscopy systems function by analyzing infrared light absorption from gas samples and comparing them with a known reference to determine the type and concentration of that particular gas. Molecules of $CO_2$ absorb infrared radiation at the specific wavelength of 4.25 $\mu m$, and this value is used to determine the concentration of the gas sample. This system operates under the Beer-Lambert law. There is an inverse linear correlation between the amount of $CO_2$ present in the sample chamber, which absorbs infrared light, and the infrared radiation that reaches the infrared detector. The advantages of infrared systems include the ability to analyze multiple gases, including $CO_2$, $N_2O$, and all of the potent inhalation agents. In addition, this type of system is relatively small, lightweight, and inexpensive. Drawbacks include water vapor interference that may result in falsely elevated readings of $CO_2$ and inhalation agents. In addition, with sidestream sampling, there is a time delay because of the length and volume of the tubing that transports the sampled gas.

Colorimetric detection is another common means of measuring $CO_2$, most typically confirming correct placement of the tracheal tube. It consists of a pH-sensitive paper within a chamber that is placed between the tracheal tube and the ventilation device. The color change is reversible and can vary from breath to breath. Several brands are marketed, but most use a similar color scale (e.g., purple, end-tidal carbon dioxide [ETCO$_2$] <4 mm Hg [<0.5% $CO_2$]; tan, ETCO$_2$ 4–15 mm Hg [0.5%–2% $CO_2$]; yellow, ETCO$_2$ >15 mm Hg [>2% $CO_2$]). Advantages include portability, low cost, and no need for other equipment. Colorimetric detection is most applicable outside of the operating room in settings where only semiquantitative results are needed.

Mass spectrometry can measure nearly every gas pertinent to anesthesia by separating gases and vapors according to differences in their mass-to-charge ratios, including $O_2$ and $N_2$, which cannot be measured by infrared spectroscopy. Mass

spectrometry also has a relatively fast response time. However, it is not used as frequently as infrared spectroscopy, likely because of the large size of most units, the need for warm-up time, and the cost.

Raman spectroscopy relies on the inelastic, or Raman, scattering of monochromatic light (e.g., a laser) by different gases, thereby providing information about the phonon modes (an excitation state, a quantum mechanical description of a special type of vibrational motion of molecules) in a system. Advantages of Raman spectroscopy include the ability to analyze multiple gases simultaneously, the accuracy of the system, and the rapid response time. However, this application is also cumbersome and expensive.

## Capnograms

Capnograms rely on time or volume to assess $CO_2$ concentration. The time capnogram is the most common, but the volume capnogram yields other unique information, such as the components of dead space and the V/Q status of the lungs. Time capnograms are further divided into slow and fast tracings, with the slow speed optimal for assessing long-term trends of ETCO$_2$ and the fast speed used for detailed waveform analysis. Normal time and volume capnograms are shown in Fig. 6.1. There is no widely accepted labeling of capnograms, but it is important to be familiar with the various normal phases and how they correspond to disease patterns, with several examples summarized in Fig. 6.2. With the use of PETCO$_2$ from the capnogram, it is possible to estimate Paco$_2$ in the

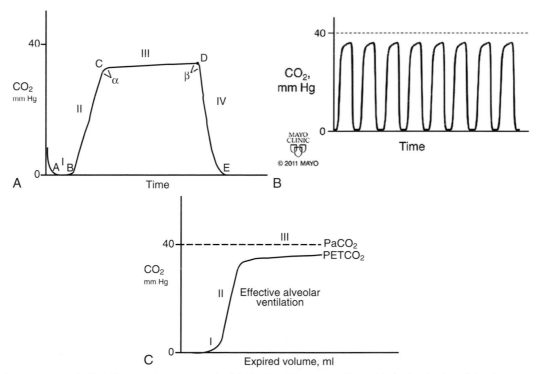

**Fig. 6.1** Normal capnograms. **A,** Fast-time capnograms can be labeled in various ways. Phase I is the beginning of dead space expiration, and the baseline value is 0. Phase II is the ascending expiratory phase, including both dead space and alveolar gas. Phase III is the alveolar plateau, which should be relatively flat in a healthy individual. The alpha angle between phase II and phase III (point C) should be 100–110 degrees; patients with obstructive lung disease will have an angle greater than 110 degrees. Point D is end-tidal $CO_2$ (PETCO$_2$) and also marks the beginning of phase IV, the start of inspiration. **B,** Slow-time capnograms are used to show trends. The PETCO$_2$ should be relatively constant. **C,** Volumetric capnograms are useful for assessing effective alveolar ventilation. Phase I contains gas from anatomic and apparatus dead space. Phase II shows increasing amounts of alveoli emptying gas. Phase III represents alveolar gas, and the highest point is PETCO$_2$. There is no inspiratory limb on a volumetric capnogram.

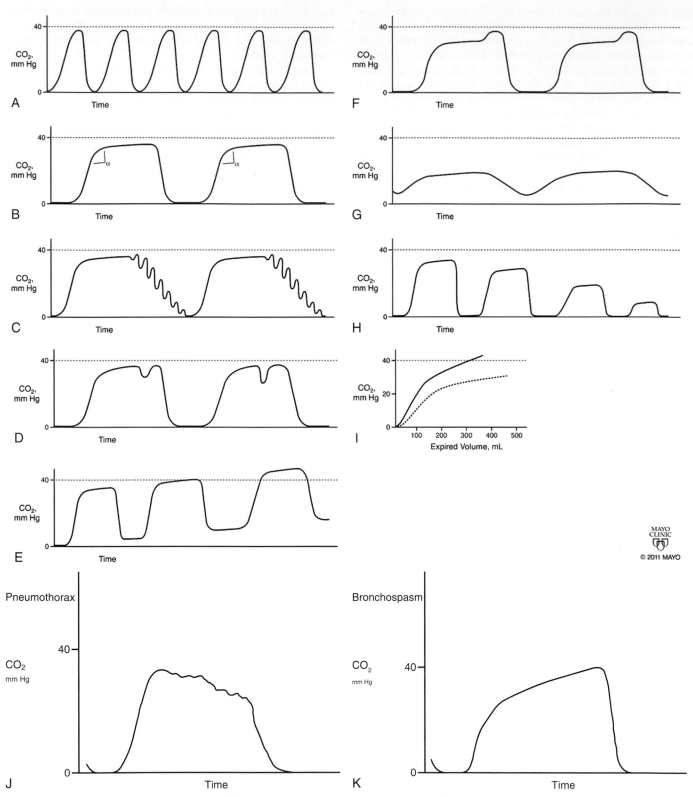

**Fig. 6.2**   Examples of various capnograms and their interpretation. **A,** Normal spontaneous breathing. **B,** Normal mechanical ventilation. **C,** Cardiogenic oscillations seen during the terminal portion of exhalation. **D,** "Curare" cleft, which is seen normally in the last part of phase III and is caused by a lack of synchrony between the diaphragm and intercostal muscles in a patient who has received neuromuscular-blocking agents and whose muscle strength is returning. **E,** Patient rebreathing $CO_2$ because of either exhausted absorbent or an incompetent inspiratory valve. The figure overdramatizes the increase in inspired $CO_2$ that will occur over time if the underlying problem is not corrected. **F,** Dual-plateau waveform because of a break in the sample line. Early during exhalation, room air is entrained, lowering $CO_2$; toward the end of exhalation, as pressure in the tubing increases, less air is entrained, and there is a second "tail." **G,** Patient with severe obstructive lung disease (forced expiratory volume at 1 second 20% or less of predicted). **H,** Increased dead space, emboli, severe bronchospasm, or obstruction in the sampling line as less air is withdrawn. **I,** Shift from right *(dotted line)* to left *(solid line)* on the volume capnogram as would occur in a patient with worsening obstructive lung disease (e.g., bronchospasm in a patient with severe chronic obstructive pulmonary disease). **J,** Possible pneumothorax, notable for loss of the alveolar plateau. **K,** Markedly increased slope of Phase III, which is characteristic of bronchospasm or chronic obstructive pulmonary disease.

blood noninvasively, with a normal $P_{ETCO_2}$:$P_{aCO_2}$ typically less than 5 mm Hg. Table 6.1 summarizes how common alterations in metabolism, circulation, and ventilation, as well as various equipment malfunctions, affect $P_{ETCO_2}$ and the $P_{ETCO_2}$:$P_{aCO_2}$ gradient. Familiarity with the characteristics of classic normal and abnormal capnograms and the associated implications for $P_{ETCO_2}$ and $P_{aCO_2}$ can help clinicians recognize and respond to ventilator and respiratory abnormalities promptly.

| TABLE 6.1 Causes of Alerted $ETCO_2$ and $P_{ETCO_2}$: $P_{aCO_2}$ Gradients | | |
|---|---|---|
| **Cause** | **$P_{ETCO_2}$** | **$P_{ETCO_2}$:$P_{aCO_2}$ Gradient** |
| **$CO_2$ OUTPUT** | | |
| Increased $CO_2$ production[a] | Increased | Normal |
| $CO_2$ insufflation | Increased | Normal |
| Hypothermia | Decreased | Normal |
| Increased depth of anesthesia | Decreased | Normal |
| **ALVEOLAR VENTILATION** | | |
| Hypoventilation | Increased | Normal |
| Chronic obstructive pulmonary disease/bronchospasm | Variable[b] | Increased |
| Hyperventilation | Decreased | Normal |
| **PULMONARY PERFUSION** | | |
| Hypertension/increased cardiac output | Increased | Decreased |
| Hypotension/hypovolemia/decreased cardiac output | Decreased | Increased |
| Pulmonary embolism | Decreased | Increased |
| Right-to-left intracardiac shunt | Decreased | Increased |
| Increased physiologic dead space | Decreased | Increased |
| **EQUIPMENT MALFUNCTION** | | |
| Rebreathing with circle system from exhausted $CO_2$ absorbent or channeling | Increased | Normal |
| Rebreathing with low fresh flow in the Mapleson system | Increased | Decreased |
| Circuit disconnection | Decreased | Increased |
| Increased apparatus dead space | Increased | Normal |
| Sampling tube leak | Decreased | Increased |
| $CO_2$ sampling rate too high or too low | Decreased | Increased |
| Poor seal around the tracheal tube | Decreased | Increased |

$P_{aCO_2}$, Partial pressure of $CO_2$ in the arterial blood; $P_{ETCO_2}$, pressure of end-tidal $CO_2$ just before inspiration.
[a]From hyperthermia, malignant hyperthermia, convulsions, tourniquet release, pain, or bicarbonate administration.
[b]Depending on the severity and compensatory mechanisms (e.g., hyperventilation), $P_{ETCO_2}$ may be decreased, normal, or increased.

## SUGGESTED READINGS

American Society of Anesthesiologists. *Standards for basic anesthetic monitoring*. Retrieved from https://www.asahq.org/standards-and-guidelines. Accessed November 21, 2021.

Barash, P. G., Cullen, B. F., Stoelting, R. K., et al. (2017). Commonly used monitoring techniques. In P. G. Barash, Cahalan MK, Cullen BF, Stock MC, Stoelting RK, Ortega R, et al., (Eds.), *Clinical anesthesia* (pp. 710–713). Philadelphia: Wolters Kluwer.

Bhende, M. S., & LaCovey, D. C. (2001). End-tidal carbon dioxide monitoring in the prehospital setting. *Prehospital Emergency Care, 5,* 208–213.

Dorsch, J. A., & Dorsch, S. E. (2007). Gas monitoring. In J. A. Dorsch, S. E. Dorsch (Eds.), *Understanding anesthesia equipment* (5th ed., pp. 685–727). Philadelphia: Lippincott Williams & Wilkins.

Kodali, B. S. *Capnography: A comprehensive educational web site*. Retrieved from www.capnography.com. Accessed November 21, 2021.

Nagler, J., & Krauss, B. (2008). Capnography: A valuable tool for airway management. *Emergency Medicine Clinics of North America, 26,* 881–897.

Thompson, J. E., & Jaffe, M. B. (2005). Capnographic waveforms in the mechanically ventilated patient. *Respiratory Care, 50,* 100–109.

# 7

# Tracheal Tubes

JONATHAN E. CHARNIN, MD

## Tracheal Tubes

Tracheal tubes, often called endotracheal tubes (ETT) are devices used to direct respiratory gases to and from the lower airways and lungs. They also allow for delivery of anesthetic gases to the patient without encroaching on the operative field. Modern tracheal tubes are round tubes usually made of polyvinyl chloride (PVC) plastic. As these are integral to the practice of anesthesia, the anesthesiologist must be familiar with all aspects of these devices.

The inner diameter, measured in millimeters, corresponds to the sizing number. Smaller tubes have a much lower cross-sectional area and therefore present higher resistance to gas flow (see Table 7.1). The outer diameter of the tube varies with the type of tube but is about 2 or 3 mm wider than the inner diameter. The tip of the tracheal tube has smoothed plastic to reduce the chance of injuries caused by a rough edge. Tracheal tubes usually have a beveled tip that is shaped to direct the tube to the right bronchus if it is inserted too deeply. Near the tip of the tracheal tube, a hole is created on the right-hand side wall of the tracheal tube called a Murphy eye, which allows gas movement if the tip of the tube is obstructed (see Fig. 7.1). Most tracheal tubes have a radiopaque line along the length of the tube to facilitate visualization of the tube on radiographs.

Near the tip of the ETT, the inflatable cuff material is attached to the outer wall of the tracheal tube. A tight seal with the trachea is created when the cuff is inflated allowing positive pressure ventilation. Most cuffs are made with enough material to be inflated to a high volume to create a seal with the inner wall of the trachea; this is called a high-volume, low-pressure cuff. This seal stops gas leaking out from the respiratory system and reduces large-volume aspiration of fluid contents in the pharynx. Folds or irregularities in this cuff material can lead to microaspiration despite cuff inflation. Different cuff designs, often changes in cuff shape, have been developed to limit the amount of aspiration that occurs around the cuff.

A small channel is manufactured into the wall of the ETT. This channel is sealed at the tip of the ETT. The side of the tube under the cuff is thinned so that the channel is open along under the cuff of the tracheal tube. The pilot balloon is connected to this thin channel, typically about two-thirds of the length of the tracheal tube from the tip. The pilot balloon houses a connector that attaches to syringes, allowing insertion and removal of gas from the cuff of the ETT. Although tactile measurement of the cuff pressure has proven to be inaccurate, the pilot balloon is squeezed after inflation by many anesthesia providers to get a sense of the pressure in the cuff.

The material of ETTs is too soft to form a good connection with the plastic components of anesthesia or ventilator circuits. A connector made of hard plastic is attached to the tracheal tube allowing tubes of different sizes to be connected to standard 22-mL respiratory systems. The tracheal tube can occasionally become disconnected at the intersection of the tube and these connector pieces, so it is important to inspect this connection to make sure it is secure prior to use.

There are several factors that may lead to changes in cuff pressure (Box 7.1). Decreased pressure in the cuff occurs with hypothermia or cardiopulmonary bypass. Increased pressure may result when pressure is created from nearby surgical procedures, at increased altitude, with a change in head position, diffusion of oxygen into the cuff, changes in muscle tone, patient coughing or straining, or with the use of certain topical anesthetic agents. Using the "feel" of the pilot balloon as a measurement of intra-cuff pressure has been proven to be unreliable in preventing overinflation of the cuff. Therefore experts recommend that cuff pressures be measured at end expiration, perhaps routinely, and certainly in operations lasting longer than 4 to 6 hours. Cuffs for patients in the intensive care unit should be routinely measured and the pressure controlled, especially for patients with long periods of intubation, like patients with COVID-19 pneumonia. Pressure measurements can be obtained by connecting the inflation tube to a manometer or to the pressure channel of a

| TABLE 7.1 | Airway Cuff Comparisons | | | |
|-----------|-------------------------|---|---|---|
| Type | Description | Advantages | Disadvantages |
| Low-volume, high-pressure cuff | Stretchy cuff material needs higher pressure to make a seal | Less cuff material, lower risk of tearing cuff during insertion, used on some tracheostomy tubes | Can lead to ischemia of the tracheal wall |
| High-volume, low-pressure cuff | Standard cuffed tracheal tube Thin and compliant and does not stretch the tracheal wall | Better for prolonged use because of decreased ischemic risk | Can tear during intubation More easily dislodged May not as effectively protect the lower airway from aspiration |

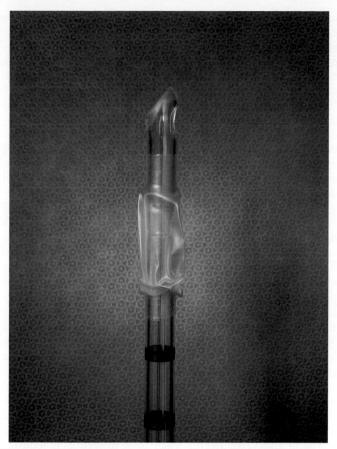

**Fig. 7.1**  Tip of an endotracheal tube, showing smoothed tip, Murphy eye, deflated cuff.

| TABLE 7.2 | Examples of Tracheal Tube Cross-sectional Area by Size | | | | | |
|---|---|---|---|---|---|---|
| Tube size (mm) | 3.0 | 5.0 | 6.0 | 7.0 | 7.5 | 8.0 |
| Tube area (mm²) | 7.1 | 19.6 | 28.3 | 38.5 | 44.2 | 50.2 |

be left in postoperatively, the cuff should be deflated and reinflated with air to prevent a leak.

Tracheal tubes contribute to airway resistance and increase the work of breathing. The internal diameter (ID) correlates with the tube cross-sectional area and is the main determinant of resistance to flow (see Table 7.2). The length of the tube also contributes to resistance. The smaller and longer the tracheal tube, the greater the resistance. Choice of tube size for adult patients varies with each patient. A 7.0-mm ID tube is adequate for most women, and an 8.0-mm ID tube is appropriate for most men; however, slightly smaller sizes may be used for short cases for patient comfort. Age is the most reliable indicator of tube size for children. A reasonable estimate for a cuffed tube in the pediatric patient is age/4 + 3.5. A tracheal tube should be inserted until the cuff is 2.25 to 2.5 cm past the vocal cords. Typically, this correlates with an insertion distance of 23 cm at the incisors for a man and 21 cm for a woman.

The cricoid cartilage is the narrowest part of the pediatric airway. Cuffless tracheal tubes can be used in children by having the tube create a seal with the cricoid cartilage, but smaller cuffed ETTs are now commonly used.

Tracheal tubes have many desirable features, such as providing a secure protected airway, the ability to be manipulated away from the surgical field, decreasing pollution in the operating room (OR) by preventing escape of anesthetic gases, and allowing for accurate monitoring of end-tidal gases, tidal volume, and pulmonary compliance. However, their use is associated with a variety of complications (Box 7.2). Emergence phenomena, such as coughing, bucking, tachycardia, and hypertension, can occur, along with the possibility of sore throat, infection, and vocal cord dysfunction. Trauma from multiple attempts to intubate the trachea, the use of excessive force, or insertion of a stylet through the Murphy eye can cause airway edema, hematoma, laceration, vocal cord avulsions and fracture, and even tracheal perforation. Tracheal tubes can also become obstructed from kinking, external compression, displacement, change in the patient's body position, material in the lumen, or a patient biting the tube.

---

**BOX 7.1   FACTORS THAT MAY LEAD TO CHANGES IN CUFF PRESSURE**

| ↓ Pressure | ↑ Pressure |
|---|---|
| Hypothermic cardiopulmonary bypass | Pressure from nearby surgical procedures |
| Cuff leak | Increased altitude |
| | Change in head position |
| | Diffusion of $N_2O$ into the cuff |
| | Coughing, straining, and changes in muscle tone |
| | Use of certain topical anesthetic agents |

---

monitor with an air-filled transducer. Cuff pressure in high-volume, low-pressure cuffs should be maintained between 20 and 30 cm $H_2O$ (15–22 mm Hg) in normotensive adults. These pressure parameters have been shown to ensure ventilation, prevent aspiration, and maintain tracheal mucosal perfusion. Complications, including subglottic stenosis, hoarseness, nerve injury, scarring, and fistula formation, have been reported with cuff pressures greater than 30 cm $H_2O$. It is noteworthy that $N_2O$ can diffuse into the cuff, leading to increased intracuff volume and pressure if the cuff is filled with air. When $N_2O$ use is discontinued, intracuff pressure decreases rapidly; therefore if the tracheal tube is to

---

**BOX 7.2   COMPLICATIONS THAT MAY OCCUR WITH THE PLACEMENT OF TRACHEAL TUBES**

- Airway edema
- Emergence phenomena (e.g., coughing, bucking, tachycardia)
- Hoarseness
- Infection
- Nerve injury
- Postoperative sore throat
- Tongue swelling
- Tracheal stenosis (often months later)
- Ulceration
- Vocal cord dysfunction

A variety of tracheal tubes are marketed. Typically, tracheal tubes are made of PVC, or less commonly, silicone, latex, red rubber, or stainless steel. They can be cuffed, uncuffed, nasal, oral, reinforced with wire, flexed, preformed (see Fig. 7.2), specialized, laser resistant (Fig. 7.3), reusable, disposable, and single lumen or multilumen.

Reinforced, armored tubes, also known as wire spirals, have a metal or nylon coil incorporated into the wall of the lumen. The tube is made of a flexible silastic material, but this spiral reinforcing coil makes the tube relatively resistant to bending,

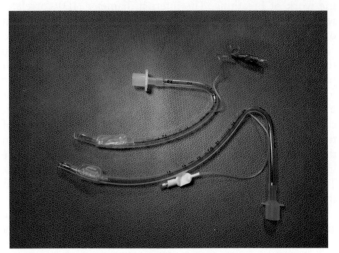

**Fig. 7.2**   Preformed tubes are commonly used during oral surgery and for operations involving the head and neck. Oral Ring-Adair-Elwin *(top)* and Nasal Ring-Adair-Elwin *(bottom)*.

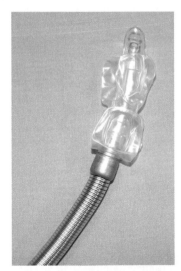

**Fig. 7.3**   A metal laser-resistant tube with a double cuff at the tip. Laser-resistant tubes can be made of malleable metal and have two cuffs at the tip. Each cuff is typically filled with 1 to 3 mL saline. The more proximal or cephalad tube sometimes contains blue dye, although many surgeons prefer not to use dye. Surgeons will know if they perforate the proximal cuff with the laser beam because they will see the saline well up in the trachea. If the saline contains dye, the dye stains tissue, making continued surgical excision difficult. If the proximal cuff is compromised, the distal cuff will continue to secure the airway. Because metal tubes reflect the laser beam, many companies have developed tubes made of either noncombustible material or polyvinylchloride wrapped in noncombustible material that will not reflect the laser beam.

compression, and kinking. This property, along with a tube connector that is firmly fixed to the tube shaft and is not detachable, makes these tubes well suited for use in tracheal procedures (see Fig. 7.1). However, the flexible nature of these tubes may make them difficult to pass nasally, without a stylet, or orally through an intubating laryngeal mask airway (LMA). If the wires of the spiral are kinked or bitten, that deformed shape will persist, and the tube may need to be replaced. Tracheal tubes that are labeled as flexible typically have a flexible, curved, and tapered tip that is designed to slide past the glottis atraumatically. Flexible tubes can also be helpful in more difficult intubations because they slide off an introducer easily and do not get caught on protruding structures in the airway.

Preformed tubes, also known as Ring-Adair-Elwin (RAE) tubes, are useful during oral surgery and for head and neck operations (see Fig. 7.2). They have a preformed bend that directs the tube away from the surgical field. A south-facing oral RAE tube rests on the patient's chin and is directed toward the chest. A north-facing nasal RAE tube is longer and directs the proximal end of the tube toward the patient's forehead. Preformed nasal tubes may not fit each patient. Smaller diameter tubes are often shorter in length, preventing the effective use of an oral 6.0 or smaller tube in the nasal position. Extended-length narrow tubes are available, and although they lack the preformed bend, they may be preferable for some patients.

Specialized tracheal tubes include one designed for head and neck procedures that has neuromonitoring electrodes embedded in the outer wall of the tube. These tubes are typically used for identification and intraoperative monitoring of recurrent laryngeal and vagus nerves when neck dissection is required (Fig. 7.4). Another specialized tube is a microlaryngoscopy tube, which has a pediatric diameter and an adult length to facilitate airway surgery. Even smaller tubes are available for jet ventilation. Jet ventilation tubes have no cuff.

Laser-resistant tubes (see Fig. 7.3) were designed to be nonflammable for use during operations in which a laser is used; however, airway fires still may occur if the laser power is great enough or if the laser application is too long. Different laser-resistant tubes vary in their compatibility with various laser types; compatibility should always be checked before use. Laser tubes can be made of stainless steel or have a PVC or rubber core that is wrapped in two layers, a foil layer to protect the tube and a nonreflective outer layer. Cuffs are not laser resistant and should be filled with 1 to 3 mL water or saline. A dye dispersant may be present to indicate cuff perforation. The dye can stain the tissue, making continued surgical excision difficult. Some tubes have two cuffs so that, if one is damaged, the other can be inflated to protect the airway, provide a seal, and prevent a leak.

Multilumen tubes are used for gas sampling, suctioning, airway pressure monitoring, fluid and drug injection, jet ventilation, and lung isolation. The double-lumen tube (DLT) is commonly used for lung isolation and can be right or left sided (Fig. 7.5). The tracheal lumen is placed above the carina, and the bronchial lumen is angled to fit into either the right or left mainstem bronchus. DLTs are sized according to the external diameter of the tracheal segment and measured in the French system. The margin of safety is greater for a left-sided tube, and therefore it is often the tube of choice, even for operations on the left lung. Almost all operations requiring differential ventilation can be accomplished with a left-side tube. Right-sided tubes could be considered in situations in which manipulation or intubation of the left main bronchus is contraindicated, such

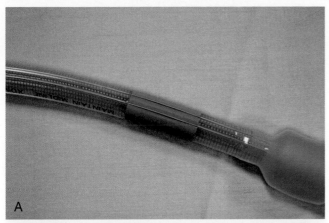

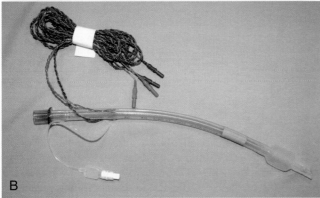

**Fig. 7.4** Intraoperative monitoring of the recurrent laryngeal nerve or vagus nerve during thyroid and parathyroid operations is possible with the use of a tracheal tube with two electrodes embedded in its side. The *blue* portion of the tracheal tube is placed between the vocal cords **(A)**, and the electrodes are connected to an appropriate monitoring system **(B).**

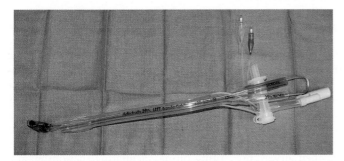

**Fig. 7.5** Left-sided double-lumen tracheal tube. The bronchial tube and its pilot balloon are color coded *blue;* the tracheal tube and its pilot balloon are made of clear polyvinylchloride.

as when the left main bronchus is narrowed or positioned too cephalad, when a stent is present, or when the left tracheobronchial tree is disrupted or a large left-sided thoracic aortic aneurysm is present. The tracheal cuff should be inflated in the same way a regular tracheal tube is inflated. The bronchial cuff should be inflated incrementally until a seal is achieved. Volumes in the bronchial cuff should be less than 3 mL. Complications associated with DLTs include difficulty with insertion and positioning, hypoxemia, obstructed ventilation, trauma, poor seal, and cuff rupture.

## Supraglottic Airways

The most commonly used supraglottic airway device is the LMA developed in the 1980s by Dr. Archie Brain. The introduction of the first-generation LMA Classic (Teleflex, Morrisville, NC) revolutionized the way general anesthetics could be delivered, and it replaced the tracheal tube in many cases. Disposable LMAs are now used more commonly than the original reusable LMAs. This airway device is less invasive than a tracheal tube and creates a hands-free seal. They may be flexible for manipulation during shared airway procedures or may have a rigid handle and be designed as a conduit for tracheal intubation, such as the LMA Fastrach (Teleflex). The newer second-generation devices include adaptations to improve performance and safety. These devices include the LMA Pro-Seal (Teleflex), the LMA Supreme (Teleflex), the i-Gel Supraglottic Airway (Intersurgical, Berkshire, Wokingham, UK), and the Laryngeal Tube Suction II Airway (VBM, Medizintechnik, Sulz, Germany). These more sophisticated supraglottic airways isolate the esophagus from the airway and provide a better seal for more effective positive pressure ventilation. The i-Gel device contains a built-in bite block. Other second-generation devices have an esophageal drain tube that directs gases away from the esophagus, thereby reducing gastric insufflation. If regurgitation occurs, this drain can shunt gastric fluids away from the airway, potentially lowering the risk of aspiration. This tube can also act as a port of access to the esophagus and stomach, where an orogastric tube or suction catheter could be inserted.

The LMA design mimics a bolus of food in the pharynx and is less noxious than a tracheal tube. The LMA is a curved tube (shaft) that is connected to an elliptical spoon-shaped mask (cup). The two flexible aperture bars where the tube attaches to the mask prevent obstruction by the epiglottis (Fig. 7.6). The LMA also has an inflatable cuff, an inflation tube, and a self-sealing pilot balloon. When placed correctly, the mask should rest on the hypopharyngeal floor, the sides should face the piriform fossae, and the upper portion of the cuff should sit behind the tongue base. Although weight-based formulas can be used for sizing, typically a man or larger adult will require a size 5 and a woman or smaller adult will require a size 4. For estimation of pediatric sizing, matching the widest part of the mask to the width of the second to fourth fingers works well.

The LMA cuff should be inflated using the minimum effective volume and pressure. Manufacturer recommendations vary, but 60 cm $H_2O$ is a common threshold and a useful guideline. As with the tracheal tube cuff, $CO_2$ and $N_2O$ can diffuse into the cuff, leading to increased intracuff pressure, which can be measured with a manometer. Elevated inflation pressures in the LMA cuffs are associated with postoperative throat pain. The traditional teaching is that leak pressure with an LMA should be greater than 20 cm $H_2O$ with positive pressure or greater than 10 cm $H_2O$ with spontaneous ventilation. The LMA can be used with mechanical ventilation, but peak inspiratory pressure should not exceed 20 cm $H_2O$ to prevent leaking, gastric distention, and pollution in the OR.

The LMA can be useful for a patient in whom mask ventilation is difficult. In fact, the use of an LMA is included in the American Society of Anesthesiologists algorithm to facilitate positive pressure ventilation or tracheal intubation for management of a difficult airway. LMAs are typically easy to insert and use, are cost-effective, and provide for a smooth awakening. The only absolute contraindications to their use are inability to

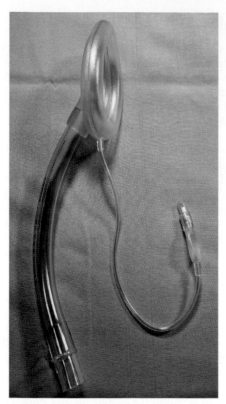

**Fig. 7.6** A laryngeal mask airway has a curved shaft connected to an elliptical cup with a pilot balloon and an inflatable cuff. The two bars at the orifice of the shaft (or tube) that connects to the cup (or mask) prevent obstruction of the mask by the epiglottis.

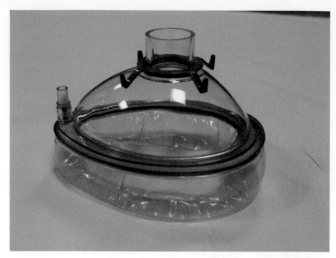

**Fig. 7.7** Facemasks include a body, a seal, and a connector and can be used to ventilate with positive pressure and to administer inhaled anesthetic gases.

open the mouth and complete upper airway obstruction. However, there are several traditionally recognized relative contraindications. These include conditions or situations that predispose the patient to an increased risk of aspiration, such as morbid obesity, pregnancy, hiatal hernia, uncontrolled diabetes or gastroesophageal reflux, neuromuscular disorders, full stomach, emergency surgery, intraabdominal or laparoscopic surgery, and surgical length greater than 3 hours. Also, if the airway must be secured definitively because of cervical trauma or disease, bleeding, restricted airway access or airway surgery, pharyngeal or laryngeal disease, tracheomalacia, perceived difficult intubation, or the need for sophisticated ventilatory support, an LMA may not be the best choice. LMAs can be used with controlled ventilation and can be used in some circumstances with neuromuscular blockers (Box 7.3).

---

**BOX 7.3   CONTRAINDICATIONS TO THE USE OF LARYNGEAL MASK AIRWAYS**

- Increased aspiration risk
- Bleeding disorder
- Cervical trauma or disease
- Hiatal hernia
- Laparoscopic or robotic surgery
- Restricted airway access
- Supraglottic trauma or disease
- Tracheomalacia

---

## Facemasks

Facemasks can be made of black rubber, clear plastic, elastomeric material, or a combination thereof. They include a body, seal, and connector (Fig. 7.7) and can be used to ventilate with positive pressure and to administer inhaled anesthetic gases. Advantages include decreased incidence of postoperative sore throat, cost-effectiveness, and decreased anesthetic requirement. Facemask anesthesia, however, is demanding of the anesthesia provider, requires higher fresh-gas flows, leads to increased pollution in the OR, causes more $O_2$ desaturation, increases the work of breathing, and can cause pressure necrosis, dermatitis, nerve injury, jaw pain, and increased movement of the cervical spine.

## Pharyngeal Airways

Pharyngeal airways are typically made of plastic or elastomeric material (Fig. 7.8). They help prevent obstruction of the laryngeal space by the tongue or epiglottis without the anesthesia provider having to manipulate the patient's cervical spine. They can also reduce the work of breathing compared with a facemask. Oropharyngeal airways (see Fig. 7.8A) include a flange, bite portion, and an air channel and are useful for maintaining an open airway, preventing biting, facilitating suctioning, and providing a pathway for inserting devices, such as a fiberscope or an endoscope, into the pharynx. This airway device is sized by measuring from the maxillary incisors to the angle of the mandible. Oropharyngeal airways can stimulate pharyngeal and laryngeal reflexes, leading to coughing or laryngospasm. Nasopharyngeal airways (see Fig. 7.8B) are better tolerated in a patient with intact airway reflexes and can be used for many of the same purposes as an oral airway. In addition, they can be used to administer continuous positive airway pressure, treat hiccoughs by stimulating the pharynx, and dilate the nasal passages for nasotracheal intubation. The appropriate size can be estimated by choosing an airway that extends from the tip of the nose to the lobe of the ear. Nasopharyngeal airways should be avoided when the patient is anticoagulated or has a basilar skull fracture, nasal deformity, nasal infection, or a history of nosebleeds requiring treatment. A vasoconstrictor can be applied topically to the patient's nasopharynx before the airway is inserted to decrease the risk of bleeding and facilitate placement by decreasing mucosal thickness, thereby enlarging the nasal passageway.

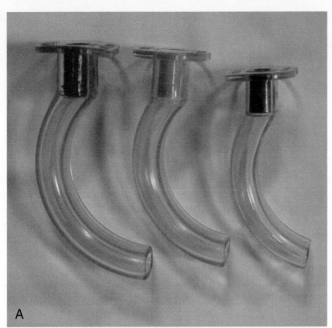

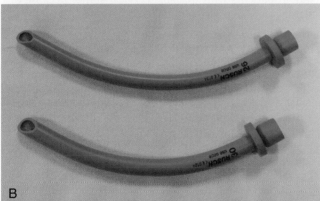

**Fig. 7.8** Pharyngeal airways. **A,** Oropharyngeal airways are available in different sizes and are frequently color coded for rapid identification of airway size. **B,** Nasopharyngeal airways also come in various sizes. They also can be color coded, but more commonly the clinician who inserts the device will size the nasopharyngeal airway, choosing a device that extends from the tip of the patient's nose to the lobe of the ear, and will then lubricate and insert the device.

## SUGGESTED READINGS

Apfelbaum, J. L., Hagberg, C. A., Connis, R. T., Abdelmalak, B. B., Agarkar, M., Dutton, R. P., et al. (2022). 2022 American Society of Anesthesiologists Practice Guidelines for Management of the Difficult Airway. *Anesthesiology, 136,* 31–81.

Dimitriou, V. K., Zogogiannis, I. D., Douma, A. K., Pentilas, N. D., Liotiri, D. G., Wachtel, M. S., et al. (2009). Comparison of standard polyvinyl chloride tracheal tubes and straight reinforced tracheal tubes for tracheal intubation through different sizes of the Airtraq laryngoscope in anesthetized and paralyzed patients: A randomized prospective study. *Anesthesiology, 111,* 1265–1270.

El-Orbany, M., & Woehlck, H. J. (2009). Difficult mask ventilation. *Anesthesia and Analgesia, 109,* 1870–1880.

Hameed, A. A., Mohamed, H., & Al-Mansoori, M. (2008). Acquired tracheoesophageal fistula due to high intracuff pressure. *Annals of Thoracic Medicine, 3,* 23–25.

Hooshangi, H., & Wong, D. T. Brief review: The cobra perilaryngeal airway (cobraPLA and the streamlined liner of pharyngeal airway (SLIPA) supraglottic airways. *Canadian Journal of Anaesthesia, 55,* 177–185.

Kim, H. Y., Kim, E. J., Shin, C. S., & Kim, J. (2019). Shallow nasal RAE tube depth after head and neck surgery: Association with preoperative and intra-operative factors. *Journal of Anesthesia, 33*(1), 118–124.

Kumar, C. M., Seet, E., & Van Zundert, T. C. (2021). Measuring endotracheal tube intracuff pressure: No room for complacency. *Journal of Clinical Monitoring and Computing, 35*(1), 3–10.

Rinder, C. S. (2008). Fire safety in the operating room. *Current Opinion in Anaesthesiology, 21,* 790–795.

Weiss, M., Dullenkopf, A., Fischer, J. E., & European Paediatric Endotracheal Intubation Study Group. (2009). Prospective randomized controlled multi-centre trial of cuffed or uncuffed endotracheal tubes in small children. *British Journal of Anaesthesia, 103,* 867–873.

Williams, D. L., Wong, S. M., Pemberton, E. J., Webb, T. G., & Alexander, K. D. (2009). A randomized, single-blind, controlled trial of silicone disposable laryngeal masks during anaesthesia in spontaneously breathing adult patients. *Anaesthesia and Intensive Care, 37,* 992–997.

# Complications of Tracheal Intubation

HELGA KOMEN, MD

Tracheal intubation is a nonsurgical technique that maintains airway patency, protects the lungs from aspiration, and permits leak-free mechanical ventilation. Use of tracheal intubation and use of other airways are associated with complications, and some of these can be life-threatening. Complications of tracheal intubation may occur during intubation, while the tracheal tube is in place, or after extubation.

## Complications That Occur During Intubation

### FACIAL SOFT TISSUE, EYES, NOSE, AND TEETH TRAUMA

Corneal abrasions may occur when an object (e.g., wristwatch), arm, or sleeve of the anesthesia provider who is performing the intubation brushes the patient's eye. Therefore patient's eyes should be protected with transparent film dressing, tape, or ointment before manipulation of the airway (ventilation, intubation). Contusions or lacerations of the upper or lower lip can occur as a result of trauma from the laryngoscope blade. Prolonged compression of the tongue by an endotracheal tube, supraglottic airway device, or an oral airway can cause venous congestion, resultant macroglossia, and potential obstruction of the airway postextubation.

Nasotracheal intubation may lead to epistaxis, which is caused when the tip of the tracheal tube traumatizes the nasal or nasopharyngeal mucosa (most frequently Kiesselbach's plexus). Locally applied vasoconstrictor drugs are used before intubation to prevent this complication. Turbinates, polyps, adenoids, and tonsils can also be traumatized. Nasal intubation is contraindicated in patients with coagulopathy, those receiving anticoagulants, or who have skull base fractures.

Dental injuries are the most common reasons for anesthesia-related malpractice claims (30%–40%). The incidence of perioperative dental injury ranges from 1:150 to 1:1500, with 75% of injuries occurring during intubation and 25% occurring with emergence. In most cases the upper incisors are involved, due to poor dentition or difficult intubation. When dental trauma occurs, the displaced tooth should be recovered to avoid aspiration, and an avulsed tooth should be placed in saline after immediate dental consultation. The details of the injury should be well documented.

### CERVICAL SPINE INJURY

Patients with cervical spine fractures, instability (atlantoaxial subluxation from rheumatoid arthritis), malformations (Down syndrome, Morquio syndrome), tumors, or osteoporosis are at increased risk of experiencing a cervical spine or spinal cord injury during intubation. In these patients, extension of the cervical spine during laryngoscopy may cause trauma to the spinal cord, which can result in severe neurologic injuries such as quadriplegia. In patients with suspected instability of the cervical spine, the head must be maintained in a neutral position by inline manual stabilization during laryngoscopy and intubation. Fiberoptic intubation is a proposed technique in these situations where endotracheal intubation should be achieved with little to no movement of unstable cervical spinal structures. In the past decade, video laryngoscopy-assisted endotracheal intubation has gained popularity for securing the airway in patients with unstable cervical spines because of its availability and high first-attempt success rate.

### PHARYNGEAL AND LARYNGEAL TRAUMA

Trauma to the pharynx can be caused by a laryngoscope blade or tube passage. Most frequently injured structures are the right tonsillar pillar and the soft palate. Trauma to the pharynx is more frequent when video laryngoscope is used, because the passage of the blade into the hypopharynx is done while observing the patient's mouth indirectly (on the screen) rather than directly. Long-term sequelae are unusual.

Laryngeal trauma during intubation is rare event. Some injuries of the larynx are vocal cord hematomas and subluxation of arytenoids (incidence of 4% and <1%, respectively). This can happen more frequently while using a flexible bronchoscope to achieve endotracheal intubation because the endotracheal tube passes through vocal cords without having a direct view.

### STIMULATION OF AIRWAY REFLEXES

Laryngoscopy can produce reflex sympathetic stimulation that results in hypertension, tachycardia, arrhythmias, and intracranial and intraocular hypertension. The magnitude of the sympathetic response is related to the duration of laryngoscopy. Patients with limited intracranial compliance or intracranial vascular anomaly may suffer serious intracranial hypertension or hemorrhage. In addition, tactile stimulation can cause cough, straining, or vomiting, which can lead to aspiration and serious pulmonary complications.

Drugs used for induction of anesthesia block the response to airway instrumentation. It is essential to give them in sufficient doses in order to avoid the aforementioned complications. Additional drugs can be used to avoid sympathetic activation, such as lidocaine (1.0 mg/kg intravenously) or a low dose of β-adrenergic antagonist. If the patient has a full stomach, rapid-sequence induction technique is used to prevent aspiration (no attempts to ventilate the patient before intubation, after all the medications are given in a rapid manner).

Stimulation of the pharyngeal or laryngeal mucosa may result in activation of vagus nerve-mediated reflexes, such as laryngospasm, bronchospasm, bradycardia, and arrhythmias. Laryngospasm may result also from attempted intubation in patient who is not anesthetized sufficiently. This must be corrected by rapidly deepening anesthesia and administering a muscle relaxant.

An endotracheal tube in place may result in reflex broncho-constriction. Bronchospasm may be especially severe in insufficiently anesthetized patients and/or patients with reactive airways; it presents clinically as wheezing. Bronchospasm may be blunted by the prior administration of anticholinergics, steroids, inhaled β₂-receptor agonists, lidocaine (topical, intravenous), or opioids.

## ESOPHAGEAL INTUBATION

Prompt recognition of esophageal intubation is vital for the patient. Unrecognized esophageal intubation is the most disastrous complication associated with intubation. The gold standard is to show the presence of expired $CO_2$. In case of absence of expired $CO_2$, the tube should be withdrawn and reintroduced. Esophageal intubation may be also recognized by gurgling sounds over the epigastrium on auscultation, the absence of breath sounds over the thorax, and abdominal distention. Esophageal intubation most frequently happens in patients with a difficult airway. It is important to properly evaluate the airway before induction and choose intubation equipment that will guarantee first-attempt success.

## BRONCHIAL INTUBATION

Bronchial intubation occurs if the tip of the tracheal tube is in one of the mainstem bronchi. In most cases, it is the right bronchus. This is more common in children because of the smaller distance between the vocal cords and the carina. Properly placed tubes may change position during head movement or repositioning of the patient and result in bronchial intubation. Bronchial intubation may be detected by monitoring flow-volume loops. The intubated lung becomes hyperinflated, receiving the entire tidal volume and predisposing to overdistension and barotrauma, whereas the unintubated lung develops atelectasis and the blood flow through that lung contributes to substantial right-to-left shunt. This results in higher peak airway pressures and arterial hypoxemia. Fiberoptic bronchoscopy is the optimal diagnostic tool to check the position of the tip of tracheal tube.

In most cases, placement of the tracheal tube 23 cm at the lips in male patients and 21 cm in female patients results in correct positioning. In children, these recommendations for tracheal tube depth should be followed (lip-to-tip distance):
Premature infant: 6 to 7 cm
Full-term infant: 8 to 10 cm
Age 1 year: 11 cm
Age 2 years: 12 cm
Age 3 to 18 years: 12 + (age/2) cm

## ESOPHAGEAL, TRACHEAL, AND BRONCHIAL PERFORATION

Perforation is more likely to happen when a stylet protrudes from the tip of the tracheal tube, when excessive force is used during intubation, or with multiple intubation attempts.

Esophageal perforation can be diagnosed soon after intubation by the presence of subcutaneous emphysema. Tracheal perforation is more frequent in patients with tracheal distortion caused by tumor or large lymph nodes, weakness in the membranous trachea, corticosteroid therapy, or chronic obstructive lung disease. Endotracheal tube changers and placement of double-lumen tracheal tubes have been associated with bronchial rupture. Signs of tracheal or bronchial perforation are subcutaneous emphysema, pneumomediastinum, and pneumothorax. Nitrous oxide should be discontinued if pneumothorax or pneumomediastinum is suspected. Chest drainage and open surgical repair may be required to treat a rupture.

# Complications That Occur With the Tracheal Tube in Place

## OBSTRUCTION

Tracheal tube obstruction can be caused by external force (e.g., biting down, kinking), internal obstruction (secretions, blood clots, foreign body, tumor tissue), or tube abnormalities. Impaction of the tip of the tube against the tracheal wall will not result in respiratory obstruction, as the Murphy eye permits airflow even if this has occurred. Herniation of the cuff over the tip of the tube may occur if the cuff is overinflated.

Obstruction of the tracheal tube can manifest with increased peak airway pressures and inability to deliver desired tidal volumes. When tracheal tube obstruction is diagnosed, visual inspection and passage of a suction catheter is indicated. If patency cannot be restored, the tracheal tube should be replaced, if necessary, over a tube exchanger.

## MIGRATION

Head flexion and head extension can advance or withdraw the tracheal tube by 2 or 5 cm, respectively. This movement can lead to bronchial intubation or tracheal extubation, which is detected by changes in peak airway pressures and capnography values. Poor fixation of the tube, excessive movement of the head during surgery, and heavy connectors producing drag on the circuit and tracheal tube may lead to dislodgement. When long-term intubation is anticipated, a chest radiograph should be obtained to verify that the tip of the tracheal tube is 3 to 6 cm above the carina.

## MUCOSAL ULCERATION OR NECROSIS

Mucosal ulceration or necrosis may occur due to ischemic injury resulting from high pressures generated when the tracheal tube or cuff presses on the mucosa.

Ulcerations or erosions of the larynx are common, even after a short duration of intubation, and progress with the length of intubation. They are most commonly found on the posterior part of the larynx corresponding to the position of the convex curve of the tracheal tube. Most heal without sequelae.

Mucosal injuries in trachea can be found in form of ulcerations or necrosis and are due to cuff pressure. Necrosis happens when mucosal blood flow is severely impeded (e.g., a combination of low perfusion pressures during hypotension and cuff pressure >25 cm $H_2O$).

Superficial ulcers heal rapidly. Deeper ulcers may result in scarring or erosion of a blood vessel and hemorrhage. It is important to inflate the cuff between 20 and 30 cm $H_2O$ and to check the pressure with a cuff manometer periodically during anesthesia.

## IGNITION

The plastic tracheal tube can ignite during airway surgery in which laser is employed. To reduce this serious hazard, specially designed noninflammable endotracheal, "laser tubes," are used. The cuffs of these tubes are inflated with saline instead of air to further decrease the risk of ignition. Inspired oxygen is kept at less than 30% because ignition requires an oxygen source. If an airway fire occurs, the surgery must immediately pause, the oxygen source must be discontinued, and the endotracheal tube must be removed. Discontinuation of the oxygen source before endotracheal tube removal is paramount because removal of the endotracheal tube with free-flowing oxygen can create a blowtorch effect, damaging even more tissue. Water and damp towels must be applied to any fire. Once the fire is extinguished, the trachea is reintubated and humidified oxygen is provided. The airway then needs examination to assess thermal injury.

## MISCELLANEOUS

Selection of a properly sized tube is necessary in adults and critically important in children to avoid excessive leak of air or resistance. In adults, a tube with an inner diameter of 7.0 mm is most commonly used in females and 8.0 mm in males. In children older than 1 year, the tube diameter can be determined with the formula:

$$\text{Tracheal tube size (mm)} = 4 + (\text{age in years}/4)$$

Microaspiration can occur if the cuff is not inflated sufficiently to occlude the tracheal lumen. The recommended pressure in the cuff is 20 to 30 cm $H_2O$.

## Complications That Occur Immediately After Extubation

### VOCAL CORD PARALYSIS

The prevalence of vocal cord paralysis is less than 1%. It can be unilateral or bilateral. Vocal cord paralysis may be secondary to surgical trauma of the vagus or recurrent laryngeal nerve. Pressure from inflated endotracheal cuffs against the thyroid lamina may cause compression injuries of the recurrent laryngeal nerve, resulting in vocal cord paralysis. This is associated with hoarseness or breathing difficulty immediately postoperatively. Bilateral vocal cord paralysis may require reintubation. Recurrent nerve injury can be prevented by avoiding overinflation of the tracheal tube cuff or careful manipulation during surgical procedures on the neck. Vocal cord paralysis, in most cases, resolves spontaneously over days to months.

## SUPRAGLOTTIC, GLOTTIC, OR SUBGLOTTIC EDEMA

Edema is the most significant complication in the early postextubation period. Contributing factors are trauma from laryngoscopy, use of an overly large tube, a malpositioned cuff that was leaning on vocal cords, excessive bucking or coughing on the tube, and current or recent respiratory infection. The strongest predictor of postextubation stridor is absence of an air leak if 30 cm $H_2O$ pressure is applied to the endotracheal tube. The use of intravenous steroids and/or nebulized racemic epinephrine has been advocated, but proof of their efficacy is not conclusive.

Sore throat may have pharyngeal, laryngeal, or tracheal sources. The prevalence of sore throat is around 27%. Risk factors for postextubation sore throat include large endotracheal tube size, high intracuff pressure, female sex, use of lubricant, and use of succinylcholine. Cuffs with a larger volume appear to cause a higher incidence of sore throat. Sore throat usually subsides within 72 hours.

## Delayed Complications

### TRACHEAL STENOSIS

Tracheal stenosis usually develops as a consequence of ischemia and eventual necrosis of the tracheal mucosa. This leads to a healing process that produces a tight fibrous stricture of the trachea. Ischemia of the tracheal mucosa can occur when the cuff of the endotracheal tube is overinflated and exceeds the capillary perfusion pressure of the tracheal mucosa of approximately 25 mm Hg.

These complications can be prevented by proper management of high-volume, low-pressure cuffs. It is important to inflate using only as much air as is required to seal the air leak during mechanical ventilation (minimal inflation technique) and to check intracuff pressure with a cuff pressure manometer (20–30 cm $H_2O$).

## SUGGESTED READINGS

Brodsky, M. B., Akst, L. M., Jedlanek, E., Pandian, V., Blackford, B., Price, C., et al. (2021). Laryngeal injury and upper airway symptoms after endotracheal intubation during surgery: A systematic review and meta-analysis. *Anesthesia and Analgesia, 132*(4), 1023–1032.

Christensen, R. E., Baekgaard, J. S., & Rasmussen, L. S. (2019). Dental injuries in relation to general anesthesia – a retrospective study. *Acta Anaesthesiologica Scandinavica, 63*(8), 993–1000.

Crosby, E. T., Duggan, L. V., Finestone, P. J., Liu, R., De Gorter, R., & Calder, L. A. (2021). Anesthesiology airway-related medicolegal cases from the Canadian Medical Protection Association. *Canadian Journal of Anaesthesia, 68*(2), 183–195.

Fornebo, I., Simonsen, K. A., Bukholm, I. R. K., & Kongsgaard, U. E. (2017). Claims compensation after injuries related to airway management: A nationwide study covering 15 years. *Acta Anaesthesiologica Scandinavica, 61*(7), 781–789.

Greer, D., Marshall, K. E., Bevans, S., Standlee, A., McAdams, P., & Harsha, W. (2017). Review of videolaryngoscopy pharyngeal wall injuries. *Laryngoscope, 127*(2), 349–353.

Joffe, A. M., Aziz, M. F., Posner, K. L., Duggan, L. V., Mincer, S. L., & Domino, K. B. (2019). Management of tracheal intubation: A closed claim analysis. *Anesthesiology, 131*(4), 818–829.

Liu, J., Zhang, X., Gong, W., Li, S., Wang, F., Fu, S., et al. (2010). Correlations between controlled endotracheal tube cuff pressure and postprocedural complications: A multicenter study. *Anesthesia and Analgesia, 111*(5), 1133–1137.

Warner, M. A., Meyerhoff, K. L., Warner, M. E., Posner, K. L., Stephens, L., & Domino, K. B. (2021). Pulmonary aspiration of gastric contents: A closed claims analysis. *Anesthesiology, 135*(2), 284–291.

# 9

# Disconnect Monitors

JONATHAN E. CHARNIN, MD

Anesthesia machines regulate the gas mixtures given and allow control over a patient's respiration when needed. Anesthesia machines are outfitted with disposable circuit components (inspiratory limb, expiratory limb, sampling tube for carbon dioxide [$CO_2$] and gas mixture), which can become disconnected. Leaks in disposable or reusable circuit components also occur. Undetected circuit disconnections during anesthesia expose patients to risk of severe harm due to hypoxia and hypercapnia. Reports of severe harm or patient death due to circuit disconnection have become less common over time, in part due to automated monitoring for circuit disconnection. Monitors to detect circuit disconnection have been recommended in the American Society of Anesthesiologists (ASA) Monitoring Guidelines since the 1980s. Disconnection alarm technologies have improved over the years using improved sensors and electronic controls in modern anesthesia machines.

None of the technologies currently used as disconnection monitors detects a physical disconnection of circuit components. Rather, sensors associated with the machine look for changes in machine performance associated with disconnections or large circuit leaks. It is hardest for the anesthesia machine to monitor for a disconnection when patients are spontaneously breathing. Vigilant monitoring for disconnections by anesthesia providers is recommended during periods of spontaneous breathing.

The first disconnection monitor introduced to clinical practice was a pressure monitor on the patient's side of the inspiratory valve that signaled when inspiratory pressures in the circuit failed to rise. This sensor was set to alarm when a specified time interval had elapsed (usually 15 seconds) without a rise in circuit pressure that crossed a set threshold. Circuit pressures rising above this threshold suggested the anesthesia circuit was competent to deliver gas at elevated pressures and that inspiration should have occurred. This type of monitoring is not helpful when the patient is spontaneously breathing. Spontaneous breathing and bag-assisted ventilation modes make detection of circuit disconnections by electronic means more difficult because the respiratory effort of the patient does not produce large pressure changes in the anesthesia circuit.

Modern anesthesia machines have sophisticated ventilator control mechanisms. For instance, pressure-limited ventilation modes (including pressure-limited assist/control ventilation or pressure-support ventilation) require sensitive pressure sensors that monitor the pressures in the circuit and use computerized control of the bellows, piston, or turbine that delivers pressure to the circuit. A natural result of the technologic sophistication supporting advanced ventilator modes is improved sensors, which are well equipped to detect and alert the user to anesthesia circuit disconnections and leaks. Increased sensitivity for disconnection also produces many alarm conditions caused by changes in performance that are not due to leaks or circuit disconnection. Therefore every user should familiarize themselves with the alarm modes of the machines they are using and identify which alarm modes signal circuit disconnection or potential circuit leak.

Three technologies are primarily used to signal disconnection: airway pressure monitors, circuit flow monitors, and $CO_2$ monitors (Table 9.1 and Box 9.1).

## Airway Pressure Monitors

The original mechanical ventilators in anesthesia machines used basic electronic controls and lacked sensors to monitor or synchronize with a patient's attempts at respiration. As technology advanced, the ASA issued recommendation guidelines that anesthesia machines be fitted with disconnection monitors.

The basic concept of airway pressure disconnect monitors is the monitoring of periodic pressure increases above a set threshold to provide evidence that the circuit can deliver positive pressure and is doing so on a regular basis. The set threshold of pressure for this monitor is often termed the low airway pressure alarm level.

All users of anesthesia machines understand the high-pressure monitors that may signal occlusion of the airway, occlusion of the circuit, or patient dyssynchrony. Pressure monitors also have the "airway pressure low" alarm level. The low airway pressure level is the set threshold of positive pressure that, when crossed, signals a successful breath in controlled

| TABLE 9.1 | Alarms Technologies Monitoring Circuit Disconnection | |
|---|---|
| **Disconnect Monitor Technology** | **Alarm Meaning** |
| Airway pressure monitor | If airway pressure is sustained below this set point and does not intermittently rise above this threshold, then the circuit may have disconnected. This is not helpful during spontaneous breathing. |
| Carbon dioxide monitor | If phasic changes in expired carbon dioxide are not measured, then circuit disconnection may be present. |
| Flow monitor | If the flow monitors detect a rapid change in compliance or inspiratory/expiratory flow imbalance, or if the direction of flow through the circuit reverses, then a circuit disconnection may be present. |

ventilation. This "airway pressure low" setting is often misunderstood. Electronic control of this alarm setting can often be automatically adjusted by the machine at the push of a button. If the airway pressure does not cross this threshold, the machine will eventually signal an apnea alarm, as the machine will infer that the inspiratory pressure threshold has not been met. Most instances of this alarm announce changes in the patient condition or poor threshold setting rather than a circuit disconnection. After longer periods without an appropriate pressure rise, anesthesia machines will announce higher priority alarms such as circuit disconnection. High levels of vigilance with these alarms should be maintained to allow early identification and correction of occult disconnections.

Patients who breathe spontaneously do not raise the circuit pressures. Unassisted breathing through the circuit does not usually have a pressure-based apnea or disconnection alarm in use.

## End-Tidal Carbon Dioxide Monitoring

End-tidal $CO_2$ monitoring itself is beyond the scope of this chapter. However, phasic changes in $CO_2$ levels are seen in effective respiration. Failure to observe phasic changes in $CO_2$ may signal to the machine that there is apnea or a circuit disconnection has occurred. Unfortunately, it is possible to have some phasic changes in $CO_2$ if the patient is spontaneously breathing even with a circuit disconnection, particularly if the disconnection happens near the Y-piece, the point where the inspiratory and expiratory limbs of the circuit connect to each other and the endotracheal tube. If there are not phasic changes in measured $CO_2$, an anesthesia machine may warn of apnea. This apnea warning should be concerning for both low levels of spontaneous breathing and possible circuit disconnection. Additionally, high-inspiratory $CO_2$ is concerning for rebreathing of exhaled gas caused by circuit disconnection.

## Flow Monitoring

Flow monitors used in anesthesia machines are sophisticated and very accurate. Because flow monitoring can be based on different technologies, it is useful to know which flow technologies are used in a machine so the anesthesiologist will be aware of potential confounding conditions (e.g., hot-wire anemometer flow meters may be ruined by nebulized medications that pass through the anesthesia circuit).

Flow monitors allow the anesthesia machine to warn of many different respiratory failures, two of which warn of circuit disconnection. First, when the anesthesia machine attempts to

deliver a controlled ventilation breath and the flow sensors detect very high flows at low pressures, the anesthesia machine is programmed to stop delivering the breath and to signal an alarm. Some machines will warn first with a lower priority alarm, such as "pressure not achieved." If the condition is not corrected, a higher priority alarm such as "circuit disconnection" will be given. Second, flow sensors detect the direction of gas flow. Because the circle system circuits used in anesthesia have unidirectional flow, flow reversal should not normally occur. If the sensors determine flow has reversed in the circuit, an alarm will be given, which should be concerning for disconnections, leaks, or valve failures.

Modern anesthesia machines have flow sensors in the inspiratory and expiratory gas pathways. These sensors allow the machine to quantitate the volumes of gas that move in inspiration and expiration. When there is an imbalance in the inspiratory and expiratory gas flows, the machine will alarm that a circuit leak is present. This may also help reveal a circuit disconnection.

## Empty Bellows Alarms

The pressure in the anesthesia machine and breathing circuit should not be lower than atmospheric pressure. Anesthesia machines are designed to prevent negative pressure from being generated in the machine because this could transmit negative pressure to the patient, leading to atelectasis or negative pressure injury. If the ventilator bellows, piston, or turbine has an insufficient amount of gas to continue delivering positive pressure breaths, one of several alarms may be produced. A low-circuit gas alarm is concerning for a circuit disconnection or occult leak.

## Disconnect Alarm Management

Prior to the induction of general anesthesia, the anesthesia machine and circuit should have a positive pressure leak check performed. This step is crucial to ensure patient safety. The airway low-pressure limit is an important setting to allow early detection of partial or complete circuit disconnections. It is recommended to set the airway low-pressure limit within 5 cm of $H_2O$ of the peak airway pressure for the patient being ventilated. Often, this alarm limit remains set in the machine from one case to the next and therefore may not be set appropriately. Alarms also need to be heard to be useful. Noisy operating rooms may require the anesthesia provider to increase the volume of the alarm so that the warnings offered by disconnection alarms can be reliably heard.

Disconnection alarms help identify leaks and disconnections that occur during the conduct of the anesthetic. Disconnections do not have to be complete to risk causing harm to a patient. Therefore early detection and correction of disconnections and circuit leaks remains a top priority. Table 9.2 lists some circuit leaks and disconnections arranged by likelihood of occurrence. A systematic approach to diagnosing disconnections is recommended (e.g., start near the patient with the endotracheal tube and Y-piece and work systematically toward the machine). Anesthesia circuit disconnections rightly belong in the same category of breathing system problems as circuit leaks, cuff leaks, and endotracheal tube holes. Whenever a machine warns of a leak, a disconnection should always be considered.

| TABLE 9.2 | **Location of Disconnections and Leaks** | |
| --- | --- | --- |
| **Source** | **Description** | **Frequency** |
| Y-piece disconnection | Endotracheal tubes, elbow pieces, flexible extensions, and various adapters attach here, and these can disconnect | Most frequent disconnection |
| Corrugated tubing disconnection | Flexible and typically disposable circuits attach to the anesthesia machine and may become disconnected | Common |
| Tube cuff leak | Can be difficult to diagnose; sometimes occurs because cuff has passed above the vocal cords or has become incompetent | Common |
| Leak at carbon dioxide absorber | Disconnection at gaskets or seals or leak in the plastic housing | Uncommon |
| Leak in tubing or anesthesia machine | Holes in the sides of the circuit tubing or cracks in the anesthesia machine | Very uncommon |
| Tube failure | Possible, especially with biting; may occur during motor-evoked potentials | Very uncommon |
| Internal gas pathway leaks | The gas pathways in the anesthesia machine are made of strong components, but leaks inside the machine remain possible | Extremely uncommon |

## SUGGESTED READINGS

Adams, A. P. (1994). Breathing system disconnections. *British Journal of Anaesthesia, 73,* 46–54.

Caplan, R. A., Vistica, M. F., Posner, K. L., & Cheney, F. W. (1997). Adverse anesthesia outcomes arising from gas delivery equipment: A closed claims analysis. *Anesthesiology, 87,* 741–748.

Dorsch, J. A., & Dorsch, S. E. (2008). *Understanding anesthesia equipment* (5th ed., pp. 731–744). Philadelphia, PA: Lippincott, Williams &Wilkins.

Gropper, M. A. (2020). *Miller's anesthesia* (9th ed., pp. 572–637). Philadelphia, PA: Elsevier.

Mehta, S. P., Eisenkraft, J. B., Posner, K. L., & Domino, K. B. (2013). Patient injuries from anesthesia gas delivery equipment: A closed claims update. *Anesthesiology, 119,* 788–795.

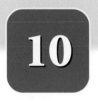

# Pulse Oximetry

KLAUS D. TORP, MD

## Technology

Oximetry involves the measurement of the oxyhemoglobin ($HbO_2$) concentration based on the Lambert-Beer law. Fractional oximetry, which measures arterial $O_2$ saturation by blood gas machine ($Sao_2$), is defined as $HbO_2$ divided by total hemoglobin (Hb). Total Hb is calculated as the sum of $HbO_2$, deoxyhemoglobin (reduced) (HHb), methemoglobin (metHb), and carboxyhemoglobin (COHb). In contrast, functional oximetry, which measures $O_2$ saturation with pulse oximetry ($SpO_2$), is defined as $HbO_2$ divided by the sum of $HbO_2$ and HHb. In clinical practice, $SpO_2$ is measured with a pulse oximeter to estimate $Sao_2$.

$$SaO_2 = HbO_2/(HbO_2 + HHb + metHb + COHb)$$
$$SpO_2 = (HbO_2/(HbO_2 + HHb))$$

Compared with $HbO_2$, HHb absorbs more light in the red band (600–750 nm), whereas $HbO_2$ absorbs more light in the infrared band (850–1000 nm). A conventional pulse oximeter probe contains two light-emitting diodes (LEDs) that emit light at specific wavelengths: one in the red band at 660 nm and one in the infrared band at 940 nm. When the probe is placed on the patient, the light emitted from the LEDs is either transmitted or reflected (depending on the site of the sensor) through the intervening blood and tissue and is detected by sensors built into the probe. The amount of transmitted light is sensed several hundred times per second to allow precise estimation of the peak and trough of each pulse waveform. At the pressure trough (nonpulsatile during diastole), light is absorbed by the intervening arterial, capillary, and venous blood, as well as by the intervening tissues. At the pressure peak (during systole), additional light is absorbed in both the red and infrared bands by an additional quantity of purely arterial blood, the pulse volume. Typical pulse amplitude accounts for only 1% to 5% of the total signal. Pulse oximeters isolate the pulsatile components from the blood volume signal (photo plethysmogram) and calculate the red/infrared ratios of the pulsatile and non-pulsatile absorbance of the light, which is then used to calculate $SpO_2$ with an algorithm based on a nomogram that is built into the software of the pulse oximeter.

Isolation and measurement of the pulsatile component allows patients to act as their own controls and eliminates potential problems with interindividual differences in baseline light absorbance.

The "calibration curve" that is used to calculate $SpO_2$ was derived from studies of healthy volunteers.

The process to identify the pulse, which is initiated with application of the probe to the subject, includes sequential trials of various intensities of light to find those that are strong enough to transmit through the tissue without overloading the sensors.

## Accuracy

The Food and Drug Administration requires a minimum accuracy for pulse oximeters to be within 3% of the root-mean-square ($A_{rms}$) difference between the $SpO_2$ and the cooximeter $Sao_2$ values across a range of different oxygen saturations (70%–100%). Sensors are calibrated to the site of application (e.g., digit, ear, and forehead). Applying a given sensor to a different site may give false $SpO_2$ readings even when an acceptable plethysmographic waveform is seen.

There are two potential problems with the accuracy of pulse oximetry at values of less than 70%. First, as stated previously, pulse oximeters have been calibrated using studies of healthy volunteers breathing different gas mixtures designed to lower the $Sao_2$ to about 70%. Therefore it is unlikely that much data have been collected for calibration at lower saturation levels. Second, the absorption spectrum of HHb is maximally steep at 600 nm. Therefore any slight variance in the light emitted from the 660-nm LED has significant potential to introduce measurement error into the system. Because decreasing levels of $SpO_2$ lead to an increasing proportion of HHb, there is the potential for decreasing accuracy as $SpO_2$ decreases. These potential problems are unlikely to be of much clinical significance. For example, it is unlikely that a treatment decision would be based on whether $SpO_2$ is 50% versus 60% at a given time. Some studies have reported poor accuracy of pulse oximeters at $SpO_2$ of less than 70%. During the COVID-19 epidemic the subject of accuracy in some, but not all, darker-pigmented individuals was raised in two observational studies, overestimating $SpO_2$ with the potential consequence of perhaps not admitting patients that should be otherwise admitted. The cause of this discrepancy is currently being investigated by the different manufacturers and investigators. Although the minimum accuracy is defined by U.S. Food and Drug Administration (FDA) regulations, and manufacturers must include 15% of dark-pigmented individuals in their supporting data, a spot-check $SpO_2$ may not be sufficient to make admission or treatment decisions, and an arterial blood gas may help if the $SpO_2$ values are close to a medical decision point. During the COVID-19 pandemic there was an unprecedented surge in the use of consumer-grade pulse oximeters, mainly because of their availability and low price. Although many of these pulse oximeters are advertised as having been manufactured to some international standards,

those standards refer to the manufacturing process and not to accuracy, which can vary widely. They are neither evaluated nor approved by the FDA to diagnose or treat diseases.

## RESPONSE TIME

Most pulse oximeters average pulse data over 5 to 8 seconds before displaying a value. Some oximeters allow for an override of this lag by providing for a shortened averaging interval or allowing a beat-by-beat display. Response time is also related to probe location and perfusion.

Desaturation response times range from 7.2 to 19.8 seconds for ear probes, from 19.5 to 35.1 seconds for finger probes, and from 41.0 to 72.6 seconds for toe probes.

## LOW-AMPLITUDE STATES

Pulse oximeters depend on a pulsatile waveform to calculate $SpO_2$. Therefore under conditions of low or absent pulse amplitude, the pulse oximeter may not reflect $Sao_2$ or may not provide a reading at all (e.g., during cardiac arrest, proximal blood pressure cuff inflation, tourniquet application, hypovolemia, hypothermia, vasoconstriction, Raynaud disease, use of a ventricular assist device, cardiac bypass). In addition, pulse oximeters are more sensitive to movement artifact during states of low pulse amplitude. Most pulse oximeters will display an index of perfusion, which can be helpful in interpreting erroneous readings.

The earlobe and forehead appear to be areas that are least sensitive to a decreased pulse pressure, probably reflecting less vasoconstriction than the digits. If the $SpO_2$ decreases without an obvious physiologic cause (e.g., low blood pressure, asystole) and changing the site of the sensor does not produce the desired result, increasing the sensitivity (if the technology permits) or changing to a different brand of pulse oximeter, with a different signal processing algorithm, may provide a reading. Accuracy of pulse oximeter readings may be negatively affected in the face of arrhythmia, in which not all electrocardiographic complexes produce a sufficient stroke volume, thus creating a pulse deficit. However, this is now fairly rare, and no relationship between pulse deficit and bias has been identified.

## DYSHEMOGLOBINS

Conventional pulse oximeters use only two wavelengths of light; therefore conventional pulse oximeters can accurately measure only $HbO_2$ and HHb. The presence of a third or fourth type of hemoglobin (e.g., metHb or COHb) can interfere with accurate measurement by causing changes in the absorbance of light in the critical red and infrared regions.

The pulse oximeter interprets COHb as a mixture of approximately 90% $HbO_2$ and 10% HHb. Thus at high COHb levels, the pulse oximeter will overestimate true $Sao_2$, as may occur in patients with recent carbon monoxide exposure (e.g., house fire, combustion engine exhaust, cigarette smoking). Those patients should benefit from a cooximeter arterial blood gas analysis.

When the heme iron is oxidized from the ferrous ($Fe^{2+}$) to the ferric ($Fe^{3+}$) state, metHb is formed. It is very dark and tends to absorb equal amounts of red and infrared light, resulting in a red/infrared ratio of 1. When extrapolated on the calibration curve, a ratio of 1 corresponds with saturation of 85%. Thus as metHb increases, $SpO_2$ approaches 85%, regardless of the true level of $HbO_2$. Drugs that cause methemoglobinemia ($>1\%$ metHb) include nitrates, nitrites, chlorates, nitrobenzenes, antimalarial agents, amyl nitrate, nitroglycerin, sodium nitroprusside, and high levels of local anesthetic agents. High levels of metHb create mitochondrial hypoxia as a result of the diminished $O_2$-carrying capacity of blood and a leftward shift in the $HbO_2$ dissociation curve.

Recent advances in pulse oximetry, some of which use more than seven wavelengths (Rainbow SET Technology, Masimo Corp., Irvine, CA), allow approximate measure of levels of COHb and metHb, but these newer pulse oximeters do not correct $SpO_2$ for COHb and metHb readings.

Pulse oximeters underestimate $SaO_2$, especially at low saturation values, in patients with anemia; however, this finding has little clinical significance because an intervention would likely occur before $SaO_2$ would reach a low level. Some new pulse oximeters can measure total hemoglobin either continuously or as a spot-check device.

## DYES AND PIGMENTS

Injections of methylene blue produce a large and consistent spurious decrease in $SpO_2$, with readings remaining below baseline for 1 to 2 minutes. Injection of indocyanine green decreases $SpO_2$ to approximately 80% to 90% for a minute or less. Injection of indigo carmine decreases $SpO_2$ the least, with the decrease lasting approximately 30 seconds.

Elevated serum bilirubin concentrations, per se, do not affect the accuracy of the pulse oximeter.

## AMBIENT LIGHT

Inaccurate $SpO_2$ readings have been reported to occur because of interference from surgical lamps, fluorescent lights, infrared light–emitting devices, and fiber-optic light sources.

## SKIN PIGMENT

Obtaining an accurate pulse oximetry reading may not be possible in very deeply pigmented patients because of a failure of LED light transmission.

## ELECTROCAUTERY

Electrocautery results in decreased $SpO_2$ readings because of interference from the wide-spectrum radiofrequency emissions that affect the pulse oximeter probe. Interference is usually of little clinical significance unless extended electrocautery occurs in patients who have decreased or unstable $SaO_2$. Some manufacturers have attenuated this problem by improving the electrical shielding of sensors and cables.

## MOTION ARTIFACT

Repetitive and persistent motion artifact of any kind tends to cause $SpO_2$ to display the local venous $SaO_2$ level. The susceptibility to motion artifacts may also depend on the signal-processing algorithm of the pulse oximeter brand.

## NAIL POLISH

Nail polish may cause a low $SpO_2$ value, especially with older models, although this effect is not constant and may be related to the color and the number of layers of polish, with the colors blue and green affecting the decreased oxygen readings the most, black being intermediate, and red and purple having the least effect on the readings. Acrylic nails usually have no significant effect, but some colors also may result in a lower $SpO_2$ reading. Placing the sensor sideways on the finger may produce a reading, but the preferred action is to remove the nail polish or choose another site.

## Other Useful Data

In addition to measuring $SpO_2$, most pulse oximeters provide plethysmography. The plethysmography waveform can provide useful information on the patient's volume status.

Variations in venous blood return (as seen with hypovolemia) change plethysmographic amplitude during the respiratory cycle, similar to changes in arterial blood pressure as measured by an arterial line (pulse pressure variation). However, because plethysmographic waveforms are highly processed and filtered, a visual estimate of the extent of the respiratory variation of pulse amplitude may not be correct. Some newer devices now provide a numeric index of that variability (which is different from the signal strength number or index of perfusion). This correlates with changes in intravascular volume status and fluid responsiveness in hypotensive patients during positive pressure ventilation similarly to variation in stroke volume or pulse pressure. Some sites, such as the forehead or the nasal ala, may be less affected by peripheral vasoconstriction, which could influence the plethysmographic reading. Some pulse oximeters also provide measurements of perfusion in a digit, and this can be used to assess a change in sympathetic tone during general or regional anesthesia or as an intraoperative indication of successful surgical sympathectomy.

## Complications of Pulse Oximetry

Complications are very rare and generally minor, including mild skin erosions and blistering, tanning of the skin with prolonged continuous use, and ischemic skin necrosis. Changing the site of the pulse oximeter probe during prolonged hospitalization should be a standard procedure.

## The Future of Pulse Oximetry

Although most pulse oximeters are displaying only the arterial saturation with a maximum of 100%, recent publications have examined the display of an oxygen reserve index (Masimo, Irvine, CA) and found good correlation and trending in a $PaO_2$ range of 100 to 200 mm Hg. Using this index could be of a possible benefit to demonstrate a rate of fall in oxygen content in apneic, preoxygenated patients before the arterial saturation drops. Although in use outside of the United States, this index is not currently approved by the FDA.

Pulse oximetry has progressed well beyond just displaying arterial saturations as shown by numerous recent publications, such as respiratory rate, plethysmographic analyses, detection of dyshemoglobinemias, total hemoglobin measurement, volume status changes, sympathetic tone, and oxygen reserve index. Although we should always remain vigilant of accuracy and clinical applicability of monitors, the noninvasive nature and simple application of a tool that dates back to the 1970s (in its "modern" form) remains an exciting field of clinical monitoring.

## SUGGESTED READINGS

Cannesson, M., Desebbe, O., Rosamel, P., Delannoy, B., Robin, J., Bastien, O., et al. (2008). Pleth variability index to monitor the respiratory variations in the pulse oximeter plethysmographic waveform amplitude and predict fluid responsiveness in the operating theatre. *British Journal of Anaesthesia, 101,* 200–206.

Chan, E. D., Chan, M. M., & Chan, M. M. (2013). Pulse oximetry: Understanding its basic principles facilitates appreciation of its limitations. *Respiratory Medicine, 107*(6), 789–799.

Fleming, N. W., Singh, A., Lee, L., & Applegate, R. L., II. (2021). Oxygen reserve index: Utility as an early warning for desaturation in high-risk surgical patients. *Anesthesia and Analgesia, 132*(3), 770–776.

Tusman, G., Bohm, S. H., & Suarez-Sipmann, F. (2017). Advanced uses of pulse oximetry for monitoring mechanically ventilated patients. *Anesthesia and Analgesia, 124,* 62–71.

Yamazaki, H., Nishiyama, J., & Suzuki, T. (2012). Use of perfusion index from pulse oximetry to determine efficacy of stellate ganglion block. *Local and Regional Anesthesia, 5,* 9–14.

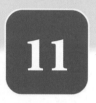

# 11

# Hemodynamic Monitoring

MONICA MYERS MORDECAI, MD

Pulmonary artery catheters (PACs), central venous catheters, and arterial catheters are invasive hemodynamic monitors that are used to obtain additional information in the care of patients. The PAC provides an invasive monitor of cardiac and respiratory function. Hemodynamic and respiratory parameters measured and calculated from PAC-derived data are combined with an assessment of the patient's clinical status to determine therapy. Some PACs have additional uses, such as the ability to provide cardiac pacing and continuous mixed venous and continuous cardiac output measurement. Central venous catheters provide a continuous measure of central venous pressure and the ability to infuse medication centrally. Arterial catheters are indicated for continuous monitoring of blood pressure and can obtain blood for laboratory testing.

## Indications for a Pulmonary Artery Catheter

PACs may be inserted in patients undergoing high-risk surgical procedures and critically ill patients who are in the intensive care unit (ICU). Patient comorbid conditions, elective versus emergency operations, and local practice settings should all be considered before placing a PAC. Many cardiac anesthesiologists place a PAC in patients undergoing cardiac surgery or ascending aorta and aortic arch procedures, in patients with poor left ventricular (LV) or right ventricular (RV) function who are undergoing any open heart or major noncardiac procedure, and for patients undergoing redo cardiac surgery.

## Insertion and Complications of Pulmonary Artery Catheters

The PAC can be inserted from any central or femoral vein, and the pressure waveform is recorded from the distal pulmonary

artery port guiding the clinician in advancing and placing the catheter. Transesophageal echocardiography can also be used to observe advancement of the PAC into the pulmonary artery. The highest success rate is typically achieved using the right internal jugular vein approach. Complications may occur during catheter insertion or while the catheter is in place (Box 11.1).

## Data and Interpretation

Central venous pressure, pulmonary artery pressure, pulmonary artery occlusion pressure (PAOP), cardiac output (CO), mixed venous oxygen saturation ($Svo_2$), and RV ejection fraction can all be measured with a PAC. In addition, several hemodynamic and oxygenation parameters can be calculated based

---

**BOX 11.1 POTENTIAL COMPLICATIONS OF A PULMONARY ARTERY CATHETER**

**DURING INSERTION**

Arrhythmias
Arterial puncture
Balloon rupture
Catheter knotting
Conduction block
Hematoma
Hemorrhage
Hemothorax
Pneumothorax
Pulmonary artery rupture
Venous air embolism

**AFTER INSERTION, LONG-TERM**

Infection
Pulmonary embolism
Pulmonary infarction
Valve injury

on PAC data. To avoid misinterpretation of the data, the pressure transducers must be leveled with the right atrium and calibrated. Mechanical ventilation, positive end-expiratory pressure (PEEP), catheter location, artifacts, and cardiac disease may affect the results of the various measurements. Incorrect measurements and misinterpretation of data can be minimized by implementation of an education program targeting physicians, nurses, and therapists (Box 11.2).

## CARDIAC OUTPUT

RV output can be measured with thermodilution. If no intracardiac shunts are present, the RV output reflects the LV output or the CO. Cardiac output provides a global evaluation of cardiovascular function. To obtain the CO measurement, a 10-mL bolus of saline (either iced or at room temperature) is injected via the proximal port of the PAC. The change in blood temperature is detected by a thermistor located 4 cm proximal to the PAC tip. The temperature change is recorded, and the data are integrated to calculate CO (modified Stewart-Hamilton equation). The thermodilution technique has become the gold standard for measuring CO.

Improvements in PAC technology have led to the development of continuous cardiac output and continuous mixed venous oximetry measurements.

Right-sided valve regurgitation and intracardiac shunt render the CO measurement unreliable. The value of measuring CO in these conditions is questionable, and the procedure should be used with caution, if at all, when the patient has right-sided valve regurgitation or an intracardiac shunt.

## PULMONARY ARTERY OCCLUSION PRESSURE

Accurate measurement of PAOP mandates that the catheter tip rest in West lung zone 3, where there is a continuous column of blood between the catheter tip and the left atrium and the effect of alveolar pressure is minimal. Pulmonary artery diastolic pressure and PAOP are indexes of LV preload and usually correlate closely with LV end-diastolic pressure and volume. However, in many clinical situations (Box 11.3), pulmonary artery diastolic pressure and PAOP either underestimate or overestimate LV end-diastolic pressure.

## MIXED VENOUS OXYGEN SATURATION

The $Svo_2$ is a global index of the balance of oxygen delivery, consumption, and extraction. It can be obtained by aspirating blood from the distal port of the PAC and subsequently analyzing the gases in this venous blood or by continuous measurement with an oximetric PAC.

The normal value of $Svo_2$ is 70% to 75%. In the presence of stable arterial oxygen saturation, oxygen consumption, and hemoglobin concentration, $Svo_2$ is a sensitive indicator of change in CO. A change in CO may reflect a hemodynamic change or a compensation for the change in other parameters. A high $Svo_2$ reading may be caused by a wedged PAC, low oxygen consumption, cyanide or carbon monoxide toxicity, hypothermia, high CO (e.g., sepsis, burns, pancreatitis), left-to-right intracardiac shunts, and the use of inotropic drugs. A low $Svo_2$ reading usually reflects inadequate oxygen delivery. Low CO is the most common cause of low $Svo_2$, but anemia and hypoxemia are other potential causes.

## RIGHT VENTRICULAR FUNCTION

Originally, central venous pressure and CO were the main parameters for assessing RV function. Measurement of central venous pressure and RV pressure has limited value in estimating RV preload. Currently, a PAC with faster thermistor response is available to calculate RV ejection fraction, stroke volume (SV), RV end-diastolic volume, and end-systolic volume. Placement of a PAC that can measure RV ejection fraction is indicated primarily in patients with RV failure, pulmonary hypertension, intrinsic lung disease, sepsis, acute respiratory distress syndrome, and heart failure.

## The Pulmonary Artery Catheter Controversy

For many years, the PAC provided valuable information and was considered the gold standard for hemodynamic monitoring and therapy. However, there is a great deal of controversy over whether a PAC improves patient outcome. A decline in the use of PACs has been documented. Several studies and meta-analyses have shown improvement, no change, or worse outcome with use of a PAC. Experienced clinicians may choose different therapies based on a review of the same clinical data, emphasizing the point that there is no "standard" or "best" practice for PACs. Several less invasive monitoring instruments that have the capability of measuring CO and calculating hemodynamic parameters are currently on the market. The PAC should be used by experienced clinicians who base their management decisions on physiologic and hemodynamic principles, modified to reflect local practice settings. Selected patient populations may benefit from the use of PACs.

## Arterial Catheters

The use of arterial catheters is classically indicated for continuous hemodynamic monitoring and obtaining blood for laboratory determinations in critically ill patients and those undergoing major surgery. The beat-to-beat visual arterial pressure wave and numerical pressure display enable prompt identification of trends or changes in blood pressure that potentially could be missed with noninvasive blood pressure monitoring. Systolic pressure variation (SPV), pulse pressure variation (PPV), and stroke volume variation (SVV) based on the arterial waveform may indicate volume status and predict fluid responsiveness. Accurate measurement of CO can be performed based on the arterial waveform. Several monitoring instruments apply this technology at the bedside.

## Equipment and Cannulation

The arterial catheter is placed in a peripheral artery or the femoral artery, and the radial artery is the most commonly used cannulation site. Arterial spasm and thrombosis, local infection and hematoma, distal ischemia, hemorrhage, and air embolism are the main complications. A 20-gauge cannula is appropriate for cannulation of a small artery, and an 18-gauge cannula is used for a larger one.

Sterile technique should always be applied. The arterial cannula is connected to a pressure transducer via high-pressure tubing. The pressure transducer should usually be located at the level of the right atrium or at the level of the external auditory meatus for the sitting patient who is undergoing a neurosurgical procedure.

## Waveform Interpretation

The arterial waveform provides valuable and continuous hemodynamic information. It changes as the measuring catheter is located more distally from the heart. The pulse pressure increases, and the dicrotic notch is delayed and then disappears. Systolic pressure is higher in a peripheral artery compared with the ascending aorta, but mean pressure is minimally affected or slightly reduced. Heart rate and rhythm can be determined from the arterial tracing. The effect of ectopic beats on arterial pressure and waveform can be evaluated. Pulse pressure may help evaluate the patient's hemodynamic status. High pulse pressure can be seen after exercise and in patients with hyperthyroidism, aortic insufficiency, peripheral vasodilation, arteriovenous malformation, increased stiffness of the aorta (most common in older patients), and mild hypovolemia. Narrow pulse pressure can be seen in patients with hypovolemia, pericardial tamponade, congestive heart failure, aortic stenosis, and shock states. The area under the arterial curve, from the onset of systole to the dicrotic notch, can estimate SV, and the systolic rise may reflect myocardial contractility. However, the arterial curve changes as the location of the arterial cannula insertion moves distally from the ascending aorta.

## Dynamic Indexes of Fluid Responsiveness

The variations derived from the arterial waveform during a mechanical breath (Fig. 11.1) are more pronounced during hypovolemia because the left ventricle operates on the steep portion of the Frank-Starling curve. Changes in RV and LV preload, which are highly sensitive to changes in intrathoracic pressure induced by a mechanical breath, cause the variation in left ventricular stroke volume. Observing the various components of SPV and PPV can establish the presence and cause of hypovolemia, with dynamic changes in the arterial waveform predicting the response to fluid challenge. They are currently the most accurate indicators of fluid responsiveness in patients in the ICU and in many surgical patients. Given that only 50% of patients in the ICU respond to fluid loading, this measurement may provide valuable data for determining which patients should be treated with fluids first and which patients may benefit from inotropic support as the first intervention to increase CO. Although simply viewing the arterial waveform on the arterial pressure tracing can provide information about respiratory variation, an accurate electronic measurement can quantify the pressure variation and its components, allowing the effect of fluid loading to be continually assessed. Spontaneous breathing, frequent arrhythmia, high PEEP, high airway pressure, high and low tidal volumes, low chest wall compliance, increased intraabdominal pressure, and vasodilators all may cause inaccurate representations of the dynamic indexes on tracings from arterial catheters.

Many studies have demonstrated the superiority of the dynamic indexes compared with the static indexes (central venous pressure, pulmonary capillary occlusion pressure, LV end-diastolic area, and global end-diastolic volume) in predicting patient response to fluid loading. The dynamic indexes of fluid responsiveness should be evaluated as a component of the entire clinical scenario for a given patient. They should not be used as a single best index for clinical decisions but should be used in the context of the other clinical parameters.

## Cardiac Output Derived From the Arterial Pressure Waveform

Arterial pressure waveform analysis is used in clinical practice with several commercially available devices that can be used to continuously measure CO, based on the arterial pressure waveform. These devices provide a CO value derived from pulse-contour measurements. This value correlates well with the value derived from the PAC thermodilution technique (a bias of 0.03–0.3 L/min), but under various clinical conditions and therapies this correlation might be disrupted. Compared with the thermodilution technique, these devices are less invasive and their use is associated with potentially fewer complications. These devices use pulse-contour analysis with various algorithms to estimate SV from the arterial waveform. SV is calculated by a mathematical computation of the area under the

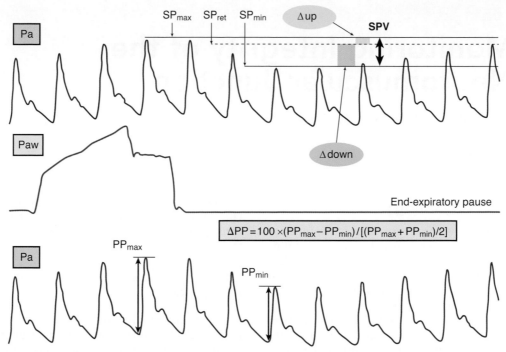

**Fig. 11.1** Analytical description of respiratory changes in arterial pressure during mechanical ventilation. Systolic pressure and pulse pressure (systolic − diastolic pressure) are maximum ($SP_{max}$ and $PP_{max}$, respectively) a few heartbeats later (i.e., during the expiratory period). Systolic pressure variation *(SPV)* is the difference between $SP_{max}$ and $SP_{min}$. Assessment of a reference systolic pressure *($SP_{ret}$)* during an end-expiratory pause allows discrimination between the inspiratory increase *(Δup)* and the expiratory decrease *(Δdown)* in systolic pressure. *Pa,* Arterial pressure; *Paw,* airway pressure; *PP,* pulse pressure; *$PP_{min}$,* pulse pressure minimum; *$SP_{min}$,* systolic pressure minimum. (Adapted from Michard, F. (2005). Changes in arterial pressure during mechanical ventilation. *Anesthesiology, 103,* 419–428.)

systolic portion of the arterial pressure waveform. The algorithm incorporates parameters such as aortic impedance, arterial compliance, and peripheral vascular resistance. They can also calculate other hemodynamic variables (e.g., static preload parameters, peripheral resistance, oxygen delivery, dynamic indexes of fluid responsiveness). The hemodynamic profile is continuously displayed, with the option to follow trends and changes during patient care.

## SUGGESTED READINGS

Bootsma, I. T., Boerma, E. C., de Lange, F., & Scheeren, T. W. L. (2022). The contemporary pulmonary artery catheter. Part 1: Placement and waveform analysis. *Journal of Clinical Monitoring and Computing, 36*(1), 5–15.

de Keijzer, I. N., & Scheeren, T. W. L. (2021). Perioperative hemodynamic monitoring: An overview of current methods. *Anesthesiology Clinics, 39*(3), 441–456.

Pinsky, M. R. (2015). Functional hemodynamic monitoring. *Critical Care Clinics, 31*(1), 89–111.

Rubin, D. S., Apfelbaum, J. L., & Tung, A. (2020). Trends in central venous catheter insertions by anesthesia providers: An analysis of the medicare physician supplier procedure summary from 2007 to 2016. *Anesthesia and Analgesia, 130*(4), 1026–1034.

Sanfilippo, F., Noto, A., Martucci, G., Farbo, M., Burgio, G., & Biasucci, D. G. (2017). Central venous pressure monitoring via peripherally or centrally inserted central catheters: A systematic review and meta-analysis. *Journal of Vascular Access, 18*(4), 273–278.

Saugel, B., Kouz, K., Meidert, A. S., Schulte-Uentrop, L., & Romagnoli, S. (2020). How to measure blood pressure using an arterial catheter: A systematic 5-step approach. *Critical Care, 24*(1), 172.

Scheeren, T. W. L., & Ramsay, M. A. E. (2019). New developments in hemodynamic monitoring. *Journal of Cardiothoracic and Vascular Anesthesia, 33* Suppl 1:S67–S72.

# Monitoring Integrity of the Neuromuscular Junction

ANDREW N. CHALUPKA, MD, MBA

## Neuromuscular Physiology

When a nerve impulse arrives at the neuromuscular junction (NMJ), voltage-gated ion channels open, leading to an influx of calcium within the terminal that causes several hundred vesicles of acetylcholine to fuse with the nerve membrane. The acetylcholine within these vesicles is released into the synaptic cleft, combining with and activating nicotinic receptors on the motor endplate, the activation of which opens ion channels on the muscle membrane and depolarizes the membrane. The release of calcium from intracellular stores stimulates an interaction between actin and myosin, resulting in muscle contraction.

## Importance of Monitoring Neuromuscular Blockade

Monitoring of neuromuscular blockade serves several functions throughout the patient's time in the operating room. At induction, it verifies suitability of intubating conditions. Intraoperatively, it facilitates surgical conditions. At emergence, it ensures return of sufficient function to allow for reversal and inform dosing of reversal agents. Prior to extubation, it evaluates the adequacy of reversal in order to minimize the likelihood of postoperative residual blockade.

Failure to properly monitor the status of the NMJ and emergence and extubation despite residual blockade may put the patient at risk for harm. Residual neuromuscular blockade, especially a TOF ratio of less than 0.9, is an important risk factor for postoperative pulmonary complications (PPCs). Up to half of all patients have residual blockade on arrival to the postanesthesia care unit (PACU). More than 75% of patients receiving a neuromuscular blocking agent (NMBA) experience PPC. Weakness can impair the patient's ability to rerecruit atelectatic lung, thereby prolonging the time to normalization of lung function. Weakness due to residual blockade is also a significant contributor to upper airway obstruction and may result in respiratory failure and reintubation. Residual blockade also increases risk of aspiration due to impaired coordination and weakness of pharyngeal and upper esophageal muscles. Airway and respiratory incidents account for about half of serious incidents in the PACU, as well as malpractice claims arising from them.

Aside from dangerous PPCs, residual blockade can cause bothersome symptoms that result in discomfort for patients: visual disturbances due to diplopia, difficulty moving or repositioning the head or extremities, and difficulty speaking and swallowing. These symptoms may occur with TOF ratios as high as 0.7 to 0.8.

Despite the consensus within the literature of the importance of monitoring, studies also show that qualitative assessment of blockade is not universally performed, and quantitative monitoring is even less frequent.

## Clinical Indicators of Neuromuscular Blockade

Although commonly used, clinical evaluation of recovery from blockade is unreliable, with poor predictive value compared with qualitative or quantitative evaluation. Clinical evaluation is often dependent on patient effort and cooperation, which are difficult to consistently attain in patients intubated and emerging from anesthesia. Effort-dependent tests, such as sustained head lift or hand grip, poorly correlate with recovery of the NMJ. Even seemingly objective respiratory parameters are of limited value. Diaphragmatic muscles regain function prior to pharyngeal muscles, so tidal volumes may appear adequate and provide false reassurance despite upper airway strength still being impaired. Weakness may not be clinically apparent until airway obstruction occurs in the recovery room.

## Qualitative Monitoring of the Neuromuscular Junction

The degree of neuromuscular blockade induced by NMBAs can be evaluated by the response induced by a supramaximal electrical stimulus delivered to a peripheral nerve via a peripheral nerve stimulator in one of the patterns described below. When a peripheral nerve is stimulated with a supramaximal stimulus, each muscle fiber innervated by that nerve responds in an all-or-nothing fashion, and the aggregate response of the whole muscle depends on the number of individual fibers that respond. Muscle fibers with nicotinic receptors that are still inhibited by NMBAs do not respond. The operator assesses the response either tactilely or visually. Qualitative monitoring, although preferable to clinical indicators, is still highly subjective. Even experienced operators tend to underestimate the degree of residual blockade when using qualitative monitoring.

### PERIPHERAL NERVE STIMULATORS

Peripheral nerve stimulators should be able to deliver several different types of stimuli, such as single-twitch, train-of-four (TOF) stimulation, tetanic stimulation, posttetanic facilitation, and double-burst stimulation (DBS). Nerve stimulators also should have polarity indicators, and most have a display that indicates the amount of current applied. Stimuli are monophasic and are delivered as a rectangular square wave with duration of 0.2 to 0.3 ms. If the duration is longer than 0.5 ms, direct muscle stimulation may result. Modern nerve simulators deliver a constant current, despite the resistance, by varying voltage to ensure that the amount of current selected is equal to the amount of current delivered.

## SITES FOR MONITORING

The ideal site for peripheral nerve stimulation is superficially located and does not overlie the muscle being used for evaluation, in order to avoid direct muscle stimulation. Ulnar nerve stimulation of the adductor pollicis meets these criteria and is commonly used but may not be accessible during surgery if arms are tucked. Posterior tibial nerve stimulation of the flexor hallucis can be useful when the patient is turned 180 degrees with respect to the anesthesiologist. Facial nerve stimulation of the orbicularis oculi may be used but carries a higher risk of direct muscle stimulation due to the proximity of the nerve and the muscle.

When interpreting response to stimulation, one must consider the variable response of different muscle groups to neuromuscular blockade. The diaphragm is more resistant to blockade, whereas the laryngeal muscles are highly sensitive to blockade. Likewise, recovery at the orbicularis oculi occurs earlier than recovery at the adductor pollicis, and use of the orbicularis oculi as the monitoring site has been linked with higher risk of residual blockade compared with the adductor pollicis.

## TYPES OF NEUROMUSCULAR BLOCK

Succinylcholine is the only commercially available depolarizing NMBA. It is an agonist at the nicotinic receptor of the NMJ and binds with a high affinity, preventing membrane repolarization and thus subsequent action potentials. Nondepolarizing NMBAs competitively inhibit the nicotinic receptor and prevent acetylcholine from binding. These blocks can be differentiated by monitoring the response to stimulation from a peripheral nerve stimulator, as described later. Of note, the response to succinylcholine may vary. Healthy patients receiving a single dose of succinylcholine exhibit so-called phase I blockade. Patients with abnormal plasma cholinesterase (pseudocholinesterase [butyrylcholinesterase] deficiency) or receiving repeated doses or an infusion of succinylcholine may exhibit phase II blockade.

## MODES OF STIMULATION

Nerve stimulators are programmed to have a variety of stimulation patterns that can be assessed visually or tactilely by the operator to subjectively monitor the presence and depth of a neuromuscular block. Each mode of stimulation has advantages and disadvantages.

### Single-Twitch Stimulation

Single-twitch stimulation is a supramaximal stimuli mode that is applied with a frequency between 0.1 and 1 Hz. The provoked responses after neuromuscular blockade are compared with a preblockade baseline. The motor response remains static until approximately 75% of the nicotinic receptors are blocked. With blockade of approximately 95% of nicotinic receptors, no response will occur.

### Train-of-Four Stimulation

TOF stimulation comprises four identical supramaximal stimuli that are delivered at 2 Hz, each of which can produce a motor response. TOF testing is one of the most common methods used for monitoring the extent of neuromuscular blockade. Unlike single-twitch stimulation, no preparalytic baseline is required.

In the absence of neuromuscular blockade, all four responses are of equal strength. With use of a nondepolarizing NMBA, responses may be all absent, all equal, or sequentially weaken (a phenomenon known as fade), depending on the degree of blockade present. When the fourth stimulus produces no twitch, approximately 80% of receptors are blocked (three twitches present); the third twitch is lost when 85% of receptors are blocked (two twitches present); and the second twitch is lost when 90% of receptors are blocked (one twitch present).

Although TOF stimulation is commonly used as a qualitative monitoring method, a notable caveat is that most clinicians are unable to visually or tactilely detect fade past a TOF ratio of 0.3 to 0.4. TOF stimulation as part of quantitative monitoring (e.g., accelerometry, described later) may better detect residual blockade.

The TOF stimulation pattern varies with succinylcholine depending on the type of blockade. Phase I blockade will produce four identical responses without fade, but the amplitude of these responses will be less than a baseline response would be in the absence of blockade. Phase II blockade produces a decremental pattern similar to that seen with nondepolarizing NMBA use.

### Tetanus

Tetanus is obtained by the delivery of repetitive stimuli, usually at 50 to 100 Hz for 5 seconds. In the absence of neuromuscular blockade, a tetanic contraction will result. With a nondepolarizing block, fade is observed (i.e., a decrease in the amplitude of force over the duration of the stimulus). Tetanus at 100 Hz is more sensitive than tetanus at 50 Hz for detecting residual blockade. Because of the potential for tetany to induce fatigue, tetanic stimulation should not be repeated more frequently than every 2 to 3 minutes.

### Posttetanic Facilitation

After tetanic stimulation, there is an abundance of acetylcholine within the NMJ. Before it dissipates, this excess can be used to facilitate a subsequent stimulus. Posttetanic facilitation testing is done with a 50-Hz tetanic stimulation for 5 seconds followed 3 seconds later by a single 1-Hz stimulus. This mode is useful in identifying early spontaneous recovery after profound neuromuscular blockade when TOF testing produces no twitch response. In this situation, if a twitch is produced with posttetanic facilitation, this indicates that 0% to 5% of receptors are unoccupied and spontaneous recovery has commenced.

### Double-Burst Stimulation

DBS involves the delivery of two short 50-Hz stimuli separated by 750 ms. In $DBS_{3,3}$, three impulses are delivered in each burst.

In DBS$_{3,2}$, three impulses are delivered followed by only two impulses. In the absence of neuromuscular blockade, the first and second groups of stimuli produce contractions of equal strength. In the presence of blockade, fade occurs: the second group of stimuli produces a contraction of lesser strength. Because the contraction produced by DBS is stronger than that produced by TOF stimulation, fade can be subjectively detected up to a TOF ratio of 0.6. Although this offers an advantage over TOF stimulation, it is still insufficient for detection of a TOF ratio of 0.9.

## Quantitative Monitoring of the Neuromuscular Junction

Whereas clinical monitoring depends on patient effort and qualitative monitoring relies on a clinician's subjective assessment, quantitative monitors allow for objective measurement of the depth of neuromuscular blockade. A recent consensus statement on standards of neuromuscular monitoring during anesthesia suggests that quantitative monitoring should be employed whenever a nondepolarizing neuromuscular blocker is used, because of the poor sensitivity of clinical or qualitative monitoring for residual blockade.

Quantitative neuromuscular monitoring encompasses multiple modalities. Acceleromyography is the most commonly used. Electromyography and kinemyography are less commonly employed, but commercially available devices are sold for clinical use. Mechanomyography and phonomyography are not routinely used in clinical practice.

### ACCELEROMYOGRAPHY

Newton's second law of motion is the foundation for acceleromyography (AMG). A piezoelectric transducer, affixed commonly to the thumb for adductor pollicis measurement, is used to measure acceleration of the stimulated muscle. Traditional acceleromyographs measured force in one direction, but newer devices can measure movement in three dimensions. AMG can be used on a variety of muscle sites and has good correlation with mechanomyography.

### ELECTROMYOGRAPHY

Electromyography measures the compound action potential from direct stimulation of a peripheral nerve. This method can be used to monitor any nerve, including those supplying laryngeal muscles and the diaphragm.

### KINEMYOGRAPHY

As with AMG, a piezoelectric sensor is used to generate an electric signal proportional to the force of the motion it experiences. In kinemyography, however, the sensor is a thin film that can be bent, rather than rigid and fixed.

### MECHANOMYOGRAPHY

Mechanomyography (MMG) is the gold standard of monitoring neuromuscular blockade because it measures the actual force of isometric contraction against a fixed resting tension with a force transducer. It is typically used on the hand (adductor pollicis) with ulnar stimulation. This is a precise mechanism, but its complexity limits its use to research.

### PHONOMYOGRAPHY

Phonomyography measures the low-frequency sounds of muscle contraction. It correlates well with MMG and can be applied to any muscle.

## SUGGESTED READINGS

Berg, S. M., & Braehler, M. R. (2020). The postanesthesia care unit. In M. A. Gropper, R. D. Miller, N. H. Cohen, L. I. Eriksson, L. A. Fleisher, K. Leslie, et al., (Eds.), *Miller's anesthesia* (9th ed., pp. 2586–2613). Philadelphia: Elsevier.

Brull, S. J., & Murphy, G. S. (2010). Residual neuromuscular block: Lessons unlearned. Part II: Methods to reduce the risk of residual weakness. *Anesthesia and Analgesia, 111,* 129–140.

Cammu, G. (2020). Residual neuromuscular blockade and postoperative pulmonary complications: What does the recent evidence demonstrate? *Current Anesthesiology Reports,* 10(2), 131–136.

Claudius, C., & Fuchs-Buder, T. (2020). Neuromuscular monitoring. In M. A. Gropper, R. D.

Miller, N. H. Cohen, L. I. Eriksson, L. A. Fleisher, K. Leslie, et al., (Eds.), *Miller's anesthesia* (9th ed., pp. 1354–1372). Philadelphia: Elsevier.

Duțu, M., Ivașcu, R., Tudorache, O., Morlova, D., Stanca, A., Negoiță, S., et al. (2018). Neuromuscular monitoring: An update. *Romanian Journal of Anaesthesia and Intensive Care,* 25(1), 55–60.

Miskovic, A., & Lumb, A. B. (2017). Postoperative pulmonary complications. *British Journal of Anaesthesia,* 118(3), 317–334.

Murphy, G. S. (2018). Neuromuscular monitoring in the perioperative period. *Anesthesia and Analgesia,* 126(2), 464–468.

Murphy, G. S., & Brull, S. J. (2010). Residual neuromuscular block: Lessons unlearned. Part I:

Definitions, incidence, and adverse physiologic effects of residual neuromuscular block. *Anesthesia and Analgesia, 111,* 120–128.

Murphy, G., De Boer, H. D., Erikkson, L. I., & Miller, R. D. (2020). Reversal (Antagonism) of neuromuscular blockade. In M. A. Gropper, R. D. Miller, N. H. Cohen, L. I. Eriksson, L. A. Fleisher, K. Leslie, et al., (Eds.), *Miller's anesthesia* (9th ed., pp. 832–864). Philadelphia: Elsevier.

Naguib, M., Brull, S. J., Kopman, A. F., Hunter, J. M., Fülesdi, B., Arkes, H. R., et al. (2018). Consensus statement on perioperative use of neuromuscular monitoring. *Anesthesia and Analgesia,* 127(1), 71–80.

# Evoked Potential Monitoring and Electromyography

BENJAMIN T. DAXON, MD | JEFFREY J. PASTERNAK, MS, MD

Evoked potential (EP) monitoring is used to assess the integrity of select neuronal pathways within the central and peripheral nervous systems whereas electromyography (EMG) is used to monitor peripheral nerves. These techniques are especially useful intraoperatively when general anesthesia otherwise limits or prevents performance of a clinical neurologic examination.

## Evoked Potential Monitoring

Evaluation of four major neuronal systems can be accomplished via EP measurements: sensory pathways via somatosensory evoked potentials (SSEP), auditory pathways via brainstem auditory evoked responses (BAER), visual pathways via visual evoked potentials (VEP), and motor pathways via motor evoked potentials (MEP). BAERs are the most resistant to the effects of anesthetic drugs, and VEPs are the most sensitive; SSEP and MEP responses are intermediate in sensitivity to the effects of anesthetic drugs.

## The Evoked Potential Waveform

All four EP techniques involve the application of a stimulus that generates a neuronal response. Typical response recordings are expressed as a graph of time (e.g., milliseconds) on the x-axis and voltage (e.g., millivolts) on the y-axis (Fig. 13.1). The responses are very low voltage and require signal averaging to enhance their quality. Therefore recorded waveforms are usually a composite of 50 to 100 or more measurements derived from multiple stimulation measurement cycles that serve to "subtract out" higher-voltage interference (e.g., electrocardiogram, electroencephalogram, and electrical noise within the operative suite). Peak and trough voltages in the measured waveform refer to positive or negative deflections, designated by a P or N, respectively.

Two major characteristics of the measured waveform are usually described: amplitude and latency.
- Amplitude refers to the voltage difference between either a successive peak or a designated reference voltage.
- Latency refers to the duration of time after stimulation in which a specific peak occurs and is usually designated as a subscript of the given positively or negatively deflected peak (i.e., $N_{20}$ is a negatively deflected peak occurring 20 milliseconds after stimulation). Interpeak latency refers to the time difference (in milliseconds) between two different peaks.

Many factors can influence the recorded waveform:
- Surgical factors: Injury to a neural pathway from compression, reduced perfusion, or transsection
- Anesthetic drugs: Variable effects depending on the EP modality and the drug

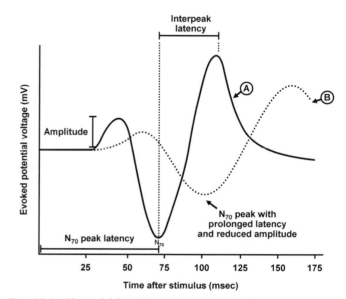

**Fig. 13.1** The *solid line* **(A)** represents a typical evoked potential waveform described in terms of latency (time from delivery of stimulus to onset of response) and amplitude (size in microvolts). Interpeak latency refers to the time difference between two peaks on the tracing. Waveform B represents a decrease in amplitude and an increase in latency compared with waveform A. This change can occur as a result of neuronal ischemia or injury, effects of various anesthetic agents, or changes in physiologic variables leading to reduced neuronal perfusion. (Modified, with permission, from Mahla ME. Neurologic monitoring. In: Cucchiara RF, Black S, Michenfelder JD, eds. *Clinical Neuroanesthesia.* 2nd ed. Churchill Livingstone; 1998.)

- Physiologic variables: Decreased oxygen delivery to the neural pathway being monitored can occur with hypotension, anemia, and hypoxia; hypothermia can also reduce the rate of neural conduction and affect recordings
- Monitoring variables: Examples include displacement of monitoring leads or changes in electrical impedance
- Positioning: Compression of a nerve due to improper patient positioning can interfere with conduction, even if the surgical site is remote (e.g., ulnar nerve compression in the prone position during spine surgery)
- Preexisting neurologic deficits: In those with preexisting neurologic deficits, the EP waveform may appear abnormal; this effect can be compounded by anesthetic drugs, making EP monitoring in patients with preexisting deficits challenging or impossible
- Age: Because the immaturity of the central nervous system, EP monitoring can be challenging in young children, often requiring an increase in the voltage required to elicit a response

| TABLE 13.1 | Effects of Anesthetic Drugs on the Amplitude and Latency of Evoked Potential Waveforms | |
|---|---|---|
| **Drug** | **Amplitude** | **Latency** |
| Etomidate | ↑ | ↑ |
| Ketamine | ↑ | ↑ |
| Opioids | – | – |
| Dexmedetomidine | – | – |
| Propofol | ↓ | – |
| Droperidol | ↓ | ↑ |
| Benzodiazepines | ↓ | ↑ |
| Nitrous oxide | ↓ | – |
| Halogenated | ↓ | ↑ |

An up arrow indicates an increase, a down arrow indicates a decrease, and a hyphen indicates no significant effect.

General principles describing the effect of anesthetic drugs on EP waveforms are summarized in Table 13.1 and include:

- Most anesthetic drugs cause an increase in the latency and a decrease in the amplitude of EP waveforms.
- Ketamine and etomidate cause an increase in both latency and amplitude of EP waveforms.
- In general, opioids have less effect on amplitude and latency of EP waveforms than do most other anesthetic drugs.
- Muscle relaxants impair motor EP monitoring but have no effect on sensory EP (i.e., SSEP, BAER, VEP).

## Brainstem Auditory Evoked Responses

BAERs allow monitoring of the integrity of the auditory pathway both peripherally and centrally. Stimuli are loud, repetitive clicks produced by a device placed over or in the auditory canals. Measurement of the response is from electrodes placed on the scalp or external ears to record contralateral and ipsilateral signals that have and have not decussated, respectively. Some anesthetic drugs may cause minor changes in amplitude or latency of recorded waveforms. However, these changes are usually very small, even with large changes in anesthetic dose. Therefore significant intraoperative BAER changes are usually indicative of a surgical trespass.

Potential indications for intraoperative BAERs include monitoring for microvascular decompression of cranial nerve V or VII, resection of tumors in the cerebellopontine angle, or resection of brainstem lesions, and BAERs may help in the declaration of brain death in the intensive care unit.

## Somatosensory Evoked Potentials

Monitoring of SSEPs permit assessment of major *afferent* neural pathways within the *dorsal column* of the spinal cord that are responsible for transmission of the sensory information of touch, vibration, and proprioception.

Stimulation and monitoring of SSEPs from the median, posterior tibial, or peroneal nerve are commonly performed. Measurement of the response can be accomplished by recording more proximally along the same nerve, over the spine, or from the contralateral scalp. The dorsal columns within the spinal cord are supplied by the posterior spinal arteries. Accordingly, SSEP measurements are generally not reliable for the detection of ischemia in regions of the cord supplied by the anterior spinal artery that include the motor pathways.

SSEP monitoring can be used for procedures involving the spine (e.g., scoliosis surgery, spinal cord tumor resection, laminectomy with fusion, vertebral fractures with instability), posterior fossa operations (e.g., tumor resection), and vascular operations (e.g., carotid endarterectomy, cerebral aneurysm clipping).

Anesthetic drugs have variable effects on recordings of SSEPs. Stimulation and measurement of potentials from peripheral nerves and subcortical regions are often minimally affected by anesthetic drugs. However, anesthetic drugs can have a significant modulatory effect on the waveforms recorded from the cortex. In general, drugs that cause increased latency and decreased amplitude include inhalation anesthetics (e.g., isoflurane, sevoflurane, desflurane), $N_2O$, propofol, benzodiazepines, and opioids. The magnitude of the effect on either latency or amplitude varies among these agents, with opioids usually having minimal effects. Increased latency or decreased amplitude can also occur with ischemia or injury to the sensory pathway. Ketamine and etomidate increase both the amplitude and latency of SSEP waveforms. As such, these drugs can actually be used to enhance signals due to their effect on amplitude. Neuromuscular blocking agents (NMBAs) have no significant effect on SSEPs.

## Motor Evoked Potentials

Unlike SSEP techniques that assess the integrity of afferent neural pathways, MEPs assess the efferent motor pathway within the corticospinal tract. Blood to the primary motor pathway in the spinal cord is derived mostly from the anterior spinal artery.

Stimulation of MEPs can be accomplished from the cerebral cortex or spinal cord by applying either an electric or magnetic stimulus. Recording can be accomplished anywhere caudal to the site stimulated; however, recording within the muscle is most commonly used.

Intraoperative recording of MEPs can be used during spine operations (e.g., scoliosis correction, spinal tumor resection) or operations involving peripheral nerves (e.g., brachial plexus or peripheral nerve reconstruction/transposition). Intraoperative MEP recording may also provide valuable information during repair of thoracoabdominal aortic aneurysms. The artery of Adamkiewicz, a branch of the aorta, often has a variable location and supplies the lower two-thirds of the anterior spinal cord; occlusion of the artery of Adamkiewicz either directly or via occlusion of the aorta at a site proximal to the artery's origin places a large portion of the spinal cord at risk and can be detected with MEP monitoring.

As with sensory EPs, MEPs are also subject to interference by anesthetic drugs and physiologic variables. Electrically induced MEPs are less sensitive to anesthetic effects than are magnetically induced MEP signals. Utilization of multipulse (versus single-pulse) electrical stimulation will further reduce the sensitivity of MEPs to the effects of anesthetic agents and will improve signal quality because of summation and recruitment of a greater number of axons to transmit the stimulus. MEPs that do not involve cerebral cortical stimulation (i.e., stimulation at the level of the spinal cord or peripheral nerve) are less sensitive to the effects of anesthetic drugs than are those involving cortical stimulation.

Complete neuromuscular blockade will result in loss of MEPs recorded from muscle. Otherwise, NMBAs should be used with caution, if at all. Inhalation anesthetic drugs, $N_2O$, propofol, barbiturates, and benzodiazepines differentially decreased signal amplitude and increased signal latency, especially when given in high doses. Ketamine, etomidate, dexmedetomidine, propofol, and opioids have minimal effects on MEPs, such that these agents can be used at moderate doses during MEP monitoring.

## Visual Evoked Potentials

VEPs allow for assessment of the integrity of the entire visual system, including the eye, optic nerve, optic chiasm, optic tracts and radiations, and visual cortex of the occipital lobe. Measurement of VEPs involves delivery of repetitive bright flashes of light through goggles or placement of contact lenses containing light-emitting diodes. Traditionally, intraoperative recording of VEPs has been attempted for resection of tumors near the optic nerve (i.e., skull-base meningioma) or optic chiasm (i.e., pituitary tumors); however, the exquisite sensitivity of VEPs to the depressant effects of anesthetic agents make them difficult for intraoperative use.

## Intraoperative Changes in Evoked Potential Signals

If EPs are being recorded intraoperatively, the clinician should have a very systematic approach to assess the reason for changes in signals. Ischemia, injury, or transection of a neural pathway will generally result in either a decrease in signal amplitude with an increase in signal latency or a complete loss of signal (i.e., isoelectricity). The following should be considered to rule out anesthetic and monitoring-based causes:

- Was a drug recently administered, or was the dose of a drug recently changed?
- Was an NMBA given during MEP monitoring?
- Is there a physiologic reason for neural ischemia or hypoxia (e.g., hypotension, hypoxia, anemia)? An increase in blood pressure, the $O_2$ content of blood, and hemoglobin concentration may all be helpful in improving $O_2$ delivery to compromised neural tissue even in the event of a surgical cause of signal decrease or loss.
- Is there significant hypothermia?
- Is there a positioning problem that may result in peripheral nerve compression?
- Is there a problem with the monitoring equipment (e.g., displacement of a monitoring lead)?

Although EPs are sensitive and valid for detecting neural injury, they often lack specificity. Once anesthetic, physiologic, and monitoring-based causes have been ruled out or corrected and the signal amplitude and latency still do not improve, surgical causes for neural compromise should be sought and corrected, if possible. This may necessitate an alteration in surgical technique or an augmentation in perfusion pressure with vasoactive drugs if nerve injury is thought to have occurred. Despite their accuracy and reliability in detecting injury, there is insufficient evidence to show that EP monitor actually alters neurologic outcomes, particularly in spinal surgery, and their use as a "standard of care" remains controversial.

## Electromyography

Unlike EPs that can be used to monitor the integrity of both the central and peripheral nervous system, EMG can only be used to monitor the integrity of peripheral nerves. EMG can be either free running or stimulated. In either case, a recording electrode is placed over a muscle or a recorded needle electrode is placed within a muscle.

During free-running EMG, when the nerve that supplies the monitored muscle is touched, stretched, heated, or injured, EMG activity in the form of a neurotonic discharge is recorded as shown in Fig. 13.2. During stimulated EMG, an electrical stimulator is used in the surgical field. When the stimulator is near the nerve that supplies the muscle of interest, EMG activity will be recorded.

EMG has broad perioperative applications. EMG can be useful during spine surgery to allow for identification of nerve roots and to warn of nerve injury, such as during pedicle screw placement. EMG is commonly used during skull-base surgery, especially during tumor resection, to assist the surgeon in identifying cranial nerves. EMG can also be useful to identify the facial nerve and its branches during parotidectomy. During thyroid gland surgery, identification of the recurrent laryngeal nerve can be accomplished with EMG. As the recurrent laryngeal nerve supplies motor function to many of laryngeal muscles, EMG activity can be monitored via a tracheal tube that contains an electrode near the distal end.

In procedures employing EMG, muscle relaxation will attenuate or prevent the detection of EMG activity and should not be used concurrently with EMG monitoring. In procedures involving laryngeal nerve monitoring, the electrode on the distal end of the tracheal tube should be placed at the level of the vocal cords.

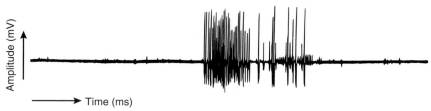

**Fig. 13.2** Example of an electromyographic neurotonic discharge.

## SUGGESTED READING

Gertsch, J. H., Moreira, J. J., Lee, G. R., Hastings, J. D., Ritzl, E., Eccher, M. A., et al. (2019). Practice guidelines for the supervising professional: Intraoperative neurophysiological monitoring. *Journal of Clinical Monitoring and Computing, 33,* 175–183.

Koht, A., & Sloan, T. B. (2016). Intraoperative monitoring: Recent advances in motor evoked potentials. *Anesthesiology Clinics, 34*(3), 525–535.

Korean Society of Neurophysiology. (2021). Clinical practice guidelines for intraoperative neurophysiological monitoring: A 2020 update. *Annals of Clinical Neurophysiology, 23,* 35–45.

Nunes, R. R., Bershot, C. D. A., & Garritano, J. G. (2018). Intraoperative neurophysiologic monitoring in neuroanesthesia. *Current Opinion in Anaesthesiology, 31,* 532–538.

Rao, S., Kurfess, J., & Treggiari, M. M. (2021). Basics of neuromonitoring and anesthetic considerations. *Anesthesiology Clinics, 39,* 195–209.

Rozet, I., Metzner, J., Brown, M., Treggiari, M. M., Slimp, J. C., Kinney, G., et al. (2015). Dexmedetomidine does not affect evoked potentials during spine surgery. *Anesthesia and Analgesia, 121,* 492–501.

# SECTION II

# Physiology

# 14

# Oxygen Transport

DAVID R. MUMME, MD

Oxygen transport is the physiologic mechanism through which oxygen in the bloodstream is delivered to tissues for metabolism. Under most circumstances, oxygen transport is critically dependent on hemoglobin, a unique protein in red blood cells that binds up to four oxygen molecules, carries oxygen to tissues, and releases bound oxygen to support tissue metabolism.

The amount of $O_2$ delivered to tissues is the arterial $O_2$ content ($CaO_2$) multiplied by the cardiac output (CO), with CO equal to stroke volume multiplied by heart rate (Fig. 14.1). Factors that affect $CaO_2$ include the concentration of hemoglobin (Hb), the amount of oxygen carried by Hb (typically, 1.39 mL/g Hb), oxygen saturation ($SaO_2$), and oxygen dissolved in the plasma ($PaO_2 \times 0.003$). The following formula is used to calculate $CaO_2$:

$$CaO_2 = (Hb \times 1.39 \times SaO_2 / 100) + (PaO_2 \times 0.003)$$

It is important to note that dissolved $O_2$ typically has little influence on $CaO_2$. Notable exceptions occur when $O_2$ carried by Hb is severely diminished (e.g., severe anemia, carbon monoxide poisoning) or if the $PaO_2$ is very high (e.g., in a hyperbaric chamber).

As an example, if Hb is 15 g/dL, $SaO_2$ is 100%, and $PaO_2$ is 100 mm Hg, then

$$CaO_2 = (15 \times 1.39 \times 1) + (100 \times 0.003)$$
$$= 20.85 + 0.3$$
$$= 21.15 \text{ mL/dL (or 211.5 mL/L)}$$

Calculating the oxygen content of mixed venous blood ($C\bar{v}O_2$) allows determination of tissue $O_2$ extraction, which is equal to the difference between $CaO_2$ and $C\bar{v}O_2$. At mixed venous $O_2$ saturation of 75% and mixed venous $O_2$ tension of 40 mm Hg, $C\bar{v}O_2$ is:

$$C\bar{v}O_2 = (15 \times 1.39 \times 0.75) + (40 \times 0.003)$$
$$= 15.64 + 0.12$$
$$= 15.76 \text{ mL/dL}$$

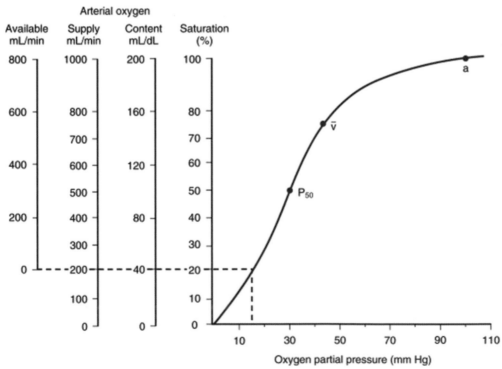

**Fig. 14.1** Oxygen-hemoglobin dissociation curve. Four different ordinates are shown as a function of oxygen partial pressure (x-axis). In order from right to left, they are arterial oxygen saturation (%), arterial oxygen content (mL of $O_2$/dL of blood), oxygen supply to peripheral tissues (mL/min), and oxygen available to peripheral tissues (mL/min), which is oxygen supply minus the approximately 200 mL/min that cannot be extracted below a partial pressure of 20 mm Hg. Three points are shown on the curve: a, normal arterial partial pressure; $\bar{V}$, normal mixed venous partial pressure; and P50, the partial pressure (27 mm Hg) at which hemoglobin is 50% saturated. (From Wilson WC, Benumof JL. Physiology of the airway. In Hagberg CA, Artime CA, Aziz MF, eds. *Hagberg and Benumof's Airway Management*. 4th ed. Elsevier; 2018:fig. 5.25.)

Oxygen delivery ($\dot{D}O_2$) to the tissues is the product of CO and $Cao_2$. For example, if CO is 5.0 L/min in the first example, then $\dot{D}O_2$ is calculated as:

$$\dot{D}O_2 = 21.15\ dL/L \times 50\ dL/min$$
$$= 1057\ mL/min\ (approx.\ 1\ L/min)$$

Oxygen consumption ($\dot{V}O_2$), approximately 250 mL/min for an adult, is CO multiplied by the difference between arterial and venous $O_2$ content (assuming no shunt). This calculation uses the Fick principle:

$$\dot{V}O_2 = CO \times C(a - \bar{v})O_2$$

For a constant $\dot{V}O_2$, a decrease in CO requires a proportionate increase in $C(a - \bar{v})O_2$, usually achieved by increasing tissue $O_2$ extraction. Conversely, if $\dot{V}O_2$ increases, CO, $C(a - \bar{v})O_2$, or both CO and $C(a - \bar{v})O_2$ must increase.

## The Oxyhemoglobin Dissociation Curve

The oxyhemoglobin dissociation curve describes the relationship between $Pao_2$ and $Sao_2$. The oxyhemoglobin disassociation curve is shifted by a variety of physiologic variables (Table 14.1). Note that shifts in the oxyhemoglobin dissociation curve can profoundly affect oxygen delivery. Also note that the P50, the position at which Hb is 50% saturated, is normally 26.7 mm Hg in adults.

Variance in the affinity of hemoglobin and oxygen can shift the oxyhemoglobin dissociation curve to the right or left. Right shifts of the curve indicate decreased affinity of hemoglobin and oxygen, and left shifts of the curve indicate increased affinity. A left shift of the curve indicates greater binding of hemoglobin and oxygen, resulting in a higher oxygen saturation at a given $Pao_2$ (e.g., fetal hemoglobin). This increased affinity of Hb for $O_2$ may require higher tissue perfusion to produce the same $O_2$ delivery (because Hb does not release oxygen to the

| TABLE 14.1 | Variables That Shift the Oxyhemoglobin Dissociation Curve | |
|---|---|
| **Left (Increased Affinity)** | **Right (Decreased Affinity)** |
| Alkalosis | Acidosis |
| Hypothermia | Hyperthermia |
| Decreased 2,3-diphosphoglycerate | Increased 2,3-diphosphoglycerate |
| Abnormal hemoglobin (e.g., fetal) | Abnormal hemoglobin |
| Carboxyhemoglobin | Hypercarbia |
| Methemoglobin | |

tissues as easily). It is important to note the marked depletion of 2,3-diphosphoglycerate (2,3-DPG) in banked blood within 1 to 2 weeks can affect $O_2$ delivery after massive transfusion.

A right shift of the curve indicates lower affinity of Hb and $O_2$, resulting in lower oxygen saturation at a given $Pao_2$. This decreased affinity of Hb and $O_2$ may compensate for decreased tissue perfusion because it promotes greater tissue unloading of $O_2$. Factors that shift the oxyhemoglobin curve to the right include increased hydrogen ions (lower pH), 2,3-DPG, and increased temperature. Shifting the oxyhemoglobin dissociation curve to the left or right has little effect on $Sao_2$ greater than 90%, at which point the curve is relatively horizontal; a much greater effect is evident for values in the steeper parts of the curve ($Sao_2 < 90\%$).

Shifts in the curve are not necessarily permanent. For instance, chronic acid-base changes cause a compensatory change in 2,3-DPG within 24 to 48 hours and restore the oxyhemoglobin dissociation curve back toward normal.

Modern multiwavelength pulse oximeters can also measure methemoglobin (metHb) and carboxyhemoglobin (COHb), leading to the term *fractional saturation*, which is the total saturation less the contributions of metHb and COHb.

## SUGGESTED READINGS

Arora, S., & Tantia, P. (2019). Physiology of oxygen transport and its determinants in intensive care unit. *Indian Journal of Critical Care Medicine, 23*(Suppl. 3), S172–S177.

Bignami, E., Saglietti, F., Girombelli, A., Briolini, A., Bove, T., & Vetrugno, L. (2019). Preoxygenation during induction of anesthesia in non-critically ill patients: A systematic review. *Journal of Clinical Anesthesia, 52*, 85–90.

Feiner, J. (2018). Clinical cardiac and pulmonary physiology. In M. Pardo, & R. D. Miller (Eds.), *Basics of Anesthesia* (7th ed., pp. 53–69). Philadelphia: Elsevier.

Scott, A. V., Nagababu, E., Johnson, D. J., Kebaish, K. M., Lipsitz, J. A., Dwyer, I. M., et al. (2016). 2,3-Diphosphoglycerate concentrations in autologous salvaged versus stored red blood cells and

in surgical patients after transfusion. *Anesthesia and Analgesia, 122*(3), 616–623.

Wilson, W. C., & Benumof, J. L. (2018). Physiology of the airway. In C. A. Hagberg, C. A. Artime, & M. F. Aziz (Eds.), *Airway management* (4th ed., pp. 110–148). Philadelphia: Elsevier.

# 15

# Blood Gas Temperature Correction

MARISSA L. KAUSS, MD  |  SARAH ARMOUR, MD

Patient temperature has a dynamic impact on blood gas measurement. An "alkaline drift" is often observed in hypothermic patients due to an inverse relationship between temperature and gas solubility ($\downarrow$ temperature, $\uparrow$ gas solubility). As temperature decreases, the dynamic equilibrium between gas solubility and partial pressure shifts, resulting in decreased $Paco_2$ as more $CO_2$ is dissolved in liquid. This lowered $Paco_2$ increases pH (alkaline drift). This drift is not apparent on routine arterial blood gas analysis because these samples are warmed to 37°C before gas tension is measured.

Acid-base management in hypothermic patients is commonly accomplished using either the pH-Stat or α-Stat method. The pH-Stat method uses temperature correction to maintain constant $Paco_2$ of 40 mm Hg and pH of 7.40 during hypothermia. The pH-Stat mechanism adds exogenous $CO_2$ to inspired gases, resulting in an increase in total $CO_2$ content. In contrast, the α-Stat approach does not correct for patient temperature. It maintains arterial pH at 7.4 and $Paco_2$ at 40 mm Hg, based on samples warmed to 37°C. The overall goal of both methods is identical: maintain arterial pH at 7.40 and $Paco_2$ at 40 mm Hg. However, these values are based on measurements obtained at different temperatures.

The principle of gas solubility ($O_2$ and $CO_2$) is addressed by Henry's law. This law states the amount of gas that will dissolve in a liquid (at a given temperature) is proportional to the partial pressure of the gas ($Paco_2$, $Pao_2$). This concept explains why hyperbaric oxygen can increase dissolved $O_2$ content in blood: increased pressure = increased dissolution into a liquid. However, this law applies only to a gas at a set temperature. Understanding how a change in temperature affects gas solubility is another important concept that anesthesia providers must understand.

The solubility of $CO_2$ is inversely proportional to patient temperature. The dynamic equilibrium between gas solubility and partial pressure will shift, resulting in decreased $Paco_2$ as more $CO_2$ is dissolved in liquid (Fig. 15.1). For example, if blood at 37°C with a $Paco_2$ of 40 mm Hg is cooled to 25°C, the $Paco_2$ would decrease to 23 mm Hg. Since plasma bicarbonate levels are not affected by temperature change, the pH will increase as $Paco_2$ decreases with hypothermia. Using the above example, the patient's pH would increase from 7.40 to 7.60.

The "alkaline drift" that is seen in patients with hypothermia can significantly affect blood gas measurements and patient management. A normal blood gas sample is heated to 37°C before it is analyzed for gas partial pressures. As a result, a sample taken from a patient with a temperature of 37°C provides an accurate assessment of arterial gas $Paco_2$, $Pao_2$, and pH. However, heating a sample from a patient with a temperature of 25°C to 37°C will show higher gas tensions and lower pH than actually are present unless these values are corrected for temperature. Two approaches are used to guide acid-base

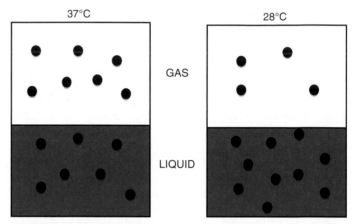

**Fig. 15.1** Representation of temperature effects on $CO_2$ solubility. $CO_2$ is represented by the black dots in the figure. At 28°C, there is more $CO_2$ dissolved in a liquid, but overall $CO_2$ content is unchanged (14 total).

management in patient with hypothermia during cardiopulmonary bypass: α-Stat and pH-Stat.

## α-Stat Method

This method is often used for patients undergoing hypothermic cardiopulmonary bypass. The name α-Stat originates from the α-imidazole ring of histidine, which provides an important pH buffer for body proteins. Charges on these rings help maintain intracellular electroneutrality and preserve normal protein function. To achieve electroneutrality, arterial pH and $Paco_2$ are maintained at 7.40 and 40 mm Hg, respectively, based on samples warmed to 37°C. There is no temperature correction or addition of $CO_2$ to the inspired gases. Total $CO_2$ content is unchanged.

## pH-Stat Method

This method, most commonly used until the 1980s, uses temperature correction to maintain constant $Paco_2$ of 40 mm Hg and pH 7.40 during hypothermia by adding exogenous $CO_2$ to inspired gases. This maintains the appropriate gas tension by increasing the total $CO_2$ content.

## pH-Stat Versus α-Stat

The goal of both approaches is to maintain arterial pH at 7.40 and $Paco_2$ at 40 mm Hg, but they are based on readings at different temperatures (Table 15.1). Each method confers physiologic advantages and disadvantages. Total $CO_2$ content is increased with pH-Stat, which leads to cerebral vasodilation and

| TABLE 15.1 | Comparison of pH-Stat and α-Stat Management, Benefits, and Disadvantages | | | | | |
|---|---|---|---|---|---|---|
| Method | Temp 28°C (In vivo/Patient) | Temp 37°C (In vitro/Lab) | $CO_2$ Added | Total $CO_2$ Content | Pros | Cons |
| pH-Stat | pH 7.40 $Paco_2$ 40 mm Hg | pH 7.27 $Paco_2$ 56 mm Hg | Yes | Increased | Increased cerebral blood flow Increased oxygenation | Increased risk of microemboli |
| α-Stat | pH 7.54 $Paco_2$ 26 mm Hg | pH 7.40 $Paco_2$ 40 mm Hg | No | Unchanged | Decreased risk of microemboli | Decreased cerebral blood flow Decreased oxygenation |

increased oxygenation (left shift of oxyhemoglobin dissociation curve). Loss of cerebral autoregulation and increased uniformity of brain cooling occur before any planned circulatory arrest. A major disadvantage of the pH-Stat strategy is increased risk of cerebral microemboli. An important theoretical consideration is "brain steal" in older patients. Global cerebral vasodilation with pH-Stat could potential shunt "steal" blood from poststenotic regions. This is important to consider given the lack of any randomized control trials in adults undergoing deep hypothermic circulatory arrest directly comparing pH-Stat to α-Stat.

There is no change in total $CO_2$ content with α-Stat management. However, as shown in Table 15.1, the lower $Paco_2$ in vivo can impair cerebral oxygenation and decrease cerebral blood flow. The major benefit of this approach, other than preservation of protein function, is decreased risk of arterial emboli to the brain. Even though α-Stat is used more commonly today, few studies indicate any significant difference in patient outcomes.

## SUGGESTED READINGS

Bergman, L., & Lundbye, J. B. (2015). Acid-base optimization during hypothermia. *Best Practice & Research Clinical Anaesthesiology, 29,* 465–470.

Broderick, D. O., Damberg, A., & Ziganshin, B. A. (2018). Alpha-stat versus pH-stat: We do not pay it much mind. Letters to the Editor. *Journal of Thoracic and Cardiovascular Surgery, 156*(1), 41–42.

Butterworth, J. F., Mackey, D. C., & Wasnick, J. D. (2018). *Morgan & Mikhail's Clinical Anesthesiology* (6th ed.). New York: McGraw-Hill.

Eastwood, G. M., Suzuki, S., Lluch, C., Schneider, A. G., & Bellomo, R. (2015). A pilot assessment of alpha-stat vs pH-stat arterial blood gas analysis after cardiac arrest. *Journal of Critical Care, 30,* 138–144.

Gravlee, G. P., Shaw, A. D., & Bartels, K. (2019). *Hensley Practical Approach to Cardiac Anesthesia* (6th ed.). Philadelphia: Lippincott Williams & Wilkins.

# 16

# Central Regulation of Ventilation

JASON M. BUEHLER, MD

Central regulation of ventilation maintains optimal and stable levels of pH, $CO_2$, and $O_2$ in the blood. This regulation depends on the respiratory center, which receives afferent input from chemical stimuli and peripheral chemoreceptors. The respiratory center is composed of a group of nuclei in four major areas within the medulla and pons (Table 16.1).

## Neural Control: Respiratory Center

### DORSAL RESPIRATORY GROUP

The dorsal respiratory group extends the full length of the dorsal medulla and functions as the site of basic respiratory drive through control of inspiration (Fig. 16.1). The neurons within the inspiratory center are located near the termination sites of afferent fibers from the glossopharyngeal (IX) and vagus (X) nerves. These neurons have intrinsic automaticity and control inspiration through the ramp effect, during which efferent activity to the diaphragm increases slowly for 2 seconds until it ceases abruptly, with a 3-second pause before initiating a new cycle. Changing the rate of increase or the duration of efferent activity alters the ramp effect.

### PNEUMOTAXIC CENTER

Located in the pons, the pneumotaxic center functions to limit inspiration by continually transmitting signals to the

| TABLE 16.1 Neurons Within the Medulla and Pons That Constitute the Respiratory Center | | | |
|---|---|---|---|
| **Center** | **Location** | **Nuclei** | **Function** |
| Dorsal respiratory (inspiratory center) | Dorsal portion of the medulla | Nucleus tractus solitarius | Results in inspiration when stimulated |
| Pneumotaxic center | Upper portion of the pons | Nucleus parabrachialis | Controls the rate and pattern of breathing; limits inspiration |
| Ventral respiratory group (expiratory center) | Anterolateral portion of the medulla (~5 mm anterior and lateral to dorsal respiratory group) | Nucleus ambiguus and nucleus retroambiguus | Primarily causes expiration; depending on which neurons are stimulated, can cause expiration or inspiration; transmits inhibitory impulses to the apneustic center |
| Apneustic center | Lower portion of the pons | | Discharges stimulatory impulses to the inspiratory center, resulting in inspiration; receives inhibitory impulses from the pneumotaxic center and stretch receptors of the lung; discharges inhibitory impulses to the expiratory center |

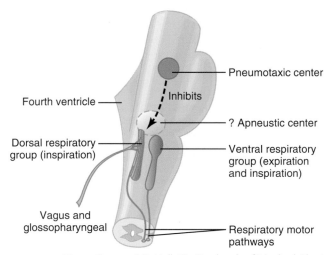

**Fig. 16.1**  Organization of the respiratory center. (From Guyton AC, Hall JE. *Textbook of Medical Physiology*. 13th ed. Elsevier Saunders; 2016: 539–548. F42-1.)

inspiratory center to turn off the ramp effect (see Fig. 16.1). A strong signal results in a short (0.5–1 second) inspiratory cycle and, consequently, a more rapid respiratory rate.

### VENTRAL RESPIRATORY GROUP

The ventral respiratory group is located in the ventral medulla and is active during periods of increased respiratory demand (see Fig. 16.1). These neurons are normally quiescent because expiration is a passive process. With increased demand, a few neurons send efferent activity to further stimulate inspiration, and the remaining neurons send efferent signals to stimulate the muscles of expiration (see Fig. 16.1).

### APNEUSTIC CENTER

The apneustic center is located in the lower pons. It antagonizes the effects of the pneumotaxic center, and it plays no role in normal respiration. In the Hering-Breuer reflex, bronchiolar stretch receptors signal the inspiratory center via the vagus nerve (X) to limit lung expansion. This reflex plays a minimal role in normal ventilation but becomes active when tidal volume exceeds 1.5 L (Fig. 16.2).

## Chemical Control

### CENTRAL

The chemosensitive area is located bilaterally in the medulla, several microns beneath the ventral surface (Fig. 16.3). This area is extremely sensitive to hydrogen ions ($H^+$). However, because these ions cross the blood-brain barrier poorly, $CO_2$ controls this region indirectly through formation of carbonic acid with dissociation to $H^+$. When stimulated, this chemosensitive area stimulates the inspiratory center to increase the rate of rise of the ramp effect and thereby increase the rate of respiration.

$$CO_2 + H_2O \rightarrow H_2CO_3 \rightarrow H^+ + HCO_3^-$$

Therefore $Paco_2$ indirectly influences the level of $H^+$ in cerebrospinal fluid and controls respiratory drive. Peak effect is reached within 1 minute. The effect begins to wane over the next several hours, and by 48 hours the effect is only one-fifth of the peak level. Compensation is caused by increased active transport of $HCO_3^-$ into the cerebrospinal fluid to neutralize the increased $H^+$.

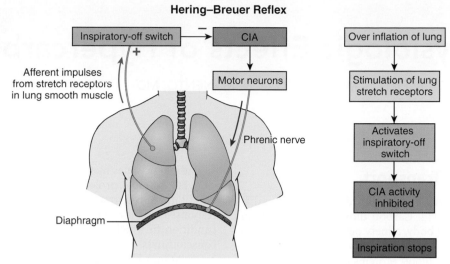

**Hering–Breuer Reflex**

Reflex activated when tidal volume is ~1500 mL (i.e., 3 × normal)

**Fig. 16.2**   The Hering-Breuer inflation reflex is triggered to prevent overinflation of the lungs. Stretch receptors in the smooth muscle of the airway respond to excessive stretching of the lung during large inspirations. When these receptors are activated, they send action potentials through the vagus nerves to the inspiratory and apneustic areas. In this way, they directly inhibit the inspiratory area and inhibit the apneustic area through inactivation of the inspiratory area, thus stopping inspiration and allowing expiration to occur. *CIA,* Central inspiratory activity.

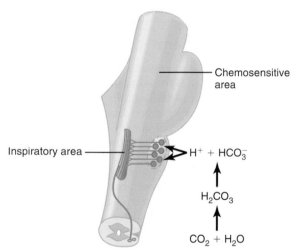

**Fig. 16.3**   Stimulation of the inspiratory area by the chemosensitive area located bilaterally in the medulla, only a few microns beneath the ventral medullary surface. $H^+$ ions stimulate the chemosensitive area, whereas mainly $CO_2$ in the fluid gives rise to the $H^+$ ions. (From Guyton AC, Hall JE. *Textbook of Medical Physiology.* 13th ed. Elsevier Saunders; 2016:539–548. F42-2.)

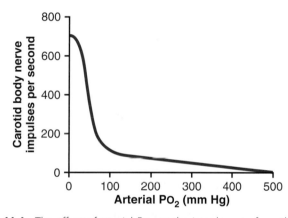

**Fig. 16.4**   The effect of arterial $Po_2$ on the impulse rate from the carotid body of a cat. (From Guyton AC, Hall JE. *Textbook of Medical Physiology.* 13th ed. Elsevier Saunders; 2016:539–548. F42-5.)

## PERIPHERAL

Peripheral chemoreceptors are located in the carotid bodies (cranial nerve IX) and aortic bodies (cranial nerve X). These areas of high blood flow are sensitive to changes in $O_2$, $CO_2$, and pH. Decreased $Pao_2$ stimulates the inspiratory center, with the greatest effect at 30 to 60 mm Hg (Fig. 16.4).

If mean arterial blood pressure drops below 70 mm Hg, respiratory drive increases. The effect of peripheral chemoreceptors in response to hypoxia is eliminated by as little as 0.1 minimum alveolar concentration of an inhaled anesthetic agent, which may be critical in patients with chronic obstructive lung disease who are dependent on hypoxic respiratory drive. Loss of the carotid body, as may occur with carotid endarterectomy, decreases the response to hypoxia, causes a 30% decrease in responsiveness to changes in $Paco_2$, and does not change the resting level of respiration.

## SUGGESTED READINGS

Guyton, A. C., & Hall, J. E. (2020). *Textbook of medical physiology* (14th ed.). Philadelphia: Elsevier Saunders.

West, J. B., & Luks, A. M. (2021). *Respiratory physiology: The essentials* (11th ed.). Philadelphia: Wolters Kluwer.

# Physiologic Effects of Hypercarbia

AMANDA R. FIELDS, MD  |  MEGAN N. MANENTO, MD

## Carbon Dioxide Transport

Normal physiologic arterial carbon dioxide tension ($Paco_2$) is between 35 and 45 mm Hg. Carbon dioxide ($CO_2$) exists in three forms in the human body. Ninety percent of all $CO_2$ is in the form of plasma bicarbonate. Five percent is bound to the terminal amino groups of blood proteins (primarily hemoglobin). The remaining 5% is dissolved in plasma and transported to the lungs for excretion. The primary synthesis of bicarbonate occurs in erythrocytes within peripheral tissue beds through the reaction:

$$CO_2 + H_2O \xleftarrow{\text{carbonic anhydrase}} H_2CO_3 \leftrightarrow H^+ + HCO_3^-$$

Physiologic changes associated with abnormal levels of $Paco_2$ in key organ systems will be reviewed.

## Central Nervous System

Carbon dioxide is a lipid-soluble molecule that freely diffuses across the blood-brain barrier and forms hydrogen ions via the aforementioned reaction within the cerebrospinal fluid (CSF). Local $H^+$ concentration in smooth muscle cells of the arteriolar walls on the brain component of the blood-brain barrier (BBB) determine the central nervous system (CNS) vascular response to $CO_2$.

$CO_2$ responsiveness of the cerebrovascular system is affected by mean arterial pressure (MAP), with abolishment of this response seen with severe hypotension (MAP <66%) (Fig. 17.1A). For $Paco_2$ levels between 20 and 80 mm Hg, each 1-mm Hg increase of $Paco_2$ increases cerebral blood flow by $1.8 \text{ mL} \cdot 100\text{g}^{-1} \cdot \text{min}^{-1}$ and increases cerebral blood volume by $0.04 \text{ mL} \cdot 100\text{g}^{-1}$. Once $Paco_2$ levels reach 25 mm Hg, this response is attenuated (Fig. 17.1B). When increased $CO_2$ crosses the BBB, as in the case of respiratory acidosis, carbonic acid ($H_2CO_3$) is synthesized and subsequently dissociates into $HCO_3^-$ and $H^+$. This causes decreased periarteriolar CSF fluid pH and rapidly triggers nitric oxide and prostaglandin ($PGI_2$)-mediated cerebral vasodilation. These changes occur rapidly within 20 to 30 seconds because $CO_2$ freely diffuses across the cerebrovascular endothelium and the BBB. The pH of the CSF then normalizes over the subsequent 6 to 8 hours as a result of active extrusion of $HCO_3^-$. Normalization of CSF pH limits the utility of hyperventilation in treating increased intracranial pressure over time and is responsible for the deleterious effects of rapid $CO_2$ normalization in settings of prolonged hypercarbia.

Of note, the $CO_2$ response in gray matter exceeds that observed in white matter because of its increased vascular density. Hypercarbia has its greatest effect on vessels less than 100 μm in diameter.

Pathologic states may decrease the CNS vascular response to $CO_2$. For example, prolonged global hypoxia, traumatic disruption of the BBB, and severe transient focal ischemia abolish $CO_2$ responsiveness for approximately 24 hours. $CO_2$ narcosis is a condition in which elevated $Paco_2$ causes a depressed level of consciousness. $CO_2$ narcosis typically occurs when $Paco_2$ exceeds 90 mm Hg but may occur at significantly lower levels in patients who are receiving opioids, benzodiazepines, or other CNS depressants.

$Paco_2$ less than 20 to 30 mm Hg induces severe vasoconstriction that leads to cerebral ischemia and electroencephalographic slowing. Severe respiratory alkalosis of this magnitude induces confusion, lightheadedness, dizziness, visual disturbances, and hypocalcemia due to increased calcium binding by albumin in the setting of alkalosis.

## Respiratory System

Hypercarbia stimulates increased minute ventilation and increases pulmonary vascular resistance through regional hypoxic pulmonary vasoconstriction. Hypocarbia, on the other hand, causes bronchoconstriction, decreased lung compliance, and inhibition of hypoxic pulmonary vasoconstriction. Maximal stimulation of minute ventilation occurs at $Paco_2$ of approximately 100 mm Hg. Any further increase in $Paco_2$ beyond 100 mm Hg often results in ventilatory depression termed $CO_2$ narcosis. In awake patients, this response is mediated about one third in part through peripheral chemoreceptors and two-thirds in part through central chemoreceptors. Under 1.0 minimum alveolar concentration (MAC) of general anesthesia, the peripheral chemoreceptor component of this response is completely abolished; however, the central chemoreceptor response remains intact. When $Paco_2$ levels exceed 15% of total inspired air, loss of consciousness and muscle rigidity can occur. $Paco_2$ levels greater than 20% induce acute convulsions.

Hypercarbia is reversible in patients undergoing mechanical ventilation and typically is the result of insufficient tidal volume, inspiratory pressure, or respiratory rate. In spontaneously breathing patients, hypercarbia is often caused by drug-induced respiratory depression. Respiratory depression is commonly seen with administration of halogenated anesthetics, sedative hypnotics, opioids, and benzodiazepines.

## Cardiovascular System

The effects of hypercarbia on the cardiovascular system result from alterations in the balance between the direct depressant effects of $CO_2$ and increased sympathetic nervous system (SNS) activity. As $CO_2$ rises, blood pressure and cardiac output usually increase in both awake and anesthetized patients. However, at very high levels (e.g., 80–90 mm Hg), hypercarbia causes a

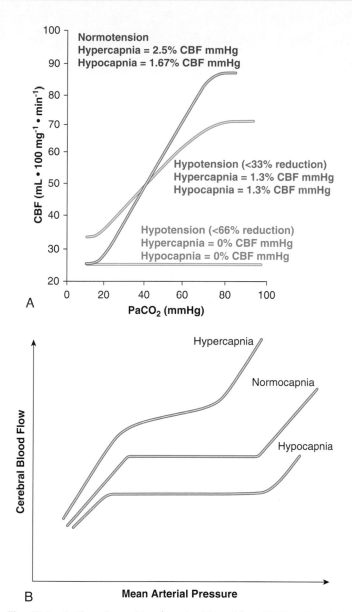

**Fig. 17.1** **A,** The relationship of cerebral blood flow *(CBF)* and partial pressure of carbon dioxide *(Paco₂)*. CBF increases with increasing Paco₂. This response is disrupted in the setting of hypotension. **B,** The relationship Paco₂ variation has on CBF and mean arterial pressure autoregulation. (Modified from Willie C.K., Tzeng Y.C., Fisher J.A., Ainslie P.N.: Integrative regulation of human brain blood flow. *J Physiol* 2014; 592: pp. 841-859 and Rickards C.A.: Cerebral blood-flow regulation during hemorrhage. *Compr Physiol* 2015; 5: pp. 1585-1621.)

reduction in cardiac output, blood pressure, and heart rate, with resultant cardiovascular collapse.

Arrhythmias may be associated with hypercarbia, especially during administration of halothane. Halothane sensitizes the myocardium to the effects of epinephrine, which is increased by activation of the SNS in the setting of hypercarbia.

Hypocarbia can cause decreased cardiac output by several mechanisms. During positive-pressure ventilation, increasing tidal volume to 10 to 20 mL/kg may impede venous return. Vasoconstriction in the CNS depresses SNS activity, which leads to decreased cardiac contractility. Respiratory alkalosis associated with hypocarbia reduces ionized calcium and decreases the inotropic state.

## Gastrointestinal System

In awake patients, hypercarbia increases hepatic and portal venous blood flow. Conversely, hypocarbia decreases hepatic and portal venous blood flow. If anesthesia depth is insufficient to completely suppress the SNS during general anesthesia, increasing Paco₂ levels will lead to splanchnic vasoconstriction and decreased hepatic blood flow. With significant SNS suppression, as occurs during deep general anesthesia, increased Paco₂ levels result in increased hepatic blood flow caused by vasodilation.

## Renal System

Chronic hypercarbia results in renal retention of $HCO_3^-$ and compensatory metabolic alkalosis. Chronic hypocarbia results in $HCO_3^-$ wasting by the kidney and compensatory metabolic acidosis. Secondary polycythemia occurs in the setting of hypercarbia as a result of elevated erythropoietin levels in response to chronic hypoxemia.

## Metabolic System

As Paco₂ rises, plasma levels of epinephrine and norepinephrine increase. Hypercarbia and respiratory acidosis lead to an increased transfer of $K^+$ from cells into the plasma. Reuptake of $K^+$ by cells is slow, and repeated episodes of hypercarbia can cause a stepwise increase in plasma $K^+$ levels. Hypercarbia is associated with fever, thyroid storm, and malignant hyperthermia, and it also may occur during laparoscopic procedures with $CO_2$ insufflation.

## Pharmacologic Effects of Changes in Carbon Dioxide

Hypercarbia and respiratory acidosis can affect the pharmacokinetics of many anesthetic agents. For example, it is the nonionized form of local anesthetic agents that readily crosses cell membranes. Because local anesthetic agents are weak bases, in the presence of acidemia the relative proportion of nonionized drug decreases, resulting in less transport across cell membranes and decreased activity.

## Effects of Changes in Carbon Dioxide on Minimum Alveolar Concentration

Paco₂ between 20 and 100 mm Hg do not affect MAC needed for surgery. Hypercarbia with Paco₂ greater than 100 mm Hg, however, does contribute to sedation and lowers the MAC of anesthetic gases. In addition, volatile anesthetics cause depression of respiratory drive and a rightward shift of the apneic threshold of the $CO_2$ response curve. Thus the MAC of volatile anesthetic at which spontaneous respirations resume under anesthesia decreases with rising Paco₂.

## Signs and Symptoms

Clinical signs and symptoms of hypercarbia are nonspecific and vary with degree of severity and chronicity (Box 17.1). Arterial blood gas analysis or end-tidal $CO_2$ monitoring are required to confirm the diagnosis.

## SUGGESTED READINGS

Adrogué, H. J., & Madias, N. E. (2010). Secondary responses to altered acid-base status: The rules of engagement. *Journal of the American Society of Nephrology, 21*, 920–923.

Azzam, Z. S., Sharabi, K., Guetta, J., Bank, E. M., & Gruenbaum, Y. (2010). The physiological and molecular effects of elevated $CO_2$ levels. *Cell Cycle, 9*(8), 1528–1532.

Barrett, K. E., Barman, S. M., Boitano, S., Brooks, H. L., & Yuan, J. X. (2015). *Ganong's Review of Medical Physiology* (25th ed.). New York: McGraw-Hill.

Curley, G., Laffey, J. G., & Kavanagh, B. P. (2010). Bench-to-bedside review: Carbon dioxide. *Critical Care, 14*, 220.

Dorrington, K. L., Balanos, G. M., Talbot, N. P., & Robbins, P. A. (2010). Extent to which pulmonary vascular responses to Pco$_2$ and Po$_2$ play a functional role within the healthy human lung. *Journal of Applied Physiology, 108*, 1084–1096.

Gropper, M. A., Miller, R. D., Cohen, N. H., Eriksson, L. I., Fleisher, L. A., Lelsie, K., et al., (Eds.), *Miller's Anesthesia* (9th ed.). Philadelphia: Elsevier Inc.

Levitzky, M. (2013). *Pulmonary Physiology* (8th ed.). New York: McGraw-Hill.

Ogoh, S., Nakahara, H., Ainslie, P. N., & Miyamoto, T. (2010). The effect of oxygen on dynamic cerebral autoregulation: Critical role of hypocapnia. *Journal of Applied Physiology, 108*, 538–543.

# 18

# Factors That Affect Pulmonary Compliance and Airway Resistance

MEGAN N. MANENTO, MD   |   RICHARD K. PATCH III, MD

Understanding pulmonary mechanics requires an appreciation of the balance between opposing forces that affect lung volume. For instance, the elastic recoil of the lung naturally works to contract the lung, resulting in lower lung volumes. The chest wall counters this force, pulling the lung outward. Thus the lung remains partially expanded even at end-respiration due to the balance forces within the closed system of the thorax. An open thoracic cage expands to a volume of approximately 1 L greater than functional residual capacity (FRC), whereas the lung contracts to minimal volumes. In a closed thorax, the lung and thorax come to rest at a volume known as the FRC. FRC is determined by the opposing lung elastic recoil of the lung, chest wall expansion force, and the resting tone of respiratory muscles. More specifically, FRC is the volume at which the lung comes to rest after passive exhalation when the respiratory muscles are their most relaxed.

At FRC respiratory muscle activity is required to either increase or decrease the size of the thoracic cage. The impedance of the respiratory system determines how the lungs respond to changes in chest wall shape, volume, and respiratory muscle strength. The five most important factors contributing to respiratory impedance are (1) elastic resistance of the lung and chest wall; (2) surface tension at the alveolar gas/liquid interface; (3) frictional resistance to airway gas flow; (4) viscoelastic tissue resistance; and (5) inertia of gas and tissue movement.

These five factors can be subdivided into elastic (factors 1 and 2) and nonelastic (factors 3, 4, and 5) respiratory system resistance. Elastic resistance is measured when gas is not actively flowing within the lung. Work stored in overcoming the elastic resistance of the lung during inspiration is stored as potential energy and used for passive exhalation during both spontaneous and mechanical ventilation.

## Compliance of the Lung and Chest Wall

Lung compliance is defined as the change in lung volume per unit change in the transmural pressure gradient (between the alveolus and the pleural space) and is typically measured in liters per centimeter of $H_2O$. Lung compliance, therefore, is also defined by the slope of the line that results from plotting lung volume against transmural pressure. In the clinical setting, lung compliance is more easily measured for the respiratory system as a unit, which includes the composite of the lung, the chest wall, or the lung and chest. The normal value for either lung or chest wall compliance is 0.2 L/cm $H_2O$. The typical compliance for the respiratory system as a whole is 0.1 L/cm $H_2O$.

Compliance is dependent both upon lung volume and time and thus has both static and dynamic components. Static compliance is determined by measuring the pressure difference when a known volume of air is inhaled and held constant starting from FRC. This can be achieved by performing an inspiratory hold during volume control mechanical ventilation while the patient is sedated and paralyzed. Dynamic compliance, on the other hand, is measured during normal tidal breathing and is derived from the slope of the line connecting the end-inspiratory and end-expiratory points of the pressure-volume loop. The difference between static and dynamic respiratory compliance reflects the time dependency of the system.

Elasticity is the reciprocal of compliance. It is the passive property of tissue that causes it to return to its resting shape after deformation by an external force. If the lung were a perfectly elastic tissue, it would obey Hooke's law. Instead, lung compliance and elastance are dependent on both time and volume. Dynamic changes in lung elastance and compliance can be graphed with a pressure-volume loop. During inhalation, lung volume at any given pressure is less than the lung volume at that same pressure during exhalation. The difference between the pressure-volume curves of inhalation and exhalation can be described as lung hysteresis and is caused by a variety of factors, including:

1. Change in surfactant activity
2. Stress relaxation
3. Gas redistribution between slow-filling and fast-filling alveoli
4. Alveolar recruitment as closed alveoli open
5. Displacement of pulmonary blood volume

## Surface Tension at the Alveolar Gas/ Liquid Interface

In 1929, von Neergaard showed that a lung completely immersed in and filled with water had an elastance that was much lower than when the lung was filled with air. This experiment shows that much of the elastic recoil of the lung is a result of alveolar surface tension. Surface tension produces an inwardly directed force that tends to reduce the size of the alveolus. The pressure within the alveoli is always higher than the surrounding pressure because of the added force of surface tension and is governed by Laplace's law.

Surface tension within the alveolar wall contributes significantly to lung recoil and impairs compliance. Laplace's law states that the pressure in a thin-walled sphere (or alveolus) is inversely proportional to its radius, such that $T = PR/2$, where P is the pressure within the bubble (dyn $\times$ cm$^{-2}$), T is the surface tension of the liquid (dyn $\times$ cm$^{-1}$), and R is the radius of the bubble (cm). Therefore smaller alveoli tend to empty into larger ones until their pressures reach equilibrium.

Pulmonary surfactant attenuates this affect and increases compliance by decreasing surface tension, particularly in smaller alveoli. Dipalmitoyl phosphatidyl choline (DPPC) is the major phospholipid that makes up surfactant and is the key factor in reducing alveolar surface tension. Its fatty acid end is hydrophobic and projects into the alveolus, and its hydrophilic end associates with the alveolar lining. DPPC molecules align in a straight monolayer or in bilayers. Surfactant is generated by type II alveolar epithelial cells, is stored in lamellar bodies within the cytoplasm, and has a half-life of 15 to 30 hours. Proteins may be required to maintain its stability and structural integrity.

Surfactant's effect on alveolar surface tension becomes more pronounced as alveoli decrease in size. This allows small alveoli to exist at the same pressure as larger alveoli. When pulmonary surfactant is lacking, increased surface tension in smaller alveoli causes them to collapse. Higher inspiratory pressures are then needed to reopen the collapsed alveoli.

## Factors That Affect Respiratory Compliance

Factors that increase FRC also increase pulmonary compliance. Emphysema, for example, increases compliance as a result of loss of the normal elastic recoil of the lungs. As another example, men have approximately 10% higher FRC and subsequently better compliance than women because men have proportionally higher lean muscle mass.

Alternatively, pulmonary compliance is reduced by factors that decrease FRC. Ascites, obesity, pleural effusion, pericardial effusion, cardiomegaly, and general anesthesia all decrease FRC through external compression or elevation of the diaphragm. Pleural, interstitial, and alveolar fibrosis will decrease FRC by decreasing the elastic properties of the lung. Atelectasis, pulmonary artery obstruction, and pneumonia decrease FRC through decreased surfactant at the alveolar/air interface. Poliomyelitis, pectus excavatum, spasticity, and kyphoscoliosis decrease FRC because of restriction of the thoracic wall. Skeletal muscle disorders decrease FRC because of diaphragmatic elevation.

Positioning and age can also affect compliance because of changes in closing capacity (CC) relative to FRC. CC is the lung volume below which small airways begin to close in the dependent lung regions. With age, CC increases at a rate that exceeds the rate of increase in FRC. CC first exceeds FRC in the supine position at the age of 44 years and then in the upright position by the age of 75 years. When CC exceeds FRC, some of the dependent alveoli cannot empty before the airways leading to them close. This contributes to increased $\dot{V}/\dot{Q}$ mismatching, A-a gradient, and hypoxemia.

Bronchial smooth muscle tone affects pulmonary compliance through increased airway resistance and thus pressure needed to expand the lung. Bronchoconstriction may increase the time-dependent properties of compliance and reduce dynamic lung compliance more than static compliance.

## Effects of Decreased Compliance

Decreased compliance results in increased work of breathing because higher pressures are needed to increase lung volume. Compensatory mechanisms to decrease the work of breathing include increased respiratory rate, decreased tidal volume, and breathing with pursed lips. Because the bronchi behave as Starling resistors, pursing the lips moves the equal pressure point away from the mouth toward the bronchi, maintaining airway patency. Smaller airways that remain closed or narrowed become underventilated despite being perfused. This leads to an increase in pulmonary shunt and increased $\dot{V}/\dot{Q}$ mismatching.

## Nonelastic Resistance

The factors contributing to nonelastic resistance include frictional resistance to airway gas flow, viscoelastic tissue resistance, and inertia of gas and tissue movement. Inertia, however, contributes very little and only really becomes a factor with very high-frequency ventilation. Thus airway and tissue resistance each typically contribute approximately 50% of respiratory system resistance.

Unlike elastic resistance, work performed to overcome nonelastic resistance is not stored as potential energy. It is unrecoverable and dissipated as heat. Because airway resistance is the major modifiable factor in clinical situations, viscoelastic tissue resistance will not be discussed further in this chapter.

## Principles of Gas Flow and Resistance

Driving pressure is the pressure necessary to move air through the airways during inspiration and expiration. During inspiration, diving pressure equals atmospheric pressure minus alveolar pressure. Ohm's law states that P = Q × R, where P is driving pressure, Q is flow rate, and R is airway resistance. Thus airway resistance equals driving pressure divided by flow. Airway resistance is created by the friction of molecules flowing gas through the airway; it is expressed in units of centimeters of $H_2O \cdot L^{-1} \cdot sec^{-1}$.

Gas flows in a laminar pattern in straight, unbranched airways during normal quiet respiration and has very little resistance. Laminar gas flow can be described as a series of concentric cylinders, with the central cylinder leading flow. The gas directly adjacent to the wall is stationary, and the gas in the center follows at the highest velocity. Laminar gas flow follows Poiseuille's law, such that resistance = $8 l\eta/\pi r^4$, where l equals the length of the airway, $\eta$ is the viscosity of the gas, and r is the radius of the airway. Resistance to flow is affected most significantly by the radius of the airway. For instance, a 50% decrement in radius increases resistance 16-fold (i.e., $2^4$).

During high gas flow rates or in conditions of high airway resistance, the flow pattern becomes turbulent and irregular. Turbulence occurs at airway branch points and with irregularities in the walls of the airways (e.g., mucus, exudates, tumor, foreign body, partial glottic closure).

Turbulent flow differs from laminar flow in that it depends on gas density, not viscosity, requires a higher driving pressure for flow, and is even more dependent on the radius of the airway. In particular, the required driving pressure in turbulent flow is proportional to the square of the flow rate and inversely proportional to the $r^5$. Turbulent flow more efficiently clears the gas content of the airway than laminar flow. Because helium has a low density and a viscosity similar to that of air, it has more of an effect on turbulent flow than on laminar flow.

The Reynolds number can be used to determine whether airflow is predominantly laminar or turbulent. If the Reynolds number is less than 2000, gas flow is typically laminar, whereas a value greater than 4000 predicts turbulent flow. The major property of a gas that affects the Reynolds number is the ratio of its density to its viscosity. The Reynolds number can be calculated from the equation:

$$\frac{\text{Linear Gas Velocity} \times \text{Tube Diameter} \times \text{Gas Density}}{\text{Gas Viscosity}}$$

## Airway Resistance

Even though an individual small airway has much greater resistance than a large airway, the aggregate cross-sectional area of all small airways is greater than that of the larger airways. Therefore airway resistance is greatest in intermediate-sized bronchi between the fourth and eighth bifurcations. Thus large changes can occur in the diameter of peripheral bronchioles before changes occur in airway resistance measured by plethysmography. These less noticeable changes may be better captured by a forced oscillation technique.

## Factors That Affect Airway Resistance

Bronchiole diameter is predominantly neurally controlled but also is affected humorally and by direct physical or chemical mechanisms. Both afferent and efferent parasympathetic nerves travel through the vagus to control bronchomotor tone through the release of acetylcholine. The sympathetic nervous system has little control over bronchomotor tone. However, bronchiole smooth muscle has an abundance of $\beta_2$-adrenergic receptors that respond to circulating concentrations of catecholamines, particularly during exercise or stress. Physical mechanisms that result in bronchoconstriction include direct stimulation by laryngoscopy, cold air, inhaled particular matter, liquids with low pH (gastric contents), and toxic gases (e.g., sulfur dioxide, ammonia).

Airway resistance is also inversely proportional to lung volume because of the associated changes in airway diameter. At lung volumes below FRC, airway collapse and air trapping further contribute to airway resistance. Even at lung volumes above FRC, smaller airways in dependent lung zones become atelectatic at volumes below closing capacity. This affect is more pronounced with older age and leads to pulmonary shunting. Shunting is responsible for the increased A-a gradient seen with aging.

Smaller airways beyond the 11th generation have little structural support to prevent collapse caused by external pressure. Reversal of the normal transpulmonary gradient during forced expiration can lead to airway collapse distal to the equal pressure point. This affect is intensified as lung volume decreases. Emphysema, for example, increases airway resistance through loss of structural support and resultant small airway collapse. Pneumothorax also increases airway resistance through alterations in the normal transpulmonary gradient.

## Major Effects of Increased Airway Resistance

Increased airway resistance increases the time needed to complete exhalation. This results in increased residual volume, FRC, and gas trapping with faster respiratory rates. In an attempt to decrease airway resistance, patients may decrease their rate of breathing to allow decreased flow velocity and greater time for exhalation. They may also exhale against pursed lips to decrease the pressure gradient within the tracheobronchial tree and move the equal pressure point proximally. Patients may also depend on active exhalation, which increases the work of breathing and alters the transpulmonary gradient. In chemically paralyzed patients who cannot actively exhale, gas trapping may severely decrease cardiac output by increasing intrathoracic pressure. The increased intrathoracic pressure both decreases preload and increases afterload.

## SUGGESTED READINGS

Lumb, A. B., & Thomas, C. (2020). *Nunn's applied respiratory physiology* (9th ed.). Philadelphia: Elsevier.

Gropper, M. A., Miller, R. D., Cohen, N. H., Eriksson, L. I., Fleisher, L. A., Lelsie, K., et al., (Eds.), (2020). *Miller's anesthesia* (9th ed.). Philadelphia: Elsevier.

Nakano, S., Nakahira, J., Sawai, T., Kuzukawa, Y., Ishio, J., & Minami, T. (2016). Perioperative evaluation of respiratory impedance using the forced oscillation technique: A prospective observational study. *BMC Anesthesiology*, *16*(1), 32.

Rehder, K., Sessler, A. D., & Marsh, H. M. (1975). General anesthesia and the lung. *American Review of Respiratory Disease*, *112*(4), 541–563.

Satoh, J. I., Yamakage, M., Kobayashi, T., Tohse, N., Watanabe, H., & Namiki, A. (2009). Desflurane but not sevoflurane can increase lung resistance via tachykinin pathways. *British Journal of Anaesthesia*, *102*, 704.

Shirai, T., & Kurosawa, H. (2016). Clinical application of the forced oscillation technique. *Internal Medicine*, *55*(6), 559–566.

Von Neergaard, K. (1929). Neue Auffassungen über einen Grundbegriff der Atemmechanik. *Ges Experimental Medicine*, *66*, 373–394.

# 19

# Pulmonary Ventilation and Perfusion

ASHLEY V. FRITZ, DO

Maximal gas exchange efficiency for $O_2$ and $CO_2$ in an ideal single-lung unit has a ventilation/perfusion ($\dot{V}/\dot{Q}$) ratio of 1 in a situation of continuous countercurrent flow of gas to blood, with a blood-to-gas exposure of 0.75 second. By contrast, the human lung is only relatively efficient, showing a range of $\dot{V}/\dot{Q}$ ratios for its many alveoli, determined by the distribution of $\dot{V}$ and $\dot{Q}$ throughout the lungs.

## Ventilation

As inspired gas flows into the lungs, it is influenced by pulmonary compliance and airway resistance. Minute ventilation is the product of tidal volume ($V_T$) and respiratory rate. Gravity interacting with posture and regional alveolar time constants for filling and emptying of lung regions interacting with the frequency of respiration are the other two major factors that determine the distribution of $\dot{V}$ within the lungs. The right lung is larger than the left lung, receiving approximately 52% of a tidal breath in the supine position, during both spontaneous breathing and mechanical ventilation. These percentages change under the influence of gravity with changes in posture. In a spontaneously breathing patient in the lateral position, the dependent lung is both better ventilated and perfused. Anesthesia, neuromuscular blockade, and mechanical ventilation cause further changes. The nondependent lung in an anesthetized patient in the lateral position is generally better ventilated independent of the ventilation mode.

At functional reserve capacity (FRC), in each slice of lung, from nondependent (apex in the sitting position, anterior lung in the supine position, nondependent lung in the lateral decubitus position) to the most dependent portion, alveolar volume decreases. Basal alveoli are one-fourth the volume of apical alveoli at end expiration. This puts the basal alveolar characteristics on a steeper portion of the pressure-volume (P-V) curve (Fig. 19.1). Although the basal alveoli are smaller than the apical alveoli at FRC, basal alveoli expand more than apical alveoli during inspiration. Therefore in an awake, spontaneously breathing patient, in all positions, ventilation per unit of lung volume is smallest at the uppermost portion (e.g., the apex in an upright patient) and increases with vertical distance down the lung.

In the supine patient, general anesthesia with paralysis and mechanical ventilation decreases the difference between ventilation of the dependent and nondependent alveoli, causing nearly uniform distribution of ventilation throughout the lung. This is attributed to decreased FRC that shifts the alveolar characteristics downward on the P-V curve (see Fig. 19.1). When the patient is in the lateral decubitus position, anesthesia reverses the distribution of ventilation so that the nondependent (upper) part of the lung receives more ventilation than does the dependent (lower) part of the lung. This arrangement holds for both spontaneous and mechanical ventilation and is clinically significant because the dependent lung has greater perfusion, which causes increased $\dot{V}/\dot{Q}$ mismatch. The change

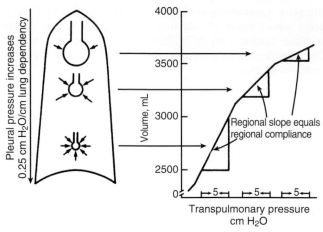

**Fig. 19.1** Pleural pressure increases 0.25 cm $H_2O$ every centimeter down the lung. The increase in pleural pressure causes a fourfold decrease in alveolar volume. The caliber of the air passages also decreases as lung volume decreases. When regional alveolar volume is translated to a regional transpulmonary pressure–alveolar volume curve, small alveoli are on a steep (large slope) portion of the curve and large alveoli are on a flat (small slope) portion of the curve. The regional slope equals regional compliance. Over the normal tidal volume range (2500–3000 mL), the pressure–volume relationship is linear. Lung volume values in this diagram relate to the upright position. (From Benumof JL. Respiratory physiology and respiratory function during anesthesia. In: Miller RD, ed. *Anesthesia.* 5th ed. Churchill Livingstone; 2000:578–618.)

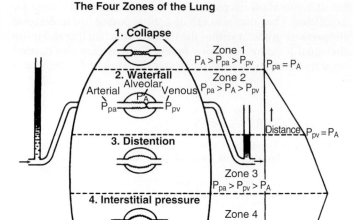

**Fig. 19.2** Distribution of blood flow in the isolated lung. In zone 1, alveolar pressure (*PA*) exceeds pulmonary artery pressure (*PPA*) and no flow occurs, presumably because collapsible vessels are directly exposed to alveolar pressure. In zone 2, arterial pressure exceeds alveolar pressure, but alveolar pressure exceeds pulmonary venous pressure (*PPV*). Flow in zone 2 is determined by the arterial–alveolar pressure difference, which increases steadily down the zone. In zone 3, pulmonary venous pressure exceeds alveolar pressure and flow is determined by the arterial–venous pressure difference (PPA − PPV), which is constant down the lung. However, pressure across the walls of the vessels increases down zone 3, so that their caliber increases, as does flow. In zone 4, flow is determined by the arterial pressure–interstitial flow (*ISF*) pressure difference (PPA − PISF) because interstitial pressure exceeds both PPV and PA. (From Benumof JL. Respiratory physiology and respiratory function during anesthesia. In: Miller RD, ed. *Anesthesia.* 5th ed. Churchill Livingstone; 2000:578–618.)

in distribution of V̇ to lung regions in the lateral decubitus position is attributed to (1) decreased FRC, causing a shift along the P-V curve (which can be partially reversed by positive end-expiratory pressure [PEEP]); (2) more compression of the dependent lung by the mediastinum and abdominal contents; and (3) increased compliance of the nondependent hemithorax.

The time constant for filling and emptying of a lung region is determined by the product of compliance and resistance of the region. If respiratory frequency does not permit complete emptying of a region before the next inspiratory effort is applied, gas trapping will occur. This is a concern when obstructive airway disease is present. Incomplete filling or emptying of lung regions also may increase V̇/Q̇ mismatching. General anesthesia may reverse bronchoconstriction and favorably affect this factor.

## Pulmonary Blood Flow

The two major determinants of pulmonary blood flow (Q̇) distribution within the lung are (1) gravity and (2) hypoxic pulmonary vasoconstriction (HPV). Pulmonary artery pressure (PPA) decreases by 1 mm Hg or 1.35 cm $H_2O$ for every 1 cm of vertical distance up the lung. Because the pulmonary circulation is a low-pressure system, this causes significant differences in Q̇ between the lower and higher regions of the lung, with greater Q̇ going to the lower lung regions. The actual Q̇ to an alveolus also depends on alveolar pressure (PALV), which opposes PPA and pulmonary venous pressure (PPV). This interaction is summarized in Fig. 19.2. All of these relationships are dynamic, varying throughout the cardiac and respiratory cycles. The lung has four defined zones of blood flow. In zone 1, at the apex of an upright lung, PALV is greater than PPA, preventing any blood flow and thereby creating alveolar dead space (VD). Zone

1 is negligible in healthy lungs. In zone 2, PPA is greater than PALV, which is greater than PPV, so that Q̇ depends only on PPA minus PALV. In zone 3, PPA is greater than PPV, which is greater than PALV, and Q̇ is a function of PPA minus PPV, independent of PALV. In zone 4, flow is determined by the difference between PPA and pressure interstitial flow (PISF). In general, decreases in PPA (e.g., hemorrhagic shock) increase the size of the upper zones (1 and 2) at the expense of the lower zones (3 and 4), whereas increases in PPA have the opposite effect. Increases in PALV (e.g., with PEEP) may recruit alveoli from lower zones into higher zones (i.e., increase the volume of zones 1 and 2).

HPV is a local response of pulmonary arterial smooth muscle to decreased regional alveolar Po2. It decreases Q̇ to underventilated regions of lung and maintains normal V̇/Q̇. HPV is effective only when there is a significant section of normally ventilated and oxygenated lung to which flow can be diverted (e.g., one-lung ventilation during thoracic operations). Intravenously administered anesthetic agents do not inhibit HPV, whereas inhaled anesthetic agents and potent vasodilators do. Therapeutically inhaled nitric oxide is a unique pulmonary-specific vasodilator that may attenuate HPV and often improves oxygenation because it is delivered only to alveoli that are already being ventilated.

## Ventilation/Perfusion Ratio

Both V̇ and Q̇ increase toward the dependent part of the lung, but at different rates (Fig. 19.3). Therefore V̇/Q̇ is greater than

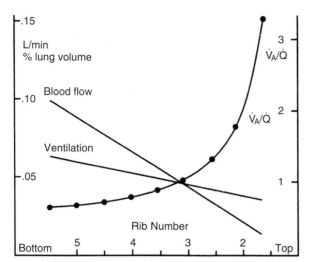

**Fig. 19.3** Distribution of ventilation and perfusion *(left vertical axis)* and the ventilation/perfusion ratio *(right vertical axis)* in the normal upright lung. Both ventilation and perfusion are expressed in L/min/percent alveolar volume and have been drawn as smoothed-out linear functions of vertical height. The *closed circles* mark the ventilation/perfusion ratios of horizontal lung slices. Cardiac output of 6 L/min and total minute ventilation of 5.1 L/min were assumed. $\dot{V}_A/\dot{Q}$, alveolar ventilation/perfusion ratio. (From West JB. *Respiratory Physiology.* 2nd ed. Williams & Wilkins; 1970.)

1 at the top, $\dot{V}/\dot{Q}$ equals 1 at the third rib in upright lungs, and $\dot{V}/\dot{Q}$ is less than 1 below the third rib. $\dot{V}/\dot{Q}$ is, of course, also affected by the factors that affect $\dot{V}$ or $\dot{Q}$ separately.

## Dead Space

$V_D$ is the volume of a breath that does not participate in gas exchange, $V_T$ is total tidal volume, and $V_D/V_T$ is the fraction of tidal volume that is composed of $V_D$ volume. Anatomic $V_D$, $V_D(AN)$, is the volume of gas that ventilates only the conducting airways. Alveolar $V_D$, $V_D(ALV)$, is the volume of gas that does not take part in effective gas exchange at the alveolar level, that is, ventilated but unperfused alveoli. Total (or physiologic) $V_D$ equals $V_D(AN)$ plus $V_D(ALV)$. Normally, the ratio of physiologic $V_D$ to tidal volume ($V_D/V_T$) equals one-third, and $V_D(AN)$ equals 2 mL/kg ideal body weight, or approximately 150 mL in a healthy, upright adult. In awake, healthy, supine patients, $V_D(ALV)$ is negligible. One mechanism that contributes to this is a bronchiolar constrictive reflex that constricts airways to unperfused alveoli.

$V_D/V_T$ may be measured by the Bohr method because all expired $CO_2$ comes from perfused alveoli and none comes from $V_D$:

$$V_D / V_T = \frac{P_{ACO_2} - \text{mixed expired } P_{CO_2}}{P_{ACO_2}}$$

Clinically, it is assumed that arterial $P_{CO_2}$ equals alveolar $P_{CO_2}$. Mixed expired $P_{CO_2}$ is the average $P_{CO_2}$ in an expired gas sample. Mixed expired $P_{CO_2}$ is not the same as end-tidal $P_{CO_2}$. During expiration, $P_{CO_2}$ increases until it reaches a steady state with the $P_{CO_2}$ of blood within the pulmonary capillaries near the end of expiration. This represents end-tidal $P_{CO_2}$.

## Factors That Affect Dead Space and Dead Space/Tidal Volume

$V_D$ and $V_D/V_T$ are affected by $\dot{V}/\dot{Q}$ and the anatomy of the conducting airways. The normal ratio of $V_D/V_T$ is 0.3. This ratio decreases with deep breathing and increases with shallow breathing. Decreased $P_{PA}$ (e.g., hemorrhage, drug effects) causes increased $V_D(ALV)$ because of an increase in zone 1 physiology.

Loss of perfusion to ventilated alveoli, despite normal or high $P_{PA}$, causes increased $V_D(ALV)$ and therefore an increase in $V_D/V_T$. These conditions may result from pulmonary emboli (including venous air embolism), pulmonary arterial thrombosis, surgical manipulation of the pulmonary arterial tree, or emphysema with loss of alveolar septa and vasculature.

Increased airway pressure (e.g., positive-pressure ventilation) causes increased $V_D(AN)$ from radial traction on conducting airways by the surrounding lung parenchyma and increased $V_D(ALV)$ from increased zone 1 physiology because of alveolar overdistention. When the patient's neck is extended and the jaw is protruded, the $V_D(AN)$ is doubled compared with a flexed neck and depressed chin. Compared with supine posture, erect posture causes increased $V_D(ALV)$ because decreased perfusion to the uppermost alveoli causes an increased volume of zone 1 physiology.

The $V_D$ of anesthesia equipment increases the $V_D/V_T$ ratio from the normal 0.3 to values of 0.4 to 0.5 with tracheal intubation and Y-piece connectors or 0.64 with facemask ventilation. Tracheostomy or intubation decreases $V_D(AN)$ by roughly half unless anesthesia equipment is added to the breathing circuit.

General anesthesia, with spontaneous or controlled ventilation, increases $V_D$ and $V_D/V_T$. The etiology is multifactorial and incompletely understood; it may be partially caused by moderate pulmonary hypotension, loss of skeletal muscle tone, or loss of bronchoconstrictor tone. Rapid, short inspirations increase $V_D$ by ventilating a greater fraction of noncompliant and poorly perfused alveoli compared with slower, deeper inspirations.

Increasing age increases both anatomic and alveolar $V_D$ because of decreased elasticity of lung tissues. Additionally, closing volume and closing capacity increase with aging.

## Shunt

Shunt ($\dot{Q}_S$) is the portion of blood flow that does not participate in gas exchange. $\dot{Q}_S/\dot{Q}_T$ is the fraction of pulmonary blood flow (total cardiac output) that is shunt. $\dot{Q}_S/\dot{Q}_T$ may be estimated with the Fick principle embodied in the shunt equation:

$$\dot{Q}_S/\dot{Q}_T = \frac{Cc'_{O_2} - Ca_{O_2}}{Cc'_{O_2} - C\overline{v}_{O_2}}$$

where $Cc'_{O_2}$ is end-capillary $O_2$ content, $Ca_{O_2}$ is arterial $O_2$ content, and $C\overline{v}_{O_2}$ is mixed venous $O_2$ content. There are anatomic contributions to shunt from the thebesian veins, bronchial veins, and any other anatomic right-to-left shunt paths that empty directly into the left side of the heart beyond the lungs. These shunts may deflect up to 5% to 7% of $\dot{Q}_T$. $\dot{V}/\dot{Q}$ mismatching may contribute a further 1% to 3% so that total shunt may be 6% to 10% of cardiac output in normal lungs. Examples of physiologic shunts include pulmonary edema and mucus plugging (Box 19.1).

## SUGGESTED READINGS

Bigatello, L., & Pesenti, A. (2019). Respiratory physiology for the anesthesiologist. *Anesthesiology, 130*(6), 1064–1077.

Gattinoni, L., Carlesso, E., Brazzi, L., & Caironi, P. (2010). Positive end-expiratory pressure. *Current Opinion in Critical Care, 16,* 39–44.

Gropper, M. A. (Ed.), (2020). *Miller's Anesthesia* (9th ed.). Philadelphia: Elsevier.

Hall, J. H. (2016). *Guyton and Hall Textbook of Medical Physiology* (13th ed.). Philadelphia: Elsevier.

Lumb, A. B. (Ed.), (2021). *Nunn and Lumb's Applied Respiratory Physiology* (9th ed.). Elsevier.

# 20

# Pulmonary Function Test Interpretation

KATHRYN S. HANDLOGTEN, MD

Basic pulmonary function tests are used to determine three types of data: (1) gas flow rates for assessment of airway diameter; (2) lung volume to assess loss of lung tissue or change induced by chest wall dysfunction; and (3) diffusing capacity for carbon monoxide (DLCO) to evaluate the efficiency of gas exchange at the pulmonary blood/gas interface.

More complex pulmonary function tests, categorized by increasing complexity, are listed in Box 20.1. Normal values for these tests vary with age (indirectly proportional), body size (directly proportional), and sex. Values for an average 40-year-old man and woman are shown in Table 20.1.

The highest prevalence of respiratory disease in surgical patients in the United States falls within two main categories: patients with obstructive disease, including asthma, bronchitis, bronchiectasis, and emphysema; and those with restrictive disease, including morbid obesity, obstructive sleep apnea, and kyphoscoliosis. The pulmonary function test results that are characteristic of obstructive and restrictive disease are outlined in Table 20.2. Although pulmonary function test results may confirm clinical diagnoses and demonstrate response to therapy, no single test reliably predicts perioperative pulmonary complications. However, predicted postoperative changes in gas flow (FEV$_1$%), DLCO, cardiovascular status, and exercise tolerance can be used to predict the risks of lung resection (Fig. 20.1).

## Tests to Measure Lung Volume

### SPIROMETRY

Spirometry measures the volume of gas passing through the airway opening. During spirometry, the patient breathes normally and then is asked to inhale maximally and exhale maximally (see Figs. 20.1 and 20.2). Measurements obtained directly by spirometry include inspiratory capacity, inspiratory reserve volume, expiratory reserve

## BOX 20.1 PULMONARY FUNCTION TESTS

**LEVEL 1 TESTS**

Spirometry/spirography
$FEV_1$
$FEV_1\%$
$FEF_{25-75}$
MVV
Response to bronchodilator
Pulse oximetry on room air or $O_2$ supplementation

**LEVEL 2 TESTS**

Arterial blood gases
$Pao_2/Fio_2$ ratio
Lung volume
TLC
FRC
RV
DLCO

**LEVEL 3 TESTS**

Flow-volume loops
Pressure-volume loops
$C_{RS}$
Pst
Respiratory muscle strength
$P_{Imax}$
$P_{Emax}$
Hypoxic and hypercapnic responsiveness
Exercise tests
Sleep studies

*CRS*, Compliance of the entire respiratory system; *DLCO*, diffusing capacity of the lung for carbon monoxide (carbon monoxide uptake from a single inspiration in a standard time, usually 10 seconds); *FEV₁*, forced expiratory volume (volume of air that can be forcibly blown out in 1 second, after full inspiration); *FEV₁%*, ratio of FEV₁ to forced vital capacity *(FVC)*, the volume of air that can forcibly be blown out in 1 second, after full inspiration; *FEF₂₅₋₇₅*, forced expiratory flow (i.e., flow [or speed] of air coming out of the lung during the middle portion of a forced expiration); *Fio₂*, fraction of inspired $O_2$; *FRC*, functional residual capacity; *MVV*, maximum voluntary ventilation, (i.e., maximum amount of air that can be inhaled and exhaled within 1 minute, usually extrapolated from a 15-second testing period); *Pao₂*, partial pressure of oxygen in arterial blood; *PEmax*, maximum expiratory pressure; *PImax*, maximum inspiratory pressure; *Pst*, static lung recoil pressure; *RV*, residual volume; *TLC*, total lung capacity (maximum volume of air present in the lungs).

## TABLE 20.1 Normal Values for a 40-Year-Old Man and Woman

| Parameter | Man[a] | Woman[b] |
| --- | --- | --- |
| VC or FVC, L | 5 | 3.5 |
| RV, L | 1.8 | 1.7 |
| TLC, L | 6.8 | 5.2 |
| FRC, L | 3.4 | 2.6 |
| FEV₁, L | 4.1 | 2.9 |
| FEV₁%, % | 82 | 83 |
| FEF₂₅₋₇₅, L/sec | 4.3 | 3.3 |
| MVV, L/min | 168 | 112 |
| DLCO, mL·min⁻¹·mm Hg⁻¹ | 33 | 24 |

[a]Height, 178 cm.
[b]Height, 165 cm.
*DLCO*, Diffusing capacity of the lung for carbon monoxide; *FEF₂₅₋₇₅*, forced expiratory flow (i.e., flow [or speed] of air coming out of the lung during the middle portion of a forced expiration); *FEV₁*, forced expiratory volume in the first second of the experiment; *FEV₁%*, ratio of *FEV₁* to forced vital capacity; *FRC*, functional residual capacity; *FVC*, forced vital capacity; *MVV*, maximum voluntary ventilation; *RV*, residual volume; *TLC*, total lung capacity; *VC*, vital capacity.
Adapted from Taylor AE, Rehder K, Hyatt RE. *Clinical Respiratory Physiology*. WB Saunders; 1989.

volume, and vital capacity. Spirometry cannot provide direct measurement of functional residual capacity (FRC), residual volume (RV), or total lung capacity (TLC); these are measured indirectly or deduced by incorporating multiple lung volumes.

## MEASUREMENT OF FUNCTIONAL RESIDUAL CAPACITY

FRC is the amount of gas in the lungs at the end of expiration during tidal breathing. Three methods can be used to measure FRC: (1) equilibration methods, in which FRC is calculated from the concentration of a tracer gas (usually helium) in a closed system in equilibrium with the patient's lungs; (2) washout methods, in which FRC is calculated from the lung washout of a tracer gas (usually nitrogen); and (3) plethysmographic methods, in which total thoracic gas volume is measured by a technique based on Boyle's law (subjects attempt to breathe against a closed airway while sitting in an airtight chamber, a

body box in which pressure and volume change can be assessed). Plethysmographic methods measure the total amount of gas in the thorax, and the other two methods measure the amount of gas in communication with the airway opening. When combined with spirometry, FRC measurements allow calculation of TLC and RV. Decreased TLC with maintained ratio of forced expiratory volume in 1 second ($FEV_1$) to forced vital capacity (FVC) and decreased RV are the hallmarks of restrictive lung disease.

## MEASUREMENT OF CLOSING VOLUME

Closing volume is the volume above RV at which airway closure, in the dependent parts of the lung, is detectable with a tracer gas. This gas may be nitrogen in a single-breath nitrogen washout after a maximal breath from RV of $O_2$, He, or Xe. This test measures the differing concentrations of tracer gas in nondependent and dependent alveoli achieved during a single maximal inspiration. It also can assess dynamic airway closure in small airways. The closing volume, if greater than FRC, will result in gas trapping and ventilation/perfusion inequality, leading to inefficient gas exchange.

# Tests of Gas Flow

## FORCED EXPIRATORY SPIROGRAPHY

In forced expiratory spirography, the subject exhales as forcefully as possible after a maximal inhalation. Expiratory flow and volume are measured with a spirometer or pneumotachograph (see Figs. 20.2 and 20.3). Maximal forced expiratory flow ($FEF_{max}$) depends on effort. Flow during continued expiration, typically measured as forced flow from 75% to 25% of forced vital capacity ($FEF_{25-75}$), is less dependent on effort.

| TABLE 20.2 | **Patterns of Lung Disease** | | | | |
|---|---|---|---|---|---|
| | **RESTRICTION** | | **OBSTRUCTION** | | |
| Parameter | Chest Wall | Parenchyma | Asthma | Bronchitis | Emphysema |
| TLC | ↓ | ↓ | ↑ | – or ↑ | ↑ |
| VC | ↓ | ↓ | – or ↓ | – or ↓ | – or ↓ |
| RV | – or ↑ | ↓ | ↑ | ↑ | ↑ |
| FRC | ↓ | ↓ | ↑ | ↑ | ↑ |
| MVV | – or ↓ | – or ↓ | ↓ | ↓ | ↓ |
| DLCO | – | ↓ | – or ↑ | – or ↓ | ↓ |
| FEV$_1$ | ↓ | ↓ | ↓ | ↓ | ↓ |
| FEV$_1$% | – | – | ↓ | ↓ | ↓ |

*DLCO*, Diffusing capacity of the lung for carbon monoxide; *FEV$_1$*, forced expiratory volume in the first second of the experiment; *FEV$_1$%*, ratio of *FEV1* to forced vital capacity; *FRC*, functional residual capacity; *MVV*, maximum voluntary ventilation; *RV*, residual volume; *TLC*, total lung capacity; *VC*, vital capacity; ↓, decreased; ↑, increased; –, normal.
Adapted from Taylor AE, Rehder K, Hyatt RE. *Clinical Respiratory Physiology.* WB Saunders; 1989.

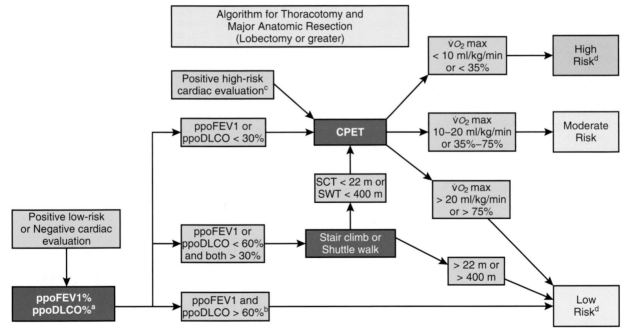

**Fig. 20.1**   Evidence-based guidelines for lung resection: physiologic assessment. *CPET*, Cardiopulmonary exercise testing; *CT*, computed tomography; *CXR*, radiograph of the chest; *DLCO*, diffusing capacity of lung for carbon monoxide; *FEV$_1$*, forced expiratory volume in the first second of the experiment; *ppo*, predicted postoperative value, calculated by estimating the percentage of lung to be removed and reducing measured FEV$_1$% (ratio of FEV$_1$ to forced vital capacity) or DLCO, accordingly; $\dot{V}o_2$ *max*, maximum O$_2$ consumption; *SCT*, stair climb test; *SWT*, shuttle walk test. (Adapted from Brunelli A, Kim AW, Berger KI, Addrizzo-Harris DJ. Physiologic evaluation of the patient with lung cancer being considered for resectional surgery: diagnosis and management of lung cancer, 3rd ed: American College of Chest Physicians evidence-based clinical practice guidelines. *Chest.* 2013;143(5 Suppl):e166S–e190S.)

The most useful parameters obtained from forced expiratory spirography are FVC and FEV$_1$. The ratio of FEV$_1$ to FVC (FEV$_1$/FVC, or FEV$_1$%) normalizes FEV$_1$ measurements for each individual's lung volume. For example, in a patient with restrictive lung disease, FEV$_1$ is low because of low lung volume, not airway obstruction. Reduced FEV$_1$/FVC is the hallmark of obstructive lung disease. FEV$_1$/FVC values of 60% to 70% indicate mild obstruction, values of 40% to 60% indicate moderate obstruction, and values of less than 40% indicate severe obstruction. Measurement results are dependent on

patient effort; they are not valid if the patient does not provide maximum effort during testing. If maximal inspiratory flows also are measured, flow-volume loops can be useful in identifying the source of airway obstruction (Fig. 20.4).

In patients with obstructive lung disease, conducting forced expiratory spirography before and after inhalation of a bronchodilator can assess the reversibility of airway obstruction and help distinguish between the diagnosis of asthma and that of chronic obstructive pulmonary disease. Improvement in FEV$_1$ of greater than 10% indicates reversibility. Inhalation of methacholine,

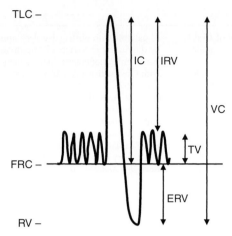

**Fig. 20.2**   Changes in lung volume over time during spirometry. *ERV,* Expiratory reserve volume; *FRC,* functional residual capacity; *IC,* inspiratory capacity; *IRV,* inspiratory reserve volume; *RV,* residual volume; *TLC,* total lung capacity; *TV,* tidal volume; *VC,* vital capacity. (Adapted from Conrad SA, George RB. Clinical pulmonary function testing. In: George RB, Light RW, Mathay RA, eds. *Chest Medicine.* Churchill Livingstone; 1984:161.)

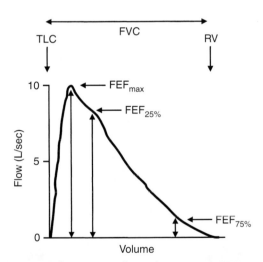

**Fig. 20.3**   Maximal expiratory flow-volume curve. *FEF_max,* Maximal forced expiratory flow; *FEF_{25%},* 25% of forced expiratory flow (FEF); *FEF_{75%},* 75% of FEF; *FVC,* forced vital capacity; *RV,* residual volume; *TLC,* total lung capacity. (Adapted from Conrad SA, George RB. Clinical pulmonary function testing. In: George RB, Light RW, Mathay RA, eds. *Chest Medicine.* Churchill Livingstone; 1984:161.)

which causes bronchoconstriction, is used to diagnose asthma in cases of intermediate pretest probability or diagnostic uncertainty. Patients with asthma have abnormally decreased flow (>15% decrease in $FEV_1$) in response to methacholine.

## MAXIMAL VOLUNTARY VENTILATION

In maximal voluntary ventilation, the subject breathes as quickly and deeply as possible through a pneumotachograph for 12 seconds. The exhaled volume is measured and multiplied by 5 to calculate maximal ventilation during 1 minute. Because this test measures patient motivation and effort and pulmonary function and mechanics, it may be a particularly useful preoperative screening test.

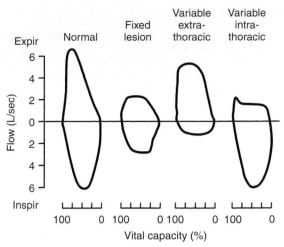

**Fig. 20.4**   Maximal inspiratory *(Inspir)* and expiratory *(Expir)* flow-volume curves used to diagnose airway obstruction. (Adapted from Taylor AE, Rehder K, Hyatt RE. *Clinical Respiratory Physiology.* WB Saunders; 1989.)

## Tests of Efficiency of Gas Exchange

Arterial blood gas and cooximeter sampling assess oxygenation, measure $CO_2$ values, and establish acid-base parameters. $O_2$ uptake and $CO_2$ clearance can be measured during rest or during exercise.

### DIFFUSING CAPACITY

Several methods are used to measure diffusing capacity, all of which measure the diffusion of carbon monoxide across the alveolar-capillary membrane. Diseases or physiologic states that reduce pulmonary blood flow (e.g., fibrosis) or alveolar mass (e.g., emphysema) decrease DLCO.

## Choosing Pulmonary Function Tests

Some of the most critical decisions made by anesthesiologists based on pulmonary function testing involve preoperative assessment of perioperative risk for lung resection. In 2007 the American College of Chest Physicians published an algorithm for this purpose, and it was updated in 2013 (see Fig. 20.1). Poor results on spirometry, symptoms of dyspnea, and diffuse chest radiographic changes indicate the need for DLCO measurement. Estimation of predicted postoperative values for $FEV_1$ (ppoFEV_1) and DLCO indicate risk and the possible need for cardiopulmonary exercise testing as a final level of assessment. The anesthesiologist must be aware of this algorithm and the risks associated with poor performance.

Common obstructive pulmonary diseases are diagnosed based on history, findings on physical examination, and bedside observation. Pulmonary function testing is reserved for assessment of disease severity and adjustment of bronchodilator therapy, but it is not indicated before routine surgery.

Obstructive sleep apnea and restrictive lung disease are increasingly common in modern anesthesia practice and are associated with morbid obesity. An anesthesiologist may be the first physician to diagnose obstructive sleep apnea. Patients should be referred for appropriate care. Although close postoperative monitoring and supportive care are mandatory in patients with obstructive sleep apnea, definitive pulmonary function testing can await specialist referral.

## SUGGESTED READINGS

Bernstein, W. K. (2012). Pulmonary function testing. *Current Opinion in Anaesthesiology, 25*, 11–16.

Bokov, P., & Delclaux, C. (2016). Interpretation and use of routine pulmonary function tests: Spirometry, static lung volumes, lung diffusion, arterial blood gas, methacholine challenge test and 6-minute walk test. *La Revue de Medecine Interne, 37*(2), 100–110.

Brunelli, A., Kim, A. W., Berger, K. I., & Addrizzo-Harris, D. J. (2013). Physiologic evaluation of the patient with lung cancer being considered for resectional surgery: Diagnosis and management of lung cancer, 3rd ed: American College of Chest Physicians evidence-based clinical practice guidelines. *Chest, 143*(Suppl. 5), e166S–e190S.

Colice, G. L., Shafazand, S., Griffin, J. P., Keenan, R., Bolliger, C. T., & American College of Chest Physicians. (2007). Physiologic evaluation of the patient with lung cancer being considered for resectional surgery. ACCP evidence-based practice guidelines. 2nd ed. *Chest, 132*(35), 161.

Gross, J. B., Bachenberg, K. L., Benumof, J. L., Caplan, R. A., Connis, R. T., Coté, C. J., et al. (2006). Practice guidelines for the perioperative management of patients with obstructive sleep apnea: A report by the American Society of Anesthesiologists Task Force on Perioperative Management of Patients with Obstructive Sleep Apnea. *Anesthesiology, 104,* 1081–1093.

Ridgway, Z. A., & Howell, S. J. (2012). Cardiopulmonary exercise testing: A review of methods and applications in surgical patients. *European Journal of Anaesthesiology, 27,* 858–865.

Siuha, P., Farwel, N. J., Singh, S., & Soni, N. (2009). Ventilatory ratio: A simple bedside test of ventilation. *Br J Anaesth, 102,* 692.

# 21

# Chronic Obstructive Pulmonary Disease and Restrictive Lung Disease

MITCHELL KERFELD, MD | MATTHEW JOHNSTON, MD

## Chronic Obstructive Pulmonary Disease

The Global Initiative for Obstructive Lung Disease defines *chronic obstructive lung (pulmonary) disease* (COPD) as "a common, preventable and treatable disease that is characterized by persistent respiratory symptoms and airflow limitation that is due to airway and/or alveolar abnormalities usually caused by significant exposure to noxious particles or gases." The definition does not include the pathologic term *emphysema* and the clinical and epidemiologic term *chronic bronchitis.*

Patients with COPD frequently have a combination of obstructive bronchiolitis or small-airway disease and parenchymal destruction or emphysema (Fig. 21.1). The ratio of forced expiratory volume in 1 second ($FEV_1$) to forced vital capacity (FVC) of less than 0.7 after administration of a bronchodilator is essential in the diagnosis of COPD. Total lung capacity, residual volume, and functional residual capacity are increased in COPD, which differs from the pattern seen with restrictive lung disease.

## CLINICAL FEATURES

The Global Initiative for Obstructive Lung Disease calculated a prevalence of COPD of 6.1% and 13.5%, respectively, after 9- and 10-year cumulative studies. In young adults, the prevalence was 2.2%, and the prevalence was 4.4% in patients 40 to 44 years of age. The primary global cause of COPD is tobacco use (with $\alpha_1$-antitrypsin deficiency as an important cause in the young). Approximately half of patients older than 60 years who have at least a 20 pack-year smoking history have spirometry results consistent with COPD. Lung parenchymal destruction

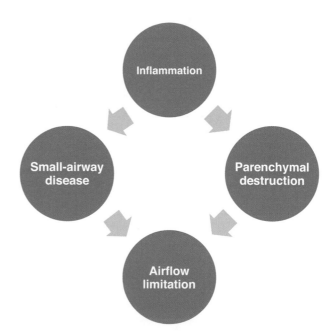

**Fig. 21.1** Patients with chronic obstructive pulmonary disease often have a combination of small-airway disease and parenchymal destruction or emphysema.

leads to loss of diffusing capacity and loss of the radial traction force on the airways. Airway inflammation produces increased mucus secretions and mucosal thickening, resulting in ventilation/perfusion mismatch and, ultimately, hypoxemia and $CO_2$ retention. Expiratory airway collapse results in air trapping,

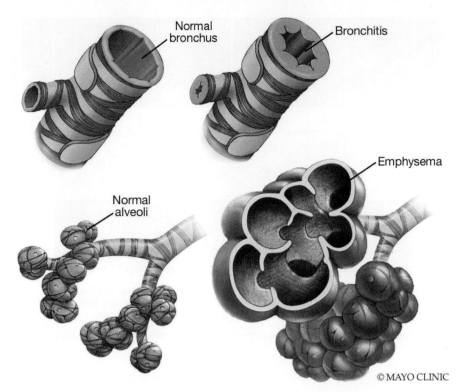

**Fig. 21.2** Continuous noxious exposure leads to pathologic changes in bronchioles and alveoli. Alveolar remodeling leads to decreased total surface area for gas exchange and increased dead space ventilation. Loss of elastic recoil in both alveoli and bronchi ultimately leads to obstruction with exhalation and increased dead space ventilation. (Used with permission of Mayo Foundation for Medical Education and Research, all rights reserved.)

| TABLE 21.1 | GOLD Classification of Severity of Chronic Obstructive Pulmonary Disease | |
|---|---|---|
| | **SPIROMETRY RESULTS** | |
| **Severity** | **FEV$_1$/FVC** | **FEV$_1$ % of Predicted Value** |
| Mild (Class 1) | <0.7 | ≥80 |
| Moderate (Class 2) | <0.7 | ≥50 and <80 |
| Severe (Class 3) | <0.7 | ≥30 and <50 |
| Very severe (Class 4) | <0.7 | <30 or <50 plus signs of respiratory or right-sided heart failure |

*FEV$_1$*, Forced expiratory volume in 1 sec; *FEV$_1$/FVC*, ratio of FEV$_1$ to FVC; *FVC*, forced vital capacity; *GOLD*, Global Initiative for Obstructive Lung Disease.

leading to dynamic hyperinflation as a result of autopositive end-expiratory pressure (Fig. 21.2).

Signs and symptoms of COPD vary significantly with disease severity. COPD severity is classified primarily by spirometry results (Table 21.1). However, the Global Initiative for Obstructive Lung Disease recently included breathlessness and a history of exacerbation to further stratify the severity of disease (Fig. 21.3). Extrapulmonary symptoms include diaphragmatic dysfunction, right-sided heart failure, anxiety, depression, and weight loss with evidence of malnutrition.

## MANAGEMENT

Smoking cessation can arrest the decline of pulmonary function associated with COPD but usually results in only a small improvement in FEV$_1$. Smoking cessation results in a subsequent rate of decline of pulmonary function that is similar to that of a nonsmoker. The concomitant use of short-acting β$_2$-adrenergic receptor agonists and anticholinergic drugs improves FEV$_1$ more than the use of either agent alone. Long-acting bronchodilators provide sustained symptomatic relief, but a mortality benefit has not been found. The use of inhaled corticosteroids is indicated for severe and repeated exacerbations but is not recommended as monotherapy. Theophylline is sometimes used in patients with severe COPD that is unresponsive to other regimens. Monitoring of theophylline blood levels is indicated to minimize potential side effects.

The Global Initiative for Obstructive Lung Disease defines an acute exacerbation of COPD as "an event in the natural course of the disease characterized by a change in the patient's baseline dyspnea, cough, and/or sputum that is beyond normal day-to-day variations, is acute in onset, and may warrant a change in regular medications in a patient with underlying COPD." Respiratory tract infections are a common cause of exacerbations. Treatment with antibiotics and steroids can shorten recovery time and decrease the rate of hospitalization associated with exacerbations of COPD. Exacerbations should prompt review of the efficacy of bronchodilator therapy, with changes as appropriate. Noninvasive mechanical ventilation should be considered as an initial approach to ventilation in patients with acute exacerbations of COPD associated with respiratory failure. If noninvasive ventilation fails, intubation with mechanical ventilation is indicated. Lung volume reduction surgery and lung transplantation have a limited role in the treatment of patients with COPD.

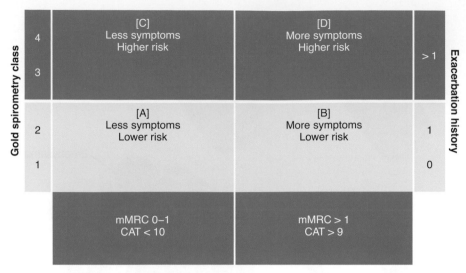

Refined ABCDE Assessment Tool takes into account breathlessness (Modified British Medical Research Council (mMRC), and COPD Assessment Test (CAT)), airflow limitation (spirometry class), and exacerbation history.

**Fig. 21.3**   GOLD Refined ABCDE Assessment Tool. *COPD,* Chronic obstructive pulmonary disease; *GOLD,* Global Initiative for Obstructive Lung Disease.

## PERIOPERATIVE CONSIDERATIONS

Intraoperative management choices of patients with COPD matter. In fact, failure of anesthesia providers to identify patients with COPD is associated with increased length of stay and trends toward increased mortality. Perioperative morbidity and mortality rates in patients with COPD are not influenced by the choice to use general versus regional anesthesia. However, excessive airway manipulation should be avoided to decrease the risk of reflex-induced bronchospasm and promote adequate airflow. Patients with severe dyspnea or acute exacerbations of symptoms should not undergo elective procedures until they are medically optimized.

Preoperative optimization of pulmonary function focuses on cessation of smoking, optimization of bronchodilator therapy, control of infections, and provision of chest physiotherapy, such as incentive spirometry, breathing exercises, and postural drainage techniques. Appropriate investigations, such as arterial blood gas analysis, electrocardiography, echocardiography, and chest radiography, provide information that is helpful in assessing the efficiency of gas exchange, evaluating right ventricular function, and diagnosing asymptomatic bullae.

Surgical patients with severe airflow limitation (severe COPD) have increased rates of postoperative pulmonary complications. Perioperative bronchodilators are associated with a reduction in postoperative pulmonary complications (PPCs) and respiratory failure in patients with COPD. Additionally, retrospective analysis identified three interventional choices associated with decreased risk of PPCs, including low tidal volume ventilation, restricted volume administration, and sugammadex reversal of neuromuscular blockade. Intraoperative monitoring of airway pressure, $O_2$ saturation, and end-tidal $CO_2$ provides useful information about the degree of airflow obstruction. Anesthetics of choice include short-acting agents, such as propofol and remifentanil, and drugs that do not stimulate histamine release. The respiratory rate of the ventilator should be decreased to allow prolonged expiration and minimize the occurrence of dynamic hyperinflation. Noninvasive positive-pressure ventilation is an attractive alternative to tracheal intubation and mechanical ventilation postoperatively.

## Restrictive Lung Disease

### CLINICAL FEATURES

Limited lung expansion or restrictive lung disease may result from several pulmonary and extrapulmonary causes, including pulmonary fibrosis, sarcoidosis, obesity, pleural effusion, scoliosis, and respiratory muscle weakness. Interstitial edema and acute lung injury are considered acute restrictive lung diseases. Spirometry can differentiate between obstructive and restrictive patterns. Total lung capacity is reduced, airway resistance is normal, and airflow is preserved in patients with restrictive lung disease. Reduced $FEV_1$ with a normal or increased $FEV_1/FVC$ suggests restrictive lung disease, but diagnosis and severity grading require measurement of decreased total lung capacity (Fig. 21.4). In patients who have an intrinsic cause of restrictive lung disease, reduced gas transfer is manifest as desaturation after exercise.

The prevalence, mortality, and morbidity associated with restrictive lung disease vary based on the underlying etiology. Idiopathic pulmonary fibrosis is diagnosed in 27 to 29 per 100,000 persons and has a median survival time of less than 3 years.

### MANAGEMENT

The treatment of restrictive lung disease is dependent on the diagnosis. For example, the primary treatment of many interstitial lung diseases includes corticosteroids in combination with immunosuppressive and cytotoxic agents. Supplemental $O_2$ therapy alleviates exercise-induced hypoxemia and improves performance.

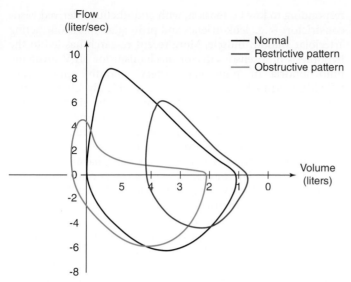

**Fig. 21.4** The physiology of obstructive and restrictive lung disease compared with a normal flow volume curve. Obstructive lung disease is characterized by an overall increase in physiologic lung volumes, much of which is physiologic dead space, with decreased speed of exhalation and incomplete emptying. Restrictive lung disease maintains a near normal $FEV_1/FVC$, but with overall decreased lung volumes and air exchange.

## PERIOPERATIVE CONSIDERATIONS

Preoperative spirometry, arterial blood gas analysis, and measurements of lung volume and gas transfer should be considered within 8 weeks before surgery to identify disease severity in patients with pulmonary lesions. Supplemental doses of corticosteroids and $O_2$ therapy may be required postoperatively, and respiratory infections should be promptly treated. Patients with extrapulmonary causes of restrictive lung disease usually breathe rapidly and shallowly, which is ineffective in clearing sputum, particularly after thoracic or upper abdominal operations. Providing vigorous chest physiotherapy and adequate analgesia is important. Patients with restrictive lung disease who require mechanical ventilation during the operative and postoperative periods typically tolerate relatively low tidal volumes and high respiratory rates.

## SUGGESTED READINGS

Agusti, A., Decramer, M., Celli, B., et al. (2021). *Global initiative for chronic obstructive lung disease. Global strategy for the diagnosis, management, and prevention of chronic obstructive pulmonary disease*. Retrieved from http://www.gold-copd.com. Accessed November 12, 2021.

Hong, C. M., & Galvagno, S. M., Jr. (2013). Patients with chronic pulmonary disease. *Medical Clinics of North America, 97*(6), 1095–1107.

Lee, A. H. Y., Snowden, C. P., Hopkinson, N. S., & Pattinson, K. T. S. (2021). Pre-operative optimisation for chronic obstructive pulmonary disease: A narrative review. *Anaesthesia, 76*(5), 681–694.

Park, S., Oh, E. J., Han, S., Shin, B., Shin, S. H., Im, Y., et al. (2020). Intraoperative Anesthetic Management of Patients with Chronic Obstructive Pulmonary Disease to Decrease the Risk of Postoperative Pulmonary Complications after Abdominal Surgery. *Journal of Clinical Medicine, 9*(1), 150.

Shin, B., Lee, H., Kang, D., Jeong, B. H., Kang, H. K., Chon, H. R., et al. (2017). Airflow limitation severity and post-operative pulmonary complications following extra-pulmonary surgery in COPD patients. *Respirology, 22*(5), 935–941.

# Measurement and Implications of the Q̇s/Q̇t

JASON M. WOODBURY, MD

A variety of factors may cause hypoxemia (Box 22.1). This chapter discusses ventilation/perfusion ($\dot{V}/\dot{Q}$) matching, hypoxic pulmonary vasoconstriction, and calculation of right-to-left shunt.

## Ventilation/Perfusion Mismatch

Ideally, pulmonary perfusion ($\dot{Q}$) and alveolar ventilation ($\dot{V}$) match at all levels of the lung. However, perfect matching of ventilation and perfusion does not occur, and the $\dot{V}/\dot{Q}$ ratio

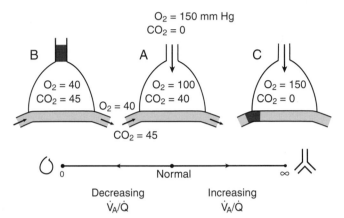

**Fig. 22.1** Effect of altering the ventilation/perfusion ratio on partial pressure of oxygen ($O_2$) and partial pressure of carbon dioxide ($CO_2$) in a lung unit from 0 **(B)** to normal **(A)** to ∞ **(C)**. (From West JB. *Respiratory Physiology: The Essentials.* 9th ed. Lippincott Williams & Wilkins; 2012:64.)

varies throughout the lung. A normal lung has a $\dot{V}/\dot{Q}$ ratio of approximately 0.8. A $\dot{V}/\dot{Q}$ ratio of 0 (i.e., a shunt) exists when perfused alveoli have no ventilation and the values for $Po_2$ and $Pco_2$ of the trapped air are equal to those of mixed venous blood ($Po_2$, 40 mm Hg; $Pco_2$, 47 mm Hg). Conversely, a $\dot{V}/\dot{Q}$ ratio of ∞ exists when ventilated alveoli have no perfusion. At sea level, the $Po_2$ and $Pco_2$ equal approximately 150 and 0 mm Hg, respectively. Alveolar dead space (nonperfused alveoli) constitutes approximately 25 to 50 mL in a healthy, spontaneously breathing, 70-kg adult. Alveolar dead space increases as regions of the lung collapse during prolonged periods of positive-pressure ventilation, as is common during general anesthesia. Fig. 22.1 depicts the progression of a $\dot{V}/\dot{Q}$ ratio from 0 to ∞; the normal idealized alveolar-capillary unit is shown as example A.

In contrast to blood vessels in all other tissues, which dilate in response to hypoxia, the blood vessels of intact lung constrict in response to hypoxia (termed *hypoxic pulmonary vasoconstriction* [HPV]). Vasoconstriction directs blood flow away from poorly ventilated regions of the lung to regions that are better ventilated. This improves the $\dot{V}/\dot{Q}$ ratio, resulting in improved blood oxygenation. HPV-related "shunting" is most effective in improving oxygenation when only small areas of lung are affected. A low $Po_2$ in the pulmonary vasculature is the predominant stimulus that provokes HPV, although a low mixed venous $O_2$ pressure ($P\bar{v}_{O_2}$) also plays a role. A $Po_2$ of less than 100 mm Hg will initiate HPV; marked vasoconstriction occurs with a $Po_2$ of less than 70 mm Hg and becomes progressively more severe as $Po_2$ levels decrease.

The mechanism for HPV is not completely understood. One hypothesis involves pulmonary vascular endothelium

responding to low $O_2$ tension, with endothelium-derived vasoconstrictors (e.g., leukotrienes and prostaglandins) contracting arteriolar smooth muscle. More recent research has led to the hypothesis of a sensor-effector mechanism for HPV involving mitochondria of pulmonary artery smooth muscle cells (PASMC). Mitochondrial sensors dynamically alter reactive oxygen species and redox couples through the electron transport chain in response to hypoxia. Multiple membrane ion channels are either inhibited or activated, resulting in PASMC depolarization causing vasoconstriction.

A variety of physiologic alterations and pharmacologic interventions alter HPV. Respiratory acidosis and metabolic acidosis enhance HPV, whereas respiratory alkalosis, metabolic alkalosis, and hypothermia attenuate it. In vitro studies have shown that volatile anesthetic agents uniformly inhibit HPV, but in vivo studies have not consistently shown clinically significant effects. Systemically administered vasodilators, such as nitroprusside and nitroglycerin, generally adversely affect HPV, which may be of consequence in patients with significant obstructive lung disease or during one-lung ventilation.

## Other Causes of Shunting

A small fraction of blood in the cardiac output, normally 2% to 5%, enters the arterial circulation without first passing through the pulmonary circulation, accounting for the normal $O_2$ alveolar-arterial gradient $P(A-a)O_2$. The causes for this type of venous admixture include (1) the thebesian veins, which drain blood from the coronary circulation directly into the left atrium and, rarely, the left ventricle; and (2) the bronchial veins, which provide nutritive perfusion to the bronchial tree and pleura. Abnormal anatomic shunts include right-to-left atrial and ventricular septal defects and pulmonary arteriovenous malformations.

Hypoxemia resulting from a physiologic or anatomic shunt does not improve with administration of supplemental $O_2$. The hemoglobin in blood that perfuses alveoli with a $\dot{V}/\dot{Q}$ ratio of 1 will readily achieve 100% saturation; increasing the partial pressure of $O_2$ in these alveoli will minimally increase the $O_2$ content. Blood that perfuses alveoli with a $\dot{V}/\dot{Q}$ ratio of 0 will not be exposed to any $O_2$ regardless of the fraction of inspired $O_2$; therefore no significant improvement in arterial oxygenation will occur (Fig. 22.2).

As previously stated, the normal shunt fraction is less than 5%. Clinically significant shunts occur at 10% to 20% of cardiac output. Shunts greater than 30% are potentially fatal. Shunts are not commonly associated with an elevated $Paco_2$. Central and peripheral chemoreceptors detect $Paco_2$ elevations and increase ventilation to compensate. The $Paco_2$ of nonshunted blood is subsequently reduced, and the overall $Paco_2$ typically remains normal.

## Calculation of Shunt Fraction

Physiologic shunting occurs when blood flow is diverted away from poorly ventilated alveoli. The fraction of cardiac output that passes through shunts (and does not participate in gas exchange) is expressed as the shunt fraction ($\dot{Q}_s/\dot{Q}_t$) and is calculated with the equation:

$$\dot{Q}s/\dot{Q}t = \left(C c_{O_2} - C a_{O_2}\right)/\left(C c_{O_2} - C \bar{v} O_2\right)$$

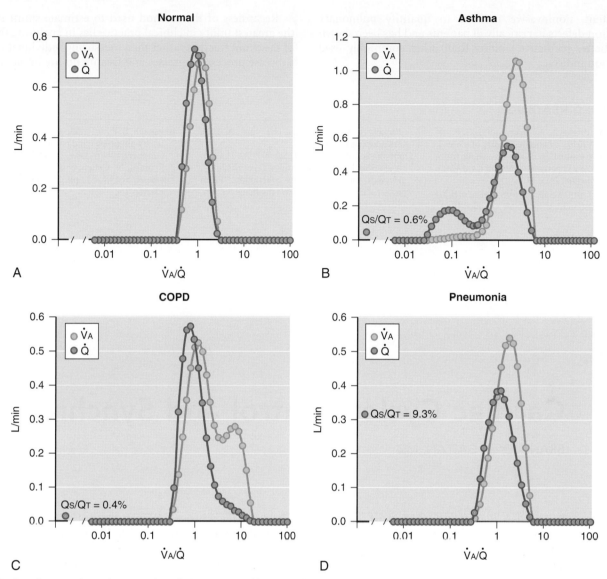

**Fig. 22.2** Distribution of ventilation and perfusion in normal lungs, asthma, chronic obstructive pulmonary disease *(COPD)*, and pneumonia. In normal lungs **(A)** there is good matching between ventilation *(orange circles)* and perfusion *(blue circles)* with a mode centered around a $\dot{V}_A/\dot{Q}$ (alveolar ventilation/pulmonary perfusion) ratio of 1. This results in near optimal oxygenation of blood and $CO_2$ removal. In asthma **(B)** there is broader distribution of $\dot{V}_A/\dot{Q}$ with some regions being ventilated well in excess of perfusion ($\dot{V}_A/\dot{Q} \geq 10$) and another mode of low $\dot{V}_A/\dot{Q}$ centered around a ratio of 0.1. This mode can be explained by collateral ventilation maintaining gas exchange in alveoli behind occluded airways. There is no shunt seen in asthma. In COPD **(C)** the pattern is similar to asthma but with an additional "high" $\dot{V}_A/\dot{Q}$ mode that adds to dead space such as ventilation. Shunt is not present, and the pattern of $\dot{V}_A/\dot{Q}$ distribution is not associated with significant hypoxemia. In lobar pneumonia **(D)** the major finding is pure shunt (consolidated, perfused, and poorly ventilated lobe); there is only minor widening of the $\dot{V}_A/\dot{Q}$ distribution. $Q_s/Q_t$, Shunt fraction. (From Kavanagh BP, Hedenstierna G. Respiratory physiology and pathophysiology. In: Gropper MA, ed. *Miller's Anesthesia.* 9th ed. Elsevier; 2020:fig. 13.26.)

where $\dot{Q}_s$ represents blood flow through the shunt and $\dot{Q}_t$ represents total cardiac output, $Cco_2$ equals the $O_2$ content of end-pulmonary capillary blood, $Cao_2$ is the $O_2$ content of arterial blood, and $C\bar{v}_2$ represents the $O_2$ content of mixed venous blood. This equation can be further simplified by substituting hemoglobin saturation values (which are easily measured by oximetry) for $O_2$ content values. Because calculating the shunt fraction (VQI) with this equation assumes perfect alveolar/capillary interface and gas exchange, the end capillary saturation ($Sc'O_2$) can be estimated as 1 (100%). The arterial blood $O_2$ saturation ($Sao_2$) can be continuously monitored by pulse oximetry, and the venous saturation of blood ($SvO_2$) can be

measured by either obtaining a mixed venous blood sample or by placing a pulmonary artery catheter capable of continuous oximetry. The resulting simplified equation is:

$$VQI = \frac{Sc'O_2 - Sao_2}{Sc'O_2 - S\bar{v}O_2} \cong \frac{1 - Sao_2}{1 - S\bar{v}O_2}$$

A normal VQI ($Q_s/Q_t$) is 0% to 4%.

Additionally, a computation model has been developed that can estimate effective shunt fraction (ES) using values from standard arterial blood gas measurements. The model provides a consistent, noninvasive method to quantify pulmonary oxygenation defects in critically ill patients and has been shown to have better predictive validity than other commonly used oxygenation indices.

Regardless of the method used to estimate shunt fraction, the greatest utility in clinical practice lies in analyzing the trend of the shunt fraction rather than measuring individual values as a disease process progresses and treatments are implemented.

## SUGGESTED READINGS

Chang, E. M., Bretherik, A., Drummond, G. B., & Baillie, J. K. (2019). Predictive validity of a novel non-invasive estimation of effective shunt fraction in critically ill patients. *Intensive Care Medicine Experimental*, 7(1), 49.

Cloutier, M. M. (2019). Ventilation (V̇), perfusion (Q̇), and their relationships. In M. M. Cloutier (Ed.), *Respiratory physiology* (2nd ed., pp. 90–100). Philadelphia: Elsevier Inc.

Dunham-Snary, K. J., Wu, D., Sykes, E. A., Thakrar, A., Parlow, L. R. G., Mewburn, J. D., et al. (2017). Hypoxic pulmonary vasoconstriction: From molecular mechanisms to medicine. *Chest*, 151(1), 181–192.

Kavanagh, B. P., & Hedenstierna, G. (2020). Respiratory physiology and pathophysiology. In M. A. Gropper, L. Eriksson, L. Fleisher, J. Wiener-Kronish, N. Cohen, & K. Leslie (Eds.), *Miller's anesthesia* (9th ed., pp. 354–383). Philadelphia: Elsevier Inc.

# 23

# Cardiac Cycle: Control and Synchronicity

BRANTLEY D. GAITAN, MD

The cardiac cycle describes the succession of atrial and ventricular events that make up a period of contraction (systole) followed by a period of relaxation (diastole) (i.e., a single heartbeat). These periods are further subdivided into phases.

The period of systole comprises *isovolumic contraction* and *ejection*. Initiation of myocardial contraction causes an abrupt increase in ventricular pressure that quickly exceeds the atrial pressure and closes the atrioventricular (AV) valves. Myocardial contraction continues with both the AV and semilunar valves closed (approximately 0.03 s) so that ventricular pressure continues to increase over a constant volume (*isovolumic contraction*). Once ventricular pressure sufficiently exceeds the pressure in either the aorta (left) or the pulmonary artery (right), the semilunar valves open and *ejection* occurs.

Immediately after systole is diastole, which comprises relaxation and ventricular filling. Diastole is further divided into four distinct phases: *isovolumic relaxation*, *rapid inflow*, *diastasis*, and *atrial systole* (Figs. 23.1 and 23.2). Relaxation of the ventricular myocardium causes the pressure within the ventricular cavity to decrease rapidly, closing the semilunar valves when the pressure falls below the pressure of the aorta and pulmonary artery. Myocardial relaxation continues with both the AV and semilunar valves closed (approximately 0.06 s) so that ventricular pressure continues to decrease over a constant volume (*isovolumic relaxation*). Once ventricular pressure drops below atrial pressure, the AV valves open and blood rapidly fills the ventricles (*rapid inflow*). The rapid myocardial relaxation creates a negative intracavitary pressure (diastolic suction) that augments the inflow of

blood into the ventricle. Once myocardial relaxation is complete, elastic distention of the ventricle begins to slow blood return (*diastasis*). This phase is followed immediately by atrial systole. Effective atrial systole contributes up to approximately 20% of ventricular filling and completes the period of diastole.

## Control

The heart contains a specialized conduction system that rhythmically generates electrical impulses (action potentials [APs]) that are transmitted rapidly through both the atria and ventricles, triggering their sequential contraction and controlling the cardiac cycle from beat to beat. Each normal cardiac cycle is initiated by spontaneous generation of an AP in the sinoatrial (SA) node of the right atrium near the opening of the superior vena cava. The AP is conducted through the atria, then through the AV node and ventricular conduction system, resulting in myocardial contraction of the atria and ventricles. Cardiac APs are the voltage changes that result from activation or inactivation of fast sodium channels, slow sodium-potassium channels, and potassium channels at different times that together create collective swings in voltage between a hyperpolarized and depolarized state. APs higher up in the conduction system have different morphologic features than those in the ventricle, which explains why control of the cardiac cycle resides in the more proximal or cephalad conducting system.

Rhythmicity of the cycle resides within the cells of the SA node because these cell membranes are inherently more "leaky" to Na+

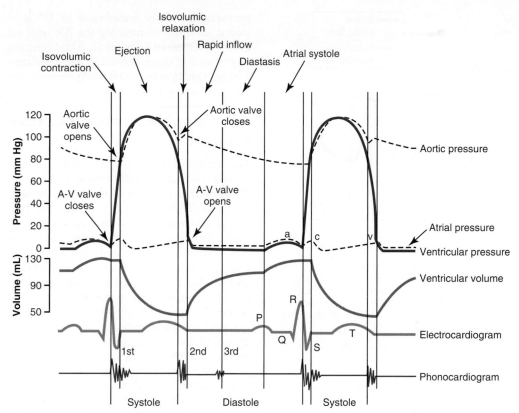

**Fig. 23.1**   The simultaneous events of the cardiac cycle for left ventricular function, showing changes in left atrial pressure, left ventricular pressure, aortic pressure, ventricular volume, the electrocardiogram, and the phonocardiogram. (From Guyton AC, Hall JE. *Textbook of Medical Physiology.* 14th ed. Elsevier; 2021.)

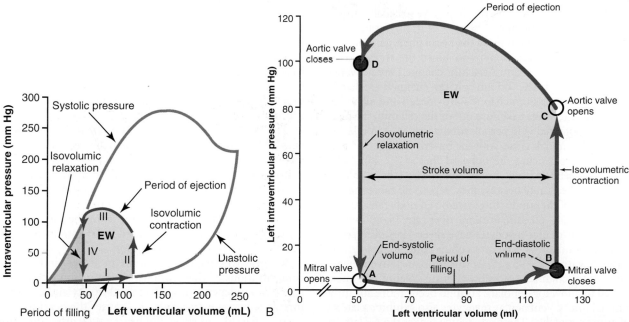

**Fig. 23.2   A,** Relationship between left ventricular volume and intraventricular pressure during diastole and systole. The diastolic pressure curve is determined by filling the heart with blood and measuring pressure immediately before ventricular contraction occurs. Until the volume of the left ventricle rises above approximately 150 mL, diastolic pressure changes minimally. However, above this volume, pressure increases rapidly because the myofibrils are stretched to their maximum. During ventricular contraction, systolic pressure increases even at low ventricular volumes and reaches a maximum pressure at volumes of approximately 150 mL. At volumes greater than 150 mL, systolic pressure may decrease because actin and myo-sin are so stretched that contraction is not optimal. Maximum systolic pressure for the left ventricle is 250 to 300 mm Hg, but it varies widely between individuals. The *heavy red lines* show the volume-pressure curve during a normal cardiac cycle. **B,** Volume-pressure curve during a normal cardiac cycle, where *EW* (shaded area) represents the net external work of the heart. The phases of systole (counterclockwise, from point *B* to point *D*) and the phases of diastole (continuing counterclockwise, from point *D* to point *B*) are labeled as are the corresponding positions of the mitral and aortic valves. *EW,* Net external work of the heart. (From Guyton AC, Hall JE. *Textbook of Medical Physiology.* 14th ed. Elsevier; 2021.)

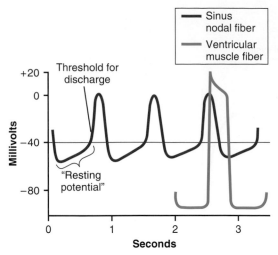

**Fig. 23.3** Action potential tracing of a sinus nodal fiber compared with that of a ventricular muscle fiber. The nodal action potential is slower in onset and offset, has less variation in membrane potential, and does not have a plateau phase, as is seen in the ventricular fiber action potential. (From Guyton AC, Hall JE. *Textbook of Medical Physiology.* 14th ed. Elsevier; 2021.)

and $Ca^{2+}$ ions than are cell membranes of the ventricular conduction system. The increased influx of $Na^+$ and $Ca^{2+}$ in these more proximal nodal fibers creates a less negative resting membrane potential ($-55$ mV), a voltage at which many of the fast sodium channels have become inactivated. Therefore depolarization is a result of activation of the slow sodium-calcium channels, and it results in a slower upslope of depolarization and a slower repolarization period compared with APs of ventricular muscle (Fig. 23.3). Passive diffusion of $Na^+$ because of its high concentration in the extracellular fluid outside the nodal fibers continues to depolarize the extracellular membrane. Once the threshold of $-40$ mV is reached, the sodium-calcium channels are activated and an AP is generated. The sodium-calcium channels are inactivated quickly, and potassium channels are opened and allow the positively charged $K^+$ ions to diffuse out of the cell until the resting membrane potential is hyperpolarized again at $-55$ mV. Finally, potassium channels close, with the inward-leaking $Na^+$ and $Ca^{2+}$ ions counterbalancing the outward flux of $K^+$ ions. The process repeats itself, eliciting another cycle. The cells in the SA node control the heart rate because they depolarize more rapidly than does the rest of the conducting system (SA node rate, 70–80/min; AV node rate, 40–60/min; Purkinje fiber rate, 15–40/min).

The APs of ventricular myocytes have several key differences compared with nodal APs. The intracellular potential is significantly more negative at $-85$ mV. At this more negative voltage, both fast sodium channels and slow sodium-calcium channels are activated to allow for depolarization to occur more abruptly than in nodal fibers. Ventricular myocytes also exhibit a plateau phase of approximately 0.2 seconds, which makes the AP last up to 15 times longer than in skeletal muscle. This plateau occurs because of the longer duration of activation of the slow sodium-calcium channels. Additionally, the membranes of ventricular myocytes become less permeable to $K^+$ ions than the cell membranes of skeletal muscle fibers. Therefore after activation, the efflux of $K^+$ is slowed and thus prevents early return of the AP voltage to its resting level. At the end of the plateau phase, the slow sodium-calcium channels are inactivated and

permeability of the membrane to $K^+$ is simultaneously restored, abruptly terminating the AP, with return of the membrane potential to its baseline. Thus ventricular APs are much more rapid in onset and offset, have a plateau phase, and have a larger variation in membrane potential compared with nodal and conducting system APs.

## Physiologic Effects on Cardiac Cycle Control

The autonomic nervous system provides control for rhythmicity and conduction of the cardiac cycle. Sympathetic nerves are distributed to all parts of the heart, especially the ventricular myocytes. These nerves (1) increase the rate of SA nodal discharge (*chronotropy*); (2) increase the rate of conduction plus excitability throughout the heart (*dromotropy, synchronicity*); and (3) increase the force of contraction of all myocytes (*inotropy*). Maximal sympathetic outflow can triple the heart rate and double the strength of contraction. Norepinephrine released at sympathetic nerve endings is believed to increase membrane permeability to $Na^+$ and $Ca^{2+}$, increasing the tendency of the membrane potential to drift upward to the threshold for excitation. Increased $Ca^{2+}$ permeability causes increased inotropic effect.

Parasympathetic preganglionic fibers are distributed mainly to the SA and AV nodes and, to a much lesser extent, the atria and ventricles through the vagus nerve. Vagal stimulation releases acetylcholine from the axonal terminus of the preganglionic fibers, which decreases (1) the rate of SA node discharge and (2) the excitability of AV junctional fibers, thus slowing impulse transmission to the ventricles. Vagal stimulation decreases heart rate, but strong vagal stimulation can completely stop SA node discharge, leading to eventual ventricular escape beats from the discharge of Purkinje fibers. Acetylcholine works by increasing the permeability of cells in the SA and AV nodes to $K^+$, thereby producing hyperpolarization (increased negativity of the resting membrane potential, $-70$ to $-75$ mV); thus conduction tissue is much less excitable and takes longer to reach threshold spontaneously.

The vasomotor center of the central nervous system (medullary-pontine area) contains neurons that affect chronotropic and inotropic responses from the heart. Vagal motor neurons that travel to the SA and AV nodes are contained within the *nucleus ambiguus*. Vagal impulses are reflexive, occurring mainly in response to carotid and aortic baroreceptor activity. Additionally, phasic input from the inspiratory center causes sinus arrhythmia: increased heart rate with inspiration, decreased heart rate with expiration.

Because APs require variation in intra- and extracellular concentrations of charged ions, alterations in electrolytes ($K^+$, $Ca^{2+}$) can independently affect rhythmicity and conduction of impulses. Excess extracellular $K^+$ causes the heart to dilate and become flaccid and slows the heart rate. Larger quantities can cause conduction delays and AV blocks. The mechanism of this effect is that high extracellular $K^+$ concentration will decrease resting membrane potential in myocytes (the membrane potential becomes less negative), which decreases the intensity of the AP and thereby decreases inotropy. Conversely, excess extracellular $Ca^{2+}$ can cause spastic contraction of the heart through the direct effect of $Ca^{2+}$ in the contraction process. A $Ca^{2+}$ deficiency can cause flaccidity.

Body temperature also influences the control of the cardiac cycle. Heat increases the permeability of myocyte membranes to ions that control the heart rate. Hyperthermia can double the heart rate, whereas hypothermia can slow the heart rate to a few beats per minute. The contractile function of the heart initially is augmented with hyperthermia, but this compensatory mechanism is soon exhausted, and the heart eventually becomes flaccid.

## Synchronicity

The AP originating in the SA node spreads through the atrium at a rate of 0.3 m/s; internodal pathways terminate in the AV node (1 m/s). The impulse reaches the AV node 0.04 s after its origin in the SA node. Delay occurs at the AV node, allowing time for the atria to empty before ventricular contraction begins. The prolonged refractory period of the AV node helps prevent arrhythmias, which can occur if a second cardiac impulse is transmitted to the ventricle too soon after the first. Purkinje fibers lead from the AV node and divide into left and right bundle branches, spreading into the apex of the respective ventricles and then back toward the base of the heart. These large fibers have a conduction velocity of 1.5 to 4 m/s (6 times that of myocytes and 150 times that of junctional fibers), allowing almost immediate transmission of cardiac impulses through the entire ventricular system. Thus the cardiac impulse arrives at almost all portions of the ventricle simultaneously, exciting the first ventricular myocytes only 0.06 seconds ahead of the last ventricular fibers (Fig. 23.4). Effective pumping by both ventricles requires this synchronization of contraction.

The AP causes myocardial myocytes to contract by a mechanism known as *excitation-contraction coupling*. The AP passes into the myocytes along the *transverse tubules*, triggering release of $Ca^{2+}$ into the cell from the

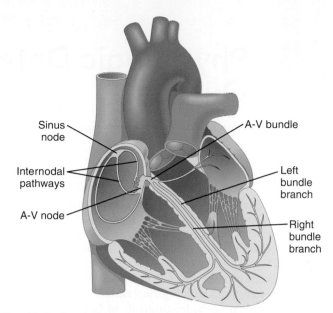

**Fig. 23.4** Conduction system of the heart, showing the sinoatrial (sinus) and atrioventricular (A-V) nodes, internodal pathways, Purkinje system, and ventricular bundle branches. (From Guyton AC, Hall JE. *Textbook of Medical Physiology.* 14th ed. Elsevier; 2021.)

sarcoplasmic reticulum and from the transverse tubules themselves. $Ca^{2+}$ ions promote the sliding of actin on myosin, creating myofibril contraction. The transverse tubules can store a tremendous amount of $Ca^{2+}$; without this store, the sarcoplasmic reticulum of myocytes would not provide an adequate supply of $Ca^{2+}$ ions to allow contraction. Availability of extracellular $Ca^{2+}$ directly affects the availability of $Ca^{2+}$ ions for release into the cellular sarcoplasm from the transverse tubules.

## SUGGESTED READINGS

Bers, D. M., & Borlaug, B. A. (2022). Mechanisms of cardiac contraction and relaxation. In P. Libby, R. O. Bonow, D. L. Mann, G. F. Thomaselli, D. L. Bhatt, & S. D. Solomon (Eds.), *Braunwald's heart disease: A textbook of cardiovascular medicine* (12th ed., pp. 889–912). Philadelphia: Elsevier.

Boulpaep, E. L. (2017). The heart as a pump. In W. F. Boron, & E. L. Boulpaep (Eds.), *Medical physiology* (3rd ed., pp. 507–532). Philadelphia: Elsevier.

Hall, J. E., & Hall, M. E. (2021a). Cardiac muscle: The heart as a pump and function of the heart valves. In A. C. Guyton, & J. E. Hall (Eds.), *Textbook of medical physiology* (14th ed., pp. 113–126). Philadelphia: Elsevier.

Hall, J. E., & Hall, M. E. (2021b). Rhythmical excitation of the heart. In A. C. Guyton, & J. E. Hall (Eds.), *Textbook of medical physiology* (14th ed., pp. 127–133). Philadelphia: Elsevier.

Lederer, W. J. (2017). Cardiac electrophysiology and the electrocardiogram. In W. F. Boron, & E. L. Boulpaep (Eds.), *Medical physiology* (3rd ed., pp. 483–506). Philadelphia: Elsevier.

Pagel, P. S., & Stowe, D. F. (2017). Cardiac anatomy and physiology. In P. G. Barash, B. F. Cullen, & R. K. Stoelting (Eds.), *Clinical anesthesia* (8th ed., pp. 276–301). Philadelphia: Lippincott, Williams & Wilkins.

# 24

# Physiologic Determinants of Cardiac Output

EDWARD J. WASHINGTON, MD

Cardiac output (CO) is defined as the volume of blood pumped by the left ventricle into the aorta during a specified interval of time and is usually stated in L/min. In the average male weighing 70 kg and with a body surface area of 1.7 m², the CO is approximately 5 to 6 L/min (10% less in females). While resting in the supine position, a person's CO decreases by ~25% and may increase by 6 to 8 times with vigorous exercise.

The major physiologic determinants of CO are stroke volume (SV) and heart rate (HR):

$$CO\ (L/min) = SV \times HR$$

## Stroke Volume

The determinants of SV are represented by the relationship between the end diastolic and the end systolic pressure-volumes. End diastolic volumes (EDVs) approximately represent preload, whereas end systolic volumes (ESVs) are dependent on afterload and contractility. This relationship is depicted in the formula SV = EDV – ESV (Fig. 24.1).

## PRELOAD

Myocardial stretch, called *preload*, is directly related to EDV (normal value is ~110–120 mL). EDV is influenced by several factors, with venous return (VR) being the most important. Venous return can be calculated by the formula VR = (Psf – RAP)/RVR, where Psf is the mean systemic filling pressure, RAP is the right atrial pressure, and RVR is the resistance to venous return. Because the circulation is a closed circuit, VR should equal CO if there is no hemorrhage or obstruction to flow. Under certain circumstances large amounts of blood can be shifted from the peripheral circulation to the central circulation. This leads to an increase in myocardial stretch resulting in a proportional increase in SV (Fig. 24.2). The average person has a SV of approximately 70 to 80 mL.

Other factors that influence preload include patient position, ventricular filling time, intrathoracic pressure, pulmonary vascular resistance, right heart function, and atrial contraction. CO measurement has traditionally required invasive techniques, such as the insertion of a pulmonary artery catheter. Recent trends have been to develop measurement instruments

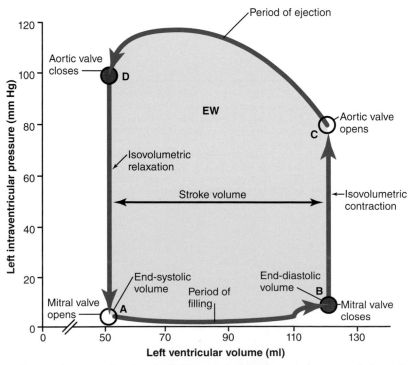

**Fig. 24.1** The volume-pressure diagram demonstrating changes in intraventricular volume and pressure during a single cardiac cycle (*red line*). The *shaded area* represents the net external work (*EW*) output by the left ventricle during the cardiac cycle. (From Hall JE. Cardiac output, venous return, and their regulation. In: Guyton AC, Hall JE. *Textbook of Medical Physiology*. 13th ed. Elsevier; 2016:118, fig. 9.10.)

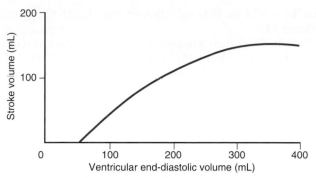

**Fig. 24.2** The Starling curve. As left ventricular end-diastolic volume (stretch of myofibrils) increases, myocardial contractility (stroke volume) increases.

that are less invasive and allow more frequent, or even continuous, measurement of CO. *Pulse contour analysis* allows for the evaluation of the arterial pulse contour that has specific values for resistance, compliance, and impedance in determining CO (e.g., FloTrac™). *Echocardiographic (transesophageal and transthoracic)* techniques have the additional advantage of evaluation of systolic and diastolic function, volume status, regional wall motion, valve function, and the presence of pericardial effusion.

## CONTRACTILITY

Although *contractility* (a determinant of ESV) is difficult to define, it can be described as the performance of the heart at a given preload and afterload (given a constant HR). Experimentally, contractility may be determined by the change in peak isometric force (isovolumetric pressure) at an initial fiber length (EDV). It is highly dependent on the presence of intracellular calcium and can be estimated by the ejection fraction (EF). Current clinical modalities used to assess EF include angiography, echocardiography, and scintigraphy.

Sympathetic nervous system stimulation can increase the maximum CO as much as twofold to threefold. During stimulation both the HR and strength of ventricular muscle contraction increase, thereby increasing the level of cardiac pumping well above normal. In addition to intracellular calcium, catecholamines and digitalis also help increase contractility. By contrast, vagal (parasympathetic) stimulation can decrease the strength of heart muscle contraction by 20% to 30%. However, these vagal fibers are mostly located in the atria of the heart and affect HR to a greater degree than the strength of contraction. Drugs such as β-adrenergic receptor blockers and calcium channel blockers decrease myocardial contractility. Acidosis, hypoxemia, and ischemia also decrease CO.

## AFTERLOAD

The load against which the left ventricle exerts its contractile force is called the *afterload*. It is the resistance to ventricular ejection and is a component of ESV. The two major determinants of afterload are myocardial wall stress and input impedance. Myocardial wall stress (P) is often described by the pressure law of LaPlace's formula:

$$P = (2 \times H \times T)/r$$

where H is wall thickness, T is tension in the LV wall, and r is ventricular radius. This law tells us that components of afterload

are ventricular transmural pressure, radius of the ventricle, and the thickness of the ventricular wall.

Ventricular cavity pressure during systole describes input impedance. The contributors include arterial compliance (aortic and peripheral), inertia of the blood column, ventricular outflow tract resistance, and arterial resistance. Systemic vascular resistance (SVR) represents the major determinant (~95%) of afterload in the form of aortic compliance. It influences the resistance to early ventricular systole and is defined by the formula

$$SVR = 80 \times (MAP - RAP)/CO$$

where MAP is mean arterial pressure and RAP is right atrial pressure. Normal SVR is 900 to 1500 dynes/sec/cm$^{-5}$.

Other factors affecting afterload include ventricular outflow tract resistance (e.g., hypertrophic cardiomyopathy and aortic stenosis), blood viscosity, length of the arterial tree, and vessel radius.

## Heart Rate

Under normal circumstances, the sinoatrial node pacemaker cells (located in the right atrium) maintain a HR between 60 and 100 beats/min. These cells are heavily influenced by venous return and neural input (Fig. 24.3).

At maximum cardiac stimulation the HR is the primary determinant of CO. Under these conditions, the SV increases by 50%, whereas the HR may increase by as much as 270% (e.g., from 50 to 185 beats/min for a marathon runner). This increase in HR leads to an increase in myocardial tension secondary to an influx of calcium into the myocardial cell cytoplasm, the Bowditch effect. However, severe tachycardia may lead to decreased diastolic filling time and lower SV. Vagal (parasympathetic) fibers are highly concentrated in the atria of the heart.

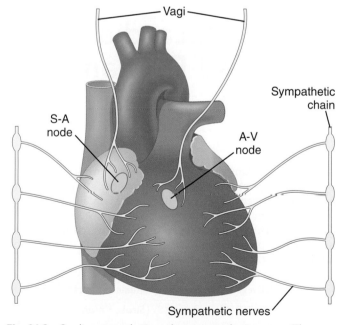

**Fig. 24.3** Cardiac sympathetic and parasympathetic nerves. (The vagus nerves to the heart are parasympathetic nerves.) *A-V*, Atrioventricular; *S-A*, sinoatrial. (From Hall JE. Cardiac output, venous return, and their regulation. In: Guyton AC, Hall JE. *Textbook of Medical Physiology.* 13th ed. Elsevier; 2016:120, fig. 9.13.)

This explains why the parasympathetic system affects HR to a greater extent than the strength of heart contraction. Maximum parasympathetic stimulation may lead to asystole; however, the myocardium usually "escapes" and beats between 20 and 40 beats/min as long as this vagal stimulation continues.

Atrial contraction contributes to the overall CO (~20%–25%). Individuals with arrhythmias such as *atrial fibrillation* may have a decrease in SV due to loss of atrial contraction. Depending on ventricular diastolic function and HR, there

may be a 30% to 40% reduction in ventricular filling and a reduced SV.

Finally, CO increases in proportion to the surface area of the body (BSA). Therefore CO can be stated in terms of the *cardiac index* (CI), represented by the formula

$$CI(L/min/m^2) = CO/BSA$$

The average 70-kg human has a BSA of 1.7 m² and a CI of approximately 3 L/min/m².

## SUGGESTED READINGS

Berne, R. M., Levy, M. N., Koeppen, B. M., & Stanton, B. A. (2006). *Principles of physiology* (4th ed., p. 250). Philadelphia: Elsevier.

Bhatt, A., Flink, L., Lu, D. Y., Fang, Q., Bibby, D., & Schiller, N. B. (2020). Exercise physiology of the left atrium: Quantity and timing of contribution to cardiac output. *American Journal of Physiology Heart and Circulatory Physiology*, *320*, H575–H583.

Flood, P., Rathmell, J. P., Shafer, S., Ramsay, J., & Larson, B. (2015). Circulatory physiology. In *Stoelting's pharmacology & physiology in anesthesia practice* (5th ed., pp. 365–391). Philadelphia: Wolters Kluwer.

Hall, J. E. (2016). Cardiac output, venous return, and their regulation. In A. C. Guyton, J. E. Hall (Eds.), *Textbook of medical physiology* (13th ed., pp. 109–122 & 245–258). Philadelphia: Elsevier.

Hou, P. C., Filbin, M. R., Napoli, A., Feldman, J., Pang, P. S., Sankoff, J., et al. (2016). Cardiac Output Monitoring Managing Intravenous Therapy (COMMIT) to treat emergency department patients with sepsis. *Shock*, *46*, 132–138.

Su, C. H., Liu, S. H., Tan, T. H., & Lo, C. H. (2018). Using the pulse contour method to measure the changes in stroke volume during a passive leg raising test. *Sensors*, *18*, 1–11.

Trentman, T. L., Gaitan, B. D., Gali, B., Johnson, R. L., Muelle, J. T., Rose, S. H., Vijitpavan, A. (2020). Physiologic determinants of cardiac output. In *Faust's anesthesiology review* (5th ed., pp. 69–72). Philadelphia: Elsevier.

Vincent, J. L. (2008). Understanding cardiac output. *Critical Care*, *12*(4), 174.

Williams, A. M., Shave, R. E., Stembridge, M., & Eves, N. D. (2016). Females have greater left ventricular twist mechanics than males during acute reductions to preload. *American Journal of Physiology Heart and Circulatory Physiology*, *311*, H76–H84.

# Myocardial Oxygen Supply and Demand

ANDREW MURRAY, MBChB

One of the fundamental concepts when considering how to protect and optimize cardiac performance is the concept of myocardial oxygen supply and demand. Maintaining an equal balance or even favoring supply serves to protect myocardial tissue and performance. Oxygen supply delivered to the myocardium is represented by the oxygen content of the blood multiplied by the cardiac output.

$$DO_2 \left(\text{Delivery of oxygen}\right) = CO\left(\text{Cardiac Output}\right) \times CaO_2$$

$$CO = HR\left(\text{Heart Rate}\right) \times SV\left(\text{Stroke Volume}\right)$$

$$CaO_2\left(\text{Arterial oxygen content}\right) =$$

$$\left(1.34 \times \left[Hb\left(\text{Hemoglobin in grams per deciliter}\right)\right] \times SpO_2\right) +$$

$$\left(0.003 \times PaO_2\left(\text{Partial pressure of oxygen in arterial blood}\right)\right)$$

*Demand* is the consumption of oxygen by the myocardium. Changes to either side of this equation that result in increased demand that is not met by increased supply have the potential to cause ischemic injury to the myocardium. Myocardial flow is estimated to be 70-80 mL/min/100gm of myocardial tissue.

The determination of the amount of blood delivered to tissue is described in a way that is analogous to the mathematical description of electrical current driven by voltage, Ohm's law, where current equals voltage divided by resistance. In the biologic blood flow model, this equates to

$$Q \text{ (flow)} = \Delta P \text{ (pressure gradient)}/R \text{ (resistance)}$$

where Q represents coronary blood flow (CBF), $\Delta P$ is the pressure gradient across the coronary vascular bed or coronary perfusion pressure (CPP), and R is the resistance to flow through the coronary vascular bed.

CPP therefore translates into the difference between aortic pressure and ventricular end-diastolic pressure. This relationship differs for each ventricle. Because of the high pressure developed in the left ventricle during systole, the subendocardial vessels are compressed during systole so that coronary perfusion only occurs during the diastolic phase. Therefore the downstream pressure in the left ventricle is the left ventricular end-diastolic pressure (LVEDP). This equates to

$$CBF = (DBP_{AO} - LVEDP)$$

where $DBP_{AO}$ represents diastolic blood pressure of the aorta. In the normal right ventricle, the normal aortic pressure is always greater than the right ventricular cavitary pressure in both cardiac phases; therefore perfusion occurs during both the systolic and diastolic phases.

## Coronary Perfusion Pressure

The combination of the high left ventricular systolic pressures along with systolic pressure changes at the coronary ostia results in CBF to the left ventricle only occurring during diastole. A further limitation to blood flow in the myocardium of the left ventricle is the high transmural pressures developed during systole. However, extremes of blood pressure may cause a greater increase in myocardial work and higher intracavitary pressures that may compromise subendocardial blood flow to a greater extent than increased flow can compensate.

The normal right ventricle, however, functions at much lower pressure that allows for CBF to occur during both phases of the cardiac cycle, resulting in more uniform phasic blood flow in the right ventricle.

Any condition that serves to decrease the diastolic blood pressure, decrease diastolic filling time, or increase the diastolic pressure of the left ventricle may result in decreased oxygen supply to the left ventricle, with resultant decreased contractility with attendant decreased stroke volume and aortic root pressure. These conditions may have a detrimental effect on left ventricle oxygen supply.

In the case of the right ventricle, hypertrophy resulting from long-standing pressure overload causes the characteristics of perfusion to begin to resemble a flow relationship that is more like that of the left ventricle, with perfusion occurring mainly during diastole. This may result in upsetting the delicate balance of supply and demand for the right ventricle.

In a similar way, if there is an acute increase in pulmonary resistance that results in decreased right ventricular performance, this may lead to poor left ventricular filling, decreased cardiac output, and consequently decreased blood pressure through both phases, further worsening the supply/demand relationship of the right ventricle.

## Vascular Resistance

Epicardial vessels are capacitance vessels and are not affected by extrinsic coronary compression to the same degree as subendocardial vessels. CPP is the difference between diastolic aortic pressure and left ventricular cavitary pressure.

Intrinsic coronary resistance plays a greater role in coronary vascular resistance than extrinsic factors and is controlled by endogenous biochemical substances and autonomic neural inputs.

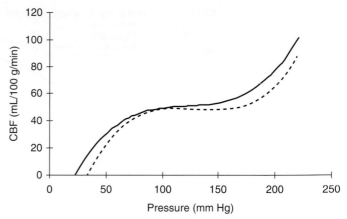

**Fig. 25.1**  Autoregulation curve. *CBF*, Coronary blood flow.

Because of the high oxygen extraction of the myocardium, the only way for the heart to preserve its oxygen supply in periods of increased need is to increase flow, and it does this over a range of mean blood pressures. Typically, this range is believed to be 60 to 140 mm Hg in healthy human beings. This is referred to as *autoregulation,* between which the flow is predominantly pressure independent. Beyond these pressures the coronary flow will be pressure dependent (i.e., the blood flow will vary along with and in the same direction as the driving pressure), representing a more linear relationship (Fig. 25.1). Additionally, fixed obstructions, like atherosclerotic plaque, can create area distal to the obstruction that are pressure dependent as they will typically develop maximal coronary vasodilation to compensate for the obstruction.

Bayliss proposed a myogenic control mechanism of vascular tone. Control of coronary autoregulation appears to be largely independent of neurohumoral inputs. Although adenosine was considered the primary mediator of this process, in fact, the process is more complex, with adenosine (acting mainly on Alpha 2a receptors) playing a redundant role alongside nitric oxide, prostaglandins, endothelin, and ATP-dependent $K^+$-channels, among others. Coronary vasodilation occurs secondary to parasympathetic input. In addition, sympathetically driven processes result in coronary vasodilation secondary to increased myocardial $O_2$ consumption and local metabolite accumulation (e.g., adenosine, nitric oxide, endothelin).

## Arterial Blood Oxygen Content

The primary determinants of arterial blood oxygen content ($Cao_2$) are hemoglobin concentration (HgB) and $O_2$ saturation ($Sao_2$). A hemoglobin molecule can bind up to four molecules of oxygen and has increasing affinity to oxygen as more molecules are added. The relationship between hemoglobin (Hb) and oxygen ($O_2$) is described by the oxyhemoglobin dissociation curve. The increasing affinity explains the steep portion of the oxyhemoglobin dissociation curve at low concentrations. Once the Hb molecules approach full saturation, the curves flatten out and the saturation cannot increase above 100%. In the same way, once the $Pao_2$ drops below 60 mm Hg, a steeper decline in saturation occurs for a given decline in $Pao_2$.

There are several factors that affect the rightward or leftward shift and the shape of the oxyhemoglobin dissociation curve. Factors that shift the curve to the right and represent decreasing

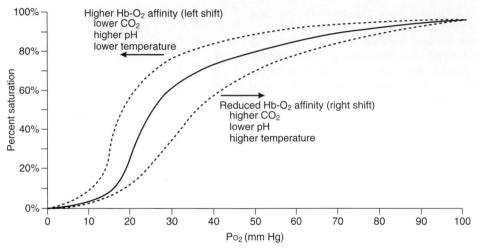

**Fig. 25.2** Oxyhemoglobin dissociation curve. $CO_2$, Carbon dioxide; $Hb$-$O_2$, oxyhemoglobin; $Po_2$, partial pressure of oxygen.

affinity of Hb to oxygen are increasing temperature, $Paco_2$, and 2,3-diphosphoglycerate, in addition to decreasing pH. These are conditions that one might expect to see in metabolically active tissues (Fig. 25.2).

## Other Factors

Several other factors also challenge myocardial oxygen supply and demand. One of the most important is atherosclerosis that serves to increase vascular resistance and decrease $O_2$ delivery. According to Poisseuille's law, long lesions can have a profound effect on effective blood flow, even if they are not critically narrow. Flow is affected by decreases in the arterial radius to the fourth power, so even small decreases can cause significant flow limitation that can impede regional myocardial blood flow significantly. Some exogenous compounds can cause vasodilation that may ease blood flow but may also induce ischemia in the steal-prone coronary anatomy. Heart rate will also have an effect on coronary blood flow as a longer diastolic time allows for the greater duration of perfusion.

## Oxygen Demand

Factors that affect oxygen demand are
1. Contractility
2. Heart rate
3. Wall tension

*Contractility* refers to the amount of oxygen that is consumed as part of contractile force generation. Ninety percent of delivered oxygen is used for contraction, and 10% is utilized for the maintenance of the tissue and the conduction system. *Contractility* or *inotropy* refers to the rapidity or velocity of the development of myocardial wall tension and has also been shown to be an important determinant of oxygen consumption, and $d$P/$d$t can be used to estimate this consumption. Heart rate is also a key component of the oxygen consumption because this determines the rate at which work is being done by the myocardium.

The systolic perfusion index correlates moderately with oxygen demand. It is determined by calculating the area under the systolic pressure versus time curve and multiplying it by the heart rate.

According to LaPlace's law, ventricular wall tension is directly proportional to the pressure in the chamber multiplied by the radius of the chamber and is inversely proportional to the wall thickness:

$$\sigma = (P \times R)/2h$$

where P is pressure, R is radius, and h is thickness of the wall of the presumed spherical object. This explains why volume overload of the ventricle can be detrimental by increasing oxygen supply. It also explains how the compensatory hypertrophy of the ventricle to pressure and volume overload serves as an attempt to lower wall tension.

## Summary

Understanding the underlying physiology is important, and this understanding must be integrated with knowledge of the effects of the individual anesthetic agents on the determinants of oxygen supply and demand. This is of paramount importance for planning an anesthetic in a manner that protects myocardial homeostasis while optimizing performance. It is also very important to remember that some drugs may have multiple effects.

## SUGGESTED READINGS

Ardehali, A., & Ports, T. A. (1990). Myocardial oxygen supply and demand. *Chest, 98,* 699–705.

Collins, J. A., Rudenski, A., Gibson, J., Howard, L., & O'Driscoll, R. (2015). Relating oxygen partial pressure, saturation and content: The haemoglobin-oxygen dissociation curve. *Breathe (Sheff), 11,* 194–201.

Guensch, D. P., Fischer, K., Jung, C., Hurni, S., Winkler, B. M., Jung, B., Vogt, A. P., et al. (2019). Relationship between myocardial oxygenation and blood pressure: Experimental validation using oxygenation-sensitive cardiovascular magnetic resonance. *PLoS One, 14*(1), e0210098.

Heusch, G. (2010). Adenosine and maximum coronary vasodilation in humans: Myth and misconceptions in the assessment of coronary reserve. *Basic Research in Cardiology, 105,* 1–5.

Odonkor, P. N., & Grigore, A. M. (2013). Patients with ischemic heart disease. *Medical Clinics of North America, 97,* 1033–1050.

Tánczos, K., & Molnár, Z. (2013). The oxygen supply-demand balance: A monitoring challenge. *Best Practice and Research. Clinical Anaesthesiology, 27*(2), 201–207.

Weber, K. T., & Janicki, J. S. (1979). The metabolic demand and oxygen supply of the heart: Physiologic and clinical considerations. *American Journal of Cardiology, 44,* 722–729.

Zong, P., Tune, J. D., & Downey, H. F. (2005). Mechanisms of oxygen demand/supply balance in the right ventricle. *Experimental Biology and Medicine, 230,* 507–519.

# 26

# Tachyarrhythmias

SOOJIE YU, MD

A tachyarrhythmia may be classified as either narrow complex tachycardia (NCT) or wide complex tachycardia (WCT), based on the width of the QRS complexes. Prompt recognition based is electrocardiographic interpretation is of clinical importance, as is the underlying arrhythmia (Fig. 26.1).

## Narrow Complex Tachycardia

NCT is defined as a rhythm with a rate greater than 100 beats/min and a QRS complex duration of less than 0.12 msec. This type of rhythm is supraventricular in origin. They can be further classified as atrioventricular (AV) node–passive or AV node–active types, based on whether the AV node is involved in the propagation and maintenance of the arrhythmia. AV node–passive tachycardia has a regular rhythm, as in atrial tachycardia or atrial flutter, or an irregular rhythm, as in multifocal atrial tachycardia, atrial flutter with varying conduction, or atrial fibrillation. With AV node reentry tachycardia (AVNRT) or accessory pathway–dependent tachycardia, the accessory pathway conduction can be orthodromic (with the AV node used as

forward conduction), with a narrow complex, or antidromic (with the accessory pathway used as forward conduction and the AV node itself used for retrograde conduction), with a wide complex.

## Treatment

NCTs can be treated medically or with cardioversion, and the strategy used should be based on the type of NCT and the degree of hemodynamic instability. Treatment of AV node–active tachycardia is typically achieved with maneuvers that prolong AV node conduction, with the goal of arrhythmia termination. These include vagal maneuvers or the administration of drugs such as adenosine (6 then 12 mg). Adenosine should be given in a central or antecubital vein. It is short acting, has a half-life of 12 to 18 seconds, and can cause flushing, bronchospasm, and chest pain.

In patients with hemodynamically stable NCT, a rate-control strategy can be used. The calcium channel blocker diltiazem (0.25 mg/kg) is preferred over β-adrenergic receptor blocking

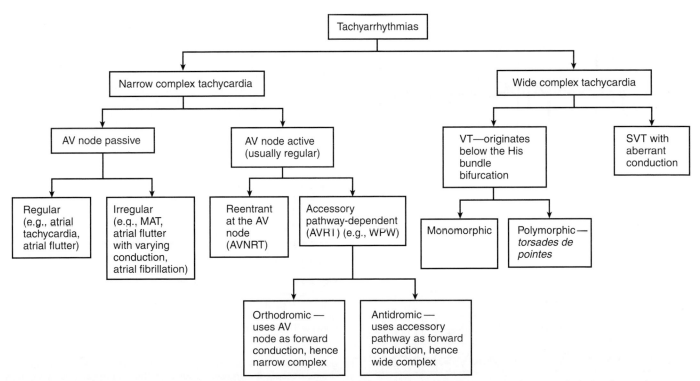

**Fig. 26.1** Classification of tachyarrhythmias into narrow complex and wide complex tachyarrhythmias and subtypes included within each category. *AV*, Atrioventricular; *AVNRT*, atrioventricular nodal reentrant tachycardia; *AVRT*, atrioventricular reentrant tachycardia; *MAT*, multifocal atrial tachycardia; *SVT*, supraventricular tachycardia; *VT*, ventricular tachycardia; *WPW*, Wolff-Parkinson-White syndrome.

agents or verapamil because diltiazem has less negative inotropy. Patients with a low ejection fraction are candidates for amiodarone administered intravenously as a bolus of 150 mg that can be repeated. Procainamide is useful as a second-line agent in this situation.

Although all NCTs can be terminated using synchronized cardioversion, the use of cardioversion should be reserved for patients in whom the arrhythmia is accompanied by hemodynamic instability.

## Wide Complex Tachycardia

WCT is defined as an arrhythmia with a QRS complex duration longer than 0.12 seconds at a rate greater than 100 beats/min. WCT is presumed to be ventricular tachycardia (VT) until proven otherwise, although supraventricular tachycardia (SVT) can present as WCT (SVT with aberrancy). Differentiating between SVT with a wide QRS complex and VT is critical because the treatment is very different (Figs. 26.2 to 26.11).

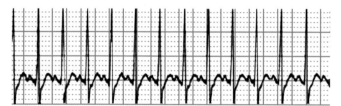

**Fig. 26.2** Atrial tachycardia originating from a single focus in the atrium. The electrocardiogram shows a regular rate of 150 to 250 beats/min. The P-wave morphologic appearance is different from that seen in sinus tachycardia.

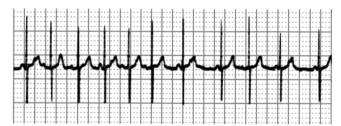

**Fig. 26.3** Multifocal atrial tachycardia (MAT) arising from multiple foci in the atria. The electrocardiogram shows an irregular rate with P waves of different morphologic appearances and varying PR intervals. MAT is not amenable to treatment with digoxin or adenosine.

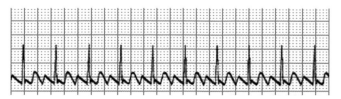

**Fig. 26.4** Atrial flutter originating in the reentry circuit in the atrium. The electrocardiogram shows sawtooth P flutter waves with variable conduction to the ventricles. The atrial rate is 250 to 300 beats/min.

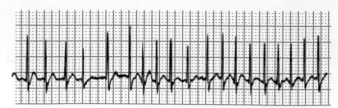

**Fig. 26.5** In atrial fibrillation, heterogeneous electrical remodeling causes multicircuit reentry in the atria, resulting in a lack of organized atrial activity and an irregular heart rhythm. Fibrillation waves can be seen in this example. P waves are absent.

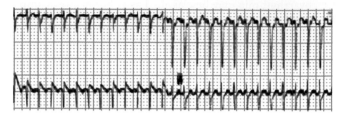

**Fig. 26.6** Atrioventricular (AV) node reentrant tachycardia (AVNRT) arises from an electrical loop involving the AV node and aberrant slower conducting tissue around the AV node. The ventricular rhythm is regular. In this example, the rate is 140 to 200 beats/min. P waves are absent or rarely seen after the QRS complex. AVNRT can be terminated with vagal maneuvers or adenosine.

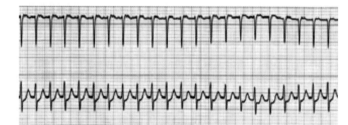

**Fig. 26.7** Atrioventricular (AV) reentrant tachycardia (AVRT), also known as reciprocating tachycardia. If conduction from the atria is through the AV node, this type of AVRT is orthodromic tachycardia (the most common variation, which has a narrow complex). If conduction is through the accessory pathway (AP), this is an antidromic tachycardia, which has a wide complex. The AP is between the atrial and the ventricular myocardium and has a faster conduction but longer refractory period than does the AV node. An example is Wolff-Parkinson-White syndrome, in which the delta wave on the QRS complex is apparent when the heart rate is normal because of conduction through the AP (preexcitation).

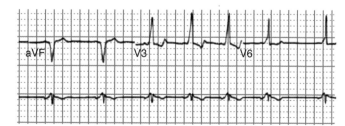

**Fig. 26.8** Wolff-Parkinson-White syndrome. In orthodromic conduction, the electrocardiogram shows narrow QRS complexes with rates of 150 to 200 beats/min and P waves that are not hidden but are present on the ST segment/T wave. Treatment of hemodynamically stable patients with tachycardia is the same as for atrioventricular node reentrant tachycardia. In 1% to 15% of patients, adenosine can cause ventricular fibrillation; thus resuscitation equipment should be readily available. Digoxin should be avoided in patients with Wolff-Parkinson-White syndrome because it increases conduction through the accessory pathway and slows the atrioventricular node. In patients with antidromic wide complex tachycardia, the use of β-adrenergic receptor blocking agents and calcium channel blocking agents should be avoided.

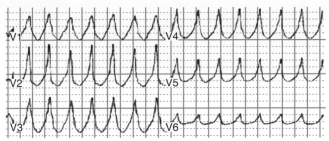

**Fig. 26.9**  Ventricular tachycardia with positive concordance.

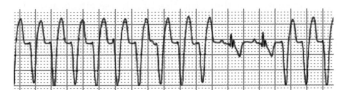

**Fig. 26.10**  Ventricular tachycardia with fusion beats and atrioventricular dissociation.

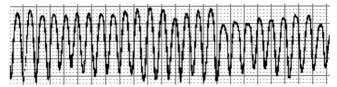

**Fig. 26.11**  Polymorphic ventricular tachycardia.

## DIAGNOSIS

For the purpose of diagnosis, WCT can be classified into four categories based on these characteristics:

1. Origin above or below the bifurcation of the His bundle.
2. Presence of an SVT with aberrant ventricular conduction. SVT with aberrancy can be caused by conduction slowing or bundle branch block. It can also be caused by anterograde conduction over an accessory AV pathway (antidromic Wolff-Parkinson-White [WPW] syndrome).
3. Presence of a wide QRS waveform generated by ventricular pacing.
4. Presence of electrolyte abnormalities, such as hyperkalemia or hypokalemia, or the use of medications, such as tricyclic antidepressants and antihistamines (sodium channel blocking drugs).

WCT associated with drug overdose usually has terminal alterations of the QRS complex with right-axis deviation (RV wave in lead aVR and S waves in leads I and aVL). The diagnosis can be made by reviewing the patient's history and electrocardiogram. VT is more likely to occur in patients with coronary artery disease and signs of AV dissociation (cannon A waves). Hemodynamic stability does not rule out a diagnosis of VT.

A diagnosis of VT is likely when, on the 12-lead electrocardiogram, the QRS complex duration is longer than 160 msec, all of the QRS complexes in the precordial leads are positive or negative (positive or negative concordance), fusion beats or capture beats are seen, and AV dissociation is present. Polymorphic VT has beat-to-beat variations in morphologic appearance as a cyclic progressive change in the cardiac axis. Polymorphic VT occurring in the setting of a prolonged QT interval is called *torsades de pointes*. VT that occurs with hyperkalemia is sinusoidal, is preceded by tall T waves, has short QT intervals, has prolonged PR intervals, and has flattened P waves. With tricyclic antidepressant toxicity, VT is characterized by a right-axis pattern with prominent S waves in leads I and aVL and an R wave in lead aVR.

## TREATMENT

Regardless of the cause of WCT, electrical defibrillation with 100 to 200 J (monophasic) or 50 to 100 J (biphasic) is the treatment of choice in patients who are hemodynamically unstable.

The use of β-adrenergic receptor blocking agents, digitalis, and calcium channel blocking agents is recommended for patients with WCT that is believed to be the result of SVT with aberrancy, but this treatment is contraindicated in patients with WPW syndrome. Procainamide and amiodarone are acceptable alternative choices because they are used to treat WCT caused by VT or SVT. Electrical cardioversion should be performed if the WCT does not respond to antiarrhythmic agents or if the patient is hemodynamically unstable. Torsades de pointes is treated with intravenously administered magnesium; the temporary use of transvenous overdrive pacing should be considered for patients with a heart rate of 100 beats/min or greater who do not respond to magnesium. Isoproterenol (1–4 μg/min in adults) can be infused with the same heart rate goal (≤100 beats/min) until pacing can be established.

Toxicity of sodium channel blocking agents, such as tricyclic antidepressants and antihistamines, should be treated with induction of alkalosis and diuresis. The administration of sodium bicarbonate infusions should be considered when the patient has persistent hypotension and arrhythmias. Hyperkalemia is treated with calcium, glucose-insulin infusions, β agonists, and sodium bicarbonate.

## SUGGESTED READINGS

Abualsuod, A. M., & Miller, J. M. (2022). Removing the complexity from wide complex tachycardia. *Trends in Cardiovascular Medicine, 32*(4), 221–225. doi:10.1016/j.tcm.2021.04.001.

Drew, B. J., Ackerman, M. J., Funk, M., Gibler, W. B., Kligfield, P., Menon, V., et al. (2010). Prevention of torsades de pointes in hospital settings: A scientific statement from the American Heart Association and the American College of Cardiology Foundation. *Circulation, 121,* 1047–1060.

Katritsis, D. G., & Josephson, M. E. (2015). Differential diagnosis of regular, narrow-QRS tachycardias. *Heart Rhythm, 12*(7), 1667–1676.

Poptani, V., Jayaram, A. A., Jain, S., & Samanth, J. (2021). A study of narrow QRS tachycardia with emphasis on the clinical features, ECG, electrophysiology/radiofrequency ablation. *Future Cardiology, 17*(1), 137–148. doi:10.2217/fca-2020-0078.

Vereckei, A. (2014). Current algorithms for the diagnosis of wide QRS complex tachycardias. *Current Cardiology Reviews, 10,* 262–276.

# 27 Bradyarrhythmias

SOOJIE YU, MD

Bradycardia is a common perioperative finding, and this chapter discusses when this arrhythmia requires treatment and the interventions currently available. The classic definition of *normal resting heart rate* is 60 to 100 beats/min. The National Institutes of Health defines bradycardia as a heart rate of fewer than 60 beats/min in adults with the exception of well-trained athletes, but population studies commonly use fewer than 50 beats/min as the lower cutoff. Bradycardia becomes problematic when the heart rate results in a decrease in cardiac output that is inadequate for a specific clinical situation. Bradyarrhythmias can be caused by pathology within the sinus node, atrioventricular (AV) nodal tissue, and the His-Purkinje conduction system.

Regardless of the presentation, bradycardia should be treated immediately in patients with hypotension or signs of hypoperfusion (e.g., acute altered mental status, seizures, syncope, ischemic chest pain, congestive heart failure). The goal of initial therapy is to administer a chronotropic drug, such as atropine, glycopyrrolate, epinephrine, or isoproterenol. Isoproterenol, a pure β-sympathomimetic agent, increases myocardial oxygen demand and produces peripheral vasodilation, both of which are poorly tolerated in patients with acute myocardial ischemia. Glucagon can be used to treat patients with symptomatic bradycardia related to an overdose of β-receptor antagonist by stimulating cyclic adenosine monophosphate synthesis independent of the β-adrenergic receptor or calcium channel blocking agents (Table 27.1). Patients with bradycardia who are unresponsive to acute medical therapy are candidates for treatment with external or transvenous pacing if hypotension or hypoperfusion persists. Pacing devices provide controlled heart rate management without the risk of adverse effects associated with medications. Temporary pacing can be transcutaneous, transesophageal, or transvenous and has its own risks including decreased patient tolerance, venous thrombosis, unstable arrythmias, and perforation.

## Heart Block or Atrioventricular Dysfunction

AV block can be classified by the site of the block into AV nodal, intra-Hisian (above the His bundle), and infra-Hisian (below the His bundle). Patients with bradyarrhythmias (including second or third degree) originating from the AV nodal level have faster and more reliable escape mechanisms (Fig. 27.1) and will generally respond to treatment with atropine and catecholamines. Patients with bradycardia due to excess vagal tone will also respond to treatment with atropine. However, in patients with Mobitz II second-degree AV block (Fig. 27.2) or new-onset wide QRS complex complete heart block (Fig. 27.3), the heart block is usually infranodal, and increased vagal tone is not a significant cause of the bradycardia. These rhythms are less likely to respond to treatment with atropine, therefore cardiac pacing is the treatment of choice.

Patients with Mobitz II second-degree AV block, even if asymptomatic, can progress without warning to complete heart block with a slow and unstable idioventricular rhythm. External pacing electrode pads or transvenous pacing electrodes should be placed prophylactically in this group of patients. Transcutaneous pacing is noninvasive but can be painful and may not produce effective mechanical capture. Transvenous (endocardial) pacing is accomplished by passing a pacing electrode into the right ventricle directly through a central vein catheter or through a pacing pulmonary artery catheter (if the catheter is already in place). The 2005 American Heart Association algorithm for bradycardia (Fig. 27.4) provides a convenient framework for managing patients with bradycardia. The recent 2020 update in the algorithm recommends starting dopamine at 5 mcg/kg/min instead of 2 mcg/kg/min.

## Intraoperative Bradycardia

Intraoperative bradycardia occurs commonly and can be hemodynamically significant, particularly in patients with preexisting heart disease. It is associated with hypotension (defined as a decrease in mean arterial pressure [MAP] of >40% from baseline or a MAP of <60 mm Hg) in approximately 60% of cases. Factors associated with bradycardia under anesthesia include (1) age (bradycardia is more prevalent with increasing age older than 50 years); (2) sex (male/female ratio of 60:40); (3) vagal stimulation (e.g., certain surgical procedures and

| TABLE 27.1 | Intravenously Administered Pharmacologic Treatment of Bradycardia |
|---|---|
| **Medication** | **Dose** |
| Atropine[a] | 0.5 mg q 3–5 min to a maximum total dose of 3 mg<br>Doses of atropine sulfate of <0.5 mg may paradoxically result in further slowing of the heart rate. |
| Dopamine | Initial: 5 $\mu g \cdot kg^{-1} \cdot min^{-1}$<br>Titrate to response |
| Epinephrine | Initial: 2–10 $\mu g/min$<br>Titrate to response |
| Isoproterenol | Initial: 2–10 $\mu g/min$<br>Titrate to response |
| Glucagon | Initial: 3 mg<br>Infusion: 3 mg/h, if necessary |

[a]Atropine administration should not delay implementation of external pacing for patients with poor perfusion.

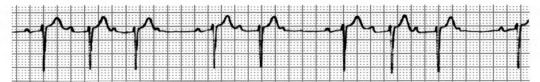

**Fig. 27.1** Second-degree atrioventricular block—Mobitz type I block.

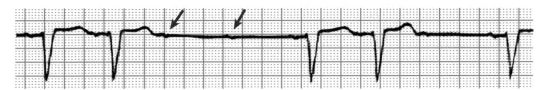

**Fig. 27.2** Second-degree atrioventricular block—Mobitz type II block. *Arrows,* P-waves.

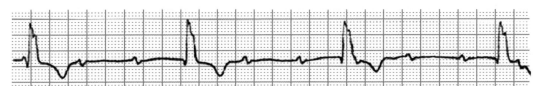

**Fig. 27.3** Complete (third-degree) atrioventricular block.

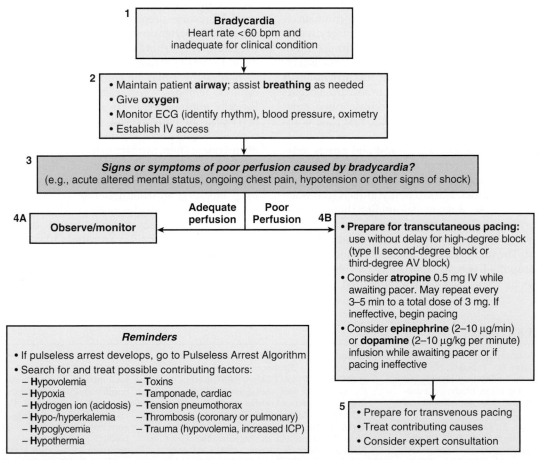

**1**
**Bradycardia**
Heart rate <60 bpm and
inadequate for clinical condition

**2**
- Maintain patient **airway**; assist **breathing** as needed
- Give **oxygen**
- Monitor ECG (identify rhythm), blood pressure, oximetry
- Establish IV access

**3**
***Signs or symptoms of poor perfusion caused by bradycardia?***
(e.g., acute altered mental status, ongoing chest pain, hypotension or other signs of shock)

Adequate perfusion | Poor Perfusion

**4A**
Observe/monitor

**4B**
- **Prepare for transcutaneous pacing:** use without delay for high-degree block (type II second-degree block or third-degree AV block)
- Consider **atropine** 0.5 mg IV while awaiting pacer. May repeat every 3–5 min to a total dose of 3 mg. If ineffective, begin pacing
- Consider **epinephrine** (2–10 µg/min) or **dopamine** (2–10 µg/kg per minute) infusion while awaiting pacer or if pacing ineffective

***Reminders***
- If pulseless arrest develops, go to Pulseless Arrest Algorithm
- Search for and treat possible contributing factors:
  - **H**ypovolemia
  - **H**ypoxia
  - **H**ydrogen ion (acidosis)
  - **H**ypo-/hyperkalemia
  - **H**ypoglycemia
  - **H**ypothermia
  - **T**oxins
  - **T**amponade, cardiac
  - **T**ension pneumothorax
  - **T**hrombosis (coronary or pulmonary)
  - **T**rauma (hypovolemia, increased ICP)

**5**
- Prepare for transvenous pacing
- Treat contributing causes
- Consider expert consultation

**Fig. 27.4** The American Heart Association algorithm for the treatment of bradycardia. Management of symptomatic bradycardia and tachycardia. *AV,* Atrioventricular; *bpm,* beats/min; *ECG,* electrocardiogram; *ICP,* intracranial pressure; *IV,* intravenous. (From 2005 American Heart Association Guidelines for Cardiopulmonary Resuscitation and Emergency Cardiovascular Care. Part 7.3: Management of Symptomatic Bradycardia and Tachycardia. *Circulation.* 2005;112:IV-67–77. Reprinted with permission of the American Heart Association.)

laparoscopic inflation of the peritoneum); (4) opioid administration; (5) administration of high doses of inhalation anesthetic agents (particularly during inhalation induction); and (6) administration of high doses of propofol.

Preoperative assessment using the 5-point multivariate "HEART" score: preoperative heart rate less than 60 beats/min or hypotension (<110/60 mm Hg), age older than 65 years, preoperative use of angiotensin-converting enzyme inhibitors/angiotensin receptor blockers or β-blockers, revised cardiac risk index greater than 3 points, and type of surgery (major surgery) can help predict increased risk of intraoperative hypotension or bradycardia.

When symptomatic bradycardia occurs, it is important to consider hypoxemia especially in infants as a cause very early in the evaluation because of its critical nature.

## IATROGENIC CAUSES OF BRADYCARDIA

Opiates, such as fentanyl and morphine, have a direct action on the sinus node in addition to central nervous system effects that result in bradycardia. Inhaled anesthetic gases (i.e., isoflurane) directly depress sinus node activity by altering the slope of phase IV depolarization, an effect that is likely related to calcium flux across the cell membrane.

Nondepolarizing neuromuscular blocking agents (NMBAs), such as vecuronium and rocuronium, lack the vagolytic effects associated with pancuronium. Succinylcholine, a depolarizing NMBA, causes bradycardia through three possible mechanisms: (1) release of choline molecules from the breakdown of succinylcholine, (2) direct stimulation of peripheral sensory receptors producing reflex bradycardia, and (3) direct stimulation of the sympathetic and parasympathetic nervous systems. Bradycardia may be observed after the first dose of succinylcholine is administered in children; however, in adults bradycardia occurs more commonly after the second dose of succinylcholine, especially if it is given 5 minutes or more after the first dose is administered.

Dexmedetomidine is a potent α-2 agonist and causes sedation through its activation of central pre- and postsynaptic α-2 receptors on the locus coeruleus. A side effect of activating α receptors is reflex bradycardia. Marked bradycardia is seen when administering a bolus dose of dexmedetomidine thought to be caused by the baroreceptor reflex from α receptor activation of vascular smooth muscles causing peripheral vasoconstriction and hypertension. The incidence of bradycardia associated with the infusion of propofol has been reported as 5% (observations from case series) to 25% (data from randomized controlled trials). Children who undergo strabismus operations and who receive propofol seem to be particularly susceptible to the activation of the ocular cardiac reflex. Bradycardia has been reported to occur in 6% to 16% of these patients, even if they are prophylactically treated with an anticholinergic drug.

## OTHER CAUSES OF BRADYCARDIA

Other causes of intraoperative bradycardia include vagal stimulation from manipulation of the oropharynx during laryngoscopy, intubation, or extubation. Insufflation for laparoscopy or thoracoscopy and surgical handling of the extraocular muscles, bronchi, peritoneum, scrotum, and rectum can give rise to autonomic reflexes that include bronchospasm, bradycardia or tachycardia, hypotension or hypertension, and cardiac arrhythmias, especially in lightly anesthetized patients or those with hypoxia or hypercapnia. The manifestations of vagal stimulation can be prevented or minimized by treatment with atropine, glycopyrrolate, topical anesthesia, intravenously administered local anesthetic agents, adrenergic blocking agents, deeper anesthesia, and vasoactive agents.

Hypothermia is known to cause bradycardia. However, the initial response to hypothermia is a transient increase in heart rate as a result of sympathetic stimulation. As temperature decreases below 34°C, the heart rate decreases proportionally. The resulting bradycardia is believed to result from the direct effect of hypothermia on the sinoatrial node. This bradycardia is not responsive to vagolytic maneuvers. Elevated intracranial pressure presenting alone—or as part of a triad of systemic hypertension, sinus bradycardia, and respiratory irregularities (Cushing syndrome)—is also a cause of bradycardia in the perioperative period.

Bradyarrhythmias are common during cardiac surgery procedures. Temporary epicardial pacing will maintain a physiologically appropriate heart rate in most patients. A smaller percentage of patients will require a permanent pacemaker, typically because of sinus node dysfunction or AV conduction disturbances after coronary artery bypass graft or valve surgery.

Bradycardia is not uncommon in the postoperative setting. The etiology is often iatrogenic; specifically, it may be caused by β-blockers, anticholinesterase reversal of neuromuscular blockade, opioids, or dexmedetomidine. Other procedure- or patient-related causes include bowel distention, increased intracranial or intraocular pressure, and spinal anesthesia. Specifically, a superiorly placed block that disrupts the cardioaccelerator fibers originating from T1 through T4 can produce severe bradycardia secondary to sympathectomy.

## SUGGESTED READINGS

Chatzimichali, A., Zoumprouli, A., Metaxari, M., Apostolakis, I., Daras, T., Tzanakis, N., et al. (2011). Heart rate variability may identify patients who will develop severe bradycardia during spinal anaesthesia. *Acta Anaesthesiologica Scandinavica*, 55, 234–241.

Cheung, C. C., Martyn, A., Campbell, N., Frost, S., Gilbert, K., Michota, F., et al. (2015). Predictors of intraoperative hypotension and bradycardia. *American Journal of Medicine*, 128(5), 532–538.

Kusumoto, F. M., Schoenfeld, M. H., Barrett, C., Edgerton, J. R., Ellenbogen, K. A., Gold, M. R., et al. (2019). 2018 ACC/AHA/HRS Guideline on the evaluation and management of patients with bradycardia and cardiac conduction delay: A Report of the American College of Cardiology/American Heart Association Task Force on Clinical Practice Guidelines and the Heart Rhythm Society. *Circulation*, 140(8), e382–e482.

Maruyama, K., Nishikawa, Y., Nakagawa, H., Ariyama, J., Kitamura, A., & Hayashida, M. (2010). Can intravenous atropine prevent bradycardia and hypotension during induction of total intravenous anesthesia with propofol and remifentanil? *Journal of Anesthesia*, 24, 293–296.

Solomon, S. C., Saxena, R. C., Neradilek, M. B., Hau, V., Fong, C. T., Lang, J. D., et al. (2020). Forecasting a crisis: Machine-learning models predicting occurrence of intraoperative bradycardia associated with hypotension. *Anesthesia & Analgesia*, 130(5), 1201–1210.

# The Autonomic Nervous System

JAMES D. HANNON, MD

The autonomic nervous system (ANS) may also be referred to as the visceral, vegetative, or involuntary nervous system. This self-controlling (autonomous) system comprises nerves, ganglia, and plexuses that innervate the heart, blood vessels, endocrine glands, visceral organs, and smooth muscle. The ANS is widely distributed throughout the body and regulates functions that occur without conscious control. However, it does not function in a completely independent fashion; rather, it responds to somatic motor and sensory input.

The ANS is typically divided functionally into the sympathetic nervous system (SNS) and the parasympathetic nervous system (PNS). A third division, the enteric nervous system (ENS), has been added in light of the complexity of the innervation of the gastrointestinal (GI) tract and because the GI tract is capable of functioning in isolation. Most visceral organs are innervated by both the SNS and the PNS, and the moment-to-moment level of activity of an individual organ represents the integration of the influences of the two systems. In addition, the actions of drugs that affect the myocardium, smooth muscle, and glandular tissue can be interpreted and classified according to their ability to modify or mimic the actions of neurotransmitters released by the ANS.

In terms of pathophysiology, the ANS is increasingly thought to contribute to the early stages of cancer development, invasion, and metastasis. In addition, overactivation of the SNS likely plays a significant role in the etiology of hypertension and has also been linked to several comorbidities commonly associated with hypertension, such as metabolic syndrome, diabetes mellitus, dyslipidemia, and sleep apnea syndrome.

## Anatomy

### SYMPATHETIC NERVOUS SYSTEM

Although the SNS is always active, an increase in its level of activity occurs in response to stresses that threaten normal homeostasis, such as intense physical activity, psychological stress, blood loss, and disease processes. Activation of the SNS dilates the pupils, decreases blood flow to the GI tract, increases cardiac output, and diverts blood flow to the skeletal muscles (fight-or-flight response).

The physical arrangement of the main parts of the peripheral ANS, including the SNS, is illustrated in Fig. 28.1. The SNS is widely distributed throughout the body. The cell bodies that give rise to the preganglionic fibers of the SNS lie in the intermediolateral columns of the thoracolumbar spinal cord from T1 to L2. Therefore the SNS system is sometimes referred to as the *thoracolumbar nervous system*. The axons of these cells are located in the anterior nerve roots, and they synapse with neurons lying in sympathetic ganglia found in three locations: paravertebral, prevertebral, and terminal. Preganglionic fibers may synapse

with multiple postganglionic fibers at ganglia higher or lower than the level of their origin from the spinal cord, resulting in diffusion and amplification of the response. The 22 pairs of paravertebral ganglia lie on either side of the vertebral column and include the superior cervical, inferior cervical, and stellate ganglia. The unpaired prevertebral ganglia lie in the abdomen or pelvis near the ventral surface of the vertebral column (celiac, superior mesenteric, and inferior mesenteric). The terminal ganglia are located near the innervated organs (adrenal medulla). The cells of the medulla are embryologically and anatomically analogous to sympathetic ganglia.

### PARASYMPATHETIC NERVOUS SYSTEM

The PNS is active during times of rest, causing the pupils to constrict, blood flow to the digestive tract to increase, and restorative processes that result in the conservation or accumulation of energy stores to predominate. The distribution of the PNS to effector organs is more limited than that of the SNS. Preganglionic fibers typically travel a greater distance than do those of the SNS, to the PNS ganglia proximal to innervated organs, and postganglionic cell bodies are located near or within innervated organs. In addition, the PNS has fewer postganglionic nerves for each preganglionic fiber and is able to produce discrete limited effects, in contrast with the diffuse mass effects characterizing SNS activation.

The preganglionic fibers of the PNS originate in the midbrain, the medulla (cranial), and the sacral part of the spinal cord. Therefore the PNS is also referred to as the *craniosacral nervous system*. Cranial parasympathetic fibers innervate the ciliary, sphenopalatine, sublingual, submaxillary, and otic ganglia. The vagus nerve (X) contains preganglionic fibers that do not synapse until they reach the many small ganglia that lie in or on the organs of the thorax and abdomen. These include the heart, lungs, stomach, intestines, liver, gallbladder, pancreas, and ureters. Indeed, 75% of the activity within the PNS is mediated through the vagus nerve. Other cranial nerves (oculomotor [III], facial [VII], and glossopharyngeal [IX]) and the second, third, and fourth sacral nerves conduct the balance of PNS efferent functions. Parasympathetic sacral outflow fibers form the pelvic nerves. These nerves synapse in ganglia near or within the bladder, rectum, and sex organs.

### ENTERIC NERVOUS SYSTEM

The ENS was originally considered a part of the PNS, and the nerves in its walls were believed to be postganglionic parasympathetic fibers. It is now known that the digestive tract contains about the same number of nerve fibers as the spinal cord and that it is capable of functioning independently of the SNS and PNS, although input from these systems is important for communication with the central nervous system.

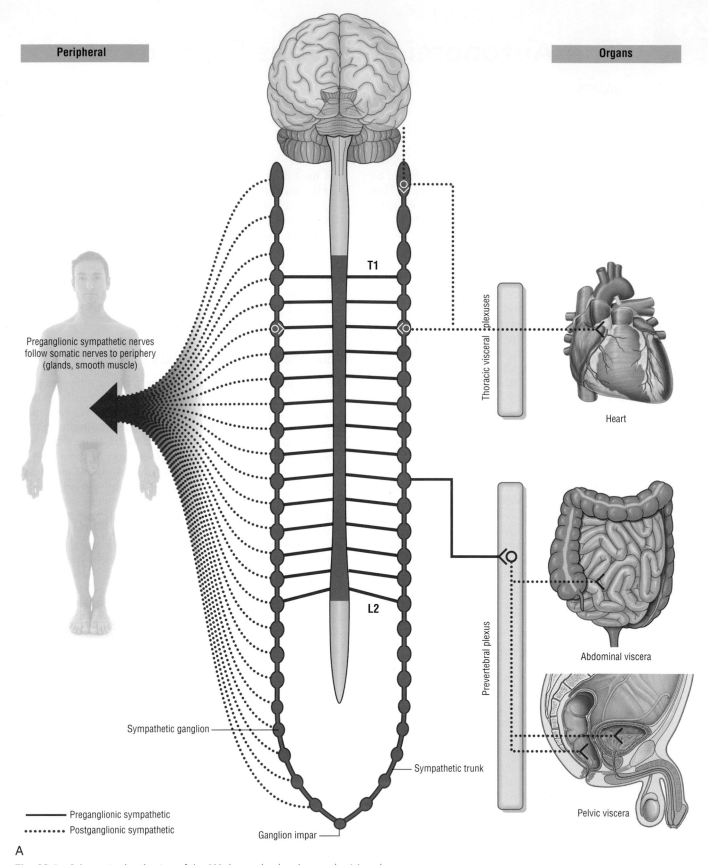

Preganglionic sympathetic nerves
follow somatic nerves to periphery
(glands, smooth muscle)

T1

L2

Thoracic visceral plexuses

Prevertebral plexus

Heart

Abdominal viscera

Pelvic viscera

Sympathetic ganglion

Sympathetic trunk

Ganglion impar

—————— Preganglionic sympathetic

·········· Postganglionic sympathetic

A

**Fig. 28.1** Schematic distribution of the **(A)** thoracolumbar (sympathetic) and

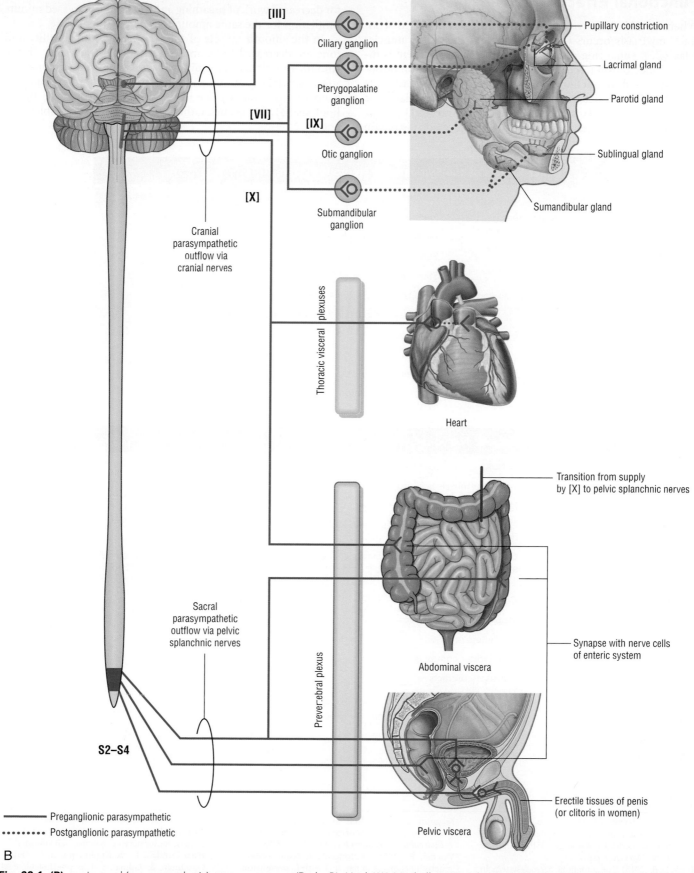

Pupillary constriction

Lacrimal gland

Parotid gland

Sublingual gland

Sumandibular gland

[III]

Ciliary ganglion

Pterygopalatine ganglion

[VII]

[IX]

Otic ganglion

[X]

Submandibular ganglion

Cranial parasympathetic outflow via cranial nerves

Thoracic visceral plexuses

Heart

Transition from supply by [X] to pelvic splanchnic nerves

Synapse with nerve cells of enteric system

Sacral parasympathetic outflow via pelvic splanchnic nerves

Prevertebral plexus

Abdominal viscera

S2–S4

Erectile tissues of penis (or clitoris in women)

Pelvic viscera

——— Preganglionic parasympathetic

········· Postganglionic parasympathetic

B

**Fig. 28.1  (B)** craniosacral (parasympathetic) nervous systems. (Drake RL, Vogl AW, Mitchell AWM, eds. The body. In: *Gray's Atlas of Anatomy.* 3rd ed. Elsevier; 2021.)

## Functional Effects

When the SNS is activated, the radial muscles of the iris contract, mydriasis occurs ($\alpha$1 receptor), and the ciliary muscles relax ($\beta$2), enhancing distant vision. In the heart, there is increased inotropism ($\beta$1), chronotropism ($\beta$1), and dromotropism (increased conduction velocity; $\beta$1). The SNS can vasodilate ($\beta$1) or vasoconstrict ($\alpha$1) the coronary arteries. Similarly, the SNS can cause vascular smooth muscles to contract ($\alpha$1) or relax ($\beta$2). In the kidney, renin is secreted ($\beta$1) and vasoconstriction occurs ($\alpha$1, $\alpha$2). Bronchial smooth muscles relax ($\beta$2), allowing for decreased work of breathing and, therefore, increased minute ventilation for the same amount of energy expenditure.

In the smooth muscle of the GI system, both motility and tone are decreased ($\alpha$2), and sphincters contract ($\alpha$1). In the smooth muscle of the genitourinary system, the trigone and sphincter ($\alpha$1) contract, and the detrusor ($\beta$2) relaxes. Glycogenolysis ($\alpha$1) takes place in the liver, and in adipose tissue, lipolysis ($\beta$1, $\beta$3) occurs. Other actions are listed in Tables 28.1 and 28.2.

**TABLE 28.1 — Other Effects of the Sympathetic Nervous System**

| Target | Action | Receptor |
|---|---|---|
| Endocrine pancreas | Inhibits production of insulin | $\alpha_2$ |
| | Inhibits release of glucagon | $\alpha_2$ |
| | Stimulates production of insulin | $\beta_2$ |
| | Stimulates release of glucagon | $\beta_2$ |
| Adrenergic nerve endings | Inhibits release of transmitters | $\alpha_2$ |
| Salivary glands | Stimulates production of thick viscous secretions | $\alpha_1$ |
| Uterus, pregnant | Contracts | $\alpha_1$ |
| | Relaxes | $\beta_2$ |
| Uterus, nonpregnant | Relaxes | $\beta_2$ |
| Sex organs, male | Promotes ejaculation | $\alpha_1$ |

**TABLE 28.2 — Actions of the Parasympathetic Nervous System**

| Target | Action | Receptor |
|---|---|---|
| Eyes | Sphincter muscles of iris contract | M2, M3 |
| | Miosis occurs | M2, M3 |
| Heart | Chronotropism, dromotropism, and inotropism decrease | M2 >> M3 |
| Vascular smooth muscle | Cerebral, pulmonary, skeletal muscle, and skin arterioles dilate | Vessels dilate because of nitric oxide production in response to muscarinic stimulation, but there is no parasympathetic nervous system innervation. |
| Bronchial smooth muscle | Contracts | M2, M3 |
| Gastrointestinal smooth muscle | Motility and tone increase | M2, M3 |
| | Sphincters relax | M3, M2 |
| | Gallbladder contracts | |
| Genitourinary smooth muscle | Detrusor contracts | M3 > M2 |
| | Trigone and sphincter relax | M3 > M2 |
| Endocrine pancreas | Insulin and glucagon secretions increase | M3, M2 |
| Salivary glands | Produce profuse watery secretions | M3, M2 |
| Sex organs, male | Penile erection | M3 |

## SUGGESTED READINGS

Barrett, K. E., Barman, S. M., Boitano, S., & Brooks (2016). Autonomic nervous system. Ganong's review of medical physiology (25th ed.). New York, NY: McGraw-Hill.

Glick, D. B. (2015). The autonomic nervous system. In R. D. Miller, L. I. Eriksson, L. A. Fleisher, J. P. Wiener-Kronish, & W. L. Young (Eds.), Miller's anesthesia (8th ed., pp. 346–386). Philadelphia: Elsevier.

Magnon, C. (2015). Role of the autonomic nervous system in tumorigenesis and metastasis. Molecular & Cellular Oncology, 2(2), e975643.

Valensi, P. (2021). Autonomic nervous system activity changes in patients with hypertension and overweight: Role and therapeutic implications. Cardiovascular Diabetology, 20(1), 170.

Westfall, T. C., Macarthur, H., & Westfall, D. P. (2017). Neurotransmission: The autonomic and somatic motor nervous systems. In Brunton, L. L., Hilal-Dandan, R., & Knollmann, B. C. (Eds.), Goodman & Gilman's: The pharmacological basis of therapeutics (13th ed.). New York, NY: McGraw Hill.

# The Sympathetic Nervous System: Anatomy and Receptor Pharmacology

JAMES D. HANNON, MD

## Anatomy

The sympathetic nervous system (SNS) is widely distributed throughout the body. Although afferent pathways are important in relaying visceral sensory information to the central nervous system, the most clearly defined elements of the SNS are the efferent preganglionic and postganglionic fibers and their associated paravertebral ganglia. The cell bodies that give rise to the preganglionic fibers of the SNS lie in the intermediolateral columns of the thoracolumbar spinal cord from T1 to L2 or L3, and the SNS is sometimes referred to as the thoracolumbar nervous system.

The short myelinated preganglionic fibers leave the spinal cord in the anterior nerve roots, form white rami, and synapse in sympathetic ganglia lying in three locations outside the cerebrospinal axis. The gray rami arise from the ganglia and carry postganglionic fibers back to the spinal nerves for distribution to the sweat glands, pilomotor muscles, and blood vessels of the skin and skeletal muscle (Fig. 29.1). The 22 sets of paravertebral ganglia are paired on either side of the vertebral column, connected to the spinal nerves by the white and gray rami communicans, and interconnected by nerve trunks to form the lateral chains. They include the upper and middle cervical ganglia;

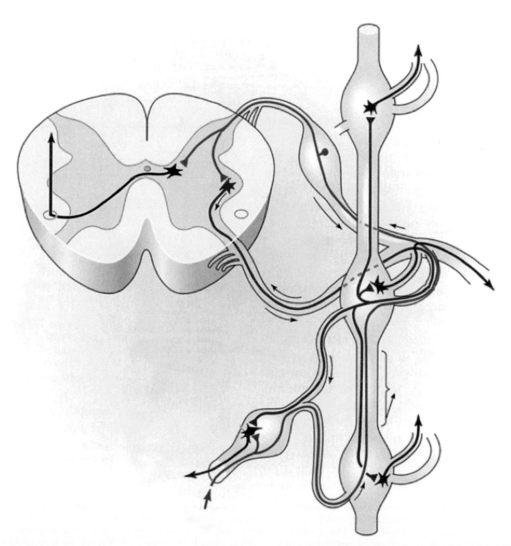

**Fig. 29.1** Anatomy of the preganglionic and postganglionic sympathetic nerve fibers and synapses. (Reprinted, with permission, from Boron WF, Boulpaep EL. *Medical Physiology*. Elsevier; 2005.)

the stellate ganglia (fusion of the inferior cervical and T1 ganglia); and the ganglia of the thoracic, abdominal, and pelvic sympathetic trunks. Unpaired prevertebral ganglia are located in the abdomen and pelvis near the ventral surface of the vertebral column. They are named according to the major branches of the aorta: for example, celiac, renal, and superior and inferior mesenteric ganglia. The terminal ganglia lie near the innervated organs (cervical ganglia in the neck, rectum, and bladder).

The cells of the adrenal medulla are analogous to sympathetic ganglia, except that the postganglionic cells have lost their axons and secrete norepinephrine, epinephrine, and dopamine directly into the bloodstream. Preganglionic fibers may pass through several paravertebral ganglia and synapse with multiple neurons in a ganglion, a characteristic that leads to a diffused output. Postganglionic fibers arising from the sympathetic ganglia may receive input from several preganglionic fibers and innervate visceral structures in the head, neck, thorax, and abdomen. They may pass to target organs through a nerve network along blood vessels or rejoin a mixed peripheral nerve.

## Receptor Pharmacology

### NEUROTRANSMITTERS

Acetylcholine is the neurotransmitter of all preganglionic sympathetic fibers, including those that innervate the cells of

the adrenal medulla. Norepinephrine is released by nearly all sympathetic postganglionic nerve endings; exceptions are the postganglionic cholinergic fibers that innervate sweat glands (sudomotor) and blood vessels in skeletal muscles (vasomotor). Increasing evidence indicates that neurons in the peripheral nervous system release two or more transmitters from individual nerve terminals when stimulated. Substances released with norepinephrine, such as adenosine triphosphate and neuropeptide Y, may function as cotransmitters or neuromodulators of the response to norepinephrine.

### SYNTHESIS, STORAGE, RELEASE, AND INACTIVATION OF NOREPINEPHRINE

The main site of norepinephrine synthesis is the postganglionic nerve terminal. Tyrosine is transported actively into the axoplasm and converted to dihydroxyphenylalanine (rate-limiting step) and then to dopamine by cytoplasmic enzymes. Dopamine is transported into storage vesicles, where it is converted to norepinephrine (Fig. 29.2). Exocytosis of norepinephrine is triggered by the increased intracellular calcium that accompanies an action potential. Active reuptake (uptake 1) of norepinephrine into the presynaptic terminal terminates the effect of norepinephrine at the effector site. This process accounts for nearly all of the released norepinephrine, which is then stored in the vesicles for reuse. Monoamine oxidase is responsible for

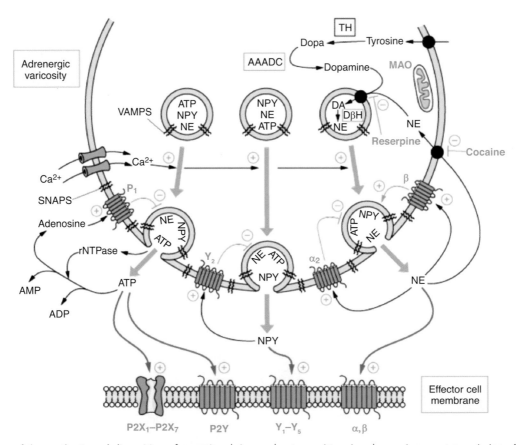

**Fig. 29.2** Diagram of the synthesis and disposition of norepinephrine and cotransmitters in adrenergic neurotransmission. *AAADC,* Aromatic l-amino acid decarboxylase; *ADP,* adenosine diphosphate; *AMP,* adenosine monophosphate; *ATP,* adenosine triphosphate; *DA,* dopamine; *DβH,* dopamine β-hydroxylase; *Dopa,* dihydroxyphenylalanine; *MAO,* monoamine oxidase; *NE,* norepinephrine; *NPY,* neuropeptide Y; *rNTPase,* RNA nucleoside triphosphatase; *SNAPS,* synaptosomal nerve-associated proteins; *TH,* tyrosine hydroxylase; *VAMPs,* vesicle-associated membrane proteins. (Reprinted, with permission, from Westfall TC, Westfall DP. Adrenergic agonists and antagonists. In: Brunton LL, Lazo JS, Parker KL, eds. *Goodman & Gilman's The Pharmacological Basis of Therapeutics.* 11th ed. McGraw-Hill; 2006.)

metabolism of the small amount of norepinephrine that enters the cytoplasm after neuronal reuptake without being taken up into vesicles. Monoamine oxidase and catechol-*O*-methyltransferase are responsible for metabolism of the norepinephrine that is not reabsorbed into neurons.

## RECEPTOR SUBTYPES

Acetylcholine activates nicotinic cholinergic receptors in the sympathetic ganglia and adrenal medulla. The primary sympathetic postganglionic neurotransmitter is norepinephrine. Epinephrine, the circulating hormone released by the adrenal medulla, and dopamine, the neurotransmitter of the less well-characterized dopaminergic system, are the other naturally occurring catecholamines that interact with peripheral adrenergic receptors. The adrenergic receptors were initially classified as $\alpha$ and $\beta$ according to their responsiveness to norepinephrine and epinephrine. Subsequent discovery of more selective agonists and antagonists allowed the $\alpha$ receptors to be subdivided into $\alpha_{1A}$, $\alpha_{1B}$, and $\alpha_{1D}$, and $\alpha_2$ and the $\beta$ receptors into $\beta_1$, $\beta_2$, and $\beta_3$. Peripheral dopamine receptors also have been discovered; these are classified as $D_1$-like ($D_1$ and $D_5$) or $D_2$-like ($D_2$, $D_3$, $D_4$). The $\alpha_1$-receptors are found in the smooth muscle of blood vessels (contraction), the genitourinary system (contraction), and the intestine (relaxation) as well as in the liver (glycogenolysis, gluconeogenesis) and heart (increased contractile force, arrhythmias). The $\alpha_2$-receptors are located in the pancreatic $\beta$ cells (decreased insulin secretion), platelets (aggregation), nerve terminals (decreased norepinephrine release), and vascular smooth muscle (contraction). The $\beta_1$-receptors are found in the heart (increased force and rate of contraction and atrioventricular node conduction) and juxtaglomerular cells (increased renin secretion). The $\beta_2$-receptors are found in the smooth muscle of the vascular, bronchial, gastrointestinal, and genitourinary systems (relaxation) as well as in skeletal muscle (glycogenolysis, uptake of potassium) and the liver (glycogenolysis, gluconeogenesis). The $\beta_3$-receptors are found in adipose tissue (lipolysis).

## RECEPTOR STIMULATION

The adrenergic receptors are coupled to regulatory proteins called *G proteins* that stimulate ($\beta_1$, $\beta_2$, $\beta_3$, $D_1$) or inhibit ($\alpha_2$, $D_2$) adenylyl cyclase or stimulate ($\alpha_1$) phospholipase C. Stimulation of adenylyl cyclase increases cyclic adenosine monophosphate, which results in protein phosphorylation. Stimulation of phospholipase C increases the production of inositol trisphosphate, which increases intracellular calcium, and diacylglycerol, which activates protein kinase C. Stimulation of presynaptic $\alpha_2$-receptors and $DA_2$ receptors suppresses the release of norepinephrine from sympathetic nerve terminals, whereas stimulation of presynaptic $\beta_2$-receptors augments it. Overactivity of the SNS has been found to play a significant role in the etiology of hypertension and has also been linked to several comorbidities commonly associated with hypertension, such as metabolic syndrome, diabetes mellitus, dyslipidemia, and sleep apnea syndrome.

## RECEPTOR MODULATION

The responsiveness of catecholamine-sensitive cells can vary over time. Multiple mechanisms are responsible for regulating this responsiveness. *Homologous regulation* describes the case in which the responsiveness is altered by the adrenergic agonists themselves (decreased receptor density or affinity). *Heterologous regulation* occurs when the responsiveness is altered by other factors. The density of receptors can be increased (upregulated) by long-term administration of $\beta$ receptor antagonists, by denervation, and by hyperthyroidism. Receptors may be downregulated by continued $\beta$ adrenergic stimulation, hypothyroidism, and possibly corticosteroids.

## Agonists

### SYMPATHOMIMETIC AMINES

The parent compound is considered $\beta$ phenylethylamine. Compounds with hydroxyl groups at positions 3 and 4 of the benzene ring are called *catechols*; *catecholamines* are catechols with an ethylamine side chain. Many directly acting sympathomimetic amines stimulate both $\alpha$ and $\beta$ receptors (Table 29.1). The ratio of activities varies among agonists along a spectrum from predominantly $\alpha$ (phenylephrine) to predominantly $\beta$ (isoproterenol). The selectivity of $\beta$ receptors is enhanced by substitution of the amine group. Table 29.2 lists the antagonists of the adrenergic receptors, and Table 29.3 lists drugs that have a unique mechanism of action within the SNS.

| TABLE 29.1 | Adrenergic Agonists | | | | | | |
|---|---|---|---|---|---|---|---|
| | **MODE OF ACTION** | | | | | | |
| **Agent** | $\alpha_1$ | $\alpha_2$ | $\beta_1$ | $\beta_2$ | $D_1$ | $D_2$ | **Dose** |
| **NATURAL** | | | | | | | |
| Norepinephrine | ++++ | +++ | ++ | +++ | − | − | 0.05–0.3 $\mu g \cdot kg^{-1} \cdot min^{-1}$ |
| Epinephrine | +++ | ++ | +++ | +++ | + | − | 0.05–0.2 $\mu g \cdot kg^{-1} \cdot min^{-1}$ |
| **DOPAMINE** | | | | | | | |
| Low dose | − | − | − | − | ++++ | ++ | 1–5 $\mu g \cdot kg^{-1} \cdot min^{-1}$ |
| Medium dose | + | ? | ++ | + | ++++ | − | 5–15 $\mu g \cdot kg^{-1} \cdot min^{-1}$ |
| High dose | +++ | ? | ++ | + | − | − | > 15 $\mu g \cdot kg^{-1} \cdot min^{-1}$ |
| **SYNTHETIC** | | | | | | | |
| Metaproterenol | − | − | + | ++++ | − | − | MDI |

*Continued*

**TABLE 29.1   Adrenergic Agonists—cont'd**

| Agent | MODE OF ACTION | | | | | | Dose |
|---|---|---|---|---|---|---|---|
| | $\alpha_1$ | $\alpha_2$ | $\beta_1$ | $\beta_2$ | $D_1$ | $D_2$ | |
| Albuterol | | | | ++++ | | | MDI |
| Terbutaline | | | | ++++ | | | MDI |
| Isoproterenol | + | | ++++ | ++++ | | | 0.01–0.2 $\mu g \cdot kg^{-1} \cdot min^{-1}$ |
| Dobutamine | + | | +++ | + | | | 2.5–15 $\mu g \cdot kg^{-1} \cdot min^{-1}$ |
| Mephentermine | ++ | ? | +++ | ? | | | 0.1–0.5 mg/kg |
| Ephedrine | ++ | ? | ++ | + | | | 0.2–1.0 mg/kg |
| Metaraminol | ++++ | ? | ++ | ? | | | 10–102 $\mu g/kg$ |
| Phenylephrine | ++++ | | + | | | | 1–10 $\mu g \cdot kg^{-1} \cdot min^{-1}$ |
| Methoxamine | ++++ | | | | | | 0.05–0.2 mg/kg |
| Dopexamine | | | ++ | | +++ | + | 1–6 $\mu g \cdot kg^{-1} \cdot min^{-1}$ |
| Fenoldopam | | | | | +++ | | 0.1–0.8 $\mu g \cdot kg^{-1} \cdot min^{-1}$ |

++++, Tremendous stimulation; +++, marked stimulation; ++, moderate stimulation; +, slight stimulation; ?, unknown; *MDI,* metered-dose inhaler.

**TABLE 29.2   Antagonists of Adrenergic Receptors**

| Receptor | Drug |
|---|---|
| $\alpha_1 = \alpha_2$ (nonselective) | Phenoxybenzamine (irreversible), phentolamine, tolazoline |
| $\alpha_1$ (nonselective) | Prazosin, terazosin, doxazosin, trimazosin |
| $\alpha_{1A}$ (selective) | Tamsulosin, silodosin, doxazosin |
| $\alpha_2$ | Atipamezole (used to reverse sedation from dexmedetomidine in animals), yohimbine (inhibits norepinephrine release) |
| $\beta_1 = \beta_2$ (nonselective) | Propranolol, timolol, nadolol, pindolol, sotalol, labetalol (weak $\alpha_1$) |
| $\beta_1$ | Metoprolol, atenolol, esmolol, acebutolol |
| $\beta_2$ | Butoxamine |
| $\beta_3$ | BRL 37344 |

**TABLE 29.3   Drugs With Unique Mechanisms of Action Within the Adrenergic System**

| Drug | Action |
|---|---|
| Labetalol | $\alpha_1$-Receptor selective antagonist and a more potent nonselective $\beta$-receptor blocker (5–10 times $\beta$ over $\alpha_1$, however, acutely lowers peripheral resistance and systemic blood pressure with little effect on heart rate) |
| Carvedilol | $\alpha_1$-Receptor antagonist selective and a more potent nonselective $\beta$-receptor blocker |
| Bretylium | Blocks norepinephrine release |
| Propafenone | $\beta$-Adrenergic receptor antagonist |
| Reserpine | Blocks vesicular uptake of norepinephrine |
| Guanethidine | Causes active release and then depletion of norepinephrine |
| Cocaine | Blocks neuronal reuptake of norepinephrine |
| Tricyclic antidepressant | Blocks neuronal reuptake of norepinephrine |
| Tyramine | Causes release of vesicular and nonvesicular stores of catecholamines |

## SUGGESTED READINGS

Glick, D. B. (2015). The autonomic nervous system. In R. D. Miller, L. I. Eriksson, L. A. Fleisher, J. P. Wiener-Kronish, N. H. Cohen, & W. L. Young (Eds.), *Miller's anesthesia* (8th ed., pp. 346–386). New York: Elsevier.

Valensi, P. (2021). Autonomic nervous system activity changes in patients with hypertension and overweight: Role and therapeutic implications. *Cardiovascular Diabetology, 20*(1), 170.

Westfall, T. C., Macarthur, H., & Westfall, D. P. (2018). Adrenergic agonists and antagonists. In L. L. Brunton, R. Hilal-Dandan, & B. C. Knollmann (Eds.), *Goodman & Gilman's: The pharmacological basis of therapeutics* (13th ed.). New York, NY: McGraw-Hill.

# 30

# Factors Affecting Cerebral Blood Flow

KIRSTIN M. ERICKSON, MD

## Cerebral Metabolic Rate

The brain consumes $O_2$ at a high rate. Although it accounts for only approximately 2% of total body weight, the brain receives 12% to 15% of cardiac output. Normal cerebral blood flow (CBF) is approximately $50 \text{ mL} \cdot 100 \text{ g}^{-1} \cdot \text{min}^{-1}$. Normal cerebral metabolic rate (CMR) for $O_2$ ($CMRo_2$) is $3.5 \text{ mL} \cdot 100 \text{ g}^{-1} \cdot \text{min}^{-1}$. Roughly 60% of the energy consumed by the brain is used for the depolarization-repolarization activity of neurotransmission. The remaining 40% is used for cellular homeostasis. Increases in regional brain activity lead to local increases in CMR that in turn lead to proportional changes in CBF. Neuronal activity directly increases CBF (in contrast to flow responding to a feedback loop). This relationship is carefully maintained and is called *neurovascular coupling* or *flow-metabolism coupling*.

Mechanisms involved are not completely defined, but appear to include local by-products of metabolism (potassium ion, hydrogen ion, lactate, and adenosine triphosphate [ATP]) along with glutamate and nitric oxide. Peptides (vasoactive peptide, substance P, and others) exert effects on nerves that innervate cerebral vessels. In addition to these chemical, metabolic, and humoral contributors, neurovascular coupling is achieved by glial, neuronal, and vascular mechanisms that are not yet well understood. Autoregulation (myogenic regulation and the relationship to mean arterial pressure [MAP]) is but one of many factors that influence cerebral blood flow. Neurogenic control of CBF occurs by sympathetic innervation and is independent of the influence of $Paco_2$.

CMR decreases during sleep, rises with increasing mental activity, and may reach an extremely high level with epileptic activity. CMR is globally reduced in coma and may be only locally impaired after brain injury.

## Autoregulation

*Autoregulation* is defined as the maintenance of CBF over a range of MAP (Fig. 30.1). Cerebral vascular smooth muscle alters cerebral vascular resistance (CVR) to maintain constant CBF. Cerebral perfusion pressure (CPP) equals MAP minus intracranial pressure (ICP). Because ICP (and therefore CPP) is not commonly available, MAP is used as a surrogate of CPP. It is now recognized that autoregulation is a complex regulatory system with a multitude of interdependent factors, and even the form of the curve may be dynamic (see Fig. 30.1).

Autoregulation occurs when MAP is between 70 and 150 mm Hg in the normal brain, although considerable interindividual variation occurs. The lower limit of autoregulation (LLA) is the point at which the autoregulation curve deflects downward and CBF begins to decrease in proportion to MAP.

CVR varies directly with blood pressure to maintain flow, taking 3 to 4 minutes for flow to be regulated after an abrupt change in blood pressure. In patients with hypertension, the autoregulatory curve is shifted to the right (Fig. 30.2). A patient with hypertension may be at risk for brain ischemia at a MAP of 70 mm Hg, for example, because the LLA will be higher than in a patient without hypertension. The curve may return to normal after blood pressure control, but the time course is not known. After significant hypotension (lower than the LLA), autoregulation is impaired, and hyperemia may occur, when MAP returns to the normal range. $CO_2$ reactivity remains intact, and inducing hypocapnia may attenuate hyperemia (Fig. 30.3). To prevent CPP from decreasing to less than the LLA and leading to ischemic injury in the traumatized brain, the Brain Trauma Foundation Guidelines suggest a target CPP of 60 to 70 mm Hg.

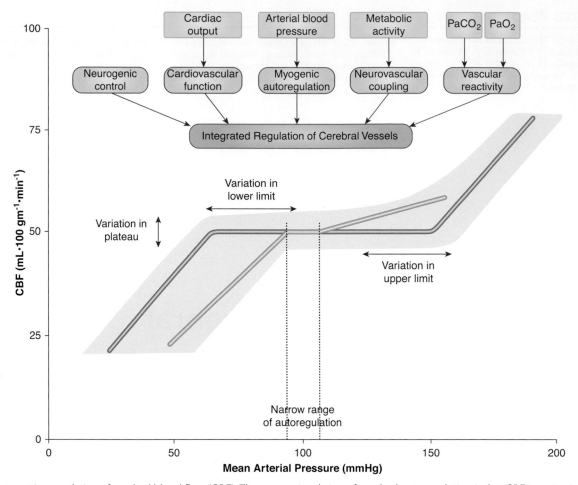

**Fig. 30.1** Integrative regulation of cerebral blood flow (*CBF*). The conventional view of cerebral autoregulation is that CBF is maintained constant with a variation in mean arterial pressure of 65 to 150 mm Hg. A more contemporary view is that cerebral autoregulation is a dynamic process that is under the influence of a number of variables including myogenic autoregulation, neurovascular coupling, arterial $CO_2$ and $O_2$ tensions, autonomic (neurogenic) activity, and cardiovascular function. Anesthetic agents in particular affect autoregulation at multiple levels: suppression of metabolism, alteration in arterial blood gas tensions, direct cerebral vasodilation, suppression of autonomic activity, and modulation of cardiovascular function. Therefore CBF at any given moment is a product of the composite of these variables. There is considerable variation in lower and upper limits, as well as the plateau of the autoregulatory curve. The conventional autoregulatory curve is depicted in *red*. The *red shaded area* represents the range of variation in CBF. The autoregulatory curve depicted in *blue* was derived from 48 healthy human subjects. In that group, the lower limit of autoregulation was approximately 90 mm Hg, and the range over which CBF remained relatively constant was only 10 mm Hg. $PaCO_2$, Arterial partial pressure of carbon dioxide; $PaO_2$, arterial partial pressure of oxygen. (From Patel PM, Drummond JC, Lemkuil BP. Cerebral physiology and the effects of anesthetic drugs. In: Miller RD, Leslie K, eds. *Miller's Anesthesia*. 9th ed. Vol. 1. Elsevier; 2019:303, fig. 11.8.)

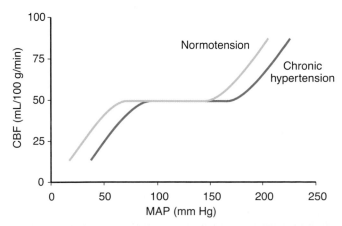

**Fig. 30.2** The relationship between cerebral blood flow (*CBF*) and mean arterial pressure (*MAP*) shows autoregulation of cerebral perfusion pressure across a range of MAP values. The curve is shifted to the right in patients with chronic hypertension. (From Erickson KM, Cole DJ. Arterial hypotension and hypertension. In: Brambrink A, Kirsch JR, eds. *Neuroanesthesia and Critical Care Handbook*. Springer; 2010.)

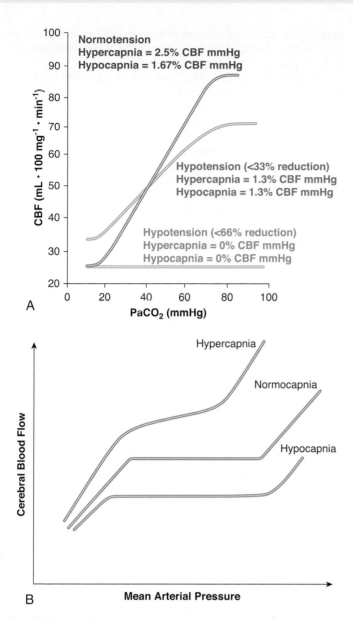

A, Normotension
Hypercapnia = 2.5% CBF mmHg
Hypocapnia = 1.67% CBF mmHg

Hypotension (<33% reduction)
Hypercapnia = 1.3% CBF mmHg
Hypocapnia = 1.3% CBF mmHg

Hypotension (<66% reduction)
Hypercapnia = 0% CBF mmHg
Hypocapnia = 0% CBF mmHg

**Fig. 30.3** **A**, Relationship between cerebral blood flow (*CBF*) and partial pressure of carbon dioxide (*Paco₂*). CBF increases linearly with increases in arterial Paco₂. Below a Paco₂ of 25 mm Hg, further reduction in CBF is limited. Similarly, the increase in CBF above a Paco₂ of approximately 75 to 80 mm Hg is also attenuated. The cerebrovascular responsiveness to Paco₂ is influenced significantly by blood pressure. With moderate hypotension (mean arterial pressure [MAP] reduction of <33%), the cerebrovascular responsiveness to changes in Paco₂ is attenuated significantly. With severe hypotension (MAP reduction of approximately 66%), CO₂ responsiveness is abolished. **B**, The effect of Paco₂ variation on cerebral autoregulation. Hypercarbia induces cerebral vasodilation and, consequently, the autoregulatory response to hypertension is less effective. By contrast, hypocapnia results in greater CBF autoregulation over a wider MAP variation. (Modified from Willie C.K., Tzeng Y.C., Fisher J.A., Ainslie P.N.: Integrative regulation of human brain blood flow. *J Physiol* 2014; 592: pp. 841-859 and Rickards C.A.: Cerebral blood-flow regulation during hemorrhage. *Compr Physiol* 2015; 5: pp. 1585-1621.)

Individual variation in autoregulation may explain why a more exact minimum CPP has not been elucidated.

Autoregulatory vasodilation may be limited by background sympathetic vascular tone. Systemic vasodilators (nitroprusside, nitroglycerin, hydralazine, adenosine, and calcium channel blockers) may extend the lower limit of tolerable hypotension

(shift the LLA to a lower pressure). Other than their effect on global cerebral perfusion pressure, β-adrenergic receptor blocking agents likely have no adverse effects on patients with intracranial pathology.

Autoregulation is impaired in areas of relative ischemia, in tissue surrounding mass lesions, after grand mal seizures, after head injury, with hemorrhage, under retractors, and during episodes of hypercarbia or hypoxemia. Fig. 30.3B shows how lost autoregulation, due to hypercapnia, may lead to dangerously low CBF. A similar phenomenon results from vasodilation with high volatile concentration. Regional or global ischemia may ensue.

## Carbon Dioxide Responsiveness

Carbon dioxide dilates cerebral arterioles. This is known as *cerebral vascular responsiveness to CO₂* (CVR-CO₂). Paco₂ levels affect CBF by changing the H⁺ concentration in the extracellular fluid surrounding smooth muscle in the arteriolar cell walls. CBF varies directly with Paco₂ (Fig. 30.3). The effect is greatest in the normal physiologic range of Paco₂. CBF changes 1 to 2 mL·100 g⁻¹·min⁻¹ for each 1-mm Hg change in Paco₂. As Paco₂ increases from 30 to 60 mm Hg, for example, CBF doubles. Below a Paco₂ level of 25, the response is attenuated.

Mild hypocapnia (Paco₂ of 30–34 mm Hg) in patients with large space-occupying lesions ("tight heads") who are undergoing craniotomy is used only selectively to facilitate surgical access. At a Paco₂ of 20 mm Hg, cerebral ischemia may occur because of a left shift in the oxyhemoglobin dissociation curve and decreases in CBF. With a Paco₂ of less than 20 mm Hg to 25 mm Hg, O₂ consumption decreases and anaerobic metabolism ensues.

MAP and Paco₂ have interrelated effects. With severe hypotension, for example, there is no observable cerebral vasoconstriction when Paco₂ is altered (Fig. 30.3A). With modest hypotension, CO₂ reactivity is mildly affected. In turn, during hypercapnia the autoregulatory response to hypertension is diminished (Fig. 30.3B). Hypocapnia increases the range of MAP over which CBF is held steady.

Changes in cerebral blood volume (CBV) due to changes in Paco₂ occur in the cerebral arterial vasculature, with greatest effect on vessels smaller than 100 μm in diameter.

The mechanism of cerebral vascular responsiveness (CVR) is secondary to changes in local H⁺ in arteriolar walls on the brain side of the blood-brain barrier. Nitric oxide and prostaglandins are mediators of hypercarbia-induced vasodilatation. Respiratory acidosis, not metabolic acidosis, leads to vasodilation because HCO₃⁻ does not cross the blood-brain barrier initially, but CO₂ does. The decreased pH of the periarteriolar cerebrospinal fluid causes vasodilation within 20 to 30 seconds. The pH of the cerebrospinal fluid normalizes with active changes in HCO₃⁻ concentration, and CBF returns to normal in 6 to 8 hours. CO₂ responsiveness in gray matter is greater than that in white matter because of increased vascular density. Pathologic states, including trauma, insulin-requiring diabetes, or ischemia, decrease CO₂ responsiveness. CVR-CO₂ is preserved in patients with intracranial pathology.

A "Robin Hood effect" may exist in which areas of focal ischemia (where CO₂ reactivity is likely lost) receive increased flow if normal vasculature is exposed to hypocapnia; however, this effect is unpredictable. Normocapnia should be maintained when regional ischemia is a risk. After a period of hypocapnia, an abrupt return to normocapnia may cause acidosis in the cerebrospinal fluid and rebound in CBF and ICP. Cerebral ischemia is a risk if intracranial elastance is poor.

## Oxygen Responsiveness

$Pao_2$ has little direct effect on CBF at values of 60 mm Hg to more than 300 mm Hg. A $Pao_2$ level below 60 mm Hg markedly increases CBF if blood pressure is maintained. A variety of factors released by deoxyhemoglobin (NO and its metabolites, and ATP) act on vascular smooth muscle to produce vasodilation. At $Pao_2$ levels above normal, up to 1 atm (760 mm Hg), only a very slight decrease in CBF has been measured.

## Hypothermia

Hypothermia (28°C–37°C) acutely reduces, but does not uncouple, $CMRo_2$ and CBF. $CO_2$ reactivity is also maintained during hypothermia. The effects of hypothermia on $CMRo_2$ are discussed in Chapter 101, Cerebral Protection.

## Effects of Anesthetic Drugs

In general, anesthetic agents, except for ketamine and $N_2O$, depress CMR.

## Intravenously Administered Anesthetic Agents

Intravenously administered anesthetic agents typically cause parallel declines in $CMRo_2$ and CBF, with preservation of $Paco_2$ responsiveness. Ketamine, however, increases both CBF and $CMRo_2$.

Propofol decreases $CMRo_2$ by approximately 50% and subsequently decreases CBF, CBV, and ICP. Autoregulation is preserved, even at propofol doses sufficient to produce burst suppression by electroencephalography. Cerebral vascular reactivity to $CO_2$ is preserved, although propofol, when used alone, promotes more vasoconstriction than do volatile anesthetics.

Thiopental decreases $CMRo_2$ and CBF in a dose-dependent manner, up to a maximum of 50% at induction of isoelectric electroencephalography tracings. No further reduction in $CMRo_2$ results when additional thiopental is given after electroencephalographic suppression. This response suggests that thiopental and other depressant anesthetic agents reduce the component of cerebral metabolism associated with electrical brain activity rather than with homeostasis. Autoregulation is preserved.

Etomidate has effects on $CMRo_2$ and CBF similar to barbiturates. However, ischemic injury can be exacerbated, and on this basis, the use of etomidate is avoided in neurologic pathology. The effects of etomidate on autoregulation have not been studied. Etomidate is epileptogenic in patients with seizure disorders.

Benzodiazepines decrease $CMRo_2$ and CBF in a dose-dependent manner. Positron emission tomographic studies have shown selective decreases in brain regions associated with attention, arousal, and memory in patients treated with benzodiazepines.

Fentanyl modestly reduces $CMRo_2$ and CBF, and $CO_2$ responsiveness and autoregulation remain intact. Sufentanil causes either a modest reduction or no change in these parameters. Alfentanil likewise causes no changes in $CMRo_2$ or CBF in dogs. Sedative doses of remifentanil can increase CBF slightly, whereas large doses suppress CBF.

Morphine depresses $CMRo_2$ and CBF by a small to moderate degree. Histamine release can cause cerebral vasodilation, and CBF and CBV will be dependent on MAP.

Dexmedetomidine reduces CBF and $CMRo_2$ in parallel. Reduction in MAP reduces the margin of safety in patients who are dependent on collateral perfusion pressure.

Mannitol causes a transient increase in CBV, which returns to normal after approximately 10 minutes.

$Paco_2$ reactivity remains intact in normal brain during anesthesia with all anesthetic medications studied.

## Inhaled Anesthetic Agents

Inhaled anesthetic agents reduce $CMRo_2$ (see Chapter 45, Effects of Inhalation Agents on the Central Nervous System of the Inhalation Agents). Decreases in $CMRo_2$ are dose dependent and nonlinear below 1 minimum alveolar concentration (MAC) of the agent; a precipitous drop is followed by a more gradual, linear decline as MAC is increased. Maximal reduction occurs with electroencephalographic suppression. Differences among the $CMRo_2$ effects of isoflurane, desflurane, and sevoflurane are minor.

Autoregulation is impaired by concentrations of volatile anesthetic agents above 1 MAC, but not at lower levels. At 0.5 MAC, CBF is reduced as a result of decreased CMR from volatile agents. At 1 MAC, the effect of decreased CMR is countered by increased vasodilation, and CBF is unchanged from the awake state. At concentrations greater than 1 MAC, vasodilation predominates. Autoregulation is impaired in a dose-dependent manner, and CBF becomes more pressure passive the higher the concentration of gas is. Sevoflurane impairs autoregulation less than does isoflurane or desflurane. This pattern follows the vasodilatory potency of each gas.

The correlation between CBF and CBV is not direct. With vasodilation induced by higher concentrations of inhalational agent, CBV increases, whereas CBF may be unchanged or reduced. Increased CBV may cause significant increases in ICP.

$CO_2$ responsiveness is preserved with the use of inhalational anesthetic agents. The effects of potent volatiles on ICP can be attenuated with simultaneous use of hypocapnia in patients with normal intracranial elastance. In patients with intracranial tumors, however, hypocapnia may not effectively block an increase in ICP caused by inhalational gas because impairments of normal brain physiology disable both $Paco_2$ responsiveness and autoregulation.

When administered alone, $N_2O$ increases $CMRo_2$, CBF, and ICP. These effects are moderated or obliterated when $N_2O$ is used in combination with intravenously administered drugs. The addition of $N_2O$ to an inhalational anesthetic agent causes a moderate increase in CBF.

## Age

In the healthy brain at 80 years of age, both CBF and $CMRo_2$ are decreased by 15% to 20%, and $CO_2$ reactivity and responsiveness to hypoxia are also mildly reduced.

## SUGGESTED READINGS

Carney, N., Totten, A. M., O'Reilly, C., Ulman, J. S., Hawryluk, G. W., Bell, M. J., et al. (2017). Guidelines for the management of severe traumatic brain injury, Fourth Edition, Cerebral perfusion pressure thresholds. *Neurosurgery, 80,* 181–190.

de-Lima-Oliveira, M., Salinet, A. S. M., Nogueira, R. C., de Azevedo, D. S., Paiva, W. S., Teixeira, M. J., et al. (2018). Intracranial hypertension and cerebral autoregulation: A systematic review and meta-analysis. *World Neurosurgery, 113,* 110–124.

Drummond, J. C. (2019). Blood pressure and the brain: How low can you go? *Anesthesia & Analgesia, 128,* 759–771.

Mariappan, R., Mehta, J., Chui, J., Manninen, P., & Venkatraghavan, L. (2015). Cerebrovascular reactivity to carbon dioxide under anesthesia: A qualitative systemic review. *Journal of Neurosurgical Anesthesiology, 27*(2), 123–135.

Rivera-Lara, L., Geocadin, R., Zorrilla-Vaca, A., Healy, R., Radzik, B. R., Palmisano, C., et al. (2020). Near-Infrared spectroscopy derived cerebral autoregulation indices independently predict clinical outcome in acutely ill comatose patients. *Journal of Neurosurgical Anesthesiology, 32*(3), 234–241.

# 31 Physiology of Neuromuscular Transmission

REKA NEMES, MD, PhD | J. ROSS RENEW, MD | SORIN J. BRULL, MD, FCARCSI (Hon)

## Neuromuscular Junction

The *neuromuscular junction* is a synapse between the tightly apposed presynaptic motor neuron terminal and the postsynaptic muscle fiber. This is where a chemical process (release of acetylcholine [ACh] from the nerve ending) leads to an electrical event (muscle membrane depolarization) that results in a mechanical effect (muscle contraction) (Fig. 31.1). Large motor nerve axons branch as they course distally within skeletal muscle. Ultimately, the axons divide into 10 to 100 smaller terminal nerve fibers and lose their myelin sheath, each nerve fiber innervating a single muscle fiber. The combination of the terminal neural fibers that originate from one axon and the muscle fibers they innervate constitutes a *motor unit.* The average number of muscle fibers innervated by a single motor neuron defines the *innervation ratio,* which in humans varies from 1:5 to 1:2000. For smaller muscles that are specialized for fine, precise movement (e.g., hand muscles, ocular muscles), the innervation ratio is low (1:5, or five muscle fibers per neuron), whereas large antigravity back muscles have very high innervation ratios (1:2000). Transmission from nerve to muscle is mediated by ACh, which is synthesized in the nerve terminal and stored in specialized vesicles; each vesicle *(quantum)* contains approximately 10,000 molecules of ACh, and about every second, one such vesicle fuses with the presynaptic neuronal cell membrane, releasing its ACh contents *(exocytosis).* This tonic release of ACh quanta maintains the postsynaptic receptors functional. Nerve terminals contain approximately 500,000 quanta, stored in a specialized region of the membrane called the *active zone.* ACh is released by exocytosis into the junctional cleft after an appropriate nerve impulse reaches the nerve terminal. ACh diffuses across the 30 to 50 nm cleft to bind *postjunctional nicotinic ACh receptors* (nAChR); this binding initiates a muscle contraction.

## Function of the Neuromuscular Junction

### ACETYLCHOLINE SYNTHESIS

ACh is synthesized from acetyl coenzyme A and choline under the catalytic influence of choline *O*-acetyltransferase enzyme in the axoplasm (Fig. 31.2). The ACh is transported into vesicles by a specific carrier-mediated system. Approximately 80% of the ACh present in the nerve terminal is in the vesicles, with the remainder dissolved in the axoplasm.

### NERVE TERMINAL DEPOLARIZATION

Depolarization of the nerve terminal follows the arrival of the nerve action potential and results from sodium influx through membrane sodium channels. The influx of sodium alters the membrane potential from $-90$ mV toward the membrane potential of sodium ($+50$ mV). However, at a membrane potential near 0 mV, potassium channels open and sodium channels begin to close, and the membrane potential reaches $+10$ mV. During depolarization, calcium ions also enter the nerve terminal, inducing the release of ACh vesicles into the synaptic cleft. The calcium influx into the axon lasts as long as the resting membrane potential is not restored. High-frequency tetanic

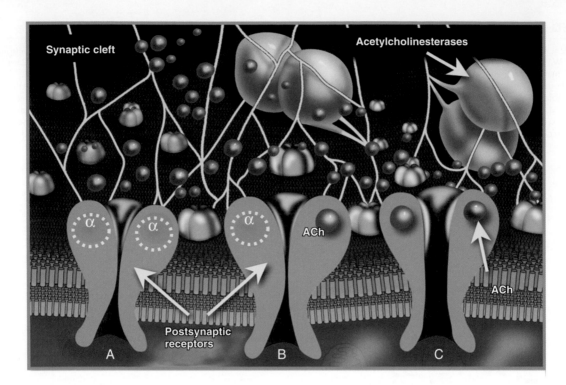

**Fig. 31.1** Normal neuromuscular junction. The synaptic cleft contains an acetylcholinesterase enzyme that hydrolyzes acetylcholine *(ACh)*. The receptors contain the ACh recognition site on the α subunits. Once both subunits are bound by ACh, the inactive (closed) receptors A and B undergo a conformational change and become active (open) by developing a central channel for cation exchange (receptor C). (Illustration courtesy Dr. Frank G. Standaert.)

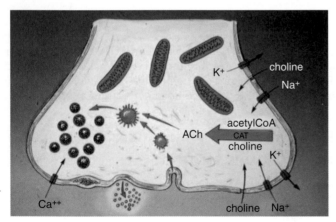

**Fig. 31.2** The nerve (presynaptic) terminal. There is no myelin sheath; acetylcholine *(ACh)* is synthesized from acetyl coenzyme A *(acetylCoA)* and choline under the catalytic influence of choline *O*-acetyltransferase *(CAT)*. Once formed, ACh is packaged into vesicles that are available for release into the cleft via exocytosis. (Illustration courtesy Dr. Frank G. Standaert.)

stimulation of the nerve results in the intracellular accumulation of calcium ions, which results in an exaggerated subsequent release of ACh into the synaptic cleft. This phenomenon is called *posttetanic potentiation.*

## ACETYLCHOLINE RELEASE

ACh is released spontaneously and tonically from the vesicles into the synaptic cleft, leading to small depolarizations (0.5 mV) at a frequency of 1 to 3 Hz, known as *miniature endplate potentials.* Each miniature endplate potential is believed to represent

the effect of the contents of a single vesicle containing 6000 to 10,000 ACh molecules, or 1 quantum. These miniature endplate potentials do not result in muscle contraction. However, a threshold action potential causes accelerated ACh release of 50 to 400 quanta by a voltage-gated calcium-dependent exocytosis process from the active zone into the synaptic cleft. The extent of calcium influx into the presynaptic neuron determines the number of ACh quanta released into the cleft and is a function of the duration of nerve depolarization. Only approximately 50% of the ACh released into the cleft reaches the postsynaptic receptors, as the rest is hydrolyzed by acetylcholinesterases within the cleft; is reuptaken into the presynaptic terminal; or diffuses out of the cleft. However, the remaining ACh is still 10 times greater than the minimum required to achieve postsynaptic ACh receptor threshold activation, and sufficient postjunctional membrane depolarization occurs to produce a threshold endplate potential and activation of the excitation-contraction sequence that results in muscle contraction.

The system of neuromuscular transmission is so effective that only 25% of the nAChRs need to be activated to produce muscle membrane depolarization and fiber contraction. This phenomenon suggests that a margin-of-safety exists when pharmacologically manipulating neuromuscular transmission. In fact, up to 75% of the nAChRs may still be occupied by neuromuscular blocking agent (NMBA) molecules while muscle fatigue is no longer detectable, either clinically or electrophysiologically.

## TRANSMITTER MOBILIZATION

The rate at which available ACh stores are replaced is termed *transmitter mobilization.* Evidence suggests that there is a positive feedback loop for ACh.

### Postjunctional Events

Released ACh diffuses across the synaptic cleft and binds to a nicotinic ACh receptor on the postjunctional membrane that forms a membrane ion channel. Two molecules of ACh must bind the receptor (one molecule to each of the two recognition sites) before the receptor undergoes the conformational change necessary to open the receptor channel to ion flow. These channels are chemically sensitive but cannot discriminate between sodium and potassium ions. Once the channels are opened, ion flow makes the immediate area more positive. Each elementary current pulse is additive and summates to produce an endplate current. The endplate current depolarizes the endplate membrane to produce the endplate potential. Once the endplate potential reaches the critical threshold, a propagating action potential is triggered that is directed away from the endplate and results in activation of a muscle fiber contraction.

### Junctional Cholinesterase

The neuromuscular junction contains two forms of acetylcholinesterase: a dissolved form in the nerve terminal axoplasm and a membrane-bound form anchored to the basement membrane of the junctional cleft by the structural proteins, rapsyn and dystrophin. This enzyme acts to rapidly hydrolyze released ACh to choline and acetate. The kinetics of this enzyme in the neuromuscular junction cause a single ACh molecule to react with a single cholinoceptor before it is inactivated by the AChE.

### Postsynaptic Receptors

The postsynaptic muscle membrane at the cleft contains multiple invaginations that markedly increase the membrane surface area. At the top of these folds are high concentrations (up to 10,000–20,000 receptors/$\mu m^2$) of nAChRs. Outside the synaptic cleft area, the concentration of receptors is at least 1000 times lower. The nAChRs are pentameric proteins consisting of two $\alpha$ subunits (protomers) and one $\beta$, $\delta$, and $\epsilon$ subunit each; the receptors are anchored to the postsynaptic muscle membrane by proteins such as agrin and rapsyn. In the adult mammal, the receptors are designated as $\alpha_2\beta\delta\epsilon$ (Fig. 31.3). Stereochemically, they are arranged in a counterclockwise order as $\alpha$, $\epsilon$, $\alpha$, $\delta$, $\beta$. Fetal nAChR is similar to that of the adult, except that fetal nAChR has a $\gamma$ protomer that is replaced in the adult by the $\epsilon$ protomer. The five subunits of nAChR form a rosette surrounding a central transmembrane pore with a diameter of approximately 0.7 nm. Each $\alpha$ subunit possesses a recognition site for ACh at the $\alpha\epsilon$ and $\alpha\delta$ subunit interfaces. When ACh binds to both $\alpha$ recognition sites, the receptor undergoes a conformational change and the central pore opens, allowing sodium flux that produces a brief (6.5-ms) current.

### Presynaptic Receptors

A second type of nicotinic receptor is found on the nerve terminal. The prejunctional nAChRs have three $\alpha$ subunits and two $\beta$ subunits. Similar to the postsynaptic receptors, they are also blocked by NMBAs but are relatively selective for calcium fluxes. They are thought to help mobilize ACh during periods of high ACh demand, such as high-frequency (tetanic) stimulation. Blockade of these receptors is thought to account for the tetanic fade produced by partial nondepolarizing blockade. Succinylcholine does not bind to prejunctional nAChRs and no (or minimal) fade is seen during depolarizing neuromuscular blockade. Beside the presynaptic nAChRs, spontaneous and activity-dependent ACh release is also modulated by different muscarinic and purinergic presynaptic ACh receptors.

## Upregulation and Downregulation

Clinical hypersensitivity and resistance to NMBAs are observed in a number of pathologic states. The concepts of upregulation and downregulation of receptor sites have been introduced to provide a cohesive theory of receptor-drug interaction that can explain a mechanism for abnormal effects of NMBAs in the clinical setting.

### UPREGULATION

An increase in the number of nAChRs develops on the postjunctional membrane in conditions involving decreased stimulation of the neuromuscular junction over time (Box 31.1). Upregulation leads to hypersensitivity to the agonists ACh and succinylcholine (SCh) and decreased sensitivity to antagonists such as nondepolarizing NMBAs. Upregulation can lead to lethal potassium release from cells after SCh administration in patients with motor neuron lesions, burns, muscle atrophy from disuse, and severe trauma and infections, as well as in those who have received NMBAs over a prolonged period in the intensive care unit. The phenomenon can develop in 3 to 5 days when there is total loss of ACh activity at the endplate. Pretreatment with

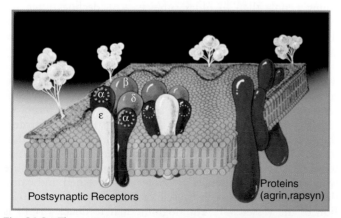

**Fig. 31.3** The postsynaptic receptors are pentameric proteins consisting of two $\alpha$ subunits and one $\beta$, $\delta$, and $\epsilon$ subunit each. They are anchored to the postsynaptic membrane by agrin and rapsyn proteins. Anticholinesterases are tethered to the basement membrane. (Illustration courtesy Dr. Frank G. Standaert.)

Labels in figure: $\alpha$, $\beta$, $\delta$, $\epsilon$, $\alpha$; Postsynaptic Receptors; Proteins (agrin, rapsyn)

---

**BOX 31.1  CONDITIONS ASSOCIATED WITH ACETYLCHOLINE UPREGULATION AND DOWNREGULATION**

**UPREGULATION: ↑ AGONIST SENSITIVITY, ↓ ANTAGONIST SENSITIVITY**

Upper and lower motor neuron lesions
Burns
Severe infection
Prolonged use of neuromuscular blocking agents
Muscle trauma
Cerebral palsy
Long-term use of anticonvulsant agents

**DOWNREGULATION: ↓ AGONIST SENSITIVITY, ↑ ANTAGONIST SENSITIVITY**

Myasthenia gravis
Organophosphate poisoning
Exercise conditioning

NMBAs does not predictably prevent SCh-induced hyperkalemia. In other conditions for which chronic anticonvulsant therapy is prescribed, such as cerebral palsy and epilepsy, resistance to NMBAs is seen without potassium release after SCh use.

## DOWNREGULATION

Increased sensitivity to antagonists (e.g., NMBAs) and decreased sensitivity to agonists (e.g., SCh) develop in conditions of chronic agonist stimulation of receptors. These effects can occur with chronic reversible (e.g., neostigmine) or irreversible (e.g., organophosphate) cholinesterase inhibitor use. Most patients with myasthenia gravis have antibodies to ACh receptors that cause the neuromuscular junction to function as if it had fewer receptors. These patients are relatively resistant to SCh but extremely sensitive to NMBAs. Downregulation is also thought to occur in muscle groups that show a greater degree of paralysis after exercise conditioning.

## SUGGESTED READINGS

Bowman, W. C. (2006). Neuromuscular block. *British Journal of Pharmacology*, 147, S277–S286.

Iyer, S. R., Shah, S. B., & Lovering, R. M. (2021). The neuromuscular junction: Roles in aging and neuromuscular disease. *International Journal of Molecular Sciences*, 22(15), 8058. doi:10.3390/ijms22158058.

Martyn, J. A., White, D. A., Gronert, G. A., Jaffe, R. S., & Ward, J. M. (1992). Up-and-down regulation of skeletal muscle acetylcholine receptors: Effects on neuromuscular blockers. *Anesthesiology*, 76, 822–843.

Nagashima, M., Sasakawa, T., Schaller, S. J., & Martyn, J. A. (2015). Block of postjunctional muscle-type acetylcholine receptors in vivo causes train-of-four fade in mice. *British Journal of Anaesthesia*, 115, 112–127.

Naguib, M., Flood, P., McArdle, J. J., & Brenner, H. R. (2002). Advances in neurobiology of the neuromuscular junction: Implications for the anesthesiologist. *Anesthesiology*, 96, 202–231.

Nishimune, H., & Shigemoto, K. (2018). Practical anatomy of the neuromuscular junction in health and disease. *Neurologic Clinics*, 36, 231–240. doi:10.1016/j.ncl.2018.01.009.

Zhai, R. G., Vardinon-Friedman, H., Cases-Langhoff, C., Becker, B., Gundelfinger, E. D., Ziv, N. E., et al. (2001). Assembling the presynaptic active zone: A characterization of an active zone precursor vesicle. *Neuron*, 29, 131–143.

# 32

# Renal Physiology

MALINPORN JAMPONG, MD  |  MANOCH RATTANASOMPATTIKUL, MD, FASN

Kidneys are essential organs for body homeostasis, especially in an organism in which cellular contents are not in continuous contact with the environment. In their vascular and tubular systems (Fig. 32.1), the kidneys regulate water and electrolyte balance, excrete waste products, reabsorb, and produce hormones. Within the smallest functional units of the kidney—the nephrons—glomerular filtration, tubular reabsorption, and tubular secretion take place.

## Renal Blood Flow

Twenty percent of the total cardiac output flows through both kidneys. Approximately 80% of renal blood flow (RBF) travels through the cortex, which accounts for filtration at the glomeruli and most of the reabsorption from proximal and distal nephron cortical tubules. Twenty percent of RBF travels to the medulla where reabsorption occurs to maintain a hypertonic interstitial gradient needed to excrete concentrated urine. RBF differs according to sex and is lower in women than in men, even when corrected for body surface area, and RBF is higher in young people than in older subjects. RBF declines after age 30 years; by the time individuals are approximately 90 years old, their RBF is about half the rate that it was when they were 20 years old.

Over a wide range of systemic blood pressure, RBF is maintained by autoregulation to keep a glomerular capillary pressure of approximately 60 to 70 mm Hg, for a constant filtration rate and thus a proportionate salt loss. Myogenic receptors regulate afferent arteriolar tone by vasoconstriction to protect the glomerulus from too high blood pressure and vasodilation to allow greater blood flow to the glomerulus in times of hypotension. Myogenic reflex increases renal perfusion pressure when arteries and afferent arterioles are stretched and cause depolarization of smooth muscle cells that promote constriction of the vessel wall. Tubuloglomerular feedback (TGF) is another mechanism of autoregulation RBF by regulatory cross-talk between distal nephron (macula densa) and afferent arteriole (juxtaglomerular apparatus) that synchronizes blood

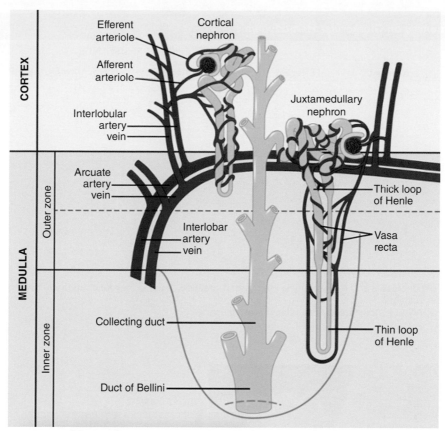

**Fig. 32.1** Schematic of relations between blood vessels and tubular structures. (From Hall JE. Guyton and Hall Textbook of Medical Physiology. 13th ed. Philadelphia: Elsevier; 2016. Figure 26-5.)

flow across networks of nephrons in response to sodium delivery. Both autoregulatory mechanisms are impaired when mean arterial blood pressure drops to less than 70 mm Hg, resulting in hypoperfusion of the cortex and oliguria. Failure of renal autoregulation is associated with progressive hypertensive renal disease.

RBF is also regulated by the renin-angiotensin-aldosterone system, natriuretic peptides, and eicosanoids. During stress, RBF is shunted from cortical to medullary areas, which are under the influence of the sympathetic nervous system and extrarenal (e.g., epinephrine, norepinephrine, vasopressin), perirenal (e.g., kinin, endothelin, adenosine), and intrarenal (e.g., nitric oxide, prostacyclin) biochemical activity. During stress, these biochemical and afferent nerve activities stimulate medullary mechanisms that increase $O_2$ consumption within the medulla, leading to conservation of water and production of concentrated urine. Functional magnetic resonance imaging studies have shown that furosemide increases $O_2$ consumption in these same areas and, depending on the adequacy of the $O_2$ supply, may create ischemic conditions. The physiologic influences on glomerular hemodynamic is demonstrated in Table 32.1.

Historically, RBF has been estimated from renal clearance of paraaminohippurate (PAH), which is both filtered at the glomerulus and actively secreted by the tubules, resulting in renal extraction of 70% to 90% from the blood. Renal plasma flow (RPF) of PAH can be calculated by

$$RPF_{PAH} = U_{PAH} \times V/P_{PAH}$$

where $U_{PAH}$ and $P_{PAH}$ are the urinary and plasma concentrations of PAH, respectively, and V is the volume of urine. Because the venous concentration of PAH is not 0, the calculated flow is referred to as *effective RPF* and approximates 600 mL/min, approximately 10% underestimation of RPF.

RBF can then be derived from this calculated RPF with a known hematocrit value:

$$RBF = RPF \, (1 - hematocrit)$$

Improved methods of RBF measurement have been introduced with laser Doppler flowmetry, video microscopy, and imaging techniques, such as positron emission tomography, high-speed computed tomography, and magnetic resonance imaging.

## Glomerular Filtration Rate

The glomerular filtration rate (GFR), an index of renal function and an initial step in urine formation, involves hydrostatic and osmotic pressure gradients between the glomerular capillaries and the Bowman space (Fig. 32.2). The hydrostatic pressure is higher than that of other vascular beds ($\approx$50 mm Hg), whereas that of the Bowman space is 10, yielding a net pressure of 40 mm Hg, which favors glomerular filtration. The ultrafiltrate has the same composition and osmolality as plasma but is protein free. The GFR of both kidneys, 120 mL/min, can increase if the glomerular capillary surface area, flow rate, or hydrostatic pressure increases. Polysaccharide or inulin concentration can be used to

| TABLE 32.1 | **Physiologic Influences on Glomerular Hemodynamic** | | | | |
|---|---|---|---|---|---|
| | **ARTERIOLAR RESISTANCE** | | | | |
| | **Afferent** | **Efferent** | **Renal Blood Flow** | **Net Ultrafiltration Pressure** | **GFR** |
| Renal sympathetic nerve | ↑↑ | ↑ | ↓ | ↓ | ↓ |
| Epinephrine | ↑ | ↑ | ↓ | ↔ | ↓ |
| Adenosine | ↑ | ↔ | ↓ | ↓ | ↓ |
| Endothelin-1 | ↑ | ↑↑ | ↓ | ↑ | ↓ |
| NSAIDs | ↑↑ | ↑ | ↓ | ↓ | ↓ |
| Prostaglandin E2, I2 | ↓ | ↓(?) | ↑ | ↑ | ↑ |
| Angiotensin II | ↑ | ↑↑ | ↓ | ↑ | ↔↓ |
| Nitric oxide | ↓ | ↓ | ↑ | ? | ↑(?) |
| Renin-angiotensin system blockade | ↓ | ↓↓ | ↑ | ↓ | a |

[a]In clinical practice, GFR initially decreases and further affects long-term protection of the kidney function (according to decline of intraglomerular pressure in diabetes mellitus patients).
*GFR,* Glomerular filtration rate; *NSAIDs,* nonsteroidal antiinflammatory drugs.

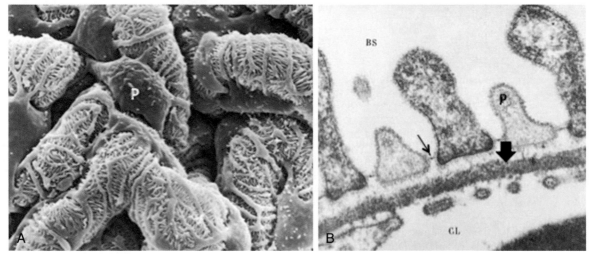

**Fig. 32.2 A,** Scanning electron micrograph of podocytes *(P)* and their processes. **B,** Electron micrograph of podocyte processes *(P),* the glomerular basement membrane, and glomerular capillaries. Slit diaphragms *(arrow)* span the podocyte processes. *Large arrow* points to the lamina densa of the glomerular basement membrane. *BS,* Bowman space; *CL,* glomerular capillary lumen. (From Brenner BM, Rector FC. The Kidney. 4th ed. Vol 1. Philadelphia: WB Saunders; 1991. Figure 19-8 & Figure 19-10).

estimate the GFR because both substances are freely filtered in glomeruli but are not secreted or reabsorbed by the renal tubules. Therefore the filtration rate equals the excretion rate, and GFR equals the concentration of inulin in urine (U) multiplied by the volume of urine production (V) divided by the concentration of inulin in plasma (P), or GFR = UV/P. The GFR is under the influence of many physiologic factors, such as the renin-angiotensin-aldosterone system, cardiac output, sympathetic innervation, hormone and vasoactive substances, and growth factors.

## Tubular Reabsorption

Nutrients, electrolytes, urea, and water are reabsorbed in the renal tubules according to the body's needs (see Fig. 32.2). Substances are passively or actively moved through the tubular epithelia, interstitium, and peritubular capillary endothelia or are moved by facilitation, pinocytosis, or solvent drag ("bulk transport") via either the transcellular or paracellular route.

Primary active transport mechanisms ($Na^+/K^+$-ATPase, $H^+$-ATPase, and $H^+/K^+$-ATPase) require high energy; other secondary transport mechanisms use energy that is released from the cotransport or countertransport of sodium, glucose, amino acids, and $H^+$. The proximal part of the renal tubule and collecting duct is the site of reabsorption of most water, whereas the loop of Henle is impermeable to water.

## Tubular Secretion

In the renal tubule, selected by-products of metabolism, such as some organic compounds bound to plasma proteins that are not filtered, are excreted. A few substances are secreted from peritubular capillaries into the tubular lumen in the energy-dependent process of active transport. Tubular secretion of $H^+$ and $NH_3$, after formation and dissociation of $NH_4^+$ ions within the collecting ducts, is important in maintaining $H^+$ homeostasis, as is secretion of excess $K^+$ in distal nephrons at the collecting duct, a process that is controlled by aldosterone.

## SUGGESTED READINGS

Chawla, L. S., & Ronco, C. (2016). Renal stress testing in the assessment of kidney disease. *Kidney International Reports, 1*, 57–63.

Johnson, R. J., & Feehally, J. (2019). *Comprehensive clinical nephrology* (6th ed.). Edinburgh: Mosby.

Post, E. H., & Vincent, J. L. (2018). Renal autoregulation and blood pressure management in circulatory shock. *Critical Care, 22*, 81.

# 33

# Renal Function Tests

RAJAT N. MOMAN, MD, MA  |  MATTHEW A. WARNER, MD

## Glomerular Filtration Rate

The glomerular filtration rate (GFR) is the amount of plasma filtered through the glomeruli per unit of time and is the single best index of functioning renal mass. Inulin is a sugar that is completely filtered by the glomerulus but is neither secreted nor reabsorbed by the tubule. Thus intravenously administered inulin cleared from the plasma can be used to calculate the GFR. However, inulin clearance is seldom used clinically because the assay is cumbersome and time consuming to perform. Creatinine (Cr) is a metabolic end product of creatine phosphate in skeletal muscle that is cleared by the kidney in a manner like inulin, albeit with limited proximal tubular secretion. Creatinine clearance (CrCl), the most clinically used measure of GFR, can be estimated with formulae such as the Cockcroft-Gault formula:

$$CrCl = \frac{(140 - age)(body\ weight\ in\ kg)}{(serum\ cratinine)(72)}$$

Body weight is multiplied by 0.85 for females in the preceding equation. More precise measurement requires timed collections (over a period of 24 h) of urine and plasma samples and requires use of the formula

$$CrCl = \frac{(UCr \times V)}{PCr}$$

where UCr is the urinary Cr concentration in mg/dL, V is the volume of urine in mL/min, and P is the plasma Cr concentration.

Normal GFR is $120 \pm 25$ mL/min/1.73m$^2$ in men and $95 \pm 20$ mL/min/1.73m$^2$ in women.

## CHRONIC KIDNEY DISEASE AND ACUTE KIDNEY INJURY

Changes in GFR and serum creatinine are often used to define the presence of chronic kidney disease (CKD) and acute kidney injury (AKI). Briefly, CKD is defined by the presence of kidney damage or decreases in kidney function that are present for at least 3 months. CKD stages of increasing severity are identified by progressive decreases in GFR. Serial GFR measurements are important in determining the severity of renal dysfunction and monitoring the progression of disease. Abrupt changes in serum creatinine (e.g., within 48 h) are commonly used to determine the presence of AKI, particularly in perioperative settings, as discussed elsewhere in this book.

## Tubular Function Tests

### FRACTIONAL EXCRETION OF SODIUM

It is useful to measure urinary sodium concentration ($U_{Na+}$) to assess volume status. $U_{Na+}$ concentration of less than 20 mEq/L suggests intravascular volume depletion. $U_{Na+}$ concentration of greater than 40 mEq/L suggests decreased ability of the renal tubules to reabsorb sodium (e.g., acute tubular necrosis [ATN]). A limitation to this test is the fact that $U_{Na+}$ does not reflect the rate of water reabsorption. Fractional excretion of sodium

($FE_{Na+}$) reflects renal tubular sodium reabsorption and can be used to distinguish the etiology of AKI. $FE_{Na+}$ describes sodium clearance as a percentage of CrCl:

$$FE_{Na+} = (sodium\,clearance/CrCl) \times 100\%$$

More commonly, $FE_{Na+}$ is calculated by the formula

$$FE_{Na+} = (U_{Na+} \times S_{Cr})/(S_{Na+} \times U_{Cr}) \times 100\%$$

$FE_{Na+}$ of less than 1% is typically seen in patients with decreased renal perfusion, often caused by hypovolemia or decreased effective circulating volume (e.g., prerenal azotemia). $FE_{Na+}$ of greater than 2% usually indicates tubular damage (e.g., ATN). $FE_{Na+}$ of 1% to 2% may be seen with either disorder or may represent postobstructive kidney injury. $FE_{Na+}$ has several limitations. $FE_{Na+}$ of less than 1% is indicative of prerenal disease only in patients with severe AKI who have greatly reduced GFR. $FE_{Na+}$ of less than 1% may also be seen in other causes of AKI (e.g., acute urinary tract obstruction, acute glomerulonephritis, ATN superimposed on chronic renal disease). Serum creatinine has a delayed uptrend increase in patients with AKI, and a single, early measurement can be misleading. Patients with CKD and those who have sodium wasting for any reason (e.g., diuretic therapy, vomiting, or nasogastric tube suction) have falsely elevated $FE_{Na+}$.

## FRACTIONAL EXCRETION OF UREA NITROGEN

Fractional excretion of urea nitrogen ($FE_{UN}$) can be used to differentiate patients with prerenal disease from those who have ATN in the context of current diuretic use. $FE_{UN}$ of 35% or less is consistent with prerenal azotemia, regardless of whether the patient is receiving diuretic therapy. $FE_{UN}$ is limited by proximal nephron function. In patients with uncontrolled diabetes, glucose-mediated diuresis inhibits proximal reabsorption, and the accuracy of this marker is reduced.

## URINE-CONCENTRATING AND URINE-DILUTING ABILITY

Urine-concentrating ability and urine-diluting ability are assessed by measuring urine osmolality (normal, 300 mOsm/kg; range, 50–1200 mOsm/kg) and can be classified as "appropriate" or "inappropriate" with respect to serum osmolality (or tonicity; normal range is approximately 278–298 mOsm/kg). Normally, as serum tonicity increases (e.g., dehydration or hypovolemia secondary to blood loss), release of antidiuretic hormone causes water conservation, and urine osmolality also increases. The normal tubular response to hypovolemia is to generate a urine-to-plasma osmolality ratio of at least 1.5 (urine osmolality is often 3–4 times plasma osmolality in dehydration). A urine-to-plasma osmolality ratio of 1.0 implies loss of tubular function and supports the diagnosis of acute renal failure. The opposite occurs with dilution of the vascular space, with water diuresis causing urine osmolality to decrease.

## URINARY ACIDIFICATION CAPACITY

The kidneys excrete nonvolatile acids produced by protein catabolism, thereby preventing systemic acidosis. For patients consuming a typical American diet, the pH of a randomly obtained urine sample is usually less than 6.5. An acidification defect can be tested by orally administering ammonium chloride. If urine pH is not less than 5.5 when serum pH is less than 7.35 and $HCO_3^-$ is less than 20 mEq/L, a renal-tubule acidification defect is present.

# Other Clinical and Laboratory Assays

## URINALYSIS

Urinalysis is a useful noninvasive diagnostic tool to assess renal function. Testing includes visual inspection (Table 33.1); dipstick determination of pH (normal, 4.5–8.0), blood, glucose,

| TABLE 33.1 | Urine Color | | |
|---|---|---|---|
| **Color** | **Endogenous Cause** | | **Exogenous Cause** |
| Red | Hemoglobinuria, hematuria, myoglobinuria, porphyria | | Beets, blackberries, chronic mercury or lead exposure, phenolphthalein, phenytoin, phenothiazines, rhubarb, rifampin, hydroxocobalamin |
| Orange | Bilirubinuria, methemoglobinemia, uric acid crystalluria secondary to gastric bypass or chemotherapy | | Carrots, carrot juice, warfarin, ethoxazene, large dose of vitamin C, phenazopyridine, rifampin |
| Brown/black | Bilirubinuria, cirrhosis, hematuria, hepatitis, methemoglobinemia, myoglobinuria, tyrosinemia | | Aloe, cascara/senna laxatives, chloroquine, copper, fava beans, furazolidone, metronidazole, nitrofurantoin, primaquine, rhubarb, sorbitol, methocarbamol, phenacetin, phenol poisoning |
| Blue, blue-green, green | Biliverdin, familial hypercalcemia, indicanuria, urinary tract infection caused by *Pseudomonas* species | | Asparagus, amitriptyline, chlorophyll breath mints, cimetidine, indomethacin, magnesium salicylates, metoclopramide, methylene blue, multivitamins, propofol, promethazine, phenol |
| White | Chyluria, phosphaturia, pyuria | | – |
| Purple | Urinary tract infection caused by *Providencia stuartii, Klebsiella pneumoniae, Pseudomonas aeruginosa, Escherichia coli,* and *Enterococcus* species; porphyria | | Beets, iodine-containing compounds, methylene blue, hydroxocobalamin |

and protein; measurement of specific gravity (normal, 1.003–1.030); and examination of urinary sediment. In patients with porphyria, urine is of normal color when fresh but discolors over time when exposed to light (which is a pathognomonic observation). The pH is rarely diagnostic but in conjunction with serum pH and bicarbonate values, it is useful in evaluating renal tubule acidification function. Dipstick determinations register glucose but not other reducing sugars; elevations in urine glucose concentrations suggest a diagnosis of hyperglycemia or a tubule defect (e.g., Fanconi syndrome or isolated glycosuria). When the plasma glucose concentration is 180 mg/dL or less, all of the glucose filtered by glomeruli is reabsorbed in the proximal tubules. Dipstick determination of glucose crudely indicates a blood glucose concentration of at least 230 mg/dL.

Hemoglobin in the urine can be detected by a dipstick because peroxidase catalyzes the reaction of peroxide and chromogen to produce a colorimetric change. False-positive results may occur if the patient has myoglobin in the urine. Hemoglobin and myoglobin can be distinguished by dissolving 2.8 g ammonium sulfate in 5 mL urine, causing hemoglobin to precipitate. The two pigments can also be distinguished by spectrophotometry, electrophoresis, immunochemical methods, or by noting the presence or absence of red blood cells on microscopic examination. Protein testing is not sensitive for albumin on dipstick analysis.

Urinary sediment is particularly useful in the diagnosis of underlying etiologies of AKI. Sediment is typically bland in prerenal azotemia apart from occasional hyaline casts. However, in AKI secondary to acute tubular injury or necrosis (ATN), renal epithelial cell casts and/or granular casts are often encountered. In acute interstitial nephritis or acute pyelonephritis, white blood cell casts may be encountered. Red cell casts are indicative of glomerular disease such as small vessel vasculitis or other causes of glomerulonephritis.

## CREATININE

Creatinine is an end product of skeletal muscle catabolism excreted solely by the kidneys. Normal serum Cr ranges from 0.8 to 1.3 mg/dL for men and 0.6 to 1.1 for women (ranges vary because of sex-specific differences in muscle mass). Because Cr production is proportional to skeletal muscle mass, elderly patients who have decreased muscle mass compared with younger patients may have normal serum Cr concentrations despite substantial reductions in renal function. The same can be seen in patients who are chronically malnourished. Although CrCl is usually used for the assessment of GFR, in progressive renal dysfunction, CrCl typically overestimates GFR because of increased proximal tubular secretion of creatinine in this setting. As mentioned previously, changes in serum creatinine are often employed to diagnose AKI.

## BLOOD UREA NITROGEN

Blood urea nitrogen (BUN) is a by-product of protein metabolism. The normal value ranges from 8 to 20 mg/dL. BUN values may increase independent of renal function as a result of dehydration, a high-protein diet, degradation of blood from a large hematoma or the gastrointestinal tract, or accelerated catabolism (e.g., a metabolic state observed in patients who have trauma, sepsis, or burns).

Both Cr and BUN values are insensitive measures of changing renal function. For example, in those with normal baseline kidney function, an initial decrease in GFR will not be adequately reflected by changes in creatinine, and patients with a GFR as low as 60 mL/min/1.73m² may still maintain creatinine levels ≤1 mg/mL. Accordingly, both are late indicators of impaired renal function. Classically, dehydration or a prerenal state is suspected in patients with a BUN/serum Cr ratio exceeding 20:1.

## CYSTATIN C

Cystatin C is a low-molecular-weight protein and a member of the cystatin superfamily that is filtered at the glomerulus and is not reabsorbed. Normal values vary by age but range from 0.6 to 1.5 mg/L. This test was initially thought to be less influenced by age, gender, or muscle mass. However, higher levels are associated with factors such as male gender and greater height and weight. The level is less affected by protein intake and likely provides a more precise estimate of kidney function than measurement of serum Cr. A recent prospective cohort study reported cystatin C has a role in identifying patients who are at risk for developing chronic kidney disease 3 months after an episode of acute kidney injury. A combined equation that uses both Cr and cystatin C yields a more accurate reflection of GFR than the use of either cystatin C or Cr alone (Table 33.2).

| TABLE 33.2 | Renal Function Tests |
| --- | --- |
| **Tubular Function Tests** | **Interpretation** |
| Glomerular filtration rate | Normal range, 120 ± 25 mL/min in men and 95 ± 20 mL/min in women |
| Urine sodium | <20 mEq/L, volume depletion; >40 mEq/L, ATN |
| Fractional excretion of sodium | <1%, prerenal disease; >2%, ATN |
| Fractional excretion of urea nitrogen | ≤35%, prerenal azotemia |
| Urine osmolality | Normal, 300 mOsm/kg (range, 50–1200 mOsm/kg) |
| Urine-to-plasma osmolality | Normal response to hypovolemia, ratio 1.5 ratio >1.5 (usually 3–4) |
| **GLOMERULAR FUNCTION TESTS** | |
| Creatinine | Normal range, 0.8–1.3 mg/dL for men and 0.6–1.1 mg/dL for women |
| Blood urea nitrogen | Normal range, 8–20 mg/dL |
| Cystatin C | Normal range (varies by age), 0.6–1.5 mg/L |

*ATN,* Acute tubular necrosis.

## SUGGESTED READINGS

Aklilu, A. M., Avigan, Z. M., & Brewster, U. C. (2021). A unique case of purple urine: A case report and literature review. *Clinical Nephrology, 95*(5), 273–277.

James, M. T., Grams, M. E., Woodward, M., Elley, C. R., Green, J. A., Wheeler, D. C., et al. (2015). A meta-analysis of the association of estimated GFR, albuminuria, diabetes mellitus, and hypertension with acute kidney injury. *American Journal of Kidney Diseases, 66*(4), 602–612.

Privratsky, J. R., Krishnamoorthy, V., Raghunathan, K., Ohnuma, T., Rasouli, M. R., Long, T. E., et al. (2022). Postoperative acute kidney injury is associated with progression of chronic kidney disease independent of severity. *Anesthesia and Analgesia, 134*(1), 49–58.

Wilson, M., Packington, R., Sewell, H., Bartle, R., McCole, E., Kurth, M. J., et al. (2021). Biomarkers during recovery from AKI and prediction of long-term reductions in estimated GFR. *American Journal of Kidney Diseases, 79*(5), 646–656.e1.

Zsom, L., Zsom, M., Salim, S. A., & Fülöp, T. (2022). Estimated glomerular filtration rate in chronic kidney disease: A critical review of estimate-based predictions of individual outcomes in kidney disease. *Toxins (Basel), 14*(2), 127.

# 34

# Acid-Base Status

RAJAT N. MOMAN, MD, MA   |   MATTHEW A. WARNER, MD

## Terminology

Normal values of pH, defined as the negative logarithm of the hydrogen ion concentration $[H^+]$ (expressed in extracellular fluids in nanoequivalents per liter), are generally defined as 7.35 to 7.45. Changes in pH are inversely related to changes in $[H^+]$: a 20% increase in $[H^+]$ decreases the pH by 0.1; conversely, a 20% decrease in $[H^+]$ increases the pH by 0.1 (Table 34.1).

The terms *acidemia* and *alkalemia* refer to the pH of blood. *Acidosis* refers to the process that either adds acid or removes alkali from body fluids; conversely, *alkalosis* is the process that either adds alkali or removes acid from body fluids. Patients can have mixed disorders that include both acidosis and alkalosis. However, they can only be diagnosed with acidemia or alkalemia because these terms are mutually exclusive. *Compensation* refers to the body's homeostatic mechanisms that generate or eliminate $[H^+]$ to normalize pH in response to acid-base disturbances. Base excess, an assessment of the metabolic component of an acid-base disturbance, quantifies the amount of acid that must be added to a blood sample to return the pH of the sample to 7.40 if the patient's $Paco_2$ was 40 mm Hg. A positive base excess value indicates that the patient has a metabolic alkalosis (acid would have to be added to the blood to reach a normal pH); a negative value indicates that the patient has a metabolic acidosis (alkali would have to be added to normalize the pH). In the perioperative setting, anesthesia professionals can often use base excess as a marker for acidosis to determine whether a patient has received adequate fluid resuscitation in relation to surgical bleeding and other fluid losses. Blood gas results are, by convention, reported as pH, $Paco_2$, $Pao_2$, $HCO_3^-$, and base excess. $HCO_3^-$ and base excess are calculated. $HCO_3^-$ is derived with the Henderson-Hasselbalch equation, which can be expressed as either of the following:

$$pH = pKa + \frac{Paco_2}{HCO_3}$$

$$[H^+] = 24 \cdot \frac{Paco_2}{HCO_3^-}$$

Tight control of pH requires a constant $Paco_2/HCO_3^-$ ratio, which allows one to check the validity of an arterial blood gas sample (Table 34.2).

## Types of Acid-Base Disorders

Acid-base disorders may be simple or mixed. Simple disorders include respiratory acid-base disorders, in which the primary

| TABLE 34.1 | pH for Given Hydrogen Ion Concentrations |
|---|---|
| **pH** | **$[H^+]$ (nEq/L)** |
| 7.2 | 64 |
| 7.3 | 50 |
| 7.4 | 40 |
| 7.5 | 30 |
| 7.6 | 24 |

| TABLE 34.2 | Examples of the Use of Henderson-Hasselbalch Equation to Calculate $H^+$ Concentration With a Known $HCO_3^-$ and $PaCO_2$ | | | | |
|---|---|---|---|---|---|
| $PaCO_2$ | $HCO_3^-$ | Predicted [$H^+$] (nEq/L) | Calculation [$H^+$] | | pH |
| 40 | 24 | 40 | $24 \times 40/24 = 40$ | | 7.4 |
| 60 | 24 | 60 | $24 \times 60/24 = 60$ | | 7.2 |
| 20 | 24 | 20 | $24 \times 20/24 = 20$ | | 7.7 |
| 40 | 16 | 60 | $24 \times 40/16 = 60$ | | 7.2 |
| 60 | 16 | 90 | $24 \times 60/16 = 90$ | | 7.05 |
| 20 | 16 | 30 | $24 \times 20/16 = 30$ | | 7.5 |

| TABLE 34.3 | Primary Change and Compensatory Response for the Primary Acid-Base Disorders | |
|---|---|---|
| Primary Disorder | Primary Change | Compensatory Response[a] |
| Respiratory acidosis | ↑ $PaCO_2$ | ↑ $HCO_3^-$ |
| Respiratory alkalosis | ↓ $PaCO_2$ | ↓ $HCO_3^-$ |
| Metabolic acidosis | ↓ $HCO_3^-$ | ↓ $PaCO_2$ |
| Metabolic alkalosis | ↑ $HCO_3^-$ | ↑ $PaCO_2$ |

[a]Homeostatic response in an attempt to maintain constant $PaCO_2/HCO_3^-$ ratio.

change in pH is secondary to changes in $PaCO_2$, and metabolic acid-base disorders, in which the primary change involves $HCO_3^-$. Mixed disorders occur when more than one acid-base disorder exists in the same patient. Acid-base disorders are simply manifestations of underlying systemic disorders. Determining why the acid-base disorder is present requires the incorporation of information from the patient's history and findings on physical examination.

A quick way to determine the cause of a simple acid-base disorder is to look at the direction of change of the pH and $PCO_2$. If both values have decreased or increased, the etiology is most likely metabolic. For example, the finding that both pH and $PCO_2$ are lower than normal suggests a simple metabolic acidosis.

## Compensatory Responses

Every primary acid-base disorder should have an appropriate compensatory response. A primary respiratory (ventilatory) disorder induces a renal response. Reabsorption of $HCO_3^-$ in the proximal tubules is altered to compensate for the change in pH that is induced by the change in $PaCO_2$. This process is slow, with completion of compensation occurring after 2 to 5 days. A primary metabolic disorder, on the other hand, induces a much faster respiratory response, with compensation occurring over 12 to 36 hours through changes in ventilation that increase or decrease $PaCO_2$ (Table 34.3). The absence of timely compensation suggests a secondary disturbance, with the caveat that patients being mechanically ventilated on a controlled mode of mechanical ventilation without spontaneous effort (i.e., in the setting of deep sedation and/or paralysis) will be unable to mount an appropriate compensatory ventilation response.

## Assessment of Acid-Base Disorders Secondary to Metabolic Disorders

### METABOLIC ACIDOSIS

Metabolic acidosis stimulates chemoreceptors that promote an increase in ventilation. When a metabolic acidosis is identified, Winter's formula should be used to calculate the expected $PaCO_2$ and determine the adequacy of respiratory compensation (Table 34.4): if the measured $PaCO_2$ is equal to the expected $PaCO_2$, the patient has a compensated metabolic acidosis. If, on the other hand, the measured $PaCO_2$ is greater than the expected $PaCO_2$, compensation is inadequate and the patient has a primary metabolic acidosis with superimposed respiratory acidosis. However, if the measured $PaCO_2$ is lower than the expected $PaCO_2$, the patient has a primary metabolic acidosis with a superimposed respiratory alkalosis.

The next step in evaluation is to determine the anion gap (AG), which one can calculate by subtracting the sum of $Cl^-$ and $HCO_3^-$ from the $Na^+$ concentration (see Table 34.4). Normal values are $12 \pm 4$ mEq/L. This gap represents the unmeasured negatively charged ions (anions) that balance the electrical charge of the positively charged ions (cations) in humans. In case of metabolic acidosis, expert guidance suggests calculating the plasma anion gap with correction for serum albumin is better than the uncorrected anion gap, where corrected anion gap (cAG) = AG + (40 − [albumin in g/L]) × 0.25. If the patient is diagnosed with a high AG metabolic acidosis, it may be useful to calculate the serum osmolal gap: measured osmoles − calculated osmoles, where calculated osmoles = 2[$Na^+$] + [glucose]/18 + [blood urea nitrogen]/2.8. A serum osmolal gap greater than 10 mOsm/kg is abnormal and suggests an underlying etiology of the high AG metabolic

| TABLE 34.4 | Key Formulas for Interpreting Acid-Base Status | |
|---|---|---|

| Formula Name | Formula | Normal Value |
|---|---|---|
| Winter's formula (for calculating compensation in metabolic acidosis) | $\text{Expected PaCO}_2 = \left(1.5 \cdot \left[\text{HCO}_3^-\right]\right) + 8 - 2$ | Compare expected $\text{PaCO}_2$ with actual $\text{PaCO}_2$ |
| Anion gap (AG) | $\text{AG} = [\text{Na}^+] - ([\text{Cl}^-] + [\text{HCO}_3^-])$ | Normal is $12 \pm 4$ mEq/L |
| Serum osmolal gap | Measured osmoles − calculated osmoles, where calculated osmoles = 2 [Na$^+$] + [glucose]/18 + [blood urea nitrogen]/2.8 | Normal serum osmolal gap is $<10$ mOsm/kg |
| Delta-delta anion gap | Delta ratio = $\Delta\text{AG}/\Delta\text{HCO}_3^-$ = (AG − 12)/ (24 − HCO$_3^-$) | $<0.4$ = non-AG metabolic acidosis<br>0.4–1 = mixed AG + non-AG metabolic acidosis<br>1–2 = pure high AG metabolic acidosis<br>$>2$ = high AG metabolic acidosis + metabolic alkalosis or preexisting respiratory acidosis |
| For calculating compensation in metabolic alkalosis | $\text{Expected PaCO}_2 = 0.7 \cdot \left(\left[\text{HCO}_3^-\right] - 24\right) + 40 - 2$ | If the measured $\text{PaCO}_2$ is equal to the expected $\text{PaCO}_2$, the patient has a metabolic alkalosis; however, if the measured $\text{PaCO}_2$ is greater than the expected $\text{PaCO}_2$, the patient has a metabolic alkalosis with superimposed respiratory acidosis; finally, if the measured $\text{PaCO}_2$ is less than the expected $\text{PaCO}_2$, the patient has a primary metabolic alkalosis with superimposed respiratory alkalosis |
| A-a gradient, at sea level (ambient air); for use in patients with respiratory acid-base disorders | $150 - \text{PaO}_2 - 1.25 \times \text{PaCO}_2$ | Normal is $\leq 10$–20 mm Hg (room air) |
| For respiratory acidosis | For every 10 mm Hg increase in $\text{PCO}_2$, $\text{HCO}_3^-$ increases by 1 mmol/L (acute acidosis) or 3 mmol/L (chronic acidosis) | Normal $\text{PCO}_2$ is considered 40 mm Hg; normal $\text{HCO}_3^-$ is considered 24 mEq/L |
| For respiratory alkalosis | For every 10 mm Hg decrease in $\text{PCO}_2$, $\text{HCO}_3^-$ decreases by 2 mmol/L (acute acidosis) or 4–5 mmol/L (chronic acidosis) | Normal $\text{PCO}_2$ is considered 40 mm Hg; normal $\text{HCO}_3^-$ is considered 24 mEq/L |

acidosis, including ethylene or propylene glycol ingestion, methanol ingestion, severe kidney disease, lactic acidosis, and/or ketoacidosis. Expert guidance suggests first applying the Henderson-Hasselbalch method using the anion gap corrected for albumin in the diagnosis of metabolic acidosis. The Stewart method can be applied in situations where the Henderson-Hasselbalch method does not explain the disorder.

## CAUSES OF AN INCREASED ANION GAP

Remembering the causes of an increase in the AG is facilitated with use of the mnemonic GOLDMARRK: glycols (ethylene and propylene), oxoproline, L-lactate, D-lactate, methanol, aspirin, renal failure, rhabdomyolysis, and ketoacidosis (diabetes, starvation, and excess alcohol intake in a malnourished patient).

## CAUSES OF A DECREASED ANION GAP

Processes that decrease the unmeasured anions or increase the unmeasured cations decrease the AG. Albumin is an anion that is responsible for approximately half of the normal AG of 12 mEq/L. If the albumin concentration is low, the AG will be lower than normal (i.e., <12 mEq/L), decreasing by approximately 2 to 3 units for every 1-g/dL decrease in serum albumin concentration. Conversely, immunoglobulins are cations, and if they increase (i.e., in paraproteinemias, such as multiple

myeloma), the kidneys retain additional chloride to maintain electrical neutrality and the AG decreases.

## CAUSES OF NON–ANION GAP METABOLIC ACIDOSIS

In metabolic acidosis without an AG, the body compensates for loss of $\text{HCO}_3^-$ by increasing chloride. Primary causes of a metabolic acidosis without an AG include gastrointestinal losses (diarrhea, small bowel fistula, ileostomy, ureterosigmoidostomy, or an ileal conduit for a ureter), urinary losses (proximal and distal renal tubular acidosis, carbonic anhydrase inhibitor therapy, hypoaldosteronism, urinary obstruction, pancreatic fistula, or the correction phase of diabetic ketoacidosis), and infusion of isotonic saline.

## DELTA ANION GAP RATIO STRATEGY

Clinicians may use the delta AG ratio strategy in patients with metabolic acidosis to detect the possibility of a superimposed metabolic alkalosis or a non-AG metabolic acidosis (see Table 34.4).

$$\text{Delta ratio} = \Delta\text{AG}/\Delta\text{HCO}_3^- = (\text{AG} - 12)/(24 - \text{HCO}_3^-)$$

If the delta ratio is less than 0.4, a hyperchloremic non-AG metabolic acidosis should be considered. If the delta ratio is

0.4 to 1, a mixed high AG metabolic acidosis and non-AG metabolic acidosis should be considered. If the delta ratio is 1 to 2, a high AG metabolic acidosis should be considered. If the delta ratio is greater than 2, a high AG metabolic acidosis in the setting of a concurrent metabolic alkalosis or a preexisting compensated respiratory acidosis should be considered.

## METABOLIC ALKALOSIS

Metabolic alkalosis can be chloride responsive or resistant. Chloride-responsive states, which are associated with urinary chloride concentrations of less than 15 mEq/L, include vomiting, continuous nasogastric suctioning, and volume-contraction states. Volume-contraction states are the most common in hospitalized postsurgical patients. Chloride-resistant disorders, associated with urinary chloride concentrations of greater than 25 mEq/L, include hypercortisolism, hyperaldosteronism, sodium bicarbonate therapy, severe renal artery stenosis, hypokalemia, and the use of diuretics, in which case patients may have high urinary chloride concentrations but the alkalosis nonetheless responds to the administration of chloride. The $Paco_2$ in patients with metabolic alkalosis can be calculated: if the measured $Paco_2$ is equal to the expected $Paco_2$, the patient has a metabolic alkalosis. However, if the measured $Paco_2$ is greater than the expected $Paco_2$, the patient has a metabolic alkalosis with superimposed respiratory acidosis. Finally, if the measured $Paco_2$ is less than the expected $Paco_2$, the patient has a primary metabolic alkalosis with superimposed respiratory alkalosis.

## Assessment of Acid-Base Disorders Secondary to Respiratory Mechanics

Although clinicians can use equations to calculate the expected change in pH for acute changes in $Paco_2$, the easiest way to assess the influences of $Paco_2$ on pH is to remember that the pH changes inversely 0.08 for every acute 10-mm Hg change in $Paco_2$. For example, if the $Paco_2$ abruptly increases to 50 mm Hg, the pH is expected to reach 7.32; if the $Paco_2$ is 30 mm Hg, the pH will be 7.48.

Acid-base disorders caused by respiratory mechanics are the most common acid-base disorders seen in otherwise "healthy" patients who are anesthetized for surgical procedures.

If respiratory disorders are more longstanding (e.g., respiratory acidosis in a patient with chronic obstructive pulmonary disease or a ventilated patient in the intensive care unit who is retaining $CO_2$), the kidneys will retain $HCO_3^-$ to minimize the change in pH.

Respiratory acidosis (see Table 34.4):
For every 10-mm Hg increase in $Pco_2$, $HCO_3^-$ increases by 1 mmol/L (acute acidosis) or 3 mmol/L (chronic acidosis).
Respiratory alkalosis (see Table 34.4):
For every 10-mm Hg decrease in $Pco_2$, $HCO_3^-$ decreases by 2 mmol/L (acute acidosis) or 4 to 5 mmol/L (chronic acidosis).

## RESPIRATORY ACIDOSIS

Causes of respiratory acidosis include airway obstruction, hypoventilation, central nervous system depression, flail chest, laryngospasm, the use of opioids or sedatives associated with hypoventilation, restrictive lung disease (kyphoscoliosis, fibrothorax), and neuromuscular diseases.

## RESPIRATORY ALKALOSIS

Causes of respiratory alkalosis include psychogenic hyperventilation, encephalitis, early pneumonia, early stages of bronchial asthma, pulmonary embolism, hepatic failure, early sepsis, and pregnancy. The lowest $Paco_2$ achieved by hyperventilation is approximately 16 mm Hg, and the pH is approximately 7.6 before renal compensatory changes occur.

## SUGGESTED READINGS

Allen, M. (2011). Lactate and acid base as a hemodynamic monitor and markers of cellular perfusion. *Pediatric Critical Care Medicine, 12*(Suppl. 4), S43–S49.

Berend, K., de Vries, A. P. J., & Gans, R. O. B. (2014). Physiological approach to assessment of acid-base disturbances. *New England Journal of Medicine, 371*(15), 1434–1445.

Jung, B., Martinez, M., Claessens, Y. E., Darmon, M., Klouche, K., Lautrette, A., et al. (2019). Diagnosis and management of metabolic acidosis: Guidelines from a French expert panel. *Annals of Intensive Care, 9*(1), 92.

Kamel, K. S., & Halperin, M. L. (2021). Use of urine electrolytes and urine osmolality in the clinical diagnosis of fluid, electrolytes, and acid-base disorders. *Kidney International Reports, 6*(5), 1211–1224.

Seifter, J. L. (2020). Anion-gap metabolic acidemia: Case-based analyses. *European Journal of Clinical Nutrition, 74*(Suppl. 1), 83–86.

# Electrolyte Abnormalities: Potassium, Sodium, Calcium, and Magnesium

DENZIL R. HILL, MD

Electrolytes are critical elements of cellular electrophysiology that are involved in a myriad of cellular enzymatic processes. This chapter will focus on anesthetic implications of alterations in several important cations. The suggested readings provide additional details on the associated pathophysiology and perioperative management.

## Potassium

The total body potassium store in a 70-kg person exceeds 3500 mEq, with less than 2% located in extracellular fluid. Potassium balance is primarily maintained by oral intake and renal elimination. Extracellular potassium is dependent on multiple factors, including acid-base balance, the activity and sensitivity of insulin, sodium-potassium adenosine triphosphate–dependent exchange channels, and blood insulin and catecholamine levels.

### HYPERKALEMIA

The most significant clinical effect of hyperkalemia involves the electrical conduction system of the heart. These changes include gradual prolongation of the PR interval (with eventual loss of the P wave), prolongation of the QRS complex, ST-segment elevation, and peaking of T waves that can ultimately lead to ventricular arrhythmias (Fig. 35.1). Cardiac conduction changes usually occur when the plasma potassium concentration exceeds 6.5 mmol/L, but they may develop at lower levels in the setting of acute hyperkalemia. Options for acute management rely on membrane stabilization and intracellular shifting of potassium and include administration of calcium chloride, sodium bicarbonate, and insulin with glucose. Membrane stabilization is a critical but temporary solution, and the underlying causes of hyperkalemia should be investigated and corrected.

### HYPOKALEMIA

For every 1-mmol/L decrease in plasma potassium concentration, the total body potassium store decreases by approximately 200 to 300 mmol. Characteristic electrocardiographic changes associated with hypokalemia include gradual prolongation of the QRS interval, with subsequent development of prominent U waves (Fig. 35.2). Hypokalemia is associated with an increased incidence of atrial and ventricular arrhythmias, and low serum potassium has also been associated with worsening outcomes in the setting of acute myocardial infarction. Hypokalemia may be associated with weakness and potentiate the effect of neuromuscular blocking agents. To treat hypokalemia, the clinician must consider the patient's total body potassium levels and the chronicity of the hypokalemia. Chronic hypokalemia is associated with a true decrease in total body potassium stores, whereas hypokalemia with normal body stores of potassium occurs more acutely. Treatment of hypokalemia involves oral or intravenous replacement of potassium. Intravenous potassium replacement should be gradual to avoid acute overcorrection and hyperkalemia. Respiratory and metabolic alkalosis should be avoided because alkalosis will worsen hypokalemia secondary to intracellular shifting.

## Sodium

Serum sodium concentration is dependent on the relationship of total body sodium levels and total body water. Therefore the treatment of abnormal serum sodium concentrations must take into account both total body sodium stores and total body

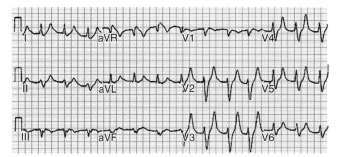

**Fig. 35.1** Marked widening of the QRS duration combined with tall peaked T waves is suggestive of advanced hyperkalemia. Note the absence of P waves, suggesting a junctional rhythm; however, in hyperkalemia, the atrial muscle may be paralyzed while the heart is still in sinus rhythm. (Courtesy Frank G. Yanowitz, MD, Professor of Medicine, University of Utah School of Medicine, Medical Director, ECG Department, LDS Hospital, Salt Lake City, UT.)

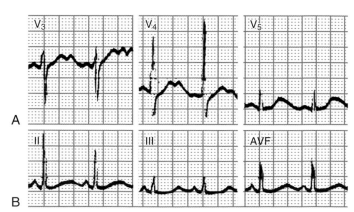

**Fig. 35.2** **A,** Note the prominent U wave in leads V₃ and V₄, giving the conjoined TU wave the appearance of a camel's hump. **B,** Note the "apparently" prolonged QT interval in leads S₂ and aVF that is explained by the fact that the T wave is actually a U wave with a flattened T wave that merges into the following U wave. (Courtesy Frank G. Yanowitz, MD, Professor of Medicine, University of Utah School of Medicine, Medical Director, ECG Department, LDS Hospital, Salt Lake City, UT.)

water. To a great extent, thirst and free water administration, sodium intake, and renal salt and water handling regulate water balance, although in many clinical situations the body's ability to regulate this relationship is impaired. When correcting sodium, changes in free water and sodium concentration are often difficult to predict; thus frequent assessment of serum sodium concentration and volume status may be required.

## HYPERNATREMIA

Hypernatremia is defined as serum sodium concentration of greater than 145 mmol/L and is often associated with a deficiency in total body water. Manifestations of hypernatremia include mental status changes, hyperreflexia, ataxia, and seizures. Free water deficit can be calculated as follows: free water deficit, in liters $= (0.6 \times \text{weight, in kg}) \times ([\text{serum sodium}/140] - 1)$. Free water is administered to correct hypernatremia, although treatment of severe central diabetes insipidus may involve the use of subcutaneously or intravenously administered desmopressin. In the setting of hypervolemic hypernatremia, diuretics may be required to allow for elimination of both water and sodium while free water is administered.

## HYPONATREMIA

Hyponatremia is a serum sodium concentration of less than 135 mmol/L. Hyponatremia may present with mental status changes, lethargy, cramps, decreased deep tendon reflexes, and seizures. A serum sodium concentration of less than 120 mmol/L is a potentially life-threatening condition, with associated mortality rates reported to be as high as 50%. However, if the correction of hyponatremia occurs too rapidly, a demyelinating brainstem lesion (central pontine myelinolysis) may cause permanent neurologic damage. In severely symptomatic patients, the recommendation is to correct sodium at a rate of 1 to 2 $\text{mmol} \cdot \text{L}^{-1} \cdot \text{h}^{-1}$ until the serum sodium concentration reaches 125 to 130 mmol/L. In hypervolemic or euvolemic hyponatremia, hypertonic (2%–3%) saline may be used to treat symptomatic patients or patients who would not tolerate additional intravascular volume. To avoid hyperchloremic metabolic acidosis, it may be desirable to administer hypertonic saline formulated as 50% sodium chloride and 50% sodium acetate. When administering solutions with a saline concentration of greater than 2%, clinicians should consider using central venous access. Management of hypervolemic hyponatremia may include administration of diuretics. After administration of diuretics, the concentration of sodium in the urine may be as high as 70 to 80 mEq/L (one-half normal saline), thus resulting in loss of free water and increasing the serum sodium concentration.

## Calcium

The total serum calcium concentration comprises three fractions: 50% protein-bound calcium (particularly to albumin), 5% to 10% anion-bound calcium, and 40% to 45% free, or ionized, calcium. Maintenance of a normal serum calcium concentration involves parathyroid hormone and calcitonin, which regulate the release and uptake of calcium and phosphorus by the kidneys, bones, and intestines through negative-feedback regulation. Ionized calcium is considered the gold standard when choosing to assess an individual's calcium status. If this is not available, a serum albumin concentration should be investigated to help determine a corrected total calcium concentration

(approximately 0.8 mg/dL or 0.2 mmol/L for every 1-g/dL fall in serum albumin).

## HYPERCALCEMIA

Common causes of hypercalcemia include hyperparathyroidism and malignancies that increase mobilization of calcium from bone. Symptoms include nausea, polyuria, and dehydration. Electrocardiographic monitoring may demonstrate prolonged PR intervals, wide QRS complexes, and shortened QT intervals as hypercalcemia worsens. Avoidance of respiratory alkalosis may be beneficial because alkalosis lowers the plasma potassium concentration, potentially exacerbating cardiac conduction abnormalities. Management of hypercalcemia includes hydration and diuresis to promote renal elimination. In acute toxicity or renal failure, hemodialysis should be considered.

## HYPOCALCEMIA

Multiple factors contribute to the development of hypocalcemia. Acquired hypoparathyroidism after neck surgery is a common cause of hypocalcemia because of decreased parathyroid hormone levels. Respiratory or metabolic alkalosis induces hypocalcemia by increasing protein binding to calcium, thereby decreasing the amount of ionized calcium. Renal failure decreases the conversion of vitamin D to 1,25-dihydroxyvitamin D, thereby decreasing intestinal and bone absorption while increasing serum phosphate levels; the phosphate then combines with calcium and precipitates as $CaPO_4$. Massive blood transfusion may also result in hypocalcemia secondary to anticoagulants (ethylenediaminetetra-acetic acid in transfused blood, which chelates calcium). Hypocalcemia is often asymptomatic, although severe hypocalcemia may be associated with a prolonged QT interval, bradycardia, peripheral vasodilation, and decreased cardiac contractility, any of which can cause hypotension. Neurologic manifestations of hypocalcemia include perioral numbness, muscle cramps, tetany, hyperreflexia, and seizures. Several factors guide calcium replacement therapy, including the absolute serum calcium level, the rapidity of the drop in serum calcium concentration, and the underlying disease process. Calcium causes vasoconstriction, and extravascular infiltration may be associated with morbidity. In patients who have no symptoms, observation may be the most appropriate treatment. Calcium chloride contains three times the amount of calcium compared with calcium gluconate.

## Magnesium

Primary determinants of total body magnesium are intake and renal excretion. Determination of magnesium deficiency is difficult because magnesium is primarily an intracellular ion and the serum magnesium concentration may not reflect tissue levels. Nonetheless, therapy for magnesium disorders, almost exclusively hypomagnesemia, is often guided by the serum magnesium concentration (normal, 1.7–2.1 mg/dL).

## HYPOMAGNESEMIA

Multiple factors may contribute to magnesium depletion, including decreased intake, impaired intestinal absorption, and increased gastrointestinal and renal losses. Hypomagnesemia is most often asymptomatic, but life-threatening neurologic and cardiac sequelae may develop. Hypomagnesemia may cause neuromuscular excitability, mental status changes, and seizures. Considerable evidence supports an association between hypomagnesemia and cardiac arrhythmias and potentiation of digoxin toxicity. Electrocardiographic changes include a prolonged QT interval and atrial and ventricular ectopy. Magnesium has been advocated as a treatment for torsades de pointes and digoxin toxicity arrhythmias, and indeed, evidence exists that a trial of $MgSO_4$ may be useful in the management of most arrhythmias. The cardiovascular effects of even rapid administration of intravenous $MgSO_4$ (4 g over 10 min) are minimal, with small decreases in blood pressure (<10%) being the most common effect. Replacement of potassium in patients with hypomagnesemia is notoriously difficult, and it is often necessary to replace both ions simultaneously.

## HYPERMAGNESEMIA

Hypermagnesemia most commonly develops in the setting of renal failure and occasionally with excessive magnesium intake (e.g., during magnesium therapy for preeclampsia). Manifestations of hypermagnesemia begin to occur when the serum magnesium concentration exceeds 5 mg/dL, and they are primarily neurologic and cardiovascular. Hyporeflexia, sedation, and weakness are common. Electrocardiographic changes are variable, but often include a widened QRS complex and a prolonged PR interval. Treatment includes enhancing renal excretion with loop diuretics and, in the setting of renal failure, dialysis. Calcium may be administered to temporarily antagonize the effects of hypermagnesemia.

## SUGGESTED READINGS

Adrogué, H. J., & Madias, N. E. (2000a). Hypernatremia. *New England Journal of Medicine, 342,* 1493–1499.

Adrogué, H. J., & Madias, N. E. (2000b). Hyponatremia. *New England Journal of Medicine, 342,* 1581–1589.

Ghali, J. K. (2008). Mechanisms, risks, and new treatment options for hyponatremia. *Cardiology, 111,* 147–157.

Lindner, G., & Funk, G. C. (2013). Hypernatremia in critically ill patients. *Journal of Critical Care, 28*(2), 216.e11–216.e20.

Pokaharel, M., & Block, C. A. (2011). Dysnatremia in the ICU. *Current Opinion in Critical Care, 17*(6), 581–593.

Thakker, R. (2006). Hypocalcemia: Pathogenesis, differential diagnosis, and management. *American Society of Bone and Mineral Research, 6,* 213.

Tommasino, C., & Picozzi, V. (2007). Volume and electrolyte management. *Best Practice and Research Clinical Anaesthesiology, 21,* 497–516.

Weisberg, L. S. (2008). Management of severe hyperkalemia. *Critical Care Medicine, 36,* 3246–3251.

# 36

# Hepatic Physiology, Preoperative Evaluation, and Planning

JORDAN S. POGU, MD  |  BRIDGET P. PULOS, MD

The prevalence of hepatic disease continues to rise in the United States, with liver cirrhosis currently ranked as the 11th leading cause of death, according to the Centers for Disease Control and Prevention's most recent National Vital Statistics System report. The most common causes of end-stage hepatic disease include viral hepatitis, alcohol-related liver disease, and nonalcohol obesity-related liver disease. Although patients with preexisting severe hepatic dysfunction are known to be at significant risk for perioperative morbidity and mortality, data on the anesthetic implications for patients with mild to moderate hepatic dysfunction remain limited. These patients may be asymptomatic when they are scheduled for elective surgery, which presents the anesthesiologist with a unique set of challenges when caring for this growing population.

Unexpected hepatic dysfunction may also develop postoperatively. Because liver function test results correlate with hepatocellular integrity rather than function, these tests are not obtained routinely in the preoperative setting. Thus some patients may have had preexisting hepatic dysfunction that was not clinically apparent. Intraoperative causes of postoperative hepatic dysfunction may be surgical or pharmacologic. Etiologies of surgical stress include traction (e.g., during gastric bypass surgery) or pneumoperitoneum (e.g., during laparoscopic surgery). From a pharmacologic perspective, all halogenated inhalational agents have the potential to cause liver injury. The mechanism of this injury is believed to be an immunogenic response to the trifluoroacetylated components produced by the metabolism of volatile anesthetics. Fortunately, although the risk of halothane-associated hepatitis was significant in the past (~1 in 15,000 on first exposure), newer volatile anesthetics (e.g., sevoflurane) carry a much lower risk.

Although liver biopsy remains the gold standard for the diagnosis, grading, and staging of liver disease, a thorough preoperative examination is critically important to identify hepatic dysfunction. All general anesthetics decrease the already low arterial pressure in patients with end-stage liver disease. Care must be taken to optimize intravascular fluid volume, minimize positive-pressure ventilation, and maintain normocapnia to ensure adequate blood flow to the hepatic artery. In terms of medication choices, there are few absolute contraindications, although it remains important to consider the potential pharmacokinetic changes in the setting of hepatic dysfunction. For example, the anesthesia provider must make dosing adjustments to account for the decrease in plasma protein.

## Hepatic Physiology

A detailed understanding of hepatic physiology and perioperative optimization allows anesthesiologists to provide the safest anesthetic possible.

### METABOLIC FUNCTION

#### Glucose Homeostasis

The liver maintains glucose homeostasis via several mechanisms: the conversion of fats and proteins to glucose by gluconeogenesis, glycogenesis (glucose $\rightarrow$ glycogen; 75 g stored in liver $\approx$ 24-h supply), and the release of glucose from glycogen by glycogenolysis. Insulin stimulates glycogenesis and inhibits gluconeogenesis and the oxidation of fatty acids. Glucagon and epinephrine have the opposite effect of inhibiting glycogenesis and stimulating gluconeogenesis.

#### Fat Metabolism

Beta oxidation of fatty acids between meals provides a substantial proportion of body energy requirements, reducing the need for gluconeogenesis.

#### Protein Synthesis

All plasma proteins are produced in the liver, except $\gamma$-globulins, which are synthesized in the reticuloendothelial system, and antihemophilic factor VIII, which is produced by the vascular and glomerular endothelium, as well as the sinusoidal cells of the liver. Most drugs administered by anesthesia providers are metabolized by the liver, with many of the metabolites excreted through the biliary system.

## Hepatic Blood Flow

Total hepatic blood flow (HBF) is approximately $100 \ mL \cdot 100 \ g^{-1} \cdot min^{-1}$. Most (75%) HBF goes through the portal vein. This blood is rich in nutrients from the gastrointestinal tract, but it is partially deoxygenated and supplies only 50% to 55% of the hepatic oxygen requirements. The hepatic artery supplies 25% of HBF but contributes 45% to 50% of the hepatic oxygen requirements.

Splanchnic vessels supplying the portal vein receive sympathetic innervation from T3 through T11. Hypoxemia, hypercarbia, and catecholamines produce hepatic artery and portal vein vasoconstriction and decrease HBF. β-Adrenergic blockade,

positive end-expiratory pressure, positive-pressure ventilation (increased intrathoracic pressure increases hepatic vein pressure, which in turn decreases HBF), inhalation anesthetic agents, regional anesthesia with a sensory level above T5, and surgical stimulation (proximity of surgery to the liver determines the degree of the reduction) can all reduce HBF.

## Preoperative Hepatic Assessment

The goal of perioperative examination of patients with hepatic dysfunction is to identify the severity and the extrahepatic manifestations of the disease. A detailed understanding of patient-specific sequelae of liver disease allows the anesthesiologist to optimize the patient preoperatively and develop an appropriate anesthetic plan.

Preoperative assessment often requires a multidisciplinary approach that includes the primary care physician, the surgical team, and the anesthesiologist. Preoperative investigations may include invasive cardiac screening, chest radiology, and cardiac ultrasonography, in addition to blood tests.

### PHYSICAL EXAMINATION

*Cardiovascular:* End-stage liver disease produces a hyperdynamic cardiac state, in which increased cardiac output compensates for chronically low systemic vascular resistance. These patients often have coexisting coronary artery disease and may have myocardial ischemia, despite the decreased workload on the left ventricle. Preoperative assessment of cardiomyopathy and cardiac risk factors is critical. This assessment often includes an electrocardiograph and echocardiogram, with potential need for subsequent stress testing, angiography, or formal cardiac consultation. The preoperative history should include a discussion of physical status, metabolic equivalents achievable, and any history of angina. Physical examination should focus on signs or symptoms of heart failure, decreased ejection fraction, or new murmurs.

*Respiratory:* Hepatic dysfunction threatens respiratory function. Primarily, ascites or pleural effusions may cause atelectasis and decreased functional residual capacity, which may then lead to hypoxia and increased risk of aspiration on induction. Perioperative optimization may involve preoperative paracentesis, and a rapid sequence induction may be chosen to reduce the risk of aspiration. Intrapulmonary shunting is another cause of perioperative hypoxemia that often develops in patients with end-stage liver disease. These patients may have clinically significant orthodeoxia, which is hypoxia relieved in the supine position. This condition is termed *hepatopulmonary syndrome*, and the gold standard for diagnosis is agitated saline testing under echocardiography. Symptoms resolve shortly after liver transplantation.

*Neurologic:* Patients should be assessed for any signs of encephalopathy as reported by the patient, the family, or medical records. Benzodiazepine premedication should be avoided given the risk of exacerbating preexisting encephalopathy in the setting of decreased hepatic clearance and prolonged medication half-life. Vitamin and nutritional deficiencies should be corrected preoperatively, such as thiamine deficiency in patients with alcohol-induced hepatitis. All other patients should continue home synthetic disaccharides and avoid excessive protein intake preoperatively.

*Gastroenterologic:* Patients should be assessed for the presence of portal hypertension, ascites, or symptoms indicative of gastric or esophageal varices. In patients with endoscopic or historical evidence of varices, it is important to avoid esophageal temperature monitoring and limit oropharyngeal suctioning. Patients with severe disease may warrant preoperative endoscopic banding. In patients with severe ascites requiring preoperative or intraoperative paracentesis, the anesthesia provider must remain vigilant to correct the subsequent decrease in plasma volume that occurs secondary to the fluid shifts of reaccumulation.

## LABORATORY INVESTIGATIONS

Routine preoperative laboratory studies for patients with liver disease should include a complete blood count, an electrolyte panel, prealbumin levels, and coagulation studies (potentially including thromboelastogram). Electrolytes often show pronounced hyponatremia due to fluid retention, which should be corrected judiciously, when appropriate, to avoid central pontine myelinolysis. Patients with severe liver disease often have anemia and thrombocytopenia. In addition, patients may have complex coagulopathies as the liver synthesizes most of the anticoagulant and procoagulant proteins. Preoperative type and screen should be considered, as transfusions of red blood cells, fresh frozen plasma, and platelets are often required during surgery.

## INDICATORS OF MORTALITY RISK

Two indices have commonly been used to assess preoperative risk in patients with underlying liver disease. The Child-Pugh score, the first scoring system used to stratify the severity of end-stage hepatic dysfunction, includes five criteria: presence of ascites, hepatic encephalopathy, international normalized ratio (INR), serum albumin, and bilirubin concentration. Patients are then stratified into three risk categories: A, minimal; B, moderate; and C, severe.

The current preferred preoperative assessment tool is the model for end-stage liver disease (MELD) score. It uses only three laboratory values to assess end-stage liver disease: INR, serum creatinine, and serum bilirubin concentration.

Patients with scores of less than 10 are acceptable candidates for elective procedures; in patients with scores of 10 to 20, surgery is associated with increased risk; in patients with scores of greater than 20, surgical procedures should be avoided unless other options have been exhausted. The MELD score is also used by the United Network for Organ Sharing to allocate cadaveric livers for transplantation.

# Regional Anesthesia and Multimodal Pain Management

The complex array of physiologic changes associated with hepatic dysfunction increases the risk of perioperative morbidity when considering not only general anesthesia but also perioperative and postoperative pain management. For example, general anesthesia is known to reduce hepatic blood flow, with potential for hepatic ischemia and subsequent exacerbation of preexisting impaired hepatic function. Postoperatively, altered metabolism and increased susceptibility to the adverse effects of pain medications, including opiates, remains a concern. Thus patients with liver dysfunction may benefit from the use of regional anesthesia. Many studies assessing regional techniques in

patients with hepatic dysfunction focus on patients undergoing hepatic resection, a procedure with an elevated risk of significant postoperative pain.

The most common regional technique employed in these patients is thoracic epidural anesthesia (TEA), which has been shown to provide superior pain relief and reduce pulmonary complications and the incidence of postoperative ileus compared with opiates. Animal models have also shown increased hepatic blood flow with TEA, a theoretical benefit in those with hepatic dysfunction, although this has not yet been demonstrated in humans. Despite these benefits, a debate remains as to the safety of regional techniques in hepatic dysfunction, with significant concern for the ramifications of a coexisting coagulopathy, including delayed catheter removal, epidural hematoma, and potential for devastating neurologic injury. The risk for epidural hematoma in the setting of coagulopathy was found to be about 1 in 315 in a large retrospective study. There is also concern that despite offering more effective pain control than opiates, TEA may reduce early postoperative mobilization due to associated hypotension and cumbersome equipment.

Although peripheral nerve blocks may also be used, there is an even greater paucity of pertinent data than that of neuraxial anesthesia. The most frequently performed technique is a subcostal transverse abduminus plane block, which has been shown to provide effective pain management in several randomized control trials, via both single injection and continuous infusion. Given the propensity for coagulopathy in these patients, it is recommended that additional care be taken when performing blocks near noncompressible vascular structures (e.g., subclavian artery for an infraclavicular block) and deep structures (e.g., lumbar plexus), which may lead to a retroperitoneal hematoma.

Another consideration in the use of regional anesthetic techniques in hepatic dysfunction is the altered metabolism of local anesthetics. Amide anesthetic metabolism is described by the hepatic extraction ratio, which demonstrates that clearance is dependent on both hepatic enzyme activity and hepatic blood flow, both of which are affected by liver disease, potentially increasing the risk of local anesthetic toxicity. It is also important to note that volume of distribution is increased in hepatic dysfunction, meaning that plasma levels in these patients may resemble those without liver disease for a single administration of local anesthetic. However, if a continuous infusion or repeated boluses are used, dose adjustment is likely necessary.

The American Society of Regional Anesthesia and Pain Medicine published consensus guidelines regarding regional techniques in the setting of anticoagulation. Although these may be of some utility in general guidance, it is important to point out that these guidelines are not specific to liver-associated coagulopathy. For example, an INR of 1.5 is often considered a marker for normal hemostasis. INR is often elevated in hepatic dysfunction due to the effects of liver disease on vitamin K–dependent clotting factor synthesis. However, in these patients the predictability of INR for hemorrhage after a bedside procedure has not been shown to be reliable. Thus utilization of a regional technique as part of a multimodal pain management strategy in patients with hepatic dysfunction often depends on a risk-versus-benefit discussion, with careful coagulation status evaluation and correction of coagulopathy when applicable.

## SUGGESTED READINGS

Dieu, A., Huynen, P., Lavand'homme, P., Beloeil, H., Freys, S. M., Pogatzki-Zahn, E. M., et al. (2021). Pain management after open liver resection: Procedure-Specific Postoperative Pain Management (PROSPECT) recommendations. *Regional Anesthesia & Pain Medicine, 46,* 433–445.

Newman, K. L., Johnson, K. M., Cornia, P. B., Wu, P., Itani, K., & Ioannou, G. N. (2020). Perioperative evaluation and management of patients with cirrhosis: Risk assessment, surgical outcomes, and future directions. *Clinical Gastroenterology and Hepatology, 18,* 2398–2414.e3.

Rahimzadeh, P., Safari, S., Faiz, S. H. R., & Alavian, S. M. (2014). Anesthesia for patients with liver disease. *Hepatitis Monthly, 14,* e19881.

Simmons, F., Pustavoitau, A., & Merritt, W. T. (2022). Diseases of the liver and biliary tract. In R. L. Hines, & S. B. Jones (Eds.), *Stoelting's anesthesia and co-existing disease* (8th ed., pp. 333–346). Philadelphia: Elsevier Saunders.

Steadman, R. H., & Braunfeld, M. Y. (2017). The liver: Surgery and anesthesia. In P. G. Barash, B. F. Cullen, & R. K. Stoelting (Eds.), *Clinical anesthesia* (8th ed., pp. 1298–1326). Philadelphia: Lippincott Williams & Wilkins.

Vaja, R., & Rana, M. (2020). Drugs and the liver. *Anaesthesia International Care Medicine, 21,* 517–523.

# 37

# Mechanisms of Hepatic Drug Metabolism and Excretion

WOLF H. STAPELFELDT, MD

*Drug clearance* is defined as the theoretical volume of blood from which a drug is completely removed within a given time interval. *Total drug clearance* ($CL_{total}$) is the sum of clearances based on a variety of applicable elimination pathways (hepatic, renal, pulmonary, intestinal, plasma, other). A drug is considered to be hepatically eliminated if hepatic clearance ($CL_{hepatic}$) assumes a large proportion of total body clearance ($CL_{hepatic} \approx CL_{total}$). This method is the case for most drugs metabolized in humans. Examples of a minority of drugs for which metabolism is independent of hepatic function include esmolol (metabolized by esterases located in erythrocytes), remifentanil (metabolized by nonspecific esterases in muscle and intestines), and cisatracurium (metabolized by Hoffman elimination in plasma). However, most drugs depend, either directly or indirectly, on adequate hepatic function for metabolism and elimination.

## Hepatic Clearance

$CL_{hepatic}$ is the volume of blood from which a drug is removed as it passes through the liver within a given time interval. Therefore $CL_{hepatic}$ is limited by the volume of blood flowing through the liver within the same time interval ($\dot{Q}_{hepatic}$). Disease-induced or anesthetic-induced reductions in total hepatic blood flow are the principal causes of diminished hepatic clearance for a majority of drugs; the elimination of these drugs is termed *flow limited*. Other factors that affect hepatic clearance include maximal hepatic metabolic enzyme activity, expressed as intrinsic clearance:

$$CL_{intrinsic} \approx V_m / k_m$$

where $V_m$ = maximal metabolic rate (mg/min) and $k_m$ (Michaelis constant) = drug concentration producing the half-maximal metabolic rate (mg/L). In this case drug elimination is termed *capacity limited*. In this situation, unlike the flow-limited condition, drug elimination may change as a function of free-drug concentration that is available for hepatic metabolism and thus may be affected by the amount of protein binding and disease-induced changes in protein binding. Whether the hepatic elimination of a drug is flow limited or capacity limited depends on the ratio of the free-plasma concentration of the drug to $k_m$ (flow limited if <0.5) and that of the $CL_{intrinsic}$ to total hepatic blood flow ($\dot{Q}_{hepatic}$) of the drug, which determines the extraction ratio (ER) of the drug (ER = $CL_{hepatic}/\dot{Q}_{hepatic}$), according to the formula (Fig. 37.1)

$$ER = CL_{intrinsic} / (\dot{Q}_{hepatic} + CL_{intrinsic})$$

Depending on these ratios, different types of hepatic ERs have been described (Table 37.1).

### HIGH–EXTRACTION RATIO ELIMINATION

$$CL_{intrinsic} \gg \dot{Q}_{hepatic}; \text{therefore ER} \approx 1, \text{and } CL_{hepatic} \approx \dot{Q}_{hepatic}$$

In drugs with a high ER elimination, $CL_{hepatic}$ is proportional to and principally limited by $\dot{Q}_{hepatic}$ (flow limited). Drug elimination is diminished by conditions of decreased $\dot{Q}_{hepatic}$ (arterial hypotension; increased splanchnic vascular resistance, including hepatic cirrhosis; hepatic venous congestion). If the drug administration rate is not adjusted for changes in hepatic

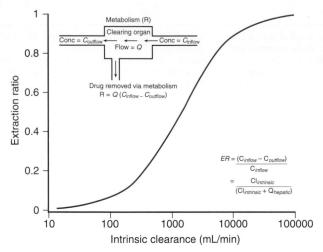

**Fig. 37.1** Relationship between intrinsic clearance (CL$_{intrinsic}$) and extraction ratio (ER), calculated for a liver blood flow of 1400 mL/min. *C, Conc, Q, R,*

clearance, resulting drug concentrations increase in a reciprocal fashion. Examples of highly extracted drugs include propofol, ketamine, fentanyl, sufentanil, morphine, meperidine, lidocaine, bupivacaine, metoprolol, propranolol, labetalol, verapamil, and naloxone.

## LOW–EXTRACTION RATIO ELIMINATION

$$\text{CL}_{\text{intrinsic}} \ll \dot{Q}_{\text{hepatic}}; \text{therefore ER} \ll 1$$

In this scenario, drug elimination is limited by the metabolic rate (capacity limited) and is thus dependent on the hepatic enzyme activity and free-drug concentration (which may be affected by disease-induced changes in plasma transport protein concentrations for drugs that are highly protein bound), whereas changes in $\dot{Q}_{\text{hepatic}}$ have minimal significance. Hepatic enzyme activity may be affected (decreased or increased) by a variety of factors, including extremes of age, genetic factors (gene polymorphisms), environmental exposure (enzyme induction), and medication history (enzyme induction by phenobarbital, polycyclic hydrocarbons, rifampin, phenytoin, or chronic alcohol consumption; enzyme inhibition by other substrates of the enzyme or by drugs, such as cimetidine). Examples of poorly extracted drugs include thiopental,

phenobarbital, hexobarbital, diazepam, lorazepam, phenytoin, valproic acid, ethanol, digitoxin, theophylline, acetaminophen, and warfarin.

## INTERMEDIATE–EXTRACTION RATIO ELIMINATION

Some drugs express an intermediate ER and variably depend on all three types of elimination ($\dot{Q}_{\text{hepatic}}$, hepatic enzyme activity, and free-drug concentration). Examples of these drugs are methohexital, midazolam, alfentanil, and vecuronium.

# Hepatic Metabolic Reactions

Hepatic drug metabolism removes drugs from the circulating plasma by enzymatically converting generally more or less lipophilic parent compounds to typically less pharmacologically active (mostly inactive), less toxic, and more water-soluble metabolites that are subject to biliary or renal excretion. Different types of reactions have been identified.

## PHASE 1 REACTIONS

Phase 1 reactions are oxidative, reductive, or hydrolytic reactions performed by more than 50 microsomal cytochrome P-450 enzymes (belonging to 17 distinct families) (Fig. 37.2) that are responsible for more than 90% of all hepatic drug biotransformation reactions. These processes act by inserting or unmasking polar OH, NH$_2$, or SH chemical groups through hydroxylation, *N*- or *O*-dealkylation, de-amination, de-sulfuration, *N*- or *S*-oxidation, epoxidation, or de-halogenation. The resulting, more hydrophilic metabolites are passively returned to blood and may serve as substrate for subsequent nonmicrosomal (phase 2) conjugation reactions. Phase 1 reactions are quite variable, exhibiting greater than fourfold differences in the maximal metabolic rate, even among healthy individuals (because of genotype and drug or environmental exposure that causes enzyme induction). They are further affected by nutrition status and hepatic disease, including a risk of oxidative stress related to the preferential centrilobular location of phase 1 reactions in zone 3, the area most vulnerable to the development of tissue hypoxia.

## PHASE 2 REACTIONS

Phase 2 reactions are conjugation reactions of drugs or metabolites with glucuronic acid, sulfate, or glycine in enzymatic processes

| TABLE 37.1 | Flow-Limited Versus Capacity-Limited Elimination of Drugs by the Liver | |
|---|---|---|
| **Type of Hepatic Elimination** | **Extraction Ratio** | **Rate of Hepatic Drug Metabolism** |
| Flow-limited elimination | High: At clinically relevant concentrations, most of the drug in the afferent hepatic blood is eliminated on first pass through the liver. | Rapid: Because drugs with a high extraction ratio are metabolized so rapidly, their hepatic clearance roughly equals their rate of transport to the liver (i.e., hepatic flow). |
| Capacity-limited elimination | Low: Hepatic elimination is determined by the plasma concentration. | Slow: When the capacity of the liver to eliminate a drug is less than the dosing rate, a steady state is unachievable; plasma levels of the drug will continue to rise unless the dosing rate is decreased. Drug clearance has no real meaning in such settings. |

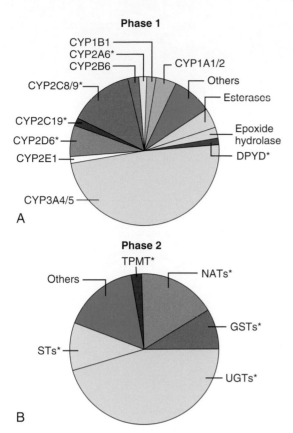

**Phase 1**

CYP1B1
CYP2A6*
CYP2B6
CYP2C8/9*
CYP2C19*
CYP2D6*
CYP2E1
CYP3A4/5
CYP1A1/2
Others
Esterases
Epoxide hydrolase
DPYD*

A

**Phase 2**

TPMT*
Others
STs*
NATs*
GSTs*
UGTs*

B

**Fig. 37.2** Proportion of drugs metabolized by major phase 1 or phase 2 enzymes. The relative size of each pie section indicates the estimated percentage of phase 1 **(A)** or phase 2 **(B)** metabolism that each enzyme contributes to the metabolism of drugs, based on literature reports. *Enzymes that have functional alleleic variants; in many cases, more than one enzyme is involved in metabolism of a particular drug. *CYP*, Cytochrome P-450; *DPYD*, dihydropyridine dehydrogenase; *GSTs*, glutathione *S*-transferases; *NAIs*, *N*-acetyltransferases; *STs*, sulfotransferases; *TPMT*, thiopurine methyltransferase; *UGTs*, uridine diphosphate glucuronosyltransferases. (Adapted from Wilkinson G. Pharmacokinetics: the dynamics of drug absorption, distribution, and elimination. In: Hardman JG, Limbird LE, Goodman GA, eds. *Goodman and Gilman's The Pharmacological Basis of Therapeutics*. 10th ed. McGraw-Hill; 2001.)

that are catalyzed by uridine diphosphate glucuronosyltransferases or several nonmicrosomal enzymes (glutathione *S*-transferase, *N*-acetyltransferase, or amino acid *N*-transferases). The resulting conjugates are typically less effective, less toxic, more hydrophilic, and more readily excreted via bile or urine. Some conjugates are

the substrate for active extrusion via phase 3 reactions. Compared with phase 1 reactions, phase 2 reactions tend to be less variable (an exception being *N*-acetyltransferase 2, which is responsible for isoniazid metabolism and is highly inducible) and less affected by advanced stages of hepatocellular disease.

## PHASE 3 REACTIONS

Phase 3 reactions are energy-dependent transmembrane transport reactions using various adenosine triphosphate–binding transport proteins to actively extrude drug conjugates into bile. These reactions tend to be well preserved into advanced stages of hepatic disease for as long as tissue oxygenation and hepatocellular energy production are maintained.

## Extrahepatic Metabolic Reactions

Hepatic disease not only may affect drug metabolism within the confines of the liver parenchyma itself but also may alter the pharmacokinetics of drugs whose metabolic products are subject to enterohepatic recirculation (such as certain antibiotics, nonsteroidal antiinflammatory drugs, hormones, opioids, digoxin, and warfarin) or distribution (and elimination) that may depend on or be affected by hepatically synthesized proteins exerting their actions extrahepatically within the plasma.

Butyrylcholinesterase (formerly called *pseudocholinesterase*) is responsible for the metabolism of drugs such as succinylcholine, mivacurium, and procaine local anesthetics. Enzyme activity is usually sufficient to terminate the action of these drugs in a clinically acceptable time frame until a very advanced stage of chronic liver disease.

The concentration of pharmacologically active free (unbound) drug that is ultimately available for systemic distribution is related not only to the effect sites of the drug but also to its sites of elimination (including in the liver) and may be affected by liver disease–induced changes in the plasma concentrations of transport proteins, such as albumin or $\alpha_1$-acid glycoprotein. To the extent that these proteins are decreased or increased, respectively, in advanced liver disease, as they frequently are, the apparent potency and elimination of highly protein-bound drugs with low hepatic extraction (e.g., thiopental bound to albumin) may be indirectly affected by concomitant changes in plasma protein binding (apparently higher potency of thiopental in the presence of hypoalbuminemia).

## SUGGESTED READINGS

Njoku, D. B., Chitilian, H. V., & Kronish, K. (2020). Hepatic physiology, pathophysiology, and anesthetic considerations. In M. A. Gropper, N. H. Cohen, L. I. Erikkson, L. A. Fleisher, K. Leslie, & J. P. Wiener-Kronish (Eds.), *Miller's anesthesia* (9th ed., pp. 420–443). Philadelphia: Elsevier.

Pan, G. (2019). Roles of hepatic drug transporters in drug disposition and liver toxicity. *Advances in Experimental Medicine and Biology, 1141*, 293–340.

Rey-Bedon, C., Banik, P., Gokaltun, A., Hofheinz, O., Yarmush, M. L., Uygun, M. K., et al. (2022). CYP450 drug inducibility in NAFLD via an in vitro hepatic model: Understanding drug-drug interactions in the fatty liver. *Biomedicine & Pharmacotherapy, 146*, 112377.

Vaja, R., & Rana, M. (2020). Drugs and the liver. *Anaesthesia International Care Medicine, 21*, 517–523.

# Pharmacology

# 38

# Molecular, Cellular, and Neural Mechanisms of General Anesthesia

CARLOS B. MANTILLA, MD, PhD

The mechanisms underlying general anesthesia are incompletely understood, despite considerable investigation and advances in the field of anesthesia. A general anesthetic state comprises *hypnosis, amnesia, analgesia,* and *lack of response to painful stimuli,* with different anesthetic drugs displaying varying potencies in attaining these behavioral and clinical end points. All general anesthetic agents cause *loss of consciousness* because of complex effects involving neural circuits in the central nervous system (CNS).

General anesthetic agents include diverse compounds, such as small molecules (e.g., nitrous oxide), alcohols, halogenated ethers, barbiturates, etomidate, and propofol. The diversity in chemical structure suggests *multiple modes of action.* Anesthetic drugs share important characteristics, including *hydrophobicity* (i.e., low water solubility, expressed as a lipid-to-water partition coefficient) and *lack of specific antagonists* capable of reversing anesthetic effects. Thus general anesthetics had been considered to act nonspecifically on lipid membranes in CNS neurons. However, it is now clear that most anesthetic drugs exert *specific* effects on membrane proteins, which depend on hydrophobic, electrostatic, and size properties. Inhaled and nonvolatile anesthetic agents affect the activity of ligand-gated ion channels and receptors that are important for neuronal excitability and synaptic transmission, acting on distinct sites in the CNS to produce the various components of the general anesthetic state. Immobility in response to painful stimuli results from effects in the spinal cord, whereas hypnosis and amnesia involve cortical and subcortical circuits regulating sleep, arousal, and memory.

A unitary hypothesis of anesthesia proposed the existence of a common mechanism for the action of all general anesthetics. The strong correlation between lipid solubility and anesthetic potency supports nonselective effects of general anesthetics on neuronal membranes (*Meyer-Overton rule*) (Fig. 38.1). According to this hypothesis, hydrophobic volatile and small-molecule anesthetics concentrate in lipid membranes, indirectly affecting the function of membrane proteins at the protein-lipid interface. Indeed, volatile anesthetics induce surgical anesthesia at remarkably similar equilibrium concentrations in the lipid bilayer. However, incomplete understanding of the basis of consciousness precludes detailed interpretation of the molecular and cellular effects of the diverse group of general anesthetic agents.

## Lipid-Based Hypotheses

Based on the Meyer-Overton rule (see Fig. 38.1A), the *lipid solubility hypothesis* suggests that anesthesia is produced when sufficient numbers of molecules disrupt neuronal lipid membranes. However, several findings are inconsistent with the lipid solubility hypothesis. First, some hydrophobic molecules, chemically similar to anesthetic drugs, are either much less potent than predicted or are altogether nonanesthetic. Second,

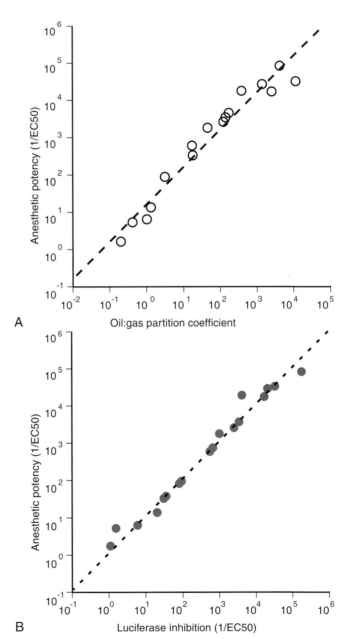

**Fig. 38.1** Anesthetic drugs exhibit a strong correlation between potency (i.e., reciprocal of the minimal alveolar concentration) and hydrophobicity **(A)**. This relationship supports the lipid solubility hypothesis of anesthetic action (Meyer-Overton rule). In addition, there is a strong correlation between the potency of different anesthetic drugs and their inhibition of the firefly enzyme luciferase **(B)**, supporting the protein-based hypothesis of anesthetic action. *EC50,* Half-maximal effective concentration. (Modified from Campagna JA, Miller KW, Forman SA. Mechanisms of actions of inhaled anesthetics. *N Engl J Med.* 2003;348:2110–2124; Franks NP. Molecular targets underlying general anaesthesia. *Br J Pharmacol.* 2006;147[Suppl 1]:S72–S81.)

application of increased pressure to membranes does not alter the lipid solubility of anesthetic agents, whereas this increased pressure antagonizes the anesthetic state (*pressure-reversal effect*). Third, n-alcohols exhibit increasing anesthetic potency and hydrophobicity as the carbon chain is elongated, but an additional carbon molecule past 12 or 13 is associated with complete loss of anesthetic action (*cutoff effect*).

Modifications of the lipid solubility hypothesis attempt to account for these phenomena by including lipid perturbation effects. The *critical volume hypothesis* suggests that anesthesia occurs when anesthetics cause lipid membrane expansion, thereby disrupting membrane protein function. At clinically relevant anesthetic concentrations, the membrane expands approximately 0.4%. This is similar to the effect of a 1°C increase in temperature, which is not associated with anesthesia. In addition, although this hypothesis would explain the pressure-reversal effect, it still fails to explain the anesthetic cutoff effect. The *lipid fluidity hypothesis* arises from the disordering effect that anesthetics exert on membranes, which could interfere with the function of membrane proteins. Anesthetic potency and cutoff correlate with the disordering effect on cholesterol membranes, and anesthetics may thus alter the lateral pressures exerted on membrane-embedded proteins, the conformation of membrane proteins, and the energy needed for proper protein, function. Increased pressure reverses anesthetic-induced changes in membrane fluidity. Nevertheless, the assumption that nonspecific changes in the lipid membrane can selectively alter the function of specific proteins lacks experimental support.

## Molecular Sites of Anesthetic Action

A large body of evidence indicates that anesthetic effects result from their actions on specific proteins, particularly *ligand-gated ion channels* such as the γ-aminobutyric acid (GABA), glycine, glutamate, and nicotinic acetylcholine receptors that are present in neuronal membranes. First, general anesthetic potency correlates well with the inhibition of several proteins (see Fig. 38.1B). Second, anesthetic binding to hydrophobic pockets in proteins explains both the correlation of potency with hydrophobicity and the anesthetic cutoff. In addition, multiple anesthetic drugs, including barbiturates, ketamine, and isoflurane, show stereoselective effects (e.g., the S-isomer is more potent than the R-isomer) consistent with protein binding. Finally, the steep dose-response curve for volatile anesthetics suggests receptor occupancy (i.e., 1 minimum alveolar concentration is effective in 50% of subjects, whereas 1.3 minimum alveolar concentration is effective in 95% of subjects).

Most evidence indicates that anesthetic drugs act specifically at ion channels (Fig. 38.2). For example, multiple anesthetic drugs (e.g., barbiturates, volatile anesthetics) potentiate GABA activity. Propofol and etomidate also act by potentiating GABA_A receptors, and mutations in the GABA_A receptor modulate anesthetic effects in vitro and in animal models. Several anesthetic agents prolong inhibitory chloride currents at GABA receptors and shift the GABA dose-response curve leftward, enhancing receptor sensitivity to GABA. All volatile anesthetics potentiate glycine receptors, the second most important inhibitory neurotransmitter after GABA. In addition, two-pore-domain K⁺ channels, which modulate baseline neuronal excitability, are activated by volatile anesthetics.

Nitrous oxide, xenon, and ketamine act by antagonism of the excitatory *N*-methyl-D-aspartate (NMDA) subtype of glutamate

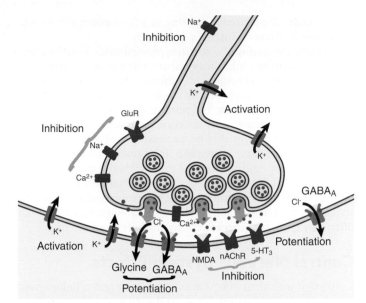

**Fig. 38.2** Potential sites of anesthetic action include presynaptic and postsynaptic targets *(large shaded areas)*. *Presynaptic* inhibition of Ca²⁺ entry in the axon terminal after the action potential and direct inhibition of neurotransmitter vesicle release can lead to decreased availability of neurotransmitter in the synaptic cleft and reduced impulse transmission. *Postsynaptic* effects are mediated by modulation of ion channels, including ligand-gated ion channel receptors. Potentiation of γ-aminobutyric acid *(GABA)* and glycine receptors enhances inhibitory neurotransmission. Activation of pre- or postsynaptic two-pore K⁺ channels causes cell hyperpolarization and reduces cellular excitability. Inhibition of glutamate (via ionotropic glutamate receptors *[GluR]*, including *N*-methyl-D-aspartate *[NMDA]* receptors), serotonin *(5-HT)* (via 5-HT₃ receptors), or acetylcholine (via neuronal nicotinic receptors *[nAChR]*) impairs excitatory neurotransmission. Anesthetic effects on ion channels likely result from specific interactions at hydrophobic pockets within transmembrane proteins, leading to altered protein function, rather than direct effects on the lipid membrane or lipid-protein interface.

receptors. Despite the effects of general anesthetics on Ca²⁺, Na⁺, and K⁺ channels at high concentrations, neuronal voltage-gated channels are largely insensitive to anesthetic drugs. However, direct effects on voltage-gated Ca²⁺ and K⁺ channels may underlie anesthetic effects in the heart, including the negative inotropic and chronotropic effects and proarrhythmogenic properties. For instance, ischemic preconditioning correlates with anesthetic effects on adenosine triphosphate–sensitive K⁺ channels. Anesthetic effects on sarcoplasmic reticulum Ca²⁺ channels (1,4,5-inositol triphosphate – IP₃ and ryanodine receptors) that mediate excitation-contraction coupling in muscle are responsible for relaxation effects on bronchial and vascular smooth muscle. A number of mutations in these channels have been implicated in malignant hyperthermia susceptibility.

## Cellular Effects

Modulation of ion channels that are present in the membranes of excitable cells, including neurons, determines the effect of an anesthetic agent. Anesthetic effects on ion channels can reduce neuronal excitability by affecting resting membrane potential, the threshold for action potential generation and input resistance. The effect of the anesthetic agent on these factors, however, will depend on the state of the specific neuron (i.e., depolarized or hyperpolarized), thus confounding interpretation of available studies. Neurons in the hippocampus, thalamus, and brainstem motor nuclei display reduced firing of action potentials despite inconsistent effects on intrinsic excitability.

*Synaptic transmission is sensitive to anesthetics.* Volatile anesthetics potentiate inhibitory neurotransmission acting on GABA or glycine receptors and inhibit excitatory transmission acting on NMDA receptors. Synaptic transmission may be affected at both presynaptic and postsynaptic sites (see Fig. 38.2). Presynaptically, anesthetics decrease neurotransmitter release to a small degree, probably by decreasing $Ca^{2+}$ entry. Postsynaptically, anesthetics potentiate inhibitory currents and/or block excitatory neurotransmission. Anesthetics may also act at extrajunctional GABA receptors and $K^+$ channels that modulate neuronal function, causing cell hyperpolarization and thus reduced neuronal excitability. However, *axonal conduction is not altered* by clinically relevant concentrations of anesthetics.

## Central Nervous System Effects

Consistent with their effects at the molecular and cellular levels, anesthetic drugs exert inhibitory and excitatory effects on various CNS structures and disrupt circuits involved in alertness, arousal, memory, and sleep. These diverse effects depend on whether synaptic transmission is blocked or enhanced at inhibitory or excitatory nuclei in the CNS. Indeed, increasing evidence from studies using clinically relevant concentrations of anesthetics suggests a selective mechanism of anesthetic action on a limited number of CNS targets. In general, anesthetics *inhibit the brainstem reticular formation*, resulting in *loss of consciousness*. Inhibitory effects at the *spinal cord* mediate the anesthetic-induced *lack of movement* in response to surgical stimuli and pain. At low concentrations, anesthetics also have excitatory supraspinal effects that result in euphoria, excitation, and hyperreflexia. The interaction between inhibitory and excitatory effects on various CNS circuits determines the behavioral, physiologic, and clinical outcomes observed during anesthesia.

Recent studies have shown differences in the electroencephalogram (EEG) "signature" of the various anesthetic agents that are likely the result of varying effects on CNS circuits. Volatile anesthetics induce dose-dependent increases in the amplitude of lower-frequency delta (0.1–4 Hz) and alpha (4–8 Hz) oscillations and induce burst suppression with alternating periods of high-amplitude activity and flat isoelectric EEG. Agents acting predominantly via GABA circuits, such as propofol, amplify alpha (8–12 Hz) oscillations with frontal predominance (not occipital, as seen in sleep) at anesthetic doses. Propofol- and benzodiazepine-induced sedation increases beta (13–30 Hz) oscillations, whereas ketamine induces higher-frequency (>30 Hz) gamma oscillations. Dexmedetomidine, an $\alpha_2$-adrenergic receptor agonist, enhances slow-delta and spindle (12–16 Hz) oscillations, similar to the EEG features of restful sleep.

In summary, anesthetic drugs act on ligand-gated ion channels and exert effects at various molecular, cellular, and circuit levels that may ultimately disrupt thalamocortical connectivity, eliminating the transmission of sensory stimuli to the cortex and depressing brainstem arousal activity. Additional, effects on cortical and subcortical circuits are important to induce loss of consciousness. Each class of anesthetic agents exerts dose- and state-dependent effects that result in specific neurophysiological signatures that may show clinical utility in evaluating anesthetic depth.

## SUGGESTED READINGS

Campagna, J. A., Miller, K. W., & Forman, S. A. (2003). Mechanisms of actions of inhaled anesthetics. *New England Journal of Medicine, 348*, 2110–2124.

Franks, N. P. (2006). Molecular targets underlying general anaesthesia. *British Journal of Pharmacology, 147*(Suppl. 1), S72–S81.

Franks, N. P. (2008). General anaesthesia: From molecular targets to neuronal pathways of sleep and arousal. *Nature Reviews Neuroscience, 9*(5), 370–386.

Herold, K. F., Sanford, R. L., Lee, W., Andersen, O. S., & Hemmings Jr., H. C. (2017). Clinical concentrations of chemically diverse general anesthetics minimally affect lipid bilayer properties. *Proceedings of the National Academy of Sciences of the United States of America, 114*(12), 3109–3114.

Mashour, G. A. (2014). Top-down mechanisms of anesthetic-induced unconsciousness. *Frontiers in Systems Neuroscience, 8*, 115.

Mihic, S. J., Ye, Q., Wick, M. J., Koltchine, V. V., Krasowski, M. D., Finn, S. E., et al. (1997). Sites of alcohol and volatile anaesthetic action on GABAA and glycine receptors. *Nature, 389*, 385–388.

Moody, O. A., Zhang, E. R., Vincent, K. F., Kato, R., Melonakos, E. D., Nehs, C. J., & Solt, K. (2021). The neural circuits underlying general anesthesia and sleep. *Anesthesia and Analgesia, 132*, 1254–1264.

Purdon, P. L., Sampson, A., Pavone, K. J., & Brown, E. N. (2015). Clinical electroencephalography for anesthesiologists. Part I: Background and basic signatures. *Anesthesiology, 123*, 937–960.

# 39

# Factors That Affect Anesthetic Gas Uptake

MOLLY B. KRAUS, MD | CHRISTOPHER BAILEY, MD

Anesthesia uptake is directly related to solubility, cardiac output, and the partial pressure difference between the alveoli and the pulmonary vein. Uptake is inversely related to barometric pressure. The relationship is expressed by the formula

$$\text{Uptake} = \lambda \cdot Q \cdot \frac{P_A - P_{\bar{V}}}{P_B}$$

where $\lambda$ is solubility, $Q$ is cardiac output, $P_A - P_{\bar{V}}$ is the alveolar-venous partial pressure difference, and $P_B$ is the barometric pressure.

$P_A$ is determined by input (delivery) minus uptake (loss) of the anesthetic agent from the alveoli into the pulmonary arterial blood. Uptake depends on solubility, cardiac output, and the alveolar-venous partial pressure difference ($P_A - P_{\bar{V}}$). Input depends on $P_I$ (inspired partial pressure of gas), alveolar ventilation, and the characteristics of the anesthetic breathing system. Highly perfused tissues (brain, heart, kidneys, and liver) account for less than 10% of body mass but receive 75% of cardiac output. Therefore they equilibrate rapidly with $P_A$, so $P_A$ can be considered as equivalent to $P_{Br}$ (partial pressure of the anesthetic in the brain). The anesthetic agent in the blood is initially distributed to the vessel-rich tissues (Table 39.1). Soon after blood returns to the lungs, depending on its blood-gas partition coefficient, it has the same partial pressure that it had on leaving the lungs ($P_I \approx P_A \approx P_{BLOOD}$). Because children have greater perfusion of the vessel-rich tissues compared with adults, $F_A/F_I$ increases more rapidly in children, so anesthesia is achieved more rapidly in these patients.

## Solubility

↑ Solubility = ↑ affinity for blood compared with the gaseous form
↓ Solubility ≅ ↓ onset of anesthesia
↑ Solubility = ↑ blood/gas coefficient
↑ Solubility = ↓ alveolar/inspired gas ratio ($F_A/F_I$)

The relative affinity of an anesthetic agent is representative of its solubility and is defined by its blood-gas partition coefficient. This coefficient at the anesthetic's equilibrium indicates the concentration in the blood compared with the concentration in the alveolus. For example, isoflurane has a blood-gas partition coefficient of 1.4. This means that, at equilibrium, the isoflurane concentration in the blood would be 1.4 times the concentration in the gas (alveolar) phase. The partial pressures of each would be the same (by definition), but the blood would contain more isoflurane. Anesthetic agents with a high blood-gas partition coefficient diffuse into the blood quickly and have

| TABLE 39.1 | Tissue Group Characteristics | | | |
|---|---|---|---|---|
| | **GROUP** | | | |
| Characteristic | Vessel-Rich Tissue | Muscle | Fat | Vessel-Poor Tissue |
| Percentage of body mass | 10 | 50 | 20 | 20 |
| Perfusion as percentage of cardiac output | 75 | 19 | 6 | 0 |

From Eger EI II. Effect of inspired anesthetic concentration on the rate of rise of alveolar concentration. *Anesthesiology.* 1963;24:153–157.

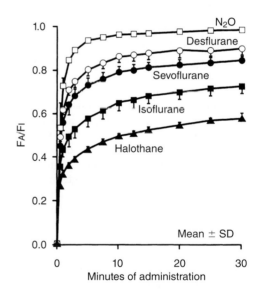

**Fig. 39.1** The pharmacokinetics of modern inhalation anesthetic agents are defined as the ratio of end-tidal anesthetic concentration *(F_A)* to inspired anesthetic concentration *(F_I)* (mean ± SD). The rate of increase of $F_A/F_I$ over time for most agents correlates inversely with the relative solubility of the anesthetic agents. *N₂O,* Nitrous oxide. (From Yasuda N, Lockhart SH, Eger EI, et al. Comparison of kinetics of sevoflurane and isoflurane in humans. *Anesth Analg.* 1991;72:316–324.)

a low alveolar/inspired gas ratio ($F_A/F_I$), resulting in a slower onset (Fig. 39.1). Also, agents with a high coefficient take longer to "fill the tank" before the partial pressure begins to rise high enough to induce anesthesia. It is not the total amount of drug in the blood but the partial pressure of inhalational agent in the blood and therefore in the brain that induces anesthesia.

| TABLE 39.2 | Partition Coefficients at 37°C |
| --- | --- |
| **Anesthetic Agent** | **Blood-Gas Partition Coefficient** |
| Desflurane | 0.45 |
| Nitrous oxide | 0.47 |
| Sevoflurane | 0.65 |
| Isoflurane | 1.4 |
| Enflurane | 1.8 |
| Halothane | 2.5 |
| Diethyl ether | 12.0 |
| Methoxyflurane | 15.0 |

Modified from Eger EI II. Effect of inspired anesthetic concentration on the rate of rise of alveolar concentration. *Anesthesiology.* 1963;24: 153–157.

The uptake of soluble gases may be increased by delivering a concentration of two to four times minimum alveolar concentration, also known as *anesthetic overpressuring*. The blood-gas partition coefficients of common inhalational anesthetics are listed in Table 39.2. Recent studies indicate blood-gas coefficients for isoflurane and, notably, sevoflurane and desflurane may be higher than previously reported.

## Cardiac Output

$\downarrow$ Cardiac output = $\uparrow$ $F_A$ (alveolar concentration) of soluble gases = faster induction

More soluble agents are affected the most by changes in cardiac output.

Blood flow through the lungs can have an impact on the physiologic movement of gases from the alveolus to the blood. For example, as cardiac output increases, more anesthetic is removed from the gas phase. This results in a lower $F_A$, thereby slowing the rate of increase of $F_A$ and slowing an inhalational induction. The more soluble anesthetic gases are affected the most significantly by changes in cardiac output. Tissue uptake affects the alveolar/venous anesthetic gradient. As tissues become more saturated, uptake in the blood ceases and this gradient approaches zero. At this point, the $F_A/F_I$ ratio approaches unity.

With decreased cardiac output, alveolar concentration increases more rapidly because less blood flows through the lungs. Again, highly soluble agents are most affected. The rate of increase of the $F_A/F_I$ ratio with less soluble agents is rapid, regardless of cardiac output. With highly soluble agents, potentially dangerous positive feedback exists in that anesthetic-induced cardiac depression decreases uptake, increases alveolar concentration, and further depresses cardiac output.

## Ventilation

$\uparrow$ Respiratory rate = $\uparrow$ $F_A/F_I$ of soluble gases
$\uparrow$ Functional residual capacity = $\downarrow$ uptake *(there is a greater volume to be filled)*

The alveolar partial pressure ($P_A$) of an anesthetic agent influences the partial pressure in the brain. The inspired anesthetic concentration ($F_I$) and the alveolar ventilation are the two factors influencing the rate at which alveolar anesthetic concentration increases. Increasing either or both will facilitate the rate of increase of the anesthetic gas in the alveoli. Other factors related to $F_A$ increase are the concentration effect and the second gas effect.

Controlled ventilation of the lung results in hyperventilation and decreased venous return, accelerating the increase in $P_A$ because of an increase in ventilation and a decrease in cardiac output. The breathing system affects anesthesia gas uptake. Increased volume in the system slows induction, and the solubility of the inhaled anesthetics in the plastic and rubber slows induction.

During hyperventilation, more anesthetic agent is delivered to the lungs, increasing the rate of $F_A/F_I$ increase. This change is more pronounced with more soluble anesthetic agents because a large portion of a highly soluble anesthetic agent delivered to the lungs is taken up by the blood. Conversely, hypoventilation results in slowed alveolar concentration.

Increased functional residual capacity results in slower uptake of the inhalation agent as a greater volume of lung must be filled, thereby slowing induction. Conversely, uptake is more rapid for patients with disease conditions that reduce functional residual capacity.

## Concentration Effect

The concentration effect describes how increasing the $F_I$ of a gas produces a more rapid rise in its alveolar concentration. This phenomenon is the sum of two components. The first is the similarly named, but different, concentrating effect; the second is the effective increase in alveolar ventilation. As the inhalation agent is taken up by the blood, total lung volume is decreased by the amount of gas taken up by the blood, concentrating the agent remaining within the lung (hence, the concentrating effect). The magnitude of this effect is influenced by the initial concentration of gas within the lung: the higher the concentration, the greater the effect. For example, when the lung is filled with 1% $N_2O$, if one-half is taken up, then the remaining concentration is 0.5% (0.5 part in 99.5 parts). If the same lung is filled with 80% $N_2O$ and one-half is taken up, then the remaining concentration is 67%, not 40% (40 parts in a total of 60). The effective increase in alveolar ventilation occurs as uptake of $N_2O$ into the blood causes a decrease in volume within the lung, causing additional gas to be drawn in via the trachea to replace $N_2O$ lost by uptake. This decreases the $F_I/F_A$ concentration difference because inspired gas (as in the second example earlier) contains 80% $N_2O$, thus further raising the alveolar concentration of $N_2O$ from 67% to 72%.

## Second Gas Effect

The phenomenon known as the *second gas effect* results from large volumes of a first gas (usually $N_2O$) are taken up from alveoli, increasing the rate of rise in the alveolar concentration of the second gas given concomitantly. For example, there is a

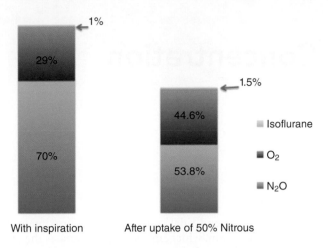

**Fig. 39.2** A lung is filled with 80% N₂O and 1% of a second gas. Uptake of 50% of the N₂O increases the concentration of the second gas to 1.5%. Restoration of the lung gas volume by addition of more of the original mixture of 80% to 1% changes the second gas concentration to 1.4%. (Reprinted, with permission, from Eger EI II. Effect of inspired anesthetic concentration on the rate of rise of alveolar concentration. *Anesthesiology*. 1963;24:153–157.)

transient increase in $P_{AO_2}$ with early-phase N₂O administration. This is based on proven pharmacokinetic principles but likely has little clinical significance. Factors that are responsible for the concentration effect also govern the second gas effect. The effective increase in alveolar ventilation should increase the alveolar concentration of all concomitantly inspired gases, regardless of their inspired concentration. Moreover, uptake of the first gas reduces the total gas volume, thereby increasing the concentration of the second gas (Fig. 39.2).

The fractional uptake of the second gas determines the relative importance of increased ventilation versus the concentrating effect. Increased ventilation plays the greater role in raising the second gas concentration when the fraction of the second gas removed by uptake into the blood is large (i.e., with more soluble second gases). The concentrating effect plays the greater role when uptake into the blood is small (i.e., with less soluble agents).

Although acknowledging the usefulness of the original description of the concentration and second gas effects for teaching purposes, It has been suggested that these explanations are too simplistic and do not consider alternative volume effects of gas uptake. The second gas effect may persist well past the phase of uptake of large volumes of N₂O. It has been reported that N₂O did not affect the alveolar or blood concentration of a second gas (enflurane) under controlled constant volume ventilation (leading the authors to conclude that the second gas effect is not a valid concept). Another study that same year with N₂O and desflurane effectively showed the predicted effects of the concentration and second gas effects.

## $\dot{V}/\dot{Q}$ Mismatch

Left → right shunt has little effect on induction
Right → left shunt slows induction

Ventilation-perfusion mismatch tends to increase the alveolar anesthetic partial pressure and decrease the arterial anesthetic partial pressure. This is most pronounced with less soluble agents. With more highly soluble anesthetic agents, blood from the relatively hyperventilated alveoli contains more anesthetic agent, which compensates for blood emerging from underventilated alveoli, resulting in less effect on the arterial partial pressure.

A left-to-right cardiac shunt in the presence of normal tissue perfusion does not affect anesthetic uptake. However, with a right-to-left shunt, a fraction of blood does not pass through the lungs and cannot take up anesthetic. This type of shunt results in a slower rate of increase in the arterial concentration of anesthetic agent and slower induction of anesthesia, with the least soluble agents affected most. Dead space (ventilation of nonperfused alveoli) does not influence the rate of induction because there is no dilutional effect produced.

## SUGGESTED READINGS

Carette, R., Hendrickx, J. F. A., Lemmens, H. J., & DeWolf, A. M. (2007). Large volume N₂O uptake alone does not explain the second gas effect of N₂O on sevoflurane during constant inspired ventilation. *Acta Anaesthesiologica Belgica, 58*, 146.

Esper, T., Wehner, M., Meinecke, C., & Rueffert, H. (2015). Blood/gas partition coefficients for isoflurane, sevoflurane, and desflurane in a clinically relevant patient population. *Anesthesia and Analgesia, 120*, 45–50.

Forman, S. A., & Ishizawa, Y. (2020). Inhaled anesthetic uptake, distribution, metabolism, and toxicity. In M. A. Gropper (Eds.), *Miller's Anesthesia* (9th ed., pp. 509–539). Philadelphia: Elsevier, Inc.

Yasuda, N., Lockhart, S. H., Eger, E. I., Weiskopf, R. B., Liu, J., Laster, M., et al. (1991). Comparison of kinetics of sevoflurane and isoflurane in humans. *Anesthesia and Analgesia, 72*, 316–324.

# Minimum Alveolar Concentration

TYLER DUNN, MD

Dosing of most drugs is based on mass of drug per kilogram of patient body weight. However, for inhalation anesthetic agents, the mass of drug and patient weight have little to do with the intensity of the drug effect. Therefore a method for quantifying the amount of inhalation agent necessary for anesthesia has been devised. *Minimum alveolar concentration* (MAC) is the alveolar concentration of an inhalation anesthetic agent at 1 atm and at steady-state concentration that is necessary to suppress a gross purposeful movement in 50% of patients in response to a skin incision.

MAC has been determined for different age groups under different conditions and for all inhalation anesthetic agents (Table 40.1), allowing for comparison of the potency of the different agents. MAC is inversely related to anesthetic potency and, therefore, to lipid solubility (Meyer-Overton theory). MAC is analogous to the pharmacologic effective dose ($ED_{50}$) of drugs.

The control of anesthesia depth to avoid awareness by measuring end-tidal anesthetic concentration is based on the MAC concept.

## Important Concepts Related to Minimum Alveolar Concentration

### ALVEOLAR CONCENTRATION

The MAC value of an inhalation anesthetic agent is expressed as a percentage of its alveolar concentration that, at steady state, should approximate the end-tidal concentration, which is measured continuously throughout anesthesia. Alveolar partial pressure of an anesthetic agent is its fractional pressure in the alveolus. The sum of the partial pressures of all components of the alveolar gas mixture equals the total ambient pressure, which is 1 atm, or 760 mm Hg at sea level. For example, if at sea level the end-tidal concentration of an anesthetic is 1%, then its partial pressure in the alveolus is 0.01 atm ≈ 7.6 mm Hg ≈ 1 kPa.

| TABLE 40.1 | Minimum Alveolar Concentration (MAC) of Inhalation Anesthetics at Ambient Pressure of 760 mm Hg | | | | |
|---|---|---|---|---|---|
| | Isoflurane | Desflurane | Sevoflurane | N$_2$O | Xenon |
| MAC in O$_2$ (vol%) | 1.3 | 6.0 | 2.1 | 105 | 71 |
| MAC in 70% N$_2$O and 30% O$_2$ (vol%) | 0.6 | 2.5 | 0.7 | – | – |

### STEADY STATE

At equilibrium, the end-tidal concentration approximates the alveolar concentration, which, in turn, approximates the anesthetic concentration at the anesthetic site of action in the central nervous system. Equilibrium is present when end-tidal, alveolar, blood, and brain anesthetic partial pressures are equal. Based on the high cerebral blood flow and low blood solubility of modern anesthetic agents, equilibration is approached after end-tidal concentration has been kept constant for 10 to 15 minutes.

### AMBIENT PRESSURE

MAC values are conventionally given as a percentage of alveolar anesthetic concentration at 1 atm. They either have been determined at sea level or, ideally, have been corrected to sea level when determined at higher altitudes. Anesthetic potency and uptake are directly related to the partial pressure of the anesthetic agent (see Table 40.1). At higher altitude, compared with sea level, the same concentration of an inhalation anesthetic agent will exert a lower partial pressure within the alveolus and, consequently, will have a reduced anesthetic effect. Modern variable bypass vaporizers compensate for this effect because, although the dials are marked in "percent," partial pressure is what is determined. At an altitude at which the pressure is one-half of sea level, a variable bypass vaporizer set to 1% would deliver 2%, although the actual partial pressure of anesthetic agent delivered would be the same. For example, at sea level, with a barometric pressure of 760 mm Hg, the partial pressure of the agent would be 7.6 mm Hg. At an altitude with a barometric pressure of 380 mm Hg, a variable bypass vaporizer set at 1% would actually deliver 2% of the agent (2% of 380 = 7.6 mm Hg partial vapor pressure). This does not apply to a desflurane vaporizer as desflurane requires an electronic vaporizer that maintains a constant temperature and vapor pressure for consistent output.

### STIMULUS AND RESPONSE

Skin incision is the standard stimulus used to define MAC in humans. As the intensity of the stimulus decreases, so too does the MAC necessary to block a defined response: intubation > skin incision > tetanic stimulation > laryngoscopy > trapezius squeeze > vocal command. A positive response, in the classic determination of anesthetic potency, is gross purposeful muscular movement of the head or extremities. Other responses can be eye-opening to command and sympathetic adrenergic reaction (increase in blood pressure and heart rate) to noxious stimuli.

## Determination of Minimum Alveolar Concentration

MAC can be determined in humans by anesthetizing them with the inhalation anesthetic agent alone in $O_2$ and allowing 15 minutes for equilibration at a preselected target end-tidal concentration. A single skin incision is made, and the patient is observed for purposeful movement. A group of patients must be tested in this fashion over a range of anesthetic concentrations that allows and prevents patient movement. The percentage of patients in groups of four or more who show a positive response to surgical stimulation is plotted against the average alveolar concentration for that group. Drawing a best-fit line through these points shows the concentration at which half of the subjects move with skin incision, thus determining MAC. Another approach is to plot the individual end-tidal anesthetic concentrations against the probability of no response by nonlinear regression analysis. This results in a typical dose-response curve, whereas the concentration that corresponds to the 0.5 probability of no response estimates the MAC value.

## Dose-Response Relationship

The dose-response curve allows for an extrapolation to that anesthetic concentration at which 95% of the patients do not respond to the applied noxious stimulus with movement. Although the $ED_{95}$ seems to be the more clinically relevant value, it is seldom used to describe anesthetic potency. The dose-response curves for inhalation anesthetic agents are steep; 1 MAC prevents skeletal muscle movement on incision in 50% of patients, whereas 1.3 MAC prevents movement in 99% of patients ($ED_{99}$). The dose-response curves for different inhalation anesthetic agents are parallel, implying that they share a common mechanism or site of action. This observation is supported by the fact that MAC values are additive. If 0.7 MAC $N_2O$ is administered with 0.7 MAC isoflurane, the resulting effect is 1.4 MAC.

## Factors That Affect Minimum Alveolar Concentration

Numerous physiologic and pharmacologic factors, disease states, and conditions can change the anesthetic sensitivity and, therefore, increase or decrease MAC (Table 40.2). Not all of the underlying mechanisms are known (e.g., decrease of MAC in pregnancy or increase in redheads). Nevertheless, anesthetic requirements seem to correlate with cerebral metabolic rate, whereas factors decreasing cerebral metabolic rate (i.e., temperature, age, severe hypoxia, hypotension, various drugs) decrease MAC.

MAC is age dependent (Fig. 40.1). The MAC value is highest in infants 3 to 6 months of age. For patients older than 1 year, MAC decreases by approximately 6% to 7% with each increasing decade of life.

MAC decreases linearly with decreasing temperature; a 1°C decrease in body temperature reduces the anesthetic requirement by approximately 4% to 5%. Factors that do not change MAC include duration of anesthesia, body size, sex, arterial blood pressure greater than 50 mm Hg, arterial $Pao_2$ greater than 50 mm Hg, arterial $Paco_2$ less than 40 mm Hg, and hematocrit greater than 10%.

| TABLE 40.2 | Effect of Pharmacologic Agents and Physiologic Factors on Minimum Alveolar Concentration (MAC) | |
|---|---|---|
| **Decreased MAC ↓** | | **MAC ↑** |
| **MEDICATIONS** | | |
| Opioids | | Inhibition of catecholamine |
| Benzodiazepines | | reuptake (amphetamines, |
| Barbiturates | | ephedrine) |
| Propofol | | |
| Ketamine | | |
| $\alpha_2$-Agonists | | |
| Intravenously administered local anesthetic agents | | |
| **ALCOHOL** | | |
| Acute ethanol ingestion | | Chronic ethanol abuse |
| **PHYSIOLOGIC CONDITIONS** | | |
| Increasing age for patients >1 year of age | | In the first months of life for infants <6 months of age |
| Pregnancy | | |
| **PATHOPHYSIOLOGIC CONDITIONS** | | |
| Hypothermia | | Hyperthermia |
| Severe hypotension | | Hyperthyroidism |
| Severe hypoxemia | | Increased extracellular $Na^+$ in |
| Severe anemia | | central nervous system |
| Acute metabolic acidosis | | |
| Sepsis | | |
| **GENETIC FACTORS** | | |
| None established[a][b] | | Genotype related to red hair |

[a]Sex does not change MAC except in the elderly Japanese population, where women may have a smaller MAC for xenon compared with men.
[b]No good data comparing MAC in different ethnic groups exist.

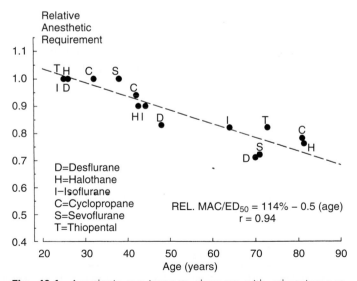

**Fig. 40.1** Anesthetic requirements decrease with advancing age. Dose is expressed as minimum alveolar concentration (*MAC*) for inhalation anesthetic agents and as the relative median effective dose (*ED50*) for intravenously administered agents. (From Muravchick S. Anesthesia for the elderly. In: Miller RD, ed. *Anesthesia*. 5th ed. Churchill Livingstone; 2000:2140–2156.)

| TABLE 40.3 | Derivatives of Minimum Alveolar Concentration (MAC) | |
| --- | --- | --- |
| MAC Derivative | MAC Value | Definition |
| Amnesia | 0.25 MAC | Blockage of anterograde memory formation in awake patients |
| Awake | 0.3 MAC | Prevention of eye-opening on verbal command |
| Intubation (IT) | 1.3 MAC | Prevention of movement and coughing in response to endotracheal intubation |
| Blockade of Autonomic Response (BAR) | 1.5 MAC | Prevention of autonomic response to skin incision |

## Derivatives of Minimum Alveolar Concentration

The classic MAC value gives a measure of the anesthetic requirement to suppress movement to skin incision. MAC derivatives (Table 40.3) have been determined in an effort to define the optimal concentrations of inhalation anesthetic agents to allow for various clinically essential stimuli, such as laryngoscopy, intubation, laryngeal mask insertion, laryngeal mask removal, and extubation. The MAC derivatives are often shown as multiples or fractions of the classic MAC value.

$MAC_{amnesia}$ is the concentration of an inhaled anesthetic to suppress anterograde memory formation in an awake patient. This value is lower than $MAC_{awake}$, which is the concentration of an inhaled anesthetic agent at which half of patients will suppress a voluntary response to verbal command such as eye-opening. These values are an index of the hypnotic potency of an inhaled anesthetic agent. Knowledge of $MAC_{amnesia}$ is helpful to prevent intraoperative awareness. $MAC_{awake}$ is approximately one-third of MAC for isoflurane, desflurane, and sevoflurane. The decrease of $MAC_{awake}$ with age is parallel to that of MAC itself. Drugs that suppress central nervous system activity (e.g., fentanyl, clonidine) reduce $MAC_{awake}$.

The MAC necessary to blunt the adrenergic or cardiovascular response in 50% of individuals who have a skin incision is known as the $MAC_{BAR}$. However, different harmful stimuli result in different degrees of hemodynamic responses, with intubation being more noxious than skin incision. Prevention of sympathetic stimulation and hemodynamic responses (heart rate and blood pressure increase) during surgery is especially important in patients with coronary heart disease. The $MAC_{BAR}$ typically is considerably greater than the classic MAC value. This creates a conundrum for the clinician; administering a $MAC_{BAR}$ to produce acceptable hemodynamic response during periods of intense surgical stimulation results in unacceptably low blood pressure during times when there is minimal stimulation. Opioids, even in small doses, and $N_2O$ markedly decrease the $MAC_{BAR}$ (see Table 40.4). This effect is the reason why $N_2O$ and opioids are frequently coadministered with halogenated anesthetics as part of a "balanced" anesthetic.

| TABLE 40.4 | Opioid Dosages for Minimum Alveolar Concentration (MAC) Reduction of Isoflurane | | |
| --- | --- | --- | --- |
| Drug | MAC Reduction | Bolus Dose | Infusion |
| Fentanyl | 50% | 3 mcg/kg | 0.02 mcg/kg/min |
| Alfentanil | 50% | 20 mcg/kg | 0.25 mcg/kg/min |
| Sufentanil | 50% | 0.15 mcg/kg | 0.003 mcg/kg/min |
| Remifentanil | 50% | 0.25 mcg/kg | 0.025 mcg/kg/min |

The anesthetic concentrations that allow laryngoscopy (LS), intubation (IT), and laryngeal mask insertion (LMI) in 50% of individuals are defined as $MAC_{LS}$, $MAC_{IT}$, and $MAC_{LMI}$. The $MAC_{IT}$ values are approximately 30% greater than the classic MAC values. The $MAC_{IT}$ and $MAC_{LMI}$ for sevoflurane have been extensively studied because inhaled sevoflurane is frequently used to induce anesthesia in children.

## Clinical Relevance

By definition, 1 MAC of an inhaled anesthetic agent alone is insufficient to provide adequate anesthesia because half of patients will respond with movement after skin incision. Nevertheless, the MAC value became the principal measure to compare the potencies of different inhalation agents. Consequently, the applied dose of an inhaled anesthetic agent often is stated in multiples or fractions of MAC. Several gas analyzers convert end-tidal concentrations of inhalation agents to MAC values; the monitor either adjusts for age and body temperature or assumes a default state of 40 years of age and normal body temperature.

Because of the many identified and unidentified factors that affect MAC (see Table 40.2), individual anesthetic requirements vary widely. It is therefore important to remember that MAC is an average value for a selected population rather than an absolute value for each individual.

## SUGGESTED READINGS

Aranake, A., Mashour, G. A., & Avidan, M. S. (2013). Minimum alveolar concentration: Ongoing relevance and clinical utility. *Anaesthesia, 68,* 512–522.

Blanchard, F., Perbet, S., James, A., Verdonk, F., Godet, T., Bazin, J. E., et al. (2020). Minimal alveolar concentration for deep sedation (MAC-DS) in intensive care unit patients sedated with sevoflurane: A physiological study. *Anaesthesia Critical Care & Pain Medicine, 39*(3), 429–434.

James, M. F. M., Hofmeyr, R., & Grocott, M. P. W. (2015). Losing concentration: Time for a new MAPP. *British Journal of Anaesthesia, 115,* 824–826.

Lobo, S. A., Ojeda, J., Dua, A., Singh, K., & Lopez, J. (2021). Minimum alveolar concentration. In: *StatPearls.* Treasure Island, FL: StatPearls Publishing.

Nguyen, V. (2014). Minimum alveolar concentration. In B. S. Freeman & J. S. Berger (Eds.), *Anesthesiology Core Review: Part One Basic Exam.* McGraw Hill.

Ni, K., Cooter, M., Gupta, D. K., Thomas, J., Hopkins, T. J., Miller, T. E., et al. (2019). Paradox of age: Older patients receive higher age-adjusted minimum alveolar concentration fractions of volatile anaesthetics yet display higher bispectral index values. *British Journal of Anaesthesia, 123*(3), 288–297.

# The Effect of Intracardiac Shunts on Inhalation Induction

EDUARDO S. RODRIGUES, MD

Cardiac shunts primarily alter the effect of uptake of the anesthetic agent by pulmonary arterial blood. The determinants of anesthetic uptake from alveoli are the blood-gas partition coefficient of the anesthetic agent, the cardiac output, and the alveolar/mixed venous partial pressure difference of the anesthetic agent (Pa − P$\overline{\text{v}}$).

The blood-gas partition coefficient is the distribution ratio of the anesthetic agent between blood and alveolar gas at equilibrium (relative solubility). For a highly soluble agent, not available in clinical practice today, it takes several passes of the blood volume through the lung before enough of the agent is absorbed that the blood is saturated to the point that the necessary Pa of the agent to achieve anesthesia is reached. A highly soluble agent, then, has a much slower induction time than a less soluble agent (see later). Assuming no change in the ventilation or inspired fraction of the anesthetic agent and normal tissue perfusion, the rate of induction is determined primarily by anesthetic solubility and adequate pulmonary blood flow.

## Right-to-Left Shunt

With a right-to-left shunt, a portion of the cardiac output (CO) bypasses the lung, slowing induction, because less anesthetic agent can be transferred from the alveoli to the systemic blood per unit of time. The rate of induction for an insoluble agent is proportional to the degree of shunting (i.e., the greater the shunt, the slower the induction). The effect of the shunt is less pronounced for a highly soluble anesthetic agent. Highly soluble anesthetics have not been available for or used in clinical practice for more than a decade, but we will use the historical inhaled anesthetic ether for the purpose of academic discussion. Ether has a blood-gas partition coefficient of 12, and 1 L of blood would have to absorb 12 times more ether than 1 L of gas. If ventilation were 5 L/min with 10% ether, 500 mL of ether would be delivered to the alveoli per minute. The entire blood volume would have to absorb 6 L of ether at equilibrium before equilibrium was reached. In this scenario, ventilation slows induction because only 0.5 L of ether is delivered to the alveoli; it would take 12 min for 6 L to be delivered to the alveoli. If there were a 50% right-to-left shunt and pulmonary blood flow was only 2.5 L (half of the "normal" 5 L/min), pulmonary blood flow would still take up the 0.5 L of ether.

However, for a poorly soluble anesthetic agent (e.g., N$_2$O, with a blood-gas partition coefficient of 0.47), if ventilation is 5 L/min with 50% N$_2$O, then 2.5 L of N$_2$O is delivered to the alveoli per minute. The entire blood volume would have to absorb approximately 1.25 L of N$_2$O before equilibrium was reached. If the patient had a 50% shunt, the 2.5 L of blood flowing through the lungs would absorb 1.25 L of N$_2$O but would then mix with the 2.5 L of blood that bypassed the lung,

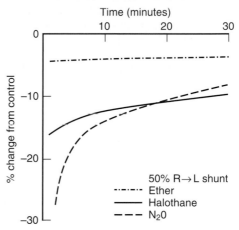

**Fig. 41.1** Decrease in the arterial-to-inspired concentration ratio caused by a 50% right-to-left (R→L) shunt from control for three anesthetic agents of different solubility (ether, halothane, and N$_2$O). (From Tanner G. Effect of left-to-right, mixed left-to-right, and right-to-left shunts on inhalation induction in children: a computer model. *Anesth Analg.* 1985;64:101–107.)

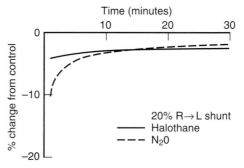

**Fig. 41.2** Decrease in the arterial-to-inspired concentration ratio from control for two anesthetic agents (halothane and N$_2$O) caused by a 20% right-to-left (R→L) shunt. (From Tanner G. Effect of left-to-right, mixed left-to-right, and right-to-left shunts on inhalation induction in children: a computer model. *Anesth Analg.* 1985;64:101–107.)

resulting in a concentration of only 0.625 L of N$_2$O. Induction time would take at least twice as long (Figs. 41.1 and 41.2).

These examples demonstrate that, with highly soluble agents, such as ether, uptake is limited primarily by ventilation. With poorly soluble agents, such as N$_2$O, uptake is determined primarily by blood flow. In a more practical example, inhalation induction with sevoflurane (blood-gas partition coefficient of 0.65) will have pharmacokinetics like $N_2O$ (with a blood-gas partition coefficient of 0.47). It will be limited primarily by blood flow because it is a relatively insoluble agent. Thus the effect of shunting is more significant with these agents of lower solubility.

## Left-to-Right Shunt

With a left-to-right shunt, no significant change occurs in the speed of induction, assuming that systemic blood flow is normal. If tissue perfusion is decreased because of the left-to-right shunt, then induction will initially be slowed because less anesthetic agent will be delivered to the brain per unit of time. CO usually increases to compensate for the shunting, and local control of vasculature maintains cerebral perfusion and minimizes the effect of the shunt (Fig. 41.3).

## Mixed Shunt (Right-to-Left and Left-to-Right)

A left-to-right shunt attenuates the slowed anesthetic induction that may occur with right-to-left shunting because of an increase in effective pulmonary blood flow.

## Clinical Practice

Inhalation induction is still frequently used in clinical practice, often in situations where inhalation induction is potentially advantageous to standard intravenous induction. Such clinical circumstances include pediatrics, difficult airway, patients with limited cardiovascular reserve, and other, less common scenarios like bronchopleural fistulas and mediastinal masses. The only potent inhaled anesthetic suitable for inhalation induction in current practice is sevoflurane, as it is nonpungent and well tolerated by patients. In an excellent publication from Hasija et al., it is well demonstrated that this agent also has a significantly slower induction time in patients with cyanotic congenital heart disease (right-to-left shunt) than in patients with no intracardiac shunt or without cyanotic congenital heart disease (left-to-right shunt). This physical concept is important to better manage and understand inhalation induction in several heterogenic clinical scenarios.

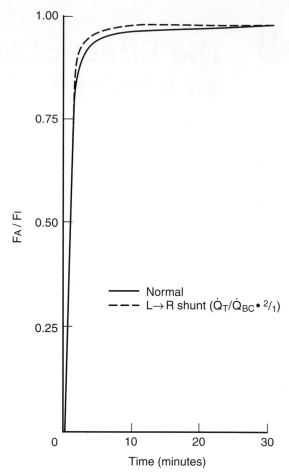

**Fig. 41.3** Arterial-to-inspired concentration ($F_A/F_I$) ratio for $N_2O$ modeled with and without a 50% left-to-right ($L{\rightarrow}R$) shunt and normal tissue perfusion. For the normal simulation, $\dot{Q}_{BC}$ = 3.0 L/min, $\dot{Q}_T$ = 3.16 L/min, $\dot{Q}_{LR}$ = 0.16 L/min, and $\dot{Q}_S$ = 0.16 L/min. For the left-to-right shunt simulation, $\dot{Q}_{BC}$ = 3.0 L/min, $\dot{Q}_T$ = 6.0 L/min, $\dot{Q}_{LR}$ = 3.0 L/min, and $\dot{Q}_S$ = 0.3 L/min. $\dot{Q}_{BC}$, Blood flow perfusing body compartments; $\dot{Q}_{LR}$, left-to-right shunt; $\dot{Q}_S$, right-to-left shunt; $\dot{Q}_T$, total cardiac output. (From Tanner G. Effect of left-to-right, mixed left-to-right, and right-to-left shunts on inhalation induction in children: a computer model. *Anesth Analg.* 1985;64:101–107.)

## SUGGESTED READINGS

Eger, E. I., II. (1974). *Anesthetic uptake and action.* Baltimore: Williams & Wilkins.

Hasija, S., Chauhan, S., Jain, P., Choudhury, A., Aggarwal, N., & Pandey, R. K. (2016). Comparison of speed of inhalational induction in children with and without congenital heart disease. *Annals of Cardiac Anesthesia, 19*(3), 468–474.

Tanner, G. (1985). Effect of left-to-right, mixed left-to-right, and right-to-left shunts on inhalation induction in children: A computer model. *Anesthesia and Analgesia, 64,* 101–107.

# Inhalation Anesthetic Agents

KEVIN T. RIUTORT, MD, MS

Inhaled anesthetics, which played a pivotal role in the development of modern surgical therapies, remain the most used agents for providing general anesthesia. The four most frequently used inhaled anesthetic agents in the United States are nitrous oxide (N$_2$O), isoflurane, sevoflurane, and desflurane. Each agent differs in its pharmacokinetic and pharmacodynamic profiles, providing unique advantages in different situations.

Originally used in 19th-century dentistry, N$_2$O, a colorless gas at room temperature, is commonly referred to as *laughing gas*. Nitrous oxide is seldom used as the sole anesthetic in modern practice, but it remains popular for use in combination with other inhaled anesthetic agents. Desflurane, sevoflurane, and isoflurane are all fluorinated inhalational anesthetic agents. Inhalational anesthetic agents that have been halogenated with fluorine demonstrate reduced flammability and greater molecular stability than historical agents, such as ether. Desflurane and sevoflurane are gradually replacing older inhalational anesthetic agents because their lower solubility results in more rapid induction and emergence from anesthesia.

## Pharmacokinetics

The pharmacokinetics of a drug refers to its absorption, distribution, metabolism, and excretion. The primary mechanism for the absorption of inhaled anesthetic agents is through the pulmonary alveoli. As these drugs are inhaled, they are exposed to the rich vascular supply of the lungs (i.e., pulmonary capillary beds) where they are absorbed and distributed systemically. The partial pressure of the inhalational anesthetic agents in the central nervous system (P$_{CNS}$) is proportional to the arterial partial pressure (P$_A$), which in turn is proportional to the alveolar pressure (P$_A$) at equilibrium. Therefore at equilibrium, P$_{CNS}$ is directly proportional to P$_A$. This is an important concept because P$_A$ can be easily measured with a gas analyzer at modern anesthesia workstations. The pharmacokinetics of inhaled anesthetics agents (and intravenous drugs) is a first-order process where the rate of change of the drug is dependent on its driving concentration gradient. Many physical processes have similar mathematics, such as heat conduction on a stove, aerodynamic drag on an aircraft, or shock absorber motion on an automobile.

## Uptake

The uptake of inhaled anesthetic agents from the lung into the bloodstream is dependent on three main factors (excluding the concentration and second gas effects). The first is the alveolar-mixed venous partial pressure difference (P$_{(A-\bar{v})}$), which is the difference between the partial pressure of the inhaled anesthetic in the alveoli and the partial pressure in the returning pulmonary capillary blood. As the anesthetic approaches equilibrium between the alveoli and the rest of the body, this gradient diminishes. The second variable is the solubility of the anesthetic agent in the blood, which is defined as the blood-gas partition coefficient ($\lambda$), and the third variable is cardiac output (CO). A simple calculation can predict the uptake of any given inhaled anesthetic agent. From this equation, it is apparent that if any of these three factors is increased, there will be greater uptake of the anesthetic agent:

$$\text{Uptake} = P_{(A-\bar{v})} \times \lambda \times CO$$

## Excretion

Excretion of inhalational anesthetic agents relies on alveolar ventilation and urinary and gastrointestinal elimination of metabolic by-products. As ventilation increases during emergence, so does the amount of anesthetic agent removed from the body. Metabolism of the inhaled anesthetic agents varies, creating variable effects on the rate of decrease of P$_A$. However, alveolar ventilation is still the primary means of excretion, even for more highly metabolized agents.

## Distribution

Body tissues vary dramatically in blood flow distribution. Tissues that receive the greatest perfusion are known as the *vessel rich group*, and these include the brain, heart, liver, and kidneys. Although the vessel-rich group makes up about 10% of the total body mass, these organs receive an overwhelming majority of CO. The muscle group has an intermediate blood flow distribution, and the fat group receives the least blood flow. The muscle and fat groups receive smaller fractions of CO, even though they make up a much larger proportion of body mass.

## Minimum Alveolar Concentration

Minimum alveolar concentration (MAC) is the concentration of an inhalational anesthetic agent that prevents movement in response to a surgical stimulus in 50% of patients. It is expressed as a percentage of the partial pressure of the anesthetic in relation to the barometric pressure. More simply stated, if the MAC of isoflurane is 1.14 at sea level, the partial pressure of isoflurane at steady state must be 0.0114 × 760 mm Hg, which is 8.66 mm Hg. For N$_2$O, with a MAC of 104, partial pressure would be 790.4 mm Hg, a partial pressure that could only be obtained under hyperbaric conditions. Using this terminology, inhalational anesthetic agents can be compared using multiples of MAC (e.g., 0.5, 1.0, 1.2) to express their relevant effects at a given concentration. It is far easier to compare inhalational anesthetic agents in terms of their MAC than their partial pressures, which can vary greatly depending on the agent, the altitude, and other factors.

| TABLE 42.1 Pharmacologic Characteristics of Inhalational Anesthetic Agents | | | | |
|---|---|---|---|---|
| | **AGENT** | | | |
| Characteristic | $N_2O$ | Desflurane | Sevoflurane | Isoflurane |
| Molecular weight | 44.02 | 168.04 | 200.05 | 184.5 |
| Minimum alveolar concentration | 104 | 6.0 | 2.05 | 1.14 |
| **PARTITION COEFFICIENT** | | | | |
| Blood-gas | 0.47 | 0.42 | 0.63 | 1.4 |
| Brain-blood | 1.1 | 1.3 | 1.7 | 1.6 |
| Muscle-blood | 1.2 | 2.0 | 3.1 | 2.9 |
| Fat-blood | 2.3 | 27 | 48 | 45 |

Just as MAC can be determined for the absence of a response to a standard surgical stimulus, MAC can also be determined for additional depths of anesthesia. For example, the MAC needed to prevent patient eye-opening on command (MAC-awake) and the MAC needed to blunt autonomic response (MAC-BAR) have been identified. The standard deviation of the MAC is approximately 10%. Therefore 1.2 MAC is roughly the concentration required to prevent response to a surgical stimulus in 97% of patients.

When fluorinated hydrocarbon agents are used in combination with $N_2O$, or when it is necessary to switch from one agent to another (i.e., isoflurane to sevoflurane), the MACs are additive. For example, if a patient inhales 0.75 MAC of $N_2O$, then only 0.25 MAC of a second inhalational anesthetic (e.g., isoflurane) is required to achieve a combined MAC of 1.0.

## Blood-Gas Partition Coefficient

The $\lambda$ value describes the relative solubility of an anesthetic agent in blood compared with its solubility in a gas (Table 42.1). Simply put, it is the concentration of anesthetic agent in the blood divided by the concentration of the agent in gas when the two phases are in equilibrium with one another.

Soluble anesthetic agents, or ones that have a high $\lambda$ value, have higher concentrations in the blood phase than in the gas phase. Therefore for a soluble anesthetic agent to exert a partial pressure in the blood phase equal to that in the gas phase, a relatively large number of molecules must be absorbed into the blood, translating into a slower rate of rise of $P_A$.

Just as the $\lambda$ value describes the solubility of anesthetic agents in blood compared with the solubility in gas, the tissue-blood coefficient is used to describe the solubility of anesthetic agents in tissue compared with their solubility in blood. Tissues with high tissue-blood coefficients (e.g., fat) require more molecules of anesthetic agent to be dissolved into them for equilibrium with the blood to be reached.

## Concentration Effect and Second Gas Effect

When anesthetic agents are combined, two phenomena, known as the *concentration effect* and the *second gas effect*, occur. The concentration effect occurs when $N_2O$ is delivered in combination with other gases. The higher the inspired $N_2O$ concentration, the faster the alveolar concentrations of $N_2O$ and the other gases will approach their respective inspired concentrations ($P_I$) (Fig. 42.1). For example, patients receiving a $P_I$ of 80% $N_2O$ will experience a more rapid increase in the $P_A/P_I$ ratio compared with patients receiving 60% $N_2O$. As pulmonary capillary blood removes $N_2O$ from the alveoli, the gases in the anatomic dead space (e.g., bronchi) will be entrained into the alveoli, which results in an even faster rise in the alveolar concentration of the agent (second gas effect).

## Shunts

Right-to-left intracardiac shunts slow the rate of increase of the anesthetic $P_A$ during induction. This delay is caused by the dilution of pulmonary blood entering the left side of the heart with venous blood that has not been exposed to the inhalational anesthetic agent within the lungs. Right-to-left intracardiac shunts therefore slow an inhalation induction.

Left-to-right intracardiac shunts deliver pulmonary blood containing inhalational anesthetic agents back to the pulmonary

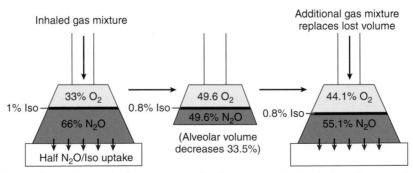

**Fig. 42.1** Concentration and second gas effects. The figure depicts alveolar gases at the beginning of an anesthetic. After an initial inspiratory breath, alveoli are filled with the gas mixture in the circuit (66% nitrous oxide [$N_2O$], 33% oxygen [$O_2$], and 1% isoflurane [Iso]) at their normal end-inspiratory volume (*left panel*). After half of the $N_2O$ and isoflurane are absorbed into pulmonary blood, the alveolar gas volume is reduced by 33.5%. At this point, the volume of $N_2O$ equals the volume of $O_2$ and the gas mixture is 49.6% $N_2O$, 49.6% $O_2$, and 0.8% isoflurane. Inflow of additional inspired gas mixture returns alveolar volume to its original value, resulting in a gas mixture of 55.1% $N_2O$, 44.1% $O_2$, and 0.8% isoflurane. The alveolar partial pressure of $N_2O$ falls much less than the fractional uptake (the concentration effect). In addition, the partial pressure of $O_2$ *increases* relative to the inspired gas $O_2$ content, and the partial pressure of isoflurane is sustained close to the inspired value, increasing its rate of uptake (the second gas effect). (From Forman SA, Ishizawa Y. Inhaled anesthetic uptake, distribution, metabolism, and toxicity. In: Gropper, MA, ed. *Miller's Anesthesia*. 9th ed. Elsevier; 2020. Fig. 20.8.)

circulation for a second pass. As a result, a smaller amount of inhalational anesthetic agent diffuses from the alveoli to capillary blood. From a clinical standpoint, the induction rate is unchanged if there is only a left-to-right shunt. However, when combined right-to-left and left-to-right shunts are present, depending on the anatomic location and size of the shunts, left-to-right shunts can affect induction times. The normally delayed induction experienced with a right-to-left shunt can be offset by a left-to-right shunt because unsaturated blood from the right side entering the left side has the opportunity to pass back to the right side, perfuse alveoli, and take up anesthetic agent.

## Alveolar-Mixed Venous Partial Pressure Difference

The relationship between the $P_A$ and the partial pressure of gases in the mixed venous blood returning to the lungs ($P_{\bar{v}}$) is known as the *alveolar-mixed venous partial pressure difference*: $P_{(A-\bar{v})}$. During induction, the $P_{(A-\bar{v})}$ is at its highest. Blood has not yet been exposed to anesthetic agents, and the high $P_A$ created by the inhaled gases leads to a large $P_{(A-\bar{v})}$. Over time, more anesthetic agent in the alveoli equilibrates with pulmonary capillary blood until, eventually, blood returning to the lungs carries back some of the anesthetic agent, resulting in a smaller $P_{(A-\bar{v})}$. As various tissues become more saturated, the $P_{\bar{v}}$ increases even further, and the amount of anesthetic agent taken up at the alveolar-capillary interface progressively declines because of the decrease in the $P_{(A-\bar{v})}$. This decrease in anesthetic uptake necessitates a decrease in the amount of anesthetic agent administered to the patient over time.

## Effect of Cardiac Output on Induction of Inhaled Anesthetic

CO plays a major role in the uptake and induction time of inhaled anesthetic agents: uptake of the inhaled anesthetic agents is directly proportional to CO. With greater CO, more blood is delivered to the pulmonary capillary tree per unit of time; more blood absorbs more anesthetic agent, slowing the rate of rise of the agent and its pressure within the alveoli ($P_A$). Similarly, in patients with a high CO, even though more anesthetic agent is absorbed, it is dissolved in a larger volume of blood, leading to a lower $P_A$ (and thus a lower $P_{CNS}$) of the inhaled agent. In patients with low CO, the opposite occurs: blood spends more time in the pulmonary circulation, allowing the anesthetic agent to equilibrate with the smaller volume of blood, and as a result, the anesthetic agent in the alveoli achieves steady state more quickly. Because the $P_A$ of the drug reaches equilibrium more quickly, so too does the $P_A$ of the blood, and as this blood is delivered to the tissues, it translates into a more rapid increase in $P_{CNS}$.

## Effects of Inhaled Anesthetic Agents on the Circulatory and Pulmonary Systems

Volatile anesthetic agents have predictable effects on the circulatory system. A common side effect is dose-dependent alterations in blood pressure, contractility, and heart rate. Blood pressure is decreased through relaxation of vascular smooth muscle. Myocardial contractility is slightly reduced with increasing concentrations of inhaled anesthetics, and the heart rate may increase modestly from baseline at approximately 1 MAC. Desflurane and, to a lesser extent, isoflurane may incite a transient but significant tachycardia. The mechanism is thought to be because of relative pungency of these agents during rapid increases in alveolar concentration, which leads to increased sympathetic tone from activation of airway receptors.

There appears to be some degree of myocardial protection associated with volatile anesthetics through the mechanism of *preconditioning*. A preconditioning stimulus, such as a brief episode of myocardial ischemia, produces an intracellular signaling cascade aimed at minimizing damage from both ischemia and reperfusion. It is thought that exposure to volatile anesthetics preconditions the heart by mimicking this process and creates a window, lasting for several hours, where the preconditioned heart better tolerates myocardial ischemia.

The pulmonary system also sees dose-dependent physiologic changes associated with the administration of inhaled anesthetics. Exposure to all the commonly used inhaled anesthetic agents results in a decrease in the ventilatory response to hypercarbia and hypoxia, and inhaled anesthetics attenuate hypoxic pulmonary vasoconstriction in animal models. The effects of inhaled anesthetic agents on pulmonary vascular resistance are much less pronounced than their effect on systemic vascular resistance, except for $N_2O$, which may lead to a small increase in pulmonary vasoconstriction and increased pulmonary arterial pressure. Spontaneously breathing patients experience increasing respiratory rates and decreasing tidal volumes with escalating concentrations of volatile anesthetics. These changes typically have minimal effect on total minute ventilation, except for higher concentrations of volatile anesthetic, which eventually lead to a reduction in minute ventilation.

Global shortages of intravenous sedatives during the COVID-19 pandemic have led to increased use of inhalation agents in the critical care setting. In ventilated patients with COVID-19 pneumonia and acute respiratory distress syndrome, inhalational volatile-based sedation has been shown to be a safe and efficacious alternative or adjunct to intravenous sedation. Isoflurane or sevoflurane is delivered either with an anesthesia machine or a critical care ventilator with an inline mini vaporizer with reflector. When used for critical care sedation, inhalation anesthetics show a reduction in extubation time compared with midazolam or propofol. Additionally, there is no significant difference in adverse events, death, or length of hospital stay when inhalation agents are used for critical sedation.

## SUGGESTED READINGS

Brioni, J. D., Varughese, S., Ahmed, R., & Bein, B. (2017). A clinical review of inhalation anesthesia with sevoflurane: From early research to emerging topics. *Journal of Anesthesia, 31*(5), 764–778.

Jerath, A., Ferguson, N. D., & Cuthbertson, B. (2020). Inhalational volatile-based sedation for COVID-19 pneumonia and ARDS. *Intensive Care Med, 46*(8), 1563–1566.

Swyers, T., Redford, D., & Larson, D. F. (2014). Volatile anesthetic-induced preconditioning. *Perfusion, 29*(1), 10–15.

Varughese, S., & Ahmed, R. (2021). Environmental and occupational considerations of anesthesia: A narrative review and update. *Anesthesia and Analgesia, 133*(4), 826–835.

Wang, Y., Ming, X. X., & Zhang, Z. F. (2020). Fluorine-containing inhalation anesthetics: Chemistry, properties and pharmacology. *Current Medicinal Chemistry, 27*(33), 5599–5652.

# 43

# Nitrous Oxide

LAYNE M. BETTINI, MD, JD

Nitrous oxide ($N_2O$), a colorless, odorless inorganic gas at room temperature, kept as a liquid under pressure (745 psig) in an E-cylinder with a capacity of 1590 L. When the cylinder pressure falls below 745 psig, 400 L $N_2O$ remain. $N_2O$ is not flammable but will support combustion as actively as does oxygen ($O_2$). It is relatively insoluble, with a blood-gas partition coefficient of 0.47, and it is the least potent inhalation anesthetic agent used in practice, with a minimum alveolar concentration of 104%. $N_2O$ is most often used in concentrations of 50% to 70% as an adjuvant to more potent inhaled anesthetic agents or in addition to intravenously administered anesthetic agents. $N_2O$ does not produce skeletal muscle relaxation but does have analgesic effects. It has been used in clinical anesthetic practice for more than 150 years. Despite this long record of use, controversy and concern continue to exist regarding its effect on cellular function via inactivation of vitamin $B_{12}$, expansion or increased pressure of air-filled spaces, effects on embryonic development, effects on postoperative nausea and vomiting, and its environmental impact.

## Systemic Effects

### RESPIRATORY SYSTEM

$N_2O$ decreases tidal volume and increases respiratory rate in spontaneously breathing patients and reduces the ventilatory response to $CO_2$ and hypoxia.

### CENTRAL NERVOUS SYSTEM

Although it is not a potent anesthetic, $N_2O$ has good analgesic properties. Maximum analgesic effects are noted at a concentration of 35%. Half of patients are unaware of their surroundings when $N_2O$ is administered at a concentration of 75%. Concentrations exceeding 60% can increase cerebral metabolic rate, cerebral blood flow, and potentially increase intracranial pressure.

### CARDIOVASCULAR SYSTEM

Compared with other inhalation agents, $N_2O$ has only minimal cardiovascular effects. The slight direct myocardial depression is usually offset by sympathetic stimulation, so that little net effect is observed. Concomitant opioids can block the sympathomimetic effects of $N_2O$. However, despite this scientific rationale, most anesthesiologists avoid the use of $N_2O$ in patients with pulmonary hypertension because of concern about sympathetic stimulation that may increase pulmonary vascular resistance.

## Metabolism

$N_2O$ is primarily excreted unchanged via the lungs, with small amounts diffusing through the skin and metabolized in the bowel.

## Postoperative Nausea and Vomiting

$N_2O$ modestly increases the incidence of postoperative nausea and vomiting. Exposure time to $N_2O$ is an important factor. In patients with a low risk for postoperative nausea and vomiting, the risk may be significantly reduced by prophylactic antiemetics.

## Toxicity

$N_2O$ inactivates methionine synthase by oxidizing the cobalt in vitamin $B_{12}$. Methionine synthase is a ubiquitous cytosolic enzyme that plays a crucial role in the synthesis of DNA, RNA, myelin, catecholamines, and other products. Decreased methionine synthase activity can result in both genetic and protein aberrations. Liver biopsies have demonstrated a 50% reduction in methionine synthase activity at 45 to 90 minutes in patients administered 70% $N_2O$.

### HEMATOLOGIC AND IMMUNE TOXICITY

Inhibition of methionine synthase may lead to megaloblastic anemia. $N_2O$ exposure for 2 to 6 hours in seriously ill patients can cause megaloblastic bone marrow changes. The elderly are particularly vulnerable to developing this complication because up to 20% of the elderly population are deficient in cobalamin. $N_2O$ has also been implicated in impairment of immune function by decreasing neutrophilic chemotaxis and mucociliary transport.

### OCCUPATIONAL EXPOSURE

Retrospective epidemiologic studies have shown an increased incidence of spontaneous abortion in women working in operating rooms. Most of these occupational exposure studies predated the modern use of scavenging and operating room ventilation. Occupational exposure limits for $N_2O$ of 25 ppm have been established. Occupational exposure limits are expressed as an 8-hour time-weighted average. No causative relationship has been proven to support a fetotoxic or genotoxic effect of $N_2O$ exposure in humans.

### NEUROLOGIC TOXICITY

Neurologic injury has been observed in patients with cobalamin deficiency, although the injury may not be apparent for several weeks. In addition, patients with unsuspected vitamin $B_{12}$ deficiency have been diagnosed with myeloneuropathy 2 to 6 weeks after they received $N_2O$ anesthesia. $N_2O$ abusers can present with altered mental status, paresthesia, ataxia, and weakness and spasticity of the legs. There are no experimental data to suggest that administering $N_2O$ causes postoperative cognitive dysfunction, although exposure to anesthesia remains a possible risk factor.

## MYOCARDIAL EFFECTS

The use of $N_2O$ has been associated with increased perioperative myocardial risks possibly secondary to increased homocysteine levels. However, a large multicenter trial (ENIGMA II) with 1-year follow-up supported the safety of $N_2O$ administration in patients with known or suspected cardiovascular disease who underwent noncardiac surgery.

# Nitrous Oxide and Closed Air Spaces

$N_2O$ can diffuse into closed air spaces with significant clinical consequences. Although relatively insoluble compared with other anesthetic agents, $N_2O$ is 30 times more soluble than $N_2$. The blood-gas coefficient of $N_2O$ is 0.47, whereas that of $N_2$ is 0.015. $N_2O$ diffuses quickly, whereas $N_2$ diffuses more slowly. As a result, at any given partial pressure, far more $N_2O$ can be carried to or removed from a closed gas space. The air space will expand, increasing volume in distensible spaces, increasing pressure in nondistensible spaces, or causing a combination of both effects.

## COMPLIANT SPACES INCREASE VOLUME

The maximum change in volume that can result is related to the concentration of $N_2O$ in the alveoli (Fig. 43.1):

$$\text{Change in volume}(\%) = FAN_2O / 1 - FAN_2O$$

$$50\% \ N_2O: \frac{0.5}{1-0.5} = 100\% \uparrow \text{in volume}$$

$$80\% \ N_2O: \frac{0.8}{1-0.8} = 400\% \uparrow \text{in volume}$$

## NONCOMPLIANT SPACES INCREASE PRESSURE

The maximum change in pressure is arithmetically related to the partial pressure of $N_2O$ in the alveoli:
50% $N_2O$ increases pressure 0.5 atm
75% $N_2O$ increases pressure 0.75 atm
These principles hold true for any anesthetic gas administered, but they are clinically relevant for $N_2O$ because of its low solubility and the high concentrations used (i.e., isoflurane would

not have a significant effect on closed air spaces because it is used at only 1%–2% concentration).

## EXAMPLES

### Bowel Gas and Bowel Obstruction

The bowel usually contains small volumes of gas, so the increase in volume is of no consequence. For example, 100 mL of bowel gas resulting from swallowing and bacteria could increase two to three times without causing clinical problems. On the other hand, the stomach and intestine can contain up to 5 to 10 L of air, and 1 to 2 L of air is not uncommon. Doubling or tripling this volume can crowd the operative field, limit movement of the diaphragm, compromise respiration, make abdominal closure difficult, and increase abdominal pressure during laparoscopy with $CO_2$ inflation. Even with obstruction, changes in volume occur slowly. Operations lasting less than 1 hour will have insignificant changes in volume.

### Pneumothorax and Communicating Blebs

Because of the high blood flow in the lungs, the effect of $N_2O$ on a pneumothorax occurs rapidly. $N_2O$ (75%) can double the size of a pneumothorax in 10 minutes and triple it in 30 minutes.

### Venous Air Emboli

The volume necessary for an air embolism to become lethal is significantly smaller in the presence of $N_2O$, owing to its potential for expansion resulting in cardiovascular collapse. If a venous air embolism is suspected, $N_2O$ should be discontinued immediately.

### Balloon-Tipped Catheters

It has been observed that when the anesthesia provider attempts to float a pulmonary artery catheter in a patient anesthetized with $N_2O$, a greater volume of air can be withdrawn from the balloon than was injected. The volume change in the catheter tip is maximal at 5 to 10 minutes, depending on the $N_2O$ mixture. This increased volume may be problematic if an occluded balloon is expanded. It is advisable to deflate the balloon and reinflate it every few minutes if $N_2O$ is being used and to deflate the balloon in all cases after the occlusion pressure has been determined.

### Tracheal Tube Cuffs

$N_2O$ can also diffuse into tracheal tube cuffs, causing increases in volume and pressure. Overexpansion of tracheal tube cuffs secondary to $N_2O$ diffusion may cause airway obstruction and glottic or subglottic trauma. The volume increase depends on the concentration of $N_2O$ and the length of time the patient is exposed to $N_2O$. Use of pure $N_2O$ (100%) for 3 hours can increase cuff volume by approximately 300%.

### Middle Ear

$N_2O$ enters the middle ear cavity, elevating middle ear pressure. Normally, any increase in middle ear pressure is vented via the eustachian tube into the nasopharynx. Narrowing of the eustachian tube by acute inflammation, scar tissue, or surgery in the vicinity of the eustachian tube impairs this venting. Increases in pressure can lead to changes in the outcome of previous middle ear operations and displacement of the tympanic membrane graft during tympanoplasty.

Alveolar nitrous oxide concentration = 50%

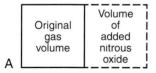

A

Alveolar nitrous oxide concentration = 80%

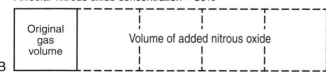

B

**Fig. 43.1** Volume changes in a compliant closed space by 100% and by 400% when the alveolar concentration of $N_2O$ is **(A)** 50% or **(B)** 80%, respectively. (From Eger EI II, Saidman LJ. Hazards of nitrous oxide anesthesia in bowel obstruction and pneumothorax. *Anesthesiology.* 1965;26:61–66.)

## Intraocular Pressure

Sulfur hexafluoride and perfluoropropane are sometimes injected into the vitreous cavity at varying concentrations during surgical management of retinal disease, including retinal detachment and macular holes. $N_2O$ is 117 times more soluble than sulfur hexafluoride. Pressure has been shown to increase by 14 to 30 mm Hg if $N_2O$ is used. This increased pressure can compromise retinal blood flow and cause retinal ischemia or infarction. Reabsorption of $N_2O$ from the ocular cavity may cause underfilling of the therapeutic gas mixtures and potentially compromise the success of the operation.

## Dural Closure

Despite concerns about $N_2O$ in closed spaces, it is not necessary to discontinue $N_2O$ before closing the dura during craniotomy to avoid expanding intracranial air and increasing intracranial pressure. However, $N_2O$ should not be initiated after dural closure because of the risk of expanding intracranial air and the development of a tension pneumocephalus.

## Environmental Impact

Like all inhalational anesthetics, $N_2O$ is a greenhouse gas. It has an atmospheric lifetime of 114 years and, on a molecule-per-molecule basis, has 300 times the warming effect of carbon dioxide. Additionally, $N_2O$ depletes the ozone layer. If $N_2O$ must be used, minimal flow anesthesia will reduce environmental harm; ideally, a total intravenous anesthetic (TIVA) technique would be preferred. It is worth noting that the multitude of single-use packaging required with TIVA is also not without consequence from an environmental impact perspective.

## SUGGESTED READINGS

Buhre, W., Disma, N., Hendrickx, J., DeHert, S., Hollmann, M. W., Huhn, R., et al. (2019). European Society of Anaesthesiology Task Force on Nitrous Oxide: A narrative review of its role in clinical practice. *British Journal of Anaesthesia, 122*(5), 587–604.

Chan, C., & Chan, M. (2021). Use of nitrous oxide in contemporary anesthesia—an ongoing tug of war. *Canadian Journal of Anaesthesia, 68,* 1597–1600.

Joshi, G., Pennant, J., & Kehlet, H. (2017). Evaluation of nitrous oxide in the gas mixture for anesthesia (ENIGMA) studies: The tale of two large pragmatic randomized controlled trials. *Anesthesia and Analgesia, 124,* 2077–2079.

Myles, P. S., Leslie, K., Chan, M. T., Forbes, A., Peyton, P. J., Paech, M. J., et al. (2014). The safety of addition of nitrous oxide to general anaesthesia in at-risk patients having major non-cardiac surgery (ENIGMA-II): A randomised, single-blind trial. *Lancet, 384*(9952), 1446–1454.

Myles, P. S., Leslie, K., Chan, M. T., Kasza, J., Paech, M. J., Peyton, P. J., et al. (2016). Severe nausea and vomiting in the evaluation of nitrous oxide in the gas mixture for anesthesia II trial (ENIGMA II). *Anesthesiology, 124,* 1032–1040.

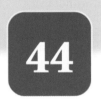

# 44

# Cardiovascular Effects of the Inhalation Agents

LINDSAY BARENDRICK, MD | GWENDOLYN RAYNOR, MD

An ideal anesthetic would produce amnesia, areflexia, analgesia, and attenuate procedural awareness—all in the setting of autonomic stability. Inhaled anesthetic agents come close to meeting these criteria. However, many inhaled anesthetics have significant, dose-dependent cardiovascular effects (Fig. 44.1).

## Systemic Vascular Resistance

The most common volatile agents in use today (desflurane, isoflurane, and sevoflurane) are all potent vasodilators, causing dose-dependent decreases in systemic vascular resistance (SVR) and blood pressure. Of these three agents, sevoflurane has demonstrated the least effect on SVR.

At greater than 1.5 minimum alveolar concentration, isoflurane and desflurane have been correlated with a significantly lower vascular resistance than sevoflurane. Although no longer in regular use within the United States, halothane had the least effect on SVR but significantly lowered systemic blood pressure due to profound negative inotropic effects (Fig. 44.2).

## Heart Rate

All modern volatile agents (desflurane, isoflurane, and sevoflurane) can increase heart rate (Fig. 44.3). Reflexive increases in heart rate are commonly seen in response to decreases in mean arterial pressure; this can occur despite the propensity of

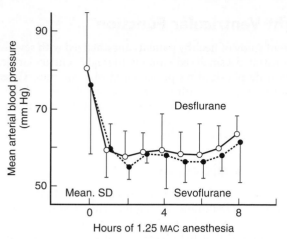

**Fig. 44.1** Mean arterial pressure decreases significantly within 1 hour of the onset of anesthesia with equivalent minimum alveolar concentration (MAC) doses of either sevoflurane or desflurane, without any difference between the two compounds. *SD,* Standard deviation. (From Eger EI, Bowland T, Ionescu P, Laster MJ, Fang Z, Gong D, et al. Recovery and kinetic characteristics of desflurane and sevoflurane in volunteers after 8-h exposure, including kinetics of degradation products. *Anesthesiology.* 1997;87:517–526.)

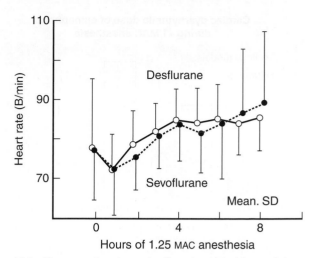

**Fig. 44.3** Heart rate increases significantly within 1 hour of the onset of anesthesia with equivalent minimum alveolar concentration (MAC) doses of either sevoflurane or desflurane, without any difference between the two compounds. *SD,* Standard deviation. (From Eger EI, Bowland T, Ionescu P, Laster MJ, Fang Z, Gong D, et al. Recovery and kinetic characteristics of desflurane and sevoflurane in volunteers after 8-h exposure, including kinetics of degradation products. *Anesthesiology.* 1997;87:517–526.)

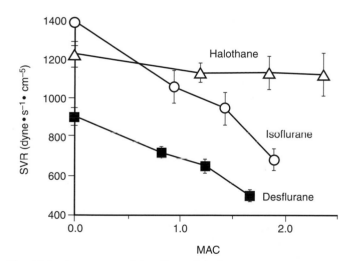

**Fig. 44.2** Comparison of the effects of desflurane with those of isoflurane and halothane on systemic vascular resistance (SVR) in healthy young men. *MAC,* Minimum alveolar concentration. (From Weiskopf RB, Cahalan MK, Eger EI II, et al. Cardiovascular actions of desflurane in normocarbic volunteers. *Anesth Analg.* 1991;73:143–156.)

| TABLE 44.1 | Cardiovascular Effects of Inhalation Anesthetic Agents | | | |
|---|---|---|---|---|
| Agent(s) | Contractility | SVR | SBP | HR |
| Halothane | ↓↓ | – | ↓ | – |
| Enflurane | ↓ | ↓ | ↓ | ↑ |
| Isoflurane, desflurane, sevoflurane | ↓ | ↓ | ↓ | ↑ |
| Xenon | – | – | – | – |
| Nitrous oxide | ↓ | – | – | – |

*HR,* Heart rate; *PVR,* peripheral vascular resistance; *SBP,* systolic blood pressure.

## Cardiac Output and Myocardial Contractility

Cardiac output is the product of stroke volume and heart rate. As previously noted, the modern volatile agents (desflurane, isoflurane, and sevoflurane) can elevate the heart rate and decrease SVR; accordingly, these agents can alter cardiac output. Halothane, which is still in use in the developing world, has less effect on SVR than modern volatile agents but pronounced depressant effects on myocardial contractility—another determinant of stroke volume. This negative inotropic action was caused by halothane's alteration of calcium release from the cardiomyocyte's sarcoplasmic reticulum. Although clinically insignificant in healthy populations, all volatile anesthetics can cause some degree of negative inotropy. A summary of the hemodynamic effects of inhaled agents compares modern and out-of-use volatile anesthetics and nonvolatile agents (Table 44.1).

volatile agents to depress the sympathetic response. Desflurane and isoflurane are more pungent and irritating to the airway (compared with sevoflurane), and as a result, stimulation-related heart rate increases may follow abrupt increases in the concentrations of these agents. Some studies have suggested that elderly patients have less heart rate lability while anesthetized with isoflurane, but it is unclear whether this is a function of age (and age-related baroceptor changes) versus anesthetic choice. Halogenated agents can also depress the baroreceptor response. Halothane was known to cause significant baroceptor impairment, but because of its sympathetic depressant effects, the heart rate either decreased or was unchanged.

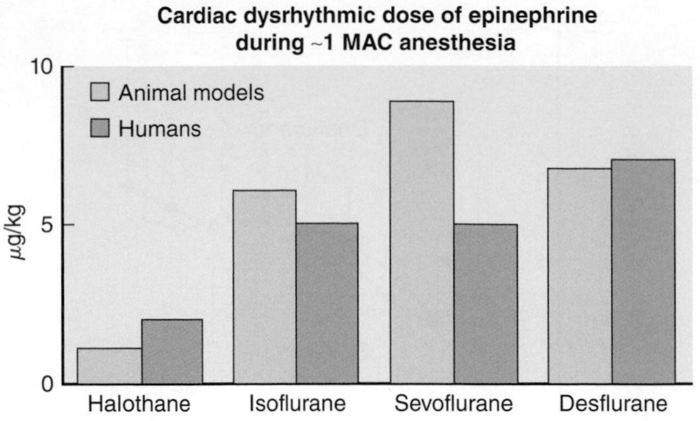

**Fig. 44.4** The dose of epinephrine associated with cardiac arrhythmias in animal and human models was lowest with halothane. The ether anesthetics (isoflurane, desflurane, and sevoflurane) required threefold to sixfold greater doses of epinephrine to cause arrhythmias. *MAC*, Minimum alveolar concentration. (Adapted from Paul Barash, Bruce Cullen, Robert Stoelting Permissions Fig. 17.18 from the 7th edition of Barash: Clinical Anesthesia with Permission)

## Arrhythmogenicity

Halogenated agents lower the arrhythmogenic threshold in adults exposed to submucosal epinephrine (halothane having been the most arrhythmogenic). Older studies defined this threshold as the amount of epinephrine needed to produce three premature ventricular contractions (PVCs). This quantity was found to be 5 μg/kg for both isoflurane and sevoflurane and 7.0 μg/kg for desflurane. Below these levels, no PVCs were seen. Given the widespread use of local anesthetics with epinephrine, a reasonable index of suspicion should be maintained for iatrogenic causes of intraoperative ectopy (Fig. 44.4).

## Coronary Vasodilation

Because of the significant vasodilating effects of volatile inhaled agents like desflurane, isoflurane, and sevoflurane, there was speculation that a coronary "steal" phenomenon could occur, whereby coronary blood flow would be diverted away from ischemic areas to previously underperfused myocardium. Several studies showed that there is no evidence to support these concerns in healthy patients.

## Anesthetic Effect on Diastolic Filling

Volatile anesthetics alter left ventricular diastolic filling, the period during which the myocardium is perfused. Although there have been disparate findings in the literature, atrial dysfunction and preload reduction have been consistently implicated. In patients with preexisting diastolic dysfunction undergoing coronary artery bypass, reductions in all transesophageal echocardiographic transvalvular velocities were observed, particularly with A wave velocities, causing an increase in the E/A ratio. Interestingly, an overall improvement of left ventricular diastolic function was seen in this population.

## Right Ventricular Function

A recent study of healthy patients anesthetized with sevoflurane demonstrated a small reduction in the right ventricular ejection fraction despite finding preserved stroke volumes. Given the negative effects of positive pressure ventilation on the right heart (e.g., increased pulmonary vascular resistance and pulmonary artery pressure), it is difficult to determine the role that sevoflurane plays in this dysfunction.

## Electrocardiogram

Prolongation of the QT interval can precipitate ventricular arrhythmias. Desflurane, isoflurane, and sevoflurane have all been shown to prolong the QTc interval, whereas several studies showed that halothane had little or no effect. Chemically inert and not in widespread clinical use, xenon has also demonstrated no perturbation of the QTc interval. Unlike inhalational agents, propofol has been found by several studies to shorten the QTc interval.

## Cardioprotection

Cardiac ischemia and ischemic reperfusion injury contribute to perioperative morbidity and mortality. A growing body of literature has demonstrated that volatile anesthetics can precondition and thereby protect the heart from devastating ischemic injury. Underlying this concept is the notion that brief periods of cardiac ischemia prior to anticipated periods of extended ischemia or can protect the heart from larger infarctions. Reactive oxygen species (ROS) and anaerobic metabolites can disrupt the intracellular pH of cardiac myocytes and impair mitochondrial function. Intracellular calcium overload and extended mitochondrial permeability transition pore opening have been directly associated with cellular death. Volatile anesthetics trigger protein kinase C, an important mediator in ischemic preconditioning pathways. Because it is difficult to predict the onset of myocardial ischemia, clinical translation of this strategy is challenging.

A related strategy is anesthetic postconditioning, which introduces brief periods of ischemia at the time of reperfusion after an ischemic insult. Myocardial ischemic reperfusion injury is mediated by many of the same mechanisms (ROS and intracellular calcium excess) seen in anesthetic preconditioning. Postconditioning may be beneficial in the setting of cardiac bypass surgery and after acute ischemic interventions.

## Nitrous Oxide

In an international randomized clinical trial, Myles and colleagues found that nitrous oxide was associated with higher, but statistically insignificant rates of perioperative myocardial infarction and death. Postulated mechanisms for nitrous oxide's role in cardiac ischemia related to its inhibition of vitamin B12. B12 is a cofactor for methionine synthase, a key enzyme in the metabolism of homocysteine back to methionine. Elevations in homocysteine can damage the endothelium and cause hypercoagulability. Nevertheless, subsequent trials have failed to prove that nitrous oxide use leads to cardiac ischemia. While its environmental and health effects continue to be studied, nitrous oxide is often utilized because of its propensity to maintain acute cardiovascular stability while contributing predictably to surgical anesthesia.

## Xenon

An inert gas, xenon has long been studied for its hypnotic, analgesic, and cardiac-stable properties. Xenon has lower blood solubility and greater anesthetic action than nitrous oxide and, like nitrous oxide, it does not decrease SVR or cause hypotension. Xenon is postulated to maintain hemodynamic stability by decreasing norepinephrine reuptake. Small studies have also shown that the agent does not prolong the QTc interval or increase the heart rate in healthy patients. Xenon's high cost has been its major barrier in clinical translation.

## SUGGESTED READINGS

Freiermuth, D., Mets, B., Bolliger, D., Reuthebuch, O., Doebele, T., Scholz, M., et al. (2016). Sevoflurane and isoflurane-pharmacokinetics, hemodynamic stability, and cardioprotective effects during cardiopulmonary bypass. *Journal of Cardiothoracic and Vascular Anesthesia, 30*(6), 1494–1501.

Jin, Z., Piazza, O., Ma, D., Scarpati, G., & De Robertis, E. (2019). Xenon anesthesia and beyond: Pros and cons. *Minerva Anestesiologica, 85*(1), 83–89.

Lemoine, S., Tritapepe, L., Hanouz, J. L., & Puddu, P. E. (2016). The mechanisms of cardio-protective effects of desflurane and sevoflurane at the time of reperfusion: Anaesthetic post-conditioning potentially translatable to humans? *British Journal of Anaesthesia, 116*(4), 456–475.

Magunia, H., Jordanow, A., Keller, M., Rosenberger, P., & Nowak-Machen, M. (2019). The effects of anesthesia induction and positive pressure ventilation on right-ventricular function: An echocardiography-based prospective observational study. *BMC Anesthesiology, 19*(1), 199.

Torregroza, C., Raupach, A., Feige, K., Weber, N. C., Hollmann, M. W., & Huhn, R. (2020). Perioperative cardioprotection: General mechanisms and pharmacological approaches. *Anesthesia and Analgesia, 131*(6), 1765–1780.

# 45

# Effects of Inhalation Agents on the Central Nervous System

MELISSA KENEVAN, MD

Inhalation anesthetic agents induce anesthesia by depressing brain function via a dose-dependent reversible mechanism that is not fully understood. Although many theories exist, it is suspected that these agents potentiate inhibitory signals and block excitatory signals throughout the central nervous system (CNS). The use of inhalational anesthetics is associated with alterations in cerebral metabolic rate (CMR), in cerebral blood flow (CBF), in cerebrospinal fluid (CSF) dynamics, on electroencephalogram (EEG), and of evoked potentials (Table 45.1). Additionally, inhalation anesthetic agents have been shown to have both neuroprotective and neurotoxic effects.

The brain depends on aerobic glucose metabolism to maintain cell function and as such has large oxygen requirements, consuming approximately 20% of total body $O_2$. Most inhalation anesthetic agents produce a dose-dependent decrease in CMR, with the exception of nitrous oxide. *Flow-metabolism coupling* is defined as matching of $O_2$ and glucose delivery (CBF) to metabolic demand (CMR). A misconception about inhalation agents is that because they increase CBF and decrease CMR, they "uncouple" flow and metabolism. In fact, although increasing concentrations of inhalation anesthetic agents result in a higher CBF for a given CMR, a coupled relationship between these variables persists (Fig. 45.1). This relationship between CMR and CBF is apparent only if adequate blood pressure is maintained.

Inhalation anesthetic agents impair autoregulation (i.e., maintenance of constant CBF during changes in arterial blood pressure) in a dose-dependent fashion (Fig. 45.2). However, inhalation agents do not inhibit $CO_2$ reactivity and, if anything, exaggerate the response. Thus in the normal brain, the cerebral vasodilation and increase in CBF that occur in response to volatile anesthetic agents (halothane > desflurane = isoflurane > sevoflurane) can be blunted, abolished, or reversed by hypocapnia. Further, many studies have confirmed that hypocapnia attenuates or blocks the increase in intracranial pressure (ICP)

| TABLE 45.1 | Physiologic Effects of Inhalation Anesthetic Agents on the Central Nervous System | | | | |
|---|---|---|---|---|---|
| | Nitrous Oxide | Halothane | Isoflurane | Desflurane | Sevoflurane |
| Cerebral blood flow* | ↑ | ↑↑ | ↑ | ↑ | ↑ |
| Cerebral metabolic rate† | ↑ | ↓ | ↓↓ | ↓↓ | ↓↓ |
| Intracranial pressure | ↑ | ↑↑ | ↑ | ↑ | ↑ |
| Electroencephalogram | ↑↓ | ↓ | ↓↓ | ↓ | ↓ |
| CSF production | N/C | ↓ | N/C | ↑ | ? |
| CSF reabsorption | N/C | ↓ | ↑ | N/C | ? |

*CSF*, Cerebrospinal fluid; *N/C*, no change; *?*, effect unknown; ↑↓, conflicting effects.
*Volume of blood (mL)/100 g brain tissue/min. Normal cerebral blood flow is 45 to 60 mL/100 g/min.
†Normal cerebral metabolic rate is approximately 3.0 to 3.8 mL $O_2$/100 g brain tissue/min.

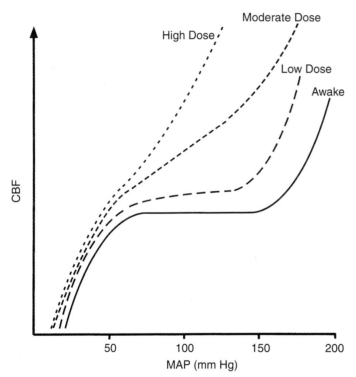

**Fig. 45.1** Regression plots of the regional cerebral metabolic rate for glucose *(CMRGlu)* versus regional cerebral blood flow *(CBF)* in the rat. As the concentration of isoflurane is increased, the slope of the regression line increases (i.e., a higher CBF for a given CMRGlu value). This indicates that isoflurane is a cerebrovasodilator in the rat brain but that it does not uncouple flow and metabolism, even at a minimum alveolar concentration *(MAC)* of 2. (From Todd MM, Warner DS, Maktabi MA. Neuroanesthesia: a critical review. In: Longnecker DE, Tinker JH, Morgan GE Jr, eds. *Principles and Practice of Anesthesiology*. 2nd ed. Vol. 2. Mosby; 1998:1607–1658. Data from Maekawa T, Tommasino C, Shapiro HM, et al. Local cerebral blood flow and glucose utilization during isoflurane anesthesia in the rat. *Anesthesiology*. 1986; 65:144–151.)

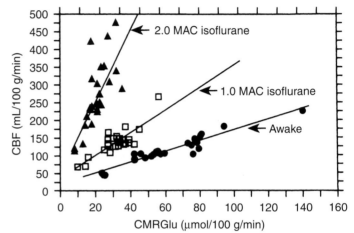

**Fig. 45.2** Schematic representation of the effect of a progressively increased dose of a typical inhalation anesthetic agent on cerebral blood flow *(CBF)* autoregulation. Both upper and lower thresholds are shifted to the left. *MAP*, Mean arterial pressure. (From Drummond JC, Patel PM. Cerebral physiology and the effects of anesthetic techniques. In: Miller RD, ed. *Anesthesia*. 5th ed. Churchill Livingstone; 2000:695–734.)

that otherwise would occur in at-risk patients. These responses may not apply, however, in the presence of abnormal intracranial anatomy or physiology.

## Effect on Central Nervous System Monitors

Anesthesia-induced EEG changes follow a common pattern. When anesthesia is induced with an inhalation agent, the frequency and amplitude of the EEG waveforms uniformly increase and the waveforms measured throughout the cortex appear to synchronize. At approximately 1 minimum alveolar concentration (MAC), the EEG slows progressively; depending on the anesthetic agent, burst suppression, an isoelectric pattern, or seizures may evolve as the anesthetic concentration increases.

The inhalation agents also affect evoked potentials, but only minimally, at concentrations below 1 MAC. All anesthetic agents tend to increase the latency and decrease the amplitude of evoked potentials at concentrations greater than 1 MAC. Evoked potentials of cortical origin are particularly sensitive to the effects of inhalation anesthetic agents; brainstem auditory evoked potentials are the most resistant. Although more sensitive to the effects of inhalation anesthetic agents, somatosensory evoked potentials can be adequately monitored at less than 1 MAC of the inhalation anesthetic agent.

## Neuroprotection Versus Neurotoxicity

Cerebral ischemia results when there is insufficient $O_2$ supply to meet the demand of cells in the brain. Volatile anesthetic agents, particularly isoflurane, have been shown to provide cerebral protection against ischemia by inducing an isoelectric EEG. This significantly decreases the CMR and therefore the brain's $O_2$ demand. Several studies have also demonstrated neuroprotective benefits of sevoflurane exposure before, during, and after hypoxic-ischemic brain injury. The mechanism of this protective effect is thought to be because of activation of antiapoptotic genes and inhibition of apoptotic pathways. In addition to the volatile agents, inhalation of the noble gas xenon recently has been shown to protect the brain from ischemic injury after hypoxic insult.

Conversely, exposure to inhaled anesthetic agents has been associated with neurotoxicity, including neuronal loss, CNS protein accumulation, and altered synapse morphology. Although the mechanism of injury related to anesthetic agents is unclear, suggested pathophysiology includes impairment of protective astrocyte function, activation of inflammatory cytokines, and alteration of gene expression. Often a decline in cognitive function can be observed in geriatric patients who have recently had surgery and anesthesia. A recent population-based cohort study demonstrated that exposure to surgery and general anesthesia was associated with a subtle decline in cognitive function that would be 0.2 standard deviations more than the expected decline because of aging. A follow-up study showed that there was no difference in cognitive decline with or without exposure to nitrous oxide ($N_2O$) during the surgery and general anesthesia event. The most common patient-related risk factors for postoperative neurocognitive dysfunction include increasing age and the presence of preexisting cognitive impairment. Other risk factors include preoperative sleep disturbances, excessive alcohol use, polypharmacy, and medical comorbidities.

In the developing brain, there are well-established data in animal models that associate anesthetic agents with neurotoxicity and neurologic dysfunction. Human studies, however, have significant limitations, and the long-term neurodevelopmental effects of anesthetic exposure in children remains unclear. Overall, the best evidence suggests that exposure to anesthesia is not associated with detrimental effects in the developing brain, and there is no clinically significant effect on academic achievement, intelligence, or a variety of other cognitive domains.

## Nitrous Oxide

### CEREBRAL METABOLIC RATE AND CEREBRAL BLOOD FLOW

Although $N_2O$ is perceived to be physiologically and pharmacologically inert, it is a cerebral vasodilator that can significantly increase CBF and therefore cerebral blood volume and ICP in patients with increased intracranial elastance. This effect on CBF is exaggerated when it is used in conjunction with volatile agents and less when it is used with intravenous induction agents other than ketamine. The effect of $N_2O$ on ICP is blocked or blunted by opioids, barbiturates, and hypocapnia. Most data suggest that $N_2O$ also increases CMR.

### ELECTROENCEPHALOGRAM

Most subjects lose consciousness at $N_2O$ concentrations of approximately 50%, when alpha activity is replaced by fast-wave activity on EEG. As the concentration of $N_2O$ approaches 75%, slow-wave activity (4–8 Hz) appears on the EEG, with some background fast-wave activity still present. If the partial pressure of $N_2O$ continues to increase (as is possible in a hyperbaric environment), fast-wave activity is abolished, with progressive slowing demonstrated on the EEG.

### EVOKED POTENTIALS

At a concentration of less than 1 atm, $N_2O$ has minimal effect on evoked potentials. Its primary effect is to decrease the amplitude of the evoked response, and it has little or no effect on latency.

### PNEUMOCEPHALUS

Pneumocephalus can occur during posterior fossa or cervical spine procedures performed with the patient in the sitting position. When the dura is open, gravity can cause the CSF to drain continuously; the CSF is subsequently replaced by air (an effect known as the inverted pop-bottle phenomenon), resulting in progressive accumulation of air in the ventricles, over the cortical surfaces, or both. If used as part of the anesthetic, $N_2O$ will equilibrate with any air-filled space in the body. Because the blood solubility of $N_2O$ is 30 times greater than that of nitrogen, a significant, albeit transient, net increase of gas molecules will occur in the air-filled space, and the volume or pressure will increase once the dura is closed. Thus $N_2O$ may cause tension pneumocephalus of sufficient significance to produce major cerebral compromise, manifested by seizures, altered consciousness, or specific neurologic deficits.

If a tension pneumocephalus is suspected, the use of $N_2O$ should be discontinued. Patients who receive a second anesthetic within the first 3 weeks after undergoing supratentorial craniotomy are at risk for developing complications if $N_2O$ is used because a number of these patients will still have significant intracranial air collection.

## Isoflurane

### CEREBRAL METABOLIC RATE AND CEREBRAL BLOOD FLOW

Of the inhalation agents, isoflurane is the least potent cerebral vasodilator. $CO_2$ reactivity and autoregulation are maintained with the use of isoflurane concentrations of less than 1 MAC. As with all of the inhalation agents, isoflurane depresses CMR; CMR decreases by 50% at 2.0 MAC of isoflurane, the point at which the EEG becomes isoelectric. Doubling the isoflurane concentration to 4.0 MAC causes no further decrease in CMR.

### INTRACRANIAL PRESSURE

The potential for isoflurane to increase ICP can be blocked by simultaneous induction of hypocapnia, although it is not necessary to induce hypocapnia before administering isoflurane. Isoflurane has no effect on CSF production, and it decreases the resistance to CSF reabsorption.

### ELECTROENCEPHALOGRAM

See the previous discussion of common EEG patterns.

## EVOKED POTENTIALS

Evoked potentials can be measured at isoflurane concentrations of less than 1 MAC.

# Desflurane

### CEREBRAL METABOLIC RATE AND CEREBRAL BLOOD FLOW

The cerebral metabolic and vascular effects of desflurane are similar to those of isoflurane. Desflurane is a cerebral arteriolar dilator, and it produces a dose-dependent decrease in cerebrovascular resistance and CMR. Similar to isoflurane, it may be used to induce controlled hypotension, but its use is more often associated with a compensatory tachycardia than is the use of isoflurane.

### INTRACRANIAL PRESSURE

As is true for all inhalation anesthetic agents, desflurane may increase ICP in certain patients, but because $CO_2$ reactivity is maintained with desflurane, the increase can be attenuated or blocked by inducing hypocapnia. However, one study in humans showed sustained elevation of lumbar CSF pressure after administration of 1 MAC desflurane, despite previous establishment of hypocapnia. Desflurane has been shown to produce an increase in CSF formation without a significant effect on CSF reabsorption in dogs.

### ELECTROENCEPHALOGRAM

Desflurane produces a dose-related depression of EEG activity. In swine, prominent burst suppression has been observed at MAC levels of greater than 1.24. Although EEG tolerance to the cerebral effects of desflurane has been observed in dogs, it has not been seen in humans.

# Sevoflurane

### CEREBRAL METABOLIC RATE AND CEREBRAL BLOOD FLOW

The effects of sevoflurane on CMR and CBF resemble those of isoflurane. In most animal models in which it has been studied, sevoflurane produces little change in global CBF, independent of $CO_2$ levels. Cerebral autoregulation and cerebrovascular responsiveness to changes in $CO_2$ are preserved in patients with cerebrovascular disease up to a concentration below 1.5 MAC.

### INTRACRANIAL PRESSURE

Institution of hypocapnia before administration of sevoflurane blocks the potential of the agent to increase ICP at concentrations up to 1.5 MAC in dogs.

### ELECTROENCEPHALOGRAM

Slowing on the EEG begins at sevoflurane concentrations of 1.2%, and burst suppression is seen at approximately 2 MAC. Therefore other agents should be used for maintenance of anesthesia if the EEG will be monitored intraoperatively. Sevoflurane has been shown to enhance epileptiform activity on EEG monitoring, making this agent useful in electrocorticographic mapping for seizure focus identification.

## SUGGESTED READINGS

Dahaba, A. A., Yin, J., Xiao, Z., Su, J., Bornemann, H., Dong, H., et al. (2013). Different propofol-remifentanil or sevoflurane-remifentanil bispectral index levels for electrocorticographic spike identification during epilepsy surgery. *Anesthesiology, 119,* 582–592.

Laitio, R., Hynninen, M., Arola, O., Virtanen, S., Parkkola, R., Saunavaara, J., et al. (2016). Effect of inhaled xenon on cerebral white matter damage in comatose survivors of out-of-hospital cardiac arrest: A randomized clinical trial. *JAMA, 315,* 1120–1128.

Schulte, P. J., Roberts, R. O., Knopman, D. S., Petersen, R. C., Hanson, A. C., Schroeder, D. R., et al. (2018). Association between exposure to anaesthesia and surgery and long-term cognitive trajectories in older adults: Report from the Mayo Clinic Study of Aging. *British Journal of Anaesthesia, 121*(2), 398–405.

Sprung, J., Abcejo, A. S. A., Knopman, D. S., Petersen, R. C., Mielke, M. M., Hanson, A. C., et al. (2020). Anesthesia with and without nitrous oxide and long-term cognitive trajectories in older adults. *Anesthesia and Analgesia, 131*(2), 594–604.

Warner, D. O., Zaccariello, M. J., Katusic, S. K., Schroeder, D. R., Hanson, A. C., Schulte, P. J., et al. (2018). Neuropsychological and behavioral outcomes after exposure of young children to procedures requiring general anesthesia: The Mayo anesthesia safety in kids (MASK) study. *Anesthesiology, 129,* 89–105.

# 46

# Hepatic Effects of the Inhalation Agents

WOLF H. STAPELFELDT, MD

Inhaled anesthetic agents have a propensity to affect hepatic function both directly and indirectly. Direct effects on hepatic parenchyma include interactions of anesthetic agents with hepatic enzymes and the generation of metabolic products with toxic or allergenic properties. Indirect effects include decreased hepatic blood flow and consequently altered hepatic drug clearance and $O_2$ delivery to hepatocytes. An understanding of the latter requires a review of the anatomy and physiology of the hepatic blood supply.

## Hepatic Blood Supply

The normal liver contains approximately 10% to 15% of the total blood volume and receives approximately 25% of the normal total cardiac output (1 mL/min of blood flow per gram of liver). Only one-third of the afferent blood supply is arterial via the hepatic artery and its branches—the remaining two-thirds come from the portal vein and its branches. However, each of these two afferent blood supply systems provides approximately 50% of the $O_2$ consumed by the liver. This dual blood supply is highly regulated via several mechanisms.

Pressure-flow autoregulation is a myogenic response of the hepatic artery that actively adjusts vascular smooth muscle tone to varying passive wall stretch to maintain blood flow in the presence of changing hepatic perfusion pressure. This mechanism appears to be operative predominantly in the postprandial state, less so in the fasted state.

Metabolic control mediates arterial vasoconstriction in response to hypocarbia or alkalemia (which is the reason why excessive hyperventilation should be avoided if hepatic perfusion is of concern), as well as vasodilation in response to hypercarbia, acidemia, or hypoxemia—direct responses that may be offset by the indirect effect of reflex increases in sympathetic vasoconstrictor tone. Therefore near normocarbia and a physiologic pH are generally considered optimal for maintaining hepatic arterial blood flow.

Hepatic arterial buffer responses provide for reciprocal (reactive) changes in hepatic arterial blood flow in response to (passive) changes in portal venous blood flow, with the goal of maintaining total hepatic blood flow. This physiologic mechanism is believed to be mediated by varying adenosine washout. It is selectively inhibited by halothane (not, however, by isoflurane, sevoflurane, or desflurane [discussed later]) and is abolished by splanchnic hypoperfusion or the presence of endotoxins.

Parasympathetic autonomic activity is mediated through the vagal nerve, whereas sympathetic autonomic control is exerted via splanchnic vasoconstrictor nerve activity (arising from T3 to T11) transmitted via hepatic arterial and venous $\alpha_1$-, $\alpha_2$-, and $\beta_2$-adrenergic receptors and portal venous $\alpha_1$- and $\alpha_2$-adrenergic receptors. $\beta$-adrenergic antagonists are being used clinically to reduce portal hypertension attributable to increased mesenteric blood flow caused by excessive $\beta_2$-adrenergic receptor activity.

Humoral control includes a profound arterial vasodilatory response to glucagon; hepatic arterial, and portal venous constrictive properties of angiotensin II; and decreased mesenteric blood flow produced by somatostatin, as well as a differential response to vasopressin, which simultaneously causes splanchnic arterial vasoconstriction and portal venous dilation, making vasopressin an effective adjuvant in the treatment of portal hypertension.

## Inhaled Anesthetic-Induced Changes in Hepatic Blood Flow

Inhaled anesthetic agents produce concentration-dependent decreases in portal venous blood flow that passively reflect their effect on arterial blood pressure, causing decreased mesenteric blood flow. To the extent that cardiac output is being maintained and hepatic arterial blood flow increased (via an intact hepatic arterial buffer response), total hepatic blood flow is maintained in the presence of isoflurane, sevoflurane, and desflurane. However, previously used anesthetics (enflurane or halothane) produced hepatic arterial vasoconstriction and obliteration of the hepatic arterial buffer response (Fig. 46.1A). The resulting anesthetic-induced net changes in hepatic arterial $O_2$ delivery (Fig. 46.1B) closely mirrored the respective anesthetic reductions in total hepatic blood flow.

## Hepatic Metabolism of Inhaled Anesthetic Agents

Although most of the total amount of modern inhaled anesthetic agent taken up by blood and tissues over the course of clinical anesthesia is ultimately eliminated unchanged through exhalation via the lungs, a fraction that is taken up by the hepatic parenchyma is subject to metabolism by members of the hemoprotein cytochrome P450 enzyme superfamily. The fractional contribution of hepatic metabolism to elimination depends on the concentration of agent in contact with hepatic enzymes subsequent to partial pressure equilibration with blood flowing through the liver, reflecting the blood solubility of the agent (isoflurane, 0.2%; desflurane, 0.01%). An exception is sevoflurane, which, despite comparatively low blood solubility, undergoes 3% to 5% metabolism. All halogenated agents principally undergo oxidative metabolism selectively catalyzed by CPY2E1, releasing fluoride anions in the process. However, only enflurane and sevoflurane cause noticeable and potentially clinically significant (>50 $\mu$M) increases in the plasma fluoride concentration; this increase typically occurs after prolonged anesthesia (several minimum alveolar concentration hours) or with prior induction of the CPY2E1 enzyme (isoniazid treatment, chronic alcohol consumption, or

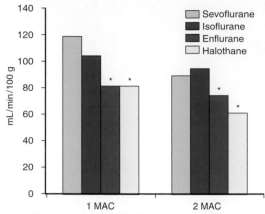

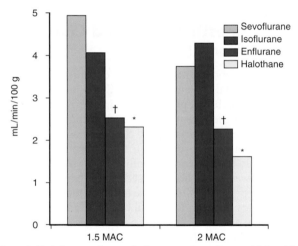

A

Impact of halothane, enflurane, isoflurane, and sevoflurane at 1.0 and 2.0 minimum alveolar concentration (MAC) on total hepatic blood flow (THBF) in dogs. THBF decreased with increasing anesthetic concentrations of each volatile agent. Sevoflurane and isoflurane were similar in their modest effect of THBF, whereas halothane caused a dramatic decrease in THBG, especially at 2-MAC exposure.

*Differs from sevoflurane and isoflurane at comparable values ($P$ <0.05).

B

Impact of halothane, enflurane, isoflurane, and sevoflurane at 1.5 and 2.5 minimum alveolar concentration (MAC) on hepatic arterial oxygen delivery in chronically instrumented dogs. Halothane produced the greatest reduction in hepatic arterial oxygen delivery, whereas sevoflurane and isoflurane had insignificant effects on oxygen delivery at any MAC level.

*Differs from isoflurane and sevoflurane at comparable MAC values ($P$ <0.05).

†Differs from sevoflurane at comparable MAC values ($P$ <0.05).

**Fig. 46.1**  Effect of inhaled anesthetics on **(A)** hepatic arterial blood flow and **(B)** $O_2$ delivery.

**Fig. 46.2**  Major by-products of oxidative and reductive halothane metabolism.

obesity). Such increases in the plasma fluoride concentration can temporarily impair renal tubular concentrating ability (temporary nephrogenic diabetes insipidus) without causing any other lasting renal compromise. Only in rare instances have the newer inhaled halogenated anesthetic agents been implicated in causing hepatic toxicity analogous to that documented for halothane. Their lesser toxicity is believed to be a result of the lesser fractional metabolism of these less soluble agents, as well as the fact that, unlike the other agents, halothane undergoes both oxidative (catalyzed by CPY2E1 and, to a lesser extent, CPY2A6) and reductive (Fig. 46.2) metabolism (within a hypoxic environment, catalyzed by CPY2A6 and CPY3A4, the most ubiquitous cytochrome P450 enzyme). In contrast with the newer anesthetic agents, halothane produces fluoride anions only as a product of reductive metabolism, whereas oxidative metabolism selectively releases

bromide anions (which may contribute to prolonged sedation after halothane anesthesia). Reductive metabolism of halothane can produce highly reactive radicals that are thought to account for hepatic toxicity that is observed primarily under hypoxic conditions. This hepatic toxicity is not to be confused with halothane hepatitis, a distinct condition that is encountered in approximately 1 in 10,000 adults or 1 in 200,000 children anesthetized with halothane. Based on factors such as previous exposure and the presence of eosinophilia, as well as demonstration of antibodies against trifluoroacetic acid acylated haptens, it is believed to represent an allergic response to oxidative (trifluoroacetic acid) metabolites.

Additional effects of inhaled anesthetics on hepatic parenchyma include the induction of insulin resistance and some degree of cellular protection against ischemia reperfusion injury, with efficacies of sevoflurane > isoflurane > desflurane.

## Extrahepatic Degradation of Inhaled Anesthetic Agents

Independent of enzymatic metabolism in the liver, inhaled anesthetic agents are also subject to spontaneous degradation in the presence of $CO_2$ absorbents (soda lime and previously Baralyme), producing potentially toxic degradation products, as well as a risk of ignition due to significant heat produced by these exothermic chemical reactions. Concerns depend on the anesthetic agent used.

Sevoflurane uniquely causes the formation of compound A, a vinyl ether with nephrotoxic properties. The threshold for renal injury appears to be approximately 150 ppm-hours of exposure, which is a potential concern only after prolonged sevoflurane anesthesia, causing glucosuria and enzymuria without any demonstrable effects on blood urea nitrogen or creatinine clearance. To limit exposure to compound A to which patients are exposed, fresh gas flows of not less than 2 L/min are recommended during sevoflurane anesthesia.

All inhaled halogenated anesthetic agents, especially desflurane, enflurane, and isoflurane (in order of decreasing propensity), can produce carbon monoxide as a result of chemical interaction with strong bases. Besides the choice of anesthetic agent (negligible risk with sevoflurane or halothane),

determining factors include the anesthetic concentration and the type (greater risk with Baralyme, which, for these reasons, has been taken off the market), temperature, and, most importantly, degree of dryness (water content) of the $CO_2$ absorbent. The risk of significant carbon monoxide production is minimized by keeping fresh gas flows low (to prevent desiccation of the absorbent) or, if necessary, replacing or rehydrating desiccated absorbent.

Both of these risks are eliminated with the use of one of the newer, calcium hydroxide–based absorbents (e.g., Amsorb, Armstrong Medical, Coleraine, Northern Ireland; Dragersorb, Drager, Lubeck, Germany), which are devoid of strong bases and thus inert with regard to the chemical reaction with inhaled anesthetic agents.

## SUGGESTED READINGS

Kim, S. P., Broussard, J. L., & Kolka, C. M. (2016). Isoflurane and sevoflurane induce severe hepatic insulin resistance in a canine model. *PLoS One*, *11*(11), e0163275.

Shiraishi, S., Cho, S., Akiyama, D., Ichinomiya, T., Shibata, I., Yoshitomi, O., et al. (2019). Sevoflurane has postconditioning as well as preconditioning

properties against hepatic warm ischemia-reperfusion injury in rats. *Journal of Anesthesia*, *33*(3), 390–398.

Toprak, H. I., Şahin, T., Aslan, S., Karahan, K., Şanli, M., & Ersoy, M. (2012). Effects of desflurane and isoflurane on hepatic and renal functions and coagulation profile during donor

hepatectomy. *Transplantation Proceedings*, *44*(6), 1635–1639.

van Limmen, J., Wyffels, P., Berrevoet, F., Vanlander, A., Coeman, L., Wouters, P., et al. (2020). Effects of propofol and sevoflurane on hepatic blood flow: A randomized controlled trial. *BMC Anesthesiol*, *20*(1), 241.

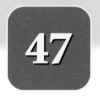

# 47

# Propofol

DANIEL A. HANSEN, MD

Propofol is an intravenous sedative-hypnotic agent used for anesthetic or sedative purposes. Chemically, propofol is an alkylphenol (2,6,-diisopropylphenol) unrelated to other hypnotic agents (Fig. 47.1). Propofol was first developed in 1976 but did not obtain U.S. Food and Drug Administration approval until 1989. Since that time, it has become the most commonly used intravenous anesthetic in the United States and Europe. Several companies manufacture propofol, but approximately 70% of the world's supply of propofol comes from Fresenius Kabi.

Because propofol is water insoluble, it must be formulated in a lipid emulsion to allow intravenous use. (Fospropofol, a water-soluble prodrug of propofol, is available, though less commonly used than propofol.) The most commonly used 1% lipid emulsion consists of 10% soybean oil, 2.25% glycerol, and purified 1.2% egg phosphatide (derived from egg lecithin). Patients with egg allergies generally have allergies to egg white antigens and not egg yolk–derived lecithin. Thus patients with egg allergies can be expected to tolerate propofol administration without sequelae. Because the lipid emulsion is a substrate

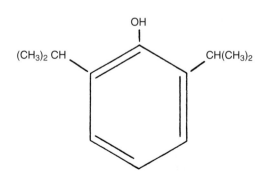

**Fig. 47.1**  Chemical structure of propofol (2,6,-diisopropylphenol).

for bacterial growth, manufacturers add an inhibitor of bacterial growth (e.g., ethylenediaminetetraacetic acid).

Since its discovery, propofol has increased in popularity as an intravenous anesthetic agent because of its rapid onset and offset, rapid redistribution, favorable side effect profile, and low cost. Thiopental was previously the most commonly used intravenous anesthetic, but because of its limited availability in some parts of the world and its less favorable pharmacologic profile, propofol has overtaken it as the intravenous anesthetic agent of choice globally.

In addition to its rapid onset and offset, propofol offers antiemetic effects and can be included as part of a multimodal antiemetic regimen. Antiemetic effects are more pronounced when propofol is administered as an infusion as the sole anesthetic agent, avoiding emetogenic volatile anesthetics; however, even small doses (10–20 mg at the time of emergence or in the recovery room) can be effective.

Compared with the other intravenously administered anesthetic agents, propofol causes the most injection site pain and the most hypotension. The prevalence of pain on injection ranges from 10% to 63%, although the incidence of thrombophlebitis is low. Pain on injection can be attenuated by the intravenous use of local anesthetic agents (e.g., lidocaine) and slow administration of propofol into a large vein with rapidly flowing intravenous fluids. Hypotension is also common with propofol administration and should be anticipated. Induction doses of propofol can cause significant decreases in both systolic and diastolic blood pressure as a result of decreased systemic vascular resistance.

Propofol infusion syndrome is a rare but potentially serious adverse effect of propofol administration. Most cases involve pediatric or younger neurosurgical patients who receive high doses of propofol for prolonged periods (e.g., $>150–200\ \mu g \cdot kg^{-1} \cdot min^{-1}$). Manifestations of the syndrome include metabolic acidosis, rhabdomyolysis, progressive bradyarrhythmias, and cardiac arrest refractory to therapy. The syndrome is associated with high mortality rates, and the precise mechanism of action remains unknown.

## Effects on Major Organ Systems

### CENTRAL NERVOUS SYSTEM

The exact mechanism of action of propofol has yet to be fully elucidated; however, stimulation of γ-aminobutyric acid (GABA) receptors is likely responsible for its anesthetic properties. GABA is the primary inhibitory compound of the human central nervous system, and activation of the ligand-gated $GABA_A$ receptors increases chloride ion permeability and inhibits further action potential generation. Additionally, recent research suggests that propofol inhibits kinesin activity. Ultimately, multiple biologic effects at multiple target sites may contribute to the pharmacologic profile of propofol. Injected intravenously as a bolus dose of 2 mg/kg, propofol induces unconsciousness in less than 1 minute, a rate that is comparable to that of thiopental, etomidate, and methohexital. Induction is smooth, with excitatory effects seen less often than with methohexital, although more often than with thiopental (though the transient pain with injection of propofol can cause a brief but pronounced sympathetic response). An induction bolus of propofol will produce anesthesia lasting approximately 4 to 5 minutes or more, a duration comparable to that of thiopental. Propofol produces electroencephalographic changes characteristic of general anesthesia with a decrease in global cerebral function and is accompanied by decreased cerebral metabolism, cerebral blood flow, and intracranial pressure.

### CARDIOVASCULAR SYSTEM

Propofol reliably causes a dose-dependent decrease in blood pressure. The decrease in blood pressure is mediated by

| TABLE 47.1 | Physiologic Changes With Propofol |
|---|---|
| Heart rate | ⟷ or ↓ |
| Mean arterial pressure | ↓↓↓ |
| Myocardial contractility | ↓ |
| Cerebral blood flow | ↓↓↓ |
| $CMRO_2$ | ↓↓↓ |
| Intracranial pressure | ↓↓↓ |
| Minute ventilation | ↓↓ |
| Ventilatory drive | ↓↓↓ |

⟷, No change; ↓, decrease; $CMRO_2$, cerebral metabolic rate of oxygen.

decreased systemic vascular resistance, though myocardial contractility decreases at higher doses, resulting in a fall in cardiac output. Propofol-induced hypotension can be attenuated by slow titration of bolus doses and/or the concomitant use of vasoactive medications such as phenylephrine to counteract the propofol induced decrease in systemic vascular resistance.

### RESPIRATORY SYSTEM

Propofol produces a dose-dependent depression of central respiratory drive that ultimately results in apnea. Largely as a result of this, propofol use is restricted to health care providers who are trained in advanced airway management. The ventilatory response to increased $Paco_2$ and hypoxia is decreased, and the effect is compounded with the addition of other respiratory depressants (e.g., opioids, benzodiazepines). Carefully titrated boluses (or low-dose infusion) for sedation can preserve spontaneous respiration; however, individual patient responses are variable. Propofol can produce bronchodilation and has minimal effects on hypoxic pulmonary vasoconstriction.

### OTHER ORGAN SYSTEMS

Propofol has little to no known clinical effect on liver function, renal function, coagulation, or steroidogenesis. Administration of propofol increases the depth but not the duration of neuromuscular blockade (Table 47.1).

## Pharmacokinetics and Pharmacodynamics

The rapid offset time of propofol after an intravenously administered bolus dose is caused by redistribution and not rapid metabolism. The concentration of propofol decreases rapidly after an intravenously administered bolus dose because of redistribution of drug (i.e., $t_{1/2\alpha} = 2–8$ min). The elimination half-life ($t_{1/2\beta} \approx$ approximately 1 h) is markedly shorter than that of thiopental ($t_{1/2\beta} \approx$ approximately 11 h). Both two-compartment and three-compartment models have been proposed to explain the rapid redistribution of propofol. The volume of distribution is large but becomes significantly smaller as the age of the patient increases with clinical implications. Thus dosages should be reduced in elderly patients because of their relative decrease in central compartment size.

Propofol is excreted as glucuronide and sulfate conjugates, primarily in the urine. Prolonged infusions can result in green urine (which is of no direct clinical significance) because of the presence of a phenolic or quinol metabolite. Because clearance of propofol exceeds hepatic blood flow, extrahepatic mechanisms have been proposed, though they remain unclear.

Blood concentrations of 2.5 to 6 μg/mL are required for patients undergoing major operations; concentrations of 1.5 to 4.5 μg/mL are adequate for minor operations. Movement on skin incision is prevented in 50% of premedicated patients (66% N₂O) by blood levels of 2.5 μg/mL propofol, though clinical measurements of blood concentration levels are generally impractical. Given our current limitations when monitoring of depth of anesthesia with propofol, increased attention is being paid to clinically applicable methods of detecting propofol-induced effects on consciousness. Bispectral index monitoring is occasionally used, and additional novel methods are being explored (e.g., exhaled gas analysis or pupillary diameter measurements).

## DOSES

The dose for induction of anesthesia is 1.5 to 2.5 mg/kg, which should be reduced in patients who are elderly, have hypovolemia, or have limited cardiac reserve. Dosing may need to be increased to 3 to 3.5 mg/kg in pediatric patients. Anesthesia can also be induced with 20 to 40 mg propofol given every 10 s until the onset of unconsciousness. Anesthesia can be maintained with frequent, intermittent 0.5-mg/kg boluses of propofol, titrated to clinical effect, or with a propofol infusion of 100 to 200 $\mu g \cdot kg^{-1} \cdot min^{-1}$. A recommended starting dose for conscious sedation is 50 $\mu g \cdot kg^{-1} \cdot min^{-1}$. As with all anesthetic agents, care must be taken when selecting the appropriate dose, and the dose should be adjusted to the individual patient.

## SUGGESTED READINGS

Asserhoj, L. L., Mosbech, H., Kroigaard, M., & Garvey, L. H. (2016). No evidence for contraindications to the use of propofol in adults allergic to egg, soy or peanut. *British Journal of Anaesthesia*, *116*(1), 77–82.

Dong, H., Zhang, F., Chen, J., Yu, Q., Zhong, Y., Liu, J., et al. (2020). Evaluating propofol concentration in blood from exhaled gas using a breathing-related partition coefficient. *Anesthesia and Analgesia*, *130*(4), 958–966.

Morgan, G. E., Mikhail, M. S., & Murray, M. J. (2006). *Clinical anesthesiology* (4th ed.). New York: McGraw-Hill.

Sabourdin, N., Meniolle, F., Chemam, S., Rigouzzo, A., Hamza, J., Louvet, N., et al. (2020). Effect of different concentrations of propofol used as a sole anesthetic on pupillary diameter: A randomized trial. *Anesthesia and Analgesia*, *131*(2), 510–517.

Schuttler, J., & Ihmsen, H. (2000). Population pharmacokinetics of propofol: A multicenter study. *Anesthesiology*, *92*, 727–738.

Shapiro, B. A., Warren, J., Egol, A. B., Greenbaum, D. M., Jacobi, J., Nasraway, S. A., et al. (1995). Practice parameters for intravenous analgesia and sedation for adult patients in the intensive care unit: An executive summary. Society of Critical Care Medicine. *Critical Care Medicine*, *23*(9), 1596–1600.

White, P. F., & Eng, M. R. (2013). Intravenous anesthetics. In P. G. Barash (Ed.), *Clinical Anesthesia* (pp. 478–500). Philadelphia: Lippincott Williams.

# 48

# Etomidate

HEIDI A. TAVEL, MD, FASA

Etomidate (R-[+]-phenylethyl-1H-imidazole-5 carboxylate sulfate) (Fig. 48.1), an intravenously administered anesthetic drug, was initially described in 1964 and was first approved for clinical use 10 years later. Its benefits include rapid onset, rapid offset, minimal cardiovascular depression, and cerebral protection. Water soluble at an acidic pH and lipid soluble at physiologic pH, it is available in the United States as a 0.2% solution with 35% propylene glycol. In this preparation, it has a pH of 6.9 and a pK of 4.2, making it a weak base. The *d*-isomer is responsible for its anesthetic effects: hypnosis and sedation, notably without analgesia. By binding to γ-aminobutyric acid (GABA_A)

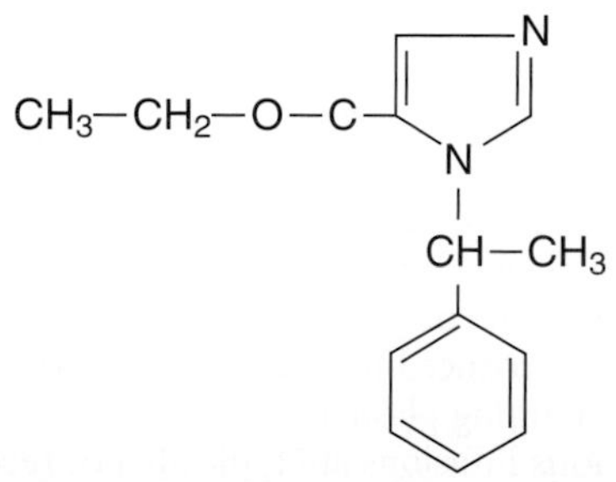

**Fig. 48.1** Chemical structure of etomidate.

| TABLE 48.1 | γ-Aminobutyric Acid Type A Subunit Binding Sites of Propofol and Etomidate | |
|---|---|
| **Subunit Binding Site** | **Drug** |
| α | Propofol |
| β₁ | Propofol |
| β₂ | Propofol, etomidate |
| β₃ | Propofol, etomidate |
| γ₂ | Propofol |

type A receptors—predominantly at the $\beta_2$ and $\beta_3$ subunits (Table 48.1)—etomidate causes neuronal hyperpolarization and subsequent depression of the reticular activating system through inhibition of neural signals. Additionally, etomidate increases the affinity of GABA receptors for the GABA molecule.

## Pharmacokinetics

### DISTRIBUTION

After an intravenous administration of a bolus dose, 99% of etomidate exists in the nonionized form in plasma, 75% of which is protein bound, primarily to albumin. Its high lipid solubility results in a fast onset of action (within 1 min of intravenous injection) and a large volume of distribution (2.5–4.5 L/kg). Redistribution is responsible for its rapid offset, due to an initial decrease in plasma concentration. Renal or hepatic disease, resulting in low plasma protein levels, can cause an increased duration of effect and a doubling of the half-life of etomidate.

### METABOLISM

Etomidate is metabolized via ester hydrolysis (both plasma and hepatic), converting the ethyl side chain into a carboxylic acid ester, rendering it water soluble and inactive.

### ELIMINATION

The majority of inactive metabolite is excreted by the kidneys, with an elimination half-life of 2.9 to 5.3 h and a clearance rate of 18 to 35 mL · kg⁻¹ · min⁻¹.

## Pharmacodynamics

### DOSING

The induction dose of etomidate typically ranges from 0.2 mg/kg to 0.6 mg/kg, with loss of consciousness occurring in the patient within 2 min after an intravenously administered bolus. A linear relationship exists between dose and duration of action. Decreased doses can be used if patients are premedicated with opioids or benzodiazepines. Elderly patients require a reduction in the dose of etomidate (typically 0.15–0.2 mg/kg) because of their smaller volume of distribution and decreased clearance rates. Maintenance of anesthesia with etomidate can be achieved via initial infusion rate of 100 μg · kg⁻¹ · min⁻¹ for 10 minutes, at which time it is reduced to rate of 10 μg · kg⁻¹ · min⁻¹ with the goal of maintaining plasma levels between 300 and 500 ng/dL, but continuous infusions are typically not recommended to due corticoadrenal suppression.

## Effects on Major Organ Systems

### CENTRAL NERVOUS SYSTEM

Etomidate provides cerebral protection by decreasing the cerebral metabolic rate, with a proportional decrease in cerebral blood flow, thus maintaining an appropriate $O_2$ supply/demand ratio. Because mean arterial pressure is unaffected, stable cerebral perfusion pressure is preserved. Intracerebral pressure is initially decreased with etomidate; however, it will later return to baseline unless high infusion rates are used.

Electroencephalographic changes that occur with the use of etomidate are similar to those seen with barbiturates, except that etomidate does not induce β waves, as do barbiturates. Epileptiform activity on the electroencephalogram (EEG), or a grand mal seizure, can be induced; etomidate is therefore avoided in patients with a history of seizure. As such, it is routinely used as an alternative general anesthetic to methohexital for electroconvulsive therapy (ECT) because of etomidate's lack of anticonvulsant properties. This compares with propofol, which is not used as a general anesthetic for ECT, as propofol increases the seizure threshold. Additionally, etomidate can be used to intentionally trigger an epileptiform focus on EEG to aid with localization during surgical interventions for seizures.

### CARDIOVASCULAR SYSTEM

Etomidate is best known for its mild cardiovascular depressant effects compared with other induction agents. Therefore it is often used in patients with hemodynamic instability, decreased ejection fraction, coronary artery disease, or valvular heart disease (Table 48.2). Although peripheral vascular resistance is decreased with etomidate, blood pressure is minimally affected; etomidate does not significantly affect cardiac output or myocardial contractility at clinical doses. Coronary blood flow will be decreased, as will the myocardial $O_2$ requirement, preserving the $O_2$ supply/demand ratio. Although etomidate is associated with the least cardiovascular depression among anesthetic medications, it can still nevertheless exacerbate underlying myocardial dysfunction, and it requires careful titration in patients with significant cardiovascular dysfunction.

### RESPIRATORY SYSTEM

Etomidate causes only minimal respiratory depression. It will decrease tidal volume, but a compensatory increase in respiratory rate is typically observed, both of which will be affected for approximatively 3 to 5 min. Apnea is typically observed when etomidate is administered at high doses and/or combined with opioids. Because of this favorable respiratory profile in patients at risk for respiratory compromise, etomidate is increasingly used for sedation in gastrointestinal endoscopic retrograde cholangio-pancreatography procedures, with decreased incidence of respiratory events, compared with propofol.

## Adverse Drug Effects

### ENDOCRINE EFFECTS

Corticoadrenal suppression is the most significant adverse effect that occurs with the use of etomidate and is the primary limiting factor. Etomidate inhibits function of 11β-hydroxylase (converts 11-deoxycortisol into cortisol), resulting in reversible, dose-dependent inhibition of cortisol and aldosterone synthesis

| TABLE 48.2 | Benefits and Adverse Drug Effects of Major Intravenously Administered Induction Agents | | | | | | | | | |
|---|---|---|---|---|---|---|---|---|---|---|
| Agent | Cardio Depressant | Decreased Intracranial Pressure | Respiratory Depression | Continuous Infusion | Analgesia | Thrombo-phlebitis | Corticoadrenal Suppression | Porphyria | Bronchorelax-ation | Myoclonus |
| Propofol | Yes | Yes | Yes | Yes | No | Yes | No | No | No | No* |
| Thiopental | Yes | Yes | Yes | No† | No | No | No | Yes | No | No |
| Midazolam | Yes | No | No | Yes | No | Yes | No | No | No | No |
| Etomidate | No‡ | Yes | No§ | No | No | Yes | Yes | Yes | No | Yes |
| Ketamine | No‡ | No¶ | No | Yes | Yes | No | No | No | Yes | No* |

*Rare reports of myoclonus.
†Used only to maintain barbiturate coma.
‡Causes cardiodepression only at high doses.
§Synergistic with opioids.
¶Increases intracranial pressure.

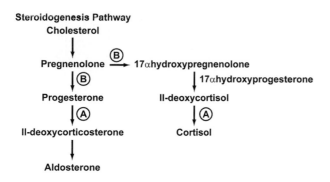

Steroidogenesis Pathway

(A) 11βhydroxylase: site of *major* enzymatic inhibition

(B) 17αhydroxylase: site of *minor* enzymatic inhibition

MAYO CLINIC

**Fig. 48.2** The major steps in the production of cortisol and aldosterone in the adrenal glands that are inhibited by etomidate.

(Fig. 48.2). The time to maximal suppression is 4 h after intravenous injection, and suppression typically resolves within 24 h. Corticoadrenal suppression was initially observed in patients receiving continuous etomidate infusions in the intensive care unit (ICU); however, the inhibition of 11β-hydroxylase can also be present with a single induction bolus dose. Therefore despite its favorable hemodynamic profile, there has been hesitation to use etomidate for ICU intubations in patients with septic shock. Nonetheless, most recent studies have shown no increase in mortality in ICU patients with sepsis who were administered a single bolus etomidate, nor was there an increase in other adverse clinical outcomes. Risks and benefits must be weighed on an individual patient basis, with an emphasis on maintenance of adequate blood pressure. Use of exogenous corticosteroids is controversial; however, long-term infusions or multiple bolus doses of etomidate should not be administered because of the proven increased risk of death. Etomidate derivatives, such as methoxycarbonyl etomidate and carboctomidate, are currently being studied but have not been approved for clinical use. The goals of these drugs would be maintenance of cardiovascular benefits of etomidate while avoiding the undesirable corticoadrenal suppression.

## PEDIATRIC EFFECTS

As with other commonly used intravenous anesthetic and sedation agents, the U.S. Food and Drug Administration has approved label changes for use in children younger than 3 years old. This warning states that exposure to these sedatives or anesthetic agents over lengthy periods or multiple surgeries may negatively affect brain development.

## ADDITIONAL EFFECTS

The effects of etomidate on the central nervous system result in an imbalance of inhibitory and stimulatory signals between the thalamus and the cortex. The resulting stimulation can produce myoclonus in 30% to 60% of patients. The risk of myoclonus may be decreased with concomitant opioid, midazolam, propofol, gabapentin, magnesium, or thiopental administration.

Etomidate causes pain with intravenous injection that can be decreased by administration of intravenous lidocaine or opioids before injection or by administration into a central venous catheter. Lipid emulsions are available in Europe as an alternative to the propylene glycol solution and are reported to decrease injection site pain. Thrombophlebitis, which can occur 24 to 48 h after the use of etomidate, affects up to 25% of patients.

The effects of etomidate on the central nervous system have been associated with increased rates of postoperative nausea and vomiting; however, a study that compared an etomidate-lipid infusion and propofol in patients with a history of postoperative nausea and vomiting showed no differences between the two drugs.

Etomidate should not be used in patients with a history of porphyria because it can induce a porphyria attack. Cases of etomidate-induced hypersensitivity are rare (1/50,000–1/450,000) and are associated with anaphylactoid reactions. Additionally, etomidate can cause postoperative hiccups and a sense of restlessness.

## SUGGESTED READINGS

Albert, S. G., & Sitaula, S. (2021). Etomidate, adrenal insufficiency and mortality associated with severity of illness: A meta-analysis. *Journal of Intensive Care Medicine, 36*(10), 1124–1129. doi:10.1177/0885066620957596.

Basciani, R. M., Rindlisbacher, A., Begert, E., Brander, L., Jakob, S. M., Etter, R., et al. (2016). Anaesthetic induction with etomidate in cardiac surgery: A randomised controlled trial. *European Journal of Anaesthesiology, 33*(6), 417–424. doi:10.1097/EJA.0000000000000434.

Bruder, E. A., Ball, I. M., Ridi, S., Pickett, W., & Hohl, C. (2015). Single induction dose of etomidate versus other induction agent for endotracheal intubation in critically ill patients. *Cochrane Database of Systematic Reviews*, (15), CD010225.

Komatsu, R., You, J., Rajan, S., Kasuya, Y., Sessler, D. I., & Turan, A. (2018). Steroid administration after anaesthetic induction with etomidate does not reduce in-hospital mortality or cardiovascular morbidity after non-cardiac surgery. *British Journal of Anaesthesia, 120*(3), 501–508. doi:10.1016/j.bja.2017.11.079.

McPhee, L. C., Badawi, O., Fraser, G. L., Lerwick, P. A., Riker, R. R., Zuckerman, I. H., et al. (2013). Single-dose etomidate is not associated with increased mortality in ICU patients with sepsis: Analysis of a large electronic database. *Critical Care Medicine, 41*(3), 774–783.

Valk, B. I., & Struys, M. M. R. F. (2021). Etomidate and its analogs: A review of pharmacokinetics and pharmacodynamics. *Clinical Pharmacokinetics, 60*(10), 1253–1269. doi:10.1007/s40262-021-01038-6.

Wagner, C. E., Bick, J. S., Johnson, D., Ahmad, R., Han, X., Ehrenfeld, J. M., et al. (2014). Etomidate use and postoperative outcomes among cardiac surgery patients. *Anesthesiology, 120*(3), 579–589. doi:10.1097/ALN.0000000000000087.

# 49

# Ketamine

MOLLY M. H. HERR, MD

Ketamine is chemically related to phencyclidine ("PCP" or "angel dust") and was introduced in the early 1960s. It was designed to become the ideal anesthetic at a time when other anesthetic agents were particularly toxic and difficult to use. Its popularity was established during the Vietnam War, where it was deemed to be an "exceptional battlefield anesthetic." Ketamine has a very high therapeutic index compared with other anesthetic medications.

Ketamine is a nonbarbiturate that is termed a *dissociative* anesthetic for two reasons. First, the patient appears "dissociated" from the environment. Effective analgesia and sedation often occur with the patient appearing awake, with slow nystagmus, whereas other reflexes remain intact (including corneal, papillary, and gag reflexes), with maintenance of laryngeal tone and muscle tension. Second, ketamine anesthesia produces an electroencephalogram showing that the thalamus is no longer synchronized with (or is "dissociated" from) the limbic system.

## Structure

The chemical structure of ketamine, 2-(2-chlorophyenyl)-2-(methylamino)-cyclohexanone, contains a chiral center within its cyclohexanone ring. Consequently, the racemic mixture consists of two optical stereoisomers, R(−) and S(+) ketamine. The S(+) isomer, which is four times more potent than the R(−) isomer, is associated with less cardiac stimulation, better analgesia, faster recovery, and has a lower incidence of psychotomimetic effects compared with the R(−) isomer. Recent studies have shown that the R(−) isomer has greater affinity as an antidepressant. In North America, ketamine is sold primarily as a racemic mixture; however, the S(+) isomer has been recently been made available as a nasal spray for use in treatment-resistant depression. Ketamine may also contain benzethonium chloride or chlorobutanol as preservative compounds.

## Mechanisms of Action

Ketamine pharmacology is complex because it is not a particularly selective drug, with multiple sites of action, including those in the central and peripheral nervous systems. The properties of ketamine are primarily mediated by noncompetitive antagonism at *N*-methyl-d-aspartate (NMDA) receptors for glutamate. Glutamate is the most prominent excitatory amino acid in the body, and its activation of NMDA receptors affects the central nervous system, the peripheral nervous system, and many other organs and tissues (e.g., lungs, inflammatory cells). NMDA receptors have been implicated in the mechanism of anesthesia, pain transmission, memory and cognitive function, neuronal toxicity, depression, and chronic neurologic diseases (e.g., Alzheimer's disease) in addition to inflammatory responses. The antagonism of ketamine at NMDA receptors is responsible for dissociative anesthesia and amnesia, inhibited sensory perception, and analgesia.

Ketamine can also act as an antagonist (inhibitor) or as an agonist (activator) at a great number of other receptors. Examples include agonistic activity at μ, δ, and κ opioid

| TABLE 49.1 | Receptor and Channel Targets of Ketamine and Clinical Effects | |
|---|---|---|
| **Receptor/Channel** | | **Clinical Effect** |
| **ANTAGONISM/INHIBITION** | | |
| N-methyl-d-aspartate receptors | | Dissociative anesthesia, amnesia, inhibited sensory perception, analgesia |
| Hyperpolarization-activated cyclic nucleotide channels | | Hypnosis |
| Calcium channels (L-type voltage dependent) | | Airway smooth muscle relaxation, dysphoria, psychosis, altered perception |
| Voltage-gated sodium channels | | Local anesthetic effects, decreased parasympathetic activity |
| Large-conductance potassium channels | | Analgesic effect on neuropathic pain |
| Monoaminergic receptors | | Sympathomimetic effects, psychotomimetic effects |
| Nicotinic receptors | | Decreased parasympathetic activity |
| Muscarinic receptors | | Hypnosis, delirium, bronchodilation, increased sympathetic tone |
| **AGONISM/ACTIVATION** | | |
| Opioid receptors | | Analgesia |
| α-Amino-3-hydroxy-5-methyl-4-isoxazolepropionic acid receptors | | Rapid antidepressant effects |
| GABA$_A$ receptors | | Anesthetic properties |

receptors, providing analgesia. It can bind to monoaminergic receptors, inhibiting uptake of the monoamines epinephrine, norepinephrine, dopamine, and serotonin and increasing sympathomimetic effects. It acts as an antagonist at voltage-sensitive sodium channels (local anesthetic effect) and inhibits L-type voltage-sensitive calcium channels (airway smooth muscle relaxation). Ketamine inhibits both muscarinic acetylcholine and nicotinic acetylcholine receptors because it produces anticholinergic symptoms (postanesthetic delirium, bronchodilation, and sympathomimetic effects). Physostigmine, an anticholinesterase, can reverse the central anticholinergic and hypnotic effects of ketamine. Table 49.1 shows the receptor and channel targets.

## Pharmacokinetics, Pharmacodynamics, and Routes of Administration

Ketamine is a lipophilic drug that easily crosses the blood-brain barrier. It is poorly bound to plasma proteins (10%–30%); therefore it has a large volume of distribution (2.5–3.5 L/kg). It is rapidly active, with a distribution half-life of 7 to 11 min and an elimination half-life of 1 to 2 h. Ketamine is a cytochrome P450–dependent drug that is metabolized by the liver to its major metabolite, norketamine, which has approximately 30% of the clinical activity of ketamine. Further metabolism of norketamine and its metabolites are then excreted in the bile and urine.

Ketamine can be administered by numerous routes: intravenous, intramuscular, oral, nasal, rectal, transdermal, subcutaneous, and epidural; recently, inhalation with preservative-free ketamine has shown to be successful. When given intravenously, the effects of ketamine occur within seconds; intramuscular injection of ketamine produces peak levels by 5 minutes. With oral administration, bioavailability is limited (20%) by hepatic metabolism, and peak levels occur in 20 to 30 minutes. Table 49.2 shows indications, administration routes, and dosage recommendations.

| TABLE 49.2 | Ketamine: Indications, Routes of Administration and Dosage Recommendations | |
|---|---|---|
| **Indication** | **Route** | **Dose** |
| Premedication | PO | 3–5 mg/kg |
| Premedication | IM | 3–5 mg/kg |
| Procedural Sedation | IV | 0.2–1 mg/kg |
| Procedural Sedation (infusion) | IV | 5–20 mcg/kg/min |
| Induction | IV | 1–4.5 mg/kg; 2 mg/kg (average) |
| Analgesia with sedation (e.g., burn dressing changes) | IM | 1–3 mg/kg |
| Analgesia with sedation (e.g., burn dressing changes) | IV | 0.5–1 mg/kg |
| Analgesia (adjunct to opioid) | IV | 0.1 mg/kg |
| Analgesia (moderate to severe) | IV | 0.2–0.3 mg/kg |
| Analgesia (infusion) | IV | 0.1–0.3 mg/kg/hr |
| Depression | IV | 0.5 mg/kg |

*IM, Intramuscular; IV, intravenous; PO, oral.*

## Systemic Effects

### CARDIOVASCULAR SYSTEM

The cardiovascular response to ketamine mimics sympathetic nervous system stimulation, causing increased blood pressure, cardiac output, myocardial $O_2$ consumption, pulmonary artery blood pressure, and tachycardia in patients with intact sympathetic and autonomic nervous systems. The action of ketamine on the cardiovascular system is a result of the inhibition of the reuptake of amines, including norepinephrine. These cardiovascular effects may be blunted with prior or concomitant administration of opioids, benzodiazepines, or inhaled anesthetics. However, at higher doses (20 mg/kg) or in the denervated or transplanted heart, there is a direct negative inotropic action effect by ketamine.

Critically ill patients occasionally respond to ketamine with unexpected decreases in blood pressure and cardiac output, which may reflect depletion of catecholamine stores and exhaustion of the sympathetic nervous system compensating mechanisms.

## RESPIRATORY SYSTEM

Ketamine alone does not induce respiratory depression, so airway patency is well maintained during ketamine anesthesia. However, if ketamine is combined with respiratory-depressing agents, such as benzodiazepines or opioids, respiratory depression and upper airway obstruction can occur. Because of its anticholinergic and adrenergic effects, ketamine induces bronchodilation by relaxing smooth muscle in the airways, and it has been administered successfully as a sedative to treat patients with asthma. Administration of an antisialagogue is often recommended (glycopyrrolate may be preferred) to decrease ketamine-induced salivary and tracheobronchial secretions.

## CENTRAL NERVOUS SYSTEM

Ketamine, a cerebral vasodilator, causes an increase in cerebral blood flow, cerebral oxygen consumption, and intracranial pressure in patients with space-occupying intracranial lesions. Elevation of intracranial pressure is minimal if ventilation is controlled.

Ketamine has multiple dose-related side effects, including hyperreflexia, transient clonus, and vestibular-type symptoms of nystagmus, vertigo, dizziness, and nausea and vomiting. Ketamine also causes an increase in intraocular pressure after administration.

Emergence delirium is reported to occur in 5% to 30% of patients who are administered ketamine as an anesthetic agent; the incidence of delirium is increased in patients older than 16 years if the dosage exceeds 2 mg/kg, if the drug is administered rapidly, or if the patient has preexisting personality problems. Emergence reactions usually occur early during emergence from anesthesia and may persist for a few hours but may last for more than 24 hours in some patients. These reactions are characterized by visual, auditory, and proprioceptive hallucinations, often with associated feelings of excitement, fear, or euphoria (schizophrenia-like reactions). The psychoactive properties of ketamine, including hallucinations and agitation, often limit its use and occur even at subanesthetic doses (0.1–0.4 mg/kg). Benzodiazepines (midazolam given intravenously approximately 5 minutes before induction with ketamine) have been proven to be most effective in preventing emergence delirium. Table 49.3 shows a summary of ketamine's physiologic effects.

## Other Side Effects, Toxicities, and Abuse

Recently urinary symptoms, including interstitial cystitis, frequency, urgency, dysuria, hematuria, detrusor overactivity, and

| TABLE 49.3 | Ketamine Effects | |
|---|---|
| **Organ System** | **Physiologic Effect** |
| Cardiovascular | ↑ HR |
| | ↑ BP |
| | ↑ CO |
| | ↑ Myocardial O$_2$ consumption |
| | ↑ Pulmonary artery pressure |
| | ↓ BP and CO in critically ill, catecholamine-depleted patients |
| Respiratory | ↑ bronchodilation |
| | No respiratory depression by itself |
| CNS | ↑ cerebral vasodilation |
| | ↑ cerebral blood flow |
| | ↑ cerebral O$_2$ consumption |
| | ↑ ICP |
| Miscellaneous | ↑ Intraocular pressure |
| | ↑ Bronchotracheal and oral secretions |

*BP*, Blood pressure; *CNS*, central nervous system; *CO*, cardiac output; *HR*, heart rate; *ICP*, intracranial pressure; *O$_2$*, oxygen.

renal impairment, have been reported in long-term ketamine users. Ketamine abuse is associated with epigastric pain, hepatic injury, and biliary dysfunction.

Although ketamine's psychedelic effects limit clinical use, they have also made ketamine a recreational drug of abuse (best known under the names *vitamin K*, *special K*, and *Kit Kat*). The annual prevalence of ketamine abuse in young adults is 1% to 2%. At subanesthetic doses it produces similar dopaminergic effects as stimulants and a number of other recreational drugs, which suggests that these dopaminergic effects may contribute to the potential for abuse. At high doses, severe schizophrenic-like symptoms occur but subside within several hours; however, with long-term use, persistent neuropsychiatric symptoms and cognitive impairment occur.

## Clinical Use

Ketamine is the only effective NMDA blocker that can be administered by several routes: intravenously, intramuscularly, subcutaneously, intranasally, sublingually, orally, rectally, and cutaneously (patches, ointment on wounds). Because of its broad range of receptor interactions, ketamine is being studied for a variety of clinical uses.

It can be used for anesthesia induction in hemodynamically unstable patients and patients with active bronchospasm. It may be given to uncooperative patients intramuscularly to allow for intravenous placement. Emergency departments have popularized its use for pediatric patients who need procedural analgesia and sedation. It also has found use in trauma medicine, including battlefield conflicts, and prehospital settings, including mass casualties, because of its analgesic effects, ease of administration, and wide therapeutic index. As an anesthetic, ketamine remains useful for short and very painful procedures performed outside the operating room where monitoring and support are limited. Burn medicine has relied on its use for repeated dressing changes and debridement.

Because NMDA antagonists have an additive or synergistic action with opioids, ketamine is being used increasingly to provide perioperative analgesia. The use of ketamine infusions has been shown to be an opiate-sparing intervention in the management of postoperative pain for abdominal, spine, thoracic, orthopedic, and gynecologic procedures, but more prominently in those who are opioid tolerant rather than the opioid-naïve patient population. Most randomized controlled trials have shown little to no preemptive effect of ketamine on persistent postoperative pain. Subanesthetic doses of ketamine (0.1 mg/kg) have been shown to help with acute pain and in limiting total opioid use in an emergency department randomized trial.

Oral ketamine and short-term intravenous ketamine infusions have also provided effective analgesia in patients with chronic and neuropathic pain. Ketamine has been used as an intravenously administered analgesic or a locally applied ointment with some success in the treatment of severe complex regional pain syndrome and in patients with phantom limb pain. Other studies have shown benefit for pain related to fibromyalgia, including muscle and referred pain; ischemic pain; migraine with aura; breakthrough pain in chronic pain states; and in patients with a history of opiate dependence and abuse. Subanesthetic ketamine infusion has been shown to improve pain in children and adolescents with complex regional pain syndrome, postural orthostatic tachycardia syndrome, and trauma-related chronic pain safely in the outpatient setting. A few studies have shown benefit with ketamine for chronic cancer pain, whereas other studies show conflicting evidence. It has been used as an oral rinse for radiation-induced mucositis. However, intolerable adverse effects, such as dissociative feelings, somnolence or insomnia, dizziness, unpleasant dreams, and sensory changes such as taste disturbances and somatic sensations, have limited its use in some situations.

Recently ketamine has emerged as a potential treatment for major depressive disorder and bipolar disorder that is unresponsive to standard therapy, with minimal short-term side effects. A single dose of 0.5 mg/kg intravenously over 40 min has been shown to have rapid (within 40 min), potent antidepressant effects. Interestingly, this also includes the acute reduction of suicidal ideation. The efficacy of ketamine as an antidepressant appears to last 1 to 2 weeks. Repeated ketamine doses may improve depressive symptoms comparably if not faster than electroconvulsive therapy (ECT). Ketamine has been used as an anesthetic for ECT for patients with high seizure thresholds. However, in a series of patients in which ketamine rather than methohexital was used for ECT, all reported a strong preference not to be given ketamine again because of its bothersome adverse effects. A newer application of ketamine shows some success in the treatment of posttraumatic stress disorder. The long-term effects of ketamine for psychiatric uses remain unclear.

Ketamine, a modulator of inflammatory responses, has been shown to be neuroprotective in several animal models of neurologic ischemia-reperfusion injury. Its hemodynamic effects may also improve cerebral perfusion and thereby influence outcomes.

Several animal studies have shown that ketamine causes apoptosis in developing brains and produces long-term cognitive impairment. This apoptotic effect of ketamine deserves attention in the field of pediatric anesthesia, especially in the organogenesis of the central nervous system from the sixth month in utero until several years after birth.

It is an exciting time in ketamine research, and many questions remain unanswered. The many effects associated with its use require balancing the beneficial actions of this pharmacologic agent with its potential adverse effects.

## SUGGESTED READINGS

Barrett, W., Buxhoeveden, M., & Dhillon, S. (2020). Ketamine: A versatile tool for anesthesia and analgesia. *Current Opinion in Anaesthesiology, 33,* 633–638.

Brinck, E., Maisniemi, K., Kankare, J., Tielinen, L., Tarkkila, P., & Kontinen, V. K. (2021). Analgesic effect of intraoperative intravenous S-ketamine in opioid-naïve patients after major lumbar fusion surgery is temporary and not dose-dependent: A randomized, double-blind, placebo-controlled clinical trial. *Anesthesia and Analgesia, 132,* 69–79.

Culp, C., Kim, H. K., & Abdi, S. (2021). Ketamine use for cancer and chronic pain management. *Frontiers in Pharmacology, 11,* 599721.

Jonkman, K., Dahan, A., de van Donk, T., Aarts, L., Niesters, M., & Velzen, van, M. (2017). Ketamine for pain [version 1; referees: 2 approved]. *F1000 Research,* 6(F1000 Faculty Rev), 1711. doi:10.12688/f1000research.11372.1.

Li, L., & Vlisides, P. (2016). Ketamine: 50 years of modulating the mind. *Frontiers in Human Neuroscience, 10*(612), 1–15.

Niesters, M., Martini, C., & Dahan, A. (2013). Ketamine for chronic pain: Risks and benefits. *British Journal of Clinical Pharmacology, 77*(2), 357–367.

Nowacka, A., & Borczyk, M. (2019). Ketamine applications beyond anesthesia: A literature review. *European Journal of Pharmacology, 860,* 172548.

Reinstatler, L., & Youssef, N. (2015). Ketamine as a potential treatment for suicidal ideation: A systematic review of the literature. *Drugs in R&D, 15,* 37–43.

Sheehy, K., Muller, E., Lippold, C., Nouraie, M., Finkel, J. C., & Quezado, Z. M. (2015). Subanesthetic ketamine infusions for the treatment of children and adolescents with chronic pain: A longitudinal study. *BMC Pediatrics, 15*(198), 1–8.

Sleigh, J., Harvey, M., Voss, L., et al. (2014). Ketamine: More mechanisms of action than just NMDA blockade. *Trends Anaesthesia Critical Care, 4,* 76–81.

# 50

# Opioid Pharmacology

HALENA M. GAZELKA, MD

According to Goodman and Gilman, "the term *opioid* refers broadly to all compounds related to opium, a natural product derived from the poppy. Opiates are drugs derived from opium and include the natural products morphine, codeine, and thebaine and many synthetic derivatives. Endogenous opioid peptide endorphins are the naturally occurring ligands for opioid receptors. Opiates exert their effects by mimicking these peptides. The term *narcotic* is derived from the Greek word for *stupor*; it originally referred to any drug that induced sleep, but it now is associated with opioids."

Opiates may be classified into three major groups based on pharmacodynamic activity: pure opioid agonists, pure antagonists (e.g., naloxone), and mixed agonists/antagonists (e.g., buprenorphine, nalbuphine). All of the opiates share common structural characteristics, and small changes in the molecular shape of these compounds can convert an agonist to an antagonist.

The clinical effects of a particular opiate depend on which specific G-protein–coupled opioid receptor type or types ($\mu_1$, $\mu_2$, $\kappa$, $\delta$, and $\sigma$) that it binds. The primary mechanism of action of opiates is via $\mu$-receptor agonism. These opioid receptor subtypes have been characterized according to their differences in affinity, anatomic location, and functional responses, as shown in Table 50.1.

The analgesic effects from systemic administration of opioids may result from receptor activity at several different nervous system sites, including the sensory neuron of the peripheral nervous system; the dorsal horn (layers 4 and 5 of the substantia gelatinosa) of the spinal cord, which inhibits the transmission of nociceptive information; the brainstem

medulla, which potentiates descending inhibitory pathways that modulate ascending pain signals; and the cortex of the brain, which decreases the perception and emotional response to pain. Opioid receptor activation inhibits the presynaptic release and postsynaptic response to excitatory neurotransmitters (glutamate, acetylcholine, and substance P).

Opioids can be administered by many routes—oral, rectal, parenteral, intramuscular, transcutaneous, subcutaneous, transmucosal, epidural, and intrathecal—making them adaptable for use in most clinical situations. The distribution half-lives of all opioids are fairly short at approximately 5 to 20 min. The highly lipid-soluble opiates, such as fentanyl and sufentanil, have a rapid onset and short duration of action.

The liver is responsible for the biotransformation of most opioids; many, including morphine and meperidine, have metabolites—morphine-6-glucoronide and normeperidine, respectively—that are equally active as the parent compound. These metabolites must be eliminated by the kidneys, and adjustment of doses of these medications is imperative for patients with renal failure. The metabolites of fentanyl, sufentanil, and alfentanil are inactive.

## Effects

### CENTRAL NERVOUS SYSTEM EFFECTS

High doses of opioids may cause deep sedation or hypnosis; however, opioids do not reliably produce amnesia. Opioids reduce the minimum alveolar concentration of inhalation anesthetic agents required during balanced general anesthesia.

Seizures can result from the neuroexcitatory effects of normeperidine, a metabolite of meperidine. Normeperidine-induced seizures are more likely to occur in patients who have received chronic meperidine therapy, have received large doses of meperidine over a short period, or have impaired renal function with decreased ability to eliminate this metabolite.

Opioids can reduce cerebral metabolic $O_2$ requirements, cerebral blood flow, and intracranial pressure if alveolar ventilation is unchanged in a healthy patient; however, fentanyl and other opioids have been shown to increase intracranial pressure in patients with traumatic brain injury, even with controlled ventilation. Opioids should not be withheld from intubation for this reason; the increased intracranial pressure associated with direct laryngoscopy without opioids would be much more detrimental. In patients in whom ventilation is not controlled, opioid-induced respiratory depression can produce hypoxemia, resulting in pupillary dilation and an increase in intracranial pressure due to hypercarbia. Opioids cause miosis by stimulating the Edinger-Westphal nucleus of the oculomotor nerve.

Opioids stimulate the chemoreceptor trigger zone located in the area postrema of the brainstem, which can result in nausea and vomiting.

| TABLE 50.1 | Opioid Receptor Subtypes, Clinical Effects, and Example Agonists | |
|---|---|---|
| Receptor | Clinical Effects | Example Agonist(s) |
| $\mu_1$ | Supraspinal analgesia<br>Bradycardia<br>Sedation<br>Pruritus<br>Nausea and vomiting | Morphine<br>Meperidine |
| $\mu_2$ | Respiratory depression<br>Euphoria<br>Physical dependence<br>Pruritus<br>Constipation | Morphine<br>Meperidine |
| $\kappa$ | Spinal analgesia<br>Respiratory depression<br>Sedation<br>Miosis | Fentanyl<br>Morphine<br>Nalbuphine |
| $\delta$ | Spinal analgesia<br>Respiratory depression | Oxycodone<br>$\beta$-endorphin<br>Leu-enkephalin |

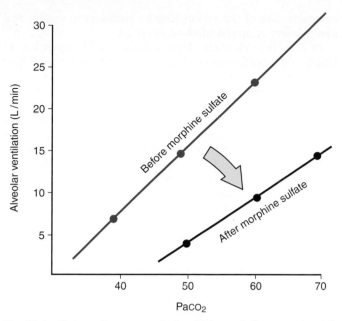

**Fig. 50.1** Opiates depress ventilation. This graph illustrates the shift of the $CO_2$ response curve down and to the right. (Modified from Nonvolatile anesthetic agents. In: Morgan GE, Mikhail MS, Murray MJ. *Clinical Anesthesiology.* 6th ed. Lange Medical Books/McGraw-Hill; 2021:195. Available at: http://www.accessmedicine.com.)

Opioids can interfere with serotonin reuptake, leading to serotonin syndrome when combined with other medications that exert a similar effect (e.g., selective serotonin reuptake inhibitors, methylene blue).

## RESPIRATORY EFFECTS

Opioid administration decreases minute ventilation by decreasing the respiratory rate (as opposed to decreasing the tidal volume). These medications have a direct effect on the respiratory centers in the medulla, producing a dose-dependent depression of the ventilatory response to $CO_2$. The $CO_2$ response curve shows a decreased slope and rightward shift when opioids are administered (Fig. 50.1). The apnea threshold, defined as the highest $Paco_2$ without ventilatory effort, is increased with the use of opioids. They also blunt the increase in ventilation in response to hypoxemia. Further, morphine and meperidine can cause histamine-induced bronchospasm.

## MUSCULOSKELETAL EFFECTS

Opioids can produce generalized skeletal muscle rigidity, a phenomenon associated with the more potent opiates (e.g., fentanyl, sufentanil, carfentanil). Loss of chest wall compliance and contraction of the laryngeal and pharyngeal muscles can be severe, resulting in ventilatory difficulty, even with positive-pressure ventilation. The mechanism of opioid-induced muscle rigidity is believed to be mediated by the μ receptors at the supraspinal level by increasing dopamine synthesis and inhibiting γ-aminobutyric acid activity. This muscle rigidity can be prevented by decreasing the rate of opioid administration or concomitantly administering a neuromuscular blocking agent and controlling ventilation.

Postoperative shivering can be attenuated with meperidine, which may act through a κ-receptor mechanism. Only 12.5 to 25 mg meperidine, administered intravenously as a slow push, is usually needed to produce this effect in an adult.

## CARDIOVASCULAR EFFECTS

At clinically relevant doses, opioids do not cause significant myocardial depression; however, opioids can cause a dose-dependent bradycardia resulting in decreased cardiac output. One exception is meperidine, which may cause tachycardia because of its structural similarities to atropine. Meperidine may also cause a decrease in myocardial contractility because it has negative inotropic effects. Most opioids exert their cardiovascular effects both by sympatholysis via vasomotor centers in the medulla and by increased parasympathetic tone via vagal pathways. Prolongation of the QT interval has been noted with both meperidine and methadone.

## GASTROINTESTINAL EFFECTS

Opioids increase nonperistaltic smooth muscle tone in the small and large bowel via vagal and peripheral mechanisms; however, this ineffective nonpropulsive activity leads to an overall increase in bowel transit time and can result in ileus. Newer medications have been developed to help combat opioid-induced constipation (e.g., methylnaltrexone, lubiprostone, naloxegol). These medications work either by increasing chloride and water secretion into the lumen via the cystic fibrosis transmembrane regulator and type 2 chloride channels or by peripheral antagonism of the μ receptor in the gastrointestinal tract. Additionally, opioids can cause contraction of the sphincter of Oddi. This contraction can mimic biliary colic, but it is responsive to antagonism of the opioids or the use of glucagon.

## HORMONE EFFECTS

Opioids decrease the stress response to pain and surgery by acting on the hypothalamus. Inhibition of gonadotropin-releasing hormone and corticotropin-releasing factor results in decreased release of endogenous cortisol. It is still uncertain whether reducing the neuroendocrine response to surgical stress results in improved clinical outcomes.

## Histamine Release

Although true allergic responses to opioids are rare, some opioids may cause a nonimmunoglobulin E–mediated release of histamine from mast cells, decreasing systemic vascular resistance, with resultant decreases in blood pressure and tachycardia, as well as possible bronchospasm. This response is most evident with meperidine and morphine.

Meperidine has fallen out of favor for use as a pain reliever because of its many associated toxicities (many of them noted previously). However, small doses of meperidine are still widely used in the management of postoperative rigors.

## Opioid-Induced Hyperalgesia

Increasing evidence suggests that opioids, which are intended to treat pain, can actually make patients more sensitive to pain and can worsen preexisting pain states. Initially, opioids provide clear analgesic effects, but then they can become associated with states of hyperalgesia (increased sensitivity to noxious stimuli). Opioid-induced hyperalgesia was first noted in patients with long-term use of these medications, but it has now been recognized in patients receiving opioids for durations as short as the length of a surgical procedure. An example is remifentanil, an ultra-short-acting opiate used as an infusion during surgical procedures. Hyperalgesia has been noted after 60- to 90-min infusions with this opioid agonist. The mechanism is thought to be secondary to increased nociceptive signal processing at the level of the spinal cord. Coadministration of ketamine abolishes the hyperalgesia induced by remifentanil, implying an underlying N-methyl-D-aspartate receptor mechanism.

## Dependence, Tolerance, and Addiction

Dependence and tolerance are two significant problems with even moderate-term administration of opioids. *Dependence* refers to the presence of withdrawal symptoms if a drug is withheld, and can be either physical or psychological. *Psychological dependence* refers to craving for a drug, whereas *addiction* is characterized by compulsive drug seeking and use, despite harmful consequences. Opioid use disorder is defined in the *Diagnostic and Statistical Manual, Fifth Edition* as *a problematic pattern of opioid use leading to clinically significant impairment or distress. Tolerance* is the need to increase the dose of an opioid over time to maintain the desired analgesic effect, reflecting desensitization of the antinociceptive pathways to opiates and upregulation of opioid-binding receptors.

In 2016, the Centers for Disease Control and Prevention released guidelines for prescribing opioids for chronic pain. These guidelines recommend that a discussion of the risks, including dependence and addiction, should occur before initiation of opioid therapy. There are risk screening tools available, but they have not been fully externally validated, and so their reliability is questionable. Diversion is a very real problem, and prescribers should be alert for concerning signs and symptoms. Providers can ensure that a reasonable number of tablets are dispensed, especially in acute settings, which may help combat excess use and diversion. A good tip for providers is to use the lowest dose possible for the shortest time interval possible.

Opioids can also be used in the treatment of addiction, and buprenorphine (a partial agonist) is one example. Buprenorphine can be combined with naloxone (a pure antagonist) for sublingual formulation to treat addiction. This combination allows the partial agonist effect of the buprenorphine to be used sublingually because naloxone has poor sublingual or oral bioavailability, but if injection of the medication is attempted, the naloxone will precipitate withdrawal. Methadone is another medication that is used in addiction. Depending on the dosing schedule of methadone, it can be used as an analgesic regimen (e.g., three times a day) or as a treatment for addiction (e.g., once a day). The pharmacodynamics properties of methadone allow these different uses.

## SUGGESTED READINGS

Brunton, L., & Knollman, B. (2022). *Goodman and Gilman's manual of pharmacology and therapeutics* (14th ed.). New York: McGraw Hill.

Dowell, D., Haegerich, T. M., & Chou, R. (2016). CDC guideline for prescribing opioids for chronic pain—United States, 2016. *MMWR Recommendations and Reports, 65*(RR–1), 1–49.

James, A., & Williams, J. (2020). Basic opioid pharmacology, an update. *British Journal of Pain, 14*(2), 115–121.

Lee, M., Silverman, S., Hansen, H., Patel, V. B., & Manchikanti, L. (2011). A comprehensive review of opioid-induced hyperalgesia. *Pain Physician, 14*, 145–161.

Strang, J., Volkow, N. D., Degenhardt, L., Hickman, M., Johnson, K., Koob, G. F., et al. (2020). Opioid use disorder. *Nature Reviews Disease Primers, 6*(1), 3.

Thiels, C. A., Ubl, D. S., Yost, K. J., Dowdy, S. C., Mabry, T. M., Gazelka, H. M., et al. (2018). Results of a prospective, multicenter initiative aimed at developing opioid prescribing guidelines after surgery. *Annals of Surgery, 268*(3), 257–268.

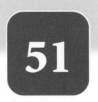

# 51

# Succinylcholine

SARAH E. DODD, MD

## Clinical Use

Succinylcholine has been the long-standing muscle relaxant of choice for laryngospasm and rapid-sequence intubation. Although higher-dose rocuronium (1.2 mg/kg) also provides rapid intubating conditions, succinylcholine was found to be clinically superior in a Cochrane Review when also considering the duration of action. Unfortunately, there are a number of considerations and side effects that are frequently encountered after succinylcholine administration. These include anaphylaxis, hyperkalemia, malignant hyperthermia, cardiac arrhythmia,

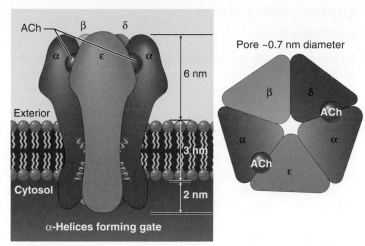

**Fig. 51.1** Nicotinic acetylcholine receptors (nAChRs) termed *adult* (because of their expression later in development) consist of five subunits: two α, one β, one δ, and one ε (denoted α2βδε). Each postsynaptic adult motor site receives neuronal input from a single motor axon, and the adult nAChRs are restricted in high concentrations (10,000/μm²) in the postsynaptic membrane but are virtually absent extrasynaptically. As with fetal nAChRs, the α subunit contains the recognition site for acetylcholine *(ACh)* and all neuromuscular blocking agents. (From Brull S, Naguib M. Review of neuromuscular junction anatomy and function. In: Mashour GA, Lydic P, eds. *The Neuroscientific Foundations of Anesthesiology.* Oxford University Press; 2011:205–210.)

prolonged apnea, phase II blockade, and postoperative myalgia, as well as increases in intraocular, intragastric, and intracranial pressures.

## Pharmacology

Succinylcholine is a neuromuscular blocking medication that depolarizes the postjunctional membrane by interacting with the alpha subunits of nicotinic acetylcholine (ACh) receptors (Fig. 51.1), causing skeletal muscle contraction. This depolarization leads to variable muscle fasciculation followed by flaccid paralysis. ACh molecules are usually metabolized quickly by acetylcholinesterase molecules, but hydrolysis of succinylcholine is comparatively slow, resulting in a sustained depolarization and muscle relaxation. The rapid breakdown of succinylcholine by butyrylcholinesterase (BChE) (also known as *plasma cholinesterase* or *pseudocholinesterase*) in plasma allows only 5% to 10% of the drug to reach the neuromuscular junction and hydrolyzes it after it diffuses away from the junction.

## Phase II Blockade

Repeated dosing or continuous infusion of succinylcholine may produce a prolonged neuromuscular blockade and a train-of-four pattern showing fade. This is called *phase II blockade*, in contrast to *phase I blockade*, which is the typical succinylcholine pattern. The mechanism is not completely known but is likely related to electrolyte shifts at the neuromuscular junction and desensitization of ACh receptors resulting in tachyphylaxis. Neostigmine may reverse phase II blockade, but this reversal is unreliable and should only be attempted if the patient has recovered a twitch after a peripheral nerve stimulator is applied.

## Succinylcholine-Associated Apnea

The effects of succinylcholine are terminated by its metabolism by BChE. However, some patients have atypical BChE enzymes, and such patients who receive a conventional dose of succinylcholine can experience a prolonged neuromuscular block. More than 30 different variants of BChE have been described, though not all of them are associated with prolonged apnea after administration of succinylcholine. Homozygotes of this atypical enzyme (approximately 1 in every 3200 patients) can have a greatly prolonged duration of succinylcholine-induced neuromuscular blockade, whereas heterozygotes (approximately 1 in every 480 patients) will experience only a modest prolongation. The most common atypical BChE can be detected with dibucaine. Dibucaine, an amide-linked local anesthetic agent, inhibits 80% of the activity of normal BChE, compared with only a 20% inhibition of the homozygote atypical enzyme. A dibucaine number of 80 (i.e., percentage of inhibition) confirms the presence of normal BChE. However, the dibucaine number does not reflect the quantity of BChE present, but rather the quality of the enzyme and its ability to hydrolyze succinylcholine. The activity of BChE refers to the number of succinylcholine molecules hydrolyzed per unit of time, expressed in international units. Fig. 51.2 illustrates the correlation between the duration of succinylcholine action and BChE activity.

Succinylcholine apnea from the various abnormal BChE phenotypes is usually of shorter duration than the surgical procedure. Skeletal muscle paralysis of excessive duration requires maintenance of mechanical ventilatory support and continuation of anesthesia or sedation, typically in the postanesthesia care unit or the intensive care unit, until neuromuscular function returns. Some have advocated transfusion of fresh frozen plasma to replace BChE, but the risks of transfusion are far higher than those associated with a few hours of mechanical ventilation. Neostigmine administration is not

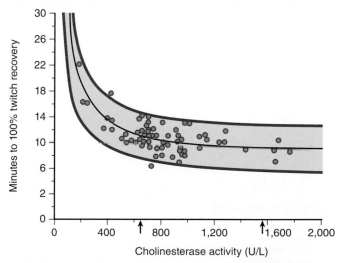

**Fig. 51.2** Correlation between the duration of succinylcholine neuromuscular blockade and butyrylcholinesterase activity. The normal range of activity lies between the *arrows*. (Modified from Viby-Mogensen J. Correlation of succinylcholine duration of action with plasma cholinesterase activity in subjects with the genotypically normal enzyme. *Anesthesiology.* 1980;517–520).

appropriate in these circumstances, as it inhibits the degradation of succinylcholine by BChE. The presence of succinylcholine interferes with both quantitative and qualitative assays; therefore it is preferable to postpone testing until the day after an episode of prolonged neuromuscular blockade associated with the use of succinylcholine to ensure accurate results.

## Variances in Butyrylcholinesterase Activity

From birth to age 6 months, the activity of BChE is 50% of that in nonpregnant adults. Activity reaches 70% of adult activity by age 6 years and normal adult levels at puberty. Pregnancy is associated with a 25% to 30% decrease in BChE activity from week 10 to postpartum week 6, and is clinically insignificant. Decreased BChE activity can also be seen in a number of disease states and with administration of various drugs. Hepatitis, cirrhosis, malnutrition, cancer, and hypothyroidism are associated with decreased BChE activity in plasma. The alteration in BChE activity may be useful as a marker of hepatic synthetic function. Certain drugs, including acetylcholinesterase inhibitors, pancuronium, procaine, hexafluorenium, and organophosphate insecticides inhibit BChE, whereas other drugs, including chemotherapeutic agents, can cause decreased BChE synthesis. BChE measurements can be used as a marker of occupational exposure to insecticides. Decreasing BChE activity to 25% of the control level, as seen in severe liver disease, prolongs succinylcholine duration of action from $3.0 \pm 0.15$ min to $8.6 \pm 0.7$ min, an increase that is usually undetectable in the clinical setting. Other diseases, such as thyrotoxicosis and nephrotic syndrome, are associated with increased BChE activity that is probably of no clinical significance (Box 51.1).

## Undesirable Effects

### HYPERKALEMIA

Depolarization of the postjunctional membrane results in extracellular movement of potassium ions. Under standard conditions, this produces an average serum potassium concentration increase of 0.5 to 1.0 mEq/L. Upregulation of junctional and extrajunctional cholinergic receptors may result in release of higher amount of potassium that is unpredictable and may result in severe hyperkalemia, to the point of cardiac arrest. This occurs in multiple clinical situations including trauma, burn, immobility, and upper motor neuron disease. The rise in potassium is not tempered by administration of a defasciculating dose of a nondepolarizing muscular blocker.

### RHABDOMYOLYSIS

Rhabdomyolysis occurs after succinylcholine administration in patients with Duchenne muscular dystrophy and has also been associated with masseter muscle rigidity. The resulting hyperkalemia may provoke cardiac arrest, and myoglobinemia may result in renal failure. It is typically advised to avoid the regular use of succinylcholine in male children younger than 5 years because of the possibility of undiagnosed Duchenne muscular dystrophy, except in cases of refractory laryngospasm or an emergent intubation.

### MALIGNANT HYPERTHERMIA

Malignant hyperthermia (MH) is a triggered by succinylcholine administration, and a known history of MH is an absolute contraindication. Clinicians should also strongly consider avoiding it in patients with a known family history or with conditions known to be associated with MH. A recent position statement

---

### BOX 51.1  CAUSES OF CHANGES IN BUTYRYLCHOLINESTERASE ACTIVITY

**INHERITED CAUSES**

Genetic variants that lead to decreased or increased activity

**PHYSIOLOGIC CAUSES**

Decreases in the last trimester of pregnancy
Reduced activity in the newborn

**ACQUIRED DECREASES**

Liver diseases
Cancer
Debilitating diseases
Collagen diseases
Uremia
Malnutrition
Hypothyroidism

**ACQUIRED INCREASES**

Obesity
Alcoholism
Hyperthyroidism
Nephropathy
Psoriasis
Electroconvulsive therapy

**DRUG-RELATED CAUSES**

Neostigmine
Pyridostigmine
Chlorpromazine
Echothiophate iodide
Cyclophosphamide
Monoamine oxidase inhibitors
Pancuronium
Oral contraceptives
Organophosphates
Hexafluorenium
Bambuterol
Esmolol

**OTHER CAUSES OF DECREASED ACTIVITY**

Plasmapheresis
Extracorporeal circulation
Tetanus
Radiation therapy
Burns

Adapted, with permission, from Whittaker M. Plasma cholinesterase variants and the anaesthetist. *Anaesthesia.* 1980;35:174–197.

by the Society for Ambulatory Anesthesia states that although succinylcholine is a known MH trigger, even outpatient surgical centers that do not stock dantrolene should still maintain an emergency-use inventory of succinylcholine for laryngospasm. This recommendation is based on the much higher incidence of laryngospasm compared with MH, and a patient given succinylcholine can be closely observed for signs of MH and transferred to a center with dantrolene if needed.

## POSTOPERATIVE MYALGIA

A 2005 metanalysis demonstrated that as many as 50% of patients have skeletal muscle myalgia at 24 hours after succinylcholine administration. Techniques that were significantly effective in reducing this rate include administration of larger doses of succinylcholine (1.5 mg/kg rather than 1 mg/kg), lidocaine, nonsteroidal antiinflammatory drugs, and nondepolarizing muscle relaxant (10%–35% of ED95) administered in advance as a defasciculating dose. This should be done with caution, however, as the study patients receiving nondepolarizing muscle relaxant had side effects including diplopia, eyelid drooping, breathing difficulties, and dysphagia.

## CARDIAC ARRHYTHMIAS

Succinylcholine has sympathetic and parasympathetic activity because of its structural similarity to ACh and may interfere with either pathway to the sinus node. This predisposes pediatric patients with higher vagal tone to bradycardia and adults with less vagal tone to tachycardia with the first dose. Subsequent doses given within 10 min may result in sinus bradycardia or junctional rhythm because of the accumulation of metabolites (primarily succinylmonocholine and choline).

## INTRAOCULAR PRESSURE INCREASE

Succinylcholine causes a modest transient increase in intraocular pressure that persists for 5 to 10 min after administration. Possible mechanisms include choroidal vascular dilatation or a decrease in drainage secondary to elevated central venous pressures. Although patients with treated glaucoma are at minimal risk, administration of succinylcholine to patients with recent ocular incisions or with penetrating eye injuries may result in vitreous expulsion and visual loss. Many case reports have been published and studies have been conducted to identify a pretreatment agent to obviate this adverse effect; results have been mixed with the use of nondepolarizing muscle relaxants, opioids, propranolol, lidocaine, and others.

## INCREASED INTRAGASTRIC PRESSURE

Succinylcholine can cause, on average, a 40-cm $H_2O$ increase in intragastric pressures, presumably as a result of abdominal muscle contraction. It has been shown that lower esophageal sphincter pressure also increases after the administration of succinylcholine, resulting in maintained gastroesophageal barrier pressures. Whether the administration of succinylcholine during induction causes increased susceptibility to esophageal reflux and possible pulmonary aspiration (secondary to increased intragastric pressures) remains debatable. Studies have shown that pretreatment with a nondepolarizing neuromuscular blocking agent decreases this rise in pressure.

## INCREASED INTRACRANIAL PRESSURE

The results of several studies have suggested that succinylcholine may increase intracranial pressure, whereas others have been unable to demonstrate this phenomenon. This ambiguity has spawned a variety of clinical recommendations and considerable debate. The proposed mechanisms include decreased venous effluent from the brain as a result of fasciculation-induced increases in intrathoracic pressure, neck muscle contraction with resultant jugular venous compression, and succinylcholine-induced increases in afferent muscle spindle activity that cause increased cerebral blood flow, cerebral blood volume, and intracranial pressure. However, succinylcholine should not be deleted from the therapeutic armamentarium for emergency airway management based solely on concerns about increased intracranial pressure.

## SUGGESTED READINGS

Joshi, G. P., Desai, M. S., Gayer, S., & Vila, H. (2017). Succinylcholine for emergency airway rescue in class B ambulatory facilities: The Society for Ambulatory Anesthesia Position Statement. *Anesthesia and Analgesia, 124*(5), 1447–1449.

Tran, D. T., Newton, E. K., Mount, V. A., Lee, J. S., Wells, G. A., & Perry, J. J. (2015). Rocuronium versus succinylcholine for rapid sequence induction intubation. *Cochrane Database of Systematic Reviews, 10*, CD002788.

# 52

# Nondepolarizing Neuromuscular Blocking Agents

PAUL A. WARNER, MD

The introduction of nondepolarizing neuromuscular blocking agents (NMBAs) into clinical practice marked a significant advance in anesthesia and surgery. The past 20 years have seen a significant evolution in nondepolarizing NMBAs, with the appearance of new drugs, free from many of the undesirable side effects of their predecessors. The most dramatic change has been the recent introduction of a novel reversal agent, sugammadex, into clinical practice in the United States. Sugammadex rapidly reverses the action of aminosteroid class NMBAs, such as rocuronium, thus providing a viable alternative to succinylcholine for rapid-onset but short-acting muscle relaxation.

## Mechanism of Action

By competing with acetylcholine (ACh) for binding to nicotinic receptor $\alpha$ subunits, nondepolarizing NMBAs cause receptor inhibition, thus resulting in skeletal muscle relaxation. The nondepolarizing NMBAs may also be capable of directly blocking the ion channel, stopping the flux of $Na^+$ through the ion pore. Some nondepolarizing NMBAs block $Na^+$ channels on prejunctional nicotinic ACh receptors, interfering with mobilization of ACh from sites of synthesis. Calcium-dependent release of ACh is not affected.

## Characteristics of Neuromuscular Nondepolarizing Blockade

Muscle relaxation caused by nondepolarizing NMBAs is characterized clinically by a train-of-four T4/T1 ratio of less than 1 (with <0.7 representing adequate surgical relaxation), tetanic "fade," posttetanic potentiation, absence of fasciculations, potentiation by other nondepolarizing NMBAs, and antagonism of the block by acetylcholinesterase inhibitors. Blockade by nondepolarizing NMBAs occurs more rapidly in the laryngeal adductors, diaphragm, and masseter than in the adductor pollicis. The $ED_{95}$ is the dose needed to produce 95% suppression of a single-twitch response evoked by a peripheral nerve stimulator in the presence of $NO_2$-barbiturate-opioid anesthesia and is used as a measure of potency. Administration of one to three times the $ED_{95}$ allows tracheal intubation. The speed of onset of blockade is inversely proportional to the potency of the NMBA.

## Alterations in Sensitivity

Enhanced NMBA effects occur with administration of inhalation anesthetics, local anesthetics, diuretics, antiarrhythmics, aminoglycosides, magnesium, and lithium. Hypothermia, acidosis, and hypokalemia also increase the potency of nondepolarizing NMBAs. Patients with myasthenia gravis are very sensitive to the effects of nondepolarizing NMBAs. In contrast, patients with burn injuries are resistant to the effects owing to proliferation of nicotinic receptors (upregulation). Administration of 10% of the intubating dose of an NMBA 2 to 4 min before the full intubating dose is given is known as *priming*. Priming may accelerate the onset of muscle relaxation to approximately 60 s.

## Chemical Structure and Pharmacokinetics

Currently used nondepolarizing NMBAs are benzylisoquinolinium and aminosteroid compounds, both of which have one or more positively charged quaternary ammonium groups (Tables 52.1 and 52.2). ACh has a single quaternary ammonium. The presence of a quaternary ammonium group on nondepolarizing NMBAs means that they are highly ionized water-soluble compounds at physiologic pH. Lipid solubility is limited, so nondepolarizing NMBAs do not easily cross lipid-membrane barriers such as the blood-brain barrier. After a single dose, the volume of distribution is similar to the extracellular fluid volume; the volume of distribution, plasma clearance, and elimination may be affected by patient age or the presence of renal or hepatic dysfunction. Although many nondepolarizing NMBAs rely on hepatic or renal clearance, or both, some are eliminated in an unusual fashion (see later discussion).

| TABLE 52.1 | Nondepolarizing Neuromuscular Blocking Agents by Duration of Action | | |
|---|---|---|---|
| Structural Class | Short-Acting Agent | Intermediate-Acting Agent | Long-Acting Agent |
| Benzylisoquinolinium | Mivacurium* | Atracurium Cisatracurium | d-Tubocurarine* Metocurine* Doxacurium* |
| Aminosteroid | Rapacuronium* | Vecuronium Rocuronium | Pancuronium |
| Asymmetrical mixed-onium chlorofumarate | Gantacurium* | – | – |

*Not available in the United States.

| TABLE 52.2 | **Characteristics of Commonly Used Neuromuscular Blocking Agents** | | | | | | | |
|---|---|---|---|---|---|---|---|---|
| **Agent** | **Intubating Dose (mg/kg)** | **Infusion Rate ($\mu g \cdot kg^{-1} \cdot min^{-1}$)** | **Onset (s)\*** | **Duration of Action** | **Vagolysis** | **Histamine Release** | **Elimination** | **Comments** |
| Succinylcholine | 1.5 | NA | 30–90 | Very short | Variable | Slight | Butyrylcholine-sterase | Depolarizing muscle relaxant |
| Mivacurium | 0.15 | 3–12 | 90–150 | Short | No | Yes | Butyrylcholine-sterase | No longer available in United States |
| Rapacuronium | 1.5 | NA | 45–90 | Short | Yes | Yes | Kidney, ester hydrolysis | No longer available |
| Rocuronium | 0.9–1.2 | 9–12 | 60–90 | Intermediate | Yes | No | Liver, kidney | – |
| Cisatracurium | 0.15–0.2 | 1–3 | 90–120 | Intermediate | No | No | Hofmann degradation | – |
| Atracurium | 0.5 | 3–12 | 90–150 | Intermediate | No | Yes | Hofmann degradation, ester hydrolysis | – |
| Vecuronium | 0.08–0.12 | 1–2 | 90–150 | Intermediate | No | No | Liver, kidney | – |
| Pancuronium | 0.08–0.12 | NA | Slow | Long | Yes | No | Kidney, liver | – |
| Gantacurium | 0.4–0.6 | NA | 90–120 | Very short | No | Yes | Cysteine adduction, ester hydrolysis | Still investigational |

*NA*, Not applicable.
*Time to intubation.

## ROCURONIUM

Rocuronium is a monoquaternary aminosteroid NMBA. When administered at three times $ED_{95}$, rocuronium has an onset of action similar to that of succinylcholine, although the laryngeal muscles are relatively more resistant to the effects of ro-curonium. Therefore rocuronium is often used as an alternative relaxant for rapid-sequence induction when the depolarizing NMBA succinylcholine is contraindicated. Doses used for rapid tracheal intubation (0.9–1.2 mg/kg) are roughly twice that of the common intubating dose (0.6 mg/kg). These larger doses typically cause neuromuscular blockade that may last for an hour or more if not antagonized by sugammadex.

## Nonrelaxant Side Effects

Nonrelaxant side effects of nondepolarizing NMBAs include histamine release and cardiovascular and autonomic effects (see Chapter 60, Vasodilators).

## Commonly Used Nondepolarizing Neuromuscular Blocking Agents

### VECURONIUM

Vecuronium is a monoquaternary aminosteroid NMBA with a structure similar to that of rocuronium. At an $ED_{95}$ of 0.05 mg/kg, its onset of action is 3 to 5 min and its duration of action is 20 to 35 min. The drug is supplied in powder form because it is unstable in solution. Vecuronium is metabolized by the liver and cleared by the kidney. Biliary excretion also plays a role in its elimination. Repeated dosing of vecuronium causes a cumulative effect that is less than that of pancuronium but greater than that of atracurium. Vecuronium has minimal, if any, cardiovascular effects. As an aminosteroid, the action of vecuronium can be reversed by sugammadex.

## ATRACURIUM

Atracurium is an intermediate-acting NMBA that is a mixture of 10 stereoisomers. At an $ED_{95}$ dose of 0.2 mg/kg, its onset and duration of action are 3 to 5 min and 20 to 35 min, respectively. Atracurium is metabolized and eliminated independent of the liver and kidney. It undergoes spontaneous nonenzymatic in vivo degradation (Hofmann elimination) at normal body pH and temperature. The drug also undergoes hydrolysis by non-specific plasma esterases, unrelated to butyrylcholinesterase. One-third of administered atracurium is degraded by Hof-mann elimination and two-thirds by ester hydrolysis. Both pathways produce laudanosine, which, although not active as an NMBA, may cause central nervous system excitation at high doses in animals. At doses of atracurium used clinically in humans, laudanosine does not appear to have significant effects. Repeated supplemental doses of atracurium do not produce a significant cumulative drug effect because of the rapid clearance of the drug from plasma. Accordingly, there is consistency of time to recovery of neuromuscular function. Atracurium causes dose-dependent histamine release, which is significant at doses greater than 0.5 mg/kg. The use of atracurium should be avoided in patients with asthma. Because atracurium is a ben-zylisoquinolinium, it will not be reversed by sugammadex.

## CISATRACURIUM

One of the 10 stereoisomers of atracurium, the 1R-cis, 1R′-cis form, makes up approximately 15% of the atracurium mixture. The purified preparation, known as *cisatracurium*, is an NMBA that is four times more potent than the parent compound. Cisatracurium does not cause histamine release and therefore has minimal cardiovascular effects. Metabolism is by Hofmann degradation, but nonspecific esterases have no role in its elimination. Like atracurium, cisatracurium is not reversed by sugammadex.

## PANCURONIUM

Pancuronium, a bisquaternary aminosteroid, is a long-acting NMBA. It has an $ED_{95}$ of 0.07 mg/kg, with onset of action of 3 to 5 min and duration of action of 60 to 90 min. The drug is mainly excreted unchanged in the urine, although there is a small component of hepatic metabolism. Renal failure may increase its duration of action. Pancuronium causes a vagolytic effect, leading to a modest increase in heart rate, blood pressure, and cardiac output. For this reason, it may be a good choice in patients undergoing cardiac operations, especially when a high-dose opioid technique is being used. Sugammadex does reverse the action of pancuronium.

## RAPACURONIUM AND MIVACURIUM

Rapacuronium, a monoquaternary synthetic steroid NMBA that has a rapid onset of action, was introduced as a replacement for succinylcholine. However, its tendency to cause life-threatening bronchospasm led to its withdrawal from clinical use. Mivacurium also has a rapid onset of action and is hydrolyzed by plasma cholinesterase at 80% of the rate of succinylcholine metabolism. Histamine-induced bronchospasm was also problematic with mivacurium, and it is no longer available in the United States.

## GANTACURIUM

Gantacurium, an NMBA under investigation in Phase 3 trials, represents a new class of nondepolarizing NMBAs known as *asymmetric mixed-onium chlorofumarates*. It is degraded by two nonenzymatic chemical reactions, cysteine adduction and ester hydrolysis. Gantacurium has a pharmacodynamic profile similar to that of succinylcholine.

## SUGAMMADEX

Perhaps the most novel drug to come to the forefront is not itself a nondepolarizing NDMA, but rather a reversal agent. Sugammadex, a modified γ-cyclodextrin, is the first selective relaxant binding agent to gain market approval. It is capable of reversing any depth of neuromuscular blockade induced by rocuronium and, to a lesser extent, vecuronium and pancuronium. The introduction of sugammadex to clinical practice has changed rocuronium from an intermediate-acting nondepolarizing NMBA to a potentially very short-acting agent. Typical dosing is based on total body weight and depends on the response to train-of-four stimulation. If spontaneous recovery of paralysis reveals two twitches on train-of-four testing, a dose of 2 mg/kg is recommended. If there is no spontaneous recovery, but there is posttetanic twitch, a dose of 4 mg/kg is recommended. To rapidly reverse paralysis, a dose of 16 mg/kg can be administered 3 min after a rapid-sequence induction dose of rocuronium. Its use in the United States was delayed for several years because of safety concerns, specifically hypersensitivity reactions. Unlike neostigmine, sugammadex has no intrinsic anticholinergic properties, eliminating the need for concomitant administration of an antimuscarinic agent. The side effects of this drug are detailed in Chapter 60, Vasodilators.

## SUGGESTED READINGS

Abrishami, A., Ho, J., Wong, J., Yin, L., & Chung, F. (2009). Sugammadex, a selective reversal medication for preventing postoperative residual neuromuscular blockade. *Cochrane Database of Systematic Reviews*, (4), CD007362.

Carron, M., Zarantonello, F., Tellaroli, P., & Ori, C. (2016). Efficacy and safety of sugammadex compared to neostigmine for reversal of neuromuscular blockade: A meta-analysis of randomized controlled trials. *Journal of Clinical Anesthesia, 35*, 1–12.

Chapter 11. Neuromuscular blocking agents. (2013). In J. F., IV. Butterworth, D. C. Mackey, & J. D. Wasnick (Eds.), *Morgan & Mikhail's clinical anesthesiology* (5th ed.). McGraw Hill. Retrieved from https://accessmedicine.mhmedical.com/content.aspx?bookid=564&sectionid=42800542. Accessed January 26, 2022.

Chapter 27. Pharmacology of neuromuscular blocking drugs. (2020). In: S. J. Brull & C. Meistelman (Eds.), *Miller's Anesthesia*. Elsevier.

Claudius, C., Garvey, L. H., & Viby-Mogensen, J. (2009). The undesirable effects of neuromuscular blocking drugs. *Anaesthesia, 64*(Suppl. 1), 10–21.

Martyn, J. A., Fagerlund, M. J., & Eriksson, L. I. (2009). Basic principles of neuromuscular transmission. *Anaesthesia, 64*(Suppl. 1), 1–9.

Naguib, M., & Brull, S. J. (2009). Update on neuromuscular pharmacology. *Current Opinion in Anaesthesiology, 22*, 483–490.

Perry, J. J., Lee, J. S., Sillberg, V. A., & Wells, G. A. (2008). Rocuronium versus succinylcholine for rapid sequence induction intubation. *Cochrane Database of Systematic Reviews*, (2), CD002788.

Stoelting, R. K., & Hillier, S. C. (2006). *Pharmacology and physiology in anesthetic practice* (4th ed., pp. 208–250). Philadelphia: Lippincott Williams & Wilkins.

# 53

# Nonrelaxant Side Effects of Nondepolarizing Neuromuscular Blocking Agents

PAUL A. WARNER, MD

In addition to their action on the neuromuscular junction, nondepolarizing neuromuscular blocking agents (NMBAs) produce a variety of nonrelaxant effects. Many of these "side effects" may be unwanted and are potentially harmful. Nondepolarizing NMBAs are commonly implicated in medication-related adverse perioperative events. Some nonrelaxant effects may be used to the advantage of the patient and the practitioner.

## Interference With Autonomic Function

Nondepolarizing NMBAs may interact with nicotinic and muscarinic cholinergic receptors in the sympathetic and parasympathetic nervous systems. The length of the carbon chain separating the two positively charged ammonium groups influences the specificity of a nondepolarizing NMBA for nicotinic receptors at autonomic ganglia (vs. nicotinic receptors at the neuromuscular junction). The so-called *autonomic margin* reflects the difference between the dose of a nondepolarizing NMBA that causes neuromuscular blockade and the dose that leads to circulatory effects. For example, blockade of autonomic ganglia leading to hypotension occurs with *d*-tubocurarine, an older nondepolarizing NMBA, at doses slightly higher than those required for blockade of the neuromuscular junction. However, the $ED_{95}$ doses for neuromuscular blockade with the use of cisatracurium, vecuronium, and rocuronium are significantly lower than the doses that cause autonomic effects, so these drugs have a wide autonomic margin.

The effects of nondepolarizing NMBAs on the parasympathetic muscarinic receptors in the heart may be clinically significant. Pancuronium, for example, produces a vagolytic action on nodal cells mediated through muscarinic receptors. This action occurs at doses used clinically for neuromuscular blockade, leading to an increase in heart rate.

The sympathetic nervous system contains at least three sets of muscarinic receptors. Blockade of these receptors on dopaminergic interneurons decreases modulation of ganglionic traffic (disinhibition), and blockade of adrenergic neurons results in removal of a negative feedback system for catecholamine release. Muscarinic blockade at sympathetic adrenergic neurons, leading to inhibition of norepinephrine uptake, represents the mechanism behind the exaggerated response that is sometimes seen with pancuronium during light anesthesia. The drug may cause norepinephrine release independent of muscarinic blockade. Thus pancuronium may cause tachycardia and a predisposition to arrhythmias because of vagal block with a shift toward adrenergic tone, indirect sympathomimetic activation, and atrioventricular nodal blockade (greater than sinoatrial nodal blockade).

## Histamine Release

The benzylisoquinolinium compounds cause nonimmunologic release of histamine and possibly other mediators from mast cells. Histamine release is a function of dose and the rate of administration. The physiologic effects of histamine include positive chronotropy (H2 receptors); positive inotropy (H2 receptors); positive dromotropy (H1 receptors); coronary artery effects (H1 receptors, vasoconstriction; H2 receptors, vasodilation); and peripheral vasodilation. Erythema of the face, neck, and torso may occur. Bronchospasm is rare but may be severe, and it has been a limiting factor in the use of some nondepolarizing NMBAs. Rapid administration of atracurium in doses greater than 0.4 mg/kg and mivacurium at doses greater than 0.15 mg/kg has been associated with histamine-related hypotension. In general, however, histamine release causes minimal effects in healthy patients. If clinical manifestations occur, they are usually of short duration (lasting 1–5 min), and the response undergoes rapid tachyphylaxis, so subsequent doses of nondepolarizing NMBAs cause little, if any, effect. Vecuronium, at doses of 0.1 to 0.2 mg/kg, may rarely cause severe bronchospasm, probably because of competitive inhibition of histamine-*N*-methyltransferase, thus inhibiting the degradation of histamine. Table 53.1 shows the approximate autonomic margins of safety of nondepolarizing NMBAs, and Table 53.2 illustrates the clinical autonomic effects of nondepolarizing NMBAs and the effects on histamine.

## Respiratory Effects

In addition to the effects of histamine on the respiratory system, nondepolarizing NMBAs may directly affect autonomic receptors in the lungs. At least three types of muscarinic receptors are found in the airways, as shown in Fig. 53.1. Nondepolarizing NMBAs have different antagonistic activities at both the M2 and M3 receptors. Blockade of M2 receptors on airway smooth muscle causes an increased release of acetylcholine, which will act on M3 receptors and cause bronchoconstriction. Blockade of M3 receptors causes bronchodilation by inhibiting vagally mediated bronchoconstriction. Rapacuronium, a nondepolarizing NMBA, blocks M2 receptors to a much greater extent than it blocks M3 receptors. Because this causes an unacceptably high incidence of bronchospasm, rapacuronium was withdrawn from the market.

| TABLE 53.1 Approximate Autonomic Margins of Safety of Nondepolarizing Neuromuscular Blocking Agents* | | | |
|---|---|---|---|
| Drug | Vagus[†] | Sympathetic Ganglia[†] | Histamine Release[‡] |
| **BENZYLISOQUINOLINIUM COMPOUNDS** | | | |
| Mivacurium | >50 | >100 | 3.0 |
| Atracurium | 16 | 40 | 2.5 |
| Cisatracurium | >50 | >50 | None |
| d-Tubocurarine[§] | 0.6 | 2 | 0.6 |
| **AMINOSTEROID COMPOUNDS** | | | |
| Vecuronium | 20 | >250 | None |
| Rocuronium | 3–5 | >10 | None |
| Pancuronium | 3 | >250 | None |

*Number of multiples of the ED$_{95}$ for neuromuscular blockade required to produce the autonomic side effect (ED$_{50}$).
[†]In the cat.
[‡]In human subjects.
[§]No longer available.
*ED*, Effective dose.
Reproduced, with permission, from Naguib M, Lien CA, Meistelman C. Pharmacology of muscle relaxants and their antagonists. In: Miller RD, Eriksson LI, Fleisher LA, et al., eds. *Miller's Anesthesia*. 8th ed. Churchill Livingstone; 2015: Table 34.8.

| TABLE 53.2 Clinical Autonomic Effects of Nondepolarizing Neuromuscular Blocking Agents | | | |
|---|---|---|---|
| Drug | Autonomic Ganglia | Cardiac Muscarinic Receptors | Histamine Release |
| **BENZYLISOQUINOLINIUM COMPOUNDS** | | | |
| Mivacurium | None | None | Slight |
| Atracurium | None | None | Slight |
| Cisatracurium | None | None | None |
| d-Tubocurarine* | Blocks | None | Moderate |
| **AMINOSTEROIDAL COMPOUNDS** | | | |
| Vecuronium | None | None | None |
| Rocuronium | None | Blocks weakly | None |
| Pancuronium | None | Blocks moderately | None |

*No longer available.
Reproduced, with permission, from Naguib M, Lien CA, Meistelman C. Pharmacology of muscle relaxants and their antagonists. In: Miller RD, Eriksson LI, Fleisher LA, et al, eds. *Miller's Anesthesia*. 8th ed. Churchill Livingstone; 2015:958–994. Table 34.9.

## Allergic Reactions

Although the development of anaphylaxis during anesthesia is rare, NMBAs are frequently implicated in such reactions. If a patient has reacted to one nondepolarizing NMBA, there is a significant risk of cross-reactivity to other NMBAs. The reactions are mediated through immunoglobulin E (IgE). NMBAs were the most common causative agents in reports from Europe and Australia. The quaternary ammonium ions found in nondepolarizing NMBAs may cross-react with other medications and other environmental factors (e.g., food, cosmetics). Interestingly, pholcodine, a morphine analog commonly used as an antitussive in several European countries and Australia, sensitizes patients to develop IgE-mediated allergic reactions to NMBAs. The availability of pholcodine (it is not approved in the United States or Canada) likely explains the geographic variation in reported rates of anaphylaxis to NMBAs. Countries that have since banned the use of pholcodine have seen a decrease in rates of NMBA-related anaphylaxis.

## Other Nonrelaxant Side Effects of Nondepolarizing Neuromuscular Blocking Agents

### TERATOGENICITY AND CARCINOGENICITY

NMBAs are highly ionized, but they and their metabolites are able to cross the placenta in small amounts. Nonetheless, at clinically relevant doses, human teratogenic effects—if they exist—are unproved. There are no data in the literature on carcinogenic effects of NMBAs.

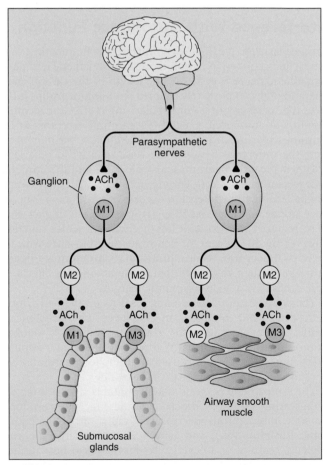

**Fig. 53.1** The muscarinic M3 receptors are located postsynaptically on airway smooth muscle. Acetylcholine *(ACh)* stimulates M3 receptors to cause contraction. M2 muscarinic receptors are located presynaptically at the postganglionic parasympathetic nerve endings, and they function in a negative feedback mechanism to limit the release of ACh. (From Naguib M, Lien CA, Meistelman C. Pharmacology of muscle relaxants and their antagonists. In: Miller RD, Eriksson LI, Fleisher LA, et al., eds. *Miller's Anesthesia*. 8th ed. Churchill Livingstone; 2015: 958–994. Fig. 34.8.)

## CRITICAL ILLNESS POLYMYONEUROPATHY

Medium-term and long-term administration of infusions of nondepolarizing NMBAs—especially those that are steroid based—in critically ill patients can lead to profound weakness, requiring prolonged periods of rehabilitation. Such weakness can occur in patients with multiorgan failure, even in the absence of NMBA use, but weakness is more likely to occur when continuous infusions of nondepolarizing NMBAs are used.

## TOXIC METABOLITES

Laudanosine is a metabolite of atracurium that causes central nervous system stimulation and possibly seizures in high concentrations. Typically administered doses of atracurium and cisatracurium, however, do not cause such problems.

## DRUG INTERACTIONS

Pancuronium inhibits butyrylcholinesterase and leads to extremely prolonged action of mivacurium.

## SUGAMMADEX

Sugammadex initially met resistance in the marketplace because of concerns for hypersensitivity reactions. Subsequent studies in healthy volunteers have demonstrated the incidence of anaphylaxis only at high doses (i.e., 16 mg/kg), with a frequency of less than 1%. Allergic reactions ranging from isolated urticarial rash to anaphylaxis have been reported in patients without prior sensitization to cyclodextrins, suggesting a non-immune phenomenon or a cross-reaction with immunoglobulins associated with unrelated chemical compounds. The most common adverse events associated with sugammadex are nausea, vomiting, pain, hypotension, and headache. In healthy volunteers, activated partial thromboplastin time and international normalized ratio were increased by up to 25% after administration of 16 mg/kg sugammadex; however, there appears to be no clinical evidence of significant coagulopathy. Because of its steroid-binding capabilities, nonhormonal contraception should be used for 7 days after administration of sugammadex because of the potential reduction of free circulating hormonal contraception.

## SUGGESTED READINGS

Carron, M., Zarantonello, F., Tellaroli, P., & Ori, C. (2016). Efficacy and safety of sugammadex compared to neostigmine for reversal of neuromuscular blockade: A meta-analysis of randomized controlled trials. *Journal of Clinical Anesthesia, 35*, 1–12.

Chapter 11. Neuromuscular blocking agents. (2013). In J. F., IV. Butterworth, D. C. Mackey, & J. D. Wasnick (Eds.), *Morgan & Mikhail's clinical anesthesiology* (5th ed.). McGraw Hill. Retrieved from https://accessmedicine.mhmedical.com/content. aspx?bookid=564&sectionid=42800542. Accessed January 26, 2022.

Chapter 27. Pharmacology of neuromuscular blocking drugs. (2020). In: S. J. Brull & C. Meistelman (Eds.), *Miller's Anesthesia.* Elsevier.

Gurrieri, C., Weingarten, T. N., Martin, D. P., Babovic, N., Narr, B. J., Sprung, J., et al. (2011). Allergic reactions during anesthesia at a large United States referral center. *Anesthesia & Analgesia, 113*, 1202–1212.

Kampe, S., Krombach, J. W., & Diefenbach, C. (2003). Muscle relaxants. *Best Practice Research in Clinical Anaesthesiology, 17*, 137–146.

Mertes, P. M., Laxenaire, M. C., & Alla, F. (2003). Anaphylactic and anaphylactoid reactions occurring during anesthesia in 1999-2000. *Anesthesiology, 99*, 536–545.

Stoelting, R. K., & Hillier, S. C. (2006). Neuromuscular blocking drugs. In R. K. Stoelting & S. C. Hillier (Eds.), *Pharmacology and physiology in anesthetic practice* (4th ed., pp. 208–250). Philadelphia: Lippincott Williams & Wilkins.

# 54

# Antagonism of Neuromuscular Block

J. ROSS RENEW, MD  |  WAYNE T. NICHOLSON, MD, PharmD  |
SORIN J. BRULL, MD, FCARCSI (Hon)

## Acetylcholinesterase Inhibitors

Neostigmine is the classic neuromuscular blockade antagonist. It acts indirectly through inhibition of the acetylcholinesterase (AChE) enzyme, which normally metabolizes acetylcholine (ACh) into choline and acetate. AChE is one of the most efficient enzymes known; a single molecule has the capacity to hydrolyze 25,000 molecules of ACh per second. When the enzyme is inhibited, the concentration of ACh in the neuromuscular junctional cleft is increased, allowing ACh to compete for ACh receptor sites from which neuromuscular blocking agents (NMBAs) have dissociated (Fig. 54.1).

The active center of the AChE molecule consists of a negatively charged subsite that attracts the quaternary group of

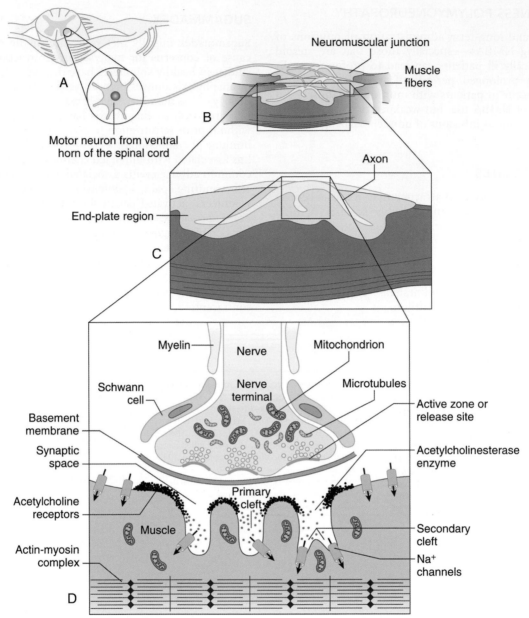

**Fig. 54.1** Structure of the adult neuromuscular junction shows the three cells that constitute the synapse: the motor neuron (i.e., nerve terminal), muscle fiber, and Schwann cell. **A,** The motor nerve originates in the ventral horn of the spinal cord or brainstem. **B,** As the nerve approaches its muscle fibers and before attaching itself to the surface of the muscle fiber, the nerve divides into branches that innervate many individual muscle fibers. **C,** Each muscle receives only one synapse. The motor nerve loses its myelin and further subdivides into many presynaptic boutons to terminate on the surface of the muscle fiber. **D,** The nerve terminal, covered by Schwann cells, has vesicles clustered about the membrane thickenings, which are the active zones, toward its synaptic side and mitochondria and microtubules toward its other side. A synaptic gutter or cleft, made up of a primary and many secondary clefts, separates the nerve from the muscle. The muscle surface is corrugated, and dense areas on the shoulders of each fold contain acetylcholine receptors. Sodium (Na⁺) channels are present at the bottom of the clefts and throughout the muscle membrane. The acetylcholinesterase and proteins and proteoglycans that stabilize the neuromuscular junction are present in the synaptic clefts. (From Jeevendra Martyn JA, Jonsson Fagerlund M. Neuromuscular physiology and pharmacology. In: Gropper MA, ed. *Miller's Anesthesia.* 9th ed. Elsevier; 2020. Fig. 12.1.)

choline through ionic forces, as well as an esteratic subsite, where nucleophilic attack occurs. Neostigmine binds to the AChE enzyme through formation of a covalent bond of a carbamoyl-ester complex at the esteratic site of the enzyme.

Neostigmine is a quaternary ammonium ion. It is poorly lipid soluble and does not effectively penetrate lipid cell-membrane barriers, such as the gastrointestinal tract or the blood-brain barrier. Neostigmine has very large volumes of distribution because of extensive tissue storage in organs such as the liver and kidneys. Renal excretion accounts for approximately 50% of the elimination of neostigmine, and its elimination half-life is 76 min. The prolongation of its elimination half-life by renal failure is similar to that affecting clearance of most NMBAs.

Although the nicotinic effects produced by the increased amounts of available ACh are desirable for reversing neuromuscular blockade, the muscarinic effects of the ACh on the gastrointestinal, pulmonary, and cardiovascular systems can be problematic. The predominant effect on the heart is bradycardia as a result of slowed conduction velocity of the cardiac impulse through the atrioventricular node. The prolongation of QTc interval in the ECG may induce ventricular arrhythmias. Hypotension may result from decreases in peripheral vascular resistance. Cholinesterase inhibitors enhance the secretion of gastric fluid and increase the motility of the entire gastrointestinal tract, probably caused by accumulated ACh at the ganglion cells of the Auerbach plexus and its effects on smooth muscle cells. However, a causal relationship between neostigmine administration and postoperative nausea and vomiting has not been confirmed. Bronchial, lacrimal, salivary, gastric, and sweat gland secretion is also increased.

To counteract these muscarinic effects, anticholinergic drugs such as atropine or glycopyrrolate are coadministered. Because of its more rapid onset of action, atropine is usually given 30 to 60 seconds after administration of neostigmine, whereas neostigmine is usually administered together with glycopyrrolate. These drugs also have side effects that need to be considered, especially atropine. Atropine is a tertiary amine, and it can cross the blood-brain barrier; in excessive doses, it can cause central anticholinergic toxicity, especially in the elderly. The typical signs include agitation, confusion, disorientation, and hallucinations, as well as dry mouth; warm, dry skin; tachycardia; and visual disturbances. Because atropine is faster in onset and more likely to cause tachyarrhythmias, which can be disadvantageous in patients with coronary artery disease, many anesthesiologists consider glycopyrrolate, with its more gradual onset of action, the better option for antagonizing the muscarinic side effects of anticholinesterases.

Large international surveys have shown that many anesthesiologists prefer not to use anticholinesterases at the end of surgery to avoid their side effects. However, residual neuromuscular blockade may pose a significant risk to patients. Respiratory insufficiency, oxygen desaturation, upper airway collapse and loss of airway patency, aspiration pneumonia, the need for emergent reintubation, and patient discomfort are well-recognized complications of residual neuromuscular blockade; the incidence of such complications can be as high as 82% when antagonists are omitted.

Factors that may delay or inhibit antagonism of neuromuscular blockade (and may therefore increase the incidence of postoperative residual neuromuscular block) include residual inhalational agent, hypothermia, respiratory acidosis (hypercarbia), the use of certain antibiotics (e.g., aminoglycosides) or opioids, hypokalemia, hypocalcemia, and hypermagnesemia. The time required to antagonize neuromuscular blockade depends on several factors: (1) the depth of block; (2) the pharmacokinetics and pharmacodynamics of the NMBA; (3) the specific antagonist used; (4) the dose of the antagonist; and (5) the type of anesthetic agents used (inhalational volatile vs. total intravenous technique). Inhalational anesthetics prolong both spontaneous recovery times and neostigmine-induced reversal of neuromuscular blockade (desflurane > sevoflurane > isoflurane > halothane > nitrous oxide).

In deep neuromuscular block, even large doses of cholinesterase inhibitors and total inhibition of the AChE enzyme are insufficient to spare enough molecules of ACh from breakdown (ceiling effect) to compete with the NMBA molecules that are still present at the neuromuscular junction. In previous studies, the time required for 70 µg/kg neostigmine to antagonize deep (Table 54.1) vecuronium or rocuronium neuromuscular block (50 min on average) was clinically comparable to spontaneous recovery times. Therefore cholinesterase inhibitors are ineffective and should not be used to antagonize neuromuscular blocks deeper than train-of-four (TOF) count 1 (Table 54.1).

In the deeper ranges of moderate neuromuscular blockade (TOF count 1–2), the effectiveness of cholinesterase inhibitors is still questionable. For this reason, their routine administration is not recommended. From the return of the third twitch of TOF stimulation (TOF count 3 and, preferably, TOF count 4), the recommended dose of neostigmine is 50 µg/kg. The dose of 70 µg/kg neostigmine (up to a maximal total dose of 5 mg) to reverse moderate neuromuscular blockade has not been conclusively shown to increase the efficacy or speed of reversal, but it can increase the likelihood of adverse events, and should no longer be used. Neostigmine can only effectively reverse shallow (from TOF count 4 to TOF ratio <0.4) and minimal levels of neuromuscular blockade (TOF ratio ≥0.4). The standard recommended dose of neostigmine for shallow block is 30 to 50 µg/kg. For minimal neuromuscular block (TOF ratio >0.4), a reduction in neostigmine dose (10–30 µg/kg neostigmine) is reasonable.

| TABLE 54.1 | Suggested Definitions of Depth (Level) of Neuromuscular Block and Recommended Reversal Regimens | | | |
|---|---|---|---|---|
| Level of Block | Depth of Block | Quantitative (Objective) Measurement at the Adductor Pollicis (Thumb) Muscle | Recommended Sugammadex Dose | Recommended Neostigmine Dose |
| Level 5 | Complete block | PTC = 0 | 16 mg/kg | Not recommended |
| Level 4 | Deep block | PTC ≥1 | 4–8[†] mg/kg | Not recommended |
| Level 3 | Moderate block | TOFC = 1–3 | 2 mg/kg | 50 µg/kg* |
| Level 2b | Shallow block | TOFR <0.4 | 1–2 mg/kg[†] | 30–50 µg/kg |
| Level 2a | Minimal block | TOFR = 0.4–0.9 | 0.22–1 mg/kg[†] | 10–30 µg/kg |
| Level 1 | Acceptable recovery | TOFR ≥0.9 | None | None |

*Reversal with neostigmine is recommended when TOFC ≥3.
[†]These doses are outside of the doses recommended in the package insert.
*PTC*, Posttetanic count; *TOFC*, train-of-four count; *TOFR*, train-of-four ratio.
Adapted from Naguib M, Brull SJ, Kopman AF, et al. Consensus statement on perioperative use of neuromuscular monitoring. *Anesth Analg.* 2018;127:71–80.

The anticholinesterase onset of action shows wide interindividual variability at every depth of neuromuscular blockade. Therefore it is recommended to allow neostigmine sufficient time to exert its action, realizing that the average duration needed for recovery from a TOF count 3 is 16 min (with a range of 7–44 min), and the recovery duration from TOF count 4 requires 10 min (range, 5–26 min). To avoid occurrence of residual weakness in slow responders (outliers), quantitative monitoring of neuromuscular function is strongly recommended. Antagonism with neostigmine in the *absence* of quantitative neuromuscular monitoring cannot reliably prevent postoperative residual neuromuscular blockade. Additionally, inappropriate use of neostigmine can further increase the prevalence of residual weakness.

Previous data showed that anticholinesterases themselves may induce genioglossus dysfunction by directly binding to nicotinic ACh receptors. For this reason, many anesthesiologists may be reluctant to administer anticholinesterases at the end of surgery to reverse shallow block. However, clinical data in this setting are contradictory because neostigmine-induced neuromuscular weakness has been reported in volunteers and patients who had not received NMBAs. On the other hand, the clinical significance of neostigmine-induced muscle weakness when antagonizing nondepolarizing neuromuscular block is questionable. Therefore routine administration of antagonists based on the depth of block is advocated unless spontaneous recovery to a TOF ratio ≥0.9 can be documented at the adductor pollicis muscle with a quantitative (objective) neuromuscular monitor.

## Sugammadex

Sugammadex is a modified γ-cyclodextrin designed to encapsulate aminosteroidal NMBA molecules. It provides fast and reliable reversal of these drugs. However, it cannot reverse the neuromuscular blockade induced by benzylisoquinolinium NMBAs or succinylcholine. The center of the ring-shaped molecule is hydrophobic, whereas the periphery is hydrophilic because of the eight side chains that are attached to the original γ-cyclodextrin molecule. Each side chain has a negatively charged carboxyl group that attracts the positively charged nitrogen ions of the aminosteroidal NMBA molecules, and the hydrophobic core encapsulates the body of the NMBA molecule. Sugammadex exerts its action in the plasma, where it forms a 1-to-1 complex with steroidal NMBA molecules. As the concentration of free NMBA molecules decreases in the plasma, free NMBA molecules leave the neuromuscular junction and move along their concentration gradient to the bloodstream, where they are encapsulated by the remaining available free sugammadex molecules.

Sugammadex was originally designed to reverse rocuronium blockade, but it has a higher affinity for pipecuronium and a lower affinity for vecuronium and pancuronium molecules. Sugammadex has an association constant that is 3.1 times lower for vecuronium than for rocuronium. Therefore reversal of vecuronium-induced blockade by sugammadex may take longer than reversal of rocuronium-induced blockade. The lower affinity for vecuronium, however, is partly offset by the greater potency of vecuronium compared with rocuronium, which leads to administration of fewer molecules of vecuronium than of rocuronium (at equivalent doses). Nonetheless, sugammadex can reverse vecuronium-induced blockade faster, more reliably, and from a deeper neuromuscular block than neostigmine.

Sugammadex is highly water soluble, and its volume of distribution approximates the extracellular fluid volume. Therefore many advocate that the dose of sugammadex be based on the actual body weight for morbidly obese patients, or at least basing the dose on ideal body weight +40%. Regardless of the dosing regimen in this at-risk population, quantitative monitoring is recommended to confirm recovery before tracheal extubation.

Sugammadex is weakly metabolized, and the sugammadex-NMBA complex is excreted unchanged almost exclusively via urine. The elimination half-life is approximately 100 minutes; therefore the majority of the complexes are excreted from the body in 8 h (assuming normal renal function). Kidney failure slightly prolongs antagonism times, and sugammadex is currently not approved for patients with end-stage renal disease. If needed, sugammadex and the sugammadex-rocuronium complex can be removed via high-flux dialysis.

Sugammadex does not influence ACh concentrations; therefore it is free of the muscarinic side effects of cholinesterase inhibitors. Early reports raised questions about potential arrhythmogenic properties, but later data did not confirm this finding. In a recent metaanalysis, sugammadex proved superior to neostigmine because it reversed the neuromuscular block faster and more reliably, with fewer adverse events. Better respiratory outcomes and higher patient satisfaction were also described in sugammadex-neostigmine comparative investigations.

Unlike cholinesterase inhibitors, sugammadex reversal is not influenced by the type of anesthesia. It is equally effective after propofol-opioid (total intravenous anesthesia) or inhalation anesthetic agents.

Sugammadex has a well-defined dosing scheme to antagonize rocuronium (and vecuronium) blockade, based on the level of neuromuscular blockade (see Table 54.1). Although anticholinesterases are contraindicated in the reversal of profound and deep neuromuscular block, sugammadex can rapidly (within 2–5 min) and reliably reverse all depths of neuromuscular blockade induced by rocuronium without major side effects. Sugammadex can be used to emergently rescue from "can't-intubate-can't-ventilate" (CICV) rapid-sequence induction situations by administering a large dose (16 mg/kg), as long as other coadministered anesthetic agents (propofol, benzodiazepines, opioids) do not prevent spontaneous ventilation. The rocuronium reversal time in this scenario is faster with sugammadex than the spontaneous recovery from succinylcholine block. However, pharmacologic reversal of neuromuscular blockade with sugammadex cannot reliably prevent hypoxic events in the CICV scenario, and appropriate interventions focusing on airway patency, oxygenation, and ventilation are still paramount. During deep neuromuscular blockade (TOF count 0, posttetanic count ≥1), treatment with 4 to 8 mg/kg sugammadex is recommended (outside the manufacturer's recommendations); after return of the first twitch to TOF stimulation (TOF count 1), a dose of 2 mg/kg sugammadex is required for antagonism (see Table 54.1). According to currently available evidence, during shallow (TOF count ≥4) and minimal (TOFR >0.40) neuromuscular block, further dose reductions (≤2 mg/kg) have been reported to be effective.

It must be emphasized that the use of sugammadex does not reliably prevent residual weakness unless the appropriate dose is chosen based on the depth of neuromuscular block assessed objectively. Quantitative monitoring should be used to guide appropriate timing and dosing of sugammadex and to confirm adequate recovery before tracheal extubation.

In addition to aminosteroid NMBAs, sugammadex binds other drugs. As a result of its interaction with hormonal-based contraceptives, patients who are using such medications should use alternative means of contraception for a week after sugammadex exposure. This is particularly important in post-menarchal adolescents, because recent data suggest that 40% of pediatric anesthesiologists use sugammadex as their primary reversal agent. Furthermore, it is advised to postpone flucloxacillin administration for 6 h after sugammadex administration to preserve its action.

In laboratory and clinical studies, sugammadex caused a transient prolongation of activated partial thromboplastin time and prothrombin time; however, no clinically significant increases in bleeding have been observed.

The introduction of sugammadex to the U.S. market was delayed by the U.S. Food and Drug Administration (FDA) because of concerns with hypersensitivity and anaphylaxis. A recent large-scale Japanese database analysis estimated the prevalence of sugammadex anaphylaxis as 0.039%, which approximates the prevalence of succinylcholine and rocuronium anaphylaxis (0.048% and 0.04%, respectively). Most case reports describe immunoglobulin-E–mediated anaphylaxis after a patient's initial exposure to sugammadex. It is theorized that this reaction occurs as patients are sensitized via exposure to cyclodextrins that are used as preservatives in food, cosmetics, and other medications. In most cases, anaphylaxis occurs within 5 min after sugammadex administration and results in profound hypotension, tachycardia, and rash. Although anaphylaxis is not dose dependent, it has been described more frequently after administration of 16 mg/kg sugammadex. Anaphylactic reactions should be treated aggressively with epinephrine and intravenous fluids.

The sugammadex-aminosteroid complex is excreted by the kidney; therefore renal impairment will alter its distribution. For patients with mild or moderate renal impairment, the usual recommended dose for the given situation should be administered. Although sugammadex will result in effective reversal, it is not currently recommended by the manufacturer for use in severe renal impairment (creatinine clearance <30 mL/min) or for patients requiring dialysis. Recent data in patients with end-stage renal disease, however, suggest that sugammadex may be considered as an alternative antagonist in this patient population.

In geriatric patients without severe renal impairment, the usual adult dose should be administered; however, recovery times may be longer. Because all doses are currently based on actual body weight, the amount required and available for use should be considered in obese patients. Sugammadex has recently been approved by the FDA for use in pediatric patients (>2 years old).

## SUGGESTED READINGS

Asztalos, L., Szabó-Maák, Z., Gajdos, A., Nemes, R., Pongrácz, A., Lengyel, S., et al. (2017). Reversal of vecuronium-induced neuromuscular blockade with low-dose sugammadex at train-of-four count of four: A randomized controlled trial. *Anesthesiology*, *127*, 441–449.

Bronsert, M. R., Henderson, W. G., Monk, T. G., Richman, J. S., Nguyen, J. D., Sum-Ping, J. T., et al. (2017). Intermediate-acting nondepolarizing neuromuscular blocking agents and risk of postoperative 30-day morbidity and mortality, and long-term survival. *Anesthesia and Analgesia*, *124*, 1476–1483.

Brull, S. J., & Kopman, A. F. (2017). Current status of neuromuscular reversal and monitoring. *Anesthesiology*, *126*, 173–190.

Brull, S. J., & Murphy, G. S. (2010). Residual neuromuscular block: Lessons unlearned. Part II: Methods to reduce the risk of residual weakness. *Anesthesia and Analgesia*, *111*, 129–140.

Herbstreit, F., Zigrahn, D., Ochterbeck, C., Peters, J., & Eikermann, M. (2010). Neostigmine/glycopyrrolate administered after recovery from neuromuscular block increases upper airway collapsibility by decreasing genioglossus muscle activity in response to negative pharyngeal pressure. *Anesthesiology*, *113*, 1280–1288.

Hristovska, A. M., Duch, P., Allingstrup, M., & Afshari, A. (2017). Efficacy and safety of sugammadex versus neostigmine in reversing neuromuscular blockade in adults. *Cochrane Database of Systematic Reviews*, *8*(8), CD012763.

Murphy, G. S., & Brull, S. J. (2022). Quantitative neuromuscular monitoring and postoperative outcomes: A narrative review. *Anesthesiology*, *136*, 345–361.

Murphy, G. S., & Brull, S. J. (2010). Residual neuromuscular block: Lessons unlearned. Part I: Definitions, incidence, and adverse physiologic effects of residual neuromuscular block. *Anesthesia and Analgesia*, *111*, 120–128.

Murphy, G. S., Szokol, J. W., Avram, M. J., Greenberg, S. B., Shear, T. D., Deshur, M. A., et al. (2018). Neostigmine administration after spontaneous recovery to a train-of-four ratio of 0.9 to 1.0: A randomized controlled trial of the effect on neuromuscular and clinical recovery. *Anesthesiology*, *128*, 27–37.

Paredes, S., Porter, S. B., Porter, I. E. II., & Renew, J. R. (2020). Sugammadex use in patients with end-stage renal disease: A historical cohort study. *Canadian Journal of Anaesthesia*, *67*(12), 1789–1797.

# 55

# Pharmacology of Atropine, Scopolamine, and Glycopyrrolate

NATHAN J. SMISCHNEY, MD, MSc

## Atropine

Atropine is a naturally occurring tertiary amine that is capable of inhibiting the activation of muscarinic receptors. These receptors are found primarily on autonomic effector cells that are innervated by postganglionic parasympathetic nerves but are also present in ganglia and on some cells. At usual doses of the drug, the principal effect of atropine is competitive antagonism of cholinergic stimuli at muscarinic receptors, with little or no effect at nicotinic receptors.

Atropine is derived from flowering plants in the family Solanaceae (e.g., deadly nightshade [*Atropa belladonna*, named for Atropos, the Fate of Greek mythology who cuts the thread of life], mandrake [*Mandragora officinarum*], or jimsonweed [*Datura stramonium*]). Venetian women dropped the juice of deadly nightshade into their eyes to produce mydriasis, which was thought to enhance beauty (hence the name *belladonna*, which, translated from Italian, is *beautiful woman*). Although atropine is used today to treat pesticide poisoning, Solanaceae plants have been used since AD 200 as biologic weapons to poison liquids for drinking (e.g., water, wine).

## PHARMACOKINETICS

### Absorption

After intravenous administration, onset of action is approximately 30 seconds with peak effect in 1 to 2 minutes. Atropine is well absorbed from the gastrointestinal tract (i.e., from the upper small intestine). It is also well absorbed after intramuscular administration or from the tracheobronchial tree after inhalation.

### Distribution

Atropine undergoes rapid distribution throughout the body and 50% is plasma protein bound. Atropine crosses the blood-brain barrier and the placenta.

### Elimination

The plasma half-life of atropine is 2 to 3 h; it is metabolized in the liver, with 30% to 50% of the drug excreted unchanged in the urine.

## PHARMACOLOGIC PROPERTIES

### Gastrointestinal System

Atropine reduces the volume of saliva and gastric secretions. The motility of the entire gastrointestinal tract, from esophagus to colon, is decreased, prolonging transit time. Atropine causes lower esophageal sphincter relaxation through an antimuscarinic mechanism.

### Cardiovascular System

The effect of atropine on the heart is dose dependent. An intravenously administered dose of 0.4 to 0.6 mg causes a transient decrease in heart rate of approximately 8 beats/min. This decrease was once believed to be caused by central vagal stimulation. However, the mechanism is not fully elucidated. Larger doses of atropine cause progressively increasing tachycardia by blocking vagal effects on $M_2$ receptors on the sinoatrial node; by the same mechanism, atropine can reverse sinus bradycardia secondary to extracardiac causes, but it has little or no effect on sinus bradycardia caused by intrinsic disease of the sinoatrial node. High doses (>3 mg) may cause cutaneous vasodilation.

### Respiratory System

Atropine reduces the volume of secretions from the nose, mouth, pharynx, and bronchi. Along with many other anticholinergic drugs (e.g., ipratropium), it relaxes the smooth muscles of the bronchi and bronchioles, with resultant decreases in airway resistance.

### Central Nervous System

Atropine is one of the few anticholinergic agents to cross the blood-brain barrier, stimulating the medulla and higher cerebral centers. Higher doses are associated with restlessness, irritability, disorientation, and delirium. Even higher doses produce hallucinations and coma. This constellation of symptoms and signs, called *central anticholinergic syndrome*, can be treated with physostigmine.

### Genitourinary System

Atropine decreases the tone and amplitude of ureter and bladder contractions, which is one of the reasons why belladonna and opium suppositories are administered to patients who have bladder spasms in response to a urinary catheter. The relaxation effect is more pronounced in neurogenic bladders. Bladder capacity is increased, and incontinence is relieved as uninhibited contractions are reduced. The renal pelves, calyces, and ureters are dilated.

### Ophthalmic Response

Atropine blocks responses of the sphincter muscle of the iris and the accommodative muscle of the ciliary body of the lens to cholinergic stimulation, resulting in mydriasis (pupil dilation) and cycloplegia (paralysis of lens accommodation). It usually has little effect on intraocular pressure except in patients with angle-closure glaucoma, in whom intraocular pressure may increase.

# Scopolamine

Scopolamine, another belladonna alkaloid, sometimes referred to as *hyoscine*, has stronger antisalivary actions and much more potent central nervous system effects than does atropine (Table 55.1). It is a strong amnesic that usually also produces sedation. Restlessness and delirium are not unusual and can make patients difficult to manage. Elderly patients who take scopolamine are at risk for incurring injury from falls when unsupervised. Scopolamine produces less cardiac acceleration than atropine, and both drugs can produce paradoxical bradycardia when used in low doses, possibly through a weak peripheral cholinergic agonist effect.

The scopolamine patch has several uses in clinical medicine. The most common are prophylaxis for postoperative nausea and vomiting, prophylaxis for excessive salvation, increased intestinal motility, amnesia as part of anesthetic induction, mania, prophylaxis for motion sickness, postencephalitic parkinsonism, preoperative sedation, spasticity, vomiting, and uveitis/iridocyclitis. The proposed mechanism for motion sickness is a disturbance in the balance between the cholinergic and adrenergic systems in the central nervous system. Because the vomiting center is activated by stimulation of cholinergic receptors in the vestibular nuclei and reticular formation neurons by impulses transmitted in response to vestibular stimulation, drugs that inhibit the cholinergic system have been proved effective in preventing motion sickness and are occasionally used to prevent or treat postoperative nausea and vomiting.

Each transdermal scopolamine patch contains 1.5 mg scopolamine base and is formulated to deliver in vivo approximately 1 mg scopolamine over 3 days. The patch is applied to the skin of the postauricular area for 3 days. It is important to wash the hands after handling the patch because blurry vision may occur as a result of a temporary increase in the size of the pupil. Because of the anticholinergic effects of scopolamine, the elderly and patients with hepatic and/or renal impairment have an increased likelihood of central nervous system effects. Urinary retention may occur, especially in the elderly and patients with urinary bladder neck obstruction.

Adverse effects of the scopolamine patch include bradyarrhythmia, hypotension, tachycardia, rash, xerostomia, confusion, dizziness, memory impairment, meningism, restlessness, somnolence, anisocoria, blurred vision, conjunctivitis, dry eye syndrome, glaucoma, eye itching, mydriasis, hallucinations, psychotic disorder, dysuria, and signs and symptoms of withdrawal. Scopolamine is no longer available in intravenous or intramuscular form.

# Glycopyrrolate

Glycopyrrolate is a synthetic antimuscarinic with a quaternary ammonium that has anticholinergic properties similar to those of atropine (see Table 55.1); however, unlike atropine, glycopyrrolate is completely ionized at physiologic pH.

## PHARMACOKINETICS

### Absorption

With intravenous injection, the typical onset of action of glycopyrrolate occurs within 1 min; with intramuscular administration, it is approximately 15 to 30 min, with peak effects occurring within approximately 30 to 45 min. Compared with atropine and scopolamine, glycopyrrolate is a more potent antisialagogue (effects persisting for up to 7 h) and has a longer duration of action (vagal blocking effects persist for 2–3 h).

### Distribution

The in vivo metabolism of glycopyrrolate in humans has not been studied.

### Elimination

After intravenous administration, the mean half-life of glycopyrrolate is 45 to 60 min, and after intramuscular administration, it is 30 to 75 min.

## PHARMACOLOGIC PROPERTIES

### Gastrointestinal System

Glycopyrrolate completely inhibits gastrointestinal motility but does not change gastric pH or the volume of gastric secretions.

### Cardiovascular System

Although not as potent as atropine on the cardiovascular system, glycopyrrolate administered at 0.1 mg intravenously, repeated every 2 to 3 minutes, can be used during surgery to counteract drug-induced or vagal reflexes and their associated bradycardia. This effect is more prolonged than that of atropine even though less potent.

### Central Nervous System

The structure of glycopyrrolate prevents it from crossing lipid barriers; therefore, unlike atropine and scopolamine, glycopyrrolate does not cross the blood-brain barrier, and the resultant effects on the central nervous system are limited.

| TABLE 55.1 | Duration of Action and Effects of Atropine, Scopolamine, and Glycopyrrolate | | | | | | |
|---|---|---|---|---|---|---|---|
| | **DURATION** | | | **EFFECT** | | | |
| Drug | IV | IM | CNS | GI Tone | Antisialagogue | HR | |
| Atropine | 5–30 min | 2–4 h | Stimulation | − − | + | + + +* | |
| Scopolamine | 0.5–1 h | 4–6 h | Sedation† | − | + + + | 0/+* | |
| Glycopyrrolate | 2–4 h | 6–8 h | None | − − − | + + + + | + | |

*May decelerate initially.
†CNS effects often manifest as sedation before stimulation.
*CNS*, Central nervous system; *GI*, gastrointestinal; *HR*, heart rate; *IM*, intramuscular; *IV*, intravenous.
Adapted with permission from Lawson NW, Meyer J. Autonomic nervous system physiology and pharmacology. In: Barash PG, Cullen BF, Stoelting RF, eds. *Clinical Anesthesia*. 3rd ed. Lippincott Williams & Wilkins; 1997:243–327.

## SUGGESTED READINGS

Renner, U. D., Oertel, R., & Kirch, W. (2005). Pharmacokinetics and pharmacodynamics in clinical use of scopolamine. *Therapeutic Drug Monitoring, 27,* 655–665.

Simpson, K. H., Smith, R. J., & Davies, L. F. (1987). Comparison of the effects of atropine and glycopyrrolate on cognitive function following general anaesthesia. *British Journal of Anaesthesia, 59,* 966–969.

Stoelting, R. K., & Hillerm, S. C. (2005). *Pharmacology and physiology in anesthetic practice* (4th ed.). Philadelphia: Lippincott Williams & Wilkins.

Takizawa, E., Takizawa, D., Al-Jahdari, W. S., Miyazaki, M., Nakamura, K., Yamamoto, K., et al. (2006). Influence of atropine on the dose requirements of propofol in humans. *Drug Metabolism and Pharmacokinetics, 21,* 384–388.

# 56

# Benzodiazepines

## TROY G. SEELHAMMER, MD

Benzodiazepines bind to the extracellular site at the interface of the alpha and gamma γ-aminobutyric acid type A (GABA$_A$) receptor to modulate the activity of the brain's major inhibitory neurotransmitter, GABA. The benzodiazepinergic enhancement of the inhibitory effect of GABA on neuronal excitability is the result of increased neuronal membrane permeability to chloride ions, leading to hyperpolarization and a less excitable neuronal state. Distinct mechanisms of action contribute to the sedative-hypnotic, anxiolytic, anterograde amnestic, and anticonvulsant effects of these drugs, although virtually all effects are mediated by binding to specific subunits of the GABA$_A$

receptor at the level of the central nervous system (CNS) (Fig. 56.1). The low aqueous solubility of most benzodiazepines means that intravenous formulations are problematic. Despite this, intravenous formulations of several benzodiazepines have been developed for procedural sedation and anesthesia. All benzodiazepines possess sedative-hypnotic properties and have displaced barbiturates for this purpose, primarily because of their remarkably low capacity to produce fatal CNS depression. Compared with barbiturates and volatile anesthetics, benzodiazepines do not produce the same degree of neuronal depression. Increasing doses progress from sedation to hypnosis to

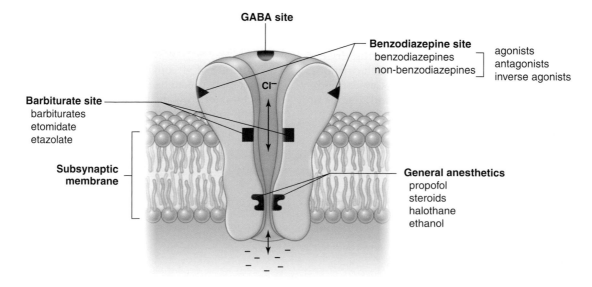

**Fig. 56.1**   Functional binding sites on the γ-aminobutyric acid receptor. (Adapted from the PACT Sedation Module European Society of Intensive Care Medicine, www.esicm.org.)

| TABLE 56.1 | **Commonly Used Benzodiazepines** | | | | |
|---|---|---|---|---|---|
| **Drug** | **Route(s)** | **Common Use(s)** | | **Comments** | **Half-Life** |
| Remimazolam | IV | Procedural sedation | | Ultrashort clinical duration of action | 18 min |
| Midazolam | Oral, IV, IM | Anesthetic premedication | | Rapid onset | 2.5 h |
| Temazepam | Oral | Insomnia | | Short-term therapy | 8.8 h |
| Alprazolam | Oral | Anxiety | | Withdrawal symptoms may be especially severe | 11.2–16.3 h |
| Lorazepam | Oral, IV, IM | Anxiety; anesthetic premedication, alcohol withdrawal | | Metabolized solely by conjugation | 14 h |
| Clonazepam | Oral | Seizure disorders; adjunctive treatment in acute mania and certain movement disorders | | Tolerance | 20–50 |
| Diazepam | Oral, IV, IM, rectal | Anxiety, status epilepticus, skeletal muscle relaxation; anesthetic premedication | | Decreases metabolism of cytochrome P450–dependent drugs | 30–60 |

*IM,* Intramuscular; *IV,* intravenous.
Modified from Mihic SJ, Harris RA. Hypnotics and sedatives. In: Brunton L, Chabner B, Knollman B, eds. *Goodman & Gilman's The Pharmacological Basis of Therapeutics.* McGraw-Hill Education; 2011.

stupor, but awareness persists (thus falling short of general anesthesia). Most benzodiazepines can be used interchangeably with therapeutic uses of a given agent, depending primarily on onset time and half-life (Table 56.1). Unique in the benzodiazepine drug class, remimazolam relies on ester metabolism (similar to remifentanil) to facilitate an ultrashort context sensitive half-time that facilitates rapid emergence from the sedative-hypnotic effects of the drug.

Benzodiazepines are used to treat insomnia, alcohol withdrawal, and seizures and are frequently used to provide sedation and amnesia in the perioperative setting. Major side effects can include lightheadedness, motor incoordination, confusion, and impairment of motor and mental functions. Benzodiazepine administration as a component of induction of general anesthesia has been associated with longer anesthesia recovery and higher rates of respiratory depression after surgery. Excess dose administration, altered pharmacodynamics, perturbation in pharmacokinetics due to tissue binding or organ dysfunction, and coadministration of respiratory depressants all can potentiate the adverse effects of this class of medications. Benzodiazepines, especially when given by infusion, have consistently been demonstrated to increase the risk of delirium in critically ill patients. Lorazepam has been identified as an independent risk factor for delirium. Midazolam, compared with dexmedetomidine or propofol, results in a higher prevalence of delirium.

## Organ Effects Outside of the Central Nervous System

The effect of benzodiazepines on respiration is generally minimal at hypnotic doses, but care must be taken in the treatment of children and those with impaired hepatic function. At higher doses, these drugs depress alveolar ventilation mediated through the suppression of hypoxic (rather than hypercapnic) drive. When administered in conjunction with opioids, benzodiazepines can cause carbon dioxide narcosis and apnea. Respiratory assistance is typically only required when benzodiazepines are coadministered with another CNS depressant. Obstructive

sleep apnea is a relative contraindication to the administration of benzodiazepines because of exacerbation of decreased muscle tone in the upper airway and an exaggerated effect of apneic episodes on alveolar hypoxia, pulmonary hypertension, and cardiac ventricular load. In clinically used doses, the effects of benzodiazepines on the cardiovascular system are minor, but a mild decrease in blood pressure and a concurrent small increase in heart rate can occur.

## Tolerance, Dependence, and Withdrawal

Tolerance to the anxiolytic effect of benzodiazepines is controversial. Even though most patients who chronically use benzodiazepines report experiencing decreased drowsiness over a few days, they do not convincingly demonstrate a tolerance to the impairment of some measures of psychomotor performance (e.g., visual tracking). On the other hand, tolerance has been demonstrated to the anticonvulsant, neuromuscular blocking, and ataxic effects of benzodiazepines. Dose escalation over time and dependence on benzodiazepines has also been reported. Abrupt discontinuation of benzodiazepines after prolonged administration of high doses may result in symptoms of withdrawal such as dysphoria, irritability, sweating, tremors, unpleasant dreams, and temporary intensification of insomnia or anxiety. Although uncommon in the perioperative setting, patients admitted to the intensive care unit receiving benzodiazepines for greater than 7 days have been reported to exhibit signs of withdrawal.

## Neonatal and Fetal Exposure

The association of benzodiazepines with teratogenic effects remains unclear, with earlier retrospective studies suggesting increased rates of congenital malformations (cleft lip and palate with first-trimester exposure), whereas more recent systematic reviews and metaanalysis of more than one million subjects showed no association with increased risk (including orofacial cleft). Benzodiazepines have been associated with preterm birth (gestational age <37 weeks) and increased risk of spontaneous abortion. Long-term exposure before delivery can cause postnatal toxicity and withdrawal, including low Apgar scores, apnea, hyperreflexia, and irritability.

# Midazolam

Midazolam is a short-acting, water-soluble benzodiazepine with sedative, anxiolytic, amnesic, and anticonvulsant properties. It may be given orally, intravenously, intramuscularly, or intranasally. Because of its rapid and reliable onset of action and short half-life and because it can be administered orally, midazolam is frequently used in the pediatric and adult perioperative setting to provide preoperative anxiolysis, conscious sedation during surgery, and induction or supplementation of general anesthesia. The safety and efficacy of oral midazolam syrup have not been established for patients younger than 6 months.

## PHARMACOLOGY

Midazolam is water soluble, making the addition of propylene glycol unnecessary. It causes virtually no local irritation after injection and can be mixed with other drugs commonly used as premedication agents. Its onset of action is among the fastest in its group (intravenous, 1–5 min; intramuscular, 15 min; oral, 15 min). Midazolam is 1.5 to 2 times as potent as diazepam, with a greater hypnotic effect because of interference with GABA reuptake. Like diazepam, it is highly bound to plasma proteins (95% protein binding). It has a rapid redistribution from the brain to other tissues, and rapid metabolism by the liver accounts for its short duration of action.

## METABOLISM

Midazolam is hydroxylated and conjugated by cytochrome P450 in the liver to two active derivatives that depend on renal excretion, and therefore patients in renal failure have prolonged pharmacodynamic effects. The elimination half-life of midazolam is 1 to 4 h and is prolonged with hepatic insufficiency, congestive heart failure, obesity, and advanced age. As mentioned, the half-life of the metabolites is prolonged in patients with renal failure, with dialysis providing only partial clearance of the parent compound and its active metabolites.

# Effects on Organ Systems

## CARDIOVASCULAR SYSTEM

An intravenously administered dose of 0.2 mg/kg midazolam causes peripheral vasodilation and a subsequent decrease in blood pressure, with an increase in heart rate; fortunately, both effects are mild and transient, but are more pronounced than with diazepam. Hypotension is more common in pediatric patients or patients with hemodynamic instability and is more prominent when the patient also has received opioids because of synergism between the opioids and benzodiazepines.

## RESPIRATORY SYSTEM

Ventilation is depressed by 0.015 mg/kg midazolam, especially in patients with chronic obstructive pulmonary disease. Transient apnea may occur, especially when large doses of midazolam are given in conjunction with opioids.

## CENTRAL NERVOUS SYSTEM

The administration of midazolam results in dose-related decreases in cerebral blood flow and cerebral $O_2$ consumption. As with most benzodiazepines, midazolam may impair either physical or mental abilities or both. Patients should not participate in activities that require mental alertness and rapid physical response time (e.g., driving) for at least 24 h after receiving midazolam.

## PLACENTA

Midazolam crosses the placenta and enters the fetal circulation. Its effects on the fetus are not known; early studies demonstrated a teratogenic risk (orofacial cleft) when midazolam was administered to pregnant patients in the first trimester, with subsequent studies showing no effect.

# Diazepam

Diazepam is a long-acting, medium-potency, water-insoluble benzodiazepine used to treat acute alcohol withdrawal and seizures, provide preoperative anxiolysis, intravenous sedation, skeletal muscle relaxation, and for maintenance of general anesthesia. Anxiolytic effects at low doses are caused by binding to the $GABA_A$ receptor in the limbic system, whereas higher doses cause myorelaxation mediated through receptors in the spinal cord and motor neurons. The safety and efficacy of diazepam in children younger than 2 years of age have not been studied.

## PHARMACOLOGY

Because of its insolubility in water, diazepam is dissolved in propylene glycol and sodium benzoate. The solution may cause pain when injected with an intravenous or intramuscular route, whereas thrombophlebitis occurs much less commonly. Diazepam is taken up rapidly into the brain because of its high lipid solubility and then redistributed extensively to other tissues. Its oral form has absorption of 85% to 100%, making this route more reliable than intramuscular administration. Diazepam is highly protein bound; therefore diseases associated with hypoalbuminemia may increase its effects.

## METABOLISM

Diazepam is metabolized by hepatic microsomal enzymes, producing two main metabolites, desmethyldiazepam and oxazepam. Desmethyldiazepam is slightly less potent than diazepam and is metabolized more slowly, contributing to sustained effects. Elimination half-life ranges from 21 to 37 h in healthy persons, increases progressively with age (approximately 1 h for each year older than 40 years), and increases markedly in the presence of hepatic insufficiency.

# Effects on Organ Systems

## CARDIOVASCULAR SYSTEM

Diazepam administered intravenously in doses of 0.3 to 0.5 mg/kg results in mild reductions in blood pressure, peripheral vascular resistance, and cardiac output. Occasionally, hypotension may occur after even modest doses of diazepam.

## RESPIRATORY SYSTEM

Diazepam causes a decreased slope of the ventilatory response to $CO_2$, but the $CO_2$ response curve is not shifted to the right as is classically described after opioid administration. Rarely, small doses of diazepam may result in apnea.

## SKELETAL MUSCLE

Diazepam reduces skeletal muscle tone through its action on the spinal internuncial neurons and at the motor cortex. This effect lends credence to the use of this agent in the treatment of spastic muscle disorders.

## ANTICONVULSANT ACTIVITY

Diazepam (0.1 mg/kg) abolishes seizure activity in status epilepticus and alcohol withdrawal, although the effect is short-lived. It also increases the threshold for local anesthetic-induced seizure activity.

## PLACENTA

Diazepam crosses the placenta easily. Long-term exposure may precipitate postnatal toxicity and withdrawal.

# Lorazepam

Lorazepam is a relatively long-acting benzodiazepine that is a more potent amnesic than diazepam or midazolam. The cardiovascular, ventilatory, and neuromuscular blocking effects of lorazepam resemble those of diazepam and midazolam. Lorazepam has proven effective as an anticonvulsant. Its elimination half-life is 10 to 20 h. Lorazepam is used clinically for preoperative sedation and anterograde amnesia, but it is seldom used for induction of anesthesia or intravenous sedation because of its slow onset of action. It is also used to treat seizures and alcohol withdrawal. Its safety has not been demonstrated in children younger than 12 years.

## PHARMACOLOGY

The onset of action is contingent upon the route of administration: intravenous, 5 min; intramuscular, 20 to 30 min; and oral, 30 to 60 min.

## METABOLISM

Lorazepam undergoes direct glucuronidation without prior cytochrome P450 metabolism to inactive compounds, which are then eliminated in urine. Because of this unique characteristic, only minor effects on the pharmacokinetics are expected with hepatic or renal dysfunction. The elimination half-life ranges from 10.5 h in older children and adults to 16 h in the elderly and 40 h in neonates. Because its metabolites are inactive, the use of lorazepam is recommended over midazolam for patients in the intensive care unit who require anxiolysis for longer than 24 h.

A concern unique to lorazepam infusions is the effect of the carrier (solvent) propylene glycol that is used to administer intravenous lorazepam. Infusions may be complicated by toxicity that is characterized by hyperosmolarity and an anion gap metabolic acidosis typically accompanied by acute kidney injury progressing to multisystem organ failure. These can occur with normal doses and renal function but typically occur with dosages greater than 0.1 mg/kg/h or with renal impairment. Treatment involves discontinuation of the offending agent and dialysis (in severe cases).

# Remimazolam

Developed to combine the typical benzodiazepine characteristics accomplished through high-affinity $GABA_A$ agonism with metabolism via esterase hydrolysis as demonstrated by the opioid remifentanil, remimazolam offers precise control of drug effect through titration of infusion or small intermittent boluses, thereby facilitating rapid recovery after dose termination. The drug offers the unique combination of rapid onset, brief half-life, small volume of distribution, and very rapid clearance that combine to achieve an ultrashort clinical duration of action. This results in reliable and predictable sedation and recovery in patients, with very low risk of pharmacokinetic drug-drug interactions. A phase III clinical study found remimazolam to be superior compared with midazolam or placebo in achieving procedural tolerance in patients undergoing colonoscopy with marked reduction in time to emergence, full recall, and postanesthesia care unit length of stay. Similarly, superiority in procedural tolerance and time to recovery of alertness compared with midazolam has been reported in patients undergoing bronchoscopy. Comparisons with propofol are awaited while clinical trial registries list multiple trials of remimazolam in general anesthesia with results pending. Remimazolam was approved for medical use in the United States in July 2020 for the induction and maintenance of procedural sedation in adults lasting 30 minutes or less.

## PHARMACOLOGY

Remimazolam is administered as an intravenous intermittent bolus or continuous infusion, offers a rapid onset time of less than 5 minutes, is hypnotic with dose-related depth, and is typified by a brief clinical duration of action (context-sensitive halftime after a 4-h infusion of 6.8 min) with full alertness regained 19 minutes after infusion cessation. The equilibration half-time between central and effect compartment is 2.7 minutes. Dose-dependent reduction in mean arterial blood pressure of up to 6% has been reported. It is important to flush the intravenous line with saline before and after remimazolam dosing, as the agent is known to precipitate in balanced salt solutions (e.g., Plasmalyte, Ringer acetate). Although preliminary data are encouraging, whether remimazolam as a hypnotic has hemodynamic advantages over volatile anesthetics or propofol remains unknown. Unlike propofol, remimazolam sedation may be completely reversed by the benzodiazepine antagonist flumazenil. As with other benzodiazepines, the carcinogenic and teratogenic potential of remimazolam remains to be fully elucidated. However, without clear evidence of harm, the risk appears low pending additional basic science and clinical research findings.

## METABOLISM

Esterase metabolism breaks remimazolam down to its carboxylic acid metabolite, CNS 7054, which is 300 to 400 times

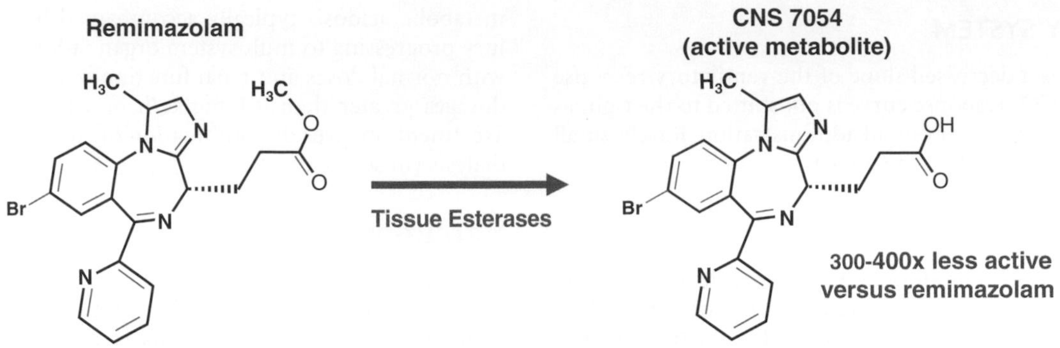

**Fig. 56.2**   Remimazolam metabolism: the parent drug is hydrolyzed by tissue esterases to the markedly less active metabolite CNS 7054.

weaker as an agonist at the $GABA_A$ receptor with terminal hepatic metabolism (terminal half-life 45 minutes) (Fig. 56.2).

## Other Benzodiazepines and Related Agents

The benzodiazepines oxazepam (Serax), clonazepam (Klonopin), flurazepam (Dalmane), temazepam (Restoril), triazolam (Halcion), and quazepam (Doral) are used most commonly to treat insomnia or anxiety. Receptor composition exhibits subunit variability that governs the interaction of allosteric modulators of these channels. The development of nonbenzodiazepine agonists (dissimilar chemical and molecular structures to benzodiazepines) that exert sedative-hypnotic effects through interaction with a subset of the benzodiazepine-binding site resulted in the creation of a class of psychoactive drugs known colloquially as "Z compounds." This group of structurally unrelated compounds (to each other and to benzodiazepines) act as positive allosteric modulators of the GABA-A receptor but are less effective as anticonvulsants or muscle relaxants. However, they have proved useful for the treatment of insomnia and include the drugs zolpidem, zaleplon, zopiclone, and eszopiclone with a variety of new compounds recently FDA approved, including alpidem and pagoclone.

## Benzodiazepine Antagonist

### FLUMAZENIL

Unconsciousness frequently develops from single-drug intoxication with benzodiazepines, but mortality is low. However, when it occurs as part of a multidrug intoxication with other drugs (opioids, ethanol), prognosis is worse and mortality has been reported. Flumazenil is a specific antagonist of the CNS effects of benzodiazepines because it binds with high affinity to specific sites on the $GABA_A$ receptor, where it competitively inhibits the binding of the neurotransmitter GABA to this receptor. Serious adverse effects have been reported in patients treated with flumazenil, including seizures, cardiac arrhythmias, and death. It remains unclear whether these incidents are related to the rapid resolution of benzodiazepine effects or from flumazenil itself.

Intravenous flumazenil has a peak effect in 6 to 10 min and is eliminated almost entirely by hepatic metabolism to inactive products. Flumazenil reliably reverses benzodiazepine-induced sedation but has complex effects on benzodiazepine-altered ventilator drive (it restores tidal volume but not respiratory rate while paradoxically decreasing the ventilator response to hypercarbia). Its clinical effects typically last 30 to 60 min, necessitating consideration for readministration should sedation reappear. Small, incremental doses are preferable to a single bolus: 1 mg flumazenil given over 1 to 3 min should abolish most effects of therapeutic doses of benzodiazepines. Patients suspected of having a benzodiazepine overdose should respond to a cumulative dose of 1 to 5 mg flumazenil administered over 2 to 10 min. If the sedated patient does not respond to 5 mg flumazenil, a cause of sedation other than benzodiazepines should be investigated. Some clinicians have successfully used flumazenil to reverse some of the sequelae of hepatic encephalopathy.

## Benzodiazepines and SARS-CoV-2 (COVID-19) Pandemic

The effects of the ongoing COVID-19 pandemic extend beyond short-term morbidity and mortality to myriad physical, cognitive, and mental health effects exacerbated by social isolation, job loss, and economic strain, with one unanticipated result being a substantial increase in prescription of benzodiazepines and Z-hypnotic agents. Global shortages in contemporary sedatives employed to achieve sedation in severe COVID-19 acute respiratory distress syndrome (ARDS) requiring mechanical ventilation have yielded a dramatic increase in utilization of midazolam and lorazepam infusions in this setting. Further, for reasons that remain unknown, patients with COVID-19 ARDS require higher doses of sedative hypnotics, including benzodiazepines, versus non-COVID-19 ARDS.

## SUGGESTED READINGS

Griffin, C. E., Kaye, A. M., Bueno, F. R., & Kaye, A. D. (2013). Benzodiazepine pharmacology and central nervous system-mediated effects. *Ochsner Journal, 13,* 214–223.

Mihic, S., Mayfield, J., & Harris, R. (2018). Hypnotics and sedatives. In L. L. Brunton, R. Hilal-Dandan, & B. C. Knollman (Eds.), *Goodman & Gilman's the pharmacological basis of therapeutics* (13th ed.). New York, NY: McGraw-Hill Education, Inc.

National Institute for Health and Care Excellence (NICE). (2014). *Antenatal and postnatal mental health: Clinical management and service guidance.* NICE clinical guideline 192. Updated Feb 2020. Retrieved from https://www.nice.org.uk/guidance/cg192/chapter/1-Recommendations. Last Accessed March 13, 2022.

Penninga, E. I., Graudal, N., Ladekarl, M. B., & Jürgens, G. (2016). Adverse events associated with flumazenil treatment for the management of suspected benzodiazepine intoxication: A systematic review with meta-analysis of randomized trials. *Basic and Clinical Pharmacology and Toxicology, 118,* 37–44.

Sneyd, J. R., & Rigby-Jones, A. E. (2020). Remimazolam for anesthesia or sedation. *Current Opinion in Anaesthesiology, 33,* 506–511.

Tapaskar, N., Hidalgo, D. C., Koo, G., et al. (2022). Sedation usage in COVID-19 acute respiratory distress syndrome: A multicenter study. *Analytical and Pharmaceutical, 56*(2):117–123.

Weingarten, T. N., Bergan, T. S., Narr, B. J., Schroeder, D. R., & Sprung, J. (2015). Effects of changes in intraoperative management on recovery from anesthesia: A review of practice improvement initiative. *BMC Anesthesiology, 15,* 54.

White, P. F., & Eng, M. R. (2013). Intravenous anesthetics. In P. G. Barash, B. F. Cullen, & R. K. Stoelting (Eds.), *Clinical Anesthesia* (7th ed., pp. 478–500). Philadelphia, PA: Lippincott Williams & Wilkins.

# 57

# Dexmedetomidine

## J. ROSS RENEW, MD

Dexmedetomidine, an intravenously administered centrally acting $\alpha_2$-agonist with sedative, analgesic, sympatholytic, and anxiolytic properties, has a unique ability to preserve respiratory drive and airway reflexes. Dexmedetomidine has been approved by the U.S. Food and Drug Administration for use in two situations: (1) as a short-term (<24 h) infusion in intubated and mechanically ventilated adults in the intensive care unit; and (2) in nonintubated adults before or during surgery or other procedures requiring sedation. Many off-label uses have also been reported (Box 57.1).

### BOX 57.1 OFF-LABEL USES OF DEXMEDETOMIDINE

As an adjunct
  To local, regional, and general anesthesia
  In labor analgesia and cesarean delivery
To facilitate awake fiberoptic intubation in patients with difficult airways
In combination with propofol, to provide anesthesia for infants undergoing microlaryngeal surgery
To alleviate preoperative anxiety and emergence delirium in children*
To blunt the cardiovascular effects of cocaine intoxication
To treat drug and alcohol withdrawal syndromes

*Administered intranasally (2 µg/kg).

A water-soluble imidazole compound, dexmedetomidine is the pharmacologically active dextroisomer (*S*-enantiomer) of medetomidine (Fig. 57.1). This highly selective $\alpha_2$-agonist has an eight times greater affinity for the $\alpha_2$-receptor than does clonidine and has $\alpha_2$:$\alpha_1$ activity of 1620:1. Presynaptic $\alpha_2$-adrenoceptor activation, primarily in the spinal cord, inhibits release of norepinephrine, terminating the propagation of pain signals. Postsynaptic $\alpha_2$-adrenoceptor activation in the central nervous system, primarily the locus coeruleus, both inhibits sympathetic activity and modulates vigilance (Fig. 57.2). Combined, these effects produce analgesia, sedation, and anxiolysis and, similar to clonidine, may decrease blood pressure and heart rate. Some have used the analgesic properties of dexmedetomidine as an opioid-sparing adjuvant for perioperative pain control. Similarly, recent metaanalyses have demonstrated perioperative use of dexmedetomidine is associated with reductions in postoperative delirium and agitation.

**Fig. 57.1** Chemical structure of dexmedetomidine.

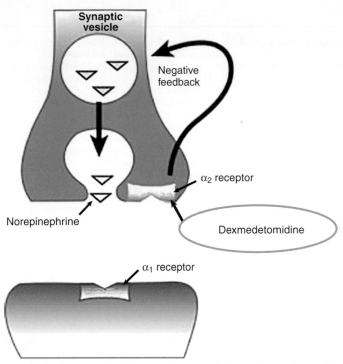

**Fig. 57.2** Proposed mechanism of action of dexmedetomidine at the synaptic cleft in the central nervous system.

## Pharmacokinetics

### DOSAGE AND ADMINISTRATION

Packaged in a glass vial containing 200 µg/2 mL (100 µg/mL) of drug, dexmedetomidine is diluted in 0.9% NaCl before administration, with a final concentration of 4 µg/mL. Premade 20-, 50-, and 100-mL preparations of 4 µg/mL concentration are also now available. For sedation in the intensive care unit, 0.5 to 1.0 µg/kg is given as a bolus over at least 10 min, followed by a maintenance infusion of 0.2 to 0.7 $\mu g \cdot kg^{-1} \cdot h^{-1}$ for up to 24 h. Omitting the loading dose minimizes the hemodynamic changes associated with the use of dexmedetomidine and has become common practice in treating critically ill patients. An infusion rate of 0.2 to 1.4 $\mu g \cdot kg^{-1} \cdot h^{-1}$ for up to 5 days has been used without the development of tolerance, rebound hypertension, tachycardia, or other adverse sequelae.

For procedural sedation, an intravenous bolus of 0.5 to 1.0 µg/kg administered over at least 10 min is followed by a maintenance infusion initiated at 0.6 $\mu g \cdot kg^{-1} \cdot h^{-1}$ and titrated to effect between 0.2 and 1.0 $\mu g \cdot kg^{-1} \cdot h^{-1}$. Infusion rates of up to 10 $\mu g \cdot kg^{-1} \cdot h^{-1}$ have been reported in the operating room.

### ONSET OF ACTION

Dexmedetomidine produces sedation within 5 min of intravenous administration and reaches its maximum effect within 15 min. The vasoconstrictive effect of dexmedetomidine occurs even sooner, with the transient increase in blood pressure beginning at 1 min and peaking within 3 min of intravenous administration.

### DURATION OF ACTION

Dexmedetomidine redistributes rapidly, with $t_{1/2\alpha}$ of 6 min and steady-state volume of distribution of 118 L. Duration of action is 4 h, with an elimination half-life ($t_{1/2\beta}$) of approximately 2 h.

### METABOLISM

Dexmedetomidine undergoes almost complete biotransformation in the liver via direct glucuronidation and cytochrome P450 metabolism, with very little excretion of unchanged drug. Therefore decreasing the dose in patients with hepatic failure may be warranted. The pharmacokinetics of the active dexmedetomidine molecule do not change in patients with renal failure; however, because 95% of dexmedetomidine metabolites are excreted in the urine, accumulation of metabolites may occur. The intrinsic activity of these metabolites is unknown.

## Systemic Effects

### CARDIOVASCULAR SYSTEM

Dexmedetomidine does not have any direct cardiac effects. A biphasic cardiovascular response to a 1-µg/kg bolus of dexmedetomidine has been described. A transient increase in blood pressure, with a decrease in baroreceptor-mediated reflex in heart rate, occurs initially; is explained by peripheral $\alpha_2$-adrenoceptor vasoconstriction; and can be attenuated by infusing the bolus over 10 min or more. The initial response lasts for 5 to 10 min and is followed by a decrease in blood pressure and a stabilization of heart rate. The final result is that both the blood pressure and heart rate fall 10% to 20% below baseline values. These effects are caused by inhibition of central sympathetic outflow and activation of the presynaptic $\alpha_2$-adrenoceptor, leading to decreased release of norepinephrine and epinephrine. Hypotension, bradycardia, and varying degrees of heart block may occur; therefore dexmedetomidine should be avoided in patients with hypovolemia, hypotension, bradycardia, fixed stroke volume, or advanced heart block. Treatment with fluid, atropine, pacing, or temporary discontinuation of the drug is usually successful.

### CENTRAL NERVOUS SYSTEM

Patients who have received therapeutic doses of dexmedetomidine appear to be asleep but are easily aroused and have preserved psychomotor function. Interestingly, dexmedetomidine produces less amnesia than do γ-aminobutyric acid receptor agonists, such as the benzodiazepines. Several other central nervous system effects have also been reported. Dexmedetomidine lowers intracranial pressure, cerebral blood flow, and cerebral metabolic $O_2$ consumption, with preservation of cerebral blood flow/cerebral metabolic $O_2$ consumption coupling. Dexmedetomidine also lowers the seizure threshold, but not to a clinically significant degree. The use of dexmedetomidine attenuates cerebrovascular reactivity to isoflurane, sevoflurane, and $CO_2$, but not to hypoxia, and may be neuroprotective under ischemic conditions.

### RESPIRATORY SYSTEM

During dexmedetomidine infusion, airway reflexes are preserved. Depression of respiratory drive is minimal and is not clinically significant. However, coadministration of dexmedetomidine with other sedatives, anesthetic agents, hypnotics, or opioids may have synergistic effects.

## MISCELLANEOUS EFFECTS

Activation of peripheral $\alpha_2$-adrenoceptors results in decreased salivation, inhibition of renin release, increased glomerular filtration rate, a mild diuretic effect, decreased intraocular pressure, and decreased insulin release from pancreatic islets, resulting in more frequent episodes of hyperglycemia in critically ill patients. Neuroprotective effects have been described in ischemic brain injury as a result of decreased inflammatory markers, such as tumor necrosis factor $\alpha$ and interleukin-6. Activation of central $\alpha_2$-adrenoceptors inhibits thermoregulatory responses and decreases the shivering threshold. Adjunctive use of dexmedetomidine during general anesthesia reduces postoperative shivering rates by 70%. Similar to the action of other $\alpha_2$-adrenoceptor agonists, dexmedetomidine prolongs neural blockade, including brachial plexus block. Although the mechanism of such prolongation is not well understood, sensory block is enhanced more than motor block, a phenomenon that facilitates earlier ambulation. Dexmedetomidine has no effect on the duration of action of neuromuscular blocking agents, adrenal steroidogenesis (compared with the suppression of steroidogenesis observed with the use of etomidate), or neutrophil function (compared with the neutrophil-inhibiting effects of $\gamma$-aminobutyric acid agonists). Dexmedetomidine crosses the placenta, but drug concentrations in the newborn are low and have no clinical effects.

## ADVERSE EFFECTS

Overall, the most common treatment-emergent adverse effects that occur in patients in the intensive care unit who receive dexmedetomidine infusion for sedation include hypotension, hypertension, nausea, bradycardia, fever, vomiting, hypoxia, tachycardia, and anemia. Recently dexmedetomidine has also been implicated as a cause of drug-induced fever when used as an infusion in the intensive care unit.

### SUGGESTED READINGS

Candiotti, K. A., Bergese, S. D., Bokesch, P. M., Feldman, M. A., Wisemandle, W., Bekker, A. Y., et al. (2010). Monitored anesthesia care with dexmedetomidine: A prospective, randomized, double-blind, multicenter trial. *Anesthesia and Analgesia, 110,* 47–56.

Coursin, D. B., Coursin, D. B., & Maccioli, G. A. (2001). Dexmedetomidine. *Current Opinion in Critical Care, 7,* 221–226.

Duan, X., Coburn, M., Rossaint, R., Sanders, R. D., Waesberghe, J. V., & Kowark, A. (2018). Efficacy of perioperative dexmedetomidine on postoperative delirium: Systematic review and meta-analysis with trial sequential analysis of randomised controlled trials. *British Journal of Anaesthesia, 121*(2), 384–397.

El-Boghdadly, K., Brull, R., Sehmbi, H., & Abdallah, F. W. (2017). Perineural dexmedetomidine is more effective than clonidine when added to local anesthetic for supraclavicular brachial plexus block: A systematic review and meta-analysis. *Anesthesia and Analgesia, 124,* 2008–2020.

Jiang, L., Hu, M., Lu, Y., Cao, Y., Chang, Y., & Dai, Z. (2017). The protective effects of dexmedetomidine on ischemic brain injury: A meta-analysis. *Journal of Clinical Anesthesia, 40,* 25–32.

Kruger, B. D., Kurmann, J., Corti, N., Spahn, D. R., Bettex, D., & Rudiger, A. (2017). Dexmedetomidine-associated hyperthermia: A series of 9 cases and a review of the literature. *Anesthesia and Analgesia, 125,* 1898–1906.

Riker, R. R., Shehabi, Y., Bokesch, P. M., Ceraso, D., Wisemandle, W., Koura, F., et al. (2009). Dexmedetomidine vs midazolam for sedation of critically ill patients: A randomized trial. *JAMA, 301,* 489–499.

# 58

# Inotropes

STEVEN T. MOROZOWICH, DO, FASE, FASA

The term *inotropy* (contractility) refers to the force and velocity of cardiac muscle contraction, and the term *inotrope* generally refers to a drug that produces positive inotropy (increased cardiac contractility). Inotropes differ from vasopressors (see Chapter 59, Vasopressors), which primarily produce vasoconstriction and a subsequent rise in systemic vascular resistance (SVR) and mean arterial pressure (MAP). However, some inotropes have vasopressor properties as well, and the predominant effect is usually dose dependent. Inotropes and vasopressors are collectively referred to as *vasoactive agents.* Vasoactive agents have been in use since the 1940s, but few controlled clinical trials have compared these drugs or documented improved patient outcomes, therefore their use is guided largely by expert opinion. Recent metaanalysis supports this practice, provided that vasoactive agent selection for the management of circulatory shock is based on correctly identifying the underlying physiologic deficit and choosing a drug with the optimal pharmacologic properties to manage it. Thus a thorough understanding of these concepts is required. In the setting of cardiogenic shock, the main clinical benefit of increasing contractility with inotropes is to increase stroke volume (SV) and thereby increase cardiac output (CO) to increase the delivery of oxygen ($\dot{D}o_2$) to vital organs until definitive therapy can be initiated. These agents are used in a supportive context with the assumption that clinical recovery will be facilitated by their temporary use.

## Physiology

*Circulatory shock* is defined as inadequate $\dot{D}o_2$ to the tissues, typically in the setting of hypotension. The current definition of hypotension varies, but systolic arterial blood pressure of less than 90 mm Hg or MAP of less than 60 to 70 mm Hg is generally accepted. For the purposes of this chapter, hypotension is defined as MAP of less than 65 mm Hg because that is currently the defined treatment target in the 2021 Surviving Sepsis Campaign guidelines.

Low CO characterizes most causes of circulatory shock. CO is the product of SV and heart rate (HR), and along with arterial oxygen content ($Cao_2$), it is a major determinant of MAP and $\dot{D}o_2$:

$$CO = SV \times HR$$
$$MAP = CO \times SVR$$
$$\dot{D}O_2 = CaO_2 \times CO \text{ (in dL/min)}$$

Thus optimizing SV will improve CO, MAP, and $\dot{D}o_2$ if HR, SVR, and $Cao_2$ remain constant. In addition to inotropy, SV and overall myocardial performance are determined by five other factors that require consideration: (1) HR and rhythm (i.e., Bowditch effect, atrioventricular synchrony); (2) myocardial blood flow; (3) preload; (4) afterload; and (5) diastolic function.

## Clinical Implications

The resuscitation goals intended to preserve organ oxygen delivery in all types of circulatory shock are (1) primary resuscitation, which involves rapidly reestablishing normal organ perfusion pressure with MAP of at least 65 mm Hg; and (2) secondary resuscitation, which involves rapidly reestablishing adequate $\dot{D}o_2$.

MAP of at least 65 mm Hg must be achieved in primary resuscitation to maintain cerebral and coronary perfusion. Because CO is a determinant of both MAP and $\dot{D}o_2$, further resuscitation focused on augmenting CO is preferred. Secondary resuscitation involves first ensuring adequate volume status (correcting hypovolemia, ideally with blood products if hemoglobin values are <8–9 g/dL) and then, if CO remains inadequate, administering vasoactive agents while monitoring resuscitation end points.

All inotropes increase CO by increasing the force of contraction of cardiac muscle, but the other determinants of myocardial performance are variably affected. For example, some inotropes directly increase HR and some indirectly decrease HR (reflex), whereas others have no effect on HR. Some inotropes increase arterial tone (i.e., SVR) and venous tone (venoconstriction), whereas others decrease vascular tone through vasodilation, and some improve diastolic function. Any given agent, therefore, may have multiple effects, many of which are dose dependent. Thus successful therapy not only depends on the ability to rapidly diagnose the etiology of circulatory shock and understand its

pathophysiology but also requires a thorough understanding of the pharmacology of vasoactive agents. The selection of a vasoactive agent is based on correcting the underlying physiologic deficits; the agent ultimately chosen probably does not matter as long as the goals are achieved.

In the example of cardiogenic shock, the failing ventricle is very sensitive to afterload, so inotropes that produce systemic vasodilation *(inodilators)* should be considered as first-line agents as long as systemic hypotension does not occur. Although supraphysiologic goals for CO have not been shown to improve outcome and may cause harm, if maximal doses of a first-line agent are inadequate to meet the previously defined goals, then an alternative drug should be considered or a second-line drug should be added. In the latter situation, consideration should be given to using agents with different mechanisms of action to maximize the potential to achieve the established goals. When assessing the effectiveness of any given agent, the anesthesia provider must monitor for side effects of these drugs with equal diligence, titrating the drug to the minimally effective dose.

## Classification

Inotropes are broadly classified here by their clinical effects as either (1) inodilators, agents that produce inotropy and vasodilation; or (2) inoconstrictors, agents that produce inotropy and vasoconstriction. Further classification of these drugs is shown in Fig. 58.1. The commonly used adrenergic agents stimulate adrenergic receptors (see Table 58.1) to produce their cardiovascular effects. The standard dosing of inotropes, their receptor binding (or mechanism of action), and their adverse effects are listed in Table 58.2.

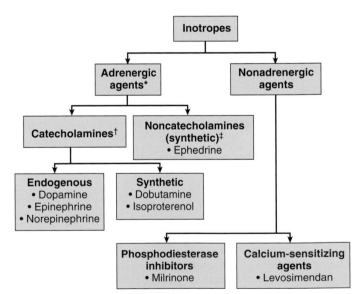

**Fig. 58.1   Inotrope classification.** *Adrenergic agents mimic sympathetic nervous system stimulation and are also termed *sympathomimetics*. †Catecholamines structurally contain a catechol group and are rapidly metabolized by catechol-O-methyltransferase (COMT) and monoamine oxidase, corresponding to their short duration of action (1–2 min), making them ideal agents for titration. ‡Noncatecholamines have a longer duration of action (approximately 5–15 min) because they are not metabolized by COMT.

<table>
<tr><td colspan="3">TABLE 58.1    **Adrenergic Receptors With Cardiovascular Effects**</td></tr>
</table>

| Adrenergic Receptor | Location | Cardiovascular Effect(s) |
| --- | --- | --- |
| $\beta_1$ | Myocardium | Inotropy (increased contractility)<br>Chronotropy (increased heart rate)<br>Dromotropy (increased conduction) |
| $\beta_2$ | Systemic arterioles<br>Pulmonary arterioles<br>Veins | Vasodilation |
| $\alpha_1$ | Systemic arterioles (receptor density*):<br>Skin (high)<br>Skeletal muscle (high)<br>Abdominal viscera/ splanchnic (moderate)<br>Kidney (moderate)<br>Myocardium (minimal)<br>Brain (minimal)<br>Pulmonary arterioles<br>Veins | Vasoconstriction |

*Vasoconstriction of the vascular beds with moderate and high $\alpha_1$-receptor density allows the redistribution of blood flow to vital organs with minimal receptor density (brain and myocardium) and is the basis for adrenergic vasopressor use (e.g., epinephrine) in advanced cardiovascular life support.

## Specific Agents

### INODILATORS

#### Isoproterenol

Isoproterenol has potent $\beta_1$-receptor and $\beta_2$-receptor activity, with virtually no $\alpha$-receptor activity, resulting in inotropy, chronotropy, and systemic and pulmonary vasodilation. Despite the inotropy of isoproterenol, the venodilation associated with its use decreases venous return (preload), resulting in a minimal increase in CO and a drop in MAP. Because of this, the use of isoproterenol is limited to situations in which hypotension and shock result from bradycardia or heart block. However, because a transplanted heart is denervated, isoproterenol has been used after cardiac transplantation to raise HR and CO.

#### Milrinone

Milrinone is a nonadrenergic agent that acts by inhibiting phosphodiesterase, which augments intracellular concentrations of cyclic adenosine monophosphate in myocytes and vascular smooth muscle cells, resulting in increased myocardial contractility and smooth muscle relaxation (i.e., vasodilation) in the pulmonary and systemic circulation. Thus milrinone improves right ventricular function in the setting of pulmonary hypertension, more so than adrenergic inodilators. In addition, milrinone uniquely improves diastolic relaxation (lusitropy). Because milrinone is a nonadrenergic agent, decreased myocardial $\beta$-adrenergic activity—whether secondary to the

<table>
<tr><td colspan="7">TABLE 58.2    **Standard Dosing, Receptor Binding (or Mechanism of Action), and Adverse Effects of Inotropes**</td></tr>
</table>

| Drug | IV Infusion Dose* | RECEPTOR ACTIVITY OR MECHANISM OF ACTION | | | | Adverse Effect(s) |
| --- | --- | --- | --- | --- | --- | --- |
| | | $\alpha_1$ | $\beta_1$ | $\beta_2$ | Dopamine | |
| Isoproterenol | $>0.15\ \mu g \cdot kg^{-1} \cdot min^{-1}$ | 0 | ++ | ++ | 0 | Arrhythmias, myocardial ischemia, hypotension |
| Milrinone | Loading dose of 20–50 $\mu g \cdot min^{-1}$, then 0.25–0.75 $\mu g \cdot kg^{-1} \cdot min^{-1}$ | Phosphodiesterase inhibitor | | | | Hypotension |
| Levosimendan | Loading dose of 12–24 $\mu g \cdot min^{-1}$, then 0.05–0.2 $\mu g \cdot kg^{-1} \cdot min^{-1}$ | Calcium sensitizer | | | | Hypotension |
| Dobutamine | 2–20 $\mu g \cdot kg^{-1} \cdot min^{-1}$ | − | ++ | + | 0 | Arrhythmias, tachycardia, myocardial ischemia, hypotension |
| Dopamine | 1–5 $\mu g \cdot kg^{-1} \cdot min^{-1}$ | − | − | − | ++ | Arrhythmias, myocardial ischemia, hypertension, tissue ischemia |
| | 5 10 $\mu g \cdot kg^{-1} \cdot min^{-1}$ | + | ++ | + | ++ | |
| | 10–20 $\mu g \cdot kg^{-1} \cdot min^{-1}$ | ++ | ++ | + | ++ | |
| Epinephrine | 0.01–0.03 $\mu g \cdot kg^{-1} \cdot min^{-1}$ | − | ++ | + | 0 | Arrhythmias, myocardial ischemia, hypertension, hyperglycemia[†], hypermetabolism/ lactic acidosis[†] |
| | 0.03–0.1 $\mu g \cdot kg^{-1} \cdot min^{-1}$ | + | ++ | + | 0 | |
| | $>0.1\ \mu g \cdot kg^{-1} \cdot min^{-1}$ | ++ | ++ | + | 0 | |
| Norepinephrine | Start 0.01 $\mu g \cdot kg^{-1} \cdot min^{-1}$ (maximum, 30 $\mu g \cdot min^{-1}$) | ++ | ++ | − | 0 | Arrhythmias, hypertension, tissue ischemia |

IV, Intravenous; ++, potent; +, moderate; −, minimal; 0, none.
*Doses are guidelines, and the actual administered dose should be determined by patient response.
†The development of hyperglycemia and lactic acidosis appears to be a $\beta_2$-mediated phenomenon unique to epinephrine. When this occurs, it is important to recognize that if the delivery of oxygen is adequate with no clinical evidence of circulatory shock, then lactic acidosis in this setting is characterized as a type B process which is not associated with the adverse outcomes seen with a type A process (i.e., lactic acidosis in the setting of circulatory shock).

use of β-adrenergic receptor blocking agents or chronic heart failure—does not diminish its effectiveness and does not produce the adverse events associated with β-receptor stimulation (see Table 58.2). However, the vasodilatory properties of milrinone limit its use in patients with hypotension, and its 30- to 60-min half-life is significantly longer than that of the adrenergic inodilators.

### Levosimendan

Levosimendan is a nonadrenergic calcium-sensitizing agent that produces inotropy by calcium sensitization of myocardial contractile proteins, without increasing intracellular calcium, and produces vasodilation within the systemic and pulmonary circulation by activation of adenosine triphosphate–sensitive potassium channels. Levosimendan produces similar clinical effects to milrinone, but it is also limited by hypotension and a long duration of action (80 h because of active metabolites). Levosimendan is not currently approved for use in the United States.

### Dobutamine

Dobutamine primarily stimulates $\beta_1$ and $\beta_2$ receptors, resulting in increased chronotropy, inotropy, and systemic and pulmonary vasodilation, which ultimately increases HR and CO and decreases SVR and pulmonary vascular resistance, with or without a small reduction in MAP. Because of these beneficial properties, dobutamine is frequently used to treat low CO after cardiac surgery. It is also currently recommended in septic shock with persistent hypoperfusion (i.e., low CO). Additionally, dobutamine may be used in early cardiogenic shock without evidence of organ hypoperfusion, but if organ hypoperfusion is present, an inoconstrictor should be used instead to restore organ perfusion pressure.

## INOCONSTRICTORS

### Epinephrine

At low doses, epinephrine increases CO because $\beta_1$ inotropic and chronotropic effects predominate, whereas the minimal $\alpha_1$ vasoconstriction is offset by $\beta_2$ vasodilation, resulting in increased CO with decreased SVR and variable effects on MAP. At higher doses, $\alpha_1$ vasoconstriction increases, producing increased SVR, MAP, and CO. Thus in the acutely failing ventricle (e.g., low CO syndrome after cardiac surgery), epinephrine maintains coronary perfusion pressure and CO. Epinephrine is used in advanced cardiovascular life support to restore coronary perfusion pressure, in the management of symptomatic bradycardia that is unresponsive to atropine or as a temporizing measure while awaiting the availability of a pacemaker, as a second-line agent in septic or refractory circulatory shock, and as the drug of choice in anaphylaxis because of its efficacy in maintaining MAP, partly as a result of its superior recruitment of splanchnic reserve (approximately 800 mL) compared with other vasoactive agents, which helps restore venous return and CO. Consequently, the degree of splanchnic vasoconstriction appears to be greater than with equipotent doses of norepinephrine or dopamine in patients with severe shock, thus limiting its liberal use. In addition, epinephrine is associated with other adverse effects (see Table 58.2) such as hyperglycemia and lactic acidosis, which appears to be a $\beta_2$-mediated phenomenon unique to epinephrine that must be recognized and thoroughly understood in order to interpret clinically.

### Norepinephrine

Norepinephrine has potent $\alpha_1$, modest $\beta_1$, and minimal $\beta_2$ activity, resulting in intense vasoconstriction and a reliable increase in SVR and MAP, but it produces a less pronounced increase in HR and CO compared with epinephrine. The increase in SVR is poorly tolerated by a left ventricle with minimal reserve; therefore caution must be used in the setting of the failing left ventricle. Reflex bradycardia usually occurs in response to the increased MAP, such that its modest $\beta_1$ chronotropic effect is mitigated and the HR remains relatively unchanged. Norepinephrine is recommended as a first-line agent in septic shock and may be the drug of choice in hyperdynamic (i.e., normal or increased CO) septic shock because of its ability to increase SVR and MAP, thus correcting the physiologic deficit in organ perfusion pressure, compared with other agents that instead increase MAP by increasing CO. Although the American College of Cardiology and the American Heart Association no longer publish detailed algorithms for the management of cardiogenic shock, norepinephrine may still be useful in the setting of left ventricular systolic dysfunction, characterized by persistent hypotension (systolic blood pressure <70 mm Hg) that is refractory to conventional treatment, because of its ability to improve MAP, thereby restoring coronary and organ perfusion pressure.

### Dopamine

Dopamine is the immediate metabolic precursor to norepinephrine and is characterized by dose-dependent effects that are a result of both direct receptor stimulation and indirect actions of norepinephrine conversion and release. Doses of less than $5\ \mu g \cdot kg^{-1} \cdot min^{-1}$ stimulate dopamine receptors and have minimal cardiovascular effects. At doses of 5 to $10\ \mu g \cdot kg^{-1} \cdot min^{-1}$, dopamine begins to bind to $\beta_1$ receptors, promotes norepinephrine release, and inhibits norepinephrine reuptake in presynaptic sympathetic nerve terminals, resulting in increased inotropy, chronotropy, and a mild increase in SVR via $\alpha_1$–adrenergic receptor stimulation. At higher doses of 10 to $20\ \mu g \cdot kg^{-1} \cdot min^{-1}$, $\alpha_1$-receptor–mediated vasoconstriction dominates. Currently, dopamine is primarily recommended for the treatment of symptomatic bradycardia that is unresponsive to atropine or as a temporizing measure while awaiting the availability of a pacemaker. Otherwise, dopamine is used less frequently than other vasopressors because of its indirect effects, significant variations in plasma concentrations in patients receiving the same dose, and a recent study that demonstrated a higher incidence of arrhythmia and a higher mortality rate in patients with cardiogenic and septic shock. Consequently, previous recommendations for its use in cardiogenic shock with systolic blood pressure of 70 to 100 mm Hg and signs or symptoms of end organ compromise, based on its $\alpha_1$ activity to correct the deficit in organ perfusion pressure, have been removed. In addition, dopamine is no longer a first-line agent for the treatment of septic shock but may still be considered for select patients with a low risk of arrhythmia who present with hypodynamic (i.e., low CO) septic shock or bradycardia, because of its inotropic and chronotropic properties.

### Ephedrine

Like epinephrine, ephedrine acts primarily on $\alpha$ receptors and $\beta$ receptors but with less potency. Ephedrine also releases endogenous norepinephrine from sympathetic neurons and inhibits norepinephrine reuptake, accounting for additional indirect α- and β-receptor effects. The combined effects of ephedrine result in increased HR, CO, and MAP. Ephedrine is a synthetic noncatecholamine, and because of its longer duration of action and its dependence on endogenous norepinephrine for its indirect effects, and therefore its potential to deplete norepinephrine, it is not ideal for use as an infusion. Therefore ephedrine is rarely used except in the setting of transient anesthetic-related hypotension.

## SUGGESTED READINGS

Evans, L., Rhodes, A., Alhazzani, W., Antonelli, M., Coopersmith, C. M., French, C., et al. (2021). Surviving sepsis campaign: International Guidelines for Management of Sepsis and Septic Shock 2021. *Critical Care Medicine, 49,* e1063–e1143.

Gamper, G., Havel, C., Arrich, J., Losert, H., Pace, N. L., Müllner, M., et al. (2011). Vasopressors for hypotensive shock. *Cochrane Database of Systematic Reviews, 2*(2), CD003709.

Morozowich, S. T., & Ramakrishna, H. (2015). Pharmacologic agents for acute hemodynamic instability: Recent advances in the management of perioperative shock—a systematic review. *Annals of Cardiac Anaesthesia, 18,* 543–554.

O'Gara, P. T., Kushner, F. G., Ascheim, D. D., Casey, D. E. Jr., Chung, M. K., de Lemos, J. A., et al. (2013). 2013 ACCF/AHA guideline for the management of ST-elevation myocardial infarction: A report of the American College of Cardiology Foundation/ American Heart Association Task Force on Practice Guidelines. *Circulation, 127,* e362–e425.

Overgaard, C. B., & Dzavik, V. (2008). Inotropes and vasopressors: Review of physiology and clinical use in cardiovascular disease. *Circulation, 118,* 1047–1056.

Vincent, J. L., & De Backer, D. (2013). Circulatory shock. *New England Journal of Medicine, 369,* 1726–1734.

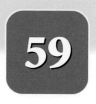

# 59

# Vasopressors

STEVEN T. MOROZOWICH, DO, FASE, FASA

*Vasopressors* are drugs that produce vasoconstriction and a subsequent increase in systemic vascular resistance (SVR) and mean arterial pressure (MAP). Vasopressors differ from inotropes (see Chapter 58, Inotropes), which primarily produce increased cardiac contractility (inotropy). However, some vasopressors have inotropic properties as well, and the predominant effect is usually dose dependent. Vasopressors and inotropes are collectively referred to as *vasoactive agents*. Vasoactive agents have been in use since the 1940s, but few controlled clinical trials have compared these drugs or documented improved patient outcomes, therefore their use is guided largely by expert opinion. A recent metaanalysis supports this practice, provided that vasoactive agent selection for the management of circulatory shock is based on correctly identifying the underlying physiologic deficit and choosing a drug with the optimal pharmacologic properties to manage it. Thus a thorough understanding of these concepts is required. Vasopressors are used in advanced cardiovascular life support (ACLS), the treatment of circulatory shock, and any clinical situation in which the goal is to increase MAP to restore organ perfusion pressure. In ACLS, vasopressors are used to constrict the peripheral vasculature, preferentially increasing coronary perfusion pressure to restore myocardial blood flow, oxygen delivery, and the return of spontaneous circulation. In circulatory shock characterized by refractory hypotension, vasopressors are used in a supportive context until definitive therapy can be initiated, with the assumption that clinical recovery will be facilitated by temporarily restoring and maintaining normal organ perfusion pressure. In certain perioperative scenarios (e.g., vasospasm rupture of a cerebral aneurysm or during cardiopulmonary bypass), vasopressors may be infused continuously to increase MAP to a predetermined level.

## Physiology

*Circulatory shock* is defined as inadequate delivery of oxygen ($\dot{D}o_2$) to the tissues, typically in the setting of hypotension. The current definition of hypotension varies, but systolic arterial blood pressure of less than 90 mm Hg and MAP of less than 60 to 70 mm Hg is generally accepted. For the purposes of this chapter, hypotension is defined as MAP of less than 65 mm Hg because that is currently the defined treatment target in the 2021 Surviving Sepsis Campaign guidelines. Depending on the underlying cause of circulatory shock, the sympathetic nervous system compensation intended to restore normal organ perfusion pressure is manifested in different ways (Table 59.1). In distributive shock (e.g., septic shock), the underlying pathophysiology prevents the compensatory increase in SVR seen in most types of circulatory shock, resulting in refractory hypotension despite normal or elevated cardiac output (CO) and $\dot{D}o_2$. Although the $\dot{D}o_2$ is normal, MAP of less than the autoregulatory range (e.g., MAP <65 mm Hg) results in

| TABLE 59.1 | Types of Circulatory Shock and Associated Clinical Picture | | | | | | | | |
|---|---|---|---|---|---|---|---|---|---|
| Type of Shock | MAP | CO | $\dot{D}O_2$ | CVP | MPAP | PAOP | SVR | Common Clinical Examples | Treatment* |
| Hypovolemic | ↓→ | ↓ | ↓ | ↓ | ↓ | ↓ | ↑ | Hemorrhage<br>Capillary leak | Volume resuscitation |
| Obstructive | ↓ | ↓ | ↓ | ↑ | ↑ | ↑→ | ↑→ | Pulmonary embolus<br>Tension pneumothorax | Inotropes[†] |
| Cardiogenic | ↓→ | ↓ | ↓ | ↑ | ↑ | ↑ | ↑ | Myocardial infarction<br>Arrhythmia | Inotropes[†] |
| Distributive | ↓ | ↑ | ↑ | ↓ | ↓ | ↓ | ↓ | Systemic inflammatory response syndrome[‡]<br>Anaphylaxis | Vasopressors[†] |

CO, Cardiac output; CVP, central venous pressure; $\dot{D}O_2$, delivery of oxygen; MAP, mean arterial pressure; MPAP, mean pulmonary artery pressure; PAOP, pulmonary artery occlusion pressure; SVR, systemic vascular resistance; ↑, increased; ↓, decreased; →, no change.
*Treatment of the underlying cause of circulatory shock is the primary objective, and pharmacologic therapy with vasopressors, inotropes, or both is used as a temporizing measure to maintain organ perfusion pressure (MAP ≥65 mm Hg) and CO while the underlying process is corrected.
[†]Adequate intravascular volume is required, especially with distributive shock, before use of a vasoconstrictor.
[‡]Includes sepsis and trauma.

impaired organ blood flow. This occurs because absolute organ perfusion pressure (or inflow pressure) is too low and the normal autoregulatory decrease in organ vascular resistance is insufficient to restore normal organ blood flow. This fluid mechanics relationship is expressed in a manner analogous to Ohm's law of electricity:

$$\text{Organ blood flow} = \frac{\text{Organ perfusion pressure}}{\text{Organ vascular resistance}}$$

Organ perfusion pressure is the difference between organ arterial (inflow) pressure and venous (outflow) pressure. Because normal organ venous pressure is typically negligible, organ perfusion pressure is usually equal to organ arterial pressure, which is MAP, thus demonstrating the direct relationship between organ blood flow and MAP:

$$\text{Organ blood flow} = \frac{\text{MAP}}{\text{Organ vascular resistance}}$$

## Clinical Implications

The resuscitation goals intended to preserve organ oxygen delivery in all types of circulatory shock are (1) primary resuscitation, which involves rapidly reestablishing normal organ perfusion pressure with MAP of at least 65 mm Hg; and (2) secondary resuscitation, which involves rapidly reestablishing adequate $\dot{D}O_2$.

MAP ≥ 65 mm Hg must be achieved in primary resuscitation to maintain cerebral and coronary perfusion. It is becoming increasingly recognized that perioperative hypotension is associated with adverse events, such as myocardial injury, kidney injury, and death. Based on this, intraoperative hypotension is a modifiable risk factor that anesthesia providers should focus on predicting and preventing based on patient, pharmacologic, and procedural factors. In this regard, quickly achieving MAP ≥65 mm Hg has recently been emphasized in critically ill patients where hypotension in a subset of comorbid patients was found to rapidly result in cardiac arrest, likely because of coronary hypoperfusion. Beyond this, because CO is a determinant of both MAP and $\dot{D}O_2$, further resuscitation

focused on augmenting CO is preferred. However, considering that MAP is the product of CO and SVR, transiently increasing SVR with vasopressors to achieve MAP ≥65 mm Hg is acceptable while secondary resuscitation is ongoing. Secondary resuscitation involves first ensuring adequate volume status (correcting hypovolemia, ideally with blood products if hemoglobin values are <8–9 g/dL) and then, if CO remains inadequate, administering vasoactive agents while monitoring resuscitation end points. The selection of a vasoactive agent is based on correcting the underlying physiologic deficits; the agent ultimately chosen probably does not matter as long as the goals are achieved.

In clinical practice, the indication for vasopressor therapy is classically demonstrated in the example of distributive shock, in which vasopressors correct the underlying deficit in SVR, thus restoring organ perfusion pressure. However, with the recent emphasis on the importance of organ perfusion pressure (i.e., MAP), vasopressors have also been recommended as secondary agents when the indication is less obvious—circulatory shock characterized by low CO and persistent hypotension refractory to conventional treatment. Historically, vasopressors were used with extreme caution in this setting to avoid the complications associated with excessive vasoconstriction (i.e., increasing SVR and organ vascular resistance beyond the normal physiologic values), such as further impairment of CO, $\dot{D}O_2$, and organ blood flow, together possibly worsening outcome. However, excessive vasoconstriction primarily occurs when vasopressors are given in the setting of inadequate volume resuscitation, with or without preexisting low CO. For this reason, patients receiving vasopressors require careful monitoring and frequent reevaluation so that these agents can be titrated to the minimum effective dose.

## Classification

Vasopressors are broadly classified here by their clinical effect as either (1) pure vasoconstrictors or (2) inoconstrictors, agents that produce inotropy and vasoconstriction. Further classification of these agents is illustrated in Fig. 59.1, and their standard dosing, receptor binding (or mechanism of action), and adverse effects are listed in Table 59.2. Although some adrenergic agents

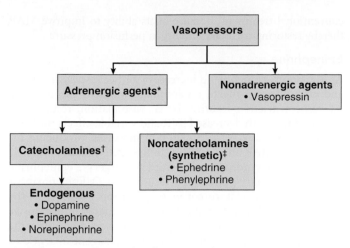

**Fig. 59.1 Vasopressor classification.** *Adrenergic agents mimic sympathetic nervous system stimulation and are also termed *sympathomimetics*. [†]Catecholamines structurally contain a catechol group and are rapidly metabolized by catechol-*O*-methyltransferase (COMT) and monoamine oxidase, corresponding to their short duration of action (1–2 min), making them ideal agents for titration. [‡]Noncatecholamines have a longer duration of action (approximately 5–15 min) because they are not metabolized by COMT.

stimulate many receptors, producing various cardiovascular effects, their vasopressor actions are mediated via $\alpha_1$ receptors, resulting in arterial and venous vascular smooth muscle contraction and an increase in SVR, pulmonary vascular resistance, and venous return. Currently, the only nonadrenergic vasopressor currently in routine clinical use is vasopressin, which exerts its vasopressor effects through $V_1$-receptor stimulation, resulting in vascular smooth muscle contraction.

## Specific Agents

### PURE VASOCONSTRICTORS

#### Vasopressin

Vasopressin (antidiuretic hormone) levels are increased in response to early shock to maintain organ perfusion, but levels fall dramatically as shock progresses. Unlike the adrenergic agents, vasopressin does not stimulate adrenergic receptors, and therefore is not associated with their adverse effects (see Table 59.2). In addition, its vasopressor effects are relatively preserved during hypoxemic and acidemic conditions, making it potentially useful in refractory circulatory shock and ACLS, specifically asystole. Further, vasopressin improves the vascular response to adrenergic agents, allowing a reduction in dosing that may reduce the adverse effects seen with adrenergic agents (i.e., an adrenergic agent–sparing effect). Although the most recent ACLS guidelines suggest that vasopressin should not be used instead of epinephrine in cardiac arrest, they acknowledge this is a weak recommendation based on low-quality evidence. Therefore the guidelines also state that those settings already using vasopressin instead of epinephrine can continue to do so. At this time, vasopressin is primarily indicated in distributive shock, usually as a secondary agent, but its ability to increase MAP and not adversely affect CO has recently been demonstrated in refractory cardiogenic shock, underscoring the physiologic importance of maintaining organ (myocardial) perfusion pressure. Perioperatively, the preemptive use of vasopressin in high-risk patients undergoing cardiac surgery has demonstrated hemodynamic stability after cardiopulmonary bypass and an adrenergic agent–sparing effect. In addition, compared with norepinephrine, vasopressin constricts the efferent arteriole, thus increasing glomerular filtration and creatinine clearance, and may prevent renal dysfunction and

| TABLE 59.2 | Standard Dosing, Receptor Binding (or Mechanism of Action), and Adverse Effects of Vasopressors | | | | | |
|---|---|---|---|---|---|---|
| | | **RECEPTOR ACTIVITY OR MECHANISM OF ACTION** | | | | |
| **Drug** | **IV Infusion Dose*** | $\alpha_1$ | $\beta_1$ | $\beta_2$ | **Dopamine** | **Adverse Effects** |
| Vasopressin | 0.01–0.04 units · min$^{-1}$ | $V_1$ receptor agonist | | | | Hypertension, excessive vasoconstriction |
| Phenylephrine | 0.15–0.75 µg · kg$^{-1}$ · min$^{-1}$ | ++ | 0 | 0 | 0 | Bradycardia, hypertension, excessive vasoconstriction |
| Norepinephrine | Start 0.01 µg · kg$^{-1}$ · min$^{-1}$ and titrate to effect (maximum, 30 µg · min$^{-1}$) | ++ | ++ | − | 0 | Arrhythmias, hypertension, tissue ischemia |
| Epinephrine | 0.01–0.03 µg · kg$^{-1}$ · min$^{-1}$ | − | ++ | + | 0 | Arrhythmias, myocardial ischemia, hypertension, hyperglycemia[†], hypermetabolism/lactic acidosis[†] |
| | 0.03–0.1 µg · kg$^{-1}$ · min$^{-1}$ | + | ++ | + | 0 | |
| | > 0.1 µg · kg$^{-1}$ · min$^{-1}$ | ++ | ++ | + | 0 | |
| Dopamine | 1–5 µg · kg$^{-1}$ · min$^{-1}$ | − | − | − | ++ | Arrhythmias, myocardial ischemia, hypertension, tissue ischemia |
| | 5–10 µg · kg$^{-1}$ · min$^{-1}$ | + | ++ | + | ++ | |
| | 10–20 µg · kg$^{-1}$ · min$^{-1}$ | ++ | ++ | + | ++ | |

*IV*, Intravenous; ++, potent; +, moderate; −, minimal; 0, none.
*Doses are guidelines, and the actual administered dose should be determined by patient response.
[†]The development of hyperglycemia and lactic acidosis appears to be a $\beta_2$-mediated phenomenon unique to epinephrine. When this occurs, it is important to recognize that if the delivery of oxygen is adequate with no clinical evidence of circulatory shock, then lactic acidosis in this setting is characterized as a type B process which is not associated with the adverse outcomes seen with a type A process (i.e., lactic acidosis in the setting of circulatory shock).

reduce renal replacement therapy when used early in the management of circulatory shock, including vasoplegia associated with cardiac surgery. Moreover, vasopressin appears to produce selective systemic vasoconstriction, with minimal effect on the pulmonary vasculature compared with adrenergic agents, such as norepinephrine. This has significant application, particularly in cardiac surgery, where vasopressin would improve right ventricular function by increasing coronary perfusion without altering right ventricular afterload, suggesting that it may be an ideal agent to optimize MAP preemptively and/or improve MAP in the setting of right ventricular dysfunction or failure. However, its 30- to 60-min duration of action is much longer than that of adrenergic agents, making titration more difficult.

### Phenylephrine

Phenylephrine stimulates only α receptors, resulting in arterial and venous vasoconstriction, clinically producing an increase in SVR, MAP, venous return, and baroreceptor-mediated reflex bradycardia. The increase in SVR (afterload) and reflex bradycardia may decrease CO, so phenylephrine should only be used transiently and with caution in patients with preexisting cardiac dysfunction (e.g., low CO). Although phenylephrine was previously considered a first-line agent in hyperdynamic (i.e., normal CO) septic shock because it restores SVR and organ perfusion pressure, it is not listed as such in the current Surviving Sepsis Campaign guidelines, but its plausible use in this setting remains. Perioperatively, phenylephrine is used to correct hypotension, improve venous return, and decrease heart rate (HR) in patients with various cardiac conditions (e.g., aortic stenosis, hypertrophic cardiomyopathy). In addition, the reflex bradycardia associated with phenylephrine may prove useful in the treatment of hypotension caused by tachyarrhythmias or when tachyarrhythmias occur in response to other vasoactive agents used in the treatment of circulatory shock.

## INOCONSTRICTORS

### Norepinephrine

Norepinephrine has potent $\alpha_1$, modest $\beta_1$, and minimal $\beta_2$ activity. Thus norepinephrine produces powerful vasoconstriction and a reliable increase in SVR and MAP but causes a less pronounced increase in HR and CO compared with epinephrine. The increase in SVR is poorly tolerated by a left ventricle with minimal reserve; therefore caution must be used in the setting of the failing left ventricle. Reflex bradycardia usually occurs in response to the increased MAP, such that its modest $\beta_1$ chronotropic effect is mitigated and the HR remains relatively unchanged. Because norepinephrine is the predominant endogenous catecholamine and sepsis can lead to its depletion, its use as the first-line agent in septic shock has been argued as intuitive. Therefore it is recommended as a first-line agent in septic shock and may be the drug of choice in hyperdynamic (i.e., normal or increased CO) septic shock because of its ability to increase SVR and MAP, thus correcting the physiologic deficit in organ perfusion pressure, compared with other agents that instead increase MAP by increasing CO. Although the American College of Cardiology and the American Heart Association no longer publish detailed algorithms for the management of cardiogenic shock, norepinephrine may still be useful in the setting of left ventricular systolic dysfunction, characterized by persistent hypotension (systolic blood pressure <70 mm Hg) that is refractory to

conventional treatment, because of its ability to improve MAP, thereby restoring coronary and organ perfusion pressure.

### Epinephrine

At low doses, epinephrine increases CO because $\beta_1$ inotropic and chronotropic effects predominate, whereas the minimal α1 vasoconstriction is offset by $\beta_2$ vasodilation, resulting in increased CO with decreased SVR and variable effects on MAP. At higher doses, $\alpha_1$ vasoconstriction increases, producing increased SVR, MAP, and CO. Thus in the acutely failing ventricle (e.g., low CO syndrome after cardiac surgery), epinephrine maintains coronary perfusion pressure and CO. Epinephrine is used in ACLS to restore coronary perfusion pressure, in the management of symptomatic bradycardia that is unresponsive to atropine or as a temporizing measure while awaiting the availability of a pacemaker, as a second-line agent in septic or refractory circulatory shock, and as the drug of choice in anaphylaxis because of its efficacy in maintaining MAP, partly as a result of its superior recruitment of splanchnic reserve (approximately 800 mL), compared with other vasoactive agents, which helps restore venous return and CO. Consequently, the degree of splanchnic vasoconstriction associated with epinephrine appears to be greater than with equipotent doses of norepinephrine or dopamine in patients with severe shock, thus limiting its liberal use. In addition, epinephrine is associated with other adverse effects (see Table 59.2) such as hyperglycemia and lactic acidosis, which appears to be a $\beta_2$-mediated phenomenon unique to epinephrine that must be recognized and thoroughly understood in order to interpret clinically.

### Dopamine

Dopamine is the immediate precursor to norepinephrine and is characterized by dose-dependent effects that are caused by both direct receptor stimulation and indirect effects of norepinephrine conversion and release. Doses of less than 5 μg · kg$^{-1}$ · min$^{-1}$ stimulate dopamine receptors and have minimal cardiovascular effects. At doses of 5 to 10 μg · kg$^{-1}$ · min$^{-1}$, dopamine begins to bind to $\beta_1$ receptors, promotes norepinephrine release, and inhibits norepinephrine reuptake in presynaptic sympathetic nerve terminals, resulting in increased inotropy, chronotropy, and a mild increase in SVR via $\alpha_1$–adrenergic receptor stimulation. At higher doses of 10 to 20 μg · kg$^{-1}$ · min$^{-1}$, $\alpha_1$-receptor–mediated vasoconstriction dominates. Currently, dopamine is primarily recommended for the treatment of symptomatic bradycardia that is unresponsive to atropine or for use as a temporizing measure while awaiting the availability of a pacemaker. Otherwise, dopamine is used less frequently than other vasopressors because of its indirect effects, significant variations in plasma concentrations in patients receiving the same dose, and a recent study that demonstrated a higher incidence of arrhythmia and a higher mortality rate in patients with cardiogenic and septic shock. Consequently, previous recommendations for its use in cardiogenic shock with systolic blood pressure of 70 to 100 mm Hg with signs or symptoms of end organ compromise, based on its $\alpha_1$ activity to correct the deficit in organ perfusion pressure, have been removed. In addition, dopamine is no longer a first-line agent for the treatment of septic shock, but it may still be considered for select patients with a low risk of arrhythmia who present with hypodynamic (i.e., low-CO) septic shock and/or bradycardia, because of its inotropic and chronotropic properties.

*Ephedrine*

Like epinephrine, ephedrine acts primarily on α receptors and β receptors but with less potency. Ephedrine also releases endogenous norepinephrine from sympathetic neurons and inhibits norepinephrine reuptake, accounting for additional indirect α- and β-receptor effects. The combined effects of ephedrine result in increased HR, CO, and MAP. Ephedrine is a synthetic noncatecholamine, and because of its longer duration of action and its dependence on endogenous norepinephrine for its indirect effects, and therefore its potential to deplete norepinephrine, it is not ideal for use as an infusion. Therefore ephedrine is rarely used except in the setting of transient anesthetic-related hypotension.

## SUGGESTED READINGS

Evans, L., Rhodes, A., Alhazzani, W., Antonelli, M., Coopersmith, C. M., French, C., et al. (2021). Surviving sepsis campaign: International Guidelines for Management of Sepsis and Septic Shock 2021. *Critical Care Medicine, 49,* e1063–e1143.

Havel, C., Arrich, J., Losert, H., Gamper, G., Müllner, M., & Herkner, H. (2011). Vasopressors for hypotensive shock. *Cochrane Database of Systematic Reviews,* (5), CD003709.

Morozowich, S. T., & Ramakrishna, H. (2015). Pharmacologic agents for acute hemodynamic instability: Recent advances in the management of perioperative shock—a systematic review. *Annals of Cardiac Anaesthesia, 18,* 543–554.

Russell, J. A. (2017). Vasopressin, norepinephrine, and vasodilatory shock after cardiac surgery: Another "VASST" difference? *Anesthesiology, 126,* 9–11.

Saugel, B., & Sessler, D. I. (2021). Perioperative blood pressure management. *Anesthesiology, 134,* 250–261.

Vincent, J. L., & De Backer, D. (2013). Circulatory shock. *New England Journal of Medicine, 369,* 1726–1734.

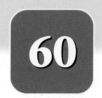

# 60

# Vasodilators

MISTY A. RADOSEVICH, MD

## Introduction

Vasodilators are an important group of medications used in the management of several conditions. A thorough understanding of each agent is vital in selecting the appropriate therapy for an individual patient. A comparison of several commonly used vasodilators is presented in Table 60.1.

## Sodium Nitroprusside

Sodium nitroprusside (NTP) is a potent, rapid-acting intravenous vasodilator used for the acute management of blood pressure. Several considerations unique to this drug are outlined in the following sections.

### MECHANISM OF ACTION

Nitroprusside exerts its effects through the action of nitric oxide (NO). Within an erythrocyte, a molecule of NO is liberated from nitroprusside via a reaction with oxyhemoglobin. It is NO that subsequently induces vasodilation by enhancing the activity of guanylyl cyclase in the production of cyclic 3′,5′-monophosphate, a mediator of several processes involved in smooth muscle relaxation. This results in both arterial and venous vasodilation.

| TABLE 60.1 | Comparison of Vasodilators | | | | | | |
|---|---|---|---|---|---|---|---|
| **Agent** | **Dose** | **Metabolism** | **Arterial Tone** | **Venous Tone** | **Inotropy** | **Heart Rate** | **Caution** |
| **Nitroprusside** | 0.5–10 µg/kg/min (no more than 10 minutes at max dose of 10 µg/kg/min) | Nitroprusside: red blood cells<br>Cyanide ions: hepatic<br>Thiocyanate: renal elimination | ↓↓↓ | ↓↓ | –/↑ | ↑ | Cyanide ion generation |
| **Nicardipine** | 5–15 mg/h | Hepatic | ↓↓↓ | ↓ | – | ↑ | |
| **Clevidipine** | 2–21 mg/h | Plasma esterases | ↓↓↓ | – | – | – | Hypoxemia due to HPV inhibition |

↓↓↓ Significant decrease; ↓↓ moderate decrease; ↓ minimal decrease; – no change; *HPV,* hypoxic pulmonary vasoconstriction.

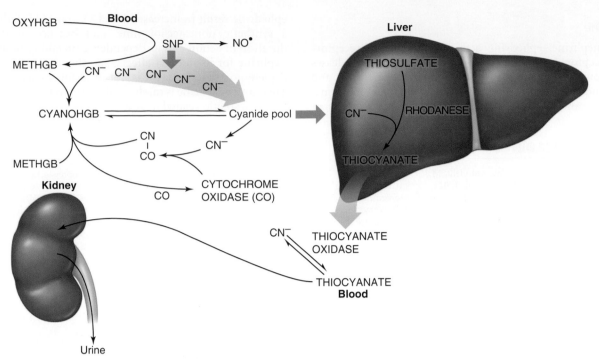

**Fig. 60.1** Metabolism of sodium nitroprusside and pathways for elimination of cyanide ions. *CYANOHGB*, Cyanmethemoglobin; *METHGB*, methemoglobin; *OXYHGB*, oxyhemoglobin; *SNP*, sodium nitroprusside.

## METABOLISM

Metabolism of nitroprusside occurs within a red blood cell, where it interacts with oxyhemoglobin. In this reaction, an electron is transferred from iron within oxyhemoglobin ($Fe^{2+} \rightarrow Fe^{3+}$) to nitroprusside. This creates an unstable molecule that breaks down into NO, five cyanide ions ($CN^-$), and methemoglobin (Fig. 60.1). These cyanide ions have one of three fates, as shown in Fig. 60.1. They may react with methemoglobin to create nontoxic cyanmethemoglobin, or the $CN^-$ may be taken up by the liver and converted to thiocyanate (100 times less toxic than cyanide, excreted in urine) from thiosulfate and vitamin $B_{12}$ via a reaction with the hepatic enzyme rhodanese. In a third pathway, $CN^-$ may bind to the $Fe^{3+}$ of mitochondrial cytochrome oxidase (a3), inhibiting the electron transport chain and oxidative phosphorylation and forcing the cell to convert to anaerobic metabolism for adenosine triphosphate production. This is the mechanism behind cellular hypoxia in cyanide toxicity. The half-life of nitroprusside is 2 min.

## DOSING

Typical dosing begins at 0.5 µg/kg/min and may be titrated up to 10 µg/kg/min in increments of 0.5 to 1 µg/kg/min (the 10 µg/kg/min dose should be used for no more than 10 minutes to limit toxicity).

## Organ System Effects

### CARDIOVASCULAR SYSTEM

Through arterial and venous vasodilation, nitroprusside reduces systemic and pulmonary vascular resistance. Reflex-mediated tachycardia and increased contractility occur, and cardiac output is often increased. Intracoronary steal has been described as a result of coronary vasodilation. Increased intracranial pressure may occur because of vasodilation of intracranial vessels and increased blood flow in the absence of hypotension. Pulmonary vasodilation may increase intrapulmonary shunt as hypoxic vasoconstriction is reversed. Nitroprusside has also been shown to reversibly impair platelet aggregation.

## TOXICITY

Cyanide toxicity is a potential serious adverse effect of nitroprusside administration when used for long periods, when given at high doses, or when given rapidly. Cyanide toxicity presents with metabolic acidosis, tachyphylaxis to the effects of nitroprusside, arrhythmias, increased mixed venous oxygen saturation, and altered mental status. At-risk populations include those with hepatic dysfunction, malnourishment, and hypothermia. Treatment involves stopping the drug, supplemental oxygen, and augmentation of the cyanide detoxification pathways. Examples include administering sodium thiosulfate (to shunt $CN^-$ to thiocyanate), 3% sodium nitrite (to generate more methemoglobin for binding $CN^-$ [do not use as first-line treatment in a patient with hypoxemia because this will further compromise oxygen delivery]), or hydroxocobalamin (to generate the nontoxic cyanocobalamin [vitamin $B_{12}$]). Additional toxicities related to nitroprusside use include methemoglobinemia (with high-dose nitroprusside or sodium nitrate) and thiocyanate toxicity in those with renal failure or high levels of thiocyanate. Thiocyanate toxicity results in central nervous system effects (fatigue, tinnitus, psychosis, seizures, coma), gastrointestinal symptoms (nausea, vomiting), hypothyroidism, hypoxia, and muscle weakness. Methemoglobinemia may be treated with methylene blue.

## Nicardipine

Nicardipine (Cardene) is a dihydropyridine calcium channel blocker used to treat hypertension and angina.

### MECHANISM OF ACTION

Nicardipine blocks calcium channels on the vascular smooth muscle and myocardium. Arterial vasodilation predominates because of the action of nicardipine on L-type calcium channels, which are more prevalent on arterial vessels. Myocardial conduction and inotropy are minimally changed. Coronary artery vasodilation results in the antianginal effects of the drug.

### DOSING

Initial intravenous dosing is 5 mg/h, increased by 2.5 mg/h every 5 to 15 min to the desired blood pressure target. Maximum recommended dose is 15 mg/h.

### METABOLISM AND DOSE ADJUSTMENTS

Nicardipine undergoes hepatic metabolism via the cytochrome P450 isoenzymes CYP3A4, 2C8, and 2D6. Onset of action is approximately 10 to 15 min, and duration of action is 15 to 20 min.

### ADVERSE EFFECTS

Adverse effects include nausea, vomiting, and hypotension.

## Clevidipine

Clevidipine (Cleviprex) is an ultrashort-acting intravenous dihydropyridine calcium channel blocker that is used for the acute treatment of hypertension.

### USE

Clevidipine has been used in blood pressure management for intracranial hemorrhage, including subarachnoid hemorrhage, and for acute ischemic stroke when systolic blood pressure is severely elevated. Additionally, it has been used after cardiac surgery and for hypertensive emergencies in the emergency department. It has been found to be noninferior to nitroprusside in achieving and maintaining target mean arterial pressure with minimal "overshoot." Time to reach target blood pressure goal is 4 to 7 minutes, faster than nicardipine or nitroprusside.

### PREPARATION

Due to poor water solubility, clevidipine is formulated in a 20% lipid emulsion containing egg yolk phospholipids and soybean oil. The standard preparation is 0.5 mg/mL. It may be administered both peripherally and centrally.

### MECHANISM OF ACTION

Clevidipine is a potent, rapidly acting arterial vasodilator that blocks calcium influx through L-type calcium channels on arterial vascular smooth muscle, including pulmonary, coronary, and internal mammary arteries, without an effect on the venous capacitance vessels. Negative inotropic effects are minimal to none.

### DOSING

Dosing is typically started at 1 to 2 mg/h, with effects seen as soon as 2 min after infusion. Because of its rapid action, the dose may be doubled every 90 sec to the desired blood pressure. A common maintenance dose is 4 to 6 mg/h. The maximum recommended dose is 21 mg/h; this limitation is based on the associated lipid dose delivered. Studies have not reviewed continuous dosing beyond 72 h.

### METABOLISM

Clevidipine has the benefit of organ-independent metabolism. It undergoes hydrolysis by blood and tissue esterases. Therefore no dose adjustment is necessary for renal or hepatic dysfunction.

The primary metabolite is carboxylic acid (inactive), which subsequently undergoes glucuronidation, oxidation, or decarboxylation before it is excreted in the urine or feces. Duration of action is approximately 5 to 15 min. The elimination half-life is 1 min (initial) to 15 min (terminal).

### ADVERSE EFFECTS

Adverse effects include hypertriglyceridemia (especially in combination with propofol), pancreatitis, rebound hypertension (not seen if an oral antihypertensive is started), infection risk (bacterial contamination), and additive antihypertensive activity with other vasodilators. Because of the soy- and egg-based lipid emulsion, clevidipine should be avoided in those with egg and soy allergies.

Hypoxemia may occur due to inhibition of hypoxic pulmonary vasoconstriction, as has been noted with other dihydropyridine calcium channel blockers. Refractory hypoxemia developing while receiving clevidipine with rapid resolution upon drug discontinuation has been documented in case reports and noted in postmarketing experience by the manufacturer.

## SUGGESTED READINGS

Hypotensive agents. (2018). In J. F. Butterworth, D. C. Mackey, & J. D. Wasnick (Eds.), *Morgan & Mikhail's clinical anesthesia* (6th ed., pp. 253–260). New York, NY: McGraw-Hill.

Keating, G. M. (2014). Clevidipine: A review of its use for managing blood pressure in perioperative and intensive care settings. *Drugs, 74*, 1947–1960.

Kourouni, I., Levy, S., Chikwe, J., & Omidvari, K. (2017). Hypoxemia caused by clevidipine complicating cardiac surgery. *American Journal of Respiratory and Critical Care Medicine, 195*, A3789.

Short, J. H., Fatemi, P., Ruoss, S., & Angelotti, T. (2020). Clevidipine-induced extreme hypoxemia in a neurosurgical patient: A case report. *A&A Practice, 14*, 60.

# 61 Nitroglycerin

CATALINA DUMITRASCU, MS, MD | MARCUS BRUCE, MD

## Mechanism of Action of Vasodilation

Nitroglycerin (glycerol trinitrate) is an organic nitrate that acts to vasodilate peripheral blood vessels through the formation of free radical nitric oxide. Specifically, nitroglycerin enters vascular smooth muscle cells and combines with sulfhydryl groups to form nitric oxide. Nitric oxide subsequently initiates a cascade that stimulates guanylate cyclase to increase the production of cyclic guanosine monophosphate in vascular smooth muscles (Fig. 61.1). Increased cyclic guanosine monophosphate leads to decreased cytosolic $Ca^{2+}$ via increased reuptake into the sarcoplasmic reticulum and movement to the extracellular space. Decreased cytosolic calcium leads to the prevention of phosphorylation of light chain myosin resulting in smooth muscle relaxation and vasodilation. Nitroglycerin has relatively greater uptake in veins compared with arteries, leading to a primarily venodilatory effect.

## Metabolism

Nitroglycerin is primarily metabolized in the liver by a reductase enzyme to glycerol and organic nitrates, which are subsequently excreted by the kidneys. The elimination half-life of the parent compound averages 2 to 3 min but can be up to 7.5 min, perhaps because of active metabolites (1,2-dinitroglycerin and 1,3-dinitroglycerin). Extrahepatic metabolism occurs in red blood cells and the vascular endothelium.

## Cardiovascular Effects

Nitroglycerin acts primarily on venous capacitance vessels, causing peripheral and splanchnic pooling of blood, decreased preload, and subsequent decreased myocardial wall tension and thus oxygen demand. With increased doses, vasodilation of arterial vessels also occurs. However, despite its effects as an arterial dilator at higher doses, it is less effective than nitroprusside in reducing afterload.

The effect of nitroglycerin on cardiac performance correlates with diastolic filling pressures via the Frank-Starling mechanism. In patients with normal or low filling pressure, cardiac output may decrease with nitroglycerin as a result of inadequate preload. In patients with high filling pressure (i.e., congestive heart failure [CHF]), cardiac output may increase as a result of (1) decreased preload, (2) reduced systolic wall tension, and, at higher doses, (3) decreased afterload promoting forward flow. Nitroglycerin is commonly used in patients with coronary artery disease because it decreases wall tension, leading to decreased myocardial oxygen demand.

Myocardial blood flow is affected both directly by coronary arterial dilation and indirectly by decreased end-diastolic pressure. Coronary perfusion increases more from low end-diastolic pressure than from improved flow during diastole. At therapeutic doses, dilation of large coronary vessels predominates over coronary arterioles, leading to improved collateral and subendocardial blood flow. At higher doses, direct arteriolar vasodilation occurs, leading to loss of coronary autoregulation and potentially coronary steal.

Nitroglycerin also has effects in the pulmonary vasculature, resulting in decreased right atrial, pulmonary arterial, and left ventricular end-diastolic pressures. For this reason, nitroglycerin may be of some benefit to patients with pulmonary hypertension and/or mitral valve regurgitation.

## Therapeutic Uses

Nitroglycerin is widely used for its antianginal properties because of its ability to reduce myocardial oxygen consumption, and it is considered a first-line agent in ischemic heart disease (Table 61.1). Doses typically range from 5 to 200 μg/min but can be transiently higher in acute heart failure. A decrease in preload leads to a reduction in left ventricular volume/systolic wall tension and thus decreased myocardial oxygen demand. Additionally, nitroglycerin dilates large coronary vessels, improving myocardial blood flow to ischemic regions of the heart. Because there is also a small degree of arterial dilation, a decrease in afterload further contributes to reduced myocardial work and thus oxygen demand. Caution must be taken in patients with right ventricular infarction (i.e., right coronary artery pathology) because nitroglycerin may cause hemodynamic compromise as a result of reduced preload to the right side of the heart. In right ventricular failure, a relatively fixed stroke volume can result, leading to downstream reduced filling of the left ventricle. An underfilled left ventricle ultimately leads to decreased cardiac output and systemic hypotension.

Many patients who have coronary artery disease are prescribed oral compounds that are closely related to nitroglycerin for prophylaxis of symptoms. Isosorbide dinitrate and isosorbide mononitrate are frequently used because these compounds have relatively longer onset of action and duration of action compared with nitroglycerin. This makes these compounds more useful than short-acting nitroglycerin in the long-term management of coronary artery disease. Oral administration of these compounds typically requires much higher doses (30–120 mg/day) than sublingual administration because of first-pass hepatic metabolism. Notably, oral isosorbide mononitrate avoids first pass metabolism, which lends to a more predictable dose response.

In the operating room, nitroglycerin is frequently used in patients who are at risk for myocardial ischemia/coronary spasm, to reduce preload in the setting of CHF, and for patients with systemic or pulmonary hypertension. The initial infusion rate is typically 5 to 10 μg/min, and it is titrated in additional increments of 5 to 10 μg/min every 10 min to effect.

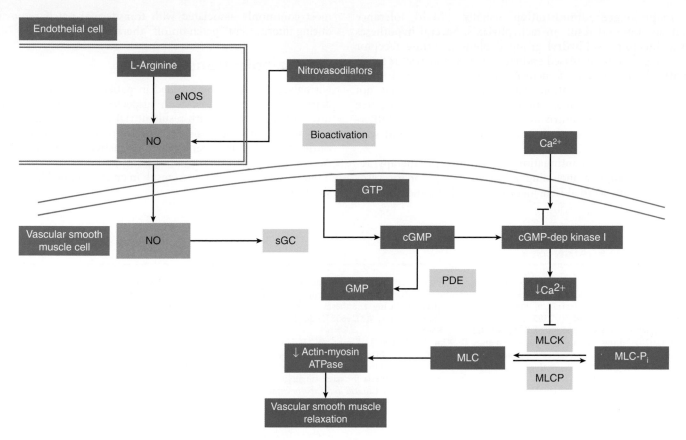

**Fig. 61.1**   Regulation of vascular tone by nitric oxide *(NO)*. NO is a powerful vasodilator that induces formation of cyclic guanosine monophosphate *(cGMP)* by activating soluble guanylyl cyclase *(sGC)* in vascular smooth muscle cells. cGMP can bind to and enhance protein kinase G activity, cGMP-gated ion channels, and cGMP-sensitive phosphodiesterases. Protein kinase G promotes reuptake of cytosolic calcium into the sarcoplasmic reticulum, the movement of calcium from the intracellular to the extracellular environment, and the opening of calcium-activated potassium channels. These changes result in reduction of vascular tone as the reduction in intracellular calcium impairs myosin light chain kinase's ability to phosphorylate myosin, resulting in smooth muscle cell relaxation. *ATPase,* Adenosine triphosphatase; *Ca$^{2+}$,* calcium ion; *cGMP-dep kinase I,* cyclic guanosine monophosphate-dependent protein kinase I; *eNOS,* endothelial nitric oxide synthase; *GMP,* guanosine monophosphate; *GTP,* guanosine triphosphate; *MLC,* myosin light chain; *MLCK,* myosin light chain kinase; *MLCP,* myosin light chain phosphatase; *MLC-P$_i$,* phosphorylated myosin light chain; *PDE,* phosphodiesterase. (From Divakaran S, Loscalzo J. The role of nitroglycerin and other nitrogen oxides in cardiovascular therapeutics. *J Am Coll Cardiol.* 2017;70(19):2393–2410.)

| TABLE 61.1 | Therapeutic Indications for Nitroglycerin Use | |
|---|---|---|
| **FDA-Approved Indications** | **Non-FDA-Approved Indications** | |
| Angina pectoris, acute and chronic | Myocardial infarction/ischemic heart disease | |
| Congestive heart failure | Pulmonary edema | |
| Perioperative hypertension | Tocolysis for uterine hypertonicity | |
| Induction of intraoperative hypotension | Gastrointestinal/biliary tract spasms | |
| Anal fissure, pain management | Preeclampsia | |
| | Dysmenorrhea | |
| | Esophageal bleeding | |

*FDA,* U.S. Food and Drug Administration.

Nitroglycerin may also be used in both hypertensive urgency and emergency to rapidly decrease blood pressure and in pulmonary edema precipitated by CHF. Off-label uses include administration for uterine relaxation during fetal delivery, control of esophageal variceal bleeding, and esophageal spasmodic disorders.

Specific tubing (i.e., polyethylene) is recommended for nitroglycerin administration because polyvinylchloride (PVC) tubing absorbs nitroglycerin. The use of PVC tubing can lead to variable dosing and requires close monitoring.

## Adverse Effects

Aside from the expected side effect of hypotension, nitroglycerin frequently causes headache (most frequent reported side effect), flushing, dizziness, and lightheadedness. These side effects are typically transient, and in all cases they improve with discontinuation of therapy. In rare cases paradoxical bradycardia is seen after nitroglycerin administration, and atropine is usually effective in treating the bradyarrhythmia. In nitroglycerin doses typically higher than 200 μg/min for longer than 48 h, methemoglobinemia can develop as a result of significant accumulation of nitrite metabolites, which oxidize the ferrous iron of hemoglobin to its ferric state. Methemoglobinemia should be suspected in patients with impaired oxygen delivery (i.e., elevated lactate value) despite adequate arterial partial pressure of oxygen. When confirmed with cooximetry, methylene blue is the treatment of choice.

In prolonged administration (usually >24 h), tolerance can develop and result in tachyphylaxis. Several hypotheses exist including sulfhydryl group depletion, nitrate receptor downregulation, increased endogenous vasoconstrictor sensitivity, altered autonomic neural function, and altered nitroglycerin biotransformation. The exact mechanism has not been elucidated. In clinical practice, when possible, drug-free intervals can allow return of clinical responsiveness. Otherwise, physiologic responsiveness can often be achieved with dose escalation.

With abrupt discontinuation of nitroglycerin therapy, rebound phenomena including hypertension, coronary vasospasm, and myocardial ischemia can occur. Rebound angina is most commonly associated with transdermal patch removal during intermittent "patch on/off" therapy.

## Contraindications

Nitroglycerin should be avoided in patients who are preload dependent, such as those with suspected acute inferior wall myocardial infarction with resultant right ventricular dysfunction, severe aortic stenosis, constrictive pericarditis, restrictive cardiomyopathy, or hypertrophic obstructive cardiomyopathy. Additionally, concomitant use of phosphodiesterase type 5 inhibitors (within 24–48 h) can result in an exaggerated hypotensive response.

## SUGGESTED READINGS

Divakaran, S., & Loscalzo, J. (2017). The role of nitroglycerin and other nitrogen oxides in cardiovascular therapeutics. *Journal of the American College of Cardiology, 70*(19), 2393–2410.

Drew, T., Jayasooriya, G., Carvalho, J. C. A., & Balki, M. (2020). Nitroglycerin use in obstetrical anesthesia: A multicentre survey of Canadian anesthesiologists. *Canadian Journal of Anaesthesia, 67*(8), 1092–1093.

Imani, F., Behseresht, A., Pourfakhr, P., Shariat Moharari, R., Etezadi, F., & Khajavi, M. (2019). Prevalence of abnormal methemoglobinemia and its determinants in patients receiving nitroglycerin during anesthesia. *Anesthesiology and Pain Medicine, 9*(3), e85852. doi:10.5812/aapm.85852.

Kim, D. H., Lee, J., Kim, S. W., & Hwang, S. H. (2021). The efficacy of hypotensive agents on intraoperative bleeding and recovery following general anesthesia for nasal surgery: A network meta-analysis. *Clinical and Experimental Otorhinolaryngology, 14*(2), 200–209.

Wakai, A., McCabe, A., Kidney, R., Brooks, S. C., Seupaul, R. A., Diercks, D. B., et al. (2013). Nitrates for acute heart failure syndromes. *Cochrane Database of Systematic Reviews,* (8), CD005151. doi:10.1002/14651858.CD005151.pub2.

Zhao, N., Xu, J., Singh, B., Yu, X., Wu, T., & Huang, Y. (2016). Nitrates for the prevention of cardiac morbidity and mortality in patients undergoing non-cardiac surgery. *Cochrane Database of Systematic Reviews,* (8), CD010726. doi:10.1002/14651858.CD010726.pub2.

# 62

# β-Adrenergic Receptor Blocking Agents

BRADFORD B. SMITH, MD

β-Adrenergic receptor antagonists are a heterogeneous group of medications widely prescribed in managing hypertension and cardiac disease. Essential to understanding their physiologic effects is knowledge of the molecular mechanism of action of the β-adrenergic receptor.

β-Receptors are divided into $\beta_1$-receptors, found primarily in the heart, and $\beta_2$-receptors, found in the smooth muscle of the vasculature and bronchi. The $\beta_1$-adrenergic receptor located on the cardiac sarcolemma is coupled to adenylyl cyclase via a G protein. When activated, adenylyl cyclase converts adenosine triphosphate to cyclic adenosine monophosphate (cAMP), a secondary intracellular messenger that stimulates protein kinase A to phosphorylate membrane calcium channels, leading to an increase in cytoplasmic $Ca^{2+}$. The result of $\beta_1$-adrenergic stimulation is positive inotropy, chronotropy, dromotropy, and lusitropic relaxant effect (the latter by increasing the reuptake of cytosolic calcium into the sarcoplasmic reticulum). Because the secondary messenger cAMP is metabolized by phosphodiesterase, phosphodiesterase inhibitors augment $\beta_1$ activity, which is manifested by sympathomimetic effects. Through inhibition of the G protein (e.g., vagal [muscarinic] stimulation), the coupling of adenylyl cyclase is interrupted, resulting in attenuation of the effects described previously (Fig. 62.1).

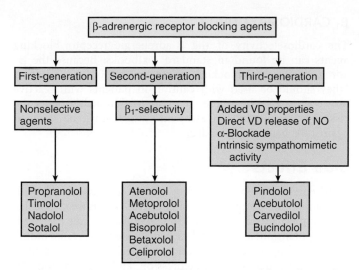

**Fig. 62.1** β-Adrenergic receptor blocking agents differ with regard to their β₁ selectivity, lipid solubility, and intrinsic sympathomimetic activity. *NO*, Nitric oxide; *VD*, vasodilatory.

β₂-Adrenergic receptors are located predominantly in the vasculature, bronchi, liver, and pancreas. The β₂-adrenergic receptor in the vasculature acts by the same mechanism as the β₁-adrenergic receptor in the cardiac sarcolemma, but increased intracellular cAMP in the vasculature promotes smooth muscle relaxation via inhibition of myosin light chain kinase. β₂-Adrenergic receptor activation in the lungs results in bronchodilation, whereas β₂-adrenergic receptor activation in the liver and pancreas promotes glycogenolysis and glucagon release, respectively.

## Indications for β-Adrenergic Receptor Blockade

Because β-adrenergic receptor-blocking agents have negative inotropy and chronotropy—decreasing myocardial oxygen demand and improving myocardial perfusion—they are used in the treatment of numerous conditions. β-Adrenergic receptor-blocking agents reduce the exercise-induced increase in contractility and blood pressure; therefore they are used to treat all classes of angina except variant or Prinzmetal angina. When β-adrenergic receptor-blocking agents are administered correctly, patients have resting heart rates of 50 to 60 beats/min and less than 100 beats/min during exercise.

β-Adrenergic receptor-blocking agents are effective in reducing the frequency of ischemic episodes in patients with myocardial ischemia or acute coronary syndrome. By decreasing both inotropy and chronotropy, β-adrenergic receptor-blocking agents reduce heart rate, contractility, afterload, and myocardial wall tension, thus optimizing myocardial O₂ supply and demand. Current recommendations for patients with acute coronary syndrome are for oral β-adrenergic receptor-blocking agents to be initiated within 24 hours unless absolute contraindications exist. The initiation of β-adrenergic receptor-blocking agents soon after acute myocardial infarction reduces infarct size and early mortality, and improves long-term survival.

β-Adrenergic receptor-blocking agents lower blood pressure by decreasing cardiac output and peripheral vascular resistance. These medications are specifically indicated to treat hypertension in patients with congestive heart failure or coronary artery disease. Patients with congestive heart failure, even without hypertension, can benefit from β-blockade; carvedilol and metoprolol have been reported to improve cardiac ejection fraction, reverse abnormal patterns of gene expression, and decrease mortality.

The inhibitory effects of β-adrenergic receptor-blocking agents on the sinus and atrioventricular nodes and other antiarrhythmic properties (Table 62.1) make these agents ideal for both acute and long-term treatment of tachyarrhythmias. They are indicated to treat supraventricular tachycardias, to control the rate in patients with atrial fibrillation and flutter, and to treat ventricular tachyarrhythmias (specifically metoprolol and sotalol [class III antiarrhythmic]). β-Adrenergic receptor-blocking agents also counteract the arrhythmogenic effects of excess catecholamine stimulation, as seen after myocardial infarction.

| TABLE 62.1 | Characteristics of Commonly Used β-Adrenergic Receptor Blocking Agents | | | | |
|---|---|---|---|---|---|
| Drug | Bioavailability (%) | Protein Binding (%) | Elimination Half-Life (H) | Major Elimination Pathway | Other Properties |
| Acebutolol | 40 | 25 | 3–4 | Hepatic | β₁ Selective |
| Atenolol | 50 | 15 | 6–9 | Renal | β₁ Selective |
| Bisoprolol | 80 | 30 | 9–12 | Equal renal and hepatic | β₁ Selective |
| Carvedilol | 30 | 95 | 7–10 | Hepatic | Antioxidant |
| Esmolol* | 100 | 55 | 0.15 | Blood esterases | β₁ Selective |
| Labetalol | 30 | 50 | 3–6 | Hepatic | α-Blocker/β-blocker ratio: 1/4 |
| Metoprolol | 50 | 10 | 3–6 | Hepatic | β₁ Selective |
| Nadolol | 30 | 30 | 14–24 | Renal | Water soluble |
| Nebivolol | 12–96 | 98 | 10–12 | Hepatic | β₁ Selective |
| Propranolol | 35 | 90 | 3–5 | Hepatic | – |
| Sotalol | 100 | 0 | 10–15 | Renal | Class III antiarrhythmic |

*Available only as intravenously administered agent.

β-Adrenergic receptor-blocking agents are recommended to treat hypertrophic obstructive cardiomyopathy to decrease systolic anterior motion of the anterior mitral valve leaflet and left ventricular outflow tract obstruction. In patients with mitral stenosis, β-blockade decreases the heart rate, which prolongs diastolic filling time and improves cardiac output. In patients with mitral valve prolapse, β-adrenergic receptor-blocking agents are recommended to treat associated arrhythmias. β-Blockade is indicated in patients with dissecting aortic aneurysms to decrease pulse pressure and sheer stress on the aortic wall.

Administration of β-adrenergic receptor-blocking agents decreases the frequency and severity of cyanotic spells associated with tetralogy of Fallot. In patients with congenital long QT syndrome, β-blockade restores the imbalance between the left and right stellate ganglia.

In patients with thyrotoxicosis, β-adrenergic receptor-blocking agents control the associated tachycardia, palpitations, and anxiety. The use of β-adrenergic receptor-blocking agents is strongly recommended to treat hypertension and tachycardia in patients with thyroid storm.

Patients presenting to the operating room may be receiving β-adrenergic receptor-blocking agents for other reasons, such as anxiety, essential tremor, neurocardiogenic syncope, open-angle glaucoma, or for prophylaxis of migraine headaches.

Of particular importance for anesthesia providers, patients with long-term use of β-adrenergic receptor-blocking agents should continue to take these agents preoperatively. In patients undergoing noncardiac surgery who are at intermediate to high risk for myocardial ischemia or undergoing high-risk surgery, it may be acceptable to initiate perioperative β-adrenergic receptor blocker therapy. A multidisciplinary discussion and an individualized approach regarding the optimal timing and risks associated with initiation of β-adrenergic receptor-blocking agents preoperatively is essential.

## Pharmacology of β-Adrenergic Receptor Blocking Agents

Multiple β-adrenergic receptor-blocking agents are available, differing in β cardioselectivity, lipid solubility, and intrinsic sympathomimetic activity (see Table 62.1).

### INTRINSIC SYMPATHOMIMETIC ACTIVITY

β-Adrenergic receptor-blocking agents with intrinsic sympathomimetic activity cause mild peripheral vasodilation without reducing cardiac output. β-Adrenergic receptor-blocking agents without intrinsic sympathomimetic activity lower blood pressure by decreasing cardiac output and inhibiting renin release and central sympathetic outflow.

### LIPID SOLUBILITY

Lipid-soluble drugs, such as propranolol, carvedilol, and nebivolol, are metabolized in the liver, have a short duration of action, and readily cross the blood-brain barrier. Metoprolol, pindolol, and timolol have intermediate lipid solubility. Atenolol, sotalol, nadolol, and betaxolol are the least lipid soluble and therefore have minimal central nervous system penetration and the longest duration of action. Esmolol, metabolized by red blood cell esterases, has a very short duration of action and is excreted in the urine.

## β₁ CARDIOSELECTIVITY

The cardioselectivity of the β-adrenergic receptor-blocking agents can be found in standard textbooks. Because the β-adrenergic receptor-blocking agents are not 100% β₁ selective, "they should be used with caution in patients with reactive airway disease." When these agents are used in such patients, the risks of precipitating an asthmatic attack must be weighed against the benefits of the drug.

## Side Effects

β-Adrenergic receptor-blocking agents are associated with symptoms that are not truly side effects but, rather, sequelae of their mechanism of action. These sequelae include bradycardia, hypotension, and central nervous system effects including sedation, fatigue (a combination of peripheral and central effects), sleep disturbances, depression, and hallucinations. In men, β-adrenergic receptor-blocking agents may increase the incidence of impotence. As mentioned previously, the use of cardioselective β-adrenergic receptor-blocking agents can still be associated with bronchospasm in patients with a history of asthma. β-Adrenergic receptor-blocking agents may mask hypoglycemic symptoms in patients with diabetes and alter triglyceride and high-density lipoprotein levels.

Abrupt discontinuation of β-adrenergic receptor-blocking agents is associated with rebound hypertension and tachycardia, which can result in myocardial ischemia or infarction. With respect to specific side effects, labetalol has been associated with an increase in the concentration of liver enzymes, an increased concentration of antinuclear and antimitochondrial antibodies, pruritus of the scalp, and false-positive results on tests for pheochromocytoma because it interferes with assays of metanephrine and catecholamines. Contraindications to the use of β-adrenergic receptor-blocking agents are listed in Box 62.1.

Anesthesia providers should use β-adrenergic receptor-blocking agents sparingly and with caution in patients taking digitalis, calcium channel blockers, propafenone, flecainide,

---

**BOX 62.1 CONTRAINDICATIONS TO THE USE OF β-ADRENERGIC RECEPTOR-BLOCKING AGENTS**

**ABSOLUTE**

- Severe bradycardia
- Sinus node dysfunction or high-grade atrioventricular block
- Overt ventricular systolic failure
- Severe asthma or active bronchospasm
- Severe peripheral vascular disease with rest ischemia
- Severe depression

**RELATIVE**

- Systolic blood pressure ≤100 mm Hg
- Raynaud phenomenon
- Insulin-dependent diabetes mellitus
- Mild asthma or severe chronic obstructive pulmonary disease
- Hyperlipidemia
- Pregnancy; may decrease placental blood flow
- Liver disease*
- Cocaine intoxication; unopposed alpha-adrenergic stimulation

*Avoid agents with high hepatic clearance (e.g., propranolol, carvedilol, timolol, nebivolol, metoprolol).

or disopyramide. Levels of β-adrenergic receptor-blocking agents metabolized by the liver (propranolol, metoprolol, carvedilol, labetalol, nebivolol) are increased by cimetidine, which decreases hepatic blood flow. In patients who have taken an accidental or intentional overdose of β-adrenergic

receptor-blocking agents, the side effects can be mitigated by atropine, glucagon 0.1 mg/kg administered intravenously over 1 min, followed by continuous infusion of 3 to 5 mg/h intravenous calcium, vasopressors, high-dose intravenous insulin with glucose, and intravenous lipid emulsion therapy.

## SUGGESTED READINGS

Baram, A. (2020). Beta-blocker exposure for short-term outcomes following non-cardiac surgery: A meta-analysis of observational studies. *International Journal of Surgery, 78*, 46–47.

Bouri, S., Shun-Shin, M. J., Cole, G. D., Mayet, J., & Francis, D. P. (2014). Meta-analysis of secure randomized controlled trials of β-blockade to prevent perioperative death in non-cardiac surgery. *Heart, 100*, 456–464.

Fleisher, L. A., Fleischmann, K. E., Auerbach, A. D., Barnason, S. A., Beckman, J. A., Bozkurt, B., et al. (2014). ACC/AHA 2014 guideline on perioperative cardiovascular evaluation and management of patients undergoing noncardiac surgery. *Circulation, 130*, e278–e333.

Lindenauer, P. K., Pekow, P., Wang, K., Mamidi, D. K., Gutierrez, B., & Benjamin, E. M. (2005). Perioperative

beta-blocker therapy and mortality after major non-cardiac surgery. *New England Journal of Medicine, 353*, 349–361.

London, M. J. (2007). Con: Beta-blockers are indicated for all adults at increased risk undergoing noncardiac surgery. *Anesthesia and Analgesia, 104*, 11–14.

Oprea, A. D., Wang, X., Sickeler, R., & Kertai, M. D. (2020). Contemporary personalized beta-blocker management in the perioperative setting. *Journal of Anesthesia, 34*(1), 115–133.

POISE Study Group. (2008). Effects of extended-release metoprolol succinate in patients undergoing non-cardiac surgery (POISE trial): A randomized controlled trial. *Lancet, 371*, 1839–1847.

Teng, L., Fang, J., Zhang, Y., Liu, X., Qu, C., & Shen, C. (2021). Perioperative baseline beta-blockers:

An independent protective factor for post-carotid endarterectomy hypertension. *Vascular, 29*(2), 270–279.

Wiesbauer, F., Schlager, O., Domanovits, H., Wildner, B., Maurer, G., Muellner, M., et al. (2007). Perioperative β-blockers for preventing surgery-related mortality and morbidity: A systematic review and meta-analysis. *Anesthesia and Analgesia, 104*, 27–41.

Wijeysundera, D. N., Duncan, D., Nkonde-Price, C., Virani, S. S., Washam, J. B., Fleischmann, K. E., et al. (2014). Perioperative beta blockade in non-cardiac surgery: A systematic review for the 2014 ACC/AHA guideline on perioperative cardiovascular evaluation and management of patients undergoing noncardiac surgery. *Circulation, 130*, 2246–2264.

# 63

# Calcium Channel Blockers

BRADFORD B. SMITH, MD

Calcium channel blockers (CCBs) are a heterogeneous group of drugs that selectively inhibit the influx of extracellular calcium through L-type voltage-gated calcium channels (VGCCs). This calcium channel plays an important role in signal transduction within excitable cells, such as myocytes and neurons. For cells to use adenosine triphosphate as an energy source, the intracellular $Ca^{2+}$ concentration must be quite low; otherwise, $Ca^{2+}$ would precipitate with phosphorus. When an action potential on the cell surface opens VGCCs, significant $Ca^{2+}$ influx into the cytoplasm occurs, and the electrical signal that depolarizes the cell membrane is thereby converted into an ion-coded signal. In this manner, $Ca^{2+}$ functions as a secondary messenger because its divalent charge is sufficient to produce conformational change in cytoplasmic proteins, including actin-myosin. VGCCs close rapidly by a voltage-dependent mechanism, and intracellular $Ca^{2+}$ quickly dissipates, allowing for precise intracellular signaling. VGCCs require either a low-voltage signal (T-type) or a high-voltage signal to open. High-voltage calcium channels are

identified as N-type (present on neurons) or L-type (present on myocytes, neurons, and endocrine cells) channels.

## Mechanism of Action

The currently available CCBs effectively inhibit the opening of L-type VGCCs, decreasing smooth muscle contraction in peripheral arterial vessels, leading to decreased systemic vascular resistance (SVR) and blood pressure. CCBs are particularly effective in dilating larger, more noncompliant arteries but have no effect on venous blood vessels.

Inotropy decreases with the use of CCBs because of the decreased amount of calcium available for each myocardial contraction. The combination of decreased SVR (afterload) and decreased inotropy optimizes myocardial $O_2$ supply and demand, decreasing the incidence and severity of angina pectoris.

In addition, CCBs decrease electrical activity in the myocardial conduction system by inhibiting VGCCs during phase 0 of the slow response in the sinoatrial and atrioventricular nodal cells and during phase 2 of the action potential of the fast-response Purkinje fibers. In combination, this produces negative chronotropic (i.e., decreased heart rate) and dromotropic effects (i.e., decreased conduction), and it is one of the reasons why CCBs are commonly used to treat atrial fibrillation and atrial flutter when heart rate control is paramount.

## Classes of Drugs

The two main types of CCBs are dihydropyridine (DHP) and nondihydropyridine (N-DHP) compounds. The DHPs and N-DHPs have distinct chemical structures, causing the two classes of drugs to bind at different sites on the L-type VGCCs, resulting in different pharmacologic effects. DHPs act primarily as vasodilators, with few chronotropic and ionotropic effects. N-DHPs slow myocardial contractility and conduction, with much less vasodilatory action.

The vasodilatory effects seen with DHPs make these agents ideal for the treatment of hypertension. Reflex tachycardia can occur with DHPs; therefore a β-adrenergic receptor blocking agent is sometimes used to counteract these effects. As a class, DHPs are approved to treat stable angina, as well as angina caused by vasospasm in the coronary arteries.

The N-DHPs have significant chronotropic and dromotropic effects for the reasons described previously. Consequently, N-DHPs increase the potential for heart block and are relatively contraindicated in patients with heart failure and reduced ejection fraction, concurrent β-blocker use, advanced atrioventricular block, and sick sinus syndrome. The N-DHP drugs have either a phenylalkylamine or a benzothiazepine chemical structure. The best-known phenylalkylamine, verapamil, is relatively selective for the myocardium and reduces myocardial $O_2$ demand and reverses coronary artery spasm. Diltiazem, the best-known benzothiazepine, has cardiac effects like those of verapamil but not as pronounced. Diltiazem has some effects on the peripheral vasculature, like those of the DHPs. It reduces SVR but does not produce the same degree of reflex tachycardia seen with the use of the DHPs.

## General Indications

All CCBs are approved to treat hypertension either as a sole agent or in combination with other medications, except for nimodipine, which is only approved to prevent or treat vasospasm associated with subarachnoid hemorrhage. CCBs have also been used (off-label) to treat Raynaud syndrome, migraines, cluster headaches, high-altitude pulmonary edema, and hypertension associated with medications, including nonsteroidal antiinflammatory agents, cyclosporine, and others. Some CCBs have been approved to treat angina and others to treat atrial arrhythmias.

### DIHYDROPYRIDINES

These drugs have a long duration of action, except for sublingual nifedipine and intravenous clevidipine. Nifedipine, nicardipine, and felodipine have some negative inotropy, whereas amlodipine and lacidipine have no, or very little, cardiac-depressant activity.

### Amlodipine

Clinically, oral amlodipine is used for the treatment of hypertension and stable or vasospastic angina. It has a slow onset (1–2 h) and a long duration of action, with an elimination half-life of 35 to 48 hrs. The principal side effect is peripheral edema, which typically occurs within 1 month of starting therapy.

### Clevidipine

Clevidipine is a lipophilic, ultrashort-acting intravenous CCB that is used for the treatment of acute hypertension. Its rapid onset (2–4 min after the start of infusion) and short duration of action (5–15 min) make it useful in the perioperative period, when rapid fluctuations in blood pressure may be seen. It is injected as a 0.25 to 0.5 mg bolus, followed by continuous infusion of 1 to 2 mg/h, titrated every 2 to 5 min to desired effect. The ECLIPSE trial showed a similar safety profile to nitroglycerine, sodium nitroprusside, and nicardipine in the treatment of acute hypertension in patients undergoing cardiac surgery. Clevidipine is formulated in a lipid emulsion; therefore hypertriglyceridemia is problematic with prolonged infusions and should be avoided in patients with soy or egg allergies.

### Nicardipine

Nicardipine is commonly administered intravenously in the perioperative period to treat acute hypertension. Nicardipine does not affect preload or heart rate and does not cause rebound hypertension on discontinuation. Onset of action is within minutes after starting continuous infusion, and duration of action is variable (30 min to 8 h). It is injected as a bolus of 0.625 to 2.5 mg, followed by a continuous infusion of 0.5 to 5 mg/h titrated every 5 to 15 min to effect. Oral nicardipine is used in the treatment of stable angina (immediate-release type only) and hypertension.

### Nifedipine

Oral nifedipine is used in the treatment of stable and vasospastic angina, hypertension (extended-release type only), and as a tocolytic. When used for preterm labor, nifedipine has been shown to improve maternal and fetal outcomes with fewer material side effects in comparison to $β_2$-adrenergic agonists. The use of immediate release nifedipine has been associated with myocardial ischemia and death when given to patients with coronary artery disease. Immediate release nifedipine may cause rapid peripheral vasodilation that decreases SVR and myocardial $O_2$ supply in addition to reflex tachycardia that results in increased myocardial $O_2$ demand. Immediate release nifedipine should not be used for acute hypertension. Because nifedipine is a potent vasodilator, its use is contraindicated in patients with aortic stenosis, hypertrophic obstructive cardiomyopathy, and severe left ventricular dysfunction. The systemic vasodilation associated with nifedipine results in its primary side effects: headaches and lower extremity edema.

### Other Dihydropyridines

Oral nimodipine is the only CCB approved for preventing and treating cerebral vasospasm after subarachnoid hemorrhage or cerebral aneurysm clipping. This drug is usually administered as 60 mg orally every 4 hrs. Oral felodipine, isradipine, and nisoldipine, all chemically similar to nifedipine, are prescribed for the treatment of hypertension and angina. These drugs are metabolized by the liver and have an elimination half-life of 7 to 12 hrs.

## NONDIHYDROPYRIDINES

### Verapamil

Verapamil, a phenylalkylamine, is indicated to treat essential hypertension, atrial arrhythmias, and stable, unstable, and vasospastic angina. Recommended doses range from 180 to 480 mg/day orally, an intravenous bolus of 2.5 to 10 mg, or a continuous infusion (5 mg/h), titrated to desired heart rate. When verapamil is administered orally, its bioavailability is only 10% to 20%, with protein binding of approximately 90%. Like the other CCBs, it has high first-pass hepatic metabolism by P450 CYP3A4, an active metabolite (norverapamil), and an elimination half-life of 3 to 7 hrs. Metabolites are excreted by the kidneys (75%) or in the gastrointestinal tract (25%).

Secondary to its mechanism of action, verapamil is contraindicated in patients with sick sinus syndrome, preexisting atrioventricular nodal disease, severe left ventricular myocardial depression, or digoxin toxicity. Patients with Wolff-Parkinson-White syndrome and concomitant atrial fibrillation are at risk for antegrade conduction through the bypass tract, manifested as wide-complex ventricular tachycardia that can rapidly deteriorate into ventricular fibrillation. Patients receiving β-adrenergic receptor blocking agents should not receive verapamil as these patients have a high risk of developing severe bradycardia.

Further side effects of verapamil include constipation, headache, facial flushing, gingival hyperplasia, and dizziness. Verapamil interacts with several drugs, increasing blood levels of digoxin, atorvastatin, simvastatin, lovastatin, ketoconazole, cyclosporine, carbamazepine, and theophylline.

CCB toxicity (including verapamil toxicity) manifesting with severe symptoms can be treated with intravenous atropine, calcium, glucagon, levosimendan, high-dose insulin and glucose, vasopressors, inotropes, and possibly lipid emulsion therapy. For patients with acute heart block that is unresponsive to pharmacologic therapy, temporary pacing should be considered.

### Diltiazem

Diltiazem, a benzothiazepine, is used to treat multiple conditions, including acute supraventricular tachycardia, atrial fibrillation or atrial flutter, stable angina, vasospastic angina, and chronic hypertension. It is often administered intravenously as a bolus dose of 0.25 mg/kg, followed by a continuous infusion of 5 to 15 mg/min for the treatment of supraventricular tachycardia or atrial arrhythmias. Recommended doses of immediate- and extended-release diltiazem range from 120 to 540 mg/day. It is approximately 80% protein bound and is metabolized in the liver to an active metabolite, desacetyl diltiazem. Metabolites are 35% excreted in urine, with the remainder excreted in the gastrointestinal tract. Infrequent side effects of diltiazem include lower extremity edema and headache. The same care should be taken when this drug is administered to patients taking β-adrenergic receptor blocking agents, and it should be used with caution, if at all, in patients with cardiomyopathy or atrioventricular nodal disease.

## Anesthetic Considerations in Patients Taking Calcium Channel Blockers

In patients undergoing noncardiac surgery, the perioperative use of CCBs reduces the risk of myocardial ischemia, supraventricular tachycardia, and death; most of these benefits are attributable to verapamil. Inhalation anesthetic agents decrease the availability of intracellular calcium, which, in turn, increases the negative inotropic, chronotropic, and dromotropic effects of CCBs. The inhibition of calcium influx into myocytes potentiates the effects of all neuromuscular blocking agents. CCBs have also been reported to impair hypoxic pulmonary vasoconstriction and, because of their vasodilating properties, to increase intracranial pressure.

## SUGGESTED READINGS

Abernethy, D. R., & Schwartz, J. B. (1999). Calcium antagonist drugs. *New England Journal of Medicine, 341*, 1447–1455.

Aronson, S., Dyke, C. M., Stierer, K. A., Levy, J. H., Cheung, A. T., Lumb, P. D., et al. (2008). The ECLIPSE trials: Comparative studies of clevidipine to nitroglycerin, sodium nitroprusside, and nicardipine for acute hypertension treatment in cardiac surgery patients. *Anesthesia and Analgesia, 107*(4), 1110–1121.

Elliott, W. J., & Ram, C. V. (2011). Calcium channel blockers. *Journal of Clinical Hypertension, 13*, 687–689.

January, C. T., Wann, L. S., Alpert, J. S., Calkins, H., Cigarroa, J. E., Cleveland, J. C., Jr., et al. (2014). 2014 AHA/ACC/HRS guideline for the management of patients with atrial fibrillation: A report of the American College of Cardiology/American Heart Association task force on practice guidelines and the Heart Rhythm Society. *Circulation, 130*, e199–e267.

O'Brien, B., Burrage, P. S., Ngai, J. Y., Prutkin, J. M., Huang, C. C., Xu, X., et al. (2018). Society of Cardiovascular Anesthesiologists/European Association of Cardiothoracic Anaesthetists Practice Advisory for the Management of perioperative atrial fibrillation in patients undergoing cardiac surgery. *Journal of Cardiothoracic and Vascular Anesthesia, 33*(1), 12–26.

Tsien, R. W., & Barrett, C. F. (2000–2013). A brief history of calcium channel discovery. In *Madame Curie Bioscience Database* [Internet]. Austin, TX: Landes Bioscience.

Varpula, T., Rapola, J., Sallisalmi, M., & Kurola, J. (2009). Treatment of serious calcium channel blocker overdose with levosimendan, a calcium sensitizer. *Anesthesia and Analgesia, 108*, 790–792.

Wijeysundera, D. N., & Beattie, W. S. (2003). Calcium channel blockers for reducing cardiac morbidity after noncardiac surgery: A meta-analysis. *Anesthesia and Analgesia, 97*, 634–641.

Wong, D., Tsai, P. N. W., Ip, K. Y., & Irwin, M. G. (2018). New antihypertensive medications and clinical implications. *Best Practice and Research. Clinical Anaesthesiology, 32*(2), 223–235.

# Renin-Angiotensin Receptor Inhibition

BRADFORD B. SMITH, MD

The renin-angiotensin-aldosterone system (RAAS) is essential for homeostasis, as it helps regulate intravascular volume and systemic vascular resistance (SVR), thereby affecting cardiac output because of its effects on preload (intravascular volume) and afterload (SVR). After RAAS activation, renal retention of sodium and water occurs, resulting in an increase in preload and in SVR via angiotensin II. Early in the development of heart failure, these compensatory mechanisms are beneficial, but over time this process becomes pathologic and leads to left ventricular remodeling. Several drug classes have been developed to modify the RAAS, including angiotensin-converting enzyme (ACE) inhibitors, angiotensin receptor blockers (ARBs), angiotensin receptor–neprilysin inhibitors (ARNIs), inhibitors of aldosterone (e.g., spironolactone), and direct renin inhibitors (e.g., aliskiren).

## Physiology

Renin, a protease, is released by juxtaglomerular cells adjacent to the afferent arterioles of renal glomeruli in response to hypotension and $\beta_1$-adrenergic receptor activation. The macula densa of distal tubules, near the juxtaglomerular cells, also release renin in response to decreased renal tubular sodium levels.

Renin released into the blood metabolizes angiotensinogen, an $\alpha_2$ globulin of hepatic origin, to angiotensin I. The vascular endothelium of many organs, but particularly within the lung, contains an enzyme, ACE, that cleaves two amino acids from angiotensin I to form angiotensin II. Angiotensin II can bind two separate receptor subtypes with different internal signaling pathways: angiotensin 1 ($AT_1$) receptors are responsible for most of the effects of angiotensin II seen in adults, and angiotensin 2 ($AT_2$) receptors are thought to be responsible for the antigrowth effects seen in the fetus. The binding of angiotensin II to $AT_1$ receptors on peripheral arterioles stimulates smooth muscle contraction, resulting in vasoconstriction and thereby increasing SVR and arterial blood pressure. Angiotensin II also stimulates the adrenal cortex to release aldosterone, which promotes the retention of sodium and free water excretion of potassium within the distal tubules of the kidney. In patients with hypertensive heart disease, the release of aldosterone may accelerate hypertrophy, fibrosis, and diastolic dysfunction. Angiotensin II has additional endocrine effects via stimulation of the posterior pituitary to release vasopressin, a potent vasoconstrictor and antidiuretic hormone. In addition, angiotensin II potentiates central and peripheral sympathetic noradrenergic activity; peripherally, the postganglionic sympathetic release of norepinephrine is enhanced, and reuptake is inhibited, thereby producing additional peripheral vasoconstriction. Through mechanisms independent of those mentioned, angiotensin II also stimulates cardiac and vascular hypertrophy.

Since the first ACE inhibitor, captopril, was marketed in 1982, several medications that affect the RAAS have been developed and marketed for an equally diverse number of indications. Most commonly, patients are prescribed ACE inhibitors for the treatment of hypertension and heart failure and, in patients with diabetes, to decrease the incidence of diabetic nephropathy. However, ACE inhibitors have been reported to be effective in multiple disease states. Patients who present for surgery may be taking drugs that alter the RAAS for a multitude of conditions that may be interrelated. Anesthesia providers should understand the pharmacokinetics and pharmacodynamics of these drugs because patients who take RAAS-modulating agents should be followed closely in the perioperative period to avoid unforeseen complications.

## Angiotensin-Converting Enzyme Inhibitors

ACE inhibitors are peripheral vasodilators that inhibit the production of angiotensin II. In patients with normal left ventricular function, ACE inhibitors decrease SVR, with minimal effect on heart rate, cardiac output, and pulmonary artery occlusion pressure. In patients with decreased left ventricular function, ACE inhibitors decrease preload, afterload, and ventricular wall tension.

These drugs are frequently used to treat hypertension in patients with heart failure, those with previous myocardial infarction, those at high risk for coronary artery disease, those diagnosed with diabetes or chronic kidney disease, and those with a history of stroke. The Heart Outcomes Prevention Evaluation Study showed that the ACE inhibitor ramipril decreased the number of cardiovascular events (e.g., death, myocardial infarction, stroke) in patients with previous cardiac events or with diabetes. The European Trial on Reduction of Cardiac Events with Perindopril in Stable Coronary Artery Disease study, in which perindopril, another ACE inhibitor, was administered to patients with stable coronary disease but no evidence of heart failure, found fewer subsequent cardiovascular events. Over time, the indications for the use of ACE inhibitors have increased. Currently, these agents are recommended for the treatment of heart failure with reduced ejection fraction, for use during the early phase of acute myocardial infarction, and for postinfarction left ventricular dysfunction (to limit adverse remodeling). ACE inhibitors also decrease the risk of nephropathy in patients with diabetes or proteinuric renal disease.

### CLASSIFICATION OF ANGIOTENSIN-CONVERTING ENZYME INHIBITORS

Oral ACE inhibitors differ in potency, bioavailability, half-life, and route of elimination (Table 64.1). Enalaprilat is the only available intravenous ACE inhibitor. It is used to treat hypertension when oral ACE inhibitor use is not practical. A dose of 0.625 to 5 mg results in onset of action within 15 min and

| TABLE 64.1 | Pharmacokinetics of Angiotensin-Converting Enzyme Inhibitors | | | | | | | |
|---|---|---|---|---|---|---|---|---|
| Drug | Usual Dose (mg) | Duration of Action (h) | Absorption (%) | Prodrug | Peak Concentration (Active Component) (h) | Route of Elimination | Plasma Half-Life (h) | Dose Reduction in Renal Disease |
| Captopril | 12.5–50 bid/tid | 6–12 | 60–75 | No | 1 | Kidney | 2 | Yes |
| Benazepril | 10–20 qd | 24 | 37 | Yes | 1–2 | Kidney/liver | 10–11 | Yes |
| Enalapril | 5–10 qd/bid | 12–24 | 55–75 | Yes | 3–4 | Kidney | 11 | Yes |
| Lisinopril | 20–40 qd | 24 | 25 | Yes | 6–8 | Kidney | 12 | Yes |
| Moexipril | 7.5–15 qd/bid | 24 | >20 | Yes | 1–2 | Kidney | 2–9 | Yes |
| Quinapril | 20–40 qd | 24 | 60 | Yes | 2 | Kidney | 25 | Yes |
| Ramipril | 2.5–20 qd/bid | 24 | 50–60 | Yes | 2–4 | Kidney/liver | 13–17 | Yes |
| Trandolapril | 2–4 qd | 24 | 70 | Yes | 4–10 | Kidney/liver | 16–24 | Yes |
| Fosinopril | 20–40 qd/bid | 24 | 36 | Yes | 3 | Kidney/liver | 12 | No |

*bid*, Twice a day; *qd*, every day; *tid*, three times daily.

| TABLE 64.2 | Pharmacokinetics of Angiotensin Receptor Blocking Agents | | | | |
|---|---|---|---|---|---|
| Drug | Usual Dose (mg) | Half-Life (h) | Bioavailability (%) | Active Metabolite | Route of Elimination |
| Losartan | 25–50 PO bid | 2 | 33 | Yes | Kidney/liver |
| Candesartan | 8–16 PO bid | 4 | 42 | Yes | Kidney/liver |
| Irbesartan | 75–300 qd | 11–15 | 70 | No | Kidney/liver |
| Valsartan | 40–80 PO bid | 6 | 25 | No | Kidney/liver |
| Telmisartan | 40–80 PO qd | 24 | 43 | No | Liver > kidney |
| Eprosartan | 400–800 qd | 5–7 | 15 | No | Liver > kidney |
| Olmesartan | 20–40 qd | 13 | 26 | Yes | Kidney/liver |
| Azilsartan | 40–80 qd | 11 | 60 | No | Feces > kidney |

*bid*, Twice a day; *PO*, by mouth; *qd*, every day.

duration of action of approximately 6 h. Enalaprilat should be avoided in patients with hemodynamically unstable heart failure, acute myocardial infarction, or suspected pregnancy.

Captopril, the original ACE inhibitor, has the shortest half-life of any of the available drugs. It is the only agent that contains a sulfhydryl group in its chemical structure (which may confer additional properties because it is the only ACE inhibitor that is also a free radical scavenger). The presence of the sulfhydryl group may also result in some of its specific side effects: skin rash, loss of taste, neutropenia, and proteinuria.

Most ACE inhibitors (enalapril, ramipril, perindopril, benazepril, cilazapril, delapril, fosinopril, quinapril, trandolapril) are prodrugs that are converted to active drugs by hepatic metabolism. In exception, lisinopril is not a prodrug and does not undergo hepatic metabolism but is water soluble and is excreted unchanged by the kidneys. Most ACE inhibitors are cleared predominantly in the kidneys, thus dosages should be monitored closely and reduced in patients with renal insufficiency.

## ANGIOTENSIN RECEPTOR BLOCKERS

ARBs, also known as *angiotensin II receptor antagonists, $AT_1$-receptor antagonists*, or *sartans*, directly block the $AT_1$ receptor and have the theoretical advantage of blocking the effects of angiotensin II formed by non-ACE pathways. ARBs have no effect on bradykinin metabolism; therefore their use is associated with a significantly reduced incidence of cough and angioedema compared with ACE inhibitors. Originally used to treat hypertension in patients intolerant of ACE inhibitors, they are now being used to treat patients with heart failure and those with hypertension and type 2 diabetes, in whom these drugs may delay the progression of diabetic nephropathy (Table 64.2). Because they have the same hemodynamic effects as ACE inhibitors, with fewer side effects, ARBs are used to treat the same conditions as the ACE inhibitors.

## SIDE EFFECTS

Several side effects are associated with RAAS-modulating agents. Some are associated with increased bradykinin levels, and others are caused by decreased angiotensin II levels. The most common side effect is a nonproductive cough, with an incidence of 5% to 20%. More worrisome are angioedema (incidence 0.3%–0.6%) and anaphylactoid reactions, both of which can be life-threatening. As might be expected secondary to their mechanism of action, ACE inhibitors and ARBs are associated with orthostatic hypotension (especially in patients with hyponatremia), hyperkalemia (more commonly seen with concomitant use of potassium-sparing diuretics or in patients with renal failure), and reversible renal failure (which can be precipitated by situations that decrease renal blood flow, such as hypotension, hypovolemia, severe congestive heart failure, severe hyponatremia, and unilateral renal artery stenosis). The use of ACE inhibitors is contraindicated in patients with bilateral renal artery stenosis, hyperkalemia, and severe renal dysfunction. ACE inhibitors and ARBs are also contraindicated in pregnant patients secondary to the teratogenic effects in the first and second trimesters and ACE inhibitor fetal nephropathy seen in the third trimester.

## ANGIOTENSIN RECEPTOR–NEPRILYSIN INHIBITORS

Neprilysin, an endopeptidase, degrades counterregulatory vasoactive peptides, such as bradykinin, adrenomedullin, and natriuretic peptides that are beneficial in the setting of heart failure. ARNIs combined with ARBs have been shown to be an alternative to the use of ACE inhibitors or single-agent ARBs in the treatment of heart failure. In patients with heart failure and reduced ejection fraction, the PARADIGM-HF trial showed that sacubitril-valsartan (ARNI/ARB) reduced rates of hospitalization and all-cause mortality compared with enalapril.

## Aldosterone Antagonists

Spironolactone and eplerenone interfere with aldosterone-dependent sodium-potassium exchange in the distal convoluted renal tubule and inhibit the harmful effects of aldosterone on the heart. These diuretics are frequently used in combination with antihypertensive agents (ACE inhibitor or ARB) and β-blockers in patients with hypertension and heart failure. Because of concern about hyperkalemia and renal failure, serum potassium and renal function tests should be monitored frequently.

## Direct Renin Inhibitors

Aliskiren is a direct renin inhibitor that is used to treat hypertension. By attaching to the S3bp binding site of renin, it inhibits the conversion of angiotensinogen to angiotensin I, lowering the plasma concentration of angiotensin II and angiotensin. Clinicians should be aware that aliskiren has been associated with increased incidence of nonfatal stroke, renal complications, hyperkalemia, and hypotension in patients with diabetes and renal impairment. Aliskiren should not be combined with ACE inhibitors or ARBs.

## Anesthetic Considerations for Patients Receiving Renin-Angiotensin-Aldosterone System Inhibitors

The decision to administer an ACE inhibitor or ARB on the morning of surgery remains controversial because refractory hypotension may develop after induction of anesthesia. Patients who take RAAS inhibitors are more likely to have decreased intravascular volume because of the mechanism of action of these medications. Hypotension is more likely to occur during major procedures with large fluid shifts, during cardiopulmonary bypass, in patients with sodium depletion, in those undergoing regional anesthesia (particularly neuraxial anesthesia), and with simultaneous diuretic use. The hypotensive episodes can be refractory to indirect-acting sympathomimetic agents and may require aggressive fluid administration, norepinephrine, or vasopressin. Most centers withhold RAAS inhibitors 24 h before elective surgery. The VISION study found that withholding long-term ACE inhibitor or ARB 24 h before noncardiac surgery led to lower rates of all-cause mortality, myocardial injury, stroke, and intraoperative hypotension compared with patients who continued to use these agents. However, there is evidence that continuing RAAS inhibitors preoperatively and postoperatively may be associated with better composite outcomes in cardiac and noncardiac surgery. Therefore the decision to continue an ACE inhibitor or ARB within 24 h of anesthesia and when to restart these medications postoperatively remains controversial and should be individualized based on the patient's history and type of surgical procedure.

Nonsteroidal antiinflammatory drugs (NSAIDs) may decrease the antihypertensive action of ACE inhibitors, an effect that is more common in the presence of low renin levels. Therefore a patient who takes NSAIDs and an ACE inhibitor or ARB may not have the same response as a patient who is not taking NSAIDs.

## SUGGESTED READINGS

Bullo, M., Tschumi, S., Bucher, B. S., Bianchetti, M. G., & Simonetti, G. D. (2012). Pregnancy outcome following exposure to angiotensin-converting enzyme inhibitors or angiotensin receptor antagonists: A systematic review. *Hypertension*, 60, 444–450.

McMurray, J. J., Packer, M., Desai, A. S., Gong, J., Lefkowitz, M. P., Rizkala, A. R., et al. (2013). Dual angiotensin receptor and neprilysin inhibition as an alternative to angiotensin-converting enzyme inhibition in patients with chronic systolic heart failure: Rationale for and design of the prospective comparison of ARNI with ACEI to determine impact on global mortality and morbidity in heart failure trial (PARADIGM-HF). *European Journal of Heart Failure*, 15, 1062–1073.

Roshanov, P. S., Rochwerg, B., Patel, A., Salehian, O., Duceppe, E., Belley-Côté, E. P., et al. (2017). Withholding versus continuing angiotensin-converting enzyme inhibitors or angiotensin II receptor blockers before noncardiac surgery: An analysis of the vascular events in noncardiac surgery patients cohort evaluation prospective cohort. *Anesthesiology*, 126, 16–27.

Solomon, S. D., Skali, H., Anavekar, N. S., Bourgoun, M., Barvik, S., Ghali, J. K., et al. (2005). Changes in ventricular size and function in patients treated with valsartan, captopril, or both after myocardial infarction. *Circulation*, 111, 3411–3419.

van Vark, L. C., Bertrand, M., Akkerhuis, K. M., Brugts, J. J., Fox, K., Mourad, J. J., et al. (2012). Angiotensin-converting enzyme inhibitors reduce mortality in hypertension: A meta-analysis

of randomized clinical trials of renin-angiotensin-aldosterone system inhibitors involving 158, 998 patients. *European Heart Journal*, 33, 2088–2097.

White, H. D. (2003). Should all patients with coronary disease receive angiotensin converting enzyme inhibitors? *Lancet*, 362, 755–757.

Yancy, C. W., Jessup, M., Bozkurt, B., Butler, J., Casey, D. E., Jr., Colvin, M. M., et al. (2016). ACC/AHA/HFSA focused update on new pharmacological therapy for heart failure: An update of the 2013 ACCF/AHA guideline for the management of heart failure: A report of the American College of Cardiology/American Heart Association task force on clinical practice guidelines and the Heart Failure Society of America. *Journal of the American College of Cardiology*, 68, 1476–1488.

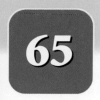

# 65 Bronchodilators

SUNEERAT KONGSAYREEPONG, MD

Three major classes of bronchodilators are used to treat bronchoconstriction: β-adrenergic receptor agonists, methylxanthines, and anticholinergic agents.

## β-Adrenergic Receptor Agonists

β-Adrenergic receptor agonists activate adenyl cyclase, converts adenosine triphosphate to cyclic adenosine 3'-5'-monophosphate (cAMP), which in turn causes relaxation of smooth muscle, resulting in bronchodilation. Selective $\beta_2$-receptor agonists, such as albuterol, terbutaline, and metaproterenol, relax the bronchioles and uterine smooth muscle without affecting the heart via $\beta_1$-receptor stimulation. Nonselective β-receptor agonists used for bronchodilation include epinephrine, isoproterenol, and isoetharine (Table 65.1). Side effects associated with the use of nonselective medications include increased heart rate, contractility, and myocardial $O_2$ consumption. Selective $\beta_2$-receptor agonists may also produce some cardiac effects, especially if administered subcutaneously or intravenously. Hypokalemia and hyperglycemia may also occur. Chronic use can be associated with tachyphylaxis.

Inhaled therapy is the preferred route with direct action on the airway, resulting in a lower amount of drug used and minimized side effects. Therapeutic aerosols may be administered, preferably with a metered-dose inhaler (MDI) or as a wet aerosol from a nebulizer containing the medication. Only particles with a diameter of 1 to 5 μm are efficiently deposited in the lower respiratory tract, which is one of the primary reasons why 13% of the output from MDIs, compared with only 1% to 5% of the output from nebulizers, reaches the lower respiratory tract. Propellants used in MDIs are blends of liquefied gas chlorofluorocarbons (CFCs), which can damage the earth's ozone layer; in addition, some patients are sensitive to these propellants, which can cause bronchospasm. Because of these concerns, some MDIs use hydrofluoroalkanes (HFAs) as the propellant. The HFA formulations of albuterol and ipratropium bromide have been shown to be equivalent to their respective CFC formulations. However, the delivered dose of HFA-formulated beclomethasone dipropionate is five times greater than the dose delivered with the original CFC formulation.

A breath-activated nebulizer, a new type of jet nebulizer, has a low dead-space volume and nebulizes only on inspiration. With this type of nebulizer, waste during exhalation should be eliminated. The delivered dose can be more than three times greater than the dose delivered with continuous nebulization.

Continuous bronchodilator therapy is sometimes necessary for the treatment of severe bronchospasm, such as for status asthmaticus. In such situations, a low dose of continuous nebulized bronchodilator (e.g., albuterol, 10–15 mg/h) should be

| TABLE 65.1 | Bronchodilators | | |
|---|---|---|---|
| Drug | Trade Name(s) | Delivery Mode/Route | Mechanism of Action |
| **β-ADRENERGIC RECEPTOR AGONISTS** | | | |
| Isoproterenol 0.05% | Isuprel | Nebulizer | Prototypical β-adrenergic receptor agonists; significant β1 side effects |
| Albuterol 0.5% | Ventolin Proventil | Oral, DPI MDI/nebulizer | $\beta_2$-Adrenergic receptor agonists; increase in cAMP |
| Isoetharine hydrochloride 1% | Bronkosol | MDI/nebulizer | $\beta_2$-Adrenergic receptor agonists; increase in cAMP |
| Metaproterenol sulfate 5% | Alupent Metaprel | MDI/nebulizer/oral | $\beta_2$-Adrenergic receptor agonists; increase in cAMP |
| Terbutaline 0.1% | | Oral/SQ/nebulizer/IV | $\beta_2$-Adrenergic receptor agonists |
| **METHYLXANTHINES** | | | |
| Aminophylline | Somophyllin | Oral/IV | Inhibition of cAMP breakdown by phosphodiesterase |
| Theophylline | Respbid, Slo-Bid, Theo-24 Theolair | Oral/IV | Adenosine antagonism |
| **ANTICHOLINERGICS** | | | |
| Atropine sulfate 2% or 5% | Abboject | SQ, IM, IV, nebulizer | Cholinergic blocker, decreased cGMP |
| Ipratropium bromide 0.02% | Atrovent | MDI/nebulizer | Cholinergic blocker, decreased cGMP |

*cAMP*, Cyclic adenosine monophosphate; *cGMP*, cyclic guanosine monophosphate; *DPI*, dry-powder inhaler; *IM*, intramuscular; *IV*, intravenous; *MDI*, metered-dose inhaler; *SQ*, subcutaneous.

used, and the patient should be continuously monitored for side effects (e.g., tachycardia, arrhythmias, hypokalemia) and worsening of symptoms.

Dry-powder inhalers (DPIs) deliver drugs in powder form to the lung. When using this type of inhaler, patients must generate sufficient inspiratory flow rate ($\geq$50 L/min). Generating this level of inspiratory flow rate may be difficult for patients to achieve if they are in acute respiratory distress, especially during a severe asthmatic attack.

Noninvasive ventilation and high-flow nasal cannula are increasingly used in patients who have acute respiratory failure postoperatively. Inhaled aerosol bronchodilator therapy can also be effectively used in combination with noninvasive ventilation or a high-flow nasal cannula without discontinuation of the system.

## CATECHOLAMINES

Catecholamines are potent and effective bronchodilators that have a rapid onset of action, reach their peak effect quickly, and have a short duration of action (0.5–3 h). These drugs are useful when rapid onset is needed.

Epinephrine has both $\alpha$-adrenergic and $\beta$-adrenergic properties. A dose of 0.3 to 0.5 mg given subcutaneously is commonly used to treat acute bronchospasm. The effects are rapid, peaking at 5 to 25 min, and improvements in pulmonary function are seen for up to 4 h. Side effects include increased heart rate, cardiac output, and systolic blood pressure and decreased diastolic blood pressure, and systemic vascular resistance.

Of the sympathomimetics, isoproterenol is the most potent $\beta$-adrenergic receptor agonist. It is effective when administered intravenously or inhaled. However, it has essentially been replaced by selective $\beta_2$-adrenergic receptor agonists.

## RESORCINOLS

Resorcinols are $\beta$-adrenergic receptor agonists with rapid onset and longer duration of action. They are well absorbed from the gastrointestinal tract and can be given orally.

Metaproterenol, a selective $\beta_2$-adrenergic resorcinol, is available as a solution for aerosol delivery, as a tablet, as a syrup, and for use in an MDI. Onset is 5 to 15 min, with a peak effect at 30 to 60 min and a duration of 3 to 4 h. As a resorcinol, metaproterenol has hydroxyl groups at the 3 and 5 positions of the phenyl ring (as opposed to catecholamines, which have them at the 3 and 4 positions). Therefore metaproterenol is resistant to metabolism by catechol-$O$-methyltransferase and has a longer duration of action than most catecholamines. It has enough structural similarities to isoproterenol, metaproterenol has substantial cardiac side effects.

Terbutaline, a selective $\beta_2$-adrenergic receptor agonist, has an onset of action of 5 to 15 min, a peak effect at 30 to 60 min, and a duration of action of 4 to 6 h. A dose of 0.25–0.5 mg administered subcutaneously is an alternative treatment for acute severe bronchospasm when the cardiac effects of epinephrine must be avoided. However, when given subcutaneously, terbutaline has some $\beta_1$-adrenergic effects and may cause ventricular arrhythmias in patients who have been anesthetized with halothane.

## SALIGENINS

Saligenins are the most recently developed $\beta$-adrenergic receptor agonists and have the most $\beta_2$-receptor specificity. Drugs in this group have a rapid onset of action and a duration of action of approximately 4 to 6 h.

Albuterol, a selective $\beta_2$-adrenergic receptor agonist, has very few side effects; cardiac effects are unlikely when the dose of albuterol is less than 400 $\mu$g. Its onset of action is 15 min, with a peak effect at 30 to 60 min and a duration of 4 to 6 h. Albuterol is available as a syrup, oral tablet, extended-release tablet, nebulizer solution, MDI, and DPI.

Salmeterol is a very lipophilic, selective $\beta_2$-adrenergic receptor agonist that must diffuse through the phospholipid membrane before reaching the receptor site. Its onset of action is very slow; therefore this drug cannot be used as a rescue medication. Salmeterol has a very long duration of action.

Formoterol is a selective $\beta_2$-adrenergic receptor agonist with a rapid onset of action (within 2–3 min) and a long duration of action (12 h). However, it cannot be used as a rescue drug because of potential toxicity.

## Methylxanthines

Theophylline is a poorly soluble methylxanthine that is found in high concentrations in tea leaves. Methylxanthines inhibit the breakdown of cAMP by phosphodiesterase. Aminophylline is the water-soluble salt of theophylline that can be administered orally (3–6 mg/kg per day, divided and given every 6–8 h) or intravenously (loading dose of 5 mg/kg, followed by 0.5–1.0 mg/kg/h). Therapeutic plasma concentrations of theophylline are between 5 and 15 $\mu$g/mL, although levels as low as 5 $\mu$g/mL have been shown to be clinically effective.

Aminophylline works in vitro by inhibiting phosphodiesterase and thereby cAMP breakdown. The in vivo mechanism of aminophylline is less clear. Antiinflammatory actions on neutrophils, sympathetic stimulation, and adenosine antagonism are possible mechanisms. The narrow therapeutic range of aminophylline and the potential for arrhythmias developing in patients with the use of this drug have made its use in the perioperative setting controversial. Theophylline is principally metabolized by the liver, and 10% is excreted unchanged in urine. Smokers metabolize the drug faster than do nonsmokers. Heart failure, liver disease, and severe respiratory obstruction all slow the metabolism of theophylline and increase the likelihood of toxicity. Metabolism is slowed by cimetidine and $\beta$-adrenergic receptor antagonists.

Theophylline improves pulmonary function and resolves obstruction, in a dose-dependent manner, in patients with reactive airway disease. The drug decreases pulmonary vascular resistance and increases cardiac output. The cardiac-stimulating effects of theophylline are still seen in the presence of $\beta$-blockade because xanthines are not receptor dependent. Theophylline has been shown to decrease the number and duration of apneic episodes in preterm infants.

Side effects with the use of theophylline are often seen when plasma levels exceed 20 $\mu$g/mL. The most frequent side effects are nausea and vomiting. Seizures may result from toxic levels and are likely to occur when plasma concentrations exceed 40 $\mu$g/mL. Tachycardia and other arrhythmias may also occur with high plasma levels. Theophylline facilitates neuromuscular transmission; thus patients receiving theophylline may require higher than normal doses of nondepolarizing neuromuscular blocking agents.

## Anticholinergic Agents

Cholinergic mechanisms play a major role in mediating reflex bronchoconstriction, and anticholinergic drugs may be used to reduce these responses. These medications may be more effective than $\beta$-adrenergic receptor agonists in some patients with chronic bronchitis and emphysema. In the management of asthma, anticholinergic agents are generally less effective than are $\beta$-adrenergic receptor agonists, but in acute asthma, a combination of the two types of agents may produce a greater response. Patients who received combined therapy were more likely to experience adverse events, such as tremor, agitation, and palpitation, than those who received $\beta$-adrenergic receptor agonists alone.

Atropine sulfate, a parasympatholytic that can relax airway smooth muscle, can also be given by nebulizer. Because atropine reduces mucociliary clearance and causes other central nervous system and cardiovascular side effects, even at low doses, this medication is not commonly used as a bronchodilator.

Ipratropium bromide, a quaternary amine delivered by nebulizer or MDI, has little systemic absorption. Its bronchodilator effects begin within minutes, with a peak effect at 1 to 2 h. Ipratropium has little or no effect on mucociliary clearance from the lung and little or no effect on heart rate, blood pressure, and the gastrointestinal tract. Ipratropium is also available in combination with albuterol.

## Antiinflammatory Agents

Antiinflammatory agents, such as cromolyn sodium, which stabilize mast cell membranes and thereby intervene in the inflammatory process, are frequently used to treat bronchospastic diseases.

Corticosteroids block both the initial immune response and the subsequent inflammatory process. Corticosteroids do not have direct effects on bronchial smooth muscle relaxation but facilitate the effects of $\beta_2$-adrenergic receptor agonists. Even though the cellular and biochemical effects are immediate, the full clinical effects take longer. The increase in $\beta$-adrenergic receptor agonist response occurs within 2 h, and $\beta$-adrenergic receptor agonist density increases within 4 h. Systemically administered steroids, such as hydrocortisone or methylprednisolone, may be required in patients with poor response to $\beta_2$-adrenergic receptor agonists over 1 to 2 h. Inhaled corticosteroids, such as beclomethasone, flunisolide, and triamcinolone, which are available as MDIs, DPIs, and nebulizer solutions, are then used to minimize systemic side effects. Symptoms usually improve in 1 to 2 weeks, with maximal response most often occurring at 4 to 8 weeks.

A combination of a corticosteroid and a long-acting $\beta_2$-agonist in one inhaler is more effective than long-acting $\beta_2$-agonists in chronic obstructive pulmonary disease.

## Adjunctive Medication

Although the exact mechanism by which $MgSO_4$ relaxes airway smooth muscle is not completely understood, it is believed to act through blockade of voltage-dependent calcium channels, thereby inhibiting $Ca^{2+}$ influx. Intravenously administered $MgSO_4$ (2 g) is a safe and effective adjunct for the treatment of acute asthma and bronchospasm in both adults and children. Nebulized $MgSO_4$ has been used, but this treatment is controversial, and in a recent metaanalysis nebulized $MgSO_4$ shown did not show significant benefits on respiratory function.

Inhalation anesthetic agents, such as isoflurane, in subanesthetic doses, have been used to relieve bronchospasm after extubation and in patients with status asthmaticus. They have also occasionally been used long-term (i.e., 2–3 days) in the intensive care unit in patients with status asthmaticus.

## SUGGESTED READINGS

Ari, A., & Fink, J. B. (2020). Recent advances in aerosol devices for the delivery of inhaled medications. *Expert Opinion on Drug Delivery, 17,* 133–144.

Bayable, S. D., Melesse, D. Y., Lema, G. F., & Ahmed, S. A. (2021). Perioperative management of patients with asthma during elective surgery: A systematic review. *Annals of Medicine and Surgery, 70,* 102874.

Fink, J., & Ari, A. (2019) Aerosol drug therapy. In R. Kacmarek, J. James Stoller, A. l. Heuer (Eds.),

*Egan's Fundamentals of Respiratory Care* (12th ed., pp. 842–884). St. Louis: Mosby.

Hess, D. R. (2015). Aerosol therapy during noninvasive ventilation or high-flow nasal cannula. *Respiratory Care, 60,* 880–891.

Kirkland, S. W., Vandenberghe, C., Voaklander, B., Nikel, T., Campbell, S., & Rowe, B. H. (2017). Combined inhaled beta-agonist and anticholinergic agents for emergency management in adults with asthma. *Cochrane Database of Systematic Reviews, 1*(1), CD001284.

Su, Z., Li, R., & Gai, Z. (2018). Intravenous and nebulized magnesium sulfate for treating acute asthma in children: A systematic review and meta-analysis. *Pediatric Emergency Care, 34,* 390–395.

Tan, D. J., White, C. J., Walters, J. A., & Walters, E. H. (2016). Inhaled corticosteroids with combination inhaled long-acting beta(2)-agonists and long-acting muscarinic antagonists for chronic obstructive pulmonary disease. *Cochrane Database of Systematic Reviews, 11,* CD011600.

# 66

# Antiemetics

CARSON C. WELKER, MD

Postoperative nausea and vomiting (PONV) occurs frequently, affecting 30% to 50% of the general surgical population and up to 80% of high-risk patients. The emetic reflex involves stimulation of the chemoreceptor trigger zone (CTZ) in the area postrema, which sends signals to the vomiting center in the brainstem. Although the CTZ is located in the central nervous system, it lacks a blood-brain barrier and is readily exposed to substances in the blood. The CTZ is susceptible to dopamine and serotonin (5-HT) in the blood and cerebrospinal fluid and also can be activated by opioids and certain anesthetic agents.

Prevention of PONV is more effective than treatment after symptoms occur. Prevention includes identification of high-risk patients and tailoring the anesthetic plan accordingly by avoiding emetogenic volatile anesthetics, nitrous oxide, and opioids. Prophylactic treatment is a pillar of PONV management alongside multimodal pain control with agents such as acetaminophen, nonsteroidal antiinflammatory drugs, and cyclo-oxygenase-2 inhibitors, all of which may reduce perioperative opioid requirements. Regional anesthesia or infiltration with local anesthetics also reduces opioid requirements and thus is similarly beneficial in PONV reduction. Adequate intravenous (IV) hydration can reduce the baseline risk of PONV, with no difference noted between crystalloid and colloid solutions. The presence of bispectral index monitoring possibly correlates with improved PONV by granting the ability to target anesthetic dosing thereby minimizing emetogenic agents. Preventions that have not been shown to be helpful include nasogastric tube placement for gastric emptying, targeting a higher fraction of inspired oxygen or specific avoidance of neostigmine.

The relatively low risk of side effects associated with the use of antiemetic drugs overall has been confirmed in several metaanalyses in commonly used antiemetics including 5-hydroxytryptamine ($5-HT_3$) antagonists, $D_2$-receptor antagonists, steroids, neurokinin-1 antagonists, and anticholinergics. One to five of every 100 people experience mild side effects, such as sedation or headache, when given an antiemetic drug. Despite decades of investigation, it is still not possible to guarantee that an individual will not experience PONV, which can result in significant surgical recovery interference extending into postdischarge nausea and vomiting (PDNV). See Table 66.1 for an overview of antiemetic drugs.

## 5-Hydroxytryptamine (Serotonin, $5-HT_3$) Receptor Antagonists

The $5-HT_3$ receptor antagonists (ondansetron, granisetron, palonosetron) bind to receptors in the CTZ and the gastrointestinal tract. Most information is based on studies of ondansetron. Studies show ondansetron to be as effective as both

| TABLE 66.1 | Antiemetic Drugs With Recommended Dosage and Timing of Administration if Established | |
|---|---|---|
| **Drug** | **Dose** | **Timing** |
| Aprepitant | 40–80 mg PO | At induction |
| Dexamethasone | 4–8 mg IV | At induction |
| Dimenhydrinate | 1 mg/kg IV | – |
| Droperidol | 0.625–1.25 mg IV | End of surgery |
| Granisetron | 0.35–3 mg IV | End of surgery |
| Haloperidol | 0.4–2 mg IV | – |
| Methylprednisolone | 40 mg IV | – |
| Ondansetron | 4 mg IV, 8 mg PO | End of surgery |
| Palonosetron | 0.075 mg IV | At induction |
| Perphenazine | 5 mg IV | – |
| Promethazine | 6.25–12.5 mg IV | – |
| Scopolamine | Transdermal | Previous evening/2 h before surgery |

*IV,* Intravenous; *PO,* oral.

droperidol and dexamethasone. In general, $5-HT_3$ receptor antagonists have greater antiemetic than antinausea effects. Palonosetron, a second-generation $5-HT_3$ receptor antagonist, has been shown to be more effective than granisetron and ondansetron in preventing PONV. Palonosetron, unlike the other $5-HT_3$ receptor antagonists, is more effective when given at the beginning of surgery, possibly because of its extended half-life of 48 h. Palonosetron may also have benefit in postdischarge nausea and vomiting. Oral granisetron, with more $5-HT_3$ affinity than ondansetron, has been shown to be just as effective as intravenous ondansetron for lowering the occurrence of PONV in laparoscopic procedures.

## SIDE EFFECTS

The $5-HT_3$ receptor antagonists besides palonosetron have the potential to affect the QTc interval. The U.S. Food and Drug Administration (FDA) recommends a single maximum dose for ondansetron of 16 mg IV. Other side effects include headache, constipation, and elevated liver enzyme levels.

## Antidopaminergic Drugs

Antidopaminergic drugs ($D_2$-receptor antagonists) include the butyrophenones (haloperidol, droperidol), phenothiazines, metoclopramide. Prophylactic low-dose droperidol (<1 mg or

15 µg/kg IV) is effective for the prevention of PONV when administered at the end of surgery. The efficacy has been shown to be similar to that of ondansetron, with low risk of adverse effects. Haloperidol reduces PONV risk at doses (0.5–2 mg intramuscularly or IV) much lower than those used to treat psychosis. The efficacy has been shown to be similar to that of ondansetron.

Prochlorperazine, a phenothiazine, and promethazine, a phenothiazine derivative, inhibit dopamine and muscarinic receptors while competing with histamine for the $H_1$ receptor. Studies show limited efficacy of these drugs, and they are not recommended as first-line agents.

Metoclopramide, a procainamide derivative, inhibits dopamine and serotonin receptors. Additionally, it enhances gastric emptying by selective peripheral cholinergic agonism. It has an antiemetic effect similar to that of ondansetron in preventing early PONV at doses larger than 20 mg. However, this dose is associated with more side effects. It is also less efficacious in late PONV.

Amisulpride is a $D_2/D_3$ receptor antagonist used in the treatment of psychosis and recently was approved by the FDA for the treatment and prevention of PONV. It has been found to be safe and effective for moderate-risk and high-risk patients in several randomized double-blind studies.

## SIDE EFFECTS

In 2001, the FDA issued a "black box" restriction on droperidol because of its propensity to prolong the QT interval. However, the doses used for PONV prophylaxis are extremely low and have not been associated with cardiovascular events. At these clinically relevant doses, studies have shown equal QTc effects of droperidol versus ondansetron and haloperidol versus ondansetron. Similarly, in 2012, the FDA issued a Drug Safety Communication regarding concerns about ondansetron and prolongation of QTc. The combination of either droperidol or haloperidol with ondansetron does not increase the risk of QTc prolongation.

Promethazine has an FDA black box label for severe tissue damage, so it should never be administered near an artery or subcutaneously.

Antidopaminergic drugs should not be used in patients with Parkinson disease, restless legs syndrome, or any other disorder in which dopaminergic drugs are used to treat the signs and symptoms of the disease. Extrapyramidal reactions, sedation, diarrhea, and orthostatic hypotension can occur with all antidopaminergic drugs.

## Anticholinergic Agents

Muscarinic antagonists (e.g., scopolamine) or anticholinergic agents act on the vomiting center and digestive tract and reduce gastrointestinal hyperreactivity. They also help in the management of motion sickness. The scopolamine patch has a 2 to 4 h onset of effect, so it is most effective if applied the night before or 2 to 4 h before surgery. The patch effectively prevents PONV and PDNV for up to 24 h. Studies have shown equal effectiveness as ondansetron or droperidol.

## SIDE EFFECTS

Adverse effects of anticholinergic medications are dry mouth, drowsiness or other mental status changes, urinary retention, and blurred vision. Scopolamine should be avoided in pediatric and older patient populations as these adverse reactions can be more pronounced.

## Steroids

Dexamethasone 4 to 8 mg IV given at the beginning of surgery is effective PONV prophylaxis. Recent studies suggest that higher doses (8 mg) of dexamethasone enhance postdischarge quality of recovery and also reduce pain. The effect of dexamethasone is similar to that of ondansetron or droperidol.

The exact mechanism of the antiinflammatory action of dexamethasone is unknown; however, it inhibits multiple inflammatory cytokines in the central and peripheral nervous systems and stabilizes plasma membranes at central and peripheral sites.

## SIDE EFFECTS

The safety concerns about dexamethasone center on the increased risk of wound infection and hyperglycemia. Most studies support the notion that a single dose of IV dexamethasone does not increase the risk of wound infection; however, it has been suggested in the literature. Increased blood glucose has been shown in healthy subjects receiving dexamethasone, so its use in patients with labile diabetes must be carefully considered. There is no concern for increased steroid-induced delirium.

## Neurokinin-1 Receptor Antagonists

The neuropeptide substance P binds to neurokinin-1 receptors and acts as a dominant mediator of vomiting, especially 12 h after a dose of chemotherapy. Aprepitant, a substance P antagonist, has a 40-h half-life and is typically given as a single 40- to 80-mg dose by mouth within 3 h before anesthesia. For the first 24 h after surgery, aprepitant is as effective as ondansetron in preventing PONV. In the 24 to 48 h after surgery, aprepitant is more effective than ondansetron in preventing PONV. Because of its high cost, aprepitant should be reserved for high-risk PONV patients or those with adverse reactions to other antiemetics. Fosaprepitant, an IV water-soluble neurokinin-1 antagonist, has been shown to more effective in preventing vomiting 48 h after surgery compared with ondansetron.

## SIDE EFFECTS

Combined use of aprepitant and hormonal contraceptives reduces the efficacy of contraceptives. Alternative methods of contraception must be used to prevent pregnancy for 1 month after the last aprepitant dose. Fatigue, nausea, hiccups, constipation, diarrhea, and abdominal pain are other side effects; neutropenia, anaphylactic reactions, and Stevens-Johnson syndrome are rarer.

## Other Antiemetics

### PROPOFOL

Propofol has antiemetic properties at subhypotic dose ranges. Studies have shown that low-dose infusions (20 µg/kg/min) reduce the risk of PONV. Additionally, the use of propofol for induction and maintenance of anesthesia reduces the incidence of PONV within the first 6 h of surgery. Propofol boluses

(20 mg) are as effective as ondansetron as rescue therapy; however, the duration of effect is likely brief.

## MIDAZOLAM

Midazolam 2 mg administered at the end of surgery has been shown to be as effective as ondansetron in preventing PONV.

## DIPHENHYDRAMINE

Diphenhydramine is an $H_1$-receptor inverse agonist that likely acts in the gastrointestinal tract to prevent vagally mediated transmission to the vomiting center. It seems particularly useful in nausea and vomiting associated with the vestibular system, such as strabismus and middle ear surgeries. It has anticholinergic properties that can result in antidyskinetic and sedative effects. Dimenhydrinate is a combination of diphenhydramine and 8-chlorotheophylline (which reduces drowsiness) and potentially has antiemetic effectiveness similar to that of both droperidol and 5-$HT_3$ antagonists. However, more data are needed on the timing of its use, dose response, and side effects.

## $\alpha_2$-AGONISTS

$\alpha_2$-Agonists, such as clonidine and dexmedetomidine, have shown weak PONV effects, possibly as a result of direct antiemetic properties or an opioid-sparing effect. Clonidine can be used both orally and through neuraxial administration and has been shown to reduce opioid consumption and decrease PONV.

## GABAPENTIN AND PREGABALIN

Studies have shown that gabapentin 600 mg given 2 h before surgery decreases PONV, likely from an opioid-sparing mechanism. However, pregabalin has not demonstrated similar effect.

## MECLIZINE

Meclizine 50 mg in combination with ondansetron has been shown to be more effective than either ondansetron or meclizine alone.

## MIRTAZAPINE

Mirtazapine is a 5-$HT_3$ receptor antagonist and noradrenergic antidepressant that has been shown to delay PONV onset when given prophylactically, especially in combination with dexamethasone.

## ANTIPSYCHOTICS

Antipsychotics such as aripiprazole, olanzapine, and risperidone are not traditionally thought of as antiemetics but have shown potential to reduce antiemetic administration in the postanesthesia care unit. This data is only based on propensity-matched scoring but deserves more investigation.

## GINGER

Ginger reduces stomach contractions and intestinal motility secondary to its anticholinergic and antiserotonergic effects. Ginger is regarded as safe and has been shown to be useful in pregnancy, chemotherapy, and reducing PONV in the operative setting.

# Nonpharmacological Prophylaxis

## USE OF A COOLING FAN AND PERIBUCCAL ISOPROPYL ALCOHOL

The use of a cooling fan in combination with peribuccal isopropyl alcohol is believed to stimulate the V2 distribution of the trigeminal nerve and olfactory nerve, respectively. According to a Cochrane review, isopropyl alcohol was more effective than a saline placebo for reducing PONV but less effective than standard antiemetic drugs.

## AROMA THERAPY

Aromatherapy, typically in the form of essential oils, has shown some benefits in reducing PONV and PDNV when used as an adjunct to standard pharmacologic therapies. However, other authors have demonstrated no difference from placebo compared with aromatherapy alone. More investigations are needed.

## AURICULAR ACUPUNCTURE AND USE OF THE WRIST P6 POINT

Many theories exist as to the mechanism of action with regard to acupuncture in treating nausea and vomiting. In a Cochrane review, compared with sham treatment, P6 acupoint stimulation significantly reduced nausea, vomiting, and the need for rescue antiemetics. There was no evidence of a difference between P6 acupoint stimulation and antiemetic drugs in the risk of nausea, vomiting, or the need for rescue antiemetics.

## COMBINATION THERAPY

The effects of different antiemetics acting on different receptors are additive (Table 66.2). For example, ondansetron has better antiemetic effects, whereas droperidol has better antinausea effects, so they work well in combination. Studies also support the use of ondansetron or droperidol with dexamethasone. However, optimal dosing regiments must be established.

| TABLE 66.2 | Recommended Combination Therapy | |
|---|---|---|
| **Recommended Combination** | | **Evidence Level** |
| Droperidol + dexamethasone | | A1 |
| 5-$HT_3$ antagonist + dexamethasone | | A1 |
| 5-$HT_3$ antagonist + droperidol | | A1 |
| 5-$HT_3$ antagonist + dexamethasone + droperidol | | A2 |

*5-$HT_3$,* 5-Hydroxytryptamine (serotonin) receptor antagonist.

## SUGGESTED READINGS

Apfel, C. C., Korttila, K., Abdalla, M., Kerger, H., Turan, A., Vedder, I., et al. (2004). A factorial trial of six interventions for the prevention of postoperative nausea and vomiting. *New England Journal of Medicine, 350*, 2441–2451.

Carlisle, J. B., & Stevenson, C. A. (2006). Drugs for preventing postoperative nausea and vomiting. *Cochrane Database of Systematic Reviews, 2006*(3), CD004125.

Gan, T. J., Diemunsch, P., Habib, A. S., Kovac, A., Kranke, P., Meyer, T. A., et al. (2014). Consensus guidelines for the management of postoperative nausea and vomiting. *Anesthesia and Analgesia, 118*(1), 85–113.

Gan, T. J., Kranke, P., Minkowitz, H. S., Bergese, S. D., Motsch, J., Eberhart, L., et al. (2017). Intravenous amisulpride for the prevention of postoperative nausea and vomiting: Two concurrent, randomized, double-blind, placebo-controlled trials. *Anesthesiology, 126*(2), 268–275.

Hines, S., Steels, E., Chang, A., & Gibbons, K. (2012). Aromatherapy for treatment of postoperative nausea and vomiting. *Cochrane Database of Systematic Reviews, *(4), CD007598.

Jabaley, C. S., Gray, D. W., Budhrani, G. S., Lynde, G. C., Adamopoulos, P., Easton, G. S., et al. (2020). Chronic atypical antipsychotic use is associated with reduced need for postoperative nausea and vomiting rescue in the postanesthesia care unit: A propensity-matched retrospective observational study. *Anesthesia and Analgesia, 130*(1), 141–150.

Lee, A., & Fan, L. T. (2009). Stimulation of the wrist acupuncture point P6 for preventing postoperative nausea and vomiting. *Cochrane Database of Systematic Reviews, *(2), CD003281.

Miller, R. D. (2010). *Miller's Anesthesia* (7th ed.). Philadelphia, PA: Churchill Livingstone/Elsevier.

Odom-Forren, J., Jalota, L., Moser, D. K., Lennie, T. A., Hall, L. A., Holtman, J., et al. (2013). Incidence and predictors of postdischarge nausea and vomiting in a 7-day population. *Journal of Clinical Anesthesia, 25*(7), 551–559. doi:10.1016/j.jclinane.2013.05.008.

Weibel, S., Schaefer, M. S., Raj, D., Rücker, G., Pace, N. L., Schlesinger, T., et al. (2021). Drugs for preventing postoperative nausea and vomiting in adults after general anaesthesia: An abridged Cochrane network meta-analysis. *Anaesthesia, 76*(7), 962–973. doi:10.1111/anae.15295.

# SECTION IV

# Colloids and Blood Products

# Albumin, Hetastarch, and Pentastarch

EDWIN H. RHO, MD

## The Colloid Controversy

For decades, medical debate has continued over the value of colloid infusion in the perioperative setting. It is important to note that in patients who are massively bleeding and require intravascular volume expansion—especially patients with trauma—first-line therapy is the use of blood products. Early colloid advocates argued that it was important to maintain normal colloid osmotic pressure to keep intravascular fluid from passing into the tissues and thereby contributing to pulmonary, cerebral, or subcutaneous edema or ascites. Albumin was the most widely used colloid before the hydroxyethyl starches were developed, and has become increasingly used again secondary to concerns of morbidity associated with hydroxyethyl starches.

## Albumin

Albumin is available in 5% and 25% concentrations, the latter being most useful in patients who cannot tolerate large volumes of fluid. Albumin is a heat-stable tightly wound protein molecule derived from human whole blood. It is heated to 60°C for 10 h to eradicate infectious organisms (both bacterial and viral). That, combined with effective donor-screening processes, minimizes the extremely remote risk of transmission of infectious diseases. Transmission of Creutzfeldt-Jakob disease has not been reported with the use of albumin, although it remains a theoretical risk.

## Hetastarch and Pentastarch

Both hetastarch and pentastarch are composed of chains of glucose molecules to which hydroxyethyl ether groups have been added to retard degradation. The glucose chains are highly branched, being derived from the starch amylopectin. One in 20 glucose monomers branches. Starch chains of various lengths are present in hetastarch, giving it an average molecular weight of 450 kD. Its number-average molecular weight is 69 kD; this term describes a simple average of the individual molecular weights and is more closely related to oncotic pressure. Approximately 80% of hetastarch polymers have a molecular weight of 30 to 2400 kD. Hetastarch is available as a 6% solution in 0.9% sodium chloride or a lactated electrolyte solution. The chemical and pharmacokinetic properties of hetastarch and pentastarch are listed in Table 67.1.

Hetastarch and pentastarch do not interfere with blood typing or crossmatching, are stable with fluctuating temperatures, and rarely cause allergic reactions. Both have been used successfully as an adjunct in leukapheresis by increasing the erythrocyte sedimentation rate to enhance granulocyte yield.

## PHARMACOKINETICS AND PHARMACODYNAMICS OF HETASTARCH AND PENTASTARCH

The colloidal properties of both hetastarch and pentastarch resemble those of 5% human albumin. Distribution is throughout the intravascular space. The principal effect after intravenous administration of any colloidal solution is plasma volume expansion secondary to the colloidal osmotic effect. In patients with hypovolemia, the prolonged plasma volume expansion causes a temporary increase in arterial and venous pressures, cardiac index, left ventricular stroke work index, and pulmonary artery occlusion pressure. The effective intravascular half-life is 25.5 h for 6% hetastarch and 2.5 h for 10% pentastarch. Both substances are eliminated by the kidney. The hydroxyethyl group is not cleared but remains attached to glucose units when excreted. Hetastarch and pentastarch molecules of less than 50,000 Da are rapidly eliminated by the kidneys. However, only 33% of an initial dose of hetastarch is eliminated within 24 h of administration, compared with approximately 70% of an initial dose of pentastarch. Up to 10% of administered hetastarch can be detected intravascularly after 2 weeks. Pentastarch is undetectable intravascularly 1 week after administration.

As a result of a lower molar substitution ratio (i.e., the number of hydroxyethyl groups per glucose unit), pentastarch is more rapidly and completely degraded by circulating amylase than is hetastarch. Hetastarch has a very long tissue retention time (a half-life of 10–15 days) because the larger molecules are stored in the liver and spleen, where they are slowly degraded enzymatically by amylase. There is a theoretical concern about impaired reticuloendothelial function caused by hetastarch. Accordingly, a pentastarch with lower molecular weight was developed to minimize this theoretical risk.

## ADVERSE EFFECTS OF HETASTARCH AND PENTASTARCH

Both hetastarch and pentastarch prolong prothrombin time, partial thromboplastin time, and bleeding times when given in large doses, most likely secondary to hemodilution. There is some evidence to suggest that platelet function may also be altered by both products. For this reason, the maximum recommended dose is 15 to 20 mL/kg. Although there are case reports of coagulopathy in neurosurgical patients after large (2 L) doses of hetastarch, the effects of hetastarch on the coagulation system seem clinically insignificant when maximum dose recommendations are not exceeded. More recently, tetrastarches have been developed to enhance degradation and minimize retention in the blood and tissues. This may be beneficial because the effects on coagulation and platelets may be decreased.

| TABLE 67.1 | Chemical and Pharmacokinetic Properties of Hetastarch* and Pentastarch | |
|---|---|---|
| Property | 6% Hetastarch | 10% Pentastarch |
| pH | 5.5 | 5.0 |
| $MW_W$ (kDa) | 450 (range, 10–1000) | 264 (range, 150–350) |
| $MW_N$ (kDa) | 69 | 63 |
| Calculated osmolar concentration (mOsmol/L) | 310 | 326 |
| Molar substitution ratio | 0.7 | 0.45 |
| Intravascular half-life (h) | 25.5 | 2.5 |
| Renal elimination | Molecules smaller than 50 kDa are rapidly excreted; <10% detected intravascularly at 2 weeks | Molecules smaller than 50 kDa are rapidly excreted; undetectable intravascularly at 1 week |
| Coagulation effects | ↑ in PT, aPTT, and clotting time; may interfere with platelet function | ↑ in PT, aPTT, and clotting time; may interfere with platelet function |
| Other miscellaneous effects | ↑ in indirect serum bilirubin levels; temporary ↑ in serum amylase concentration | Temporary ↑ in serum amylase concentration |

*In 2010 to 2011, several medical journals retracted articles describing studies examining the use of hetastarch. However, the data presented here are accurate.

*aPTT*, Activated partial thromboplastin time; *MW_N*, number-average molecular weight; *MW_W*, weight-average molecular weight; *PT*, prothrombin time.

Both hetastarch and pentastarch have been reported to produce rare hypersensitivity reactions, such as wheezing and urticaria. However, neither substance has been shown to stimulate antibody formation.

Transient increases in serum amylase and indirect bilirubin levels have occurred after hetastarch and pentastarch administration. However, no association with pancreatitis or biliary injury has been reported.

## Clinical Usefulness of Colloids

Multiple authors have studied the importance of colloids in perioperative fluid therapy and attempted to determine the value of colloid solutions in comparison with inexpensive crystalloid solutions. Colloids have not been proven to prevent the extravascular accumulations that lead to edema in the lungs, pleura, brain, abdomen, and soft tissues of critically injured and ill patients. In the past, clinical trials failed to show a difference in outcome for patients receiving colloid versus crystalloid solutions. More recent studies have suggested that hydroxyethyl starches may be associated with an increased risk of mortality, acute kidney injury, renal replacement therapy, or a combination compared with crystalloid solutions. Albumin may be associated with higher mortality rates in critically ill patients with traumatic brain injury compared with normal saline. Nonetheless, colloids may be useful in patients who cannot tolerate large volumes of intravenous fluids yet need preload expansion.

## Contraindications to the Use of Colloid Solutions

Hetastarch and pentastarch are contraindicated in patients with known hypersensitivity to hydroxyethyl starch, as well as critically ill adults, including those with severe sepsis/septic shock, coagulopathy, congestive heart failure in which volume overload may pose a problem, or renal disease. In response to evidence of hydroxyethyl starch solutions increasing mortality, acute kidney injury, and excessive bleeding, the U.S. Food and Drug Administration has issued a boxed warning and recommended use only when adequate alternative treatments are not available.

## Acknowledgment

The author and editors would like to thank Ronald J. Faust, MD, for his work on this chapter in previous editions.

## SUGGESTED READINGS

Allen, C. J., Valle, E. J., Jouria, J. M., Schulman, C. I., Namias, N., Livingstone, A. S., et al. (2014). Differences between blunt and penetrating trauma after resuscitation with HES. *Journal of Trauma and Acute Care Surgery, 77*(6), 859–864.

Barron, M., Wilkes, M., & Nvickis, R. (2004). A systematic review of the comparative safety of colloids. *Archives of Surgery, 139,* 552–563.

Bellomo, R., Morimatsu, H., Presneill, J., French, C., Cole, L., Story, D., et al. (2009). Effects of saline or albumin resuscitation on standard coagulation tests. *Critical Care and Resuscitation, 11,* 250–256.

He, B., Xu, B., Xu, X., Li, L., Ren, R., Chen, Z., et al. (2015). Hydroxyethyl starch versus other fluids for non-septic patients in the intensive care unit: A meta-analysis of randomized controlled trials. *Critical Care, 19*(1), 92.

Lagny, M. G., Roediger, L., Koch, J. N., Dubois, F., Senard, M., Donneau, A. F., et al. (2016). Hydroxyethyl starch 130/0.4 and the risk of acute kidney injury after cardiopulmonary bypass: A single-center retrospective study. *Journal of Cardiothoracic and Vascular Anesthesia, 30*(4), 869–875.

Myburgh, J. A., Finfer, S., Bellomo, R., Billot, L., Cass, A., Gattas, D., et al. (2012). Hydroxyethyl starch or saline for fluid resuscitation in intensive care. *New England Journal of Medicine, 367,* 1901–1911.

Pensier, K., Deffontis, L., Rolle, A., Aarab, Y., Capdevila, M., Monet, C., et al. (2022). Hydroxyethyl starch for fluid management in patients undergoing major abdominal surgery: A systematic review with meta-analysis and trial sequential analysis. *Anesthesia and Analgesia, 134*(4), 686–695. doi:10.1213/ANE.0000000000005803.

Westphal, M., James, M., Kozek-Langenecker, S., Stocker, R., Guidet, B., & Van Aken, H. (2009). Hydroxyethyl starches. *Anesthesiology, 111,* 187–202.

Zarychanski, R., Abou-Setta, A. M., Turgeon, A. F., Houston, B. L., McIntyre, L., Marshall, J. C., et al. (2013). Association of hydroxyethyl starch administration with mortality and acute kidney injury in critically ill patients requiring volume resuscitation: A systematic review and meta-analysis. *JAMA, 309,* 678–688.

# 68

# Type, Screen, and Crossmatch of Red Blood Cells

MICHAEL D. GODBOLD, MD  |  ROBERT M. CRAFT, MD

An ABO-incompatible red blood cell (RBC) transfusion is defined as the transfusion of RBCs that contain A and/or B antigens to a recipient with the corresponding antibodies. This transfusion reaction is the second most common cause of death from blood transfusion and is almost exclusively caused by clerical error. Therefore all blood banks routinely type, screen, and crossmatch RBCs (Table 68.1) to attenuate, if not eliminate, these transfusion reactions. Recently physicians have developed the Maximum Surgical Blood Ordering Schedule (MSBOS) to help advise providers about which patients require a preoperative type and screen versus type and cross. The MSBOS was developed to help better allocate and use the limited blood availability.

## Type

The type (group) test determines whether the A, B, and RhD antigens are present on the patient's RBCs. The type test is divided into two steps. In the first step, commercially available antibodies to A, B, and RhD antigens are mixed with the patient's RBCs to check for agglutination. A second confirmatory test is then performed by mixing commercially available cells containing the A or B antigen with the recipient's serum to test for the presence of anti-A or anti-B antibodies in the serum. This test uses the fact that almost all individuals will have antibodies to the ABO antigens not present on their RBCs (i.e., a Type A patient would have anti-B antibodies). O Rh⁻ patients will have RBCs that do not contain A, B, or RhD antigens and will have serum that contains anti-A and anti-B antibodies. Thus O Rh⁻ patients are universal donors because their RBCs have an absence of ABO antigens. AB Rh⁺ patients are considered universal recipients because their serum lacks anti-A, anti-B, and anti-D antibodies. The anti-D antibody is only formed after exposure to Rh-D⁺ RBCs, usually from a previous transfusion or pregnancy with an Rh-D⁺ child (Table 68.2).

## Screen

The screen test is performed to determine whether the recipient has "unexpected" antibodies to the approximately 20 clinically significant antigens on RBCs found in various groups, such as Rh (C, E, c, e), Diego (Diᵃ, Diᵇ, Wrᵃ), Duffy (Fyᵃ, Fyᵇ), MNS (S, s), Kell (K, k, Ku), and Kidd (Jkᵃ, Jkᵇ, Jk3). Commercially available type O cells with these 20 antigens are mixed with the plasma from the recipient to check for agglutination. If agglutination takes place, then the presence of unexpected antibodies in the recipient's plasma is known and will require additional testing (sometimes several hours in duration) to identify which antibodies are present. Most antibodies discovered at screening are either immunoglobulin (Ig)G alloantibodies, which develop as the result of previous transfusions or pregnancy, or naturally occurring cold-reactive IgM antibodies, which are usually clinically insignificant.

## Crossmatch

A crossmatch can be performed by computer or serologically to ensure compatibility between the donor's RBCs and the recipient's plasma. For a computer-generated crossmatch, if the recipient does not have antibodies (i.e., negative antibody screen), then a program can electronically match the ABO-RhD type of the recipient with a compatible donor unit. This requires that ABO-RhD type has been confirmed twice (on the current sample, by comparison with previous records, on a second current sample, or a second time on the same sample). Advantages of computerized crossmatching include more rapid availability

| TABLE 68.1 | Purposes and Preparation of Blood/Blood Product for Transfusion | | | |
|---|---|---|---|
| Procedure | Purpose | Time Required (min)* | Description |
| Type | ABO RhD determination | 5 | Patient's RBCs are mixed with commercial anti-A, anti-B, and anti-D antibodies |
| Screen | Detection of unexpected antibodies in patient's serum | 45 | Patient's serum is mixed with commercial O cell with known antigen panel |
| Crossmatch | Trial transfusion | 45 | Donor's RBCs are mixed with the patient's serum to determine compatibility |

*For preparation of 1 unit of blood/blood product and the recipient does not have antibodies.
*RBC,* Red blood cell.

| TABLE 68.2 | Blood Types and Their Frequency in U.S. White Population | |
|---|---|---|
| **Blood Type** | **Frequency (%)** | |
| O Rh$^+$ | 37 | |
| A Rh$^+$ | 36 | |
| B Rh$^+$ | 9 | |
| O Rh | 7 | |
| A Rh | 6 | |
| AB Rh$^+$ | 3 | |
| B Rh | 2 | |
| AB Rh | 1 | |

of blood for transfusion, decreased workload in the blood bank, increased flexibility in managing blood stores, and decreased waste of blood product.

A serologic crossmatch is required to ensure ABO compatibility if unexpected antibodies are present or in the absence of computer crossmatch technology. The serologic crossmatch is essentially a trial transfusion of the donor's RBCs with the recipient's plasma. This consists of two phases: immediate spin phase and incubation/antiglobulin phase. The immediate spin phase rechecks for ABO incompatibility and the presence of antibodies to MNS and Lewis group antigens; this phase requires 1 to 5 min to complete. During this initial abbreviated crossmatch, the patient's serum is mixed with the donor's RBCs at room temperature, centrifuged, and then assessed for macroscopic agglutination. This abbreviated crossmatch is 99.9% effective in detecting transfusion reactions. Next, in the incubation/antiglobulin phase, salt solution or albumin is added to the mixture of recipient plasma and donor RBCs, which are then incubated at 37°C. In the incubation stage, antibodies to certain RBC antigens will attach to the specific antigen but will lack the strength to cause agglutination. However, the addition of antiglobulin allows the incomplete recipient antibodies attached to the donor RBC antigens to cause agglutination and, thus, detect recipient antibodies to antigens found in groups such as Duffy, Kell, and Kidd.

## Incompatibility Risk and Emergency Transfusion

The most common cause of a fatal hemolytic transfusion reaction (with an occurrence rate of 1 in 1.8 million in the United States) is a clerical error in which the wrong unit is given to the patient. The overall incompatibility risk of immediate-spin type-specific blood (ABO-compatibility checked twice) is 1 in 1000 if the recipient has never received a transfusion. This risk rises to 1 in 100 if the recipient has previously received a transfusion. The so-called universal donor, O Rh$^-$ blood is routinely used as the first choice for emergency transfusions. Packed RBCs are preferred to whole blood to decrease the transfusion of IgM anti-A and anti-B antibodies commonly found in type O serum.

Because approximately 85% of the population in the United States is RhD$^+$, the use of O Rh$^+$ packed RBCs as an alternative to the traditional O Rh$^-$ "universal donor" blood is appropriate in emergency transfusion if the recipient is not a woman of childbearing age. O Rh$^+$ RBCs should not be given to women of childbearing age because she may develop an anti-D antibody. The presence of anti-D antibodies significantly increases her risk of having a child with hemolytic disease of the newborn, essentially a transfusion reaction in utero between mother and Rh-D$^+$ baby.

## SUGGESTED READINGS

American Red Cross. (January 2021). *A compendium of Transfusion Practice Guidelines* (4th ed.).

Demirkan, F. (2013). A new method for electronic crossmatch: ABO/Rh blood group confirmation and antibody screening concomitantly with serologic crossmatch. *Blood, 122*(21), 4833.

Mazer, C. D., Whitlock, R. P., Fergusson, D. A., Belley-Cote, E., Connolly, K., Khanykin, B., et al. (2018). Six-month outcomes after restrictive or liberal transfusion for cardiac surgery. *New England Journal of Medicine, 379*(13), 1224–1233.

Wong, K. F. (2011). Virtual blood bank. *Journal of Pathology Informatics, 2*(1), 6.

# 69

# Red Blood Cell and Platelet Transfusion

BRIAN S. DONAHUE, MD, PhD

## Red Blood Cells: Collection, Storage, and Administration

Whole blood is collected as 450-mL aliquots to which 150 mL of an anticoagulant preservative containing citrate, phosphate, and dextrose is added. Red cells are then isolated by centrifugation and preserved with 100 mL of a solution consisting of adenine, dextrose, saline, and mannitol. Adenine and dextrose are substrates, respectively, for adenosine triphosphate formation and glycolysis, and phosphate buffer extends viability of the unit to 42 days. The U.S. Food and Drug Administration (FDA) defines a viable unit as one from which 70% of transfused red cells are present in the recipient's circulation after 24 h. Stored red cells also develop a progressive intracellular acidosis, extracellular hyperkalemia, and decreased concentration of intracellular 2,3-diphosphoglycerate (2,3-DPG). Intracellular $K^+$ levels rise in red cells shortly after transfusion, but intracellular 2,3-DPG levels remain below normal for at least 24 h.

Increased acidity, decreased 2,3-DPG levels, and defects in deformability associated with older red cell units has been summarily termed the *red cell storage lesion*. Awareness of this phenomenon has fueled the clinical tendency to avoid transfusion of older red cell units, which is supported somewhat by retrospective observations that the use of older blood was associated with increased morbidity. Yet the same conclusion is not supported by prospective evidence: 13 randomized trials directly comparing older with fresher red cell units all failed to show any improvement in outcome associated with fresher blood. Both the American Association of Blood Banks (AABB) and the American Society of Anesthesiologists (ASA) Task Force for Perioperative Blood Management have thus recommended standard issue of red cells without regard to storage duration.

Rare red cell phenotypes are frozen and are stored in glycerol to prevent lysis, better preserving 2,3-DPG levels. Upon thawing, the red cells are washed in saline to remove the glycerol, which also decreases the leukocyte count and the incidence of febrile reactions. Disadvantages include cost and a short (24-h) expiration time after thawing.

In the past, red cells were infused through line filters to remove microaggregates of red cells, fibrin, and platelets because these components were thought to cause transfusion-related acute lung injury (TRALI). Filters are not routinely used now because we have a better understanding of the cause of TRALI and because of the widespread use of leukocyte-reduced products, which have fewer microaggregates.

## Red Cell Transfusion in Practice

The sole reason to transfuse red cells is to increase the content of $O_2$ in the blood, thereby increasing $O_2$ delivery ($Do_2$), which is a product of hemoglobin concentration, arterial $O_2$ saturation, and cardiac output. A specific hematocrit value may sustain adequate $Do_2$ if cardiac output is adequate but may be insufficient when cardiac output is limited or when arterial saturation is impaired by the presence of a transpulmonary shunt. Therefore the decision to transfuse should take into consideration the current hemoglobin level, estimated blood loss, cardiac reserve, vital signs, likelihood of ongoing hemorrhage, and risk of tissue ischemia. The dynamic nature of surgical hemorrhage requires a more aggressive approach to blood replacement in the operating room, compared with sites elsewhere in the hospital. In patients with chronic anemia, increased 2,3-DPG levels make $O_2$ transport (see Chapter 14, Oxygen Transport) more efficient; in acute anemia, cardiovascular mechanisms of compensation (e.g., increased cardiac output, heart rate, myocardial $O_2$ consumption) are more important.

Massive transfusion, or the administration of a volume of allogenic blood product greater than the patient's blood volume, represents an important problem for blood conservation and patient morbidity. In recent years, massive transfusion protocols have been developed among leading trauma centers and are based primarily on ratios of red cells to other blood products, usually plasma and platelets. The 2015 ASA Task Force guidelines for transfusion now specifically recommend use of a massive transfusion protocol when available, as a means to optimize transfusion therapy. These specific issues are addressed in Chapter 70, Massive Transfusion.

## Autologous Blood Transfusion and Directed Transfusion

Transfusion of red cells carries specific risks: hemolytic, infectious, immunomodulatory, economic, and others. Most of these risks are outlined in other chapters of this book. An awareness of these risks constitutes the major drive to reduce transfusion, and most efforts to decrease transfusion have been associated with improved morbidity. *Autologous blood donation* before a scheduled surgical procedure and retransfusion to the patient during surgery is one mechanism that has been proposed to decrease the need for allogeneic blood products. Although autologous donation has been shown to decrease allogeneic exposure in routine cardiac and orthopedic surgery, it does not always eliminate the need for allogeneic blood, nor is it necessarily less expensive than the use of allogeneic blood. Likewise, *cell salvage*, or autotransfusion at the site of care, may reduce allogeneic transfusion but may not necessarily offer a cost advantage. The most recent guidelines from the ASA Task Force recommend cell salvage as a means of reducing allogenic transfusion, when appropriate.

Acute normovolemic hemodilution (ANH) is an autologous transfusion technique where a patient's blood is diluted preoperatively by exchange of whole blood for an equal volume of crystalloid or colloid. The whole blood is then reserved for later during the operation when transfusion is indicated. Supporting evidence for ANH exists mostly for surgical populations at high risk for transfusion (cardiac, major orthopedic, liver). The ASA Task Force recommends that ANH be considered as a means for reducing allogenic transfusion, if possible.

Directed donation is the process in which a patient or patient's family selects blood that comes from an identified donor, often a relative of the patient. Interestingly, directed donation may be associated with increased infection risk because the donor who responds to a specific request to donate is no longer an anonymous volunteer; an element of coercion is present. Directed donation does not eliminate the risk of alloimmunization or immunomodulation, because the blood is allogenic. Blood transfusion from a related donor also significantly increases the risk of transfusion-acquired graft-versus-host disease, necessitating irradiation of the unit.

## Synthetic Hemoglobins

The use of hemoglobin-based $O_2$ carriers (HBOCs) has been hampered by difficulty in defining meaningful clinical end points, safety parameters, and risk/benefit ratios. All HBOCs rapidly bind nitric oxide, resulting in increased vascular resistance and interference with other functions of nitric oxide. Increased levels of inflammatory cytokines, increased platelet reactivity, and decreased organ blood flow are thought to be responsible for the pancreatitis, esophageal spasm, myocardial injury, pulmonary hypertension, and acute lung injury associated with the use of HBOCs. Recombinant hemoglobin-based products have the advantages of $O_2$-binding characteristics more similar to those of native hemoglobin but are unstable in solution, scavenge nitric oxide, and release free iron into circulation. Reactive $O_2$ species, resulting from free iron release, may mediate renal and central nervous system injury. A 2008 metaanalysis found an increase in death and myocardial infarction associated with the use of HBOCs, and the FDA responded by halting all HBOC trials because of this safety concern. A single phase 2 study by one manufacturer was later approved, but the company terminated its operations in 2013.

### PERIOPERATIVE ANEMIA AND RISK

The association of perioperative anemia with organ injury and perioperative morbidity is strong. For example, Turan and colleagues observed a consistent, stepwise increase in postoperative nonfatal myocardial infarction (MI) and all-cause mortality for each 1 g/dL reduction in postoperative hemoglobin concentration in their cohort of 7227 subjects from the Perioperative Ischemic Evaluation-2 (POISE-2) trial. In a survival analysis of 1011 hospitalized patients refusing transfusion,

Guinn and colleagues reported a greater than 50% increase in hazard ratio for death associated with anemia, independent of other risk factors. In a 2011 retrospective analysis of more than 227,000 subjects from the surgical NSQIP database, logistic regression revealed an independent association of perioperative anemia with 30-day morbidity, including mortality. This association was even observed for what was defined as mild anemia (hematocrit 29–39 for males, 29–36 for females).

Physiologically, otherwise healthy patients can make extraordinary adaptations to maintain $Do_2$ in the face of varying levels of anemia, but those with cardiovascular and cerebrovascular disease have limited ability to compensate for acute anemia. Organ ischemia is often silent and is not always related to the heart rate and blood pressure. Furthermore, anemia and transfusion are strongly correlated with each other, and this coupling has made it difficult to separate the intrinsic risks associated with each.

Optimal patient management therefore can be accomplished by appreciation of the data from prospective trials and adoption of a comprehensive blood management program. Such a blood management program necessarily considers case-specific considerations and thus includes identification of patients at risk, appropriate iron and erythropoietin supplementation, coagulation management, acute normovolemic hemodilution, cell salvage, and laboratory monitoring throughout the perioperative period.

## Moving From Evidence to Action: Thresholds for Transfusion of Red Blood Cells

The relevant question, then, is at what level of hemoglobin is transfusion justified by evidence? This question is complicated by practice history, because red cell transfusion has been practiced for decades with little objective evidence for specific transfusion thresholds. Yet we are in a better position to answer this question now than we have ever been, after several recent prospective trials. Excluding neonates and patients with cardiovascular disease, the preponderance of data indicates that a restrictive transfusion threshold (hemoglobin 7–8 g/dL) is associated with either improved outcome or at least no worse outcome than a more liberal threshold (hemoglobin 9–10 g/dL). The following studies involve intensive care unit (ICU) and cardiac surgery patients—higher-risk populations—but the reader should at least be familiar with their relevant findings.

- The TRACS trial was a 2010 single-center randomized controlled noninferiority study of restrictive (hematocrit >24) versus liberal (hematocrit >30) transfusion practices in 502 consecutive cardiac surgery patients. Researchers observed no statistically significant difference between the two groups in terms of 30-day morbidity, defined as cardiac, respiratory, neurologic, infectious, or bleeding complications; ICU length of stay; or hospital length of stay. Notably, the number of transfused red cell units was a significant risk factor for worse outcome, regardless of the treatment group assignment.
- The Titer2 trial, published in 2015, compared a hemoglobin transfusion trigger of 90 g/L with 75 g/L in 2003 cardiac surgery patients at 17 UK institutions and observed

no differences in their primary outcome (major organ morbidity at 90 days) between the two groups. However, 90-day mortality was statistically higher (4.2% vs. 2.6%, $P = 0.045$) in the restrictive transfusion group.

- The TRISS trial was an international (northern European) study of restrictive (hemoglobin 7 g/dL) versus liberal (hemoglobin 9 g/dL) transfusion strategies in 998 patients with septic shock admitted to the ICU. Primary outcome (90-day mortality) was no different (43% vs. 45%) between the groups. Secondary outcomes included ischemic events and use of life support (pressors and mechanical ventilation) and showed no statistical difference between the groups, even after adjusting for presence of hematologic malignancy.

- The TRICS-III trial, originally published in 2017, was the largest prospective randomized noninferiority study of liberal versus restrictive red cell transfusion practices for adults with moderate to elevated risk undergoing cardiac surgery. Interestingly, with respect to the composite end point of death, MI, stroke, or new-onset renal failure, the results suggested strongly that patients of age 75 or older likely benefit from the restrictive strategy, whereas those younger than 75 benefit from a more liberal strategy. The TRICS-IV study is now underway to test the hypothesis that a liberal transfusion strategy may be beneficial in younger patients undergoing cardiac surgery (NCT 04754022).

Although many other prospective noninferiority studies share similar conclusions regarding the safety of lower transfusion thresholds, not all reports share this finding. For instance, a recent single-center retrospective review of patients admitted with pneumonia found a significant association between mortality and lower transfusion triggers across three treatment groups.

Accordingly, the ASA Task Force and the AABB have issued guidelines that specify transfusion thresholds. The current recommendation from the AABB is a threshold of 7 g/dL for stable adults undergoing nonorthopedic and noncardiac surgery, and 8 g/dL for orthopedic or cardiac surgery. Both guidelines are considered strong recommendations, with moderate quality of evidence. These guidelines also list patient groups where a more liberal threshold is recommended: acute coronary syndromes, thrombocytopenia in hematology patients at risk for bleeding, and chronic transfusion-dependent anemia. These guidelines are also supported by a recent metaanalysis and systemic review, and a Cochrane review.

## Platelet Transfusions: Platelet Preparation and Storage

Platelet concentrate is prepared by centrifugation of freshly drawn donor blood to separate red cells from platelet-rich plasma (PRP). The PRP is then transferred to a satellite bag and is recentrifuged to separate the platelets from the plasma. Each unit of platelet concentrate contains about 50 mL of plasma and approximately $5.5 \times 10^{10}$ platelets. Platelet concentrate is the preferred source of platelets for transfusion because these platelets provide a more rapid therapeutic effect with less volume, compared with fresh whole blood or PRP. The platelet count of an adult should increase $5 \times 10^9$/L to $10 \times 10^9$/L for each unit of platelet concentrate transfused. Multiple units of platelets can be drawn from a single donor

using pheresis techniques. A continuous-flow centrifuge is used to separate platelets from plasma and red cells. These elements are then returned to the donor. Although this technique is more costly, its advantages include decreased infectious risk and the capability of selecting compatible platelet donors for patients with multiple antiplatelet antibodies. A standard 170-$\mu$m filter is recommended for platelet administration to remove microaggregates.

Platelets are stored at room temperature with gentle agitation to minimize aggregation and increase mixing of the platelet concentrate with oxygen passing through the wall of the platelet pack. New plastics introduced in the mid-1980s increased the shelf life of platelet concentrate by allowing better oxygen transfer to the contained cells. Current FDA standards require that in vivo platelet recovery be greater than 66% for a platelet unit to be considered viable.

Two time-dependent processes limit the duration of storage for platelets. The first is the increased risk for bacterial contamination. The second is a functional artifact of handling and storage, known as the *platelet storage lesion*. During storage, platelets gradually become activated and lose their ability to aggregate and to adhere to the extracellular matrix. Transfused platelets are viable in the blood for only 4 to 5 days, approximately half their normal life span of 7 to 10 days, probably due to loss of sialic acid residues on platelet membrane glycoproteins.

## Platelet Matching

Platelets are not routinely matched for ABO compatibility, because expression of the A and B antigens on platelets is believed to be of little significance. However, recent evidence indicates that ABO-incompatible platelet transfusions have decreased efficacy and can precipitate hemolytic transfusion reactions. Therefore ABO matched platelets, or administration of low-titer anti-A/anti-B platelets, is now suggested if available. Although platelets do not express Rh antigens, platelet transfusions are matched for Rh compatibility. That is, Rh-positive platelets are administered only to Rh-positive recipients because a small number of red cells are invariably present in platelet concentrates and could theoretically alloimmunize an Rh-negative recipient. Despite this theoretical concern, recent studies of Rh-incompatible platelet transfusions have shown that this is probably not a significant risk.

## Indications for Platelet Transfusion

Box 69.1 summarizes the indications for platelet transfusion listed in the most recent guidelines from the AABB. In most cases, the authors attempted to arrive at specific transfusion thresholds based on platelet count. It is notable that many of the new guidelines are based on low quality of evidence and/or carry weak recommendations. Patients with abnormal platelet function or thrombocytopenia are likely to benefit from platelet transfusions if the platelet disorder is thought to induce or exacerbate their bleeding. The ASA Task Force recommends assessment of platelet count, and if possible platelet function, prior to transfusion of platelets.

For surgical procedures it is desirable to increase the platelet count to $50 \times 10^9$/L, and prophylactic administration of platelet transfusions is indicated. Platelet transfusion is not indicated simply to increase platelet count in patients who are neither bleeding nor about to undergo interventional procedures with platelet counts above the listed thresholds. Patients with immune thrombocytopenic purpura should not receive platelet transfusions unless they have life-threatening bleeding. These patients produce autoantibodies that react against all human platelets, thus they derive little to no benefit from a platelet transfusion. After cardiopulmonary bypass (CPB), most patients develop both thrombocytopenia and a functional platelet impairment. Although the correlation between platelet counts and the extent of bleeding in these patients is poor, transfusing based on algorithms using platelet count or function as an indication for platelet transfusion reduces the need for platelet transfusion.

## PLATELET TRANSFUSION GUIDELINES FOR PEDIATRIC PATIENTS

The Pediatric Critical Care Transfusion and Anemia Expertise Initiative–Control/Avoidance of Bleeding (TAXI-CAB) has very recently issued numerous detailed statements to guide practitioners in pediatric plasma and platelet transfusion for various clinical settings: noncardiac surgery and procedures outside the operating room (OR); trauma, brain injury, and intracranial hemorrhage (ICH); malignancy, liver failure, and sepsis; and cardiopulmonary bypass and extracorporeal membrane oxygenation (ECMO). The resulting consensus statements are numerous and are specific to each of these patient groups. Although not a substitute for reading the guidelines, the following summary points for pediatric patients may be concluded:

1. For patients undergoing CPB or ECMO, critically ill patients undergoing procedures outside the OR, critically ill oncology or stem cell transplant patients, critically ill patients with liver failure or post–liver transplant, or patients with sepsis or disseminated intravascular coagulation (DIC), insufficient evidence exists for recommending specific indications or transfusion strategies.
2. For patients undergoing cardiac surgery with cardiopulmonary bypass, trauma, traumatic brain injury (TBI), or

nontraumatic ICH, viscoelastic testing may supplement standard coagulation tests to guide platelet transfusion.
3. Institution-specific algorithms may be considered to reduce blood product use.
4. For cardiac surgery patients and neurologically stable critically ill patients with severe trauma, moderate or severe TBI, and/or ICH, in the absence of bleeding, there is unlikely benefit from platelet counts greater than $100 \times 10^9$/L.
5. If an ICP monitoring device must be inserted in a neurologically deteriorating critically ill pediatric patient with TBI and/or ICH, platelet transfusion might be considered if the platelet count is less than $100 \times 10^9$/L.
6. In critically ill patients undergoing elective lumbar puncture, prophylactic platelet transfusion may be considered when the platelet count is below $20 \times 10^9$/L; it is uncertain whether there is benefit to prophylactic platelet transfusion when the count is between 20 and $50 \times 10^9$/L.
7. In patients who are undergoing noncardiac surgery and who have minimal or no bleeding, platelet transfusion may be considered when platelet count is less than $20 \times 10^9$/L. If moderate bleeding is present, platelet transfusion may be considered when platelet count is less than $50 \times 10^9$/L. The risk of platelet transfusion should be balanced against the clinical condition, timing from surgery, type of surgery, pattern or trajectory of bleeding, site of bleeding and associated risk, and other coagulation parameters.
8. In critically ill oncology or stem cell transplant patients, platelet transfusion may be considered when the platelet count is below $10 \times 10^9$/L.
9. In critically ill oncology or stem cell transplant patients, therapeutic platelet transfusions might be considered for moderate or severe bleeding.
10. In critically ill patients with liver failure, post–liver transplant, or with sepsis or DIC, prophylactic platelet transfusion may not be beneficial in the absence of moderate or severe bleeding.
11. In critically ill patients with sepsis or DIC, in the absence of moderate or severe bleeding, platelet transfusion might be considered when platelet count is less than $10 \times 10^9$/L. With moderate bleeding in such patients, platelet transfusion may be considered when platelet count is less than $50 \times 10^9$/L.
12. In critically injured pediatric patients in hemorrhagic shock after trauma, a resuscitation strategy of red cells, plasma, and platelets in ratios between 2:1:1 and 1:1:1 might be considered.

Functional platelet disorders are encountered less frequently than thrombocytopenia. CPB, uremia, liver disease, myeloproliferative disorders, and dysproteinemias can cause platelet dysfunction, but the most common cause is antiplatelet drugs. Aspirin, nonsteroidal antiinflammatory drugs, P2Y12 receptor inhibitors, glycoprotein inhibitors, theophyllines, tricyclic antidepressants, and some antibiotics cause functional platelet disorders that may or may not become clinically significant. Inherited functional platelet disorders include Glanzmann thrombasthenia, Bernard-Soulier syndrome, gray platelet syndrome, and dense granule deficiency syndrome.

# Platelet Alloimmunization and Platelet Refractoriness

Platelets have dozens of known glycoproteins on their surfaces, and polymorphic variants have been identified in almost all of these. Platelets also express HLA antigens. As a result, platelets from nonidentical donors are antigenic, and 24 immunologic platelet-specific antigens have been defined serologically. Sensitization to platelet antigens is common in patients who have received multiple platelet transfusions. Patients who are sensitized to these antigens or to HLA antigens will rapidly destroy transfused platelets, decreasing the therapeutic effectiveness of the platelet transfusion. In sensitized patients, only type-specific matched platelets are effective. Leukodepletion is effective in reducing platelet alloimmunization.

# Other Risks of Platelet Transfusion

The other major risks associated with platelet transfusion overlap with the risks associated with the transfusion of red cells: febrile transfusion reactions, allergic reactions, and transmission of infectious disease. Although platelet concentrates are drawn from single donors, many units are usually given at a time, increasing the risk of complications. Platelet transfusions also contain more donor plasma and are more likely to cause lung injury. Bacteria can proliferate in platelet concentrates because they are stored at room temperature; they are often implicated in septic transfusion reactions.

## SUGGESTED READINGS

Carson, J. L., Guyatt, G., Heddle, N. M., Grossman, B. J., Cohn, C. S., Fung, M. K., et al. (2016). Clinical Practice Guidelines from the AABB: Red blood cell transfusion thresholds and storage. *JAMA, 316*(19), 2025–2035.

Cholette, J. M., Muszynski, J. A., Ibla, J. C., Emani, S., Steiner, M. E., Vogel, A. M., et al. (2022). Plasma and platelet transfusions strategies in neonates and children undergoing cardiac surgery with cardiopulmonary bypass or neonates and children supported by extracorporeal membrane oxygenation: From the transfusion and anemia EXpertise initiative-control/avoidance of bleeding. *Pediatric Critical Care Medicine, 23*(Suppl. 1 1S), e25–e36.

Goodnough, L. T., & Panigrahi, A. K. (2017). Blood transfusion therapy. *Medical Clinics of North America, 101*(2), 431–447.

Guinn, N. R., Cooter, M. L., & Weiskopf, R. B. (2020). Lower hemoglobin concentration decreases time to death in severely anemic patients for whom blood transfusion is not an option. *Journal of Trauma and Acute Care Surgery, 88*(6), 803–808.

Hare, G. M. T., & Mazer, C. D. (2021). Anemia: Perioperative risk and treatment opportunity. *Anesthesiology, 135*(3), 520–530.

Kaufman, R. M., Djulbegovic, B., Gernsheimer, T., Kleinman, S., Tinmouth, A. T., Capocelli, K. E., et al. (2015). Platelet transfusion: A clinical practice guideline from the AABB. *Annals of Internal Medicine, 162*(3), 205–213.

Lieberman, L., Karam, O., Stanworth, S. J., Goobie, S. M., Crighton, G., Goel, R., et al. (2022). Plasma and platelet transfusion strategies in critically ill children with malignancy, acute liver failure and/or liver transplantation, or sepsis: From the transfusion and anemia EXpertise initiative-control/ avoidance of bleeding. *Pediatric Critical Care Medicine, 23*(Suppl. 1 1S), e37–e49.

Practice guidelines for perioperative blood management: An updated report by the American Society of Anesthesiologists Task Force on Perioperative Blood Management*. (2015). *Anesthesiology, 122*(2), 241–275.

Tobian, A. A., Heddle, N. M., Wiegmann, T. L., & Carson, J. L. (2016). Red blood cell transfusion: 2016 clinical practice guidelines from AABB. *Transfusion, 56*(10), 2627–2630.

Tucci, M., Crighton, G., Goobie, S. M., Russell, R. T., Parker, R. I., Haas, T., et al. (2022). Plasma and platelet transfusion strategies in critically ill children following noncardiac surgery and critically ill children undergoing invasive procedures outside the operating room: From the transfusion and anemia EXpertise initiative-control/avoidance of bleeding. *Pediatric Critical Care Medicine, 23*(Suppl. 1 1S), e50–e62.

Turan, A., Rivas, E., Devereaux, P. J., Bravo, M., Mao, G., Cohen, B., et al. (2021). Association between postoperative haemoglobin concentrations and composite of non-fatal myocardial infarction and all-cause mortality in noncardiac surgical patients: Post hoc analysis of the POISE-2 trial. *British Journal of Anaesthesia, 126*(1), 87–93.

Warner, M. A., Shore-Lesserson, L., Shander, A., Patel, S. Y., Perelman, S. I., & Guinn, N. R. (2020). Perioperative anemia: Prevention, diagnosis, and management throughout the spectrum of perioperative care. *Anesthesia and Analgesia, 130*(5), 1364–1380.

### ICU and Cardiac Surgical Studies
#### TRACS
Hajjar, L. A., Vincent, J. L., Galas, F. R., Nakamura, R. E., Silva, C. M., Santos, M. H., et al. (2010). Transfusion requirements after cardiac surgery: The TRACS randomized controlled trial. *JAMA, 304*(14), 1559–1567.

#### TRICS III
Mazer, C. D., Whitlock, R. P., Fergusson, D. A., Hall, J., Belley-Cote, E., Connolly, K., et al. (2017). Restrictive or liberal red-cell transfusion for cardiac surgery. *New England Journal of Medicine, 377*(22), 2133–2144.

Mazer, C. D., Whitlock, R. P., Fergusson, D. A., Belley-Cote, E., Connolly, K., Khanykin, B., et al. (2018). Six-month outcomes after restrictive or liberal transfusion for cardiac surgery. *New England Journal of Medicine, 379*(13), 1224–1233.

Mazer, C. D., Whitlock, R. P., & Shehata, N. (2018). Restrictive versus Liberal transfusion for cardiac surgery. *New England Journal of Medicine, 379*(26), 2576–2577.

#### Titer 2
Murphy, G. J., Pike, K., Rogers, C. A., Wordsworth, S., Stokes, E. A., Angelini, G. D., et al. (2015). Liberal or restrictive transfusion after cardiac surgery. *New England Journal of Medicine, 372*(11), 997–1008.

# Massive Transfusions

WOLF H. STAPELFELDT, MD

Transfusion of the equivalent of more than 10 to 12 units of blood may be necessary to maintain a patient's hemoglobin concentration within the guidelines promulgated by the American Society of Anesthesiologists. Accordingly, red blood cell (RBC) transfusion is almost always advocated if the patient's hemoglobin concentration is less than 6 g/dL and is recommended at a hemoglobin concentration of less than 10 g/dL whenever a patient's compensatory capacity for maintaining $O_2$ delivery may be compromised (e.g., in the presence of coronary artery disease) such that a diminished ability to increase cardiac output may no longer support adequate regional blood flow sufficient to meet metabolic needs, reflected in a rise in plasma lactate. Ongoing blood loss may be caused by surgical or gastrointestinal medical hemorrhage, disease-induced or drug-induced coagulopathy, or very often a combination of these factors. Causes for bleeding diatheses include inherited coagulopathies (hemophilias A, B, and C; platelet disorders such as idiopathic thrombocytopenic purpura, Glanzmann thrombasthenia, von Willebrand disease, or Bernard-Soulier syndrome; or vascular disorders such as Ehlers-Danlos syndrome); comorbid conditions (liver disease, disseminated intravascular coagulopathy, or uremia); the effects of anticoagulant drugs (warfarin, heparin, fibrinolytic or antiplatelet medications); drug-induced thrombocytopenia (heparin-induced thrombocytopenia [in 5% of patients within 5 days]); or platelet dysfunction. Last, coagulopathy commonly ensues over the course of massive transfusions. Although some patients may fare well and may be extubated as early as in the operating room, providing that homeostasis has been effectively maintained (hemodynamic stability, adequate oxygenation and hemoglobin concentration, normal acid-base status, electrolyte balance, normal coagulation status, good urine output, stable core temperature) and the underlying problem successfully remedied (e.g., in liver transplantation). Patients requiring massive amounts of blood products are typically at an increased risk of morbidity and mortality caused by a variety of intraoperative and postoperative transfusion-related complications. Patient outcome is further adversely affected by patient age and the range of comorbidities. Predictors of particularly poor outcome include a plasma lactate level greater than 10 mmol/L and a pH less than 7.0, especially in elderly patients (>65 years).

## Intraoperative Complications

Transfusion reactions range from minor allergic or febrile responses, which occur in approximately 1% of blood product transfusions, to often lethal acute hemolytic reactions caused by the administration of ABO-incompatible RBCs or fresh frozen plasma (FFP) in up to 1 in 12,000 transfusions, a major cause of intraoperative death. Ten times less frequent are delayed hemolytic responses, which often only become apparent postoperatively (after days to weeks).

Hemolytic reactions need to be expected in approximately 1 of every 1000 emergency transfusions of RBCs or FFP that have not been crossmatched and in 1 of every 100 transfusions in patients who have been pregnant or previously received blood transfusions. Other reactions include anaphylactic (in patients with hereditary immunoglobulin [Ig]A deficiency) or anaphylactoid reactions, which are another rare cause of intraoperative death (1 in 25,000 to 1 in 50,000). More common, and the most important cause of postoperative death, is transfusion-related acute lung injury (TRALI) in response to RBC, FFP, or platelet transfusion, presumably due to antibodies contained in the donor plasma. The treatment of acute transfusion reactions includes immediate discontinuation of the transfusion, pharmacologic support of the circulation if necessary, and alkalinization of the urine to prevent the precipitation of hematin and red blood cell stroma in renal tubules, depending on the extent of hemolysis. Coagulopathy often ensues, either as part of the primary underlying pathophysiology or iatrogenic subsequent to volume resuscitation (dilutional coagulopathy). The former includes hepatic disease (clotting factor deficiency, thrombocytopenia, primary fibrinolysis) or clinical conditions associated with disseminated intravascular coagulopathy and resulting secondary fibrinolysis (Box 70.1), including trauma, hypotension, and tissue hypoxia. Dilutional coagulopathy may result from iatrogenic dilution of circulating clotting factors to less than 20% to 30% of normal (usually after loss of approximately 1.5 blood volumes) or thrombocytopenia (after loss of 2–3 blood volumes). Hypothermic coagulopathy may be manifested by an approximately 50% prolongation of the actual temperature-adjusted prothrombin time (PT), partial thromboplastin time

---

### BOX 70.1 CAUSES OF DISSEMINATED INTRAVASCULAR COAGULOPATHY

Sepsis (gram-positive or gram-negative organisms)
Viremias
Obstetric conditions
    Amniotic fluid embolism
    Fetal death in utero
    Abruptio placentae
    Preeclampsia
Extensive tissue damage
    Burns
    Trauma
Liver failure
Extensive cerebral injury
    Head injury
    Cerebrovascular injury
Extensive endothelial damage
    Vasculitis
Hemolytic transfusion reaction
Metastatic malignancies
Leukemia
Snake venoms

(PTT), or thromboelastogram (TEG) reaction times, as well as hypothermic thrombocytopenia. Except during initial damage control, resuscitation with ideally either whole blood or respective components at near equivalent ratios (FFP:RBC:PLT close to 1:1:1) for any ongoing hemorrhage, not however, mere crystalloid solution, treatment of residual or ensuing coagulopathy should not generally be prophylactic, but instead should as soon as feasible be specifically directed as indicated by results of selective coagulation tests performed in the presence of continuous oozing, lack of clot formation, and/or persistent hemorrhage despite of ostensible achievement of surgical control. The therapeutic options are discussed later.

Hypotension may result from intravascular hypovolemia, decreased blood viscosity (low hematocrit), or diminished vascular tone caused by vasodilatory mediators, such as bradykinin (particularly in the presence of angiotensin-converting enzyme inhibitors) or ionized hypocalcemia (see later discussion). The treatment goals include maintenance of intravascular euvolemia, adequate cardiac output, and systemic vascular resistance to maintain mean arterial pressure sufficient to preserve vital organ perfusion. The latter may require the judicial use of α-adrenergic agonists, inotropes, vasopressin, calcium chloride, and/or some combination thereof.

Hypothermia predictably develops if fluids (room temperature) or blood products (4°C) are administered without being warmed. Other contributing conditions may include hepatic failure or severe splanchnic hypoperfusion, each of which may compromise the approximate 20% contribution of hepatic metabolic activity to normal body heat generation. Preventive (and corrective) means to treat severe hypothermia include the use of fluid warmers, convective heating blankets, warm irrigation of open body cavities (abdomen), and raising the ambient temperature in the operating room.

Tissue hypoxia may be caused by hemorrhagic or septic shock and may be further exacerbated by a left shift of the oxyhemoglobin dissociation curve due to the decreased 2,3-phosphodiglycerate content of transfused RBCs, subnormal (core or regional tissue) temperature, or both. Therapeutic goals are maintenance of tissue oxygenation by supporting the circulation (euvolemia, normal to increased cardiac output) while maintaining an adequate blood $O_2$ content (hematocrit and $O_2$ saturation) and preventing or treating severe hypothermia.

Metabolic acidemia may progressively develop subsequent to tissue hypoxia in conjunction with the continued administration of fluids and blood components featuring a less than physiologic pH (normal saline, pH 5.5; packed RBCs, pH 6.5), particularly in the presence of abnormal hepatic (liver disease, splanchnic hypoperfusion) or renal function. Treatment options are identical to those aimed at correcting tissue hypoxia. Severe acidemia (pH <7.1) may require the administration of sodium bicarbonate or tromethamine (to prevent a potentially harmful increase in sodium concentration and the associated risk of central pontine myelinolysis, especially in patients starting out with low sodium concentrations as is often the case in patients with advanced liver disease) with the goal of maintaining enzymatic hemostasis and restoring sufficient pharmacologic efficacy of endogenously released or exogenously administrated catecholamines.

Hyperkalemia may occur with rapid administration of packed RBCs ($K^+$ >20 mEq/L) if infused at a rate exceeding 90 to 120 mL/min, especially in the context of worsening metabolic acidemia and less than normal renal function (chronic renal insufficiency, acute renal failure, hepatorenal syndrome). It may manifest itself as a prolonged PR interval, widened QRS complex, and peaked T waves on the electrocardiogram and warrant treatment with hyperventilation; administration of calcium chloride, sodium bicarbonate, β-adrenergic agonists, glucose, and/or insulin; or a combination of several of these approaches. Refractory hyperkalemia may require the institution of venovenous hemofiltration or intraoperative hemodialysis.

Hypocalcemia may result from the reaction of the patient's ionized calcium with sodium citrate contained in whole blood, packed RBCs, or FFP (if transfused at a rate exceeding 1 unit every 5 min). Clinical signs include hypotension and narrow pulse pressure, as well as elevated left ventricular end-diastolic and central venous pressures. The electrocardiogram may exhibit a widened QRS complex, prolonged QT interval, or flattened T wave. Hypomagnesemia may cause ectopic rhythms and pose an increased risk for the development of ventricular tachycardia or fibrillation, including torsades de pointes. Either electrolyte abnormality should be treated by correcting its underlying plasma concentration with the administration of calcium chloride or magnesium chloride, respectively.

## Postoperative Complications

Patients receiving massive transfusions are at an elevated risk for developing a host of complications attributable to the administration of blood products. Major causes of postoperative death include sepsis caused by bacterial infection of blood products, particularly of platelets, which are stored at room temperature prior to being transfused. This risk is greatly diminished with the routine use of leukocyte reduction filters, which has become the recommended practice. Millipore filters (40 μm) are used to prevent microaggregate injury caused by cell-saver blood. TRALI may be diagnosed in the postoperative period as a cause of persisting noncardiogenic pulmonary edema and may be associated with 5% to 8% mortality rate, the leading cause of transfusion-related death. The age of donor erythrocytes has been inculpated as a possible cause for increased risk of postoperative morbidity and death, although the results of more recent studies have been controversial. Last, despite significant risk reductions due to improved testing and donor selection, viral infection remains a small but persistent threat after the transfusion of blood products (hepatitis B in 1:350,000; hepatitis C in 1:2 million; HIV in 1:2 million; human T-lymphotropic virus type I in 1:2.9 million). The risk of transmission of cytomegalovirus (present in donor leukocytes) to cytomegalovirus-negative immunocompromised recipients is reduced by using leukocyte-reduction filters, single-donor apheresis, or platelet irradiation.

Another possible consequence of massive transfusion is an increased risk of thromboembolism. Hypercoagulable states are to be avoided in the course of massive transfusion to reduce this risk.

## Treatment of Coagulopathy

In an effort to minimize transfusion risks, beyond a phase of damage control resuscitation with a balanced mix of blood components (FFP:RBC:PLT near 1:1:1, supplemented with cryoprecipitate as needed), the administration of blood products should not be prophylactic but should be instituted, as soon as possible, as specifically indicated by the results of coagulation tests in symptomatic patients. Commonly used tests include PT, PTT, activated coagulation time, platelet count, fibrinogen, fibrin split products, D-dimers (elevated in disseminated intravascular coagulation, not primary fibrinolysis), and the TEG. Additional tests are available for special circumstances, such as platelet function tests (platelet dysfunction), reptilase time (patients on heparin), euglobulin lysis time (to detect fibrinolysis), ecarin clotting time (patients on direct thrombin inhibitors), or specific clotting factor assays (isolated factor deficiencies).

FFP (increased PT, TEG reaction time), platelets (low platelet count; TEG maximum amplitude <50), cryoprecipitate (low fibrinogen; low factor VIII, factor XIII, or von Willebrand factor), or prothrombin complex concentrate (to reverse the effect of warfarin) may be administered as specifically indicated. Available adjunct treatment modalities not associated with the risk of blood product transfusion include desmopressin (to treat von Willebrand disease types 1 and 2A; platelet dysfunction caused by antiplatelet medications, ethanol, or uremia; mild hemophilia A); recombinant factor VIIa (to treat factor VII deficiency and to promote thrombin formation independent of the intrinsic pathway boost and in the absence of disseminated intravascular coagulopathy or antifibrinolytic treatment); serine protease enzyme inhibitors (to treat primary, but not secondary, fibrinolysis and/or prevent cardiopulmonary bypass–induced platelet dysfunction); and protamine (to treat heparin-caused increase in activated coagulation time, PTT, or heparinase-sensitive TEG reaction time). An example of a diagnostic and treatment algorithm used for the differential diagnosis and management of coagulopathy as routinely encountered during liver transplantation in over 1000 patients is shown in Fig. 70.1.

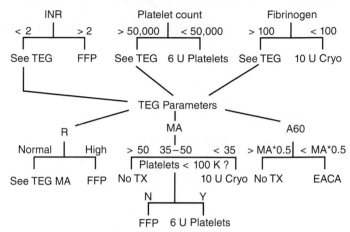

**Fig. 70.1** Algorithm for the perioperative assessment and treatment of coagulation abnormalities in patients undergoing orthotopic liver transplantation. *A60*, TEG amplitude 60 min after the time of MA; *Cryo*, cryoprecipitate; *EACA*, ε-aminocaproic acid; *FFP*, fresh frozen plasma; *INR*, international normalized ratio; *MA*, TEG maximal amplitude; *R*, TEG reaction time; *TEG*, thromboelastogram; *TX*, treatment. (Adapted from Stapelfeldt WH. Liver, kidney and pancreas transplantation. In: Murray MJ, Coursin DB, Pearl RG, Prough DS, eds. *Critical Care Medicine: Perioperative Management*. 2nd ed. Lippincott, Williams & Wilkins; 2002.)

## SUGGESTED READINGS

Al-Jeabory, M., Szarpak, L., Attila, K., Simpson, M., Smereka, A., Gasecka, A., et al. (2021). Efficacy and safety of tranexamic acid in emergency trauma: A systematic review and meta-analysis. *Journal of Clinical Medicine, 10*(5), 1030.

American Society of Anesthesiologists Task Force on Perioperative Blood Transfusion and Adjuvant Therapies. (2006). Practice guidelines for perioperative blood transfusion and adjuvant therapies: An updated report by the American Society of Anesthesiologists Task Force on perioperative blood transfusion and adjuvant therapies. *Anesthesiology, 105*, 198–208.

Bradburn, E. H., Ho, K. M., Morgan, M. E., D'Andrea, L., Vernon, T. M., & Rogers, F. B. (2021). Massive transfusion protocol and subsequent development of venous thromboembolism: Statewide analysis. *American Surgeon, 87*(1), 15–20.

Cole, E., Weaver, A., Gall, L., West, A., Nevin, D., Tallach, R., et al. (2021). A decade of damage control resuscitation: New transfusion practice, new survivors, new directions. *Annals of Surgery, 273*(6), 1215–1220.

Delaney, M., Stark, P. C., Suh, M., Triulzi, D. J., Hess, J. R., Steiner, M. E., et al. (2017). Massive transfusion in cardiac surgery: The impact of blood component ratios on clinical outcomes and survival. *Anesthesia and Analgesia, 124*(6), 1777–1782.

Jones, A. R., Patel, R. P., Marques, M. B., Donnelly, J. P., Griffin, R. L., Pittet, J. F., et al. (2019). Older blood is associated with increased mortality and adverse events in massively transfused trauma patients: Secondary analysis of the PROPPR Trial. *Annals of Emergency Medicine, 73*(6), 650–661.

Lo, B. D., Merkel, K, R., Dougherty, J. L., Kajstura, T. J., Cruz, N. C., Sikorski, R. A., et al. (2021). Assessing predictors of futility in patients receiving massive transfusions. *Transfusion, 61*, 2082–2089.

Moore, H. B., Tessmer, M. T., Moore, E. E., Sperry, J. L., Cohen, M. J., Chapman, M. P., et al. (2020). Forgot calcium? Admission ionized-calcium in two civilian randomized controlled trials of prehospital plasma for traumatic hemorrhagic shock. *Journal of Trauma and Acute Care Surgery, 88*(5), 588–596.

Park, Y. H., Ryu, D. H., Lee, B. K., & Lee, D. H. (2019). The association between the initial lactate level and need for massive transfusion in severe trauma patients with and without traumatic brain injury. *Acute Critical Care, 34*(4), 255–262.

Rijnhout, T. W. H., Duijst, J., Noorman, F., Zoodsma, M., van Waes, O. J. F., Verhofstad, M. H. J., et al. (2021). Platelet to erythrocyte transfusion ratio and mortality in massively transfused trauma patients. A systematic review and meta-analysis. *Journal of Trauma and Acute Care Surgery, 91*(4), 759–771.

Taylor, J. R., III, Fox, E. E., Holcomb, J. B., Rizoli, S., Inaba, K., Schreiber, M. A., et al. (2018). The hyperperfibrinolytic phenotype is the most lethal and resource intense presentation of fibrinolysis in massive transfusion patients. *Journal of Trauma and Acute Care Surgery, 84*(1), 25–30.

# 71

# Hemolytic Transfusion Reactions

KIP D. ROBINSON, MD  |  ROBERT M. CRAFT, MD

## Introduction

Allogeneic blood transfusions (ABTs) have well-known risks. Over the past decade, nucleic acid testing has significantly reduced the risk of transfusion-transmitted infections. Therefore noninfectious serious hazards of transfusions have become a more prominent concern (see Table 71.1). In a 10-year study in New York, the U.S. Food and Drug Administration (FDA) reported death rates caused by hemolytic transfusion reactions were more than double the rate of all combined infectious transmissions. Hemolytic transfusion reaction, transfusion-related acute lung injury (TRALI), and transfusion-associated sepsis (TAS) make up the majority of transfusion-related deaths. Of the transfusion-related deaths in the United States reported to the FDA between 2014 to 2018, 26% were attributed to TRALI, 18% to hemolytic transfusion reaction, and 14% to TAS. Whereas TRALI carries its greatest risk with the transfusion of products containing plasma (most commonly fresh frozen plasma), TAS is at highest risk in transfusion of platelets (since March 2004, TAS deaths have been cut in half by introduction of bacterial detection methods of apheresis platelets). Hemolytic transfusion reactions occur most often in patients receiving red blood cells (RBCs). Hemolytic transfusion reactions caused by ABO incompatibility resulted in 13 deaths in the United States between 2014 and 2018. Hemolytic transfusion reaction caused by ABO incompatibility has become one of the least common fatal complications of transfusion, estimated at 1:1,972,000 red-cell units transfused in 2016. Acute hemolytic transfusion reactions in trauma management using non–cross-matched blood is estimated to occur in 1:2000 transfusions.

## Pathophysiology

Hemolysis related to transfusion can be immune mediated or nonimmune mediated. Non-immune-mediated hemolysis may occur because of coadministration of incompatible fluids such as 5% dextrose solution, incorrect storage of the blood, or inappropriate administration sets. Immune-mediated hemolytic transfusion reactions are further classified as acute hemolytic transfusion reaction (AHTR) and delayed hemolytic transfusion reaction. An immune-mediated response to transfusion of blood products incompatible with the recipient's blood is the mechanism for the immune-mediated hemolytic transfusion reaction. Incorrect blood component transfusion can be innocuous, mildly symptomatic, life-threatening, or fatal. (see Fig. 71.1.) Severity of reaction depends on amount of antigen transfused and intensity of complement activation and cytokine release.

Acute hemolytic transfusion reactions occur primarily with mistransfusion or incorrect blood-component transfusion. This is typically a clerical or administrative error, and when

| TABLE 71.1 | Noninfectious Serious Hazards of Transfusion | |
|---|---|
| **Immune Mediated** | **Nonimmune Mediated** |
| Hemolytic transfusion reaction (acute/delayed) | Septic transfusion reaction |
| Febrile nonhemolytic transfusion reaction | Nonimmune hemolysis |
| Allergic/urticarial/anaphylactic transfusion reaction | Mistransfusion |
| Transfusion-related acute lung injury (TRALI) | Transfusion-associated circulatory overload |
| Transfusion-associated graft versus host disease (TA-GVHD) | Metabolic derangements |
| Microchimerism | Coagulopathic complications from massive transfusion |
| Alloimmunization | Complications from red cell storage lesions Over-/undertransfusion Iron overload |

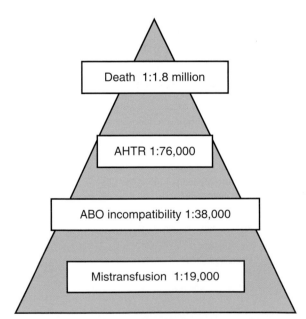

**Fig. 71.1  Risk of Death From Mistransfusion.** Risk of mistransfusion, ABO incompatibility, acute hemolytic transfusion reaction (AHTR), and death related to mistransfusion as result of a 10-year study in New York State. (From Linden JV, Wagner K, Voytovich AE, et al. Transfusion errors in New York State: An analysis of 10 years' experience. Transfusion 2000; 40:1207–1213).

found suggests the importance of tracking the error. Because patients and blood components are often matched in pairs, a mismatched unit should suggest the possibility of a second patient at risk for the same. An overwhelming majority of these reactions have been caused by incompatible RBC transfusion. There are reported cases, however, of hemolysis due to incompatible plasma or intravenous immunoglobulin. These rare cases are unusual and rarely fatal.

In the case of transfused RBCs, antibodies present in the recipient recognize foreign antigens on the surface of donor cells. Most often this is due to ABO incompatibility (preformed immunoglobulin [Ig]M anti-A, anti B), but complement-fixing IgG alloantibodies such as anti-P, anti-Vel, Lewis, Kidd (anti-Jk$^a$, anti-Jk$^b$), and Kell (anti-K1) have also been implicated. Destruction of the circulating RBCs occurs by two distinctive mechanisms. Intravascular destruction occurs by complement activated lysis, initiated by preformed antibodies (mainly IgM). Intravascular hemolysis is a distinctive characteristic of ABO-incompatible transfusion and is most often what is referred to when discussing hemolytic transfusion reactions. Intravascular hemolysis can destroy more than 200 mL of RBCs within an hour. A drop in measured hemoglobin (Hb) by 5 g/dL can occur within hours and can be life-threatening or fatal. Extravascular destruction occurs by monocytes or macrophages recognizing IgG or complement proteins on the RBC surface, binding and altering the RBC. Fragmented or phagocytosed RBCs are destroyed and removed primarily in the liver and spleen. Extravascular destruction is a much slower process as it is limited by the capacity of the reticuloendothelial system (RES). Free Hb is released into the intravascular space resulting in acute tubular necrosis and renal failure. Mast cell activation and release of proinflammatory cytokines, bradykinin, and kallikrein promotes a systemic inflammatory response.

Delayed hemolytic transfusion reactions typically occur over 3 to 10 days posttransfusion. This can occur as a slower developing primary immune response but is typically an anamnestic response after reexposure to antigens previously encountered during prior transfusion, pregnancy, or transplantation. These circulating antibodies are at undetectable levels and rapidly increase after antigen reexposure. Antigens frequently implicated include anti-D (Rh), Duffy (Fy$^a$), and Kidd (Jk$^a$). IgG antibody–coated cells are marked for destruction by phagocytic cells in the spleen and other areas of the RES. This extravascular hemolysis results in mild jaundice (elevated unconjugated bilirubin), increased reticulocytosis, and spherocytosis. Patients like those with sickle cell disease who require frequent transfusions are at particular risk for this phenomenon. A hemolytic transfusion reaction can often precipitate sickle crisis. Likewise, pain, dyspnea, fever, and chest pain that can be caused by a delayed transfusion reaction can easily be misdiagnosed as a sickle crisis. Additional measures including extended red cell antigen phenotyping prior to initiating transfusion therapy can significantly reduce this risk.

## Signs and Symptoms

Signs and symptoms of acute hemolytic transfusion reaction can be seen in Table 71.2. The classic triad of fever, flank pain, and red/brown urine is rarely seen. Unfortunately, signs and symptoms are nonspecific, and many are masked by general anesthesia, leaving a definitive diagnosis difficult to make in a timely manner. This is of particular concern because severity of reaction

| TABLE 71.2 | Signs/Symptoms of Acute Hemolytic Transfusion Reaction |
|---|---|
| **Signs/Symptoms of Acute Hemolytic Transfusion Reaction** |
| Fever |
| Chills/rigors |
| Chest, back, or abdominal pain |
| Pain at infusion site |
| Sense of impending doom |
| Nausea/vomiting |
| Dyspnea |
| Hypotension |
| Hemoglobinuria |
| Oliguria/anuria |
| Diffuse bleeding |

and mortality risk are linked to volume transfused. During general anesthesia, fever, hypotension, tachycardia, hemoglobinuria, and diffuse bleeding are the best clues. If these signs occur after initiating blood transfusion, AHTR should be suspected.

## Complications

Inflammatory cytokines, histamines, bradykinin, vasoactive amines, and anaphylotoxins are generated during the complement activation process. Fever, wheezing, hypotension, and disseminated intravascular coagulation (DIC) can occur as a result, leading to shock, renal failure, respiratory failure, and death. Renal failure is a result of acute tubular necrosis, initially thought to be predominantly from tubular damage from circulating free Hb. Both free Hb and antibody-coated red cell stroma have renal vasoconstricting properties. Ischemic renal failure is a result of renal vasoconstriction and systemic hypotension. Tissue factor released from hemolyzed RBCs can be a trigger for DIC.

## Prevention

Primary prevention of hemolytic transfusion reactions begins with avoiding unnecessary ABT. Use of cell-salvaging devices and avoidance of unnecessary transfusion will reduce patient risk. Information systems and transfusion protocols have significantly reduced clerical error, thereby reducing mistransfusion and ABO-incompatible ABT. Machine-readable blood component containers and multiple patient identifiers, including unique blood band number attached to the patient, further reduce the risk of clerical error. Between 1976 and 1985 there were 158 AHTR-related deaths reported to the FDA. Mortality risk from AHTR was estimated at 1:250,000 units transfused. With current preventative measures, risk of death is now estimated to be approximately 1:1.8 million units transfused.

## Treatment

Treatment of hemolytic transfusion reaction is supportive. Because of its nonspecific signs and symptoms, vigilance and high index of suspicion are critical in identifying an acute hemolytic reaction.

| TABLE 71.3 | Treatment for Acute Hemolytic Transfusion Reaction |
|---|---|

1. Stop blood transfusion
2. Identify patient and blood labeling for error in compatibility
3. Return any unused blood product to blood bank
4. Maintain systemic blood pressure
   a. Volume
   b. Vasopressors (as needed)
   c. Inotropes (as needed)
5. Preserve renal function
   a. Promote urine output (>1 mL/kg/hr)
   b. Maintain renal perfusion
   c. Maintain volume
   d. Diuretics (consider mannitol and/or furosemide)
   e. Consider alkalization of urine (sodium bicarbonate)
6. Prevent DIC
   a. Maintain cardiac output
   b. Prevent hypotension
   c. Appropriate component therapy if DIC manifests
7. Obtain blood and urine samples
   a. Repeat blood type and crossmatch
   b. DAT, also known as Coombs test
   c. Haptoglobin
   d. Plasma and urine-free hemoglobin
   e. Bilirubin
   f. Baseline coagulation tests: PT/PTT, fibrinogen and fibrinogen split products, monitor for change
   g. Brief centrifugation (simple rapid test for hemolysis)
   h. Monitor renal function (blood urea nitrogen, creatinine)

*DAT,* Direct antiglobulin test; *DIC,* disseminated intravascular coagulation; *PT,* prothrombin time; *PTT,* partial thromboplastin time.

Treatment for AHTR is outlined in Table 71.3. Transfusion should immediately cease. Supportive care should target management goals of maintaining systemic perfusion, preserving renal function, and preventing DIC. Appropriate component therapy should be given if DIC manifests. Patient and blood product containers should be reidentified, and remaining blood product should be returned to the blood bank. Blood and urine samples should be sent to the lab for analysis to include repeat cross match. Hemoglobinuria, hemoglobinemia, and elevated indirect bilirubin are evidence of hemolysis but are nonspecific, and they can be seen with nonimmune mechanisms of hemolysis (mechanical, thermal, osmotic, drug related). The direct antiglobulin test, also known as the indirect Coombs test, is the definitive test to verify an immune-mediated hemolytic process. Additional RBC administration may be necessary, particularly if intravascular hemolysis with a rapid drop in Hb occurs. With practitioners transfusing less and allowing patients to have lower Hb values to initiate transfusion, critically low Hb values can occur quickly in the event of intravascular hemolysis.

## SUGGESTED READINGS

Delaney, M., Wendel, S., Bercovitz, R. S., Cid, J., Cohn, C., Dunbar, N. M., et al. (2016). Transfusion reactions: Prevention, diagnosis, and treatment. *Lancet, 388,* 2825–2836.

Eder, A. F., & Chambers, L. A. (2007). Noninfectious complications of blood transfusion. *Archives of Pathology and Laboratory Medicine, 131,* 708–718.

Flegel, W. (2015). Pathogenesis and mechanisms of antibody-mediated hemolysis. *Transfusion, 55,* S47–S58.

Goel, R., Tobian, A., & Shaz, B. H. (2019). Noninfectious transfusion-associated adverse events and their mitigation strategies. *Blood, 133*(17), 1831–1839.

Hendrickson, J. E., & Hillyer, C. D. (2009). Noninfectious serious hazards of transfusion. *Anesthesia and Analgesia, 108,* 759–769.

Linden, J. V., Wagner, K., Voytovich, A. E., & Sheehan, J. (2000). Transfusion errors in New York State: An analysis of 10 years' experience. *Transfusion, 40,* 1207–1213.

Panch, S. R., Montemayor-Garcia, C., Klein, H. G. (2019). Hemolytic transfusion reactions. *New England Journal of Medicine, 381,* 150–162.

Stainsby, D., Jones, H., Asher, D., Atterbury, C., Boncinelli, A., Brant, L., et al. (2006). Serious hazards of transfusion: A decade of hemovigilance in the UK. *Transfusion Medicine Reviews, 20*(4), 273–282.

Stainsby, D., Jones, H., Wells, A. W., Gibson, B., Cohen, H., & SHOT Steering Group. (2008). Adverse outcomes of blood transfusion in children: Analysis of UK reports to the serious hazards of transfusion scheme 1996-2005. *British Journal of Haematology, 141,* 73–79.

Vamvakas, E. C., & Blajchman, M. A. (2009). Transfusion-related mortality: The ongoing risks of allogeneic blood transfusion and the available strategies for their prevention. *Blood, 113,* 3406–3417.

Wu, Y. Y., Mantha, S., & Snyder, E. L. (2008). Transfusion reactions. In *Hematology: Basic principles and practice* (5th ed.). Elsevier Churchill Livingstone.

# 72

# Nonhemolytic Transfusion Reactions

ALLAN M. KLOMPAS, MB, BCh, BAO

Blood transfusion is one of the most common procedures performed in the United States, and, with many of these occurring in the perioperative setting, anesthesia providers are frequently involved in the decision to transfuse and monitor for clinical and/or pathologic response. Although blood products have become incredibly safe and most transfusions are uncomplicated, many patients experience new signs and symptoms around the time of transfusion that can be directly attributed to the blood product (overall morbidity 4.91/100,000, mortality 1.05/100,000). These reactions are important to recognize because they have the potential to lead directly to patient harm, affect the safety of future patients if products from the same donors continue to be used, and have regulatory consequences for the hospital and transfusion service. Newly implemented systemic reporting of transfusion reactions has improved our understanding of the true risks of transfusion and trends over time. The following are the most common nonhemolytic transfusion reactions (NHTR) as defined by the Centers for Disease Control and Prevention (CDC), covering the spectrum from mild to severe. See Table 72.1 for a summary of the common reactions and their relative frequencies. Of note, each blood product has a different propensity to cause transfusion reactions based on whether the mechanism is predominantly cell mediated (red blood cells [RBCs], leukocytes) or plasma mediated (fresh frozen plasma [FFP], cryoprecipitate, and platelets). The figure concluding the chapter (Fig. 72.1) highlights a simplified algorithm for the acute management of a transfusion reaction.

## Febrile Nonhemolytic Transfusion Reaction

Fever is one of the most common and sensitive indicators of an acute hemolytic transfusion reaction and therefore demands a full investigation; however, simple febrile reactions are very common. Using the CDC definitions, fever is defined as an increase in body temperature (usually ≥1°C) within 4 h of transfusion, is usually mild, and is quickly responsive to treatment.

Associated symptoms can include chills, rigors, cold, headaches, nausea, and vomiting. Remarkably, despite the title, fever is not actually required to be present if other inflammatory symptoms are observed. While generally well tolerated and responsive to antipyretic agents, they have been associated with subsequent chest imaging, blood cultures, and hospital admissions and thus contribute to the burden on the patient and care team. Although premedication with acetaminophen and/or diphenhydramine is commonly performed, its efficacy at preventing NHTRs remains questionable.

These reactions are most often associated with transfusion of cellular components (e.g., red blood cells, platelets, and granulocytes), but have also been observed with transfusion of noncellular components (e.g., FFP or cryoprecipitate). Although the etiology has yet to be fully elucidated, it is hypothe-

sized that recipient *alloimmunization* (i.e., antibody production in response to a previous transfusion or pregnancy) toward donor white blood cells (WBCs) or platelets triggers release of leukocyte-derived or platelet-derived pyrogenic cytokines (e.g., interleukin [IL]-1β, IL-6, IL-8, tumor necrosis factor α, CD40L) that increase the hypothalamic thermoregulatory set point. Alternatively, fever may occur in response to direct transfusion of pyrogenic cytokines or other inflammatory mediators that accumulate during the storage of blood products such that the greater the interval between collection and transfusion, the higher the frequency of febrile NHTR. Leukocyte reduction techniques have been liberally applied to blood products in many blood centers and act to reduce the frequency of febrile reactions. By reducing the WBC burden in the blood product immediately after collection, it is thought that fewer cytokines are released into the unit during storage and following transfusion into the patient, both of which reduce the likelihood of producing febrile reactions.

## Mild Allergic Reactions

Mild allergic reactions are the second most common NHTR, occurring with a frequency of 0.5% to 3%, with plasma-based components (FFP, cryoprecipitate, apheresis platelets) being more common. Signs and symptoms are usually mild and include urticarial rash and generalized pruritus as a result of immunoglobulin (Ig)E-mediated histamine release from degranulated mast cells and basophils in response to foreign substances (e.g., transfused plasma proteins) found in any plasma-containing blood products. Despite usually being mild, clinically these present in a spectrum to anaphylaxis at its most severe, and the transfusion must therefore be stopped until progressive symptoms have been ruled out. Following assessment with the blood product stopped, patients who do not show signs of having an anaphylactic reaction should be treated symptomatically with diphenhydramine, and the transfusion may be continued. **This is the only circumstance where a blood product can be restarted following an acute reaction!**

## Anaphylactic Reactions

Anaphylaxis, which represents the most severe end of the allergic spectrum, occurs in 6.9/100,000 transfusions (about 7.5% of all allergic reactions). Transfusion of any blood product may result in an anaphylactic response; however, this type of reaction is far more common with plasma-containing products. Signs, symptoms, and treatment do not differ from those of other anaphylactic reactions and include pruritus, urticaria, angioedema, bronchospasm, hypotension/shock, tachycardia, arrhythmias, loss of consciousness, nausea, vomiting, and so on.

Reactions may be caused by any molecule present in the blood product, and in many cases a confirmed cause is never

| TABLE 72.1 | Summary of Transfusion Reactions | | | | | |
|---|---|---|---|---|---|---|
| | **Frequency per 100,000** | | | | | |
| **Transfusion Reaction** | **RBC** | **Plt** | **FFP** | **Mechanism** | **Able to Restart the Unit** | |
| Simple allergic | 87–3000 (based on broad definition) | | | IgE antibodies from recipient to foreign donor proteins or donor IgE to recipient proteins | Yes | |
| Anaphylactic | 2–7 | | | Recipient IgE antibodies toward substance in donor blood product | No | |
| Febrile nonhemolytic transfusion reaction | 111.7 | 115.3 | 14.6 | Cytokine mediated from donor leukocytes released either in storage or after transfusion | No | |
| Hypotensive transfusion reaction | 3.5 | 4.2 | 2.1 | Transfusion of vasoactive substances in the blood product, especially bradykinin in patients taking ACEI | No | |
| TACO | 0.1 | 0.1 | 0 | Includes simple cardiogenic pulmonary edema due to volume overload and biologic/inflammatory mediators | No | |
| TRALI | 0.6 | 1.4 | 0.2 | Classically, donor antineutrophil antibodies attack and sequester/activate recipient leukocytes in the lungs | No | |
| Transfusion-associated dyspnea | 4.3 | 4.8 | 2 | Diagnosis of exclusion with new respiratory distress within 24 h and not explained by TACO, TRALI, or allergic reaction | No | |
| Posttransfusion purpura | 1–2 | | | Recipient antiplatelet antibodies lead to destruction of both transfused and native platelets | No | |
| TA-GVHD | Very rare | | | Donor lymphocytes attack an immunosuppressed recipient's tissues | No | |
| Bacterial contamination | 40–70 | | | Bacterial contamination from collection, processing, storage, or transfusion is introduced into the patient | No | |
| Immunomodulation | | | | | N/A | |
| Frequencies extracted from CDC NHSV Hemovigilance module, 2013–2018 | | | | | | |

Frequencies extracted from CDC National Healthcare Safety Network Hemovigilance Module, 2013–2018.

*ACEI*, Angiotensin-converting enzyme inhibitors; *CDC*, Centers for Disease Control and Prevention; *FFP*, fresh frozen plasma; *IgE*, immunoglobulin E; *Plt*, platelets; *RBC*, red blood cells; *TACO*, transfusion-associated circulatory overload; *TA-GVHD*, transfusion-associated graft versus host disease; *TRALI*, transfusion-related acute lung injury.

found. One of the more common causes of anaphylactic reactions occurs in patients with hereditary IgA deficiency, which is relatively common (1 in 700 persons of European descent). During exposure to "foreign" IgA from a previous transfusion or pregnancy, patients become alloimmunized (i.e., recipients develop IgE directed against donor IgA). IgE elicits an immune response by binding to Fc receptors on the surface of mast cells and basophils, resulting in degranulation and release of vasoactive mediators (e.g., histamine, leukotrienes, and prostaglandins) culminating in an anaphylactic reaction. Although IgA deficiency accounts for about half of anaphylactic transfusion reactions, the cause in the remaining half is usually not identified. In those of Asian ethnicities, IgE antibodies toward haptoglobin are more frequently the cause.

The diagnosis of an anaphylactic transfusion reaction is clinical. In those cases with IgA deficiency, the presence of anti-IgA may be found in recipient plasma; however, it is important to recognize that an IgA-deficient patient may have a normal IgA level, because subtypes of IgA exist; simply measuring IgA levels may therefore be misleading. Levels of serum β-tryptase, a marker for mast cell degranulation, may be measured or a basophil activation test performed; however, these laboratory studies are often time-consuming and may not be readily available. Thus once a diagnosis of anaphylactic transfusion reaction is suspected, the transfusion should be stopped immediately and the patient supported as in other forms of anaphylaxis. If blood transfusion must be continued, the blood bank should be contacted for support, as blood products may require modifications (e.g., blood from donors known to be IgA deficient or washed red blood cells and platelets) before release. Importantly, the washing process is time-consuming (often 1–3 h) and decreases the yield of the RBC or platelet product with loss of 20% of RBC and 40% to 50% of platelets.

Both mild allergic and IgA anaphylactic reactions usually begin within 45 min after blood transfusion is started but may be delayed for as long as 1 to 3 h. Shorter onset times tend to be associated with more severe reactions, with anaphylactic reactions occurring after the transfusion of a few milliliters of blood product.

# Hypotensive Transfusion Reactions

Hypotension is common in the perioperative period and is often a contributing factor for deciding to transfuse blood products. There is, however, an association between the transfusion of some blood products and a "clinically significant" acute drop in blood pressure that usually occurs within minutes and resolves almost immediately upon stopping the transfusion. The true incidence of these reactions is unknown (most recent estimate 3.1/100,000), but it is likely underreported because of the broad differential diagnosis for hypotension around the time of transfusion. Per the CDC criteria, diagnosis requires a drop in blood pressure of more than 30 mm Hg within 1 h of transfusion with **ALL other causes of hypotension excluded.**

The mechanism is still unknown but has been hypothesized to be related to transfusion of vasoactive substances, with bradykinin being most frequently implicated because it can be produced when blood is passed through some of the filters used in the manufacture of blood products. Supporting this theory are case reports of these reactions being more frequent in patients taking angiotensin-converting enzyme inhibitors that prevent the breakdown of bradykinin. Treatment involves stopping the transfusion and supportive care.

# Transfusion-Related Acute Lung Injury

Transfusion-related acute lung injury (TRALI) is a noncardiogenic form of pulmonary edema that is difficult to distinguish from acute respiratory distress syndrome (ARDS) or other causes of acute lung injury. TRALI, a diagnosis of exclusion, occurs within 6 h of blood product transfusion and is characterized by acute respiratory distress, radiograph evidence of bilateral pulmonary infiltrates, severe hypoxemia ($PaO_2/FiO_2$ <300 mm Hg), and no evidence of a cardiogenic cause; however, the criteria for ARDS have recently changed and no longer include acute lung injury. Similarly, a 2019 consensus redefinition of TRALI now recognizes two subtypes: type I TRALI occurs in patients without coexisting risk factors for TRALI, whereas in type II TRALI, the patient either has coexisting risk factors *or* a prior diagnosis of ARDS (formerly transfused ARDS). Despite this change, remaining differences in how TRALI is diagnosed and reported based on which criteria are used means TRALI is likely underdiagnosed and underreported. However, it is estimated to occur in 0.02% to 1.12% of all transfusions, but up to 8% in intensive care unit patients. Although any product is capable of inducing TRALI, plasma-based products are more frequently implicated. Treatment is supportive, and depending on the severity of TRALI, the patient may require tracheal intubation, oxygenation, and mechanical ventilation.

The pathogenesis of TRALI is incompletely understood but is likely multifactorial. In 65% to 90% of patients who develop TRALI, donor WBC (including human leukocyte antigens [HLAs] or neutrophil-specific) antibodies that bind recipient WBC antigens can be identified in donor plasma, whereas in the remaining 10% the antibody is present in the recipient and "attacks" donor WBCs. Another explanation for the development of TRALI may be the two-hit theory: an initial insult (e.g., infection, surgery, or trauma) attracts and "primes" neutrophils that adhere to pulmonary vascular endothelium. A subsequent "activating stimulus" (e.g., transfusion of plasma containing biologically active mediators) causes these marginated neutrophils to release oxidases, $O_2$ free-radical species, and proteases, resulting in endothelial damage and extravasation of intravascular fluid into lung parenchyma. A recent proposal of "perioperative" TRALI recognizes the third hit of perioperative factors that may directly contribute to developing ARDS.

Although transfusion of any blood product containing plasma can cause TRALI, the vast majority of implicated donors are multiparous women who have been alloimmunized to paternal neutrophil antigens (HLAs or human neutrophil antigens) (reported to occur in up to 25% women with >3 pregnancies). This association has led to the widespread minimization of collecting plasma-containing products from female donors, and many centers will test female donors for HLA antibodies before collecting any plasma-based products. These strategies have reduced the rates of TRALI in the United States by more than half. Because the blood product itself is often implicated, it is imperative to alert the blood bank of a suspected TRALI so other blood products manufactured from the donor can be sequestered and the donor deferred from future donations, thereby protecting other patients.

The mortality from TRALI continues to be very high (10%–50% depending on comorbidities) and remains one of the leading causes of transfusion-related death in the United States; however, most patients with TRALI improve clinically, physiologically, and radiographically within 48 to 96 h.

# Transfusion-Associated Circulatory Overload

It has long been known that transfusion of blood products can result in cardiogenic pulmonary edema, but recently there has been a greater appreciation for how common and injurious transfusion-associated circulatory overload (TACO) can be. Despite this recent resurgence of interest and recognition, it is very likely to remain underdiagnosed. Incidence may be as low as 1% to as high as 11% in critically ill patients. In contrast to TRALI, TACO lacks clear consensus on diagnostic criteria, but the diagnosis centers around cardiogenic pulmonary edema resulting in dyspnea and orthopnea, hypoxemia, tachycardia, and elevated brain natriuretic peptide. It is most common in patients with underlying predisposition to fluid overload (children and the elderly) or heart failure but can occur in anyone. Management is supportive and similar to other forms of cardiogenic edema and hypoxemia.

The pathogenesis of TACO is complex. The traditional model suggests a typical overload of Starling's forces producing increased accumulation of fluid in the lung parenchyma and associated dyspnea, in a patient already at risk of volume intolerance. Alternative models have been proposed that involve biologic mediators and lipids, glycocalyx-induced endothelial dysfunction, cell free hemoglobin, and red cell storage lesions all contributing to pulmonary edema, suggesting that there may be a larger inflammatory role than previously thought.

Although often thought of as benign fluid overload by clinicians, TACO is associated with significant morbidity and mortality. In data from the US hemovigilance module, mortality from TACO now rivals TRALI in both absolute number and frequency per transfusion. Similarly, other countries have seen TACO overtake TRALI as the number-one cause of transfusion-related death. Despite the recent improvement in recognition, TACO remains an underappreciated cause of transfusion-associated morbidity and mortality.

## Transfusion-Associated Dyspnea

Transfusion-associated dyspnea is a catch-all category that is a diagnosis of exclusion. It is defined as the onset of new respiratory distress and dyspnea within 24 h of transfusion that cannot be explained as TACO, TRALI, allergic reaction, or another reaction category. Despite the unfamiliarity, it now constitutes 2% of all reported transfusion reactions with approximately 4/100,000 transfusions. This category incorporates a broad differential and may be particularly convenient for the anesthesia provider to ignore because of the frequency of respiratory symptoms in the perioperative period. For this reason, it requires a high index of suspicion and should be reported to the blood bank.

## Posttransfusion Purpura

Posttransfusion purpura (PTP) is a rare complication of blood transfusion that results in a sudden and severe thrombocytopenia (often <10,000/$\mu$L) that usually occurs 5 to 10 days following transfusion. It can occur with any blood product but is more common with RBCs or whole blood. Although the true frequency is unknown, it is proposed that it occurs in 0.1 to 1/100,000 transfusions. The mechanism is not completely understood; however, often a platelet-specific antibody is formed (most commonly anti-HPA-1a) that results in the destruction of both transfused platelets and the patient's own native platelets, often producing *profound* thrombocytopenia. Treatment is supportive and includes intravenous immunoglobulin, plasma exchange, and corticosteroids, although steroids have the weakest evidence. In the absence of life-threatening bleeding, transfusion of additional platelets is not recommended, as it may worsen the situation. Despite the severity of disease, prognosis is usually good with mortality ranging from 0% to 13%; however, it can recur with subsequent transfusions. Hence, a history of PTP should be reported to the blood bank so that suitable products can be given in the perioperative period to minimize the risk of recurrence.

## Transfusion-Associated Graft-Versus-Host Disease

Although very rare, transfusion-associated graft-versus-host disease (TA-GVHD) is one of the most serious complications of transfusion and is usually fatal. This most often occurs in a patient with profound cellular immunosuppression when viable donor lymphocytes attack recipient tissues, although *half* of TA-GVHD occurs in those not predicted to be at risk. Mortality is estimated at greater than 90%. At-risk populations should have blood products irradiated before transfusion. Rather than remove the donor lymphocytes, this modification limits their ability to replicate and prevents expansion/cell destruction in the recipient.

## Transfusion-Transmitted Infection

Although blood products have become incredibly safe in the past several decades because of improved recruiting, screening, and testing practices, many patients are still aware of the risk of transmission of pathogenic viruses, parasites, and bacteria that were prevalent in the past. It is essential for anyone consenting to the transfusion of blood products to understand the risks of various infectious diseases.

In the United States all blood donations are tested for past or present infection with hepatitis B and C, HIV, HTLV, WNV, syphilis, Chagas, and, most recently, Zika virus. Other pathogens may also be transmitted by blood products (e.g., CMV, EBV, parvovirus) but are not currently tested for. Although prion diseases are not technically infectious pathogens, there is still a risk of transmission, and anyone with a family history of CJD is not eligible to donate. The recent COVID-19 pandemic has raised the question of whether respiratory viruses can be transmitted via transfusion. Although trace amounts of viral particles may be found in blood from coronavirus-positive donors, there have been zero confirmed transmissions via blood transfusion; therefore blood donations are not routinely tested for respiratory viruses.

It is critical for anyone suspecting a transfusion-transmitted infection to report this to the blood bank to ensure the safety and security of future transfusions and to allow follow-up with the potentially infected donor.

## Bacterial Contamination

All blood products provide excellent growth media for various bacteria. Although blood products are collected and stored using processes to minimize the risk of contamination, it is impossible to eliminate this risk, although emerging pathogen reduction technologies continue to reduce the risk further. When transfused, a contaminated product can produce a typical septic reaction including high fevers, leukocytosis, hypotension/shock, and disseminated intravascular coagulation. Although all products are capable of transmitting bacteria, historically platelets are most frequently implicated (>80% of bacterial contaminations) because of their room temperature storage in comparison to most other products being stored at refrigerated temperatures. The risk of platelet contamination has been estimated between 0.1/1000 and 7.4/1000; however, these rates are likely to decrease with the widespread introduction of novel pathogen reduction technologies. Management is supportive as in other cases of septic shock. As with other transfusion reactions, communication to the blood bank is critical to ensure additional contaminated products do not get issued for transfusion.

## Immunomodulation

Blood transfusion can significantly improve (in a dose-dependent manner) allograft survival after renal transplantation, yet it worsens tumor recurrence and mortality rate after resection of many cancers (e.g., breast, colorectal, gastric, head and neck, hepatocellular, lung, prostate, renal, soft-tissue sarcoma) compared with patients who do not receive transfusions or individuals who receive leukocyte-reduced blood transfusions. In either case, alterations in patient outcome have been attributed to transfusion-mediated immunomodulation, referred to as a "tolerogenic effect." Although the full mechanisms are not yet elucidated, such an effect may be a result of upregulation of humoral immunity (i.e., B-cell function and antibody production), downregulation of cell-mediated immunity (i.e., T-cell function), or both.

Despite improved renal allograft survival in transfused transplant recipients, routine perioperative blood transfusion is *not* indicated because of the effectiveness and safety of immunosuppressant drugs (e.g., cyclosporine) and concerns about transfusion-related infection.

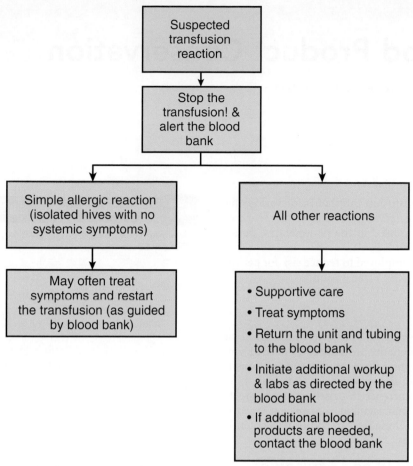

**Fig. 72.1** Flowchart of steps to take in the event of a transfusion reaction.

## SUGGESTED READINGS

Annual Shot Report 2020. (2021). *UK: The Medicines and Healthcare Products Regulatory Agency (MHRA).* Retrieved from https://www.shotuk.org/wp-content/uploads/myimages/SHOT-REPORT-2020.pdf. Accessed December 9, 2021.

Bulle, E. B., Klanderman, R. B., Pendergrast, J., Cserti-Gazdewich, C., Callum, J., & Vlaar, A. P. J. (2022). The recipe for TACO: A narrative review on the pathophysiology and potential mitigation strategies of transfusion-associated circulatory overload. *Blood Reviews, 52,* 100891.

CDC. *National Healthcare Safety Network Biovigilance Component Hemovigilance Module Surveillance Protocol.* Published March, 2021. Retrieved from https://www.cdc.gov/nhsn/pdfs/biovigilance/bv-hv-protocol-current.pdf. Accessed December 9, 2021.

Kracalik, I., Mowla, S., Basavaraju, S. V., & Sapiano, M. R. P. (2021). Transfusion-related adverse reactions: Data from the National Healthcare Safety Network Hemovigilance Module - United States, 2013-2018. *Transfusion, 61*(5), 1424–1434.

Popovsky, M. A. (2012). *Transfusion reactions* (4th ed.). Bethesda, MD: AABB Press.

Shaz, B., & Hillyer, C. D. et al. (2013). *Transfusion medicine and hemostasis: Clinical and laboratory aspects.* Amsterdam: Elsevier Science.

Vlaar, A. P. J., Toy, P., Fung, M., Looney, M. R., Juffermans, N. P., Bux, J., et al. (2019). A consensus redefinition of transfusion-related acute lung injury. *Transfusion, 59*(7), 2465–2476.

# Blood Product Conservation

GREGORY JAMES MICKUS, MD

## Questions

What are acceptable transfusion thresholds for various patients undergoing surgery?

How are patients best assessed in the perioperative period for risk of transfusion?

Which measures may be employed to reduce risk for perioperative red blood cell (RBC) transfusion?

## Background

RBC transfusions are administered to a variety of surgical patients and are more prevalent in procedures associated with acute blood loss (Table 73.1). Multiple studies suggest transfusions impair the immune system, increase infection rates, and lead to early cancer recurrence in patients with colorectal cancer. Appropriate RBC management remains an essential perioperative concern given these risks in addition to potential high-mortality complications.

## Transfusion Threshold and Strategies

### LIBERAL VERSUS CONSERVATIVE STRATEGIES

RBC management strategies have emerged from the evaluation of perioperative transfusion thresholds by multiple studies. Under ideal circumstances with adequate preoperative

| TABLE 73.2 | Allowable Blood Loss Calculation |
|---|---|

Average blood volume (Men 75 mL/kg, Women 65 mL/kg, Obesity 50–55 mL/kg)

Estimated blood volume = weight in kg × average blood volume

$$\text{Allowable blood loss in mL} = \frac{EBV \times (Hgb_i - Hgb_t)}{Hgb_i}$$

$Hgb_i$ – Initial hemoglobin
$Hgb_t$ – Target hemoglobin

planning and calculation of allowable blood loss (Table 73.2), transfusions may be avoided in the intraoperative setting. When planning is paired with a restrictive transfusion strategy (hemoglobin [Hgb] 7–8 g/dL) discussed openly before surgical incision, similar rates of mortality, complications, and length of stay have been observed with fewer RBC transfusions compared with liberal approaches (Hgb >9 g/dL). Some notable exceptions include ongoing massive or high-rate hemorrhage, as well as clinical or laboratory indicators of impending organ ischemia.

### CORONARY ARTERY DISEASE

Several studies have evaluated transfusion triggers for patients with preexisting coronary artery disease, which substantiate no difference between liberal (Hgb 9–10 g/dL) or conservative (Hgb 7.5–8 g/dL) strategies for infections, ischemic events, morbidity, or 30-day mortality. In one study, however, 90-day mortality was significantly higher in the conservative group. Overall, the data suggests a more conservative strategy is beneficial for this at-risk patient population.

### PRONE SPINAL SURGERY

Classical teaching is to maintain hemoglobin greater than 10 g/dL with the goal to reduce risk of posterior ischemic optic neuropathy. Newer literature alternatively suggests liberal transfusion strategies increase morbidity and hospital length of stay. Debate among anesthesiologists remains because of insufficient data, with a majority in agreement of Hgb greater than 9 g/dL being ideal. Other mainstays of therapy should include continuous blood pressure monitoring, maintenance of appropriate mean arterial pressures, and judicious intravascular volume repletion with crystalloid fluids or 5% albumin.

| TABLE 73.1 | High-Bleeding-Risk Surgical Procedures | |
|---|---|---|
| **System** | **Surgery** | |
| Neurologic | Intracranial Kyphoscoliosis repair Multilevel laminectomy + fusion | |
| Cardiovascular | Open heart Pacemaker/ICD insertion Major vascular (open aortic, iliac/femoral bypass) Thoracic | |
| Abdominal | Liver resection Splenectomy Partial nephrectomy | |
| Gastrointestinal | Colonic polyp excision (>1 cm) Sessile polyp | |
| Urologic | TURP Tumor ablation | |
| Miscellaneous | Cancer/mass excision Reconstructive plastic surgery Major trauma | |

*ICD,* Implantable cardioverter defibrillator; *TURP,* transurethral resection of the prostate.

## SEPSIS AND SEPTIC SHOCK

Administration of hemoglobin through packed RBC transfusion has the ability to manipulate the Fick equation through an increase in oxygen delivery, and thus an indirect increase in mixed venous oxygen saturation ($Svo_2$), which is generally important for overall tissue perfusion. Although this effect appears theoretically beneficial, no significant benefit has been shown with liberal RBC transfusion in septic patients. In this population, a generally accepted strategy is a trigger of Hgb less than 7 g/dL, an ideal range between 7 to 9 g/dL, and only aims for Hgb greater than 10 g/dL if the $Svo_2$ is low within the first 6 hours of a septic shock diagnosis (serum lactate >2 mmol/L and requiring vasopressor support).

## Preoperative Assessment

Preoperatively, both patient and surgical factors require assessment, with the aim to limit intraoperative RBC transfusion. At-risk patients include but are not limited to coagulopathy (Table 73.3), history of thromboembolism (deep vein thrombosis/pulmonary embolism [DVT/PE]), and anemia of any cause. Identification of patients who refuse blood products in addition to those at risk for adverse reactions to blood components (i.e., history of prior/serial blood transfusions, known blood antibodies, prior transfusion reaction) is important. Surgical procedures associated with acute blood loss and transfusions are identified in Table 73.1.

Patients who refuse blood products or those with preexisting anemia may benefit from preoperative erythropoietin +/− oral iron therapy, if sufficient time allows, especially in the case of iron-deficiency anemia. Ensuring blood components are readily available for a patient undergoing surgical procedures with anticipated large volume blood loss is ideal, and preoperative autologous donation may be of benefit if performed in a timely manner with erythropoietin therapy.

In general, discontinuation of anticoagulant and antiplatelet agents is made on a case-by-case basis, with members of the perioperative team considering the nature/invasiveness of the

| TABLE 73.3 | Conditions and Pharmacologic Agents Associated With Coagulopathy | | |
|---|---|---|
| **Conditions** | **Medications** | **Supplements** |
| Hemophilia A/B<br>Von Willebrand disease<br>Chronic renal failure<br>Vitamin K deficiency (biliary tract disease, celiac disease, Crohn disease, cystic fibrosis, end-stage liver disease, gallbladder disease) | Aspirin<br>Clopidogrel<br>Prasugrel<br>Ticlopidine<br>Ticagrelor<br>Warfarin<br>Unfractionated heparin<br>Enoxaparin<br>Direct factor Xa inhibitors (-xaban)<br>Indirect factor Xa inhibitors (-aparinux)<br>Direct thrombin inhibitors (-gatran, -rudin) | Black cohosh (contains salicylate)<br>Chamomile (additive effects w/warfarin because of coumarin)<br>Feverfew (inhibits platelet aggregation, additive with antiplatelet agents and warfarin)<br>Fish oil (dose-dependent risk >3 g/day)<br>Garlic (inhibits platelet aggregation)<br>Ginkgo (inhibits PAF [platelet activating factor])<br>Ginseng (inhibits platelet aggregation)<br>Saw palmetto (unknown mechanism of action, associated with excessive intraoperative bleeding) |

| TABLE 73.4 | Risk Stratification for Perioperative Anticoagulation Bridge Therapy | | |
|---|---|---|
| **High** | **Intermediate** | **Low** |
| Mechanical prosthetic valve<br>Recent ATE/VTE (<3 months)<br>Prior ATE/VTE when warfarin held<br>Chronic AF with CHADS$_2$ ≥5<br>Prothrombotic state (protein C/S deficiency, antithrombin 3 deficiency, antiphospholipid syndrome)<br>Rheumatoid valvular disease plus AF | New-generation (bileaflet) prosthetic aortic valve plus CHADS$_2$ ≥1<br>Bioprosthetic aortic valve <3 months from replacement surgery<br>Chronic AF plus CHADS$_2$ 3 or 4<br>VTE >3 or <12 months | New-generation (bileaflet) prosthetic aortic valve plus CHADS$_2$ = 0<br>Chronic AF plus CHADS$_2$ ≤2<br>VTE >12 months |

*AF*, Atrial fibrillation; *ATE*, arterial thromboembolism; *CHADS$_2$*, score for stroke risk in atrial fibrillation; *VTE*, venous thromboembolism.

surgical procedure, indication for anticoagulation, risk of perioperative thrombosis versus hemorrhage, and necessitation of bridge therapy (Table 73.4).

## Intraoperative Considerations

The following techniques are often used to limit intraoperative blood component transfusions.

### TRANSFUSION PROTOCOLS

Protocols involving transfusion algorithms or institution-specified criteria have shown remarkable benefit, especially when based on thromboelastography (TEG) versus traditional coagulation profile testing. TEG offers a significant reduction in overall transfusion rates and exists as an important consideration when large-volume blood loss is expected. In cases such as trauma where blood component transfusion is absolutely necessary, massive transfusion protocols play an important role by improving ratios of products administered (i.e., RBC:FFP:PLT 1:1:1) to mitigate dilutional coagulopathy compared with higher-ratio strategies. Furthermore, during massive transfusion, it is imperative to consider calcium chloride administration after every several blood component units transfused to reduce risk of life-threatening hypocalcemia from citrate, an anticoagulant agent used to preserve stored blood components.

### MONITORS AND LABORATORY TESTS

At the present juncture, no isolated monitor or laboratory value is solely used in the setting of continued hemorrhage or coagulopathy, and instead many factors play a unique role in the evaluation of the bleeding patient. Although current evidence is lacking on the effectiveness of visual surgical field assessment, to ignore warning signs such as large sanguineous volumes in surgical collection canisters or numerous saturated lap sponges would be extremely controversial. Likewise, information obtained from standard clinical monitors alone or routine hemoglobin-hematocrit measurements do not appear useful, and instead their utility holds greater value to the anesthesiologist when paired with clinical context and other monitors.

Technological advancement has refined echocardiography (transesophageal/transthoracic) for left ventricular end-diastolic volume assessment, as well as cerebral oximetry for tissue perfusion analysis, to aid clinical decision-making in combination with other measures. In addition to TEG, the use of rotational elastometry has increased and shown reduction in blood component transfusions versus situations where traditional coagulation profile testing (prothrombin time/international normalized ratio [PT/INR], partial thromboplastin time, fibrinogen) was solely used. Knowledge of these tests and the ability to interpret their results is essential for the modern-day anesthesiologist.

## ACUTE NORMOVOLEMIC HEMODILUTION

Acute normovolemic hemodilution (ANH) is the process of pre-incision blood removal/collection, intraoperative replacement with crystalloid or colloid fluids, and subsequent administration of collected blood after surgical completion. ANH is unique, as it employs a rarely used "whole blood" transfusion strategy, is extremely cost-effective, and has shown significant reduction in blood volume transfusion during high-risk bleeding procedures when paired with intraoperative blood salvage. Cautious patient selection is important because patients with preexisting anemia may not tolerate further reductions in Hgb concentration to potentially critical levels, risking organ ischemia.

## ANTIFIBRINOLYTIC AGENTS

Antifibrinolytic agents aminocaproic acid and tranexamic acid appear to play an important role in cardiac, liver transplantation, and elective orthopedic surgeries when given preoperatively and/or intraoperatively, accounting for lower rates of perioperative blood loss and overall transfusion. Significant controversy surrounds the use of tranexamic acid for major trauma surgery in modernized trauma centers, with unclear effects on overall mortality or transfusion rates, and risk of seizure, venous thrombosis, or acute kidney injury. Aminocaproic acid has shown benefit versus placebo in perioperative blood loss for major cardiac and liver surgeries, and both have shown benefit in total knee and hip arthroplasty.

## ARGON PLASMA COAGULATION

One method used by surgeons is the argon beam coagulator, a monopolar electrosurgical tool that involves high-frequency electrical current conducted via an ionized argon gas stream that results in superficial coagulation to several millimeters of tissue. Of note, an electrosurgical grounding pad must be appropriately placed before argon beam use, and extreme caution must be exercised in patients with automatic implantable cardioverter-defibrillators for the risk of inadvertent shock, as well as pacemaker-dependent patients, to minimize risk of device interference and lethal arrhythmias.

## BLOOD SALVAGE

Surgical blood loss collection, then processing blood cells using filters, centrifugation, with or without ultrafiltration, offers an appealing opportunity to reduce allogenic transfusions in select patient populations. The methodology is routinely employed in cardiac surgery, especially with cardiopulmonary bypass; however, versatility in other situations for high-risk bleeding patients is apparent. Direct blood salvage transfusion is the most cost-effective option and has not shown any increased risk in coagulopathy or blood loss compared with centrifugation or ultrafiltration strategies. It is important to note that centrifugation of salvaged blood removes plasma and may put patients at risk for coagulopathy if multiple units are transfused without concomitant factor or platelet administration. As opposed to centrifugation, ultrafiltration uses hydrostatic pressure differences across a membrane to filter salvaged blood, preserving plasma proteins, providing whole blood for readministration, and reduces the risk of coagulopathy when employed. Once an established blood salvage program is in place at an institution, the cost of each blood salvage unit is significantly less than an allogenic transfusion and poses an additional long-term institutional benefit; however, it still remains more expensive than ANH.

Historically, the debate over blood salvage use in cancer patients undergoing surgery has limited or precluded its use in those situations. Multiple observational studies, however, have shown no difference in long-term outcomes or metastatic spread of malignancy after use of cell salvage in cases of malignancy. To the contrary, studies have noted poorer outcomes and greater recurrence of malignancy when cancer patients receive allogenic transfusions, at least in part attributable to the immunosuppressive effect of allogenic transfusions. Methods employed to reduce tumor burden in salvaged blood include radiation and leukocyte depletion filters, although recirculated tumor burden has not been proven to have any clinical prognostication.

## DESMOPRESSIN

As a synthetic analog of arginine vasopressin, desmopressin has multiple clinical applications including diabetes insipidus, hemophilia A, quantitative types of von Willebrand disease, uremia, and nocturnal enuresis. Its mechanism of action in hematologic dysfunction involves vasopressin-2 receptor agonism on the vascular endothelium and resultant release of von Willebrand factor, which then interacts with factor VIII to improve platelet adherence and overall clot strength via several mechanisms. Strong evidence supports desmopressin use to reduce perioperative blood loss, which likely provides particular benefit when used in the setting of hemophilia A, quantitative von Willebrand disease, or uremia.

## HEMOSTATIC AGENTS

Use of topical hemostatic agents such as silver nitrate, oxidized regenerated cellulose (Surgicel), or absorbable gelatin (Surgifoam, Gelfoam), has become commonplace in the operating room for control of minor surgical bleeding. Newer agents including highly absorbent clot-promoting dressings, human fibrin glue, and combination thrombin gel with absorbable gelatin (Thrombi-Gel) have shown promise in situations where significant bleeding is encountered. Both human fibrin glue and thrombin gel significantly reduce perioperative blood loss compared with traditional hemostasis measures. Anesthesiologists must be aware that these agents are not compatible with blood salvage circuits because of the risk of systemic thrombosis upon reinfusion, and concomitant use must be avoided.

## RECOMBINANT FACTORS AND PROTHROMBIN COMPLEX CONCENTRATES

Certain circumstances and disease states call for the utilization of factor concentrates to promote substantial hemostasis. For example, hemophilia A (factor VIII deficiency) may be treated with desmopressin to indirectly increase circulating factor VIII in minor procedures, or factor VIII concentrate transfusion for major/emergent procedures, and patients with hemophilia B (factor IX deficiency) would benefit from factor IX administration. Unfortunately, because of the likelihood of prior concentrate exposure in these patient populations, some will develop antibodies and refractory disease that require the addition of either recombinant factor VIIa or four-factor prothrombin complex concentrates (PCCs) including factors II, VII, IX, and X. In patients with hemophilia, recombinant factor VIIa promotes greater local tissue coagulation compared with the higher rate of systemic thrombosis with PCCs and affords a lower risk of anaphylactoid reactions. Extreme caution must be exercised with use of recombinant factor VIIa in patients without hemophilia, because the rate of generalized thrombosis (pulmonary embolism, cerebrovascular accident, myocardial infarction), and therefore the risk of morbidity or mortality, is significantly higher. Use of prothrombin complex concentrates for major bleeding in the general population provides a reduction in perioperative blood loss, and in patients with major bleeding on vitamin K antagonists, rapid normalization of the PT/INR provides a unique opportunity to mitigate morbidity or mortality.

## RED BLOOD CELLS: NEW VERSUS OLD

Multiple studies have evaluated the differences between complications and outcomes for patients receiving newer ($<8$–10 days) versus older RBCs. As RBCs age during storage, multiple changes occur causing shape deformation, reduction in oxygen-carrying capacity, and an increase in vascular adhesiveness. No difference in morbidity or mortality has been attributed to the age of transfused blood products, based on low and moderate certainty of evidence respectively. For reasons that are still unclear, data has suggested a slight increase in nosocomial infections with transfusions of newer RBCs.

## SUGGESTED READINGS

Ferraris, V. A., Brown, J. R., Despotis, G. J., Hammon, J. W., Reece, T. B., Saha, S. P., et al. (2011). 2011 Update to The Society of Thoracic Surgeons and The Society of Cardiovascular Anesthesiologists Blood Conservation Clinical Practice Guidelines. *Annals of Thoracic Surgery, 91,* 944–982. doi:10.1016/j.athoracsur.2010.11.078.

Bennett, S., Baker, L., Shorr, R., Martel, G., & Fergusson, D. (2016). The impact of perioperative red blood cell transfusions in patients undergoing liver resection: A systematic review protocol. *Systematic Reviews, 5,* 38. doi:10.1186/s13643-016-0217-5.

Cardone, D., & Klein, A. (2009). Perioperative blood conservation. *European Journal of Anaesthesiology, 26*(9), 722–729. doi:10.1097/EJA.0b013e32832c5280.

*Herbal Medicines: Anticoagulation effects.* Retrieved from https://www.openanesthesia.org/herbal_medicines_anticoagulation_effects. Accessed November 14, 2021.

Lyu, X., Qiao, W., Li, D., & Leng, Y. (2017). Impact of perioperative blood transfusion on clinical outcomes in patients with colorectal liver metastasis after hepatectomy: A meta-analysis. *Oncotarget, 8*(25), 41740–41748. doi:10.18632/oncotarget.16771.

Manjuladevi, M., & Vasudeva-Upadhyaya, K. (2014). Perioperative blood management. *Indian Journal of Anaesthesia, 58*(5), 573–580. doi:10.4103/0019-5049.144658.

Ferraris, V. A., Ferraris, S. P., Saha, S. P., Hessel, E. A., II, Haan, C. K., Royston, B. D., et al. (2007). Perioperative blood transfusion and blood conservation in cardiac surgery: The Society of Thoracic Surgeons and The Society of Cardiovascular Anesthesiologists Clinical Practice Guideline. *Annals of Thoracic Surgery, 83,* S27–S86. doi:10.1016/j.athoracsur.2007.02.099.

Practice Guidelines for Perioperative Blood Management: An updated report by the American Society of Anesthesiologists Task Force on Perioperative Blood Management. (2015). *Anesthesiology, 122*(2), 241–275. doi:10.1097/ALN.0000000000000463.

Quraishy, N., Bachowski, G., Benjamin, R., Borge, D., Dodd, R., Eder, A., et al. (2021). *A Compendium of Transfusion Practice Guidelines* (4th ed.). Washington, DC: American Red Cross.

Shander, A., & Javidroozi, M. (2015). Blood conservation strategies and the management of perioperative anaemia. *Current Opinion in Anaesthesiology, 28*(3), 356–363. doi:10.1097/ACO.0000000000000179.

Theusinger, O., & Spahn, D. (2016). Perioperative blood conservation strategies for major spine surgery. *Best Practice & Research Clinical Anaesthesiology, 30*(1), 41–52. Retrieved from https://doi.org/10.1016/j.bpa.2015.11.007.

# Preoperative and Postoperative

# Principles of Preoperative Evaluation

FRANCES HU, MD

## Preoperative Evaluation and Risk Assessment

An effective preoperative evaluation should consist of an individualized assessment of patient- and surgery-specific risk factors to formulate an overall patient- and surgery-specific assessment of perioperative morbidity and mortality risk. The results of the combined risk stratification should guide perioperative testing and management decisions, including appropriate surgical center assignment, available staff expertise and level of care, and patient disposition.

Major components of the preoperative evaluation include a review of significant medical comorbidities, functional capacity and psychosocial assessment, medication review, and screening for personal and family history of anesthetic complications, bleeding and thrombotic risk, and sleep apnea. A focused physical exam should be performed, relevant test results reviewed, and targeted preoperative testing ordered when medically or surgically indicated. Vulnerable populations such as older adults may benefit from additional targeted preoperative assessments.

Risk stratification results and management recommendations should be documented and communicated to the patient and surgical team, including details about proposed preoperative testing and consultations, medication management, and specific risk mitigation strategies.

The appropriate timing of the preoperative evaluation is influenced by factors such as degree of surgical invasiveness and concurrent medical disease burden and severity. When possible, a patient undergoing highly invasive surgery or with high burden of coexistent disease should be evaluated far enough in advance of planned surgery to allow for additional necessary testing, comorbidity optimization, and risk reduction interventions. Patients with limited and stable comorbid conditions undergoing surgical procedures with low invasiveness could feasibly undergo preoperative evaluation either on or before the day of surgery.

## Surgical Urgency and Risk

Surgical risk is influenced by the intrinsic invasiveness of the planned surgical procedure and processes that augment or modulate the stress response. An understanding of the urgency of the planned surgery (Table 74.1) is essential to guide appropriate perioperative assessment and management strategies (Fig. 74.1). The 2014 ACC/AHA Guideline distinguishes between emergency, urgent, time-sensitive, and elective surgery. With *emergency surgery* (life or limb threatened if not taken to the operating room [OR] typically within 6 h), there is very limited time for preoperative clinical evaluation. With *urgent surgery* (life or limb threatened if not taken to the OR typically within 6–24 h), there may be time for limited clinical assessment and interventions before surgery. *Time-sensitive surgery* refers to a procedure where a delay of >1–6 weeks adversely affects outcomes. *Elective surgery* can generally be delayed up to 1 year.

## Patient-Specific Risk Assessment

Unstable medical conditions (e.g., acute coronary syndrome, decompensated heart failure, unstable cardiac dysrhythmias, severe symptomatic aortic/mitral valve stenosis) require additional

| TABLE 74.1 | Surgical Urgency Categories | | |
|---|---|---|---|
| Surgical Urgency Category | Description | Typical Timing of Necessary Surgical Intervention | Examples |
| Emergency | Life or limb-threatening condition requiring immediate surgical intervention | Within 6 h | AAA rupture<br>Abdominal or extremity compartment syndrome<br>GSW to chest/abdomen |
| Urgent | Life or limb-threatening condition | Within 6–24 h | Necrotizing fasciitis<br>Knee dislocation with neurovascular compromise<br>Femoral neck fracture |
| Time Sensitive | Condition where additional surgical delay for evaluation or change in management would adversely affect outcome | Within 1–6 weeks | Cancer resection surgeries<br>Carotid endarterectomy for symptomatic carotid stenosis<br>Spinal cord decompression for myelopathy |
| Elective | Non-life-threatening condition<br>Typically scheduled in advance | Up to 1 year | Total joint arthroplasty for OA<br>Brain resective surgery for drug-refractory epilepsy |

*AAA,* abdominal aortic aneurysm; *GSW,* gunshot wound; *OA,* osteoarthritis.

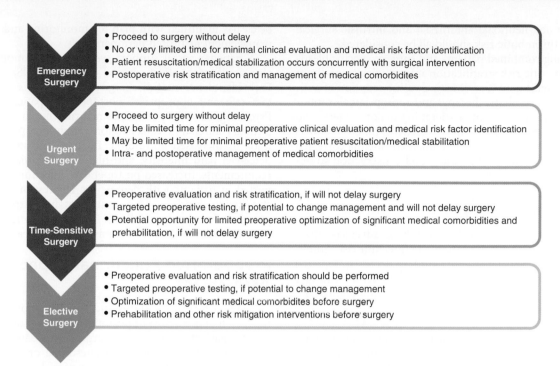

**Emergency Surgery**
- Proceed to surgery without delay
- No or very limited time for minimal clinical evaluation and medical risk factor identification
- Patient resuscitation/medical stabilization occurs concurrently with surgical intervention
- Postoperative risk stratification and management of medical comorbidites

**Urgent Surgery**
- Proceed to surgery without delay
- May be limited time for minimal preoperative clinical evaluation and medical risk factor identification
- May be limited time for minimal preoperative patient resuscitation/medical stabilization
- Intra- and postoperative management of medical comorbidities

**Time-Sensitive Surgery**
- Preoperative evaluation and risk stratification, if will not delay surgery
- Targeted preoperative testing, if potential to change management and will not delay surgery
- Potential opportunity for limited preoperative optimization of significant medical comorbidities and prehabilitation, if will not delay surgery

**Elective Surgery**
- Preoperative evaluation and risk stratification should be performed
- Targeted preoperative testing, if potential to change management
- Optimization of significant medical comorbidites before surgery
- Prehabilitation and other risk mitigation interventions before surgery

**Fig. 74.1** Surgical urgency management approach.

evaluation and stabilization before proceeding with elective non-cardiac surgery. Similarly, diagnoses associated with a high risk of perioperative complications (e.g., myocardial infarction [MI] without revascularization within 60 days, recent percutaneous coronary revascularization, venous thromboembolism [VTE] within 90 days, ischemic stroke/transient ischemic attack [TIA] within 6–9 months) should prompt deferral of nonurgent surgery during these highest-risk time frames.

## Medical Comorbidities

Significant medical comorbidities should be identified, with disease severity and stability assessed. Poorly controlled medical conditions that affect surgical outcomes (e.g., diabetes, heart failure, chronic obstructive pulmonary disease) should be optimized before proceeding with elective surgery.

Cardiovascular system conditions such as ischemic heart disease, heart failure, pulmonary hypertension, valvulopathies (especially severe aortic and mitral stenosis), left ventricular outflow tract obstructions, uncontrolled arrhythmias, and conduction system disorders are associated with an increased risk of perioperative cardiovascular complications including major adverse cardiac event (MACE) and death. Recent ischemic stroke or TIA is associated with an increased risk of perioperative stroke, independent of surgical risk classification. Details of coronary stents and cardiac implantable electrical devices with stent/device indication, device dependency status, and most recent device interrogation report should be obtained and documented. Management of antiplatelet and other antithrombotic therapy is individualized based on combined bleeding and thrombotic risk stratification.

Postoperative pulmonary complications (PPCs) occur at least as commonly as cardiac complications after noncardiac surgery and are associated with higher morbidity, mortality, length of stay (LOS), and cost, and account for almost 25% of deaths that occur in the first postoperative week. Postoperative pneumonia is responsible for 4% of readmissions and predicts long-term mortality in patients over age 70 years. Patient-specific PPC risk factors include increasing age, smoking, chronic obstructive pulmonary disease, poorly controlled asthma, obstructive sleep apnea, heart failure, pulmonary hypertension, functional status dependency, malnutrition, recent respiratory infection (within 30 days), and higher American Society of Anesthesiologists (ASA) physical status class. Surgery-associated risk factors include surgical site proximity to the diaphragm, longer duration of surgery (>3 h), general versus regional anesthesia, residual neuromuscular block, and emergency surgery.

The status and severity of other coexistent medical conditions with potential effect on surgical/anesthesia outcome (e.g., diabetes/endocrinopathies, neuromuscular disorders, kidney and liver disease, immune deficiencies and hematologic conditions including coagulopathies, thromboembolic history, and anemia) should also be detailed. Specific discussion of perioperative management of individual medical comorbidities is beyond the scope of this chapter.

## Bleeding/Thrombotic Risk Assessment

Patient and surgery-specific factors should be incorporated into an individualized risk assessment for bleeding and thrombotic complications. Personal and family history of bleeding diatheses and thrombophilia; clinical history of bleeding and thrombotic events; relevant medical comorbidities (e.g., coronary stents, mechanical heart valves, active malignancy diagnosis, systemic lupus erythematosus, nephrotic syndrome, inflammatory bowel disease, quantitative platelet disorders, significant liver dysfunction, alcohol use disorder); medications/therapies that increase bleeding or thrombotic risk (and indication for therapy); planned neuraxial anesthesia; and intrinsic surgical bleeding and thrombotic risk should all be considered.

The resulting combined patient- and surgery-specific bleeding and thrombotic risk stratification informs decisions about medication management (continuation vs. interruption of antiplatelet and antithrombotic therapy) and appropriate thromboprophylaxis strategies. Patients undergoing major surgery who have beliefs precluding them from receiving blood products should have their wishes clearly documented, anemia corrected prior to surgery when possible, and blood conservation strategies prioritized.

## Psychosocial History

Cigarette smoking and hazardous drinking adversely affect wound healing and increase surgical site infection risk. Smoking is additionally associated with skin flap necrosis, impaired bone healing, increased PPCs, venous thromboembolism and cardiovascular complication risk, and higher postoperative pain intensity and narcotic requirements.

Hazardous drinking ($\geq$3 alcohol equivalents [AEs]/day) has also been associated with increased bleeding complications, cardiopulmonary and neurologic complications, unplanned intensive care unit transfers, and increased LOS; surgical complications are increased as much as twofold to fourfold in patients who drink 5+ AEs/day.

Vaping/electronic cigarette products contain numerous ingredients such as flavorings and preservatives and are associated with increased airway inflammation and hyperreactivity, as well as e-cigarette and vaping associated lung injury and deaths.

In the United States as of March 2022, recreational adult cannabis use has been legalized in 18 states, the District of Columbia, and two U.S. territories; medical cannabis use is legal in 37 states, the District of Columbia, and four U.S. territories.

Cannabinoids exert dose-dependent effects on the sympathetic and parasympathetic nervous systems and cardiovascular system (affecting heart rate, blood pressure, myocardial contractility, and myocardial and cerebral blood flow); alter central thermoregulation; and impair endothelial and platelet function. Perioperative complications in cannabis users includes cardiac arrhythmias, myocardial and cerebral ischemia, airway hyperreactivity (smokers), intraoperative hypothermia/severe postoperative shivering, and impaired hemostasis. Chronic users may experience prolonged anesthetic effects and require significantly higher doses of anesthetics and postoperative analgesics.

Patients on high doses of chronic opioids or taking medications for opioid use disorder (e.g., methadone, buprenorphine, intramuscular naltrexone) may benefit from formal pain service consultation for perioperative pain management recommendations prior to undergoing elective surgery with significant anticipated postoperative pain; multimodal analgesia strategies and optimization of opioid-sparing analgesic techniques should be employed.

Screening for tobacco, alcohol, substance and opioid use, and vaping/e-cigarette use should be performed prior to all elective surgeries. Patients should be counseled on risks, with smoking and hazardous alcohol cessation advised for at least 4 to 8 weeks preoperatively when feasible. PPC and other risk mitigation measures should also be employed perioperatively. High-risk patients may benefit from referral for intensive intervention. Patients at risk for alcohol or drug withdrawal should

be clearly identified with plan for monitoring and appropriate management instituted perioperatively.

A patient's social support system and emotional state can also significantly affect surgical outcomes, LOS, and recovery. Early identification of discharge planning needs can help facilitate safe and appropriate postoperative patient disposition. Psychological stress potentiates neurohormonal hypothalamic-pituitary-adrenal axis activation. High preoperative anxiety leads to increased autonomic fluctuations, augmentation of perceived pain intensity, and higher anesthesia and analgesic requirements. Increased postoperative infections have been reported in patients with depression. Depression, anxiety, catastrophizing mindsets, fear of surgery, high stress levels, and poor social supports are all risk factors for central pain sensitization and development of persistent postoperative pain.

## Preoperative Functional Capacity Assessment

Dependent functional status and poor functional capacity are independent predictors of postoperative morbidity and mortality. All patients undergoing surgical procedures other than minor procedures under local anesthesia or sedation should undergo an assessment of their functional capacity as part of their preoperative evaluation. Evaluation of functional capacity using a standardized, multi-item validated functional capacity assessment tool such as the Duke Activity Status Index appears to correlate better with cardiopulmonary exercise testing results than does subjective provider assessment (Measurement of Exercise Tolerance before Surgery trial) and has additional predictive value for perioperative MI and death.

## Sleep Apnea Screening

Preoperative sleep apnea screening using a standardized, validated sleep apnea risk assessment tool is advised for all surgical patients without a preexisting diagnosis of sleep apnea. Patients with moderate or severe sleep apnea on sleep apnea treatment (positive airway pressure therapy or dental appliance) should generally be advised to bring their device on the day of surgery and perioperative risk mitigation measures and monitoring employed.

## Focused Physical Examination

A focused preoperative physical exam should include a minimum of an airway evaluation, heart and lung exam, and documentation of vital signs. A general assessment of cognitive and mobility status (including use of mobility aids) and documentation of focal neurologic deficits and medical implantable electronic devices and vascular access devices are also suggested. Other specific physical examination elements should be directed by individual medical history and systems review.

## Ancillary Testing

Preoperative testing and recommendation for additional specialty consultation, if any, should be individualized and guided by inherent surgical risks, patient comorbidities, and medication and disease monitoring considerations.

Low-value testing (e.g., obtaining "routine" preoperative laboratory testing and electrocardiograms prior to low-risk outpatient surgeries in the absence of independent medical indications), where results are not anticipated to significantly influence perioperative management, adds unnecessarily to medical costs and may lead to further invasive testing with potential harm and surgical delays and should be avoided (ABIM Choosing Wisely campaign). High-risk patients and patients undergoing highly invasive surgeries may benefit from additional preoperative testing for further risk stratification or diagnostic purposes.

Symptoms or clinical findings warranting additional medical evaluation independent of the planned surgery (e.g., new unexplained chest pain or dyspnea; physical exam findings suggestive of advanced liver disease in a pre–hip arthroplasty patient; acute nontraumatic unilateral leg swelling in a patient undergoing a lobectomy for lung cancer) should be investigated appropriately before proceeding with nonurgent surgery.

## Preoperative Medication Management

An accurate, updated list of all medications taken (including over the counter, supplements, and as-needed medications) should be obtained in all surgical patients. Use of medications that increase surgical site infection/delayed wound healing risk, bleeding or thrombosis risk, perioperative respiratory insufficiency, urinary retention, falls and neurocognitive dysfunction, or are otherwise high risk (e.g., monoamine oxidase inhibitors, buprenorphine, opioids, benzodiazepines) should be specifically noted. Polypharmacy should be reduced prior to surgery when possible, and a specific plan for perioperative management of each medication detailed and provided to the patient in writing.

## Anemia and Nutrition

Preoperative anemia is an independent risk factor for perioperative morbidity, LOS, readmission, and increased 30-day mortality in both cardiac and noncardiac surgeries. Preoperative anemia should be identified, investigated, and treated when feasible prior to major surgery and blood conservation strategies employed to reduce the need for perioperative red blood cell transfusion (RBCT) (see Table 74.2).

Malnutrition and undernutrition are common in hospitalized patients, and the prevalence in the general population rises with increasing age. Malnutrition is an independent risk factor for morbidity and mortality after major surgery, including wound, infectious, and pulmonary complications and increased LOS. Preoperative screening for malnutrition is recommended in patients undergoing major surgery; at-risk patients may benefit from preoperative nutritional intervention (oral/enteric nutritional supplementation) to promote a positive net protein balance during the surgical period. Prolonged preoperative fasting should be avoided and oral/enteric intake resumed early in the postoperative period.

## Special Populations—Geriatrics

Thirty-five percent of inpatient surgical procedures in the United States are performed now on individuals aged 65 and older. Biologic age, rather than chronologic age, with higher burden of accumulated disease in addition to age-related physiologic decline in organ function, is associated with higher rates of adverse postoperative outcomes.

In recognition of the special needs of our rapidly growing geriatric surgical population, the American Geriatrics Society and the American College of Surgeons (ACS) National Surgical Quality Improvement Program (NSQIP) Geriatrics Surgery Task Force jointly developed best-practices guidelines on the optimal preoperative evaluation and perioperative care of the geriatric surgical patient. In addition to other usual components of the preoperative evaluation, they recommend that the older surgical patient evaluation include assessment of age-related at-risk domains, including cognitive, functional, and mobility status; nutritional status; psychosocial assessment; perioperative neurocognitive dysfunction and fall risk assessments; and frailty screening.

Frailty is a geriatric syndrome characterized by accumulated deficits in multiple domains (including functional status, mobility, nutrition, cognition, psychosocial/emotional, disease burden, strength, and balance), which results in diminished physiologic reserves, loss of resiliency, and increased vulnerability to stressors. Frailty better predicts postoperative complications than chronologic age and is an independent risk factor for perioperative morbidity and mortality, including postoperative delirium and other complications, failure to rescue, increased LOS, 30-day readmission, non-home discharge, reduced functional recovery, and early and 1-year postoperative mortality.

Geriatric patients undergoing intermediate and high-risk elective procedures should undergo frailty screening as part of their preoperative assessment. Patients identified as frail and pre-frail should be considered high-risk from a surgical standpoint.

## Risk Stratification and Mitigation

Patient- and surgery-specific risks are factored into multivariate risk analyses to calculate combined risk assessments. The ACS NSQIP Surgical Risk Calculator has broad clinical applicability and incorporates 20 individual patient- and surgery-specific variables to calculate the patient's estimated and comparative risk for 13 specific surgical outcomes (with 4 additional optional geriatric outcomes). Other risk calculators have been developed for use in specific patient or surgical populations (e.g., Geriatric-Sensitive Perioperative Cardiac Risk Index, Vascular Quality Initiative risk calculators), or outcomes of interest (e.g., MACE risk, PPCs, VTE), and can be useful for additional risk stratification purposes.

Risk reduction strategies should focus on modifiable risk factors and optimization of comorbid medical conditions. The extent and intensity of preoperative risk mitigation measures should be individualized based on overall patient- and surgery-specific risk (Table 74.2) and considering the implications of surgical delay on clinical outcomes in the case of urgent or time-sensitive surgery. Decisions to proceed with or delay surgery should be made on a case-by-case basis as part of a shared decision-making process involving the patient and surgical and medical care teams.

| TABLE 74.2 | Preoperative Risk Assessment and Mitigation Strategies |
| --- | --- |
| **Preoperative Risk Factor Assessment** | **Potential Preoperative Risk Mitigation Strategies** |
| Identification of comorbid conditions, severity, stability<br>Cardiac and pulmonary risk stratification<br> • ACC/AHA Guideline, ESC/ESA Guideline, CCS Guideline<br> • RCRI, ACS NSQIP MICA risk calculator (Gupta), ACS NSQIP Surgical Risk Calculator, cardiac biomarker screening<br> • ARISCAT Risk Index, Arozullah Respiratory Failure Index, Gupta Postop Pneumonia and Postop Respiratory Failure risk calculators | Comorbidity optimization<br>Consider initiation of statin therapy in high risk patients<br>Antiplatelet/antithrombotic therapy management plan<br>Inspiratory muscle training<br>Perioperative MINS monitoring |
| Medication reconciliation | Detailed medication management instructions<br>De-prescribe unnecessary medications<br>Avoidance of Beers criteria PIMs<br>Pharmacogenomic testing |
| Sleep apnea screening<br> • STOP-Bang, Sleep Apnea Clinical Score, Berlin Questionnaire, ASA OSA Checklist<br> • BMI ≥30 + elevated serum $HCO_3$ (possible OHS) | Perioperative risk mitigation strategies<br>Consider referral for sleep testing pre- or postop<br>Opioid sparing techniques<br>Consider appropriateness of planned surgery location (e.g., free-standing ASC vs. hospital-based), monitoring capabilities, postoperative pain requirements |
| Smoking, alcohol, substance use screening<br> • Single-screen question, AUDIT-C, TAPS | Preoperative counseling<br>Smoking and alcohol cessation (≥4–8 weeks)<br>Referrals for substance abuse counseling/treatment<br>Monitoring for withdrawal syndromes |
| Opioid use disorder identification | Consider pain service consultation<br>Multimodal analgesia strategy<br>Optimize opioid-sparing therapies |
| Bleeding, thrombotic risk stratification<br> • Caprini RAM, Rogers RAM<br> • ASCO Clinical Practice Guideline Update, ACC Expert Consensus Decision Pathway, ASH Guideline, ACCP Perioperative Guideline | Perioperative management plan for medications that increase bleeding/thrombotic risk<br>Smoking cessation<br>Perioperative thromboprophylaxis recommendations |
| Wound healing/SSI risk factors | Perioperative management plan for biologic disease modifying therapies, sirolimus, systemic chemotherapy/immunotherapy<br>Preoperative reduction of long-term daily GC dosing, when possible<br>Smoking and alcohol cessation |
| Functional capacity<br> • DASI, modified DASI<br>Functional status dependency | Prehabilitation: aerobic/resistance training |
| Fall risk | Fall precautions, access to mobility aids<br>Prehabilitation |
| Nutritional screening | Oral nutritional supplementation, increased protein intake<br>Avoid prolonged preoperative fasting |
| Anemia | IV/oral iron, ESA<br>Blood conservation strategies |
| Neurocognitive dysfunction risk<br>Cognitive screening<br> • Mini-Cog test | Access to assistive devices, glasses, hearing aids<br>Reduce polypharmacy, avoidance of Beers criteria PIMs<br>Correction of anemia, electrolyte imbalances; avoidance of dehydration |
| Frailty screening<br>FRAIL scale, Edmonton Frailty Index, others<br>+/− cognitive screening (Mini-Cog test) | Multimodal prehabilitation (physical (aerobic/resistance/ +/− ROM) training, nutritional support, psychological preparation)<br>SDM, goals of care discussion<br>Comprehensive geriatric assessment<br>Specialized/geriatric care pathways, geriatrics comanagement<br>Geriatrics/palliative care consultation |
| Psychosocial assessment | Early involvement of case management for discharge planning<br>Nonpharmacologic anxiety/stress management |

*ACC/AHA*, American College of Cardiology/American Heart Association; *ESC/ESA*, European Society of Cardiology/Euroean Society of Anaesthesiology; *RCRI*, Revised Cardiac Risk Index; *ACS NSQIP*, American College of Surgeons National Surgical Quality Improvement Program; *MICA*, Gupta Perioperative Myocardial Infarct or Cardiac Arrest; *ARISCAT*, Assess Respiratory Risk in Surgical Patients in Catalonia Tool; *STOP-Bang: Snoring*, Tiredness, Oserved Apnea, Pressure, BMI, Age, Neck Circumference, Gender; *ASA OSA*, American Society of Anesthesiology Obstructive Sleep Apnea; *BMI*, body mass index; *AUDIT-C*, Alcohol Use Disorders Identification Test; *TAPS*, Tobacco, Alcohol, Prescription Medication, and other Substance Tool; *RAM: Risk Assessment Model*; *ASCO*, American Society of Clinical Oncology; *ACC*, American College of Cardiology; *ASH*, American Society of Hematology; *ACCP*, American College of Chest Physicians; *DASI*, Duke Activity Status Index; *FRAIL*, Fatigue, Resistance, Ambulation, Illness, and Loss of weight; *MINS*, Myocardial Injury after Noncardiac Surgery; *PIMs*, Potentially Inappropriate Medications; *ASC*, Ambulatory Surgical Center; *GC*, Glucocorticoid; *IV*, intravenous; *ESA*, Erythrpoiesis-stimulating agents; *ROM*, range of motion; *SDM*, shared decision making.

## SUGGESTED READINGS

ABIM Foundation Choosing Wisely Campaign. Retrieved from https://www.choosingwisely.org/?s=surgery. Accessed December 2021.

ACS NSQIP Surgical Risk Calculator. Retrieved from http://riskcalculator.facs.org/RiskCalculator/. Accessed December 2021.

Alvarez-Nebreda, M. L., Bentov, N., Urman, R. D., Setia, S., Huang, J. C., Pfeifer, K., et al. (2018). Recommendations for preoperative management of frailty from the Society for Perioperative Assessment and Quality Improvement (SPAQI). *Journal of Clinical Anesthesia, 47,* 33–42.

Benesch, C., Glance, L. G., Derdeyn, C. P., Fleisher, L. A., Holloway, R. G., Messé, S. R., et al. (2021). Perioperative neurological evaluation and management to lower the risk of acute stroke in patients undergoing noncardiac, nonneurological surgery: A scientific statement from the American Heart Association/American Stroke Association. *Circulation, 143,* e923–e946.

Chow, W. B., Rosenthal, R. A., Merkow, R. P., Ko, C. Y., Esnaola, N. F., American College of Surgeons National. (2012). Optimal preoperative assessment of the geriatric surgical patient: a best practices guideline from the American College of Surgeons National Surgical Quality Improvement Program and the American Geriatrics Society. *Journal of the American College of Surgeons, 215*(4), 453–466.

Goodman, S. M., Springer, B.D., Chen, A.F., Davis, M., & Fernandez, D.R., et al. (2022). 2022 American College of Rheumatology/American Association of Hip and Knee Surgeons guideline for the perioperative management of antirheumatic medication in patients with rheumatic diseases undergoing elective total hip or total knee arthroplasty. *Journal of Arthroplasty,* 37, 1676–1683. doi:https://doi.org/10.1016/j.arth.2022.05.043. 35732511.

Institute for Clinical Systems Improvement (ICSI). *Health care guideline: Perioperative* (6th ed.). January 2020. Retrieved from https://www.icsi.org/wp-content/uploads/2021/11/Periop_6th-Ed_2020_v2.pdf.

Mayo Clinic Proceedings. *Thematic review on perioperative medicine* (mayoclinicproceedings.org) 2020 – 2021. Retrieved from https://www.mayoclinicproceedings.org/perioperative_med; Mayo Clinic Proceedings. Society for Perioperative Assessment and Quality Improvement (SPAQI) Medication Management consensus statements. Accessed December 2021.

Mohanty, S., Rosenthal, R. A., Russell, M. M., Mohanty, S., Rosenthal, R. A., & Russell, M. M. (2016). Optimal perioperative management of the geriatric patient: A best practices guideline from the ACS NSQIP/American Geriatrics Society. *Journal of the American College of Surgeons, 222*(5), 930–947.

# 75

# Preoperative Evaluation of the Patient With Cardiac Disease for Noncardiac Operations

J. ROSS RENEW, MD   |   HARISH RAMAKRISHNA, MD, FACC, FESC, FASE

Cardiovascular disease is one of the leading causes of death worldwide and the chief cause of death in the United States. Cardiac complications following noncardiac operations account for the majority of the morbidity and mortality risks in the perioperative period, with incidences ranging from 1.5% in the unselected population to 4% in patients at risk for or with cardiovascular disease to as high as 11% in patients with multiple risk factors. The key role of the anesthesiologist as perioperative physician when confronted with a patient with cardiovascular disease for a noncardiac operation is to effectively identify patients with modifiable conditions and those at risk for experiencing cardiac events in the perioperative period. The risk stratification that follows is the basis for safe perioperative management of patients with cardiovascular disease. The key issues that need to be addressed are based on the American College of Cardiology/American Heart Association (ACC/AHA) Guidelines on Perioperative Cardiovascular Evaluation for Noncardiac Surgery. The revised guidelines also include recommendations for the management of patients with coronary artery stents and the perioperative use of β-adrenergic receptor blocking agents.

## Defining Comorbid Conditions

The clinician should identify any active cardiac conditions (Table 75.1) or clinical risk factors that have been associated with adverse outcomes. Active cardiac conditions are defined as unstable coronary syndromes, decompensated systolic or diastolic heart failure, significant arrhythmias, and severe valvular heart disease. Clinical risk factors are independent risk factors that are associated with poor outcomes and include history of ischemic heart disease (suggestive history, symptoms, or Q waves on electrocardiogram), history of prior or compensated heart failure (suggestive history, symptoms, or examination findings),

| TABLE 75.1 | Active Cardiac Conditions That Mandate Preoperative*Evaluation and Treatment | |
|---|---|---|
| **Condition** | **Examples** | |
| Unstable coronary syndromes | Unstable or severe angina[†] (CCS class III or IV)[‡]<br>Recent MI[§] | |
| Decompensated HF (NYHA functional class IV; worsening or new-onset HF) | | |
| Significant arrhythmias | High-grade AV block<br>Mobitz type II AV block<br>Third-degree AV block<br>Symptomatic ventricular arrhythmias<br>Supraventricular arrhythmias, including AF, with uncontrolled ventricular rate (HR >100 beats/min at rest)<br>Symptomatic bradycardia<br>Newly recognized ventricular tachycardia | |
| Severe valvular disease | Severe aortic stenosis (mean pressure gradient >40 mm Hg, aortic valve area <1.0 cm$^2$, or symptomatic)<br>Symptomatic mitral stenosis (progressive dyspnea on exertion, exertional presyncope, or HF) | |

*Before noncardiac operations.
[†]According to Campeau L. Letter: grading of angina pectoris. *Circulation.* 1976;54:522–523.
[‡]May include "stable" angina in patients who are sedentary.
[§]The American College of Cardiology National Database Library defines "recent" MI as occurring >7 days but ≤30 days previously.
*AF,* Atrial fibrillation; *AV,* atrioventricular; *CCS,* Canadian Cardiovascular Society; *HF,* heart failure; *HR,* heart rate; *MI,* myocardial infarction; *NYHA,* New York Heart Association.
Reprinted, with permission, from Fleisher LA, Fleischmann KE, Auerbach AD, et al. ACC/AHA 2014 guidelines on perioperative cardiovascular evaluation and management of patients undergoing noncardiac surgery: a report of the American College of Cardiology/American Heart Association Task Force on practice guidelines. *J Am Coll Cardiol.* 2014;64(22):e77–137.

history of stroke or transient ischemic attack, insulin-dependent diabetes mellitus, and renal insufficiency (serum creatinine concentration >2 mg/dL).

## Assessing Surgical Risk

Evaluation of surgical risk is crucial during preoperative assessment. Surgical procedures have been classified as low-risk, intermediate-risk, and high-risk vascular operations (Table 75.2).

| TABLE 75.2 | Surgical Risk* Stratification for Patients With Preexisting Cardiac Disease | |
|---|---|---|
| **Level of Risk** | **Procedure Examples** | |
| High (vascular procedures)[†] | Aortic and other vascular operations<br>Peripheral vascular operations | |
| Intermediate[‡] | Intraperitoneal and intrathoracic operations<br>Carotid endarterectomy<br>Head and neck operation<br>Orthopedic operations<br>Prostate operations | |
| Low[§] | Endoscopic procedures<br>Superficial procedures<br>Cataract operations<br>Breast operations<br>Ambulatory operations | |

*Combined incidence of cardiac death and nonfatal myocardial infarction.
[†]Reported cardiac risk often >5%.
[‡]Reported cardiac risk generally 1%–5%.
[§]Reported cardiac risk generally <1%. These procedures do not generally require further preoperative cardiac testing.

Understandably, procedures with differing levels of stress (alterations in heart rate, blood pressure, intravascular volume, blood loss, and pain) are associated with differing levels of morbidity and mortality risks. Ophthalmologic and superficial procedures represent the lowest risk and very rarely result in morbidity and death. The intermediate-risk category (includes endovascular abdominal aortic aneurysm repair and carotid endarterectomy) represents procedures with associated morbidity and mortality risks that vary depending on the surgical location and extent of procedure. Major vascular procedures are the highest risk procedures and mandate further investigation.

## Evaluating Functional Status

Assessment of functional status in the patient with cardiovascular and pulmonary disease is important because $O_2$ uptake is considered to be the best measure of cardiovascular reserve and exercise capacity. Functional status is measured using metabolic equivalents (METs) (Table 75.3). One MET represents the $O_2$ consumption of a person at rest (3–5 mL · kg$^{-1}$ · min$^{-1}$). A functional capacity of four METs is considered the minimum requirement for a patient undergoing a major surgical procedure. Consequently, patients who are unable to meet a minimum of 4-MET demand during daily activities are at higher risk for developing perioperative cardiovascular and pulmonary complications. Those patients with multiple medical comorbid conditions that limit activity will need to be formally tested to objectively determine cardiopulmonary reserve.

| TABLE 75.3 | Energy Requirement for Various Activities |
|---|---|
| **Energy Expenditure** | **Can You ...** |
| 1 MET ↓ | Take care of yourself? Eat, dress, or use the toilet? Walk indoors around the house? Walk a block or two on level ground at 2–3 mph (3.2–4.8 kph)? |
| 4 METs ↓ | Do light work around the house, like dusting or doing dishes? Climb a flight of stairs or walk up a hill? Walk on level ground at 4 mph (6.4 kph)? Run a short distance? Do heavy work around the house, like scrubbing floors or lifting or moving heavy furniture? |
| >10 METs | Participate in moderate recreational activities, like golf, bowling, dancing, doubles tennis, or throwing a football or baseball? |

*kph,* Kilometers per hour; *MFT,* metabolic equivalent; *mph,* miles per hour.
Reprinted, with permission, from Fleisher L, Beckman J, Brown K, et al. ACC/AHA 2007 guidelines on perioperative cardiovascular evaluation and care for noncardiac surgery: a report of the American College of Cardiology/American Heart Association Task Force on practice guidelines. *J Am Coll Cardiol.* 2007;50:e159–241.

# Applying the Revised American College of Cardiology/American Heart Association Guidelines

Once the clinician has performed a history and examination, a stepwise approach outlined by the ACC/AHA can then be used for risk stratification and determination of the need for additional cardiac testing (Fig. 75.1).

Step 1. Is the noncardiac operation emergent? If so, the patient is taken to the operating room without delay, with the focus being appropriate intraoperative and postoperative cardiac surveillance.

Step 2. Does the patient have acute coronary syndrome? If so, evaluate and treat according to goal-directed medical therapy.

Step 3. Based on combined clinical/surgical risk, is the perioperative risk low? Recognizing that the risk for perioperative cardiac complications in low-risk operations is less than 1% even in high-risk patients, the guidelines state that the patient may proceed to surgery without further testing.

Step 4. If the patient demonstrates good functional capacity (being able to perform >4 METs of activity without cardiopulmonary symptoms), the patient may proceed to surgery.

Step 5. Patients with poor or indeterminate functional capacity for intermediate-risk or high-risk procedures require further testing if the results will affect clinical decision-making or their perioperative care. The key issue here is the number of clinical predictors (derived from the Revised Cardiac Risk Index). Patients with no clinical risk factors may proceed to surgery. Patients with one or two risk factors may proceed to surgery with heart rate

control; noninvasive testing may be considered only if it will change management. Patients with three or more clinical risk factors warrant more scrutiny. These patients scheduled for vascular operations should be considered for noninvasive testing—if it will change management. On the other hand, even those with three or more risk factors scheduled for intermediate-risk operations should proceed to surgery with perioperative heart rate control. Noninvasive testing for this group should, again, be considered only if it will change management.

## Perioperative β-Adrenergic Receptor Blockade

The issue of the use of β-adrenergic receptor blocking agents in the perioperative period is controversial, largely because of limited and conflicting data from studies performed in the surgical setting, determinations of the ideal target population, type of β-adrenergic receptor blocking agent, route of administration, and duration of preoperative drug titration. Nevertheless, the latest guidelines state that perioperative β-adrenergic receptor blockade is indicated for patients already on β-adrenergic receptor blocking agents for the treatment of angina, hypertension, symptomatic arrhythmias, or congestive heart failure or for patients undergoing vascular operations who are at high cardiac risk because of ischemia (as was shown on preoperative testing).

Unless contraindicated, β-adrenergic receptor blocking agents should be considered for patients with coronary artery disease who are undergoing vascular or intermediate-risk to high-risk operations. They may be considered for any patient undergoing a vascular operation or those at intermediate to high cardiac risk who are undergoing intermediate-risk to high-risk operations. Their usefulness is uncertain in patients undergoing either intermediate-risk procedures or vascular operations with one or no clinical risk factors. Patients with absolute or relative contraindications to the use of β-adrenergic receptor blocking agents—such as decompensated heart failure, nonischemic cardiomyopathy, severe valvular heart disease, and elevated stroke risk in the absence of flow-limiting coronary disease or severe bronchospastic disease—should not receive them. If β-adrenergic receptor blocking agents are going to be started in the preoperative period to mitigate cardiovascular risk, this therapy should not be initiated the day of surgery as to allow enough time for careful titration. Statins should ideally be continued through the perioperative period for all patients.

## Patients With Prior Percutaneous Coronary Interventions

Nonelective operations in patients who have undergone percutaneous coronary interventions (PCIs), with or without coronary artery stenting, present significant risks in the perioperative period. An increasing number of these patients require noncardiac operations within a year of stenting, and this puts them at high risk of developing stent thrombosis, which is associated with significant morbidity and mortality risks (significantly higher with drug-eluting stents compared with bare metal stents). The reasons for the perioperative hypercoagulability of these patients are multifactorial and include the prothrombotic state associated with surgery,

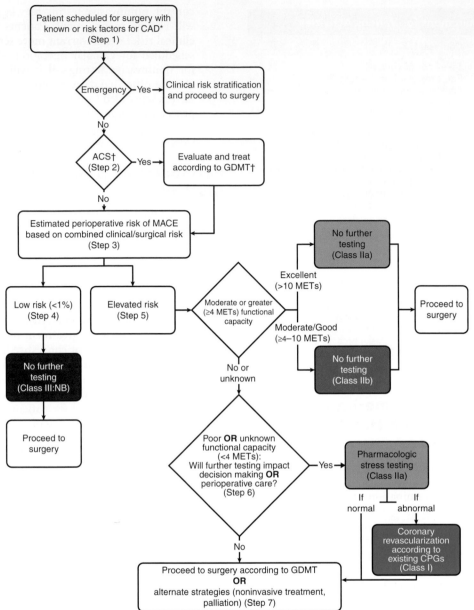

**Fig. 75.1** Stepwise approach to perioperative cardiac assessment for coronary artery disease *(CAD)*. Step 1: In patients scheduled for surgery with risk factors for or known CAD, determine the urgency of surgery. If an emergency, then determine the clinical risk factors that may influence perioperative management and proceed to surgery with appropriate monitoring and management strategies based on the clinical assessment. Step 2: If the surgery is urgent or elective, determine whether the patient has an acute coronary syndrome *(ACS)*. If yes, then refer patient for cardiology evaluation and management according to guideline-directed medical therapy *(GDMT)* according to the UA/NSTEMI and STEMI clinical practice guidelines *(CPGs)*. Step 3: If the patient has risk factors for stable CAD, then estimate the perioperative risk of a major adverse cardiac event *(MACE)* on the basis of the combined clinical/surgical risk. This estimate can use the American College of Surgeons NSQIP risk calculator (http://www. surgicalriskcalculator.com) or incorporate the RCRI with an estimation of surgical risk. For example, a patient undergoing very low-risk surgery (e.g., ophthalmologic surgery), even with multiple risk factors, would have a low risk of MACE, whereas a patient undergoing major vascular surgery with few risk factors would have an elevated risk of MACE. Step 4: If the patient has a low risk of MACE (<1%), then no further testing is needed, and the patient may proceed to surgery. Step 5: If the patient is at elevated risk of MACE, then determine functional capacity with an objective measure or scale such as the DASI. If the patient has moderate, good, or excellent functional capacity (≥4 metabolic equivalents *[METs]*), then proceed to surgery without further evaluation. Step 6: If the patient has poor (<4 METs) or unknown functional capacity, then the clinician should consult with the patient and perioperative team to determine whether further testing will affect patient decision-making (e.g., decision to perform original surgery or willingness to undergo CABG or PCI, depending on the results of the test) or perioperative care. If yes, then pharmacologic stress testing is appropriate. In those patients with unknown functional capacity, exercise stress testing may be reasonable to perform. If the stress test is abnormal, consider coronary angiography and revascularization depending on the extent of the abnormal test. The patient can then proceed to surgery with GDMT or consider alternative strategies, such as noninvasive treatment of the indication for surgery (e.g., radiation therapy for cancer) or palliation. If the test is normal, proceed to surgery according to GDMT. Step 7: If testing will not affect decision-making or care, then proceed to surgery according to GDMT or consider alternative strategies, such as noninvasive treatment of the indication for surgery (e.g., radiation therapy for cancer) or palliation. *CABG,* Coronary artery bypass graft; *DASI,* Duke Activity Status Index; *PCI,* percutaneous coronary intervention; *RCRI,* Revised Cardiac Risk Index; *STEMI,* ST-elevation myocardial infarction; *UA/NSTEMI,* unstable angina/non–ST-elevation myocardial infarction. (From Fleisher LA, Fleischmann KE, Auerbach AD, et al. ACC/AHA 2014 guidelines on perioperative cardiovascular evaluation and management of patients undergoing noncardiac surgery: a report of the American College of Cardiology/American Heart Association Task Force on practice guidelines. *J Am Coll Cardiol.* 2014;64(22):e77–137.)

incomplete stent reendothelialization, and premature discontinuation of dual-antiplatelet therapy. As per the revised ACC/AHA guidelines, patients who have undergone PCIs without stent placement should have elective operations delayed for at least 2 weeks to allow for healing of vessel injury at the balloon inflation site. Patients who have had bare metal stents implanted should have elective operations delayed for at least 30 days while being on dual-antiplatelet therapy to reduce the incidence of stent thrombosis. Drug-eluting stents pose a particular challenge because of the highly delayed reendothelialization that is a hallmark of these stents, markedly increasing the risk of early and late stent thrombosis in patients in whom drug-eluting stents have been placed.

The ACC/AHA guidelines have recently been updated for the management of dual-antiplatelet therapy in patients with drug-eluting stents. Such patients should have elective noncardiac surgery delayed until at least 3 months after implantation. In patients with stable ischemic heart disease, dual-antiplatelet therapy can be stopped after 6 months, and elective surgery can proceed. Between 3 and 6 months after drug-eluting stent implantation, clinicians must weigh the risks of stent thrombosis versus the risk of delaying surgery.

## Patients With Cardiac-Rhythm Management Devices

Patients with cardiac-rhythm management devices (pacemakers and implantable cardioverter-defibrillators [ICDs]) are another group of high-risk patients who need special attention. These patients should have their devices interrogated within 3 to 6 months after undergoing an operation. The risk of device malfunction is high perioperatively owing to electromagnetic interference. Reliance on a magnet is not recommended, except for emergencies. Preoperatively, the pacemaker should be reprogrammed to asynchronous mode if electrocautery is being used and the surgical site is above the umbilicus. In the case of ICDs, the antitachyarrhythmia function should be turned off by reprogramming or by use of a magnet in an emergency. Defibrillator pads should be considered whenever the antitachyarrhythmia function is turned off, in case the patient experiences a perioperative ventricular arrhythmia. Postoperatively, the function of the device should be interrogated, especially if an electrosurgical unit has been used, and in the case of ICDs, tachyarrhythmia function must be restored.

## SUGGESTED READINGS

Auerbach, A., & Goldman, L. (2006). Assessing and reducing the cardiac risk of noncardiac surgery. *Circulation, 113*, 1361–1376.

Feringa, H. H., Bax, J. J., Boersma, E., Kertai, M. D., Meij, S. H., Galal, W., et al. (2006). High-dose beta-blockers and tight heart rate control reduce myocardial ischemia and troponin T release in vascular surgery patients. *Circulation, 114*(Suppl. 1), s344–s349.

Fleisher, L. A., Fleischmann, K. E., Auerbach, A. D., Barnason, S. A., Beckman, J. A., Bozkurt, B., et al. (2014). 2014 ACC/AHA guideline on perioperative cardiovascular evaluation and management of patients undergoing noncardiac surgery: A report of the American College of Cardiology/American Heart Association task force on practice guidelines. *Journal of the American College of Cardiology, 64*, e77–e137.

Lee, T. H., Marcantonio, E. R., Mangione, C. M., Thomas, E. J., Polanczyk, C. A., Cook, E. F., et al. (1999). Derivation and prospective validation of a simple index for prediction of cardiac risk of major noncardiac surgery. *Circulation, 100*, 1043–1049.

Levine, G. N., Bates, E. R., Bittl, J. A., Brindis, R. G., Fihn, S. D., Fleisher, L. A., et al. (2016). 2016 ACC/AHA guideline focused update on duration of dual antiplatelet therapy in patients with coronary artery disease: A report of the American College of Cardiology/American Heart Association task force on clinical practice guidelines. *Journal of Thoracic and Cardiovascular Surgery, 152*, 1243–1275.

Nishimura, R. A., Otto, C. M., Bonow, R. O., Carabello, B. A., Erwin, J. P., III, Fleisher, L. A., Jneid, H., et al. (2017). 2017 AHA/ACC focused update of the 2014 AHA/ACC guideline for the management of patients with valvular heart disease: A report of the American College of Cardiology/American Heart Association Task Force on Clinical Practice Guidelines. *Circulation, 135*(25), e1159–e1195.

POISE Study Group. (2008). Effects of extended release metoprolol succinate in patients undergoing noncardiac surgery (POISE Trial). *Lancet, 371*, 1839–1847.

Poldermans, D., Bax, J. J., Schouten, O., Neskovic, A. N., Paelinck, B., Rocci, G., et al. (2006). Should major vascular surgery be delayed because of preoperative cardiac testing in intermediate-risk patients receiving beta-blocker therapy with tight heart rate control? *Journal of the American College of Cardiology, 48*, 964–969.

Smilowitz, N. R., Gupta, N., Ramakrishna, H., Guo, Y., Berger, J. S., & Bangalore, S. (2017). Perioperative major adverse cardiovascular and cerebrovascular events associated with noncardiac surgery. *JAMA Cardiology, 2*, 181–187.

Spertus, J. A., Kettelkamp, R., Vance, C., Decker, C., Jones, P. G., Rumsfeld, J. S., et al. (2006). Prevalence, predictors, and outcomes of premature discontinuation of thienopyridine therapy after drug-eluting stent placement: results from the PREMIER registry. *Circulation, 113*, 2803–2809.

Vicenzi MN, Meislitzer T, Heitzinger B, Halaj M, Fleisher LA, Metzler H. (2006). Coronary artery stenting and non-cardiac surgery: A prospective outcome study. *British Journal of Anaesthesia, 96*, 686–693.

Xu-Cai, Y. O., Brotman, D. J., Phillips, C. O., Michota, F. A., Tang, W. H., Whinney, C. M., et al. (2008). Outcomes of patients with stable heart failure undergoing elective noncardiac surgery. *Mayo Clinic Proceedings, 83*, 280–288.

# 76

# Tobacco Use in Surgical Patients

YU SHI, MD, MPH

Approximately 14% of adults in the United States smoke cigarettes, and each year an estimated 10 million smokers undergo surgical procedures. Chronic and acute exposures to cigarette smoke cause profound changes in physiology that increase perioperative risks of cardiovascular, pulmonary, and wound-related complications (Fig. 76.1). Thus the knowledge of how smoking and abstinence from cigarettes affect perioperative physiology is of practical importance. This chapter will review (1) why smokers should maintain perioperative abstinence from smoking for as long as possible, (2) why surgery provides a good opportunity to quit smoking permanently, and (3) how anesthesiologists can help their patients quit smoking.

## Smoking Abstinence and Perioperative Outcomes

Although some of the effects of smoking are irreversible (e.g., airway damage in chronic obstructive pulmonary disease [COPD]), abstinence from smoking can improve the function of many organ systems and reduce the risk of perioperative complications. The amount of time needed for the body to recover from the reversible effects of smoking varies widely. However, the effects of many smoke constituents are transient. For example, because nicotine has a short half-life (~1–2 h), plasma nicotine levels are very low after 8 to 12 h of abstinence.

### CARDIOVASCULAR OUTCOMES

Smoking is a major risk factor for cardiovascular diseases. In the long term, abstinence from smoking decreases the risk for all-cause mortality in smokers with coronary artery disease by approximately one-third. Smoking a cigarette acutely increases myocardial oxygen consumption by increasing heart rate, blood pressure, and myocardial contractility. These effects are likely mediated primarily by nicotine, which both increases sympathetic outflow and directly contracts some (but not all) peripheral vessels. The carbon monoxide in cigarette smoke binds to hemoglobin and shifts the oxyhemoglobin dissociation curve to the left, interfering with oxygen release. These effects all contribute to an increased risk of myocardial ischemia. During anesthesia, the frequency of ischemia as assessed by the electrocardiogram is well correlated with exhaled carbon monoxide levels. This suggests that smoking in the immediate preoperative period increases acute cardiovascular risk, and that even brief preoperative abstinence may benefit the heart, as carbon monoxide values fall rapidly after abstinence from smoking (within about 12 h). As the effects of nicotine and carbon monoxide dissipate, the risks of acute ischemia may also quickly decrease as myocardial oxygen demand decreases and oxygen supply increases. After 12 h of abstinence, maximum exercise capacity, a measure of overall cardiovascular function, is significantly increased.

### RESPIRATORY OUTCOMES

Smoking is a major cause of pulmonary diseases. For example, COPD develops in about 15% of smokers. Even those smokers who do not develop clinical lung disease show acceleration in the normal age-related declines in pulmonary function. Smoking induces an inflammatory state in the lung, causing goblet cell hyperplasia, smooth muscle hyperplasia, fibrosis, and structural epithelial abnormalities. Smoking affects both the volume and composition of mucus and decreases mucociliary clearance. All these abnormalities predispose smokers to a greater frequency of pulmonary infections and reactive airway diseases. Smoking status is a consistent risk factor for several perioperative pulmonary complications, including bronchospasm and pneumonia. Even relatively low-level exposure to smoke has clinical consequences; for

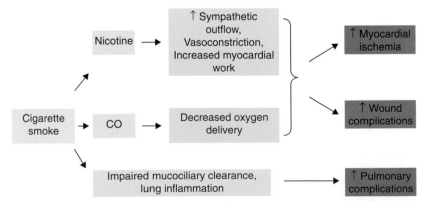

**Fig. 76.1** Mechanisms of how cigarette smoking increases perioperative risk. *CO*, Carbon monoxide.

example, children exposed to secondhand smoke have an increased rate of upper airway complications. Despite the inflammatory response induced by cigarette smoke, important elements of lung defenses against infection are impaired during anesthesia to a greater degree in smokers compared with nonsmokers. Lung recovery from chronic smoke exposure is a complex process. Symptoms of cough and wheezing decrease within weeks of abstinence. Goblet cell hyperplasia, mucus production, and mucociliary clearance also improve. As a result of this recovery, abstinence decreases the risk of perioperative pulmonary complications, but it appears that several months of abstinence are required for maximal benefit. However, it is *not* true that brief abstinence from smoking prior to surgery increases the risk of pulmonary complications. This belief was based on the idea that quitting produces a transient increase in cough and mucous production, which is also not true. Thus although the longer the duration of preoperative abstinence the better, smokers should never be discouraged from quitting at any time, even if only briefly before surgery.

## WOUND AND BONE HEALING OUTCOMES

Smokers are more likely to develop postoperative wound-related complications, such as dehiscence and infection, especially in procedures that require undermining of the skin, such as plastic surgery. This is likely caused in part by smoking-induced decreases in tissue oxygenation, which is an important determinant of wound healing. Cigarette smoke may also directly affect the function of fibroblasts and immune cells, which play an important role in the healing process. Microvascular disease caused by smoking may also interfere with angiogenesis via impaired release of substances, such as nitric oxide, that are important for wound repair. For this reason, some surgical specialties (especially plastic surgeons) refuse to perform cosmetic procedures unless their patients at least temporarily stop smoking. Smoking has significant effects on bone metabolism and is a major risk factor for osteoporosis. Smoking increases the risk for nonunion of spinal fusions, and the healing of fractures and ligaments may also be impaired in smokers. There is now strong evidence that abstinence can reduce wound-related complications such as wound infections. The duration of preoperative abstinence required for benefit is not known. However, because tissue oxygenation is a primary determinant of risk, and because tissue oxygenation improves quickly with the cessation of smoking, there is good reason to believe that even brief periods of abstinence would be beneficial. It is important for patients to maintain postoperative abstinence for the first week after surgery to allow for the initial stages of the healing process to occur.

## Surgery Represents an Excellent Opportunity for Smoking Cessation

As discussed earlier, even brief abstinence from smoking before surgery may decrease the risk for perioperative complications. A metaanalysis suggests that intensive preoperative intervention on smoking cessation reduces postoperative complications (risk ratio, 0.42; 95% CI, 0.27–0.65). Another reason that patients should try to quit smoking around the time of surgery is that surgery is a "teachable moment" that motivates

individuals to change smoking behavior: undergoing a major surgical procedure doubles the rate of spontaneous quitting. Also, studies suggest that symptoms of nicotine withdrawal do not consistently occur in the perioperative period. For example, smokers do not report greater increases in stress over the perioperative period compared with nonsmokers. Whether because of opioids and other medications given postoperatively, or the fact that patients are out of their normal environments that usually provide cues for smoking, this suggests that patients can be encouraged to maintain perioperative abstinence from cigarettes, without fearing that this will contribute to the stress caused by the surgical experience itself. Because smoking is the most common preventable cause of premature death, surgery is an excellent opportunity to promote long-term health of surgical patients.

## Helping Patients Quit Smoking

Treatment of tobacco dependence involves both behavioral counseling (to address the habit of smoking) and pharmacotherapy (to address nicotine addiction) (Fig. 76.2). Even brief advice to stop smoking offered by a physician increases quit rates. More intensive counseling further increases quit rates. It may not be practical for anesthesiologists to deliver intensive behavioral interventions, as most are not trained to do so and time is limited in busy clinical practices. However, anesthesiologists can refer patients to other existing services such as telephone quitlines, which are available in all states (1-800-QUIT-NOW) and provide low- or no-cost assistance and follow-up to smokers attempting to quit. Pharmacotherapy helps smokers treat symptoms of nicotine withdrawal, including cravings for cigarettes. Nicotine replacement therapy (NRT) in the forms of gum, inhaler, patch, and lozenges is effective in promoting abstinence, with many forms available without prescription. NRT does not produce adverse cardiac effects in healthy smokers and is safe in patients with cardiovascular diseases. There is no evidence that a therapeutic dose of NRT in humans affects wound healing, so current evidence supports the safety of NRT for surgical patients.

## E-cigarettes

Vaping nicotine may also have deleterious effects on surgical patients. The vaporization process produces other pharmacologically active compounds beyond nicotine and may cause injuries to the lungs. Although more studies are needed to elucidate the risk of vaping cigarettes in the perioperative period, patients should be advised on stopping vaping for surgery. E-cigarettes are not recommended as a means of NRT.

## Summary

Smoking increases the risk of perioperative complications. Although patients should stop smoking for as long as possible both before and after surgery, even brief preoperative abstinence may be beneficial (and is not harmful). Anesthesiologists should consistently ask their patients about tobacco use, advise them to quit smoking, and refer them to resources such as telephone quitlines that can provide support for quit attempts (1-800-QUIT-NOW).

**Methods to help patients quit**

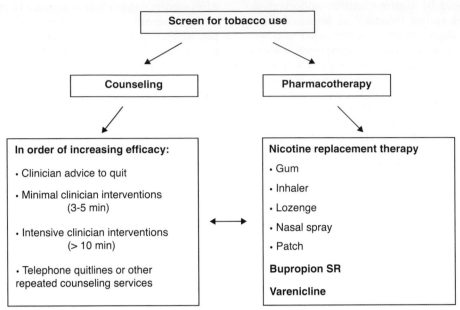

**Fig. 76.2** Summary of methods to help patients quit smoking. (Modified from Warner DO. Helping surgical patients quit smoking: why, when, and how. *Anesth Analg.* 2005;101:481–487, with permission.)

## SUGGESTED READINGS

Rusy, D. A., Honkanen, A., Landrigan-Ossar, M. F., Chatterjee, D., Schwartz, L. I., Lalwani, K., et al. (2021). Vaping and e-cigarette use in children and adolescents: Implications on perioperative care from the American Society of Anesthesiologists Committee on Pediatric Anesthesia, Society for Pediatric Anesthesia, and American Academy of Pediatrics Section on Anesthesiology and Pain Medicine. *Anesthesia and Analgesia, 133*(3), 562–568.

Shi, Y., & Warner, D. O. (2010). Surgery as a teachable moment for smoking cessation. *Anesthesiology, 112*, 102–107.

Thomsen, T., Villebro, N., & Moller, A. M. (2014). Interventions for preoperative smoking cessation. *Cochrane Database of Systematic Reviews, 3*, CD002294.

Warner, D. O. (2006). Perioperative abstinence from cigarettes: Physiologic and clinical consequences. *Anesthesiology, 104*, 356–367.

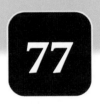

# 77

# Obstructive Sleep Apnea

MANDEEP SINGH, MBBS, MD, MSc, FRCPC  |
FRANCES CHUNG, MBBS, MD, FRCPC

## Introduction

Obstructive sleep apnea (OSA) is a common type of sleep-related breathing disorder characterized by repeated episodes of partial or complete upper airway (UA) obstruction leading to frequent nocturnal arousals and arterial oxygen desaturation with or without hypercapnia. This condition can also coexist with obesity hypoventilation syndrome, pulmonary hypertension, and other respiratory conditions such as chronic obstructive lung diseases.

# Epidemiology

The prevalence of OSA is estimated at 13% of adult men and 6% of adult women, whereas the estimates are even higher in older adults and those who are overweight. The prevalence may be higher in surgical patients, reaching up to 70% in patients undergoing bariatric surgery. Moreover, between 60% and 90% of surgical patients with moderate to severe OSA remain undiagnosed preoperatively.

# Pathophysiology

The UA from the hard palate to the larynx has evolved as a multipurpose complex structure. UA collapsibility and patency are dependent on an interaction between collapsing and expanding forces. The airways of patients with OSA are narrow and more prone to collapse (Fig. 77.1). These individuals are more dependent on increased tone of the airway dilator muscles during wakefulness to maintain airway patency. Decreased tone at the onset of sleep, especially in those patients who are highly dependent on increased muscle tone during wakefulness, can result in airway obstruction. Arousal from sleep helps OSA patients restore normal respiratory patterns, but the result is poor-quality fragmented sleep. The UA collapse and obstructive events occur more frequently and for longer duration under the influence of sedative and anesthetic medications. Complete or partial UA obstruction episodes and worsening of OSA may persist for up to one to three nights after surgery, hence necessitating increased vigilance.

## CLINICAL DIAGNOSIS

Overnight polysomnography is the gold standard for OSA diagnosis. Polysomnography determines the number of abnormal respiratory events such as hypopneas (partial obstruction) or apneas (complete cessation) per hour of sleep. The Apnea-Hypopnea Index (AHI) corresponds to the average number of abnormal breathing events per hour of sleep. Different AHI cutoffs are used to classify the severity of OSA (mild OSA: AHI >5 to <15 events/h; moderate OSA: AHI >15 to <30 events/h; severe OSA: AHI ≥ 30 events/h). The clinically important definition of OSA syndrome requires either an AHI of 15 or more, or an AHI greater than or equal to 5, with symptoms such as excessive daytime sleepiness, unintentional sleep during wakefulness, unrefreshing sleep, loud snoring reported by a partner, or observed obstruction during sleep.

## OBSTRUCTIVE SLEEP APNEA AND COMORBID CONDITIONS

Surgical patients with OSA often have multiple relevant comorbidities including obesity, metabolic syndrome, insulin resistance, gastroesophageal reflux, cardiovascular morbidity (myocardial ischemia, heart failure, arrhythmias), and cerebrovascular disease. The mechanism of increased cardiovascular risk in patients with OSA has not been entirely delineated but appears to involve the sustained sympathetic activation, oxidative stress, and resulting vascular inflammation that occur with the repetitive episodes of hypercarbia and hypoxia. Demographic factors (male sex, age >50 years), lifestyle factors (e.g., smoking, alcohol consumption), UA deformities (e.g., large tongue, micrognathia, midfacial hypoplasia), and endocrine problems (e.g., exogenous steroids, hypothyroidism, Cushing disease) are potential risk factors associated with OSA.

## OBSTRUCTIVE SLEEP APNEA AND POSTOPERATIVE COMPLICATIONS

A diagnosis of OSA increases the risk for perioperative complications such as difficult airway, respiratory failure requiring noninvasive or mechanical ventilation, aspiration pneumonia, pulmonary embolism, delirium, atrial fibrillation, and intensive care unit transfer. Patients with severe OSA (AHI ≥30) or undiagnosed

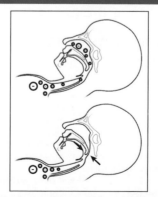

**Obstructive Sleep Apnea (OSA)**

- **Episodes of upper airway obstruction**

- **Apnea or hypopnea periods during sleep**

- **Continuation of breathing efforts or snoring**

- **Recurrent EEG arousals and oxygen desaturations with or without hypoventilation**

| OSA severity | Apnea-hypopnea Index (AHI), events/h |
|---|---|
| Mild | >5 to <15 |
| Moderate | ≥15 to <30 |
| Severe | ≥30 |

**Fig. 77.1** Obstructive sleep apnea: definition and classification of severity. (Data from Berry RB, Budhiraja R, Gottlieb DJ, et al. Rules for scoring respiratory events in sleep: update of the 2007 AASM manual for the scoring of sleep and associated events. *J Clin Sleep Med.* 2012;8(5):597–619.)

OSA have a two- to threefold increased risk of postoperative respiratory and cardiovascular complications. However, surgical patients with OSA on positive airway pressure (PAP) treatment have fewer postoperative complications than untreated OSA patients.

## Anesthetic Management of Patients With Obstructive Sleep Apnea

### SCREENING FOR OBSTRUCTIVE SLEEP APNEA

The guidelines of the American Society of Anesthesiologists and the Society of Anesthesia and Sleep Medicine state that adult patients at risk of OSA should be identified before surgery. A number of validated screening tests can be used to identify patients at risk of OSA, with the STOP-Bang questionnaire being the most validated screening tool for surgical patients. The STOP-Bang questionnaire consists of eight questions related to the clinical features of OSA (**S**noring, **T**iredness, **O**bserved apnea, high blood **P**ressure, **B**MI, **A**ge, **N**eck circumference, and male **G**ender). A positive answer results in 1 point to a maximum score of 8. Patients are at low risk of OSA with a score of 0 to 2, intermediate risk with a score of 3 or 4, and high risk with a score of 5 to 8). A score of 5 or higher is predictive of more severe OSA and is associated with higher postoperative complications.

### PATIENTS WITH DIAGNOSED OBSTRUCTIVE SLEEP APNEA

For patients with OSA, severity and PAP device setting should be determined before surgery. OSA patients who are poorly adherent to PAP therapy and have uncontrolled conditions with impaired ventilation or gas exchange (e.g., hypoventilation syndromes, severe pulmonary hypertension, resting hypoxemia not attributable to other cardiopulmonary disease) should receive further optimization.

In the presence of optimized comorbid conditions, OSA patients, including those who are untreated, may undergo surgery as long as strategies for mitigation of postoperative complications are implemented (Table 77.1). Postoperative use of home PAP therapy can reduce postoperative complications. Patients should bring their PAP therapy device to the hospital and use it during hospitalization. Home PAP settings are usually sufficient but may require further postoperative adjustment by respiratory therapists.

Patients with mild OSA may be at similar risk as the general population, and requirements for PAP therapy and postoperative monitoring may not be that strictly enforced. Clinical judgment should be exercised and thorough discussion should take place with the surgical team, as patients having surgery of the head and neck, or thoracic cavity may be more at risk of UA collapse and gas exchange issues.

### PATIENTS WITH SUSPECTED OBSTRUCTIVE SLEEP APNEA

There is insufficient evidence to support cancelling or delaying elective surgery to formally diagnose OSA. However, patients suspected of OSA should have a focused history and physical for OSA symptoms and signs and undergo screening with the STOP-Bang questionnaire. Identification and optimization of coexisting major comorbidities should be done, especially uncontrolled systemic conditions with ventilation or gas exchange (see earlier). In these cases, non–life-threatening surgery should be delayed until medically optimized. Otherwise, patients with suspected OSA should be assumed high-risk and strategies to reduce postoperative complications should be adopted (Table 77.1). Because OSA carries long-term cardiovascular risk, screen-positive patients should be advised to follow up with their primary care provider and be referred for further evaluation and treatment.

### PERIOPERATIVE CONSIDERATIONS AND RISK MITIGATION STRATEGIES

Patients with OSA present several anesthetic challenges that require careful planning to obviate these risks (Fig. 77.2, Table 77.1). OSA may induce physiologic changes like arterial hypoxemia, polycythemia, hypercapnia, and pulmonary hypertension. In the presence of pulmonary hypertension, care

| TABLE 77.1 | Considerations for Perioperative Management of Patients With Obstructive Sleep Apnea | | |
|---|---|---|---|
| **Before Surgery** | **Inside the Operating Room** | **After Surgery** | |
| • Identify suspected OSA (STOP-Bang questionnaire) or diagnosed OSA<br>• Confirm severity of OSA (sleep study data, if available)<br>• Evaluate type of treatment (CPAP, dental appliance, positional therapy), treatment compliance<br>• Consider optimization before surgery, if possible (SASM guidelines):<br>  • Obesity-hypoventilation syndrome (serum $HCO_3^-$ ≥ 28 mmol/L)<br>  • Severe pulmonary hypertension<br>  • Resting hypoxemia in the absence of other cardiopulmonary cause<br>  • Associated significant or uncontrolled systemic disease | • Opioid sparing techniques<br>• Local or regional anesthesia technique, if applicable<br>• Light sedation<br>• Low threshold for respiratory monitoring<br>• May use OSA treatment inside the OR, such as CPAP under sedation<br>• If deep sedation needed, consider securing airway<br>• Head elevation<br>• Airway adjuncts<br>• Short-acting agents<br>• Lung recruitment and PEEP<br>• Complete reversal of neuromuscular blockade | • Opioid sparing techniques and multimodal analgesia<br>• Avoid sedatives or hypnotic<br>• PACU observation to ensure no recurrent respiratory events<br>• Enhanced respiratory monitoring and/or CPAP therapy, if untreated or noncompliant, recurrent respiratory events, or requiring increased parenteral opioid medications | |

*CPAP*, Continuous positive airway pressure; *OR*, operating room; *OSA*, obstructive sleep apnea; *PACU*, postanesthesia care unit; *PEEP*, positive end-expiratory pressure; *SASM*, Society of Anesthesia and Sleep Medicine.

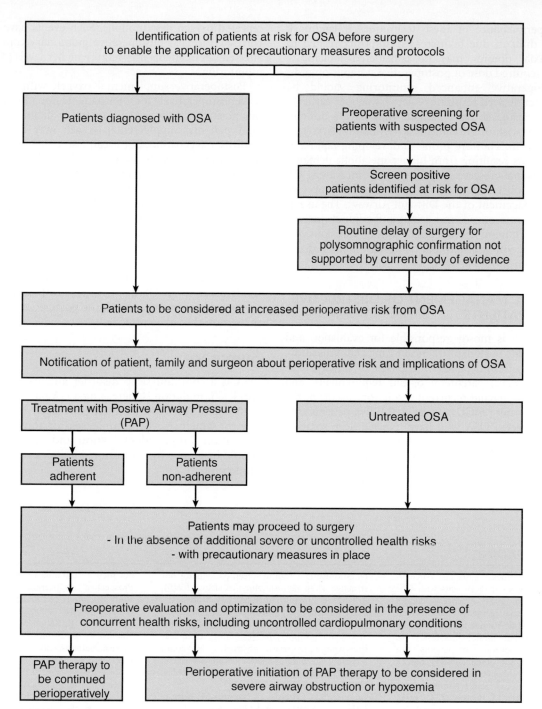

**Fig. 77.2** Recommendations for the preoperative management of obstructive sleep apnea (OSA) from the Society of Anesthesia and Sleep Medicine and the American Society of Anesthesiologists Task Force on Perioperative Management of Patients with OSA. (From Cozowicz C, Memtsoudis SG. Perioperative management of the patient with obstructive sleep apnea: a narrative review. *Anesth Analg.* 2021;132(5):1231–1243.)

should be taken to prevent elevation of pulmonary artery pressure by avoiding hypercarbia, hypoxemia, hypothermia, and acidosis. OSA patients should have well-controlled hypertension and glucose homeostasis, and any dyslipidemia or gastroesophageal reflux should be treated. Unfortunately, these patients with complex conditions often present on the day of surgery. Management of these patients consists of two elements: optimizing the medical conditions often seen in conjunction with OSA and developing the least invasive anesthetic plan.

OSA patients may have increased sensitivity to respiratory depressants. The safest anesthetic is local anesthesia with minimal or no sedation. Patients on home PAP therapy may continue using their PAP device during procedures under mild to moderate sedation. A secured airway is preferred for procedures requiring deep sedation. If local anesthesia is not feasible, the anesthesia provider should consider using regional anesthesia. Peripheral nerve block and neuraxial anesthesia may be successfully employed with minimal sedation. Use of ultrasound can facilitate performance of these techniques if landmark techniques are difficult due to increased adiposity related to obesity. Neuraxial opioids may be considered judiciously to decrease the required dose of postoperative systemic opioids; however, postoperative enhanced monitoring should be arranged to detect delayed respiratory depression (see earlier).

For general anesthesia, OSA patients may have a difficult airway with higher risk of difficult mask ventilation, laryngoscopy, and intubation. They are prone to developing rapid and severe desaturations resulting from higher metabolic demand, decreased functional reserve capacity, and increased UA collapsibility and obstruction of the pharyngeal airway (see Chapter 148, Management of the Difficult Airway). The use of opioids should be minimized, and nonopioid adjuncts including continuous peripheral nerve blocks, epidural infusions of a local anesthetic agent, nonsteroidal antiinflammatory drugs and acetaminophen should be used.

## POSTOPERATIVE MANAGEMENT OF OBSTRUCTIVE SLEEP APNEA PATIENTS

The anesthesiologist is mostly responsible for evaluation and planning for adequate postoperative monitoring and disposition. Postoperative disposition depends on the type of surgery, OSA severity and treatment, parenteral opioid requirements, and whether patients are having recurrent respiratory events in the postanesthesia care unit (PACU). It is advisable that patients with diagnosed or suspected OSA who have received deep sedation or general anesthesia be monitored for an extended period in the PACU. OSA patients in the PACU should be observed carefully for signs of respiratory depression (e.g., apnea, bradypnea, repeated oxygen desaturation). Such events have been strongly correlated to later postoperative pulmonary complications and affected OSA patients may require higher levels of postoperative monitoring.

Postoperative supplemental oxygen without PAP is often used postoperatively for OSA patients nonadherent to continuous positive airway pressure or newly diagnosed or suspected OSA patients. Supplemental oxygen may decrease AHI and improve oxygenation, but it can also contribute to respiratory depression in patients receiving opioids. Empiric PAP therapy may be required for patients with recurrent obstructive events with significant hypoxemia, but this therapy should be continued postoperatively to the final destination. Auto-titrated continuous positive airway pressure (APAP) therapy for OSA automatically adjusts pressure by continuous analyses of flow profiles. It is an effective treatment that is increasingly being used postoperatively. APAP therapy has been shown to decrease postoperative AHI and improve oxygenation in patients with moderate to severe OSA. For patients who decline PAP therapy, enhanced monitoring, nonsupine posture, and oxygen supplementation should be provided.

## Summary

OSA is a common sleep disorder and its prevalence in the surgical population is increasing. OSA patients are associated with significant comorbidities, increased risk of postoperative consequences, therefore increasing the cost and resource utilization. Proper identification and optimal management should be guided by institutional policies and evidence-based guidelines.

## SUGGESTED READINGS

American Society of Anesthesiologists Task Force on Perioperative Management of Patients with Obstructive Sleep Apnea. (2014). Practice guidelines for the perioperative management of patients with obstructive sleep apnea: An updated report by the American Society of Anesthesiologists Task Force on Perioperative Management of patients with obstructive sleep apnea. *Anesthesiology, 120*(2), 268–286. doi:10.1097/ALN.0000000000000053.

Chung, F., Memtsoudis, S. G., Ramachandran, S. K., Nagappa, M., Opperer, M., Cozowicz, C., et al. (2016). Society of Anesthesia and Sleep Medicine Guidelines on preoperative screening and assessment of adult patients with obstructive sleep apnea. *Anesthesia and Analgesia, 123*(2), 452–473. doi:10.1213/ANE.0000000000001416.

Chung, F., Yegneswaran, B., Liao, P., Chung, S. A., Vairavanathan, S., Islam, S., et al. (2008). STOP Questionnaire: A tool to screen patients for obstructive sleep apnea. *Anesthesiology, 108*(5), 812–821. doi:10.1097/ALN.0b013e31816d83e4.

Gali, B., Whalen, F. X., Schroeder, D. R., Gay, P. C., & Plevak, D. J. (2009). Identification of patients at risk for postoperative respiratory complications using a preoperative obstructive sleep apnea screening tool and postanesthesia care assessment. *Anesthesiology, 110*(4), 869–877. doi:10.1097/ALN.0b013e31819b5d70.

Memtsoudis, S. G., Cozowicz, C., Nagappa, M., Wong, J., Joshi, G. P., Wong, D. T., et al. (2018). Society of anesthesia and sleep medicine guideline on intraoperative management of adult patients with obstructive sleep apnea. *Anesthesia and Analgesia, 127*(4), 967–987. doi:10.1213/ANE.0000000000003434.

Seet, E., Chung, F., Wang, C. Y., Tam, S., Kumar, C. M., Ubeynarayana, C. U., et al. (2021). Association of obstructive sleep apnea with difficult intubation: Prospective multicenter observational cohort study. *Anesthesia and Analgesia, 133*(1), 196–204. doi:10.1213/ANE.0000000000005479.

Singh, M., Liao, P., Kobah, S., Wijeysundera, D. N., Shapiro, C., & Chung, F. (2013). Proportion of surgical patients with undiagnosed obstructive sleep apnoea. *British Journal of Anaesthesia, 110*(4), 629–636. doi:10.1093/bja/aes465.

Subramani, Y., Singh, M., Wong, J., Kushida, C. A., Malhotra, A., & Chung, F. (2017). Understanding phenotypes of obstructive sleep apnea: Applications in anesthesia, surgery, and perioperative medicine. *Anesthesia and Analgesia, 124*(1), 179–191. doi:10.1213/ANE.0000000000001546.

# 78

# Postoperative Nausea and Vomiting

CARSON C. WELKER, MD

## Introduction

Postoperative nausea and vomiting (PONV) is a frequent side effect that occurs after exposure to anesthetic agents, occurring in 30% to 50% of the general surgical population and up to 80% in high-risk patients. PONV results in increased health care costs from prolonged postanesthesia care unit (PACU) stays, unanticipated hospitalization, or postdischarge nausea and vomiting (PDNV) which can persist up to 7 days postoperatively.

## Physiology

The vomiting center of the brain, in the reticular formation, receives input from the chemotactic trigger zone, gastrointestinal tract, vestibular portion of the eighth cranial nerve, and pharynx. Important neurotransmitter receptor sites documented, or suspected, to be associated with PONV include serotonin, dopamine, histamine, neurokinin-1, opioid, acetylcholine, and muscarinic receptor sites (see Chapter 66, Antiemetic Agents).

### RISK FACTORS

In 2014, the Society for Ambulatory Anesthesia published consensus guidelines for the management of PONV. The development of PONV involves the presence of anesthetic factors in a susceptible individual (Table 78.1). Patient-specific risk factors include female gender (strongest predictor), history of PONV, nonsmoking status, history of motion sickness, and younger age. Anesthesia-related predictors include the use of volatile anesthetics (strongest), duration of anesthesia, postoperative

| TABLE 78.1 | Risk Factors Associated With Increased Incidence of Postoperative Nausea and Vomiting |
|---|---|
| **RISK FACTORS FOR PONV IN ADULTS** | |
| Female gender | |
| History of PONV | |
| History of motion sickness | |
| Nonsmoker | |
| Younger age | |
| General vs. regional anesthesia | |
| Use of volatile anesthetics | |
| Use of nitrous oxide | |
| Postoperative opioids | |
| Duration of anesthesia | |
| Type of surgery (cholecystectomy, laparoscopic, gynecologic) | |

*PONV,* postoperative nausea and vomiting.

opioid use, and nitrous oxide use. Fig. 78.1 illustrates a risk score from Apfel et al. for PONV in adults. When 0, 1, 2, 3, and 4 risk factors are present, the associated risks of PONV are approximately 10%, 20%, 40%, 60%, and 80%, respectively. The effects of volatile anesthetics on PONV are dose dependent and often present 2 to 6 h after surgery. Postoperative opioids are also dose dependent with the effect persisting for the duration of their use.

PDNV is an additional concern for anesthesiologists. Risk factors for PDNV include female gender, young age, history of PONV, PACU opioid use, and PACU PONV. The risk score for PDNV from Apfel et al. is found in Fig. 78.2. When 0, 1, 2, 3, 4, and 5 risk factors are present, the associated risks for PDNV are approximately 10%, 20%, 30%, 50%, 60%, and 80%, respectively.

Risk factors for postoperative vomiting (POV) in children include longer surgery (>30 min), age 3 years or older, strabismus surgery, and history of POV/PONV in relatives.

Identification of high-risk patients will allow a more effective and cost-efficient prophylactic treatment program to be established, whereas low-risk patients (i.e., most general surgical patients) would be spared the added expense and possible side effects of treatment. However, studies have found that anesthesia providers routinely and greatly underestimate risk for PONV, and some have advocated near-universal PONV prophylaxis.

### TREATMENT

The first step in treating PONV is to reduce baseline risk. A lower incidence of PONV is associated with (1) using regional anesthesia compared with general anesthesia, (2) using propofol for induction and maintenance of anesthesia, (3) avoiding the use of nitrous oxide, (4) minimizing perioperative opioids, and (5) providing adequate hydration.

The most important step in preventing PONV is to identify high-risk patients and administer an effective prophylactic program to them (see Fig. 78.3). Chapter 66, Antiemetics, discusses each agent in further detail. Intraoperatively, any underlying cause of hypotension or cerebral hypoxia should be identified and corrected. For patients who develop PONV, rescue therapy is warranted. Rescue therapy should consist of an antiemetic drug from a different class than the prophylactic antiemetic, if one was given. Readministering a drug from the same class can be considered if it has been more than 6 h since the last dose. Dexamethasone and scopolamine should not be redosed. Additionally, nonpharmacologic measures like acupressure or aromatherapy can be considered.

## Conclusion

Further investigation is required to ultimately eliminate the problem of PONV; however, advances have been made to significantly lower the incidence of PONV through preoperatively identifying high-risk patients and providing appropriate treatment.

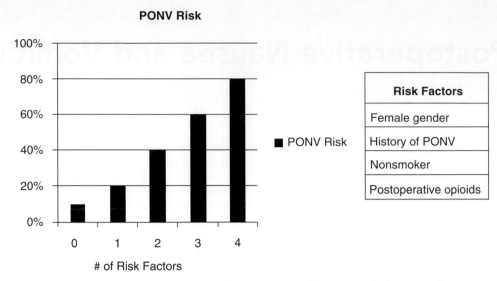

**Fig. 78.1** Simplified postoperative nausea and vomiting *(PONV)* risk score. (From Apfel, C. C., Heidrich, F. M., Jukar-Rao, S., Jalota, L., Hornuss, C., Whelan, R. P., et al. (2012). Evidence-based analysis of risk factors for postoperative nausea and vomiting. *British Journal of Anaesthesia, 109*(5), 742–753. doi:10.1093/bja/aes276.)

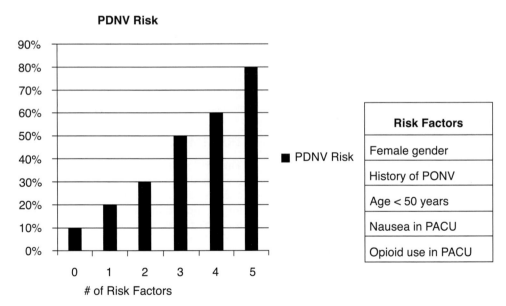

**Fig. 78.2** Simplified postdischarge nausea and vomiting *(PDNV)* risk score. *PACU,* Postanesthesia care unit; *PONV,* postoperative nausea and vomiting. (From Apfel, C. C., Heidrich, F. M., Jukar-Rao, S., Jalota, L., Hornuss, C., Whelan, R. P., et al. (2012). Evidence-based analysis of risk factors for postoperative nausea and vomiting. *British Journal of Anaesthesia, 109*(5), 742–753. doi:10.1093/bja/aes276.)

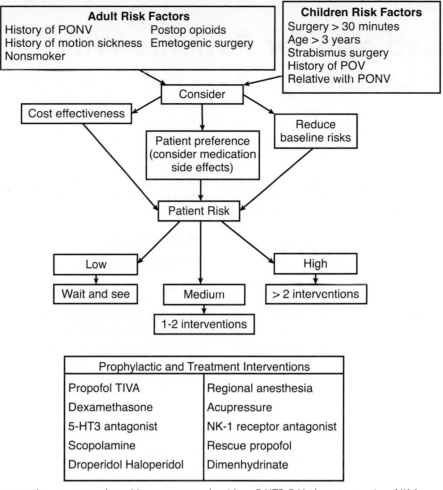

**Fig. 78.3** Example of postoperative nausea and vomiting treatment algorithm. *5-HT3*, 5-Hydroxytryptamine; *NK-1*, neurokinin-1; *POV*, postoperative vomiting; *PONV*, postoperative nausea and vomiting; *TIVA*, total intravenous anesthesia.

## SUGGESTED READINGS

Apfel, C. C. (2010). Postoperative nausea and vomiting. In R. D. Miller (Ed.), *Miller's anesthesia* (7th ed., pp. 2947–2973). Philadelphia: Churchill Livingstone/Elsevier.

Apfel, C. C., Korttila, K., Abdalla, M., Kerger, H., Turan, A., Vedder, I., et al. (2004). A factorial trial of six interventions for the prevention of postoperative nausea and vomiting. *New England Journal of Medicine, 350*, 2441–2451.

Apfel, C. C., Läärä, E., Koivuranta, M., Greim, C. A., & Roewer, N. (1999). A simplified risk score for predicting postoperative nausea and vomiting: Conclusions from cross-validations between two centers. *Anesthesiology, 91*, 693–700.

Apfel, C. C., Philip, B. K., Cakmakkaya, O. S., Shilling, A., Shi, Y. Y., Leslie, J. B., et al. (2012). Who is at risk for postdischarge nausea and vomiting after ambulatory surgery? *Anesthesiology, 117*, 475–486.

Elvir-Lazo, O. L., White, P. F., Yumul, R., & Cruz Eng, H. (2020). Management strategies for the treatment and prevention of postoperative/postdischarge nausea and vomiting: An updated review. *F1000Research*, 9, F1000 Faculty Rev-983.

Gan, T. J., Diemunsch, P., Habib, A. S., Kovac, A., Kranke, P., Meyer, T. A., et al. (2014). Consensus guidelines for the management of postoperative nausea and vomiting. *Anesthesia and Analgesia, 118*, 85–113.

Odom-Forren, J., Jalota, L., Moser, D. K., Lennie, T. A., Hall, L. A., Holtman, J., Hooper V, & Apfel, C. C. (2013). Incidence and predictors of postdischarge nausea and vomiting in a 7-day population. *Journal of Clinical Anesthesia, 25*(7), 551–559. doi:10.1016/j.jclinane.2013.05.008.

Skolnik, A., & Gan, T. J. (2014). Update on the management of postoperative nausea and vomiting. *Current Opinion in Anaesthesiology, 27*(6), 605–609.

Weibel, S., Schaefer, M. S., Raj, D., Rücker, G., Pace, N. L., Schlesinger, T., et al. (2021). Drugs for preventing postoperative nausea and vomiting in adults after general anaesthesia: An abridged Cochrane network meta-analysis. *Anaesthesia, 76*(7), 962–973. doi:10.1111/anae.15295.

# 79

# Anesthesia for Patients Who Are Lactating

SARAH E. DODD, MD

The provision of human milk to infants is the recommended method of infant feeding worldwide. In addition to providing nutrition, lactation offers additional benefits for the infant and the lactating patient including reduced rates of infectious and chronic health conditions. It is important for individual and public health that lactating patients are supported by the health care system, even when they present outside of the obstetric context. Maternal medications and illness are two of several risk factors for early or unintended weaning that are relevant to anesthesiologists. The American Society of Anesthesiologists and the Association of Anaesthetists in the United Kingdom have released guidelines that support the continuation of lactation around the time of surgery by providing patients with a compatible anesthetic and recommending that lactation not be interrupted.

## Preoperative

The first step to appropriately care for lactating patients who present for anesthesia care is to elicit lactating status on routine perioperative interview. This can be accomplished by the addition of a routine question about breastfeeding or lactating when asking other demographically appropriate screening questions.

For patients who are breastfeeding and wish to continue beyond the perioperative encounter, there are multiple considerations, and a complete perioperative plan of care should be developed with the surgical team and support staff. If the infant is premature or acutely or chronically ill, a discussion with the infant's pediatrician is prudent. Blanket recommendations to express and discard breast milk should not be provided to lactating patients.

### REGULAR EMPTYING OF BREASTS

Lactation is induced after delivery by hormonal changes, and then a dynamic supply is maintained by the demand created when regular expression or direct feeding occurs. The patient will typically be able to describe the schedule on which they routinely feed their infant or empty their breasts (typically every 2–6 hours, depending on the age of the infant). Complete breast emptying is important for the maintenance of the milk supply, for comfort, and for prevention of complications such as mastitis.

The patient should be encouraged to feed their infant or pump in the preoperative area as close to the time of surgery as possible. The time that the patient will be separated from the infant or unable to pump should be accurately estimated. If the time of separation is longer than the patient's usual pumping interval, a plan for intraoperative milk expression may be necessary and should be discussed with the patient. If available, a consultation with a lactation professional may be offered.

## Intraoperative

### MEDICATIONS

Although some components of breast milk are actively transported across the cellular membranes, the primary process of medication transfer is passive diffusion. In general, ideal lactation-compatible medications are short-acting and do not easily cross the plasma membrane. Any medications present in breast milk will be taken orally by the infant; therefore the oral bioavailability of the medication is also relevant.

During the development of new medications and trials involving existing medications, lactating patients are often excluded, and randomized control data in this population and their infants are limited. However, existing pharmacologic and clinical practice evidence has supported that most perioperative medications are compatible with uninterrupted lactation, and the risks of trace medications present in milk are outweighed in most cases by the benefits to the patient and the infant (Table 79.1).

A lactation-compatible anesthetic plan should be developed and discussed with the patient. Special attention should be paid to multimodal analgesia, rapid recovery, and prevention of postoperative nausea and vomiting. Multiple reference books and online databases are maintained to assist in evaluating additional medications for breastfeeding compatibility, and some offer mobile phone applications.

### FLUID MANAGEMENT

Lactation typically requires an additional 200 to 500 mL per day in fluid intake, and this should be considered when calculating replacement and maintenance fluids. Volume overload should also be avoided, as interstitial fluid accumulation can lead to compression of the ducts, making milk expression more difficult and causing painful engorgement.

### POSITIONING AND INTRAOPERATIVE MILK EXPRESSION

The breasts should be positioned free from pressure. If intraoperative pumping is planned, it should be performed by an experienced provider and only after appropriate discussion with the patient or surrogate decision-maker in the case of an emergent or unexpectedly long operation.

| TABLE 79.1 | Lactation Compatibility of Common Anesthesia Medications | | |
|---|---|---|---|
| **Class** | **Compatible** | **Limited Evidence** | **Recommend Avoiding** |
| **Analgesics** | Acetaminophen, ibuprofen, ketorolac, low-dose ketamine, morphine, oxycodone*, hydrocodone, fentanyl, neuraxial opioids, remifentanil | Hydromorphone | Codeine, tramadol, meperidine |
| **Anesthetics** | Propofol, midazolam, dexmedetomidine, etomidate, volatile agents, nitrous oxide, lidocaine, bupivacaine, liposomal bupivacaine | Induction-dose ketamine | Diazepam |
| **Antiemetics** | Ondansetron, dexamethasone, metoclopramide, haloperidol, scopol-amine† | Droperidol | |
| **Miscellaneous** | Succinylcholine, NDMR, neostigmine, glycopyrrolate, sugammadex‡, gadolinium and iodinated contrast | | |

*Recommend ≤30 mg total per day of oxycodone because of oxymorphone metabolite accumulation.
†May affect milk production and should be weighed against risk of dehydration caused by postoperative nausea and vomiting.
‡Society for Obstetric Anesthesia and Perinatology Statement on Sugammadex during pregnancy and lactation recommends the use of alternative NDMR reversal in early postpartum if lactation is not yet fully established.
**NDMR,** Nondepolarizing muscle relaxant.

## Postoperative

Following anesthesia, the patient may directly breastfeed or express milk intended for infant consumption as soon as awake, alert, and able. The level of alertness of the patient corresponds to low plasma levels and therefore low breast milk levels of anesthetic medications. Patients should be offered multimodal analgesia beginning with nonopioid medications and regional techniques, followed by opioid medications as needed for breakthrough pain. The patient and caregiver should be given instructions to monitor the baby for any changes and contact information for any concerns.

## SUGGESTED READINGS

American Society of Anesthesiologists. (2019). *Statement on resuming breastfeeding after anesthesia.* Retrieved from https://www.asahq.org/standards-and-guidelines/statement-on-resuming-breastfeeding-after-anesthesia.

Bartick, M., Hernández-Aguilar, M. T., Wight, N., Mitchell, K. B., Simon, L., Hanley, L., et al. (2021). ABM clinical protocol #35: Supporting breastfeeding during maternal or child hospitalization. *Breastfeeding Medicine, 16*(9), 664–674.

Cobb, B., Liu, R., Valentine, E., & Onuoha, O. (2015). Breastfeeding after anesthesia: A review for anesthesia providers regarding the transfer of medications into breast milk. *Translational Perioperative and Pain Medicine, 1*(2), 1–7.

*Drugs and lactation database (LactMed)* [Internet]. (2006). Bethesda (MD): National Library of Medicine (US). Retrieved from https://www.ncbi.nlm.nih.gov/books/NBK501922/

*Hale's medications & mothers' milk.* Retrieved from https://www.halesmeds.com/.

Mitchell, J., Jones, W., Winkley, E., & Kinsellaz, S. M. (2020). Guideline on anaesthesia and sedation in breastfeeding women 2020: Guideline from the Association of Anaesthetists. *Anaesthesia, 75*(11), 1482–1493.

Reece-Stremtan, S., Campos, M., & Kokajko, L. (2017). Academy of Breastfeeding Medicine. ABM clinical protocol #15: Analgesia and anesthesia for the breastfeeding mother, revised 2017. *Breastfeeding Medicine 12*(9), 500–506.

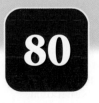

# 80

# Acute and Chronic Alcoholism and Anesthesia

JULIAN NARANJO, DO

Ethyl alcohol (ethanol, ETOH) is an addictive central nervous system depressant. Chronic and acute exposure to alcohol can affect multiple organ systems. Alcohol-related deaths have been attributed to trauma, cardiac arrhythmias, cardiomyopathy, cirrhosis, bleeding from gastritis or esophageal varices, hepatitis, malnutrition, pancreatitis, and psychiatric disorders.

Alcohol use disorders (AUDs) significantly affect all aspects of health care worldwide. Excessive alcohol use is the third leading cause of preventable death in the United States behind tobacco and poor diet and physical inactivity. The latest data from the National Institute of Alcohol Abuse and Alcoholism and the National Survey on Drug Use and Health indicate that, in the United States in 2019, almost 14.5 million people aged 12 and older or 5.3% of this group were considered to have an AUD. This number includes 9.0 million men (6.8% of men in this age group) and 5.5 million women (3.9% of women in this age group). Additionally, 414,000 adolescents aged 12 to 17 are considered to have an AUD. This number includes 163,000 male adolescents (1.7% of males in this age group) and 251,000 female adolescents (2.1% of females in this age group). The traditional prevalence of AUDs is higher in men (6.8%) than in women (3.9%); however, that gap is narrowing, especially among younger women. The rate of all alcohol-related emergency department (ED) visits increased 47% between 2006 and 2014. Alcohol contributes to 18.5% of all ED visits and 22.1% of overdose deaths related to opioids. Furthermore, at the start of the COVID-19 pandemic, suppression efforts coupled with the relaxation of alcohol sales restrictions were immediately followed by substantial increases in alcoholic beverage sales. In a survey of 993 individuals conducted in May 2020, respondents in all sociodemographic subgroups surveyed reported consuming more drinks, exceeding recommended drinking limits more often, and more binge drinking. In 2008, a study conducted in Germany suggested that anesthesiologists do a poor job of preoperatively identifying patients with AUDs, particularly among women and younger patients, compared with older men.

## Metabolism

ETOH is quickly absorbed through the gastrointestinal tract. It is highly diffusible, with rapid distribution to all aqueous compartments. Because women, compared with men, have a smaller aqueous compartment and decreased gastric alcohol dehydrogenase activity, they may have a higher blood alcohol concentration (BAC) after consuming the same quantity of ETOH as do men of similar height and weight. Ninety percent of alcohol ingested is metabolized in the liver via the alcohol dehydrogenase pathway. The remaining 10% is eliminated by direct pulmonary diffusion or through perspiration and urine. Twelve ounces of beer, 1.5 ounces of spirits, or 5 ounces of wine all contain approximately the same amount of alcohol. Alcohol is metabolized in the body at a rate of approximately 15% of the BAC per hour.

$$\left(C_2H_2O\right) \text{ ethanol} \xrightarrow[\text{NAD} \to \text{NDH}]{\text{alcohol dehydrogenase}}$$

$$\left(C_2H_4O\right) \text{ accetaldehyde}$$

$$\xrightarrow[\text{NAD} \to \text{NADH}]{\text{acetaldehyde dehydrogenase}} CO_2 + H_2O + \text{acetate}$$

## Acute Central Nervous System Effects

At low to moderate BAC, ETOH binds to γ-aminobutyric acid type A (GABA$_A$) receptors, resulting in relaxation, decreased anxiety, sedation, ataxia, increased appetite, and decreased inhibition, which is occasionally manifested as violent and risky behavior. As blood alcohol levels rise, ETOH begins to act as an antagonist to N-methyl-D-aspartic acid (NMDA) receptors, decreasing learning ability and memory. Opioid, dopamine, and cannabinoid receptors are also influenced by ETOH.

| TABLE 80.1 | Central Nervous System Effects Related to Blood Alcohol Concentration |
|---|---|
| **BAC (mg/dL)** | **Effects** |
| 50 | Decreased mental activity<br>Depression of higher cortical centers<br>Disinhibition<br>Impaired judgment<br>Increased emotional excitability |
| 150 | Ataxia<br>Emotional imbalance<br>Slurred speech |
| >350 | Coma<br>Lethargy<br>Stupor |
| >400 | Potential death* |

*Death may result from cardiac or respiratory depression or aspiration-related asphyxia.

*BAC,* Blood alcohol concentration.

Progressive central nervous system effects are seen as BAC increases (Table 80.1); 80 mg/dL is the typical legal limit for intoxication.

## Chronic Alcoholism

Alcoholic liver disease progresses in stages. Initially, elevated liver transaminases and increased mean red blood cell volume may be the only clues to the presence of parenchymal damage. Fatty liver disease, or hepatic steatosis, typically manifests as hepatomegaly but is otherwise not associated with any symptoms and is an early finding that will resolve if ETOH ingestion is stopped. With continued ETOH intake, however, alcoholic hepatitis (steatohepatitis)—a combination of a fatty liver, diffuse inflammation, and liver necrosis—ensues. Up to 35% of people with AUDs develop steatohepatitis, which carries an increased nonsurgical mortality rate between 25% and 60% per year, and 40% to 50% of patients with steatohepatitis develop alcoholic cirrhosis within 5 years; cirrhosis and portal hypertension are the final sequelae of alcoholic liver disease (associated with a 40% 5-year mortality rate) with a 25% to 30% per decade probability of clinical manifestation development. Although liver biopsy and histopathological examination is the gold standard for confirming hepatic fibrosis, noninvasive fibrosis tests (NITs) such as simple serum tests (e.g., Fibrosis Score 4), complex serum tests (e.g., N-terminal propeptide of type 3 collagen); sonographic and magnetic resonance elastography; lipidomic, proteomic, and gut microbiome profiles; and microRNA signatures overcome many limitations of liver biopsy and are either currently being incorporated into specialist practices or are being investigated for future use. Nutritional, cardiovascular, pulmonary, gastrointestinal, central nervous system, hematologic, renal, and immunologic abnormalities may be associated with alcoholic cirrhosis (Table 80.2).

## Anesthetic Management of Patients With Alcohol Use Disorders

Patients with alcoholic cirrhosis may exhibit an unpredictable response to the induction of general anesthesia. For example, cross-tolerance with benzodiazepines, propofol, isoflurane,

| TABLE 80.2 | Abnormalities Associated With Alcoholic Cirrhosis |
|---|---|
| **System or Function** | **Abnormalities** |
| Cardiovascular | Hyperdynamic state* |
| Central nervous system | Asterixis<br>Encephalopathy |
| Gastrointestinal | Cholelithiasis<br>Fetor hepaticus<br>Gastroesophageal varices<br>↓ Gastroesophageal sphincter tone<br>Pancreatitis<br>Peptic ulcer disease<br>Portal vein hypertension<br>Splenomegaly |
| Hematologic | Anemia<br>Coagulopathy† |
| Immunologic | Suppressed immune-defense mechanisms |
| Nutrition | ↓ Albumin concentration<br>Megaloblastic anemia‡<br>↓ Vitamin K absorption<br>Hypoglycemia§ |
| Pulmonary | Hypoxia‖<br>Intrapulmonary arteriovenous shunting<br>Right-to-left shunting#<br>Pneumonia** |
| Renal†† | ↑ Aldosterone secretion<br>↑ Angiotensin production<br>↓ Glomerular filtration rate<br>↓ Renal blood flow<br>↑ Renin production |

*Characterized by increased cardiac output, arteriovenous shunting, increased intravascular volume, decreased blood viscosity secondary to anemia, cardiomyopathy, and congestive heart failure.
†Secondary to decreased synthesis of clotting factors (except factor VIII), resulting in increased prothrombin time and activated partial thromboplastin time; ethyl alcohol suppresses platelet function and survival (splenic sequestration) and enhances fibrinolysis.
‡Requires vitamin $B_{12}$ and folate replacement.
§Caused by decreased gluconeogenesis or decreased glycogen stores.
‖Secondary to extrinsic restrictive lung disease resulting from ascites-induced cephalad displacement of the diaphragm.
#Secondary to portal vein hypertension.
**Secondary to decreased pulmonary phagocytic activity or aspiration of gastric contents.
††Abrupt oliguria with concomitant cirrhosis (hepatorenal syndrome) is associated with a 60% mortality rate.

nitrous oxide, local anesthetics, and barbiturates has been reported. Ketamine has been demonstrated to have an altered effect on patients with AUDs. Accordingly, anesthetic doses may need to be increased.

However, if the patient's nutrition status is poor, a decrease in serum albumin may increase the amount of free drug and potentiate the myocardial-depressant effect of the drug. Patients with chronic alcoholism are at risk for aspirating gastric contents for the following reasons: increased gastric acid secretion, decreased gastric motility, ascites-induced changes in the angle of the gastroesophageal junction, and increased intragastric pressure.

The minimum alveolar concentration (MAC) of an anesthetic agent is decreased in patients after acute ETOH ingestion. In contrast, MAC is increased in patients with a history of chronic alcoholism. Patients with alcoholic cardiomyopathy may be exquisitely sensitive to the myocardial-depressant effects of anesthetic drugs. Opioids and benzodiazepines may have prolonged half-lives because patients with chronic alcoholism may have impaired hepatic biotransformation. A retrospective study has suggested that patients with a history of frequent alcohol consumption required more opioids for postoperative pain control.

Patients with alcoholism may appear to be resistant to the effects of nondepolarizing neuromuscular blocking agents (NMBAs). Increased volume of distribution is reflected in the prolonged elimination half-lives of the long-acting nondepolarizing NMBAs. Elimination half-lives of vecuronium (in doses <0.1 mg/kg), atracurium, and cisatracurium are unaffected by hepatic disease. Atracurium and cisatracurium have a theoretic advantage in these patients because it has a pathway for nonmetabolic elimination (Hofmann elimination). All NMBAs should be titrated to effect using transcutaneous nerve stimulation.

Plasma cholinesterase synthesis may be decreased in patients with cirrhosis, although prolongation of apnea after succinylcholine administration would usually not be clinically noticeable. Regional anesthesia may be used in patients with chronic alcoholism. Relative contraindications to the use of regional anesthesia include coagulopathy, peripheral neuropathy, and decreased intravascular volume. Monitoring should include periodic monitoring of neuromuscular blockade, measurement of urine output, and periodic measurement of serum glucose and electrolyte concentrations. Postoperative complications may include poor wound healing, bleeding, infection, and hepatic dysfunction.

## Liver Disease and Cirrhosis

Excessive intraoperative and postoperative bleeding is one of the most common and feared complications of surgery. In the setting of impaired clotting factor synthesis and/or thrombocytopenia, hemostasis becomes an increased concern. Patients with AUD and suspected or known liver disease (hepatitis, jaundice, persistent bleeding, frequent bruising, cirrhosis) would benefit from preoperative evaluation to assess hepatic function and any additional workup prior to elective surgery. Routine serologic testing of hepatic function is not currently recommended in the absence of heightened clinical suspicion on the basis of symptoms or relevant medical history. For those patients for which additional workup is indicated based on symptoms or medical history, prothrombin time (PT/INR) along with platelet count are valuable tools to screen for potential hemostatic complications. Prothrombin time is one of the best indicators of hepatic synthetic function. Based on a study of 1135 patients with end stage liver disease undergoing tooth extraction, it was discovered that INR less than 2.5 and platelet count greater than $40 \times 10^3/\mu L$ portended a bleeding risk comparable to healthy individuals, whereas lab values outside of these thresholds were correlated with a 40% increase in bleeding risk requiring surgical intervention.

Perioperatively, decreased protein binding of administered drugs may lead to increased circulating unbound active medication. In addition, clearance of hepatically metabolized medications will be slowed in the face of liver disease. This combination may result in prolonged duration of action, oversedation, and delayed awakening, especially with infusions or repeated boluses of sedating medication. For example, most benzodiazepine and opioid elimination half-lives and durations of action can be expected to increase as liver disease progresses. Doses should be titrated to clinical effect, which in this case would almost certainly result in a reduction of the dose administered.

## Acetaminophen

Despite the documented risk for acute hepatotoxicity, acetaminophen is still strongly recommended for the management of mild to moderate pain. Hepatotoxicity in healthy individuals takes place at doses close to 10 g per day. In patients with confirmed cirrhosis there was no evidence of hepatotoxicity or accumulation after administration of 4 g per day for 14 days. Current recommendations limit acetaminophen in patients with known liver disease to 2 g per day and recommend avoiding it altogether in patients with severe hepatitis or acute liver injury. Caution is advised in patients who are actively and chronically consuming alcohol as the induction of the CYP450 system may increase production of toxic metabolites.

## Nonsteroidal Antiinflammatory Drugs

Nonsteroidal antiinflammatory drugs (NSAIDs) should be used with caution in patients with moderate liver disease and are contraindicated in the setting of advanced liver disease and cirrhosis. NSAIDs have the potential to increase variceal bleeding, decrease renal function, and promote the development of diuretic resistant ascites.

## Delirium Tremens

Patients with AUDs may show signs of withdrawal 6 to 8 h after their last drink. Onset of delirium tremens typically occurs 24 to 72 h after cessation of drinking. Mortality rate can be as high as 10%. Signs and symptoms of delirium tremens include tremulousness, disorientation, hallucinations, autonomic hyperactivity (diaphoresis, hyperpyrexia, tachycardia, and hypertension), hypotension, and grand mal seizures. Laboratory findings include hypomagnesemia, hypokalemia, and respiratory alkalosis. Treatment includes the use of benzodiazepines, β-adrenergic antagonists (propranolol or esmolol), protection of the patient's airway, supplemental thiamine (for the treatment of Wernicke encephalopathy), and correction of electrolyte abnormalities (especially magnesium and potassium).

## Alcoholic Abstinence

Patients may present to the operating room on medications designed to promote abstinence.

Disulfiram (Antabuse) is a medication intended to alter the metabolic consequences of alcohol and cause a severe aversive reaction by blocking the conversion of acetaldehyde by acetaldehyde dehydrogenase. With alcohol ingestion, acetaldehyde levels increase rapidly and cause nausea, vomiting, tearing, and potential bronchoconstriction and cardiac arrhythmias. The half-life of disulfiram is 1 to 2 weeks. Disulfiram can inhibit the enzyme necessary for conversion of dopamine to norepinephrine (dopamine β-hydroxylase), resulting in perioperative hypotension (decreased cardiovascular response to indirect-acting sympathomimetic amines). Disulfiram can also potentiate benzodiazepines via decreased clearance, alter the metabolism of warfarin via inhibition of hepatic microsomal enzymes, and cause drowsiness. If possible, disulfiram should be discontinued 10 days before surgery.

Naltrexone is a μ-opioid receptor antagonist that has been shown to reduce alcohol ideation. In some situations, the use of naltrexone has decreased the incidence of relapse in recovering patients with alcoholism. Naltrexone increases the threshold dose of opioid required to produce euphoria. A patient receiving naltrexone during the perioperative period will have an increased opioid requirement to achieve analgesia. Conversely, withdrawal of naltrexone or other μ-receptor antagonists may result in increased sensitivity to opioids because of upregulation of μ-receptors. Naltrexone should be stopped 3 days before elective operations.

Carbamazepine, valproate, and gabapentin are antiepileptics thought to attenuate neural hyperexcitability caused by alcohol abuse. Carbamazepine and other antiepileptics hasten recovery from intermediate and long-acting nondepolarizing muscle relaxants by enhancing the clearance of these drugs, increasing plasma concentrations of $\alpha_1$-acid glycoprotein, and producing proliferation of postsynaptic acetylcholine receptors. Acamprosate is an amino acid derivative that also reduces neural hyperexcitability via inhibition of NMDA receptors and activation of $GABA_A$ receptors. The anesthetic implications of acamprosate therapy are unknown.

## Selective Serotonin Reuptake Inhibitors

Selective serotonin reuptake inhibitors (SSRIs) appear to reduce drinking in alcoholics with concomitant depression and may also prevent relapse in recovering patients with anxiety and other affective disorders. Profound bradycardia and hypotension have been reported in patients treated with SSRIs, though it is very rare.

## SUGGESTED READINGS

Chen, G., Cheung, R., & Tom, J. W. (2017). Hepatitis: Sedation and anesthesia implications. *Anesthesia Progress, 64*(2), 106–118. doi:10.2344/anpr-64-02-13.

Diehl, A. M. (2002). Liver disease in alcohol abusers: Clinical perspective. *Alcohol, 27*(1), 7–11.

Fassoulaki, A., Farinotti, R., Servin, F., & Desmonts, J. M. (1993). Chronic alcoholism increases the induction dose of propofol in humans. *Anesthesia and Analgesia, 77*(3), 553–556.

Frezza, M., di Padova, C., Pozzato, G., Terpin, M., Baraona, E., & Lieber, C. S. (1990). High blood alcohol levels in women: The role of decreased gastric alcohol dehydrogenase activity and first-pass metabolism. *New England Journal of Medicine, 322*(2), 95–99.

Grameniz, A., Caputo, F., Bisselli, M., Kuria, F., Loggi, E., Andreone, P., et al. (2006). Alcoholic liver disease: Pathophysiological aspects and risk factors. *Alimentary Pharmacology & Therapeutics, 24*, 1151–1161.

Retrieved from https://pubs.niaaa.nih.gov/publications/AlcoholFacts&Stats/AlcoholFacts&Stats.htm. Last Accessed February, 2022.

Kao, S. C., Tsai, H. I., Cheng, C. W., Lin, T. W., Chen, C. C., & Lin, C. S. (2017). The association between frequent alcohol drinking and opioid consumption after abdominal surgery: A retrospective analysis. *PLoS One, 12*(3), e0171275.

Kip, M. J., Neumann, T., Jugel, C., Kleinwaechter, R., Weiss-Gerlach, E., Guill, M. M., et al. (2008).

New strategies to detect alcohol use disorders in the preoperative assessment clinic of a German University Hospital. *Anesthesiology, 209,* 171–179.

Krystal, J. H., Petrakis, I. L., Limoncelli, D., Webb, E., Gueorgueva, R., D'Souza, D. C., et al. (2003). Altered NMDA glutamate receptor antagonist response in recovering ethanol-dependent patients. *Neuropsychopharmacology, 28*(11), 2020–2028.

Loomba, R., & Adams, L. A. (2020). Advances in non-invasive assessment of hepatic fibrosis. *Gut, 69*(7), 1343–1352.

May, J. A., White, H. C., Leonard-White, A., Warltier, D. C., & Pagel, P. S. (2001). The patient recovering from alcohol or drug addiction: Special issues for the anesthesiologist. *Anesthesia and Analgesia, 92,* 1601–1608.

National Institute on Alcohol Abuse and Alcoholism. *Alcohol facts and statistics.* Retrieved from https://www.niaaa.nih.gov/publications/brochures-and-fact-sheets/alcohol-facts-and-statistics. Accessed December, 2021.

Spies, C. D., & Rommelspacher, H. (1999). Alcohol withdrawal in the surgical patient: Prevention and treatment. *Anesthesia and Analgesia, 88,* 946–954.

Stahre, M., Roeber, J., Kanny, D., Brewer, R. D., & Zhang, X. (2014). Contribution of excessive alcohol consumption to deaths and years of potential life lost in the United States. *Preventing Chronic Disease, 11,* 130293.

Tsuchiya, H. (2016). Anesthetic effects changeable in habitual drinkers: Mechanistic drug interactions with neuro-active indoleamine: Aldehyde condensation products associated with alcoholic beverage consumption. *Medical Hypotheses, 92,* 62–66.

# 81

# The Evaluation and Management of Prolonged Emergence From Anesthesia

THOMAS M. STEWART, MD

Recovery from anesthesia occurs on a continuum: the patient initially responds to noxious stimuli and then to oral command, though the patient remains amnestic; motor control returns gradually; finally, in 15 to 45 min, the patient is able to converse rationally. Wakefulness requires diffuse cortical activation (arousal) elicited by afferent stimuli from the reticular formation in the brainstem. Within 15 min of admission to the postanesthesia care unit (PACU), 90% of patients regain consciousness. Delayed awakening after general anesthesia (i.e., 45–60 min after admission to the PACU) is secondary to a diverse number of causes and can be broadly classified as pharmacologic, metabolic, or neurologic (Box 81.1).

Delayed emergence from anesthesia should be evaluated in a systematic fashion by the anesthesia provider (Box 81.2) while simultaneously managing the patient's preoperative comorbid conditions and medications. Consideration should be given for the type of operation, the type and doses of anesthetic drugs, drugs administered by the surgical team, and the duration and complications of anesthesia. Importantly, delayed emergence may be associated with the patient's inability to protect his or her airway, airway obstruction, and respiratory failure. Many of the causes of delayed emergence are overlapping and may coexist.

## Pharmacologic Causes of Delayed Emergence

### ANESTHETIC AGENTS

The rate of emergence from general anesthesia correlates with the timing, half-life, and total dose of anesthetic agents used, as well as an individual's biovariability. Residual effects of drugs administered during the perioperative period are the most frequently cited cause for delayed awakening. The cumulative effects of multiple drugs, some of which may be synergistic, may result in a relative drug overdose. Nonanesthetic medications may potentiate anesthetic effects, such as in the case of a lidocaine infusion used to treat cardiac arrhythmia. Patients given scopolamine or atropine may develop central anticholinergic syndrome. The highly soluble inhalation agents may be implicated when high concentrations are delivered for long periods of time or when hypoventilation slows emergence, prolonging recovery.

Opioids decrease the response to hypercarbia, resulting in hypoventilation and subsequent decreased clearance of inhalation agents. Benzodiazepines, droperidol, haloperidol, gabapentin or pregabalin, dexmedetomidine, scopolamine, and

## BOX 81.1 CAUSES OF DELAYED POSTOPERATIVE AROUSAL

**PHARMACOLOGIC CAUSES**

Residual drugs, overdose
  Medications administered during the perioperative period by
    personnel other than anesthesia providers
  Benzodiazepines
  Opioids
  Anesthetic agents—induction, inhalation, or intravenous
  Neuromuscular blockade
  Decreased metabolism, excretion, or protein binding of drugs
Pharmacokinetic factors
  Age
  Malnutrition
  Drug interactions
  Underlying renal, hepatic, CNS, or pulmonary disease
  Biologic variability
  Hypothermia
  Decreased cardiac output-hypoperfusion, hypovolemia

**METABOLIC CAUSES**

Hypothyroidism
Adrenal insufficiency
Hypoxemia
Hypoglycemia
Hyperosmolar hyperglycemic nonketotic coma

Hyponatremia, SIADH, TURP syndrome
Sepsis

**NEUROLOGIC CAUSES**

Hypoperfusion
  Low cardiac output, occlusive cerebrovascular disease
  Embolism
  Thrombus
  Air-venous, paradoxical
Intraoperative retraction, resection
  Thrombus-atrial fibrillation
Hypertension
  Hyperperfusion
  Intracerebral hemorrhage
Elevated intracranial pressure
  Subdural or epidural hematoma
  Cerebral edema
  Malfunctioning shunt
  Pneumocephalus
Seizure
Factitious disorder
Psychogenic unconsciousness
Head injury

*CNS,* Central nervous system; *SIADH,* syndrome of inappropriate antidiuretic hormone secretion; *TURP,* transurethral resection of the prostate.

## BOX 81.2 MANAGEMENT OF DELAYED EMERGENCE

I. AIRWAY, BREATHING, CIRCULATION
  a. Maintain and protect airway; reintubate if necessary
  b. Ventilate to maintain normal arterial $CO_2$
  c. Assess heart rate, blood pressure, perfusion, and urine output
II. DRUGS
  a. Review all medication that the patient has received perioperatively
  b. Persistent neuromuscular blockade
    i. Assess train-of-four with a peripheral nerve stimulator
    ii. Assess for phase II block in patients who received succinylcholine
  c. Opioids
    i. Check for pinpoint pupils and slow respiratory rate
    ii. Administer naloxone in 40-$\mu$g increments, titrating to effect
    iii. Reexamine the patient on a regular basis; the duration of intravenously administered naloxone is approximately 17 min
  d. Benzodiazepines
    i. Provide supportive management
    ii. Consider administering a benzodiazepine antagonist, flumazenil, in 0.1- to 0.2-mg increments (maximal dose, 1 mg); arrhythmias, hypertension, and convulsions are potential side effects
  e. Provide active warming if necessary
III. ELECTROLYTES
  a. Check blood glucose concentration
  b. Check serum sodium concentration
  c. Check magnesium, calcium, and phosphate concentrations
IV. FAILURE TO FIND CAUSE OF DELAYED EMERGENCE
  a. Consider the potential for a neurologic event to have occurred
  b. Perform focused neurologic exam
  c. Consider consulting a neurologist for evaluation
  d. Order neurologic imaging studies

ketamine—when given as premedication or as part of the anesthetic—may potentiate other general anesthetic agents, delaying arousal. Awakening may be delayed because of the timing of drug administration (e.g., agents administered shortly before emergence) or the route of administration (e.g., oral, rectal, or intramuscular have delayed absorption). Large doses of barbiturates or benzodiazepines may overwhelm lean tissue distribution and subsequent liver metabolism, thereby prolonging drug effects. Monoamine oxidase inhibitors potentiate the effects of opioids, barbiturates, and benzodiazepines. Both diagnosis and treatment of opioid overdose are accomplished by carefully titrating naloxone intravenously in 40-$\mu$g increments, up to 400 $\mu$g. Complete opioid reversal is undesirable because it might lead to severe pain or withdrawal symptoms. Benzodiazepines can be reversed by administration of flumazenil intravenously in 0.2-mg increments up to 1.0 mg, and physostigmine can reverse the effect of some sedatives, especially the central effects of anticholinergic agents such as scopolamine.

## NEUROMUSCULAR BLOCKADE

Muscle weakness, whether from inadequately reversed neuromuscular blocking agents or pseudocholinesterase deficiency, may result in hypoventilation, hypercarbia, and incomplete washout of inhalation anesthetic agents. Acidosis, hypermagnesemia, or certain drugs (clindamycin, gentamicin, neomycin, and furosemide) accentuate the effects of neuromuscular blocking agents and may interfere with reversal of these agents. Patients may be conscious but may be unable to mount a motor response to noxious stimuli when they have muscle weakness and therefore appear as though they are still anesthetized. Residual neuromuscular blockade should be evaluated with a peripheral nerve stimulator and response to train-of-four ratio (should be ≥0.9). Treatment for residual blockade includes allowing for more time to elapse, giving additional cholinesterase inhibitors (without exceeding maximum recommended dose) or sugammadex (only for rocuronium or vecuronium) to reverse the blockade.

## Pharmacokinetic and Pharmacodynamic Factors

Low cardiac output can reduce perfusion to the lungs, kidneys, and liver, thus reducing metabolism and excretion of anesthetic agents. Decreased protein binding of anesthetic agents from hypoproteinemia or competition of binding sites with other drugs (e.g., intravenously administered contrast dyes, sodium acetrizoate, sulfadimethoxine) results in higher blood levels of the active drug.

Renal failure and azotemia are associated with altered acid-base status, decreased protein binding (more likely due to hypoproteinemia than to acidosis), delayed or reduced excretion of drugs or their metabolites, and electrolyte changes, all of which contribute to delayed emergence. It is hypothesized that changes in permeability of the blood-brain barrier may increase sensitivity to hypnotics in patients with renal failure or azotemia.

Liver metabolism of anesthetic agents is decreased in malnourished patients, in patients at extremes of age (through immature or decreased enzyme activity), in the presence of hypothermia (below 33–34°C), or during simultaneous administration of drugs dependent on liver microsomal detoxification (e.g., ethanol or barbiturates). Ketamine administration in patients with liver dysfunction delays anesthetic emergence. Patients with liver disease and a history of hepatic coma develop central nervous system (CNS) depression after the administration of small amounts of opioids; cimetidine may also cause mental status changes in such patients. Although increased sensitivity to barbiturates has been reported in animals with hepatectomy or liver damage, such sensitivity has not been demonstrated in humans with these same conditions.

Hypothermia not only reduces the metabolism of drugs by the liver but also directly depresses CNS activity (cold narcosis) and increases the solubility of inhalation anesthetic agents, which, in turn, slows their transfer from blood into alveoli. Central respiratory depression and increased sensitivity to anesthetic agents are diagnoses of exclusion. Any anesthetic agent may cause central respiratory depression. Biologic variability in sensitivity to anesthetic drugs follows a bell-shaped gaussian distribution; sensitivity in older adults, compared with younger adults, is not equally distributed on such a curve. Anesthetic requirements diminish with age and in patients who are hypothermic or hypothyroid.

## Metabolic Disturbances of Delayed Emergence

### ACID-BASE DISORDERS

Mental status changes occur with a cerebrospinal fluid pH of less than 7.25. During acute hypercapnia, CNS activity is depressed because hydrogen ions cross the blood-brain barrier more quickly than do bicarbonate ions. Hypoxia and hypercapnia accentuate residual anesthetic effects and the effects of preexisting conditions (e.g., hepatic encephalopathy). Metabolic encephalopathies, per se, sensitize patients to the effects of CNS depressants.

### ENDOCRINE DISORDERS

Certain endocrine disorders (e.g., hypothyroidism, adrenal insufficiency) are associated with prolonged anesthetic emergence. The stress of anesthesia and surgery generally increases blood glucose concentrations. Sepsis, systemic inflammatory response syndrome (SIRS), uremia, pancreatitis, pneumonia, burns, and administration of hypertonic solutions or mannitol can trigger hyperosmolar hyperglycemic nonketotic coma, which can cause delayed anesthetic emergence.

Hypoglycemia can occur secondary to perioperative administration of antiglycemic drugs, after manipulation of insulin-producing tumors and retroperitoneal carcinomas, or in patients with severe liver disease who have decreased gluconeogenesis. Hypoglycemia is associated with several CNS side effects ranging from irritability to seizures and coma.

### ELECTROLYTE ABNORMALITIES

Electrolyte disorders—such as hypoosmolality and hyponatremia due to absorption of large volumes of hypotonic fluids (e.g., during transurethral resection of the prostate) or from the syndrome of inappropriate antidiuretic hormone secretion—may delay emergence. Other electrolyte abnormalities to consider when evaluating a patient with delayed emergence include hypercalcemia, hypocalcemia, hypermagnesemia, and hypomagnesemia.

### NEUROLOGIC CAUSES OF DELAYED EMERGENCE

Delayed arousal after anesthesia may be caused by global or regional ischemia from cerebral hypoperfusion or hyperperfusion, hypoxia, elevated intracranial pressure, cerebral hemorrhage, traumatic brain injury, seizure or postictal state, or, more rarely, factitious disorder or psychogenic unconsciousness. Certain neurosurgical procedures and cerebral hypoperfusion from reduced cardiac output, obstruction to flow, or decreased systemic vascular resistance (systemic shock) have the potential to delay emergence from anesthesia. Arterial compression from retraction or improper positioning of the head and neck are other causes of hypoperfusion.

Hypotension occurring perioperatively may result in cerebral ischemia and stroke and occurs most often in patients with preexisting cerebrovascular disease. Thromboembolic events may be observed in patients undergoing cardiac, vascular, and invasive neck procedures or in patients with atrial fibrillation or hypercoagulable states. Venous air embolism can occur in cases in which the surgical site is higher than the heart; if patients have a patent foramen ovale, they are at increased risk for developing a paradoxical venous air embolism from even small amounts of entrained air. Stage II hypertension or a cerebrovascular accident from hemorrhage or hematoma can precipitate cerebral hyperperfusion, which can delay emergence. Intracranial pressure may increase from hyperperfusion or from intracerebral or subdural hemorrhage or hematoma. Cerebral edema, pneumocephalus, or a malfunctioning shunt or drain are also causes. Delayed emergence caused by regional ischemia is manifested by hemiplegia or other focal signs, also known as differential awakening. In theory, focal areas of underperfused or previously injured brain tissue may have trapping or increased sensitivity to anesthetic agents. Physical examination looking for focal neurologic disturbances, urgent neurology consultation, and imaging with computed tomography scan are all indicated if a primary neurologic cause for delayed awakening is suspected, or if other causes have been ruled out.

Seizures in the perioperative period have been linked to hypoxia, metabolic/electrolyte disturbances, fever, or CNS disease. Seizures may be nonconvulsive, making identification in the perioperative setting difficult. Neurology consultation and use of multichannel electroencephalogram recording may be helpful in identifying subclinical status epilepticus and in ruling out other causes for delayed awakening. Treatment includes benzodiazepines and antiepileptics such as phenytoin and carbamazepine. Patients in a postictal state may also remain unresponsive in the perioperative period and could be a potential cause for a delay in arousal after anesthesia.

Factitious disorder is the intentional production of physical or psychological symptoms in order to assume the sick role. It is a diagnosis of exclusion, only after more serious causes of delayed emergence have been eliminated. Psychogenic unconsciousness, a diagnosis of exclusion, is a dissociative psychiatric disorder with sustained amnesia and unexplainable delayed emergence from anesthesia. Many patients who present with factitious disorders have underlying psychiatric and psychological illnesses. Current recommendations are to provide supportive care and reassurance, whereas repeated noxious stimuli are not humane and not advocated.

## SUGGESTED READINGS

Cascella, M., Bimonte, S., & Di Napoli, R. (2020). Delayed emergence from anesthesia: What we know and how we act. *Local and Regional Anesthesia*, *13*, 195–206.

Evered, L. A., Chan, M. T. V., Han, R., Chu, M. H. M., Cheng, B. P., Scott, D. A., et al. (2021). Anaesthetic depth and delirium after major surgery: A randomised clinical trial. *British Journal of Anaesthesia*, *127*(5), 704–712.

Garcia, A., Clark, E. A., Rana, S., Preciado, D., Jeha, G. M., Viswanath, O., et al. (2021). Effects of premedication with midazolam on recovery and discharge times after tonsillectomy and adenoidectomy. *Cureus*, *13*(2), e13101. doi:10.7759/cureus.13101.

Maheshwari, K., Ahuja, S., Mascha, E. J., Cummings, K. C., III, Chahar, P., Elsharkawy, H., et al. (2020). Effect of sevoflurane versus isoflurane on emergence time and postanesthesia care unit length of stay: An alternating intervention trial. *Anesthesia and Analgesia*, *130*(2), 360–366.

Shapses, M., Tang, L., Layne, A., Beri, A., & Rotman, Y. (2021). Fatty liver is an independent risk factor for delayed recovery from anesthesia. *Hepatology Communications*, *5*(11), 1848–1859.

Wu, Y. M., Su, Y. H., Huang, S. Y., Lo, P. H., Chen, J. T., Chang, H. C., et al. (2021). Recovery profiles of sevoflurane and desflurane with or without m-entropy guidance in obese patients: A randomized controlled trial. *Journal of Clinical Medicine*, *11*(1), 162. doi:10.3390/jcm11010162.

# 82

# Delirium in the Postanesthesia Care Unit

LAYNE M. BETTINI, MD, JD

Postoperative delirium is the acute onset of altered or fluctuating mental status combined with significant inattention that can present in multiple ways and represents acute brain failure. Although often thought to include one or more of the following manifestations—hyperarousal, agitation, hyperactivity, and even frank psychosis—postoperative delirium more often exhibits as hypoactivity, which may include flat affect, withdrawal, and lethargy.

Postoperative delirium occurs more frequently at the extremes of age, occurring in 5% to 50% of older patients. In children, delirium is relatively common (with a reported incidence of approximately 30%), manifesting as emergence excitement or agitation (e.g., inconsolable crying or disorientation) occurring within the first 10 min of postanesthesia care unit (PACU) arrival and resolving within an hour. If children are not yet conscious when brought to the PACU, they can experience agitation later in their PACU stay.

## Predisposing and Perioperative Risk Factors

Risk factors for postoperative delirium are summarized in Box 82.1. Patients with no risk factors have a 9% chance of developing postoperative delirium. For those with one or two risk factors, the chance increases to 23%, and for those with three or four risk factors, the chance jumps to 83%. Multiple hypotheses exist as to why certain individuals are at risk for developing delirium. The primary risk factors include old age, American

## BOX 82.1   PREDISPOSING AND PERIOPERATIVE FACTORS ASSOCIATED WITH INCREASED RISK FOR DELIRIUM IN POSTANESTHESIA CARE UNIT

| Predisposing Factors | Perioperative Factors |
|---|---|
| Abnormal glycemic control | Airway obstruction |
| Age >65 y | Bladder distention |
| ASA score ≥3 | Duration of operation >1 h |
| BUN/Cr >18 | Duration of preoperative fluid fasting* |
| Cognitive dysfunction or dementia† | Electrolyte imbalance |
| Depression | Emergent vs. elective procedure |
| Excessive alcohol use | High-risk operation |
| Illicit drug use or use of ≥3 prescription drugs | Hypocapnia or hypercapnia |
| Immobility | Hypoxia |
| Intracranial injury | Orthopedic operation |
| Male sex | Pain |
| Metabolic derangements | Prolonged mechanical ventilation |
| Neurologic disease‡ | Sensory overload |
| Sensory impairment, particularly visual | Use of specific drugs for anesthesia and analgesia§ |
| Sepsis | |
| Sleep-disordered breathing | |
| Use of β-adrenergic receptor blocking agents | |

*Duration of preoperative fluid fasting ≥6 h, compared with 2 to 6 h, increases the risk for development of postoperative delirium.
†Particularly impairment in executive function.
‡Alzheimer disease and Parkinson disease.
§Drugs administered perioperatively that have been associated with an increased risk for development of postoperative delirium include anticonvulsants, atropine, benzodiazepines, corticosteroids, droperidol, fentanyl (larger doses), H₂-receptor antagonists, ketamine, meperidine, metoclopramide, and scopolamine.
*ASA*, American Society of Anesthesiologists; *BUN/Cr*, blood urea nitrogen/creatinine ratio.

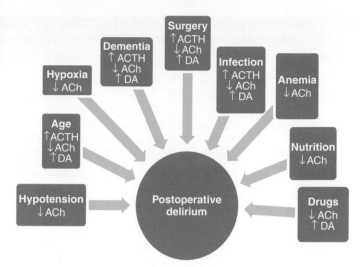

**Fig. 82.1**   Decreased levels of acetylcholine (*ACh*) and increased levels of dopamine (*DA*) or cortisol (*ACTH*) can lead to postoperative delirium.

involved; cytokines are released in response to surgical stress and are associated with neuronal death. Hemodynamic and ventilatory management may also play a role with some evidence that intraoperative hypocapnia and hypotension are associated with postoperative delirium. Given this information, some studies suggest that regional anesthesia may be associated with less postoperative delirium than general anesthesia, as regional anesthesia typically uses fewer sedatives, opioids, and other anesthetic drugs. There is also debate as to whether depth of anesthesia contributes to a higher incidence of postoperative delirium, but studies yield inconsistent results.

Acetylcholine is important for maintenance of arousal, attention, and memory, whereas dopamine has an opposing effect. Thus perioperatively administered medications that decrease levels of acetylcholine or increase levels of dopamine can lead to delirium (Fig. 82.1). Central anticholinergic syndrome, caused by blockade of muscarinic cholinergic receptors in the central nervous system, manifests as decreased heart rate and contractility, bronchial constriction, decreased salivary secretions, intestinal and bladder contraction, relaxation of sphincters, and delirium. Sedatives, such as benzodiazepines and opioids (especially meperidine because it is structurally similar to the anticholinergic drug atropine) are prime contenders. Corticosteroids, H₂-receptor antagonists, and anticonvulsants have also been implicated. Renal and hepatic dysfunction compromise clearance of these medications causing further exacerbation of delirium.

In children, the highest incidence of postoperative delirium occurs in those too young (i.e., aged 2–4 years) to communicate in words when awakening from anesthesia, thereby making the differentiation between delirium and pain more difficult. Treating preoperative anxiety likely has some beneficial effect. Using desflurane for maintenance of anesthesia after a sevoflurane induction may reduce the severity of emergence delirium, compared with sevoflurane induction and maintenance. Propofol decreases the risk of emergence agitation when used throughout anesthesia and for maintenance after sevoflurane induction.

## Diagnosis

Screening tools have been developed and adapted for use in the PACU to assess patients for the presence of delirium

Society of Anesthesiologists physical status III or higher, hypoalbuminemia, intraoperative hypotension, perioperative blood transfusion, and history of excessive alcohol use. In elderly patients, contributing factors include smaller brain mass (atrophy), decreased number of neurons, and decreased neurotransmitter (acetylcholine, serotonin, and dopamine) production and receptor density. Accordingly, the elderly appear to have limited "cognitive reserve." Therefore, even minor disturbances can lead to postoperative delirium. Specifically, severe illness (including psychiatric illness), cognitive impairment with or without dementia, dehydration, and substance abuse have been shown to be predisposing risk factors. Preexisting diminished executive function, decreased functional status, and depression are independent predictors of postoperative delirium. Additionally, in older patients, sleep-disordered breathing, such as obstructive and central sleep apnea, has been associated with cognitive impairment.

Other perioperative risk factors also include high-risk surgical procedures (cardiac, thoracic aortic, noncardiac thoracic, orthopedic), breast and abdominal procedures, and prolonged operations. Many of these high-risk operations are associated with embolic phenomena (e.g., air, thrombus, cement), large fluid shifts, and substantial rates of blood transfusion. The incidence of postoperative delirium after total joint arthroplasties may be as high as 10%, with variability as a result of the different tools used to diagnose delirium. Inflammation may also be

| TABLE 82.1 | Tools Used to Score Delirium in Postanesthesia Care Unit | | | |
|---|---|---|---|---|
| Feature | CAM | DDS | Nu-DESC | PAED |
| Number of questions | 4 | 5 | 5 | 5 |
| Responses | Yes/No | 0–2 scale | Weighted score for each of 4 possible responses | 0–4 scale |
| Domains measured | Acute onset or fluctuating course, inattention, disorganized thinking, altered level of consciousness | Disorientation, inappropriate behavior, inappropriate communication, illusions or hallucinations, psychomotor retardation | Orientation, hallucinations, agitation, anxiety, paroxysmal sweating | Eye contact, purposeful actions, awareness, restlessness, consolability |

*CAM*, Confusion Assessment Method; *DDS*, Delirium Detection Score; *Nu-DESC*, Nursing Delirium Screening Scale; *PAED*, Pediatric Anesthesia Emergence Delirium.

(Table 82.1). The Nursing Delirium Screening Scale appears to be the most sensitive in detecting postoperative delirium, which is largely a diagnosis of exclusion. Common metabolic derangements that are associated with delirium include hyponatremia, hypoglycemia or hyperglycemia, hypokalemia or hyperkalemia, hypercalcemia, hypermagnesemia, lactic acidemia, hypothermia, hypothyroidism, and adrenal insufficiency. Arterial hypoxemia and alveolar hypoventilation are potential respiratory-associated causes of delirium. Postoperative nausea and vomiting and infection (e.g., urinary tract infection, pneumonia, or septicemia) should also be considered in patients who exhibit signs of postoperative delirium.

## Prevention

Because the treatment of postoperative delirium is largely symptom management, the best approach to treatment is prevention. A Cochrane review evaluated six randomized clinical trials regarding interventions to prevent delirium and concluded that evidence to support pharmacologic prevention is inadequate. It has been suggested that melatonin, donepezil, and olanzapine administered perioperatively may decrease the incidence of postoperative delirium. However, identifying high-risk patients by means of a thorough preoperative assessment, including administering tests that measure depression and cognitive flexibility or executive function, may be helpful in planning the anesthetic and analgesic management. The preoperative assessment should also seek to discern and address potentially modifiable risk factors (see Box 82.1). This should include preoperative screening for sleep-disordered breathing using a screening tool such as the STOP-Bang questionnaire.

## Treatment

The goal of treatment is ensuring patient safety. For violent or severely agitated patients, this may include the use of restraints. The initial intervention—verbal support to provide reassurance and reorientation—includes voicing the patient's name and current location, the surgeon's name, and the time of day. Physiologic causes of delirium should be considered, including distended bladder, nausea, uncomfortable positioning, or the possibility of the patient lying on a foreign object. Sleep-disordered breathing should be considered and ruled out. If it is in the differential diagnosis, consider continuous pulse oximetry, supplemental oxygen, and continuous positive airway pressure. Thereafter, treatment becomes more aggressive beginning with the reversal of any potentially lingering anesthetic agents via intravenous administration of flumazenil (0.2-mg increments), naloxone (0.04-mg increments), or physostigmine (1–2 mg). Physostigmine remains controversial but is currently indicated for the treatment of central anticholinergic syndrome. Haloperidol (2.5–5 mg every 5 min) has been reported to decrease the severity—but not the incidence—of delirium. Adding quetiapine helps resolve delirium more quickly than haloperidol alone (1 day vs. 4.5 days).

A multitude of drugs have been used in children undergoing surgical procedures to prevent or treat emergence delirium. The most commonly used agents include clonidine, dexmedetomidine, propofol, and opioids. Intraoperative administration of $\alpha_2$-adrenergic agonists reduces the incidence of emergence delirium in children. A 2-mcg/kg dose of clonidine administered after induction of anesthesia has been shown to reduce the severity of emergence delirium. Dexmedetomidine (0.5 mcg/kg) administered 5 min before the end of the surgical procedure is also effective. Prophylactic propofol at the end of surgery is also effective in reducing the incidence and severity of agitation upon emergence. Intravenous fentanyl administered 10 to 20 min before the end of surgery decreases agitation on emergence and does not appear to increase duration of PACU stay or postoperative nausea and vomiting.

## Outcomes and Long-Term Consequences

Emergence delirium, especially if it leads to postoperative delirium, can be costly in terms of staffing, increased hospital length of stay, and increased morbidity (self-extubation, pulling out tubes, lines, drains) and mortality risks. Delirious patients can also harm others should they become physically violent. If delirium in the PACU progresses to prolonged delirium, there is an increased likelihood that the patient will be discharged to a skilled care facility.

## SUGGESTED READINGS

Kim, N., Park, J. H., Lee, J. S., Choi, T., & Kim, M. S. (2017). Effects of intravenous fentanyl around the end of surgery on emergence agitation in children: Systematic review and meta-analysis. *Paediatric Anaesthesia, 27*, 885–892.

Lam, W. K., Chung, F., & Wong, J. (2017). Sleep-disordered breathing, postoperative delirium, and cognitive impairment. *Anesthesia and Analgesia, 124*, 1626–1635.

Li, Y., Li, H., Li, H., Zhao, B. J., Guo, X. Y., Feng, Y., et al. (2021). Delirium in older patients after combined epidural–general anesthesia or general anesthesia for major surgery: A randomized trial. *Anesthesiology, 135*(2), 218–232.

Lu, X., Jin, X., Yang, S., & Xia, Y. (2018). The correlation of depth of anesthesia and postoperative cognitive impairment: A meta-analysis based on randomized controlled trials. *Journal of Clinical Anesthesia, 45*, 55–59.

Mutch, W., El-Gabalawy, R., Girling, L., Kilborn, K., & Jacobsohn, E. (2018). End-tidal hypocapnia under anesthesia predicts postoperative delirium. *Frontiers in Neurology, 9*, 678.

Nazemi, A. K., Anirudh, K. G., Carmouche, J. J., Kates, S. L., Albert, T. J., & Behrend, C. J. (2017). Prevention and management of postoperative delirium in elderly patients following elective spinal surgery. *Clinical Spine Surgery, 30*, 112–119.

The American Geriatrics Society Expert Panel on Postoperative Delirium in Older Adults. (2015). *Journal of the American College of Surgeons, 220*, 136–148.

Wildes, T., Mickle, A., Abdallah, A., Maybrier, H. R., Oberhaus, J., Budelier, T. P., et al. (2019). Effect of electroencephalography-guided anesthetic administration on postoperative delirium among older adults undergoing major surgery. The ENGAGES randomized clinical trial. *JAMA, 321*(5), 473–483.

# Specialty Anesthesia: Regional Anesthesia

# Local Anesthetic Agents: Mechanism of Action and Pharmacology

STEVEN R. CLENDENEN, MD

The mechanism of action of local anesthetic (LA) agents is to prevent the transmission of nerve impulses generated by a chemical, mechanical, or electrical stimulus that triggers an action potential.

## Anatomy of a Nerve Cell

Nerve cells communicate with each other through axons, which are elongations of the cell body, and by dendrites. The cell membrane is a hydrophobic lipid bilayer that incorporates ion channels composed of lipoproteins. In contrast to the nerve cells of the central nervous system, many peripheral nerves are enveloped in myelin produced by Schwann cells. Gaps known as nodes of Ranvier, located approximately 1 mm apart in the myelin sheath, have a high concentration of $Na^+$ channels, facilitating saltatory transmission between sequential nodes and increasing the speed of electrical conduction along the axon.

## Nerve Cell Membrane and Depolarization

The cell membrane creates a barrier between the $Na^+$-rich extracellular fluid and the $K^+$-rich intracellular fluid, creating a resting membrane potential of $^-60$ to $^-90$ mV (Fig. 83.1). There is constant movement of $Na^+$ ions through $Na^+$ channels that spontaneously open and close; active transport of $Na^+$ out of the cell maintains the resting membrane potential. When an appropriate stimulus of adequate magnitude opens a sufficient number of $Na^+$ channels, the surrounding membrane depolarizes (becomes less negative), recruiting additional channel openings—a cascade of open channels allows more $Na^+$ to enter the cell, with $K^+$ diffusing out of the cell through $K^+$ channels to the point that the entire membrane depolarizes, producing an all-or-nothing electrical signal (action potential) that is propagated along the axon. Once the

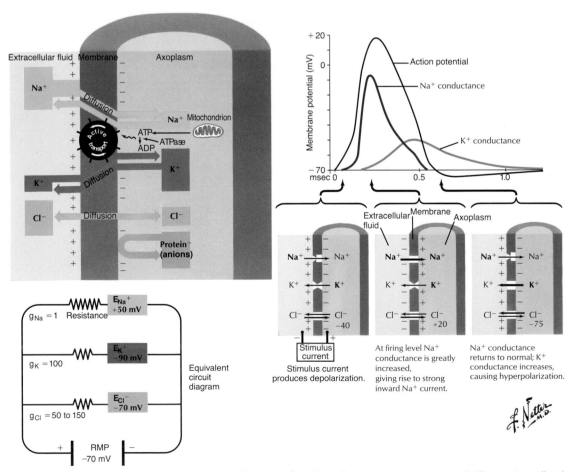

**Fig. 83.1** Resting membrane and action potentials. (Netter illustration from http://www.netterimages.com. © Elsevier Inc. All rights reserved.)

action potential passes, an energy-dependent mechanism reestablishes the concentrations of $Na^+$ and of $K^+$, restoring the resting membrane potential.

## Structure of Local Anesthetic Agents

Molecules of LA agents contain an aromatic lipophilic end, which is connected by an intermediate chain to a hydrophilic tertiary amine (weak base). The intermediate chain is either an amide or an ester linkage; this linkage is the basis for the two different classes of LA agents (esters and amides), which have similar mechanisms of action but different metabolic pathways. Because the nonionized form of the molecule crosses the cell membrane, compounds that are more lipophilic have a faster onset of blockade. And because LA agents are weak bases, compounds with a $pK_a$ close to physiologic pH will have a faster onset of blockade as more molecules remain in the nonionized state. Clearance of the drug from the site of injection and protein binding of LA agents by $\alpha_1$-acid glycoprotein also affect the duration of action because it is the concentration of free drug that is available to diffuse across the membrane that determines blockade (Fig. 83.2, Table 83.1).

## Action of Local Anesthetic Agents

Intracellular pH is typically less than 7; therefore once molecules of the LA agent cross the cell membrane, many molecules will dissociate into the ionized form of the molecule. These ions have affinity for the $\alpha$ subunits of the $Na^+$ channels. The ionized molecule of the LA agent enters a $Na^+$ channel from within the cell, binding with the $\alpha$ subunit and ultimately rendering the $Na^+$ channel inactive. If $Na^+$ cannot traverse the membrane, the cell cannot depolarize, and an action potential would not be generated. Myelinated nerves require blockade of three consecutive nodes of Ranvier to ensure impulse extinction.

Local anesthetics work by blocking sodium conductance through voltage-gated sodium channels. The cause of LA failure is unknown; however, a genetic defect has been proposed as a potential mechanism. A genetic variant that is associated with LA resistance in the gene encoding a variant form of voltage-gated sodium channel has been identified, explaining a plausible reason for LA failure. A large number of patients with Ehlers-Danlos syndrome and joint hypermobility syndrome are resistant to local anesthesia, which is often identified during dental procedures. Further research is needed to identify the genetic causes of local anesthetic resistance.

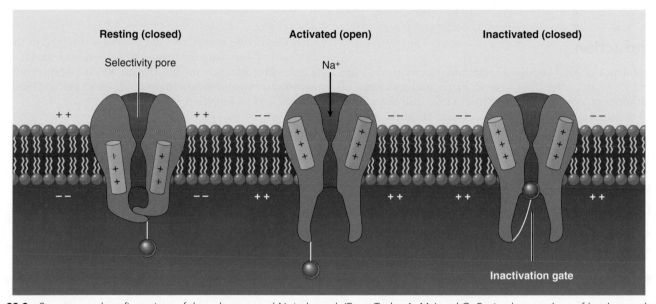

**Fig. 83.2**  Structure and configurations of the voltage gated $Na^+$ channel. (From Taylor A, McLeod G. Basic pharmacology of local anaesthetics. *BJA Educ.* 2020;20(2):34–41.)

| TABLE 83.1 | Chemical and Physical Properties of the Most Commonly Used Local Anesthetic Drugs | | | | |
|---|---|---|---|---|---|
| Property | Lidocaine | Mepivacaine | Bupivacaine | Ropivacaine | Levobupivacaine |
| Molecular weight | 234 | 246 | 288 | 274 | 288 |
| $pK_a$ | 7.7 | 7.6 | 8.1 | 8.1 | 8.1 |
| Liposolubility* | 4 | 1 | 30 | 2.8 | 30 |
| Partition coefficient | 2.9 | 0.8 | 28 | 9 | 28 |
| Protein binding (%) | 65 | 75 | 95 | 94 | 95 |
| Equipotency (%) | 2 | 1.5 | 0.5 | 0.75 | 0.5 |

*Liposolubility of each of the local anesthetic agents, compared with mepivacaine (e.g., lidocaine is four times more lipid soluble than mepivacaine).

## SUGGESTED READINGS

Clendenen, A., Cannon, A., Porter, S., Robards, C. B., Parker, A., & Clendenen, S. (2016). Whole-exome sequencing of a family of local anesthesia resistance. *Minerva Anestesiologica, 82,* 1089–1097.

Scholz, A. (2002). Mechanism of (local) anaesthetics on voltage-gated sodium and other ion channels. *British Journal of Anaesthesia, 89,* 52–61.

Schubart, J. R., Schaefer, E., Janicki, P., Adhikary, S. D., Schilling, A., Hakim, A. J., et al. (2019). Resistance to local anesthesia in people with the Ehlers-Danlos Syndromes presenting for dental surgery. *Journal of Dental Anesthesia and Pain Medicine, 19*(5), 261–270.

Taylor, A., & McLeod, G. (2020). "Basic pharmacology of local anaesthetics." *BJA Education, 20*(2), 34–41. doi:10.1016/j.bjae.2019.10.002.

# 84

# Toxicity of Local Anesthetic Agents

ALI AKBER TURABI, MD | GIFTY A. DOMINAH-AGYEMANG, MD

## Introduction

The incidence of local anesthetic systemic toxicity (LAST) has become lower since the 1980s due to better understanding of the pathophysiology of local anesthetics (LAs) and the utilization of methods such as ultrasound guidance. However, it is still imperative that one recognize the proper dosing, pharmacologic properties, presentation of symptoms, and management of LAST, as major events can be detrimental.

## Factors Influencing Blood Levels of Local Anesthetic Agents

The site of and route of injection (Table 84.1), the specific drug properties, the dose of the drug used, the coadministration of vasoconstricting agents, and the pathways involved in the metabolism of the drug determine blood levels of an LA agent. These affect not only the speed with which blood levels of LA agents rise but also the duration of the effect and the likelihood that toxicity will develop.

### SITE OF ADMINISTRATION

Absorption of LA agents is dependent on the blood supply at the site of injection. (See Fig. 84.1.) Highly vascular areas are at greatest risk for uptake. Administration of LA to topical areas, especially mucosal membranes in high doses or in repeated amounts, can result in LAST. For instance, the use of topical lidocaine for bronchoscopy has been shown to result in high blood levels of the drug and have even led to cardiac arrest.

| TABLE 84.1 | Pharmacokinetics and Maximum Dose and Duration of Commonly Used Local Anesthetic Agents | | | | | | | |
|---|---|---|---|---|---|---|---|
| | | | | DURATION (h) | | MAX DOSE (mg/kg) | |
| Class | Drug | pKa | Onset | W/o epi | W/ epi | W/o epi | W/ epi |
| Amide | Lidocaine 1–5% | 7.9 | Rapid | 2 | 4 | 5 | 7 |
| Amide | Etidocaine 0.5–1.5% | 7.7 | Rapid | 4 | 8 | 2.5 | 4 |
| Amide | Mepivacaine 1.5% | 7.6 | Medium | 3 | 6 | 5 | 7 |
| Amide | Ropivacaine 0.5% | 8.1 | Medium | 3 | 6 | 2 | 3 |
| Amide | Prilocaine 4% | 7.9 | Medium | 1.5 | 6 | 5 | 7.5 |
| Amide | Bupivacaine 0.25–0.75% | 8.1 | Slow | 4 | 8 | 2.5 | 3 |
| Ester | Procaine 0.5–1% | 8.9 | Rapid | 0.75 | 1.5 | 8 | 10 |
| Ester | Chloroprocaine 2–3% | 8.7 | Rapid | 0.5 | 1.5 | 10 | 15 |
| Ester | Tetracaine 0.1–0.5% | 8.5 | Slow | 3 | 10 | 1.5 | 2.5 |

Different drugs have different properties that affect absorption through the cell membrane, effect onset, and duration. Knowing maximum doses is important in avoiding LAST.

Route of Administration of Local Anesthetic With Relative Rapidity of Absorption

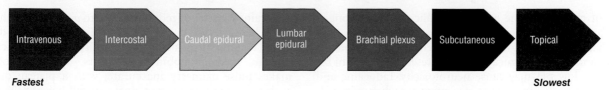

**Fastest**                                                                                    **Slowest**

**Fig. 84.1** The fastest route of administration of local anesthetic (LA) with relation to drug absorption is intravenous. The slowest is topical, yet local anesthetic systemic toxicity can still occur with high doses or frequent readministration of topical LA.

## LOCAL ANESTHETIC AGENT PROPERTIES
### (SEE TABLE 84.1)

Lipid Solubility: Increased lipid solubility results in greater potency as it allows for more of the drug to penetrate the cellular lipid bilayer. A lower dose of this drug may be required to achieve analgesic effects and may lead to LAST.

Protein Binding: A high degree of protein binding to alpha-1-acidic glycoprotein (AAG) and albumin relates to a lesser likelihood of developing LAST. The protein binding acts as a reservoir for the drug and decreases the levels of free local anesthetic systemically.

pKa: the pKa of the LA in comparison to the surrounding pH plays a large role in the potency of the drug. Having a lower pKa means that more of the drug is in its uncharged state and therefore can pass more readily through the lipophilic cellular membranes.

Volume of Distribution: A large volume of distribution (prilocaine) results in lower systemic blood levels.

### METABOLISM

Absorption and delivery to the site of metabolism (for amides, the liver; for esters, the plasma) is necessary for LA metabolism to occur. Chloroprocaine is metabolized within 45 seconds by plasma cholinesterase. Because of its short plasma half-life, episodes of reported LAST events with chloroprocaine are usually very brief, lasting less than 40 seconds. On the other hand, bupivacaine is metabolized in the liver and has a half-life of about 8 hours.

### DOSE OF LOCAL ANESTHETIC AGENT

The higher the concentration of the LA agent, the more likely that toxicity will occur. For example, transversus abdominis plane blocks often require a large volume of local anesthetic (>20 mL) to ensure adequate spread and are often performed bilaterally.

### COADMINISTRATION OF VASOCONSTRICTORS

The effect of the addition of epinephrine or phenylephrine to the LA agent depends on the local blood supply at the injection site and the vasoconstrictive or dilating properties of the specific LA agent. In general, the addition of vasoconstricting agents lowers the peak blood levels and increases the time to achieve the peak blood levels of LA agents. Additionally, epinephrine can be used as a test of potential LAST toxicity when administering epidural LA, as it will increase the heart rate by 10 bpm or more and the systolic blood pressure by 15 mm Hg or more if it enters the intravascular system.

## Clinical Presentation of Systemic Toxicity (Box 84.1)
### MECHANISM OF ACTION

LAs impede pain signal transmission by blocking voltage-gated sodium channels on sensory neurons, thus preventing sodium influx and therefore generation of action potentials. This effect is nonspecific to sensory neurons, however, and other sodium channels can also be blocked, leading to toxicity. Central nervous system (CNS) abnormalities are the first manifestation of LAST, whereas cardiac abnormalities result from higher concentrations of LA agents.

## Central Nervous System Toxicity

The initial symptoms and signs of LA-induced CNS toxicity are tinnitus, blurred vision, dizziness, tongue paresthesia, metallic taste, and perioral numbness. Excitatory phenomena (nervousness, restlessness, agitation, and muscle twitching) result from selective blockade of inhibitory pathways and often precede CNS depression and tonic-clonic seizures. The presence of hypercarbia (secondary to CNS depression and decreased ventilatory drive) lowers the seizure threshold because the hypercarbia increases cerebral blood flow, and the associated respiratory acidosis decreases protein binding, making more active drug available.

---

**BOX 84.1   CLINICAL SIGNS AND SYMPTOMS OF LOCAL ANESTHETIC SYSTEMIC TOXICITY**

| Brain | Heart |
|---|---|
| • Dizziness | • Tachycardia |
| • Tinnitus | • Bradycardia/heart block |
| • Blurred vision | • Hypotension |
| • Tongue paresthesia | • Ventricular tachycardia or fibrillation |
| • Metallic taste | • Asystole |
| • Perioral numbness | |
| • Excitatory phenomena | |
|   • Nervousness | |
|   • Restlessness | |
|   • Agitation | |
|   • Muscle twitching | |
|   • Shivering | |
|   • Tonic-clonic seizure | |
|   • Obtundation | |
|   • Coma | |

Neurologic signs tend to precede cardiac signs; however, they can overlap. For example, dizziness and blurred vision can be accompanied by tachycardia and hypotension.

## Peripheral Nervous System Toxicity

The use of chloroprocaine has been implicated in prolonged sensory and motor deficits in some patients. Studies have shown that although chloroprocaine itself is not neurotoxic, large amounts of chloroprocaine in the presence of sodium bisulfite and a low pH may cause neurotoxicity. Lidocaine and other LA agents also may cause neurotoxicity when administered in high doses.

## Cauda Equina Syndrome

Prolonged neurologic injury with motor paralysis and sensory changes (including pain) is a rare complication that occurs when LA agents are used to induce spinal anesthesia. Although preservatives or other contaminants administered with the LA agent have been cited as the cause of this complication, neural toxicity has been described after injection of high concentrations and doses of certain LA agents, including chloroprocaine and lidocaine, independent of the preservative used. A number of cases were reported in the 1990s after the use of microcatheters for continuous spinal anesthesia with high-dose lidocaine, presumably because catheter placement allowed a high concentration of the drug to accumulate near sacral nerve roots.

## Transient Neurologic Symptoms

Lidocaine is not often used in spinal anesthesia because of its association with transient neurologic symptoms. Severe pain radiating down both legs is the most described symptom. Associated factors include surgical position (specifically lithotomy), early ambulation, and obesity. This poses a special problem when spinal anesthesia is chosen for short procedures because there are few alternatives for outpatient regional anesthesia. Alternatives to lidocaine include procaine, mepivacaine (which has also been associated with transient neurologic syndrome), very-low-dose lidocaine (25 mg) with fentanyl (25 μg), and very-low-dose bupivacaine (4–7 mg) with fentanyl (10–25 μg). Recently bisulfite-free chloroprocaine has seen a rebirth in use for spinal anesthesia considering the faster return to ambulation and shorter times to meet hospital discharge criteria compared with low-dose, but still longer-acting, bupivacaine. Thus chloroprocaine perhaps may be the best-suited LA for outpatient spinal anesthesia.

### CARDIOVASCULAR SYSTEM TOXICITY

All LA agents cause a dose-dependent depression in myocardial contractility and also exhibit vasodilating properties (with the exception of cocaine, a vasoconstrictor). Like CNS toxicity, myocardial depression is proportional to the potency of the LA agent. The use of bupivacaine has also been associated with a higher-risk profile for cardiac toxicity. Compared with lidocaine, bupivacaine is more cardiotoxic because it binds more strongly to resting or inactivated sodium channels, and bupivacaine dissociates from sodium channels during diastole more slowly than does lidocaine. It is associated with cardiac arrhythmias having the lowest cardiovascular collapse to CNS ratio (CC:CNS ratio) of the commonly used LAs.

## Methemoglobinemia

Prilocaine is metabolized in the liver to *o*-toluidine, which oxidizes hemoglobin to methemoglobin. In general, doses of about 600 mg of prilocaine are required before clinically significant methemoglobinemia occurs. Methemoglobinemia makes pulse oximetry inaccurate, with a plateau occurring such that the $O_2$ saturation does not fall below 84% to 86%, regardless of true oxygenation and even if methemoglobin constitutes more than 35% of the total hemoglobin. Methemoglobinemia may be treated by intravenous administration of methylene blue (1 mg/kg).

## Diagnosis, Prevention, and Treatment of Toxic Reactions

Most toxic reactions to LA agents can be prevented through safe performance of neural blockade, including careful selection of the dose and concentration of the LA agent. Use of a test dose and incremental injections with intermittent aspiration decrease the risk of systemic toxicity. Ultrasound guidance aids in reducing the risk of LAST by allowing for visualization of extravascular injection. Patients should be closely monitored for signs of intravascular injection (i.e., increased blood pressure and heart rate in the presence of epinephrine) or signs/symptoms of CNS toxicity. Of note, patients who are sedated and paralyzed will not show initial signs of CNS toxicity such as tinnitus, perioral numbness, or even seizure, thus delaying recognition and treatment time of LAST. Although the tonic-clonic motions are inhibited in a patient given a neuromuscular blocking agent, seizure activity will still be present on an electroencephalographic tracing.

Treatment of toxic reactions caused by LA agents is like the management of other medical emergencies, focusing on ensuring adequate airway, breathing, and circulation. Once an airway is established, 100% $O_2$ should be administered. Hypoxia and hypercarbia must be avoided. If convulsions occur, a small amount of a benzodiazepine will rapidly terminate the seizure without causing cardiovascular compromise. If only propofol available, use a low dose (e.g., 20-mg increments). Should intubation be required to secure the airway, succinylcholine may be administered.

Certain modifications to advanced cardiac life support should be considered when treating LAST.

1. Ventricular arrhythmias should be treated with amiodarone instead of lidocaine.
2. Avoid vasopressin, β-blockers, calcium channel blockers, and LAs as all are associated with adverse outcomes in LAST.
3. Reduce epinephrine dose to 1 mcg IV or less.

Additionally, a 20% lipid emulsion should be administered (>70 kg: 100 mL over 2–3 min followed by a continuous infusion 250 mL over 15–20 min; if patient remains unstable repeat bolus and double infusion; <70 kg: 1.5 mL/kg bolus over 1 min followed by a continuous infusion at 0.25 mL/kg/min) because lipid emulsions have been associated with rapid recovery from LA toxicity. There are several theories for the mechanism action for lipid emulsion therapy, but positive results may be multifactorial. The prevailing current theory is that the lipid binds the LA and removes it from effective circulation. Although propofol is formulated in a lipid emulsion, the formulation is only 10% lipid; therefore propofol should not be used as a substitute for lipid emulsion in this circumstance because the lipid content is too low to provide benefit and the cardiovascular suppression associated with the use of propofol may worsen the ability to resuscitate the patient. In some cases, patients have been placed on cardiopulmonary bypass or extracorporeal membrane oxygenation until cardiac toxicity resolves.

Though most patients require only sustained cardiopulmonary resuscitation, repeated cardioversion may be necessary and high doses of epinephrine are often required for circulatory support.

## Special Populations

### PREGNANCY

AAG and albumin are reduced during pregnancy, which increases the free fraction of LA in pregnant patients. Additionally, increased cardiac output and epidural venous engorgement will increase absorption.

### INFANTS

Low AAG levels and immature hepatic clearance increase risk of LAST in infants.

### LIPOSUCTION

When liposuction is performed, large amounts of dilute LA agent are used; therefore the total dose of LA agent administered may be quite high. The American Academy of Dermatology has published guidelines for the performance of liposuction that recommend a maximum safe dose of lidocaine of 55 mg/kg. Because the absorption of lidocaine can be delayed in adipose tissue, toxicity is more likely to occur between 6 and 12 h after the procedure, rather than immediately after the procedure.

## SUGGESTED READINGS

Hoegberg, L. C., Bania, T. C., Lavergne, V., Bailey, B., Turgeon, A. F., Thomas, S. H., et al. (2016). Systematic review of the effect of intravenous lipid emulsion therapy for local anesthetic toxicity. *Clinical Toxicology, 54,* 167.

Macfarlane, A. J. R., Gitman, M., Bornstein, K. J., El-Boghdadly, K., & Weinberg, G. (2021). Updates in our understanding of local anaesthetic systemic toxicity: A narrative review. *Anaesthesia, 76*(Suppl. 1), 27–39.

Neal, J. M., Neal, E. J., & Weinberg, G. L. (2021). American Society of Regional Anesthesia. Checklist for treatment of local anesthetic toxicity: 2020 version. *Regional Anesthesia and Pain Medicine, 46,* 81–82.

Weinberg, G., & Barron, G. (2016). Local Anesthetic Systemic Toxicity (LAST): Not gone, hopefully not forgotten. *Regional Anesthesia and Pain Medicine, 41,* 1.

# 85

# Regional Analgesia Adjuvants, Liposomal Bupivacaine

JASON K. PANCHAMIA, DO

The etymology for adjuvant is from Latin, *adjuvāre,* which means "to help."

The duration of action of our currently available local anesthetics is limited to less than 24 hours after single-injection peripheral nerve blocks. Peripheral nerve block catheter devices can extend the duration of analgesia by delivering a continuous infusion of local anesthesia solution; however, some drawbacks include increased procedure time, concern for intravascular migration, and infection risk. In general, clinical doses of local anesthetics for regional anesthesia are considered safe.

Conversely, it is important to recognize that local anesthetics are inherently neurotoxic because of their numerous effects at the cellular level, and abnormal elevated plasma levels may produce central nervous system (CNS) and cardiovascular systemic (CVS) toxicity.

The ideal local anesthetic would include a fast onset of action, prolonged analgesic duration of action, minimal effects on motor function, and a low risk of adverse events. Although it is unknown whether different combinations of perineural adjuvants with local anesthetics provide an additive or synergistic benefit, the potential for a single-injection solution to achieve all of these advantages has generated great research interest. Alternatively, liposomal bupivacaine (extended-release bupivacaine) has gained popularity for its use in surgical wound infiltration, fascial plane blocks, and interscalene brachial plexus nerve blocks.

Some of the adjuvants listed in this chapter are not approved for use with peripheral nerve blocks by the U.S. Food and Drug Administration; therefore perineural administration is considered off-label and should be used judiciously. Further, the use of perineural adjuvants should be weighed against the risk of prolonged motor blockade, which may affect postoperative rehabilitation. The next section highlights regional anesthesia adjuvants, organized from those commonly used in clinical practice to those used within emerging research protocols. The last section provides a brief overview of liposomal bupivacaine, primarily discussing mechanism of action, compatibility, analgesic efficacy, and patient safety.

## Regional Anesthesia Adjuvants

### EPINEPHRINE

Epinephrine administration around neural structures limits blood flow to the surrounding area because of local or perineural vasoconstriction. When epinephrine is combined with local anesthetics, there is a decrease in the systemic absorption of the local anesthetic solution. As a result, a greater amount of local anesthetic remains focused at the targeted neural tissue producing a greater duration of action.

Coadministration of epinephrine prolongs the duration of sensory and motor blockade for many local anesthetics. Ropivacaine is considered an exception because of its intrinsic vasoconstrictive properties, which limits any further clinical benefit. Also, the addition of epinephrine serves as a protective feedback mechanism for unintended intravascular injections (i.e., "test dose"), thereby allowing the proceduralist to quickly detect and minimize risk of local anesthetic systemic toxicity.

There are some concerns with the use of epinephrine as an additive. Vascular uptake of epinephrine could result in undesirable effects such as tachycardia, hypertension, and electrocardiogram changes, which can be detrimental to patients with a history of cardiovascular disease. Another issue is the potential for neurotoxicity. Because local anesthetics are inherently neurotoxic, coadministration with epinephrine may potentiate this risk by reducing blood flow to the nerves. Although it is rare to observe neurotoxicity in healthy patients, the concern predominantly arises in patients with preexisting, but perhaps subclinical, neural compromise such as diabetes mellitus, history of peripheral neuropathy, and patients on particular chemotherapeutic medications (e.g., platinum chemotherapy drugs).

Perineural epinephrine is associated with lower local anesthetic peak plasma levels and increased time to maximum plasma concentration because of the delayed clearance of local anesthetics into the systemic circulation. Consequently, higher doses of local anesthetics (mainly intermediate-acting local anesthetic) may be safely administered in a mixture with epinephrine. An example would be lidocaine's suggested maximum dose of 4.5 mg/kg without epinephrine compared with 7 mg/kg with epinephrine. Perineural epinephrine is considerably important at sites with higher vascular uptake (e.g., intercostal nerve blocks) where high local anesthetic serum levels can rapidly be obtained, thereby increasing the risk for CNS or CVS toxicity.

### SODIUM BICARBONATE

Local anesthetics exist in nonionized and ionized forms. The nonionized form is responsible for diffusion into the lipid membrane of the nerve to target the intracellular sodium channel receptors. Synthetic local anesthetic solutions are acidic and contain more ionized to nonionized molecules. Alkalization of the local anesthetic solution with sodium bicarbonate will increase the availability of the nonionized form and hasten the onset of action.

The addition of sodium bicarbonate to mepivacaine has shown to decrease the onset of nerve blockade (albeit of minor benefit). The results have been inconsistent with lidocaine and show trivial clinical value with long-acting local anesthetics.

One major concern for sodium bicarbonate and local anesthetic combinations is the risk for solution precipitation. Typically, 1 mEq of sodium bicarbonate is added to 10 mL of intermediate-acting local anesthetic (e.g., lidocaine or mepivacaine). Sodium bicarbonate–induced precipitation can occur at lower doses when combined with long-acting local anesthetics, especially ropivacaine. Extreme caution is advised when mixing, or consider avoiding sodium bicarbonate altogether.

The greatest value for the addition of sodium bicarbonate to local anesthetics (specifically intermediate-acting local anesthetics) appears to be in the obstetric population, where obtaining surgical anesthesia during emergent situations is time-sensitive.

### DEXAMETHASONE

The analgesic mechanism of action for dexamethasone remains unclear but is perceived to involve a combination of its systemic antiinflammatory properties and direct inhibitory action on the nociceptive C fibers. Compared with local anesthetics alone, the combination of perineural dexamethasone admixed with local anesthetics improves duration of analgesia and prolongs sensory and motor blockade. Similarly, intravenous administration of dexamethasone also prolongs peripheral nerve blocks, thus raising the question if some of the analgesic effect of perineural dexamethasone is a result of systemic absorption.

Perineural dexamethasone use as an adjuvant with local anesthetics for peripheral nerve blockade has become a controversial topic, particularly compared with intravenous administration. Published clinical trials evaluating postoperative analgesic outcomes between perineural and intravenous dexamethasone have reported conflicting results because of study variability (administered dose, local anesthetic volume, injection site), with recent evidence suggesting a marginal benefit in favor of the perineural route. In addition to prolonging the duration of analgesia, both routes have been shown to provide antiemetic effects.

Irrespective of route of injection, there are a few concerns with dexamethasone. Clinically, dexamethasone appears to be safe, with numerous studies reporting no increased rate of neurologic complications or evidence of neurotoxicity. In contrast, in vitro studies have demonstrated perineural dexamethasone-induced neurotoxicity. Dexamethasone administration can elevate blood glucose levels, which has been postulated to be harmful in some populations (e.g., patients with diabetes mellitus). However, literature would suggest the clinical relevance of dexamethasone improves rather than hinders recovery after orthopedic surgery even in patients with diabetes mellitus. Last, it is unclear if the analgesic effect and associated adverse effects of dexamethasone are dose dependent; the optimal dose of dexamethasone remains unknown. Given the potential neurotoxic risk, off-label use, and questionably relevant analgesic benefit over intravenous route, perineural dexamethasone administration should be considered on a case-by-case basis.

## ALPHA-2 AGONISTS: CLONIDINE AND DEXMEDETOMIDINE

Perineural administration of clonidine or dexmedetomidine prolongs peripheral nerve block duration by preventing C fibers (pain), A-delta fibers (pain), and A-alpha fibers (motor) from restoring their resting membrane potential from the previous hyperpolarized state. As a result, additional action potentials cannot be generated. The combination of clonidine with intermediate- and long-acting local anesthetics for peripheral nerve blockade can extend the duration of postoperative analgesia by about 2 hours and prolong sensory and motor blockade. Clinical trials evaluating dexmedetomidine admixed with a long-acting local anesthetic, particularly for brachial plexus nerve blockade, appear promising. In general, dexmedetomidine improves brachial plexus nerve block sensory and motor onset time, prolongs sensory and motor block duration, and prolongs duration of analgesia. These results may not extrapolate to other regional anesthetic blocks.

Adverse events associated with perineural clonidine and dexmedetomidine are presumed to be caused by systemic absorption and commonly include hypotension, bradycardia, and sedation. Perineural administration of these alpha-2 agonists should be done carefully for surgical operations associated with fluctuating blood pressure, such as shoulder surgery performed in the beach-chair position. Because these unwanted effects are dose dependent, it is advised to limit clonidine doses to 0.5 to 1.0 mcg/kg, up to a maximum dose of 150 mcg. Similarly, perineural dexmedetomidine dosing is 0.5 to 1.0 mcg/kg with a reported optimal dose of 50 to 60 mcg.

## BUPRENORPHINE

Buprenorphine is a partial mu-opioid receptor agonist. Doses reported for perineural buprenorphine range from 150 to 300 mcg. Buprenorphine exhibits local anesthetic-like features by binding to voltage-gated sodium channels, which may explain the prolonged duration of peripheral nerve blockade when administered via the perineural route.

Multiple clinical studies demonstrate a substantial increase in duration of analgesia after perineural buprenorphine and local anesthetic mixtures for a variety of peripheral nerve blocks. Further, buprenorphine appears to provide superior analgesia via the perineural route compared with the intramuscular route, signifying that its analgesic properties are at the level of the neuron rather than systemic uptake. There is a risk for postoperative nausea and vomiting reported in the dose ranges above.

## OTHER

Other local anesthetic adjuvants currently being examined via perineural route include tramadol, ketamine, and midazolam.

Given the paucity of available data evaluating analgesia and safety, their use as perineural adjuvants is not recommended at this time.

## Liposomal Bupivacaine

Liposomal bupivacaine, an extended-release bupivacaine formulation (currently marketed as Exparel; Pacira Pharmaceuticals, Inc., Parsippany, NJ), is indicated for single-dose surgical wound infiltration in patients 6 years and older and was recently approved for single-injection interscalene brachial plexus nerve block in adults. At this time, liposomal bupivacaine is not recommended for other peripheral nerve blocks, neuraxial procedures, and certain vulnerable populations (e.g., pregnancy and patients younger than 6 years old).

Liposomal bupivacaine consists of bupivacaine housed in multiple, nonconcentric aqueous chambers contained within lipid-based particles. These multivesicular liposomes will dissolve slowly and release bupivacaine over time, thus providing a longer analgesic effect (up to 72 hours) than standard bupivacaine hydrochloride (HCl). Liposomal bupivacaine is supplied in a 10- or 20-mL vial containing either 133 or 266 mg (1.3%; 13.3 mg/mL), respectively. In view of the slow-releasing technology, bupivacaine HCl and liposomal bupivacaine are not bioequivalent, and dose conversion is not possible. Safeguards should be applied to prevent a medication error with propofol given the similar appearance in solution, and maximum dose administration should conform to manufacturer recommendations: 266 mg for surgical site infiltration in adults, 4 mg/kg (up to maximum of 266 mg) in patients aged 6 to 17 years, and 133 mg for interscalene brachial plexus nerve block in adults.

Disruption to the structural integrity of liposomal bupivacaine may result in abnormal increased levels of free bupivacaine, thereby affecting safety, clinical efficacy, and properties of its slow-release delivery system. Fortunately, liposomal bupivacaine has shown to be compatible with various solutions and materials that may be involved at the surgical site, such as commonly used implantable products (e.g., silicone, titanium) and medications (e.g., epinephrine, antibiotics). Liposomal bupivacaine should not be in direct contact with surgical prep solutions (e.g., povidone iodine); consequently, disinfecting solutions must be dried completely if applied as skin prep, or the surgical site should be rinsed clear if it is used as an irrigation solution. In addition, liposomal bupivacaine should only be diluted with normal saline 0.9% or lactated Ringer injection up to a maximum volume of 300 mL. There are a few special considerations when coadministering liposomal bupivacaine with other local anesthetics. Nonbupivacaine-based local anesthetics display a stronger affinity toward the liposome matrix, causing bupivacaine displacement and subsequent elevated serum levels. Lidocaine is the only recommended nonbupivacaine local anesthetic that can safely be administered into the same area as liposomal bupivacaine; however, 20 minutes or more must elapse between injections. Bupivacaine HCl may be coadministered separately with liposomal bupivacaine or admixed in the same syringe provided that the bupivacaine HCl to liposomal bupivacaine dose ratio is 1:2 or less (i.e., bupivacaine HCl dose does not exceed 50% of liposomal bupivacaine dose administered). Additional bupivacaine HCl administration should be withheld for at least 96 hours after surgical wound infiltration and 120 hours after interscalene brachial

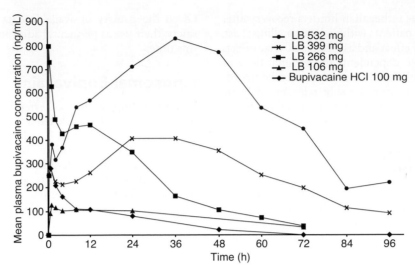

**Fig. 85.1** Plasma bupivacaine concentration versus time for liposome bupivacaine 106, 266, 399, and 532 mg, and bupivacaine HCl 100 mg. *LB*, Liposome bupivacaine. (Obtained with written permission from Hu D, Onel E, Singla N, Kramer WG, Hadzic A. Pharmacokinetic profile of liposome bupivacaine injection following a single administration at the surgical site. *Clin Drug Investig.* 2013;33(2):109–115.)

plexus nerve block because of bupivacaine systemic plasma levels persisting within this time frame.

Liposomal bupivacaine exhibits a bimodal plasma concentration-time profile. The initial peak occurs within 1 hour of administration and is attributed to a small percentage of unencapsulated bupivacaine found within the solution. A second peak occurs between 12 and 36 hours, which is characteristic for its slow-release properties (Fig. 85.1). Clinically, the immediate analgesic effect is variable and dependent on the total drug amount administered, location of administration, and vascularity of surgical site. Bridging this analgesic "gap" with a mixture of bupivacaine HCl and liposome bupivacaine has been advocated to obtain both a quicker onset and longer duration of analgesia.

Presently, there is a limited number of investigations evaluating the utility of liposomal bupivacaine in regional anesthesia. Although liposomal bupivacaine may provide analgesic benefit compared with placebo, current evidence fails to support the routine use of liposomal bupivacaine over standard local anesthetics for surgical wound infiltration and peripheral

nerve blocks in a variety of surgical procedures. Liposomal bupivacaine appears to exhibit a safety profile comparable to standard bupivacaine HCl for both surgical wound infiltration and peripheral nerve blocks, and there is no evidence to date suggesting harm with its use. Generally, adverse events are mild to moderate in severity and commonly entail nausea, constipation, and vomiting. Furthermore, the incidence of cardiovascular-related adverse events is low, with the most common cause being dysrhythmias (e.g., tachycardia, bradycardia). CNS and CVS toxicity are considered rare events and supported by pharmacokinetic studies demonstrating plasma levels below CNS and CVS toxic threshold values at approved doses. Local anesthetic systemic toxicity after liposomal bupivacaine administration should be managed similar to any local anesthetic–induced CNS or CVS toxicity. This includes the use of 20% lipid emulsion therapy, resuscitative measures (advanced cardiac life support), and adhering to the local anesthetic systemic toxicity checklist established by the American Society of Regional Anesthesia and Pain Medicine.

## SUGGESTED READINGS

Hussain, N., Brull, R., Sheehy, B., Essandoh, M. K., Stahl, D. L., Weaver, T. E., et al. (2021). Perineural liposomal bupivacaine is not superior to nonliposomal bupivacaine for peripheral nerve block analgesia: A systematic review and meta-analysis. *Anesthesiology, 134,* 147–164.

Ilfeld, B. M., Eisenach, J. C., & Gabriel, R. A. (2020). Clinical effectiveness of liposomal bupivacaine administered by infiltration or peripheral nerve block to treat postoperative pain. *Anesthesiology, 134,* 283–344.

Ilfeld, B. M., Viscusi, E. R., Hadzic, A., Minkowitz, H. S., Morren, M. D., Lookabaugh, J., et al. (2015). Safety and side effect profile of liposome bupivacaine (Exparel) in peripheral nerve blocks. *Regional Anesthesia and Pain Medicine, 40,* 572–582.

Vorobeichik, L., Brull, R., & Abdallah, F. W. (2017). Evidence basis for using perineural dexmedetomidine to enhance the quality of brachial plexus nerve blocks: A systematic review and meta-analysis of randomized controlled trials. *British Journal of Anaesthesia, 118,* 167–181.

# 86

# Multimodal Analgesia

ROY A. GREENGRASS, MD, FRCP

## Multimodal Analgesia

Multimodal analgesia is an analgesic regimen using multiple analgesic agents, which work at multiple sites along nociceptive pathways. Multimodal analgesia accords enhanced analgesia with fewer side effects than any unimodal analgesic therapy. Most contemporary enhanced recovery after surgery (ERAS) protocols use multimodal analgesic methodologies.

When multimodal agents were first introduced into clinical practice their efficacy was often measured by subsequent reduction in opioid consumption. Perhaps more useful is the concept of number needed to treat (NNT), where a specific dose of an analgesic is evaluated to determine how many patients are needed to accord a 50% reduction in maximal pain for 4 to 6 hours. Agents currently used for multimodal analgesia include nonselective and cyclooxygenase selective (COX-2 selective) nonsteroidal antiinflammatory drugs (NSAIDs), steroids, local anesthetics, α2-receptor agonists, ketamine, α2δ ligands, and opioids (Fig. 86.1).

## NSAIDs

Cyclooxygenase receptors produce prostaglandins that promote inflammation. Additionally, COX-1 receptors produce prostaglandins that protect the gastric mucosa and activate platelets. COX-1 receptors are everywhere in the body (constitutional), whereas COX-2 receptors are increased by stress (inducible). NSAIDs decrease inflammation by blocking COX receptors.

NSAIDs have been determined to decrease opioid requirements by 30%. NSAID effects on NNT vary by dose and specific agent but are very effective (ibuprofen 400 mg and celecoxib 400 mg have an NNT of 2.7). Etoricoxib (a COX-2 used in Europe) has an NNT of 1.7. NSAIDs have a ceiling effect for analgesia but not for side effects. Nonselective NSAIDs may result in gastric erosions, particularly in the elderly. All NSAIDs decrease renal blood flow and are contraindicated in patients with significant renal dysfunction. There is little evidence in the literature that nonspecific NSAIDs cause significant surgical bleeding; however, many surgeons remain reluctant to use them perioperatively. COX-2 NSAIDs have little effect on platelets and result in a 50% decrease in gastric erosions. Both nonspecific and COX-2 NSAIDS are currently available both orally and parenterally.

## Acetaminophen

Acetaminophen has minimal antiinflammatory or peripheral activity. Its antipyretic and analgesic properties are thought to emanate from two possible mechanisms: stimulation of central inhibitory pathways or inhibition of central COX-3 (COX-3 being a variant of COX-2) pathways. Published trials evaluating acetaminophen have demonstrated opioid-sparing effects in the range of 20%, less than that of NSAIDs. Similarly, NNTs for acetaminophen are higher than NSAIDs, which are in the range of 3.7. Interestingly, higher doses of acetaminophen do not accord better analgesia, suggesting a ceiling effect for efficacy. The NNTs for 500, 650, and 1000 mg of acetaminophen are similar. Long used in Europe, intravenous acetaminophen is currently being used in the United States. NNTs for intravenous acetaminophen are the same as oral administration; thus intravenous use should be restricted to analgesic rescue situations including patients without a functioning gastrointestinal tract.

## Steroids

Steroids have potent antiinflammatory and immunosuppressive effects, which decrease the inflammatory response at the site of surgery, thereby decreasing nociceptive input into the spinal cord. A direct effect of steroids decreasing signal transmission in nociceptive C fibers has also been demonstrated. A single dose of glucocorticoids has been demonstrated to inhibit the synthesis and release of proinflammatory and antiinflammatory mediators in major abdominal and cardiovascular operations. Among the steroids, glucocorticoids are preferred for perioperative antiinflammatory use because of enhanced efficiency and avoidance of mineralocorticoid effects of fluid retention and edema. Suppression of the hypothalamic pituitary adrenal axis after single-dose steroid therapy is not an issue. Additionally, there is no evidence in the literature that single-dose steroid administration will increase the risk of wound infection. It appears that the hyperglycemic response to surgical stress is no greater in patients who receive steroids, even those with type 2 diabetes. Recent implementation of stringent perioperative glucose control protocols should limit hyperglycemia whether steroids are used or not. Analgesic doses of steroids are higher than those used for nausea and vomiting prophylaxis (0.1–0.15 mg/kg of dexamethasone or equivalent).

## Local Anesthetics and Regional Anesthesia

Regional anesthesia is without parallel in providing superior perioperative analgesia. Central and peripheral nerve blocks decrease or prevent nociceptive signals from reaching central processing centers, with implications for both acute and chronic pain reduction. Systemic local anesthetic administration decreases inflammation and directly depresses both peripheral and central neuronal excitability. Studies on some abdominal procedures have demonstrated similar analgesic effects of intravenous local anesthetics to that associated with epidural administration.

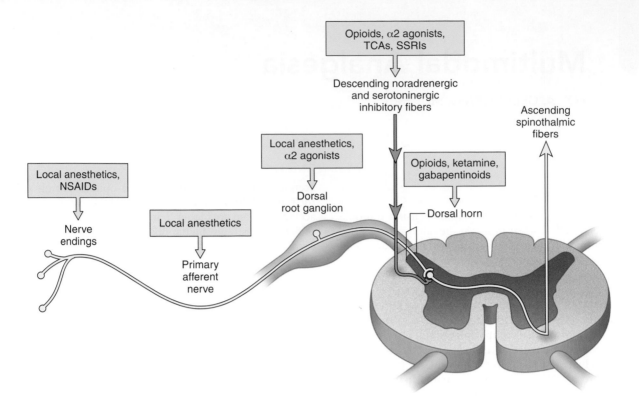

**Fig. 86.1** Sites of action of multimodal agents. *NSAID,* Nonsteroidal antiinflammatory drug; *SSRI,* selective serotonin reuptake inhibitor; *TCA,* tricyclic antidepressant.

## α2-Receptor Agonists

α2-Receptor agonists have effects at peripheral, spinal, and brainstem loci. Prototypes, such as clonidine, appear to work by hyperpolarizing neurocircuits, both peripherally and centrally, rather than by an α2-receptor block. Clonidine has also been demonstrated to enhance analgesia in peripheral nerve blocks, particularly with intermediate-duration local anesthetic agents. The ability of clonidine to enhance the quality of analgesia with long-acting local anesthetic agents is controversial.

Dexmedetomidine, a much more selective α2 agonist, is currently used for many applications including awake intubation, intensive care sedation, and as an adjunct for many surgical procedures. Recent investigations of low-dose dexmedetomidine, 30 to 50 μg, added to local anesthetic for nerve blocks have demonstrated earlier onset of block and prolonged block duration with minimal side effects.

## α2δ Ligands

α2δ Ligands, such as gabapentin and pregabalin, bind to the α2δ subunit of voltage-gated calcium channels, preventing release of nociceptive neurotransmitters. Sites of action include peripheral sites, primary afferent neurons, spinal neurons, and supraspinal sites. Studies of gabapentin reveal poor efficacy at low dose (NNT for 300-mg gabapentin is 9.2). Unfortunately, more efficacious analgesic doses are associated with significant incidences of sedation, dizziness, and nausea.

## Ketamine

Ketamine is a phencyclidine derivative that was previously used to produce general anesthesia, particularly in high-risk groups such as trauma patients with hypotension. Unfortunately, dose-dependent side effects of dysphoria and hallucinosis generally preclude the use of ketamine as a primary anesthetic agent. However, under certain circumstances it can be a useful adjuvant. Although NNT studies are not available for ketamine, studies using analgesic doses in opioid-naive patients have demonstrated a minor benefit only. On the contrary, patients on large doses of opioids preoperatively experience significant benefits of low-dose ketamine, which is felt to be a direct result of N-methyl-D-aspartate receptor blockade. Doses of ketamine commonly used in surgery for patients on chronic opioids include a bolus dose of 0.5 mg/kg after induction followed by an infusion of 5 to 20 mg/h in adults. In many centers the infusion is continued in postoperative recovery and on surgical wards.

## Opioids

The tragedy of the opioid epidemic has resulted in increased scrutiny of opioid use in contemporary practice. It appears that perioperative prescriptions of oral opioids, not intraoperative opioids, are mainly implicated in the risk of opioid abuse. The use of NSAID and acetaminophen combinations have been found to be more successful in pain control and associated with fewer side effects than oral opioids in many surgeries, including simple breast and gynecologic surgeries, which has resulted in many surgical centers of excellence abandoning the use of oral opioid prescriptions. For major and painful surgeries where regional anesthesia cannot be applied, opioids remain an important component of intraoperative care. Unfortunately, compassionate attempts to limit opioid abuse by providing opioid-free anesthesia have in many circumstances resulted in enhanced patient morbidities.

A novel G protein–biased opioid ligand, oliceridine, has recently been released with promise of less nausea, vomiting, and respiratory depression compared with contemporary opioids. Its lack of active metabolites additionally makes it an attractive alternative in patients with renal failure and other comorbidities.

## Conclusion

Multimodal analgesia is an ideal evidence-based method of analgesia administration that accords excellent analgesia, allowing significant reduction or avoidance of unimodal analgesic modalities such as opioids.

## Appendix

A reasonable perioperative multimodal regimen for adults is:
- Celecoxib 400 mg by mouth followed by scheduled dosing of 200 mg by mouth two times a day.
- Acetaminophen 1g by mouth followed by scheduled dosing of 1g by mouth four times a day
- Dexamethasone 10 mg intravenous. A second dose of intravenous dexamethasone may be administered the next day.
- Intravenous lidocaine 1.5 to 2.0 mg/kg bolus followed by 1.2 to 2.0 mg/kg per h.

Doses of all medications are reduced in the elderly and pediatric patients. For all procedures local anesthetic administered by the surgeon, given intravenously, or utilized via single injection or continuous, regional anesthesia should be utilized.

## SUGGESTED READINGS

De Oliveira, G. S., Jr., Almeida, M. D., Benzon, H. T., & McCarthy, R. J. (2011). Perioperative single dose systemic dexamethasone for postoperative pain: A meta-analysis of randomized controlled trials. *Anesthesiology, 115*(3), 575–588.

Hussain, N., Grzywacz, V. P., Ferreri, C. A., Atrey, A., Banfield, L., Shaparin, N., et al. (2017). Investigating the efficacy of dexmedetomidine as an adjuvant to local anesthesia in brachial plexus block: A systematic review and meta-analysis of 18 randomized controlled trials. *Regional Anesthesia and Pain Medicine, 42*(2), 184–196.

Loftus, R. W., Yeager, M. P., Clark, J. A., Brown, J. R., Abdu, W. A., Sengupta, D. K., et al. (2010). Intraoperative ketamine reduces perioperative opiate consumption in opiate-dependent patients with chronic back pain undergoing back surgery. *Anesthesiology*, 2010;*113*(3):639–646.

Moore, Andrew, R, Derry, Sheena, Aldington, Dominic, & Wiffen, Philip (2020). Single dose oral analgesics for acute postoperative pain in adults- an overview of Cochrane reviews. Cochrane Dtabase of Systemic Reviews.

Murphy, G. S., Szokol, J. W., Avram, M. J., Greenberg, S. B., Shear, T., Vender, J. S., et al. (2014). The effect of single low-dose dexamethasone on blood glucose concentrations in the perioperative period: A randomized, placebo-controlled investigation in gynecologic surgical patients. *Anesthesia and Analgesia, 118*(6), 1204–1212.

Richman, J. M., Liu, S. S., Courpas, G., Wong, R., Rowlingson, A. J., McGready, J., et al. (2006). Does continuous peripheral nerve block provide superior pain control to opioids? A meta-analysis. *Anesthesia and Analgesia, 102*(1), 248–257.

Shanthanna, H., Ladha, K. S., Kehlet, H., & Joshi, G. P. (2021). Perioperative opioid administration: A critical review of opioid-free versus opioid-sparing approaches. *Anesthesiology, 134*(4), 645–659.

# 87

# Needle Blocks of the Eye

ADAM PAUL ROTH, MD

Local anesthesia of the eye was pioneered in 1884 when Carl Koller successfully used topical cocaine for cataract surgery. The first retrobulbar block was performed that same year by Herman Knapp when cocaine was injected into the retrobulbar space for an enucleation. Despite this initial success, retrobulbar blocks fell out of favor until the 1930s when alternative local anesthetics became available. Recent changes in surgical technique have shifted the paradigm back to the application of topical anesthetics for ocular procedures involving the anterior chamber, especially cataract surgery. Nonetheless, regional blocks of the eye remain commonplace for a variety of ophthalmologic operations; therefore the anesthesiologist must be familiar with them and their associated side effects.

## Anatomy

The ciliary ganglion, a parasympathetic ganglion that measures 1 to 2 mm in diameter, is located between the optic nerve and lateral rectus muscle 1.5 to 2 cm posterior to the globe. Preganglionic parasympathetic fibers originating from the Edinger-Westphal nucleus in the rostral midbrain course along the oculomotor nerve (CN III) to synapse in the ciliary ganglion with postganglionic parasympathetic fibers exiting via 8 to 10 short ciliary nerves to innervate the sphincter pupillae and ciliaris muscles. Postganglionic sympathetic fibers originating from the superior cervical ganglion innervate the dilator pupillae muscle. Sensory innervation to the cornea, iris, and ciliary body is supplied by the nasociliary nerve, a branch of the ophthalmic nerve (CN $V_1$). Sympathetic and sensory fibers enter the eye via two pathways: (a) merging with long ciliary nerves (branches of the nasociliary nerve) and (b) traversing the ciliary ganglion to run within the short ciliary nerves (Fig. 87.1).

## Terminology

Although the terms *retrobulbar* and *peribulbar* identify various blocks used in ophthalmologic procedures, these terms are often confusing and quite imprecise. More precise and anatomically correct terms are *intraconal* and *extraconal*, which refer to the orbital space within or outside of the muscular cone delineated by the four rectus muscles with an anterior base and posterior apex.

## Local Anesthetic Agents

Choice of local anesthesia depends on clinician preference and desired duration of effect. Commonly employed agents include

**Fig. 87.1** Orbital anatomy. **A**, Diagram illustrating a lateral view of a dissected orbit revealing the relations of the orbital nerves and extraocular muscles (vessels have been excluded for the purposes of clarity). **B**, Dissection of the orbit similar to the previous diagram except that lateral rectus has not been cut and the course of the orbital nerves within the cavernous sinus is also shown (by removal of the lateral dural wall). • The lateral wall has been removed and the infratemporal fossa has been dissected to expose the pterygomaxillary fissure and pterygopalatine fossa. • The cranial cavity has been opened to reveal the dura (reflected) covering the frontal lobe. • The lateral rectus has been divided and reflected to expose the optic nerve and other cranial nerves entering the orbit through the tendinous ring. Note the abducent nerve entering its bulbar surface. • The ciliary ganglion lies between the lateral rectus and the optic nerve. Note the motor root and sensory root as seen in the superior view. The nerve to inferior oblique (NIO) is a useful landmark for finding the ciliary ganglion. The short ciliary nerves emerge from the ganglion and enter the globe around the optic nerve. • Note the three nerves that enter the orbit outside the tendinous ring: lacrimal, frontal and trochlear. • The nerve to superior rectus (branch of superior division of III nerve) pierces the muscle and enters the levator palpebrae superioris, which it supplies, from below. • Branches of the pterygopalatine ganglion (PTG) enter the orbit through the inferior orbital fissure and contribute to the formation of the retrobulbar plexus (not shown). • Inferior oblique passes backwards, laterally and superiorly beneath the inferior rectus. • Orbitalis (Müller's muscle), a band of smooth muscle, covers the inferior orbital fissure. ICA, Internal carotid artery; IO, inferior oblique; ION, infraorbital nerve; LR, lateral rectus; MA, maxillary artery; MS, maxillary sinus; PCA, posterior communicating artery; PC, posterior cerebral artery; PSA, posterior superior alveolar nerves; SR, superior rectus; TG, trigeminal ganglion; V 1, V 2, V 3, divisions of the trigeminal nerve; IV, trochlear nerve. Arrow, nerve to superior oblique branch of oculomotor nerve (III). (From Forrester J, Dick A, McMenamin P, Roberts F, Pearlman E. *The Eye: Basic Sciences in Practice*. 5th ed. Elsevier; 2021.)

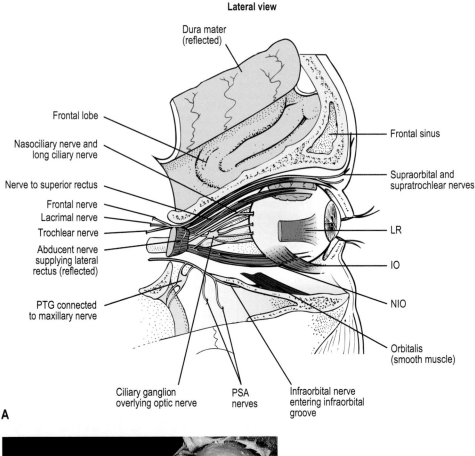

**Lateral view**

Dura mater (reflected)

Frontal lobe

Nasociliary nerve and long ciliary nerve

Nerve to superior rectus

Frontal nerve

Lacrimal nerve

Trochlear nerve

Abducent nerve supplying lateral rectus (reflected)

PTG connected to maxillary nerve

Frontal sinus

Supraorbital and supratrochlear nerves

LR

IO

NIO

Orbitalis (smooth muscle)

Ciliary ganglion overlying optic nerve

PSA nerves

Infraorbital nerve entering infraorbital groove

**A**

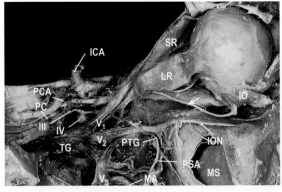

**B**

2% lidocaine or a 1:1 mixture of 2% lidocaine with 0.375% to 0.75% bupivacaine. The addition of hyaluronidase, first described by Atkinson in 1949, helps facilitate the spread of local anesthetic within the orbital space and is now used by many clinicians in varying concentrations for retrobulbar, peribulbar, and sub-Tenon blocks. Epinephrine can be used to improve block duration and minimize bleeding but is controversial in that it can cause problems related to vasoconstriction of the retinal vasculature.

## Types of Eye Blocks

### RETROBULBAR BLOCK

Historically considered the gold standard for eye blocks, retrobulbar anesthesia consists of an intraconal block that involves the ciliary ganglion; short and long ciliary nerves; and CN II, III, and VI. Because of its extraconal location, CN IV is sometimes, but not always, blocked via diffusion of local anesthetic within the orbit. In 1936, the classic Atkinson technique for retrobulbar block was first described in the *Archives of Ophthalmology* and, though effective, its "up-and-in" gaze position places the optic nerve along the intended needle path and increases the risk of optic nerve injury; hence, this technique has largely been supplanted by a "forward-looking" position (described in Box 87.1, Fig. 87.2*A–C*). Quite commonly, the ipsilateral facial nerve is also blocked to prevent blinking via the Van Lindt or modified Van Lindt technique. A 38-mm (1.5-inch) 23-gauge needle with rounded point (Atkinson) is preferred to

---

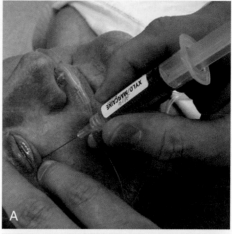

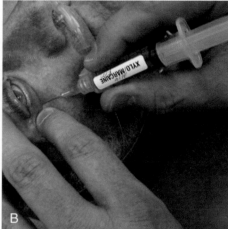

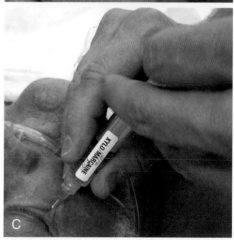

**Fig. 87.2** Retrobulbar block placement. Administering a retrobulbar block. See Box 87.1 for further explanation of technique shown. **A,** Needle placement. **B,** Needle advancement. **C,** Entering the muscle cone and injecting.

---

> **BOX 87.1   TECHNIQUE COMMONLY EMPLOYED TO PERFORM A RETROBULBAR BLOCK**
>
> **Anesthetic Preparation.** Connect a 5–10 mL syringe containing the desired anesthetic solution to a 38-mm (1.5-inch) 23-gauge needle with rounded point (Atkinson).
>
> **Patient Position.** An assistant should hold the patient's head securely and assist with retraction of the upper lid, allowing the globe to be visualized throughout block placement.
>
> **Needle Placement.** With the patient looking forward, the lower eyelid should be cleansed with an alcohol swab. The needle tip, bevel down, is advanced parallel to the orbital floor, entering at the junction between the medial two-thirds and lateral one-third of the inferior orbital margin.
>
> **Needle Advancement.** Resistance to advancement will be noted when the orbital septum is reached. Once the needle has passed the equator of the globe (halfway point of the needle is at the level of the iris), the needle is angled superior and slightly medial toward the muscular cone.
>
> **Entering the Muscle Cone and Injecting.** Resistance and relief can be detected as the needle enters the muscle cone. After gentle aspiration to rule out intravascular placement, 3–4 mL of local anesthetic can be injected with an additional 1–2 mL injected during needle withdrawal.
>
> **Assessment.** Ask the patient to close the eye. Gentle pressure should be applied for 2–4 min to help facilitate diffusion of the injectate.
>
> If worsening proptosis, hemorrhagic chemostasis, or increasing posterior pressure is noted during surgery, retrobulbar hemorrhage must be ruled out.
>
> ---
>
> Recently, ophthalmologists have cautioned against the conventional upward and inward positioning of the eye because this places the routine needle path close to the optic nerve and the ophthalmic artery and vein.
> Brown, DL. *The Atlas of Regional Anesthesia.* 3rd ed. Elsevier Health Sciences; 2005.

increase sensory feedback and reduce the potential for injury to ocular structures, as opposed to a sharp-pointed needle. Total injectate is normally 3 to 5 mL.

### PERIBULBAR BLOCK

An extraconal block involving injections above and below the orbit results in local anesthetic diffusing throughout the orbit, including the intraconal space. Because of the larger volumes required (6–12 mL), anterior spread results in blockade of the orbicularis oculi muscle, negating the need for a facial nerve block. Furthermore, the risk of intraocular or intradural injection, intraconal (retrobulbar) hemorrhage, and direct optic nerve injury is decreased because the anesthetic is deposited outside the muscle cone. Although some sources claim this block frequently needs supplementation and/or yields inadequate akinesia of the medial rectus muscle, a 2008 Cochrane Database Review found no significant differences in success rate or complications between peribulbar and retrobulbar blocks.

## PARABULBAR (SUB-TENON) BLOCK

The sub-Tenon block involves the insertion of a flexible, blunt-tipped cannula or curved, blunt-tipped needle into the sub-Tenon space, which extends from the corneal limbus anteriorly to the optic nerve posteriorly, and subsequent infusion of variable volumes of local anesthetic. Avoiding the hazards of a sharp needle, this technique obviates the risk of globe penetration, retrobulbar hemorrhage, and trauma to the optic nerve. However, this block does require a small incision through the conjunctiva and sub-Tenon capsule to gain access to the sub-Tenon space.

# Contraindications

Eye blocks are not used in procedures that are anticipated to last longer than 90 min or in patients younger than 15 years. Any factor that precludes the patient from following commands or lying still during the procedure, or that increases the patient's bleeding risk, is also a contraindication to the use of an eye block (Box 87.2).

# Complications

## RETROBULBAR HEMORRHAGE

The most common complication, retrobulbar hemorrhage, occurs secondary to puncture of vessels within the retrobulbar space. It is characterized by a tense, hard orbit within seconds to minutes of block placement and associated proptosis, ptosis, and a marked increase in intraocular pressure. Because of the potential for globe ischemia and blindness, the surgeon should be notified immediately so that the orbit can be surgically decompressed, if warranted, and the intraocular pressure can be reduced.

---

**BOX 87.2  CONTRAINDICATIONS TO THE USE OF AN EYE BLOCK**

Procedure is anticipated to last >90–120 min
Patient has:
    Uncontrolled cough, tremor, or convulsive disorder
    Excessive anxiety or claustrophobia
    Bleeding or coagulation disorder
    Perforated globe
    Language barrier
Patient is:
    Deaf
    Disoriented
    Cognitively impaired
    Unable to lie flat
    Younger than 15 years

---

## OCULOCARDIAC REFLEX

The oculocardiac reflex is manifested by bradycardia, arrhythmias, and even periods of cardiac asystole when pressure or traction is applied to orbital contents because of profound parasympathetic outflow. It may occur acutely with block placement or expanding retrobulbar hemorrhage. The latter may occur several hours after a retrobulbar hemorrhage, as additional blood extravasates. Treatment includes the immediate cessation of noxious stimuli and/or intravenous atropine (0.01 mg/kg).

## DIPLOPIA

The incidence of diplopia after retrobulbar block for cataract surgery is reported to be between 0.1% and 4%, depending on the experience of the clinician performing the block. The cause of diplopia is multifactorial, but injection of local anesthetic into the small intraocular muscles with subsequent hemorrhage and scarring is felt to disturb the normal balance among these muscles. These patients may subsequently present for repair of their iatrogenic strabismus.

## CENTRAL RETINAL ARTERY OCCLUSION

Retrobulbar hemorrhage can result in central retinal artery occlusion that, if not treated promptly, may result in total loss of vision. This potential complication can also occur if the dura around the optic nerve is violated and local anesthetic is injected into the subarachnoid space.

## PUNCTURE OF THE GLOBE

Perforation of the globe can occur during any needle block of the eye but is most seen with retrobulbar injection, particularly in patients with severe myopia because of their elongated globe. Signs and symptoms include immediate ocular pain, restlessness, and possible intraocular hemorrhage and retinal detachment.

## PENETRATION OF THE OPTIC NERVE

Optic atrophy and permanent loss of vision may occur even in the absence of retrobulbar hemorrhage. The postulated mechanisms include direct injury to the optic nerve, injection into the nerve sheath with compressive ischemia, and intramural sheath hemorrhage.

## INADVERTENT BRAINSTEM ANESTHESIA

Accidental injection into the cerebrospinal fluid can occur during performance of ocular blocks secondary to puncture of the meningeal sheaths surrounding the optic nerve. This rare complication is more common with sharp-needle techniques, especially retrobulbar blocks, but can occur with any ocular block. Signs are variable, but the patient is likely to experience disorientation or unconsciousness within seconds to minutes of block placement. Convulsions and respiratory or cardiac arrest may ensue, necessitating careful patient monitoring. In one large series, the incidence of central nervous system spread was shown to be 0.13%.

## SUGGESTED READINGS

Alhassan, M. B., Kyari, F., & Ejere, H. Q. (2008). Peribulbar versus retrobulbar anaesthesia for cataract surgery. *Cochrane Database of Systematic Reviews, 3,* CD004083.

Eichel, R., & Goldberg, I. (2005). Anaesthesia techniques for cataract surgery: A survey of delegates to the congress of the international council of ophthalmology, 2002. *Clinical & Experimental Ophthalmology, 33,* 469–472.

Kandavel, R. (2009). Local anesthesia for cataract surgery. In D. M. Colvard (Ed.), *Achieving excellence in cataract surgery a step-by-step approach* (pp. 1–9). Los Angeles.

Kumar, C. M. (2011). Needle-based blocks for the 21st century ophthalmology. *Acta Ophthalmologica, 89,* 5–9.

Palte, H. D. (2015). Ophthalmic regional blocks: Management, challenges, and solutions. *Local and Regional Anesthesia, 8,* 57–70.

Scholle, T. M. (2020 Fall). Anesthesia for ocular surgery. *International Ophthalmology Clinics, 60,* 41–60.

# 88

# Spinal Cord Anatomy and Blood Supply

KAIYING ZHANG, MD   |   ADRIAN W. GELB, MBChB, FRCPC

## Anatomy

The vertebral column encompasses the spinal cord and comprises 33 vertebrae—24 of which articulate (7 cervical, 12 thoracic, 5 lumbar) and 9 of which are fused (5 sacral and 4 coccygeal)—and four curvatures. Anteriorly, the cervical and lumbar curves are convex, whereas in the thoracic and sacral areas the vertebral column is concave (Fig. 88.1). The vertebral body, the pedicles, the lamina, and the spinous processes form the bony structure surrounding and protecting the spinal cord. The stability and elasticity of the vertebral column is achieved via several ligaments, intervertebral discs, and the articular surfaces on the pedicles (Fig. 88.2). During spinal anesthesia with a midline approach, the needle will pass through skin, subcutaneous tissue, the supraspinous ligament, the interspinous ligament, the ligamentum flavum, the epidural space, the dura mater, the arachnoid mater, and the subarachnoid space.

## Vertebrae

The pedicles form the intervertebral foramina that contain a superior and inferior vertebral notch through which the spinal nerves exit the spinal cord (see Fig. 88.2). The C1 vertebra is also called the *atlas*. It does not have a body or a spinous process. The atlas and the *axis*, or C2 vertebra, form the atlanto-axial joint. This joint can become unstable, for example, in patients with rheumatoid arthritis. Vertebral arteries run upward through the transverse foramina of the C2 through C6 vertebrae. The C7 and T1 spinous processes are prominent and

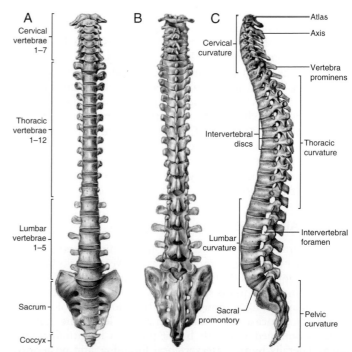

**Fig. 88.1**  Anterior, lateral, and posterior views of the spinal cord showing the curvatures and the angulation of the spinous processes. (Reproduced with permission from Mahadevan V. Anatomy of the vertebral column. *Surgery (Oxford).* 2018;36(7):327–332.)

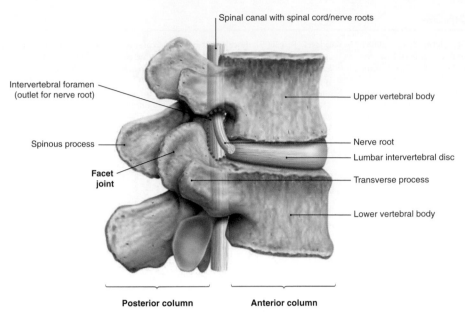

Spinal canal with spinal cord/nerve roots

Intervertebral foramen
(outlet for nerve root)

Spinous process

**Facet
joint**

Upper vertebral body

Nerve root

Lumbar intervertebral disc

Transverse process

Lower vertebral body

**Posterior column**   **Anterior column**

**Fig. 88.2** Expanded view of the lumbar vertebra demonstrating how the pedicles form the intervertebral foramina that the nerves pass through. The relatively straight spinous processes favor access to the epidural and subarachnoid spaces. (Reproduced with permission from Hombach-Klonisch S. Back and spine. In: Hombach-Klonisch S, Klonisch T, Peeler J., eds. *Sobotta Clinical Atlas of Human Anatomy.* Elsevier; 2019:39–82.)

easily palpable on the back of the neck. The spinous processes in the lumbar region are approximately horizontal in contrast to those in the thoracic region, which are angled downward and therefore grant easier access for neuraxial anesthesia (see Fig. 88.1). In the pediatric population, the S5 vertebra is not fused and has a sacral hiatus that is used for caudal epidural anesthesia.

## LIGAMENTS

The supraspinous ligament is a band of longitudinal fibers interconnecting the tips of the spinous processes from the sacrum to C7. It is continuous with the interspinal ligament at all levels and with the ligamentum nuchae cephalad. The interspinous ligament is a thin, membranous band that connects adjacent spinous processes and extends from the supraspinal ligament posteriorly to the ligamentum flavum anteriorly. The ligamentum flavum, the strongest of the ligaments, runs from the base of the skull in front of and between the laminae to the sacrum. The anterior and posterior longitudinal ligaments are the primary ligaments that provide vertebral column stability by binding the vertebral bodies.

## EPIDURAL SPACE

The epidural space surrounds the spinal meninges and contains fat, alveolar tissue, nerve roots, and extensive networks of arteries and venous plexuses (Fig. 88.3). This space extends from the foramen magnum to the sacral hiatus and is widest in its posterior dimension. L2 is thought to be the widest part of the epidural space, measuring 5 to 6 mm at this level. The epidural space is bounded anteriorly by the posterior longitudinal ligament, laterally by the intervertebral foramina, and posteriorly by the ligamentum flavum.

## MENINGES

The spinal meninges are three individual membranes that surround the spinal cord (see Fig. 88.3): (1) The dura is the tough, fibroelastic, outermost membrane extending from the foramen magnum superiorly to the lower border of S2 inferiorly, where it is pierced by the filum terminales (i.e., the distal end of the pia mater). (2) The arachnoid is the middle membrane that is closely attached to the dura. This layer is very thin and avascular. (3) The pia is a highly vascular membrane that lies close to the spinal cord. The space between the arachnoid and pia is the subarachnoid space. This space contains the spinal nerves and cerebrospinal fluid, as well as numerous delicate trabeculae that intertwine within this space. Lateral extensions of the pia mater, the denticulate ligaments, help support the spinal cord by binding to the dura.

The spinal cord begins at the level of the foramen magnum and ends as the conus medullaris. At birth, the cord extends to L3, but it moves to its adult position at the lower border of L1 by age 1 year; however, it may be found as low as L2 in some individuals.

## SPINAL CORD

The spinal cord is a cylindrical structure composed of white and gray matter with a central canal filled with cerebrospinal fluid (CSF) (Fig. 88.4). The gray matter contains cell bodies of neurons and is divided into different segments. The dorsal horn contains sensory nuclei and the ventral horn contains motor neurons; the intermediate column and the lateral horn have autonomic neurons innervating visceral organs. Thirty-one pairs of spinal nerves exit the spinal cord, each composed of an anterior motor root and a posterior sensory root.

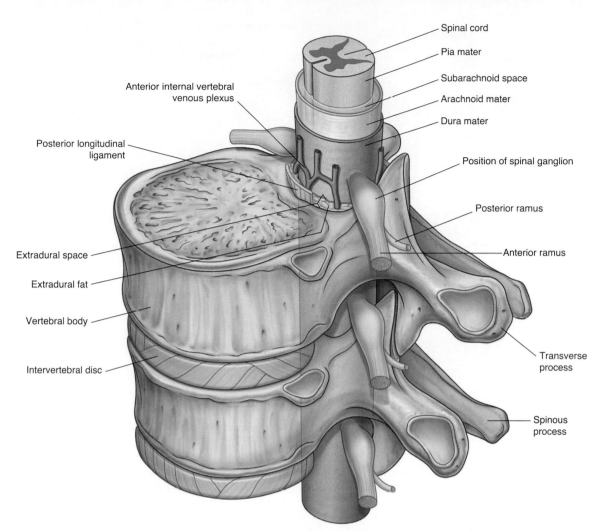

**Fig. 88.3**  The spinal cord is enveloped in bone, ligament, dura, arachnoid, cerebrospinal fluid, and the thin, tightly adherent pia. Veins in the epidural space may be injured during epidural or spinal puncture. (Reproduced with permission from Drake RA, Vogl W, Mitchell A. The body. In: *Gray's Anatomy for Students*. 3rd ed. Churchill Livingston; 2015:59.)

## Blood Supply

The spinal cord is supplied by one anterior spinal artery and two posterior spinal arteries (see Fig. 88.4). Throughout their length, these three spinal arteries receive contributions from radicular branches of intercostal arteries. The anterior spinal artery, which lies in the anterior median sulcus of the spinal cord, is formed at the level of the foramen magnum by the union of two radicular rami of the vertebral arteries. Although the anterior spinal artery is often considered to be a continuous structure, this is not the case; 8 to 12 medullary arteries join the anterior spinal artery through its course to the conus medullaris, and each forms an arborization pattern (Fig. 88.5). Contributing to the anterior spinal artery system is a group of 8 to 12 radicular arteries. In the cervical region, these arteries derive from the cervical branches of the vertebral and ascending cervical arteries. In the superior thoracic cord, contributions arise from the ascending and deep cervical arteries. The medullary arteries augmenting blood flow to the middle and lower thoracic cord are less prominent. The most caudal medullary artery is usually the largest, the arteria medullaris magna anterior (artery of Adamkiewicz). This artery has a variable origin along the spinal cord, arising between T5 and T8 in 15% of patients, between T9 and T12 in 60%, and between L1 and L5 in 25%. Spinal cord perfusion via anterior spinal artery could be compromised during thoracoabdominal aortic surgery, CSF drainage is often used to decrease CSF pressure to improve spinal cord perfusion pressure.

The posterior spinal arteries arise from the vertebral or posterior inferior cerebellar arteries and descend as two branches, one anterior and the other posterior to the dorsal nerve root. These arteries are segmentally reinforced with radicular collaterals from the vertebral, cervical, and posterior intercostal arteries, and they provide better vascular continuity than does the anterior spinal arterial system.

The peripheral border of the spinal cord receives its blood supply from ventral and dorsal penetrating vessels. Collateral circulation of the peripheral cord is adequate. However, within the spinal cord itself, there are no anastomoses, and the penetrating vessels are essentially end arterioles.

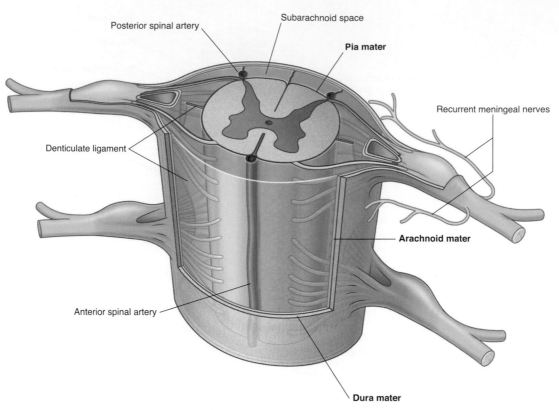

**Fig. 88.4**   Spinal cord blood supply showing the single anterior and two posterior spinal arteries in relation to the spinal cord and nerve roots. (Reproduced with permission from Drake RA, Vogl W, Mitchell A. The back. In: *Gray's Anatomy for Students*. 3rd ed. Churchill Livingston; 2015:103.)

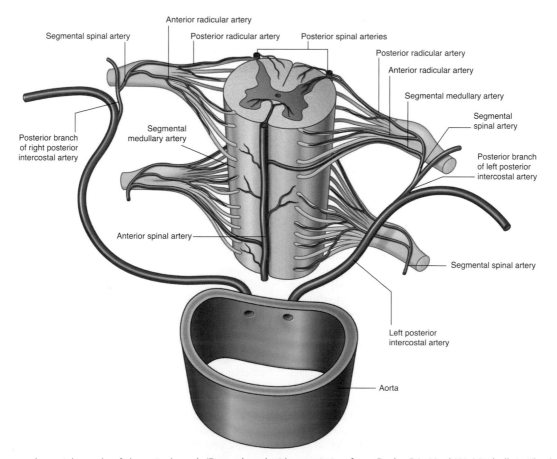

**Fig. 88.5**   Segmental arterial supply of the spinal cord. (Reproduced with permission from Drake RA, Vogl W, Mitchell A. The back. In: *Gray's Anatomy for Students*. 3rd ed. Churchill Livingston; 2015:101.)

## SUGGESTED READINGS

Brull, R., MacFarlane, A. J. R., & Chan, V. W. S. (2020). Spinal, epidural, and caudal anesthesia. In *Miller's anesthesia* (9th ed., pp. 1413–1449). Philadelphia: Michael AG, Elsevier.

Cramer, G. D., & Darby, S. A. (2021). *Clinical anatomy of the spine, spinal cord, and ANS* (3rd ed.). Philadelphia: Elsevier.

Drake, R. A., Vogl, W., & Mitchell, A. (2015). *Gray's anatomy for students* (3rd ed.). Philadelphia: Churchill Livingston.

Hombach-Klonisch, S. (2019). Back and spine. In *Sobotta clinical atlas of human anatomy* (1st ed., pp. 39–82).

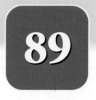

# 89

# Spinal Anesthesia

LOPA MISRA, DO

## Introduction

Although the first spinal block was performed in the 1880s, spinal anesthesia did not gain popularity in the United States until the 1940s. However, because of reports of toxicity and neurologic concerns, there was a decline in the number of blocks performed until the 1980s when a large study performed by Clergue and colleagues demonstrated the relative paucity of such complications. When used in appropriate patients, advantages of spinal blocks include a decrease in thromboembolic events, cardiac morbidity and mortality, bleeding, and subsequent transfusion requirements. In addition, subarachnoid blocks have been shown to decrease vascular graft occlusion and postoperative pulmonary compromise. Benefits of spinal anesthesia are multifactorial, including decreased hypercoagulable state, increased tissue blood flow, increased oxygenation, increased peristalsis, and decreased stress response. The mechanism of action of spinal anesthesia is attributed to the bathing of nerve roots within the subarachnoid space with local anesthetic. Effects of local anesthetics depend on size and myelin content of nerve fibers, concentration of agent, and duration of contact between the nerve and the local anesthetic. Loss of autonomic function occurs before sensory loss, which occurs before motor loss. This is because heavy myelinated fibers present in motor nerves are the most resistant to effects of local anesthetics. Autonomic block is two or more dermatomes *above* the level of skin analgesia, and motor block is two or more levels *below* the level of skin analgesia (Fig. 89.1).

## Anatomy

Traditionally, anatomic landmarks have been identified by palpation, most commonly using a line connecting the iliac crests that represents the interspace between the fourth and

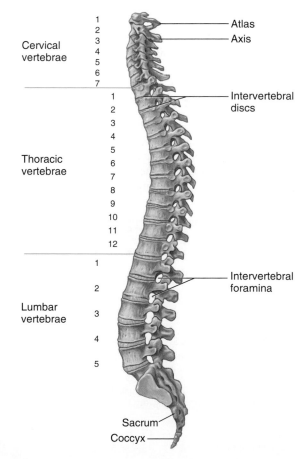

**Fig. 89.1**  The spinal column is seen from a lateral view. All of the vertebrae, intervertebral discs, and intervertebral foramina are shown.

fifth interspace. However, a recent review noted palpation technique may not be as accurate compared with the use of plain radiographic films for landmark identification. Another technique proposed by Jung and colleagues, which uses the 10th rib line, is believed to be a more reliable method of identifying the lumbar vertebral level. Radiopaque markers are placed with the aid of plain films, and the 10th rib line is used to detect the L2 spinous process, thereby reducing the risk of needle insertion at a cephalad level with potential for cord injury.

Other approaches such as ultrasound and fluoroscopic imaging may enhance accuracy. Particularly, the use of real-time ultrasound lowered the number of puncture attempts, in addition to lowering the number of interspaces attempted for puncture and needle manipulations. Alternatively, fluoroscopy has been successfully used for anatomic identification in technically challenging and morbidly obese individuals. Disadvantages of fluoroscopy include credentialing of training, time commitment, and additional radiation exposure for patients and providers.

## Factors Affecting Block Level

Important factors affecting block level are baricity, patient positioning during and after placement, and local anesthetic dose. Additionally, specific gravity of local anesthetic compared with the specific gravity of cerebrospinal fluid determines which direction the local anesthetic will travel. For instance, hyperbaric local anesthetics travel "down," or assisted by gravity, whereas hypobaric local anesthetics travel "up," or against gravity. Typically, isobaric solutions remain at the site of injection or have been shown in vivo to behave similar to hypobaric solutions. Other potential determinants of block height are injection site level, patient height, spinal anatomy, and direction of needle bevel (Table 89.1).

## Spinal Anesthetic Agents

The most used solutions are hyperbaric or isobaric bupivacaine (12–15 mg). However, tetracaine, ropivacaine, procaine, and 2-chloroprocaine have also been used. Historically, lidocaine had been used for spinal anesthesia. However, in the 1990s, several case reports of cauda equina syndrome (hallmark signs

of bowel or bladder dysfunction) after the use of 5% lidocaine through microcatheters were documented. Later, transient neurologic symptoms (TNSs)—a painful condition of the buttocks and thighs with possible radiation to the lower extremities beginning as soon as a few hours after spinal anesthesia and lasting as long as 10 days—were also linked to lidocaine use within spinal anesthesia. It should be noted that all local anesthetics can cause TNS. However, lidocaine and mepivacaine both have a relative risk for TNS that is seven times that of bupivacaine, prilocaine, and procaine.

Contemporary total hip and total knee arthroplasty practice, with its focus on multimodal analgesia and early ambulation, has led to a renaissance in short- and intermediate-use local anesthetics including mepivacaine and lidocaine. Schwenk and colleagues have shown patients receiving mepivacaine ambulated earlier and were more likely to be discharged the same day as surgery compared with both hyperbaric and isobaric bupivacaine, without an increased incidence in TNS. It has been postulated that the common use of nonsteroidal antiinflammatory drugs for joint arthroplasty multimodal analgesia may be treating or perhaps preventing TNS.

Previously, 2-chloroprocaine was formulated with sodium metabisulfite (an antioxidant), which was associated with lower extremity paralysis and sacral nerve dysfunction. Thus it was changed to a formulation that contained the preservative ethylenediaminetetraacetic acid (EDTA). However, EDTA was associated with extreme back pain and lumbar muscle spasms. Recently, 2-chloroprocaine has been reformulated once again and is now antioxidant and preservative free. It has reemerged as a spinal anesthetic for use in ambulatory surgical populations (e.g., outpatient orthopedics, nonobstetric surgery) because of a shorter duration of action than bupivacaine, lidocaine, or mepivacaine. Quality and duration of blocks may be enhanced by adding vasoconstrictors (e.g., epinephrine) and opioids. Less commonly, clonidine, magnesium, and neostigmine have also been trialed; however, the benefits of increased onset time and time to recovery of spinal block need to be balanced against potential dose-related side effects or potential for drug error from the use of these adjuvants.

## Cardiovascular Effects

Spinal anesthesia results in a sympathectomy, which in turn leads to hypotension and bradycardia in addition to reduced cardiac contractility. Treatment includes fluids, vasopressors, and atropine.

The risks for bradycardia (<50 beats/min) are:

- Baseline heart rate less than 60 beats/min
- American Society of Anesthesiologists (ASA) I physical status
- β-Blockers
- Sensory level above T6
- Age less than 50 years
- Prolonged PR interval

## Pulmonary Effects

Pulmonary effects, although uncommon, may also occur as a result of spinal blocks despite gas exchange being a relatively passive process. The diaphragm is innervated by the phrenic nerve, which is composed of C3–C5 fibers typically unaffected by spinal blockade. However, in cases of high thoracic spinal levels, there is a reduction in vital capacity because of

| TABLE 89.1 | Determinants of Local Anesthetic Spread in the Subarachnoid Space |
|---|---|

**PROPERTIES OF LOCAL ANESTHETIC SOLUTION**
Baricity
Dose
Volume
Specific gravity

**PATIENT CHARACTERISTICS**
Position during and after injection
Height (extremely short or tall)
Spinal column anatomy
Decreased CSF volume (increased intraabdominal pressure caused by increased weight, pregnancy, etc.)

**TECHNIQUE**
Site/level of injection
Needle bevel direction

*CSF,* Cerebrospinal fluid.
Courtesy NYSORA.COM.

the loss of abdominal and accessory respiratory muscle function despite the tidal volume remaining unchanged. In severe chronic lung disease, patients rely on accessory muscles for respiration. Therefore caution is advised in this group when considering spinal anesthesia. In general, all patients should be on supplemental oxygen because acute airway closure, hypoxia, and atelectasis may occur. In cases of total spinal or high spinal, the resulting apnea and hypotension are usually caused by brainstem hypoperfusion and *not* direct local anesthesia blockade. Treatment includes supporting blood pressure with vasopressors, fluids, and securing the airway if needed.

## Gastrointestinal Effects

Because of the resultant sympathectomy accompanying spinal blocks, a small, contracted gut with peristalsis ensues. This is a result of enhanced vagal activity. Additionally, hepatic blood flow may be reduced secondary to a decrease in mean arterial pressure.

## Genitourinary Effects

There is minimal effect on renal blood flow from spinal blockade because renal blood flow is autoregulated. If a spinal is placed at the lumbar or sacral level, one can see loss of autonomic control of bladder function resulting in urinary retention, which resolves when the block dissipates.

## Cerebral Blood Flow

Cerebral blood flow is maintained during spinal anesthesia. However, if mean arterial pressure is less than 60 mm Hg, cerebral blood flow will decrease, resulting in hypoxia, nausea, and vomiting. In these episodes of "spinal-induced hypotension," a head-down/Trendelenburg position may help increase mean cerebral arterial pressure (however, use caution with hyperbaric solutions). In addition, fluids and vasopressors (e.g., phenylephrine as a bolus or an infusion) may be used to restore blood pressure to adequate values.

## Contraindications to Spinal Anesthesia

Absolute contraindications include coagulopathy, elevated intracranial pressure (except in those with pseudotumor cerebri), unclear neurologic disease, severe hypovolemia, infection at the injection site, and patient refusal. Sepsis away from site of puncture and unclear surgical duration are considered relative contraindications to subarachnoid blocks.

## Emerging Concerns in Neuraxial Anesthesia

With routine practice of postoperative deep vein thrombosis prophylaxis with heparin and warfarin, and, more recently, the advent of newer direct oral anticoagulants (DOACs), there is an additional layer of complexity in choosing spinal anesthesia. This may be attributed to lack of familiarity with newer agents and the intricacies of individual medical pharmacokinetics. Four DOACs are in use both in the United States and in other countries: dabigatran, apixaban, edoxaban, and rivaroxaban. Currently, dabigatran (a direct thrombin inhibitor) is the lone DOAC with a reversal agent; however, renal clearance of dabigatran makes this DOAC less ideal for those patients with renal insufficiency. Hence, familiarizing oneself with their pharmacokinetics of DOACs, warfarin, and heparin formularies is of utmost importance when considering surgery with or without spinal anesthesia. In general, specialty groups such as the American Society of Regional Anesthesia and Pain Medicine have recommended waiting two to three half-lives after the last dose of oral anticoagulants when performing neuraxial anesthesia in low-risk patients. In high-risk patients, waiting five half-lives is recommended.

## SUGGESTED READINGS

Horlocker, T. T., Wedel, D. J., Rowlingson, J. C., Enneking, F. K., Kopp, S. L., Benzon, H. T., et al. (2010). Regional anesthesia in the patient receiving antithrombotic or thrombolytic therapy: American Society of Regional Anesthesia and Pain Medicine evidence-based guidelines (third edition). *Regional Anesthesia and Pain Medicine*, *35*, 64–101.

Levy, J. H., ALbaladejo, P., Samama, C. M., Spyropoulos, A. C., Hunt, B., & Douketis, J. (2017). Perioperative management of the new anticoagulants: Novel drugs and concepts. *APSF Newsletter*, *32*, 1–6.

Li, J., & Halaszynski, T. (2015). Neuraxial and peripheral nerve blocks in patients taking anticoagulant or thromboprophylactic drugs: Challenges and solutions. *Local and Regional Anesthesia*, *28*, 21–32. Retrieved from NYSORA.com. Accessed June, 2017.

Pollock, J. E. (2007). Transient neurologic symptoms. In J. M. Neal, J. P. Rathmell (Eds.), *Complications in regional anesthesia & pain medicine* (pp. 119–124). Philadelphia: WB Saunders.

Schwenk, E. S., Kasper, V. P., Smoker, J. D., Mendelson, A. M., Austin, M. S., Brown, S. A., et al. (2020). Mepivacaine versus Bupivacaine spinal anesthesia for early postoperative ambulation. *Anesthesiology*, *133*, 801–811.

Vadhanan, P. (2021). Recent updates in spinal anesthesia: A narrative review. *Asian Journal of Anesthesiology*, *59*, 41–50.

# Epidural Anesthesia

ROCHELLE J. POMPEIAN, MD | EMILY E. SHARPE, MD

Epidural anesthesia has clinical applications in three main areas: surgery, obstetrics, and chronic pain relief.

## Applied Anatomy of the Epidural Space

The epidural space, a potential space surrounding the spinal meninges, contains fat, nerve roots, and vascular plexuses. The anatomy of the spine, ligaments, meninges, and blood flow throughout the spinal cord are described in detail in Chapter 88. Knowledge of surface anatomy (Fig. 90.1) and key anatomic features of the cervical, thoracic, and lumbar spinal regions (Box 90.1) is critical to the performance of safe and reliable epidural placement.

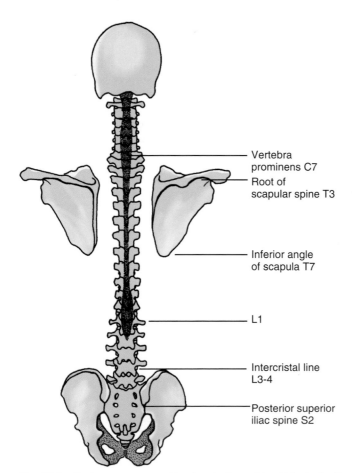

Vertebra prominens C7

Root of scapular spine T3

Inferior angle of scapula T7

L1

Intercristal line L3-4

Posterior superior iliac spine S2

**Fig. 90.1** Surface anatomy and landmarks for epidural blockade. Termination of the spinal cord is at L1 in adults. The dural sac terminates at S2. Needle placement between C7 and T1 is different because of the narrow epidural space. Between T1 and T7, a paramedian approach is recommended to bypass angled spinous processes. Below T7, needle placement becomes progressively similar to that for L2–L3. (Modified from Bromage PR. *Epidural Analgesia*. WB Saunders; 1978:8.)

> **BOX 90.1 ANATOMIC FEATURES OF CERVICAL, THORACIC, AND LUMBAR SPINE REGIONS**
>
> **LUMBAR SPINE**
>
> The epidural space is widest (i.e., 5–6 mm).
> Needle insertion below L1 (in adults) avoids the spinal cord.
> The ligamentum flavum is thickest in the midline in the lumbar area.
> The spinous processes have only slight downward angulation.
> The epidural veins are prominent in the lateral portion of the epidural space.
>
> **THORACIC SPINE**
>
> The epidural space is 3 to 5 mm in the midline, narrow laterally.
> The ligamentum flavum is thick but less so than in the midlumbar region.
> The spinous processes have extreme downward angulation; the paramedian approach is recommended.
>
> **CERVICAL SPINE**
>
> The epidural space is narrow, only 2 mm at C3–6.
> The ligamentum flavum is thin.
> The spinous process at C7 is almost horizontal.

All segments of the spinal canal, from the base of the skull to the sacral hiatus, are accessible to epidural injection. Epidural anesthesia, provided either alone or in combination with general anesthesia, may be adapted to almost any surgical procedure that takes place below the level of the patient's chin. Ideally, needle and catheter placement should occur at the dermatomal level of the surgical incision (e.g., lumbar placement for lower extremity operations and thoracic placement for thoracic/abdominal operations) to allow for block of only the parts of the body that fall within the surgical field. However, a lumbar technique may be used for even upper abdominal procedures, although it would result in a complete sympathectomy, including potentially blocking the cardiac accelerator fibers. Assessment of the dermatomal sensory level enables the anesthesiologist to determine approximate level of sympathectomy and anticipate the resulting hemodynamic effects (Table 90.1).

## Identification of the Epidural Space

The epidural space may be accessed using a midline or a paramedian approach (Fig. 90.2). The epidural space is identified by the passage of the needle from an area of high resistance (ligamentum flavum) to an area of low resistance (epidural space). After the needle is positioned in the ligamentum flavum, a syringe with a freely movable plunger is attached and pressure is applied to the plunger. If the needle is positioned correctly in the ligament, the syringe should not inject when pressure is applied to the plunger. As the needle passes into the epidural

| TABLE 90.1 | Sensory Level of Epidural Blockade Required for Surgical Procedures | | |
|---|---|---|---|
| Cutaneous Landmark | Segmental Level | Type of Operation | Significance |
| Fifth finger | C8 | | All cardioaccelerator fibers (T1–T4) blocked |
| Nipple line | T4–T5 | Upper abdominal | Possibility of cardioaccelerator blockade |
| Tip of xiphoid | T6 | Lower abdominal | Splanchnics (T5–L1) blocked |
| Umbilicus | T10 | Hip | Sympathetic blockade to lower extremities |
| Lateral aspect of foot | S1 | Leg and foot | No lumbar sympathectomy |
| Perineum | S2–S4 | Hemorrhoidectomy | |

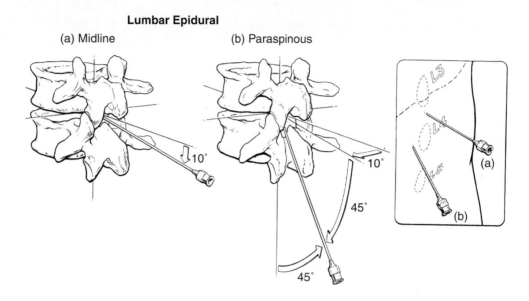

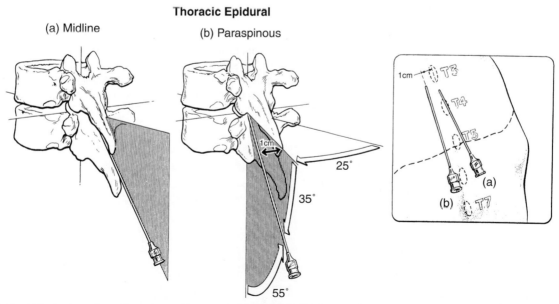

**Fig. 90.2** Epidural block: sites of needle insertion. *Upper panel:* Lumbar epidural: *(a)* midline—note insertion closer to the superior spinous process and with a slight upward angulation; *(b)* paraspinous (paramedian)—note insertion beside caudad edge of "inferior" spinous process, with 45-degree angulation to long axis of spine below. *Lower panel:* Thoracic epidural: *(a)* midline—note extreme upward angulation required in midthoracic region—paramedian approach may be technically easier; *(b)* paramedian—note needle insertion next to caudad tip of the spinous process above interspace of intended level of entry through ligamentum flavum—upward angulation is 55 degrees to long axis of spine below, and inward angulation is 10–15 degrees.

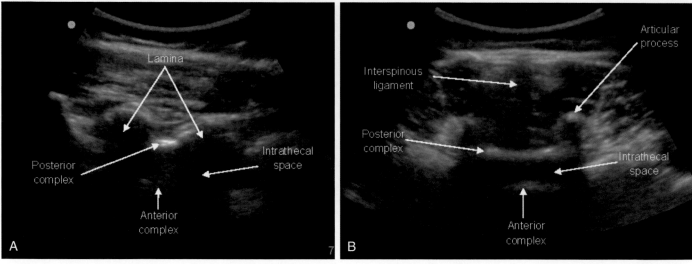

**Fig. 90.3**   Ultrasound paramedian sagittal oblique **(A)** and midline **(B)** views of the lumbar spine. In the paramedian sagittal oblique view, the ultrasound probe is placed parallel and slightly lateral to the midline of the spine. In this view, the lumbar laminae appear as hyperechoic structures in a classic "sawtooth" pattern. The ligamentum flavum, posterior epidural space, and dura are often not individually distinguishable, appearing as a single hyperechoic structure, referred to as the posterior complex. Similarly, the anterior complex also appears as a single hyperechoic structure and is composed of the anterior epidural space, anterior dura, posterior longitudinal ligament, and posterior aspect of the vertebral body.

space, a sudden loss of resistance in the plunger will be felt, and the air or fluid will easily inject. At this point, a flexible nylon catheter may be advanced 3 to 5 cm through the needle into the epidural space to allow repeated and incremental injections or infusions. Preinsertion ultrasound imaging has been demonstrated to accurately identify the level of the vertebrae and to estimate the depth of the epidural space (Fig. 90.3).

A test dose containing either a local anesthetic alone or a combination of a local anesthetic and epinephrine (typically 3 mL of lidocaine 1.5% and epinephrine 1:200,000) is then injected to detect inadvertent intravascular or subarachnoid placement. An increase in systolic blood pressure of at least 15 mm Hg or an increase in heart rate of at least 10 beats/min raises suspicion for intravascular injection (because of systemic uptake of the epinephrine in the test dose), whereas a change in lower extremity sensation (with or without a decrease in blood pressure) may represent subarachnoid injection.

## Selection and Dose of Local Anesthetic Agent

When injected in the epidural space, local anesthetics act primarily at the level of the spinal nerve roots, where the dura is relatively thin. Only a small amount of local anesthetic agent diffuses across the dura into the subarachnoid space.

A local anesthetic agent, and dosing thereof, should be selected on the basis of indication (analgesia, primary anesthetic, or supplementation to general anesthesia), desired speed of onset, degree of motor blockade required, and duration of the surgical procedure (Table 90.2). Local anesthetic dose may be calculated by the following formula: dose equals 1 to 1.5 mL of local anesthetic agent per segment blocked. The dose may need to be significantly reduced in parturients and in obese and elderly patients because of altered local anesthetic metabolism. Incremental dosing is an effective method of avoiding serious

| TABLE 90.2 | Clinical Effects of Local Anesthetic Solutions Commonly Used for Epidural Blockade | | |
|---|---|---|---|
| Drug | Time Spread to ± 4 Segments ± 1 SD (min) | Approximate Time to 2-Segment Regression ± 2 SD* (min) | Recommended Top-up Time From Initial Dose* (min) |
| Lidocaine, 2% | 25 ± 5 | 100 ± 40 | 60 |
| Prilocaine, 2%–3% | 15 ± 4 | 100 ± 40 | 60 |
| Chloroprocaine, 2%–3% | 12 ± 5 | 60 ± 15 | 45 |
| Mepivacaine, 2% | 15 ± 5 | 120 ± 150 | 60 |
| Bupivacaine, 0.5%–0.75% | 18 ± 10 | 200 ± 80 | 120 |
| Ropivacaine, 0.75%–1% | 20.5 ± 7.9 | 177 ± 49 | 120 |
| Levobupivacaine, 0.5%–0.75% | 20 ± 9 | 200 ± 80 | 120 |

*Note that top-up time is based on duration ±2 SD, which encompasses the likely duration in 95% of the population. In a conscious cooperative patient, an alternative is to use frequent checks of segmental level to indicate the need to top up. All solutions contain 1:200,000 epinephrine.
Reprinted with permission from Veering BT, Cousins MJ. Epidural neural blockade. In: Cousins MJ, Carr DB, Horlocker TT, Bridenbaugh PO, eds. *Neural Blockade in Clinical Anesthesia and Management of Pain.* 4th ed. Lippincott Williams & Williams; 2009:241–295.

complications. A second dose of approximately 50% of the initial dose will maintain the original level of anesthesia if injected when the blockade has regressed one or two dermatomes (see Table 90.2).

The addition of epinephrine can prolong the duration of lidocaine up to 50%. Less dramatic results are usually observed when bupivacaine or ropivacaine is used. The addition of vasoconstricting agents reduces blood flow in the richly vascularized epidural space, reducing systemic absorption; because more of the drug remains in proximity to the nerve, the onset of blockade is quicker and the duration of action is longer. Confirmation of this concept comes from studies demonstrating that the peak plasma levels of various agents are lower when epinephrine is present. Epinephrine also acts on α-adrenergic receptors located in the central nervous system, modulating central pain processing at those sites.

## Complications

One of the most common complications of epidural analgesia is a postdural puncture headache (PDPH), which may occur when the dura is inadvertently punctured during placement.

The risk of an unintentional dural puncture is approximately 1%. Of those who suffer an accidental dural puncture, 50% to 75% may develop a PDPH. Risk factors for PDPH include young age, female sex, pregnancy, larger-gauge needle, cutting needles, and multiple dural punctures.

The risks of severe or disabling neurologic complications are rare with the use of epidural anesthesia; however, reported rates vary widely depending on the study methodology and patient population studied. A review of 1.7 million neuraxial blocks found a total of 62 severe neurologic complications; risk was higher for patients with coagulation abnormalities, concurrent spinal stenosis, or preexisting neurologic disease (0.3–1.1%, compared with 0.001%–0.07% in healthy patients). Spinal anesthesia was associated with a greater risk for peripheral neuropathy than epidural anesthesia. Epidural anesthesia had a higher risk of spinal hematoma; the risk was higher in patients undergoing orthopedic surgery (1:22,000) than in pregnant patients (1:200,000).

Absorption of excessive amounts of local anesthetics can lead to local anesthetic systemic toxicity. Lipid emulsion (20%) therapy (bolus 100 mL in patients >70 kg and 1.5 mL/kg in patients <70 kg) should be available whenever regional blocks are performed.

## SUGGESTED READINGS

Brull, R., Alan, M., & Chan, V. W. S. (2020). Spinal, epidural, and caudal anesthesia. In M. A. Gropper, R. D. Miller, N. H. Cohen, L. I. Eriksson, L. A. Fleisher, K. Leslie, et al., (Eds.), *Miller's anesthesia* (9th ed., pp. 1413–1449). Philadelphia: Elsevier Saunders.

Chin, K. J., Karmakar, M. K., & Peng, P. (2011). Ultrasonography of the adult thoracic and lumbar spine for central neuraxial blockade. *Anesthesiology, 114,* 1459–1485.

Guay, J. (2009). The epidural test dose: A review. *Anesthesia and Analgesia, 108,* 1232–1242.

Neal, J. M., Barrington, M. J., Brull, R., Hadzic, A., Hebl, J. R., Horlocker, T. T., et al. (2015). The second ASRA practice advisory on neurologic complications associated with regional anesthesia and pain medicine: Executive summary 2015. *Regional Anesthesia and Pain Medicine, 40*(5), 401–430.

Veering, B. T., & Cousins, M. J. (2009). Epidural neural blockade. In: M. J. Cousins, D. B. Carr, T. T. Horlocker, P. O. Bridenbaugh (Eds.), *Neural blockade in clinical anesthesia and management of pain* (4th ed., pp. 241–295). Philadelphia: Lippincott, Williams & Williams.

# 91

# Combined Spinal-Epidural Blockade

KATHRYN CLARK, MB, BCh, BAO | LINDSAY WARNER, MD

Combined spinal-epidural (CSE) blockade was first described in 1937 but was not commonly used until the early 1980s. CSE blockade combines the rapid onset and reliability associated with subarachnoid blocks with the flexibility of dosing, duration, and analgesic-level control of an indwelling epidural catheter. CSE block is used primarily for obstetric analgesia and anesthesia, but its use has been described for a variety of applications, including general surgery, orthopedic and trauma surgery of the lower limb, urologic surgery, and gynecologic surgery.

## Applied Anatomy

The essence of a CSE block is single-shot administration of intrathecal anesthetic or analgesic agents along with placement of a catheter into the epidural space (Fig. 91.1). The applied

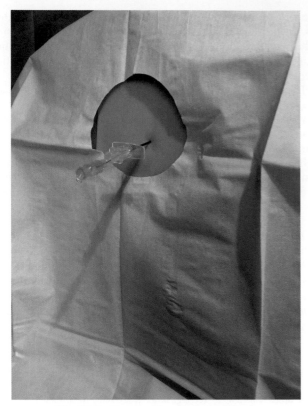

**Fig. 91.1** The combined spinal epidural.

| TABLE 91.1 | Absolute and Relative Contraindications to Neuraxial Anesthesia/Analgesia | |
|---|---|---|
| **Absolute** | **Relative** | |
| Patient refusal | Preexisting neurologic disease | |
| Bacteremia/sepsis | Severe psychiatric disease or dementia | |
| Increased intracranial pressure | Aortic stenosis | |
| Infection at needle insertion site | Left ventricular outflow tract obstruction | |
| Shock or severe hypovolemia | Various congenital heart conditions (absolute contraindication if severe) | |
| Coagulopathy or therapeutic anticoagulation | Deformities or previous surgery of the spinal column | |

anatomy of a CSE block is the same as that for subarachnoid and epidural blockade (see Chapter 90, Epidural Anesthesia, Fig. 90.1).

## Indications

CSE blockade can be used in patients in whom a neuraxial technique is indicated and would benefit from combining the density of block and rapid onset achieved with spinal anesthesia/analgesia with the ability to provide prolonged anesthesia/analgesia (as is usually done with a continuous infusion of medication through an epidural catheter). In obstetric anesthesia, CSE is used for both labor analgesia and cesarean anesthesia.

A common application for labor analgesia is a multiparous parturient at an advanced cervical dilation requesting neuraxial pain relief. The intrathecal fentanyl (typically about 15 mcg) provides a rapid onset of visceral pain relief. The intrathecal bupivacaine (typically about 2.5 mg) provides coverage of the sacral nerve roots, thereby providing relief from the intense somatic pain of second stage. The catheter can provide epidural analgesia if the parturient is still laboring after the spinal dose wears off or can provide anesthesia if the parturient proceeds to cesarean delivery.

CSE for cesarean anesthesia would be a consideration in a patient presenting for a complex cesarean delivery that may require prolonged surgical time. In these cases, intrathecal medication administration, with a full surgical intrathecal dose, provides density and reliability, and the epidural catheter

can be used if the length of the surgery outlasts the spinal block.

## Contraindications

Contraindications for CSE block are the same as those for all neuraxial blocks (Table 91.1).

## Advantages

Some studies have indicated that catheters placed during a CSE technique are less likely to fail than are epidural catheters placed during an epidural-only technique, because the epidural space is verified by the return of cerebrospinal fluid through the spinal needle. However, a systematic review comparing CSE and epidural labor analgesia found no evidence for differences in the rate of epidural catheter replacement or the rate of epidural top-ups (Heesen et al., 2014). The CSE technique, however, does offer some benefits for labor analgesia:

- The onset of anesthesia or analgesia is faster.
- The total dose of local anesthetic agent required to achieve analgesia/anesthesia is smaller than the dose necessary with an epidural-only technique, thus reducing the risk of local anesthetic toxicity. This may ultimately result in lower systemic and fetal (if used for labor and delivery) concentrations of local anesthetic agents.
- Intrathecal opioids can be administered as the sole agent, without the addition of local anesthetic drugs, providing about 90 min of analgesia for the first stage of labor with no motor block. This can be beneficial for high-risk cardiac patients to avoid a rapid sympathectomy or a decrease in systemic vascular resistance and allows time for careful titration of local anesthetic.
- Placement of labor analgesia can be more difficult in obese women and women with anatomic variations of the spine. A CSE has the added benefit of visualization of cerebrospinal fluid return, which can help confirm appropriate placement of the epidural.
- Subsequent epidural dosing may provide greater sacral nerve root coverage and a lower incidence of unilateral block.

- More rapid cervical dilation is associated with the use of CSE versus epidural labor analgesia.
- In anesthesia for cesarean delivery, a CSE (with a full surgical intrathecal dose) results in lower incidence of block failure necessitating general anesthesia and greater maternal comfort than an epidural-only technique, and if the epidural catheter is left in place, it provides an option for providing continued postoperative analgesia.
- In anesthesia for external cephalic version (ECV), a CSE can increase the success rate of version with the added benefit of the option to extend the block in the case of emergency cesarean delivery.

## Disadvantages

Possible disadvantages of using a CSE technique, in comparison with an epidural technique, include the following:
- Determination of the reliability of the epidural catheter for surgical anesthesia may be delayed.
- Intrathecally administered opioids can cause pruritus.
- Theoretically, the risk of infection may be increased because the subarachnoid space is accessed.
- When used for labor analgesia, intrathecally administered opioid medications may increase the incidence of postanalgesia uterine tachysystole and fetal heart rate decelerations; however, this disadvantage is controversial, and the complex discussion is beyond the scope of this chapter.

## Equipment and Technique

CSE blockades are typically performed via a needle-through-needle technique with traditional epidural and spinal needles. When the needle-through-needle technique is performed, a sterile field is created at the procedure site, the skin and subcutaneous tissue are infiltrated with a local anesthetic agent, and an epidural needle is inserted into the *ligamentum flavum*. Loss of resistance with air or saline is used to identify the epidural space. A spinal needle is then advanced through the epidural needle into the subarachnoid space. The spinal needle must be longer than the epidural needle to allow dural puncture, projecting 13 to 17 mm beyond the tip of the epidural needle. After the appearance of cerebrospinal fluid, the intrathecal anesthetic or analgesic agent is injected, and the spinal needle is removed. Finally, a catheter is advanced through the epidural needle into the epidural space, and the epidural needle is removed.

Another CSE technique involves performing separate passes, either in the same or different interspaces, for the spinal followed by the epidural. This technique can be used for parturients who are in such distress from labor pain that they are unable to stay still for the epidural needle insertion. Performing the spinal first to increase comfort may allow for optimal patient positioning and may decrease the risk of an inadvertent dural puncture with a large gauge needle. A disadvantage of this technique is the patient may be exposed to the remote risks associated with performing a neuraxial technique on nerves that are surrounded by local anesthetic agent. If the epidural catheter is inserted first, then there may be the very remote risk of damaging the epidural catheter with the spinal needle.

## Epidural Test Doses

The timing of the epidural test dose in a CSE technique is controversial. If a local anesthetic agent has been injected into the intrathecal space, detecting an intrathecal catheter with injection of a test dose of local anesthetic agent through the catheter may be difficult. Furthermore, a successful test dose does not guarantee a properly placed epidural catheter because the catheter could conceivably migrate after the test dose is administered but before the catheter is loaded. On the other hand, it may not be convenient to wait until the spinal block from the initial intrathecal injection of drug has worn off before administering a test dose through the catheter. Many anesthesiologists recommend the early use of test doses of local anesthetic agents with epinephrine to confirm catheter position.

## Complications

In comparison with an epidural technique alone, the CSE technique is not associated with an increased frequency of anesthetic complications, including postdural puncture headache (PDPH). Potential complications of the CSE technique are the same as those for spinal and epidural techniques and include PDPH, total spinal anesthesia, hypotension, bradycardia, meningitis, spinal abscess and hematoma, intravascular injection, intrathecal catheter migration, and nerve injury and, when used for labor analgesia, fetal bradycardia.

## Dural Puncture Epidural

A modification of the CSE technique is the dural puncture epidural (DPE) technique. Like a CSE, a dural perforation is created with a spinal needle; however, no intrathecal medication is administered. The spinal needle is then removed, and the epidural catheter is inserted via the Tuohy needle, after which the epidural is then dosed with the conventional epidural solution mix. A benefit of this technique include improvement in caudal spread, thought to be attributed to translocation of the epidural medication into the intrathecal space through the dural hole. Compared with the traditional epidural technique, the DPE technique provides significantly faster and bilateral blockade, although not as rapid as the CSE technique. As the DPE technique does not involve direct administration of opioids into the intrathecal space, there is a lower incidence of uterine tachysystole and hypertonus compared with the CSE technique. DPE may improve the speed to onset compared with the traditional epidural technique, in addition to improving caudal spread, without the side effects observed with the CSE technique. Like CSE, DPE has not been shown to have an increase incidence of PDPH compared with the traditional epidural technique.

## SUGGESTED READINGS

Bi, Y., & Zhou, J. (2021). Spinal subdural hematoma and subdural anesthesia following combined spinal-epidural anesthesia: A case report. *BMC Anesthesiology, 21*(1):130. doi:10.1186/s12871-021-01352-3.

Cappiello, E., O'Rourke, N., Segal, B., & Tsen, L. (2008). A randomized trial of dural puncture epidural technique compared with the standard epidural technique for labor analgesia. *Anesthesia and Analgesia, 107,* 1646–1651.

Chau, A., Bibbo, C., Huang, C. C., Elterman, K. G., Cappiello, E. C., Robinson, J. N., et al. (2017). Dural puncture epidural technique improves labor analgesia quality with fewer side effects compared with epidural and combined spinal epidural techniques: A randomized clinical trial. *Anesthesia and Analgesia, 124*(2), 560–569.

Gambling, D., Berkowitz, J., Farrell, T. R., Pue, A., & Shay, D. (2013). A randomized controlled comparison of epidural analgesia and combined spinal-epidural analgesia in a private practice setting: Pain scores during first and second stages of labor and at delivery. *Anesthesia and Analgesia, 116,* 636–643.

Heesen, M., Van de Velde, M., Klohr, S., Lehberger, J., Rossaint, R., & Straube, S. (2014). Meta-analysis of the success of block following combined spinal-epidural vs epidural analgesia during labour. *Anaesthesia, 69,* 64–71.

Murata, Y., Yamada, K., Hamaguchi, Y., Yamashita, S., & Tanaka, M. (2021). An optimal epidural catheter placement site for post-cesarean section analgesia with double-space technique combined spinal-epidural anesthesia: A retrospective study.

*JA Clinical Reports, 7*(1), 3. doi:10.1186/s40981-020-00405-9.

Simmons, S., Taghizadeh, N., Dennis, A., Hughes, D., & Cyna, A. M. (2012). Combined spinal-epidural versus epidural analgesia in labour. *Cochrane Database of Systematic Reviews, 10*(10), CD003401.

Wong, C. A. (2020). Epidural and spinal analgesia/anesthesia for labor and vaginal delivery. In D. H. Chestnut, C. A. Wong, L. C. Tsen, W. D. Ngan Kee, B. Beilin, J. M. Mhyre, et al., (Eds.), *Chestnut's obstetric anesthesia* (6th ed., pp. 474–539). Philadelphia: Elsevier Saunders.

**92**

# Neuraxial Anesthesia and Anticoagulation

TERESE TODDIE HORLOCKER, MD   |   SANDRA L. KOPP, MD

The actual incidence of neurologic dysfunction resulting from hemorrhagic complications associated with neuraxial blockade is unknown; however, recent epidemiologic studies suggest the incidence is increasing. In a review of the literature between 1906 and 1994, Vandermeulen and colleagues reported 61 cases of spinal hematoma associated with epidural or spinal anesthesia. In 87% of patients, a hemostatic abnormality or traumatic/difficult needle placement was present. More than one risk factor was present in 20 of 61 cases. Importantly, although only 38% of patients had partial or good neurologic recovery, spinal cord ischemia tended to be reversible in patients who underwent laminectomy within 8 h of onset of neurologic dysfunction.

It is impossible to conclusively determine risk factors for the development of spinal hematoma in patients undergoing neuraxial blockade solely through review of the case series, which represent only patients with the complication and do not define those who underwent uneventful neuraxial analgesia. However, large inclusive surveys that evaluate the frequencies of complications (including spinal hematoma) and identify subgroups of patients with higher or lower risk enhance risk stratification. In the series by Moen and colleagues, involving nearly 2 million neuraxial blocks, there were 33 spinal hematomas. The methodology allowed for calculation of frequency of spinal hematoma among patient populations. For example, the risk associated with epidural analgesia in women undergoing

childbirth was significantly less (1 in 200,000) than that in elderly women undergoing knee arthroplasty (1 in 3600, $P < 0.0001$). Likewise, women undergoing hip fracture surgery under spinal anesthesia had an increased risk of spinal hematoma (1 in 22,000) compared with all patients undergoing spinal anesthesia (1 in 480,000).

Overall, these series suggest that the risk of clinically significant bleeding varies with age (and associated abnormalities of the spinal cord or vertebral column), the presence of an underlying coagulopathy, difficulty during needle placement, and an indwelling neuraxial catheter during sustained anticoagulation (particularly with standard heparin or low-molecular-weight heparin [LMWH]). They also consistently demonstrate the need for prompt diagnosis and intervention.

## Vitamin K Antagonists (Warfarin)

Clinical experience with patients who, congenitally, are deficient in factors II, IX, or X suggests that a factor activity level of 40% for each factor is adequate for normal or near-normal hemostasis. Bleeding may occur if the level of any clotting factor is decreased to 20% to 40% of baseline. The prothrombin time (PT) is most sensitive to the activities of factors VII and X and is relatively insensitive to factor II. During the first few days of therapy, the PT reflects primarily a reduction of factor VII, the half-life of which is approximately 6 h. After a single dose, marked prolongation of the international normalized ratio (INR) may occur, although adequate factor levels are still present. However, with additional doses, an INR greater than 1.4 is typically associated with factor VII activity less than 40% (and the potential for inadequate clotting).

The management of patients receiving warfarin perioperatively remains controversial. Recommendations are based on warfarin pharmacology, the clinical relevance of vitamin K coagulation factor levels/deficiencies, case series, and the case reports of spinal hematoma.

Preoperatively, warfarin is typically discontinued for at least 5 days before a neuraxial procedure is performed and normalization of the INR is documented. Few data exist regarding the risk of spinal hematoma in patients with indwelling epidural catheters who are anticoagulated with warfarin. Neuraxial injections and removal of epidural catheters appear to be safe when done within 24 h after warfarin was initiated. Although it does not appear to increase risk to remove epidural catheters 12 to 24 h after warfarin was given, the risk of removing epidural catheters at 48 h is not guaranteed. This is because adequate activities of clotting factor VII are not assured and the activities of factors IX and X also start to decline. Thus not only the INR but also the duration of warfarin therapy must be considered, and prolongation within the first 48 h may represent a significant increase in risk.

## Intravenous and Subcutaneous Standard (Unfractionated) Heparin

The safety of neuraxial techniques in combination with intraoperative heparinization is well documented, providing no other coagulopathy is present. The safety of indwelling spinal and epidural catheters during systemic heparinization was demonstrated in a study involving over 4000 patients undergoing vascular surgery. However, the heparin was administered at least 60 min after catheter placement, the level of anticoagulation was closely monitored, and the indwelling catheters were removed at a time when circulating heparin levels were relatively low. A subsequent study in the neurologic literature stated there were seven spinal hematomas in 342 patients (2%) who underwent a diagnostic lumbar puncture and subsequent heparinization. Traumatic needle placement, initiation of anticoagulation within 1 h of lumbar puncture, and concomitant aspirin therapy were identified as risk factors in the development of spinal hematoma in anticoagulated patients. Subsequent studies using similar methodology have verified the safety of this practice, provided the monitoring of anticoagulant effect and the time intervals between heparinization and catheter placement/removal are maintained.

Low-dose subcutaneous (SQ) standard (unfractionated) heparin (UFH) is administered for thromboprophylaxis in patients undergoing major thoracoabdominal surgery and in patients at increased risk of hemorrhage with oral anticoagulant or LMWH therapy. There are nine published series totaling over 9000 patients who have received this therapy without complications, as well as extensive experience in both Europe and the United States without a significant frequency of complications. However, the majority of patients received twice-daily dosing with doses of 5000 U SQ UFH.

The safety of neuraxial blockade in patients receiving doses greater than 10,000 U UFH daily or more than twice-daily dosing of UFH has not been established. Although the use of thrice-daily UFH may lead to an increased risk of surgical-related bleeding, it is unclear whether there is an increased risk of spinal hematoma. If thrice-daily unfractionated heparin is administered, techniques to facilitate detection of new/progressive neurodeficits (e.g., enhanced neurologic monitoring and neuraxial solutions to minimize sensory and motor block) should be applied and additional hemostasis altering medications (e.g., ketorolac) avoided.

Management of the patient receiving perioperative SQ UFH is dependent on dosing schedule and total daily dose. Delay needle placement for 4 to 6 h from last dose of 5000 U SQ UFH dose with twice-daily or thrice-daily administration. Preoperative "higher-dose" SQ UFH for *thromboprophylaxis* (e.g., individual heparin dose of 7500–10,000 U twice-daily or a daily dose of ≤20,000 U) delay neuraxial block for 12 h after subcutaneous heparin administration *and* assessment of coagulation status. For preoperative *therapeutic* SQ UFH (e.g., individual dose >10,000 U SQ per dose, or >20,000 U total daily dose), delay neuraxial block for 24 h after subcutaneous heparin administration *and* assessment of coagulation status.

## Low-Molecular-Weight Heparin

Extensive clinical testing and utilization of LMWH in Europe suggested there was not an increased risk of spinal hematoma in patients undergoing neuraxial anesthesia while receiving LMWH thromboprophylaxis perioperatively. However, in the first 5 years after the release of LMWH for general use in the United States in May 1993, over 60 cases of spinal hematoma associated with neuraxial anesthesia administered in the presence of perioperative LMWH prophylaxis were reported to the manufacturer. Many of these events occurred when LMWH was administered intraoperatively or early postoperatively to patients undergoing continuous epidural anesthesia and analgesia. Concomitant antiplatelet therapy was present in several cases (Box 92.1). The apparent difference in incidence in Europe compared with the United States may be a result of a

---

**BOX 92.1   PATIENT, ANESTHETIC, AND LOW-MOLECULAR-WEIGHT HEPARIN DOSING VARIABLES ASSOCIATED WITH SPINAL HEMATOMA**

**PATIENT FACTORS**

Female sex
Increased age

**ANESTHETIC FACTORS**

Traumatic needle/catheter placement
Epidural (compared with spinal) technique
Indwelling epidural catheter during LMWH administration

**LMWH DOSING FACTORS**

Immediate preoperative (or intraoperative) LMWH administration
Early postoperative LMWH administration
Concomitant antiplatelet or anticoagulant medications
Twice-daily LMWH administration

---

*LMWH,* Low-molecular-weight heparin.
Adapted from Horlocker TT, Wedel DJ. Neuraxial block and low-molecular-weight heparin: balancing perioperative analgesia and thromboprophylaxis. Reg Anesth Pain Med. 1998;23:164–177.

difference in dose and dosage schedule. For example, in Europe the recommended dose of enoxaparin is 40 mg once daily (with LMWH therapy initiated 12 h preoperatively), rather than 30 mg every 12 h. However, timing of catheter removal may also have an impact. It is likely that the lack of a trough in anticoagulant activity associated with twice-daily dosing resulted in catheter removal occurring during significant anticoagulant activity. The incidence of spinal hematoma in patients undergoing neuraxial block in combination with LMWH has been estimated at 1 in 40,800 spinal anesthetics and 1 in 3100 continuous epidural anesthetics.

Indications for thromboprophylaxis, as well as treatment of thromboembolism or myocardial infarction, have been introduced. These new applications and corresponding regional anesthetic management warrant discussion. Several off-label applications of LMWH are of special interest to the anesthesiologist. LMWH has been demonstrated to be efficacious as a "bridge therapy" for patients chronically anticoagulated with warfarin, including parturients, patients with prosthetic cardiac valves, a history of atrial fibrillation, or preexisting hypercoagulable condition. The doses of LMWH are those associated with deep vein thrombosis treatment, not prophylaxis, and are much higher. An interval of at least 24 h is required for the anticoagulant activity to resolve.

## New Oral Anticoagulants

The new oral anticoagulants (dabigatran, rivaroxaban, apixaban, and edoxaban) are used in the primary prevention of venous thromboembolism (VTE) after elective total hip replacement surgery, the prevention of stroke and systemic embolism in adult patients with nonvalvular atrial fibrillation, and the prevention and treatment of (recurrent) VTE and pulmonary embolism. These drugs are at least as effective anticoagulants as the vitamin K antagonists but seem to be safer in terms of bleeding, have a rapid onset of action, a short half-life, and are devoid of the need for routine laboratory monitoring. Until recently, any specific antidotes were lacking.

### DABIGATRAN

Dabigatran etexilate is a prodrug that specifically and reversibly inhibits both free and clot-bound thrombin. The drug is absorbed from the gastrointestinal tract with a bioavailability of 5%. Once absorbed, it is converted by esterases into its active metabolite, dabigatran. Plasma levels peak at 2 h. The half-life is 8 h after a single dose and up to 17 h after multiple doses. It is likely that once-daily dosing will be possible for some indications because of the prolonged half-life. Because 80% of the drug is excreted unchanged by the kidneys, it is contraindicated in patients with renal failure. Dabigatran prolongs the activated partial thromboplastin time (aPTT), but its effect is not linear and reaches a plateau at higher doses. However, the ecarin clotting time (ECT) and thrombin time (TT) are particularly sensitive and display a linear dose response at therapeutic concentrations.

Idarucizumab is a monoclonal antibody fragment that binds to dabigatran and reverses its anticoagulant effects both in vitro and in vivo in rats. Idarucizumab completely reversed the anticoagulant effect of dabigatran within minutes in patients with bleeding or requiring urgent surgery. In October 2015, idarucizumab was approved by the U.S. Food and Drug Administration to be used in adult patients treated with dabigatran when rapid reversal of its anticoagulant effects is required in situations of emergency surgery/urgent procedures or life-threatening, uncontrolled bleeding. The recommended dose is 5 g via an intravenous (IV) infusion/injection. The 2022 cost of reversal was approximately $4000.

There is limited experience with dabigatran and neuraxial anesthesia, and none with the use of indwelling epidural catheters. Given the prolonged half-life and the uncertainty of an individual patient's renal function, dabigatran should be discontinued a minimum of 5 days before neuraxial block. Consider documentation of reversal of anticoagulant effect (assessment of a TT or ECT) if less than 5 days have elapsed since discontinuation.

### RIVAROXABAN

Rivaroxaban is a potent selective and reversible oral activated factor Xa inhibitor, with an oral bioavailability of 80%. After administration, the maximum inhibitory effect occurs in 1 to 4 h; however, inhibition is maintained for 12 h. Rivaroxaban is cleared by the kidneys and gut. The terminal elimination half-life is 9 h in healthy volunteers and may be prolonged to 13 h in the elderly due to a decline in renal function (hence a need for dose adjustment in patients with renal insufficiency and contraindicated in patients with severe liver disease).

Rivaroxaban prolongs the INR in a dose-dependent way, but the results are not always reliable because of an important interassay variability dependent on the reagent used. At best, the PT can give some qualitative information. The aPTT is even less sensitive, has a nonlinear dose-dependent prolongation and an important interassay variability, and is not suited to qualitatively and quantitatively assess the effects of rivaroxaban. The best method to assess rivaroxaban is the use of chromogenic anti-Xa assays developed for the measurement of direct factor Xa inhibitors using specific rivaroxaban calibrators.

There are minimal clinical data on the use of neuraxial anesthesia in rivaroxaban-treated patients. Indwelling neuraxial catheters are contraindicated because of the "boxed warning." Likewise, indwelling neuraxial catheters should be removed 6 h before initiation of rivaroxaban therapy postoperatively.

### APIXABAN

Apixaban inhibits platelet activation and fibrin clot formation via direct, selective, and reversible inhibition of free and clot-bound factor Xa. After administration, the maximum inhibitory effect occurs in 3 to 4 h; however, inhibition is maintained for 12 h. Apixaban is cleared mainly by the liver; less than 30% is by renal excretion. The terminal elimination half-life is 12 h in healthy volunteers and may be prolonged in patients with renal impairment.

Both the PT and the aPTT are not suited to qualitative and quantitative assessment of the effects of apixaban. These tests produce unreliable results because of a low sensitivity for apixaban and a large interassay variability dependent on the reagents used. The aPTT also displays a nonlinear dose-dependent prolongation. Chromogenic anti-Xa assays developed for the measurement of direct factor Xa inhibitors and using specific calibrators for apixaban are the monitoring tests of choice.

There are very little prospective data concerning the use of neuraxial blocks in apixaban-treated patients. There should be at least a 26 to 30 h time interval between the last dose of prophylactic dose of apixaban (2.5 mg twice daily) and the subsequent neuraxial puncture and/or catheter manipulation/removal. If a dose of 5 mg twice daily is used and/or in patients with a serum creatinine 1.5 mg/dL or greater and aged 80 years or older, or a body weight 60 kg or less, a time interval of 72 h should be observed. The absence of any remaining apixaban activity can be documented using a chromogenic anti-Xa assay calibrated for apixaban. The next dose of apixaban should be administered at least 6 h after the neuraxial puncture or withdrawal of the neuraxial catheter.

## EDOXABAN

Edoxaban also is a highly selective reversible factor Xa inhibitor. After oral ingestion, maximum plasma levels are reached within 1 to 2 h. The kidney clears about 50% of the administered dose, and metabolism and biliary/intestinal excretion accounts for the remainder. The elimination half-life after oral administration is 10 to 14 h in healthy patients. In the presence of mild, moderate, and severe renal insufficiency, the total exposure to edoxaban is increased by 32%, 74%, and 72% resulting in an elimination half-life of 8.4, 9.45, and 16.9 h, respectively.

The PT and aPTT should not be used to assess the anticoagulant activity of edoxaban, as the compound behaves in much the same way as apixaban. Edoxaban is best assessed using specific chromogenic anti-Xa assays. The use of neuraxial anesthetic techniques in edoxaban-treated patients should be cautiously considered, as there are no data. A minimum of 3 days should elapse between discontinuation of apixaban and neuraxial block. Indwelling neuraxial catheters are contraindicated and should be removed 6 h prior to initiation of edoxaban therapy postoperatively.

## Reversal of Direct Oral Anticoagulants

Andexanet alfa (or andexanet) was released for general use in 2019. Andexanet alfa is indicated for anticoagulation reversal in life-threatening or uncontrolled bleeding in patients treated with rivaroxaban or apixaban *only*. Andexanet alfa is an engineered variant of factor Xa, whose similarity to the human form allows it to bind factor Xa inhibitors with high affinity. There are two dosing regimens. The low-dose regimen consists of a 400 mg IV bolus followed by a 2-h IV infusion at a rate of 4 mg/min. The high dose is an 800 mg IV bolus followed by a 2-h IV infusion at a rate of 8 mg/min. The recommended regimen for a particular patient is based on the factor Xa inhibitor used, the dose of factor Xa inhibitor, and the time since the last dose of factor Xa inhibitor. The 2022 cost varied between $27,500 and $49,500.

## Antiplatelet Medications

Antiplatelet medications are seldom used as primary agents of thromboprophylaxis. However, many orthopedic patients report chronic use of one or more antiplatelet drugs. Although Vandermeulen and colleagues implicated antiplatelet therapy in 3 of the 61 cases of spinal hematoma occurring after spinal or epidural anesthesia, several large studies have demonstrated the relative safety of neuraxial blockade in obstetric, surgical, and pain clinic patients receiving these medications.

Ticlopidine and clopidogrel are also platelet aggregation inhibitors. These agents interfere with platelet-fibrinogen binding and subsequent platelet-platelet interactions. The effect is irreversible for the life of the platelet. Platelet dysfunction is present for 5 to 7 days after discontinuation of clopidogrel and 10 to 14 days with ticlopidine.

Prasugrel is a new thienopyridine that inhibits platelets more rapidly, more consistently, and to a greater extent than do standard and higher doses of clopidogrel. In the United States, the only labeled indication is for acute coronary syndrome in patients intended to undergo percutaneous coronary intervention. After a single oral dose, 50% of platelets are irreversibly inhibited, with maximum effect 2 h after administration. Platelet aggregation normalizes in 7 to 10 days after discontinuation of therapy. The labeling recommends that the drug "be discontinued at least 7 days prior to any surgery."

Ticagrelor represents a new class of nonthienopyridine platelet inhibitors designed to address the limitations of current oral platelet drugs. Ticagrelor completely *reversibly* inhibits ADP-induced platelet activation, unlike the thienopyridines (e.g., clopidogrel, prasugrel). Ticagrelor has been studied in acute coronary syndrome in combination with aspirin. Maintenance doses of aspirin above 100 mg decreased the effectiveness and should be avoided. The labeling recommends that, when possible, ticagrelor should "be discontinued at least 5 days prior to any surgery."

Platelet glycoprotein IIb/IIIa receptor antagonists, including abciximab, eptifibatide, and tirofiban, inhibit platelet aggregation by interfering with platelet-fibrinogen binding and subsequent platelet-platelet interactions. Time to normal platelet aggregation after discontinuation of therapy ranges from 8 h (eptifibatide, tirofiban) to 48 h (abciximab). Increased perioperative bleeding in patients undergoing cardiac and vascular surgery after receiving ticlopidine, clopidogrel, and glycoprotein IIb/IIIa antagonists warrants concern regarding the risk of anesthesia-related hemorrhagic complications.

## The Anticoagulated Parturient

The incidence of spinal hematoma after neuraxial blockade (with or without altered hemostasis) in the obstetric patient is very difficult to determine, although it is widely reported these patients have a significantly lower incidence of complications than their elderly counterparts. Until 2011, all case reports of neuraxial hematomas in obstetric patients with altered hemostasis have occurred in parturients with a preexisting coagulopathy (e.g., thrombocytopenia, hemorrhage, preeclampsia, thrombocytopenia, HELLP [hemolysis, elevated liver enzymes, and low platelet count]) either at the time of epidural placement or removal. With the introduction of more aggressive thromboprophylaxis peripartum (and administration of LMWH and higher dose SQ UFH), several cases of spinal hematoma involving anticoagulation and neuraxial anesthesia in obstetric patients have been reported.

The peripartum management of the anticoagulated parturient represents a significant clinical challenge to both the obstetrician and the anesthesiologist. In the event of unforeseen labor or urgent cesarean delivery, the choice of analgesia and/or anesthesia should weigh the risks of general anesthesia and benefits of neuraxial anesthesia in the setting of the anticoagulant type, dose,

| TABLE 92.1 | **Recommendations for Management of Patients Receiving Neuraxial Blockade and Anticoagulant Drugs** |
|---|---|
| Warfarin | Discontinue chronic warfarin therapy 4–5 days before spinal procedure and evaluate INR. INR should be within the normal range at time of procedure to ensure adequate levels of all vitamin K–dependent factors. Postoperatively, daily INR assessment with catheter removal occurring ideally with INR <1.5; catheters may be maintained with caution with 1.5 < INR < 3. |
| Antiplatelet medications | No contraindications with aspirin or other NSAIDs. Clopidogrel and ticagrelor should be discontinued 5–7 days, prasugrel 7–10 days, and ticlopidine 14 days before procedure. Glycoprotein IIb/IIIa inhibitors should be discontinued to allow recovery of platelet function before procedure (8 h for tirofiban and eptifibatide, 24–48 h for abciximab). |
| Thrombolytics/fibrinolytics | There are no available data to suggest a safe interval between procedure and initiation or discontinuation of these medications. Follow fibrinogen level and observe for signs of neural compression. |
| LMWH | Delay procedure at least 12 h from the last dose of thromboprophylaxis LMWH dose. For "treatment" dosing of LMWH, at least 24 h should elapse before procedure. LMWH should not be administered within 24 h after the procedure. Indwelling epidural catheters should be maintained only with once-daily dosing of LMWH and strict avoidance of additional hemostasis-altering medications, including ketorolac. |
| Unfractionated SQ heparin | Delay procedure for 4–6 h from last dose of 5000 U SQ dose with twice-daily or thrice-daily administration. For higher *prophylaxis* dosing regimens, delay 12 h and check aPTT. For *therapeutic* SQ dosing, delay 24 h and check aPTT. |
| Unfractionated IV heparin | Delay needle/catheter placement 2–4 h after last dose; document normal aPTT. Heparin may be restarted 1 h after procedure. Sustained heparinization with an indwelling neuraxial catheter associated with increased risk; monitor neurologic status aggressively. |
| Dabigatran | Discontinue 5 days before procedure; for shorter time periods, document normal TT. First postoperative dose 24 h and 6 h after catheter removal (whichever is later). |
| Rivaroxaban, apixaban, and edoxaban | Delay needle placement 3 days after discontinuation. Avoid neuraxial catheters during rivaroxaban therapy. First dose 24 h postoperatively and 6 h after catheter removal (whichever is later). |

*aPTT*, Activated partial thromboplastin time; *INR*, international normalized ratio; *IV*, intravenous; *LMWH*, low-molecular-weight heparin; *NSAID*, nonsteroidal antiinflammatory drug; *SC*, subcutaneous; *TT*, thrombin time.

time of administration, and pertinent laboratory values. The plan for reinitiating anticoagulation postpartum must also be considered. Given the limited pharmacologic data on antithrombotic agents in pregnancy and in the absence of a large series of neuraxial techniques in the pregnant population receiving prophylaxis or treatment for venous thromboembolism, it is suggested that existing guidelines be applied to parturients. However, noting that for maternal or fetal indications, the risk of general anesthesia may be greater than neuraxial anesthesia, exceptions/modifications of these guidelines may be appropriate.

## Anesthetic Management of the Anticoagulated Patient

The decision to perform spinal or epidural anesthesia/analgesia and the timing of catheter removal in a patient receiving thromboprophylaxis should be made on an individual basis, weighing the small though definite risk of spinal hematoma with the benefits of regional anesthesia for a specific patient. Alternative anesthetic and analgesic techniques exist for patients considered to be at an unacceptable risk. The patient's coagulation status should be optimized at the time of needle/catheter placement, and the level of anticoagulation carefully monitored during the period of epidural catheterization (Table 92.1). Indwelling catheters should not be removed in the presence of a significant coagulopathy. In addition, communication between clinicians involved in the perioperative management of patients receiving anticoagulants is essential in order to decrease the risk of serious hemorrhagic complications. If spinal hematoma is suspected, the treatment is typically immediate decompressive laminectomy. Recovery is unlikely if intervention is postponed for more than 10 to 12 h.

## SUGGESTED READINGS

Horlocker, T. T., Vandermeulen, E., Kopp, S. L., Gogarten, W., Leffert, L. R., & Benzon, H. T. (2018). Regional anesthesia in the patient receiving antithrombotic or thrombolytic therapy: American Society of Regional Anesthesia and Pain Medicine evidence-based guidelines (fourth edition). *Cochrane Database of Systematic Reviews, 43*, 263–309.

Kietaibl, S., Ferrandis, R., Godier, A., Llau, J., Lobo, C., Macfarlane, A. J., et al. (2022). Regional anaesthesia in patients on antithrombotic drugs: Joint ESAIC/ESRA guidelines. *European Journal of Anaesthesiology, 39*, 100–132.

Leffert, L., Horlocker, T., & Landau, R. (2019). Don't throw the baby out with the bathwater: Spinal-epidural hematoma in the setting of obstetric thromboprophylaxis and neuraxial anesthesia. *International Journal of Obstetric Anesthesia, 39*, 7–11.

Moen, V., Dahlgren, N., & Irestedt, L. (2004). Severe neurological complications after central neuraxial blockades in Sweden 1990 to 1999. *Anesthesiology, 101*, 950–959.

Shaw, J. R., Kaplovitch, E., & Douketis, J. (2020). Periprocedural management of oral anticoagulation. *Medical Clinics of North America, 104*, 709–726.

Vandermeulen, E. P., Van Aken, H., & Vermylen, J. (1994). Anticoagulants and spinal-epidural anesthesia. *Anesthesia and Analgesia, 79*(6), 1165–1177. doi:10.1213/00000539-199412000-00024.

# 93

# Brachial Plexus Anatomy

ADAM W. AMUNDSON, MD

A firm understanding of the brachial plexus is important to be proficient in regional anesthesia of the upper extremity. This chapter describes the anatomy of the brachial plexus and important branching neural structures.

## Anatomy of the Brachial Plexus

The brachial plexus is formed by the ventral rami of the fifth to eighth cervical nerves and the greater part of the ramus of the first thoracic nerve. Additionally, small contributions to the brachial plexus may come from the fourth cervical and second thoracic nerves (Fig. 93.1). The complexity of the brachial plexus occurs as the ventral rami emerge from between the middle and anterior scalene muscles until they end in the five terminal branches to the upper extremity: the axillary, musculocutaneous, median, radial, and ulnar nerves (see Fig. 93.1).

After the roots pass between the scalene muscles, they reorganize into the superior, middle, and inferior trunks and continue toward the first rib. At the lateral edge of the first rib, these trunks undergo a primary anatomic division into anterior and posterior divisions. This anatomic division is significant because nerves destined to supply the originally ventral part of the upper extremity separate from those that supply the dorsal

part (Fig. 93.2). As these divisions course under the clavicle and enter the axilla, the divisions become three cords. The posterior divisions of all three trunks unite to form the posterior cord, the anterior divisions of the superior and middle trunks form the lateral cord, and the medial cord is the anterior division of the inferior trunk. These cords are named according to their relationship to the second part of the axillary artery.

At the lateral border of the pectoralis minor muscle, the three cords reorganize to give rise to the peripheral nerves of the upper extremity. The branches of the lateral and medial cords are all "ventral" nerves to the upper extremity. The posterior cord, in contrast, provides all "dorsal" innervation to the upper extremity. Posterior cord terminal nerves include the axillary nerve, which provides innervation to several shoulder muscles, and the radial nerve, which innervates all the dorsal musculature in the upper extremity below the shoulder. From the lateral cord, the musculocutaneous nerve supplies muscular innervation in the arm while providing cutaneous innervation within the forearm. In contrast, the median nerve (from the lateral and medial cords) and the ulnar nerve (the terminal branch of the medial cord) are nerves of passage in the arm, but in the forearm and hand they provide motor innervation to the ventral musculature. These nerves can be further characterized,

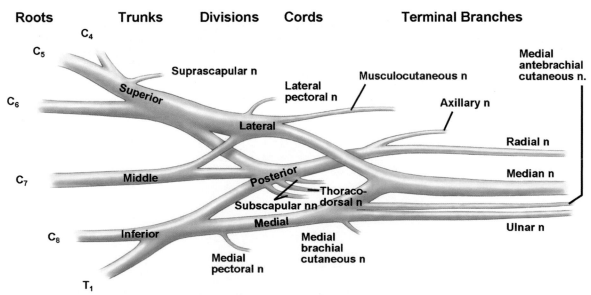

**Fig. 93.1** Brachial plexus schema showing the ventral rami of the spinal nerves branching from the five main roots into three trunks, then six divisions, then three cords, and finally into terminal branches. (From Torsher LC, Smith HM & Jacob AK. Chapter 10: Interscalene Blockade. In: Hebl JR & Lennon RL, editors. Mayo Clinic Atlas of Regional Anesthesia and Ultrasound-Guided Nerve Block. New York: Oxford University Press, 2010, p. 192; used with permission of Mayo Foundation for Medical Education and Research, all rights reserved.)

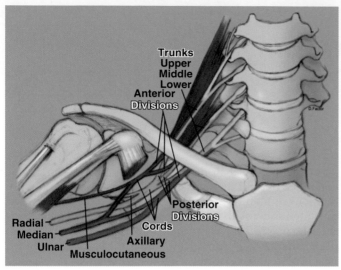

**Fig. 93.2** Anatomic relationships of the brachial plexus as it is formed from medial to lateral.

with the median nerve innervating primarily the forearm, and the ulnar nerve innervates more heavily in the hand. See Chapter 94, Upper Extremity Blocks, for details about the brachial plexus and upper extremity peripheral nerve blocks.

## Anatomy of the Brachial Plexus With Clinical Correlations

The phrenic nerve is formed from branches of the third, fourth, and fifth cervical nerves, and it passes through the neck on the ventral surface of the anterior scalene muscle, descending through the superior thoracic aperture, and eventually runs between the mediastinal pleura and the pericardium. It is often sonographically viewed next to the fifth cervical nerve when performing an interscalene nerve block. Caution or even contraindication to interscalene nerve blockade should be considered in patients with moderate to severe obstructive lung disease as the phrenic nerve, which innervates the diaphragm, is commonly anesthetized with this block. Further, the dorsal scapular (C5 with frequent contribution from C4) and long thoracic nerves (C5, C6, and C7) both branch off of the brachial plexus at the level of the nerve roots and descend into the belly of the middle scalene muscle. Cases have been reported where both have been injured during interscalene nerve blockade when the needle trajectory to the plexus passed through the middle scalene muscle. Injury to the long thoracic and dorsal scapular nerves are clinically relevant complications causing *winged scapula*, or disruption to shoulder muscle stabilization, with marked consequences to postoperative rehabilitation.

Knowledge of the anatomy of the brachial plexus can be invaluable for selective regional anesthesia techniques for key nerves to the upper extremity and thorax. For instance, the long thoracic, medial pectoral, and lateral pectoral nerves innervate a significant portion of the anterior chest wall that can be purposely blocked for surgical cases such as mastectomy or pacemaker placement. Also, the suprascapular nerve (C5, C6) branches from the superior trunk and covers up to 70% of innervation to the shoulder, and the axillary nerve (C5, C6) covers approximately 20% of shoulder innervation. This anatomic knowledge is useful when an interscalene block is contraindicated, as described earlier, secondary to potential pulmonary compromise, because both nerves can be individually blocked more distally and may still be of value for pain management after shoulder surgery.

## SUGGESTED READINGS

Brown, D. L. (2006). Upper extremity block anatomy. In D. L. Brown (Eds.), *Atlas of regional anesthesia* (3rd ed., pp. 25–36). Philadelphia: Elsevier Saunders.

Hebl, J. R., & Lennon, R. L. (Eds.), (2009). *Mayo Clinic atlas of regional anesthesia and ultrasound-guided nerve blockade.* Rochester, MN: Mayo Clinic Scientific Press.

Kessler, J., Schafhalter-Zoppoth, I., & Gray, A. T. (2008). An ultrasound study of the phrenic nerve in the posterior cervical triangle: Implications for the interscalene brachial plexus block. *Regional Anesthesia and Pain Medicine, 33*, 545–550.

Neal, J. M. (2009). The upper extremity: Somatic blockade. In M. J. Cousins, D. B. Carr, T. T. Horlocker, P. O. Bridenbaugh (Eds.), *Cousins and Bridenbaugh's neural blockade in clinical anesthesia and pain medicine* (4th ed., pp. 316–342). Philadelphia: Lippincott Williams & Wilkins.

# 94

# Upper Extremity Blocks

ADAM W. AMUNDSON, MD  |  SANDRA L. KOPP, MD

## Interscalene Brachial Plexus Block

The interscalene approach to the brachial plexus (Fig. 94.1), at the level of the roots/trunks, is best suited for operations on the shoulder (Fig. 94.2). At this level, blockade of the inferior trunk (C8–T1) (Table 94.1) is often incomplete, requiring supplementation of the ulnar nerve for adequate anesthesia of the forearm and hand. Advantages of this block include easily obtainable sonographic imaging of the brachial plexus and the ability to perform the block with the patient's arm in any position, which is especially relevant for cases involving upper extremity trauma or other painful conditions.

## TECHNIQUE

The patient is positioned supine with the head elevated at approximately 30 degrees and turned toward the contralateral shoulder. This block is commonly performed with the use of ultrasound guidance and/or nerve stimulator to accurately place the local anesthetic solution next to the nerves. It is easiest to obtain a sonographic supraclavicular view (see description later) of the subclavian artery and brachial plexus and then track the plexus proximal until the plexus roots/trunks are visualized as hypoechoic structures between the anterior and medial scalene muscles (Fig. 94.3A, B). A 22-gauge, 4- to 5-cm

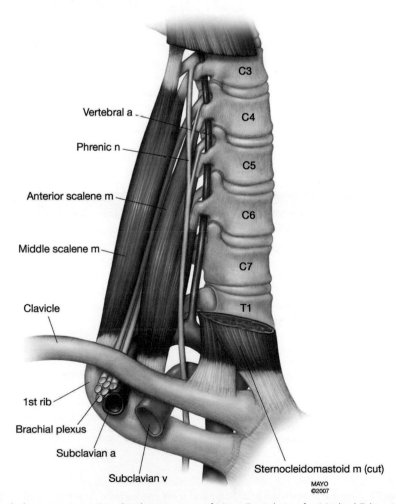

Vertebral a
Phrenic n
Anterior scalene m
Middle scalene m
Clavicle
1st rib
Brachial plexus
Subclavian a
Subclavian v

C3
C4
C5
C6
C7
T1
Sternocleidomastoid m (cut)

MAYO
©2007

**Fig. 94.1** Brachial plexus anatomy. (Used with permission of Mayo Foundation for Medical Education and Research.)

**303**

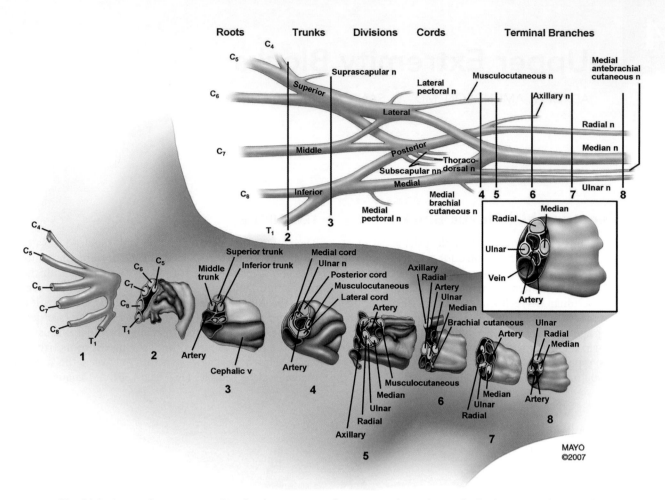

**Fig. 94.2**   Interscalene anatomy. (Used with permission of Mayo Foundation for Medical Education and Research.)

| TABLE 94.1 | Regional Anesthetic Techniques for Upper Extremity Operations | | | |
|---|---|---|---|---|
| Brachial Plexus Technique | Level of Blockade | Peripheral Nerves Blocked | Surgical Applications | Comments |
| Axillary | Distal branches | Radial, ulnar, median; musculocutaneous unreliably blocked if only using nerve stimulator | Operations of the forearm and hand | Unsuitable for proximal humerus or shoulder surgery Requires patient to abduct the arm |
| Infraclavicular | Cords | Radial, ulnar, median, musculocutaneous, axillary | Operations of the midhumerus, elbow, forearm, and hand | Can be a deep block, easier to perform if the arm is abducted |
| Supraclavicular | Divisions | Radial, ulnar, median, musculocutaneous, axillary | Operations of the midhumerus, elbow, forearm, and hand | Risk of pneumothorax requires caution in ambulatory patients Phrenic nerve paresis in up to 30% of cases |
| Interscalene | Roots/trunks | Radial, median, musculocutaneous, axillary; spares ulnar nerve | Surgery to shoulder, proximal and mid humerus | Phrenic nerve paresis in up to 100% of patients for duration of the block Unsuitable for patients unable to tolerate a 25% reduction in pulmonary function |

Adapted from Kopp SL, Horlocker TT. Regional anaesthesia in day-stay and short-stay surgery. *Anaesthesia.* 2010;65(suppl 1):84–96.

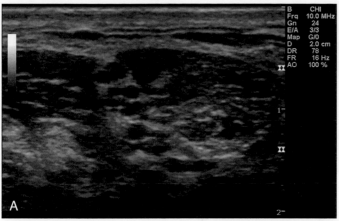

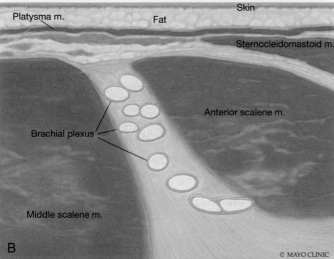

**Fig. 94.3**  Ultrasound-guided interscalene block. **A**, Ultrasound image. **B**, Corresponding anatomy. (Used with permission of Mayo Foundation for Medical Education and Research.)

short-bevel needle is advanced near the plexus in a short-axis view with the needle advanced in an out-of-plane or in-plane approach to a depth of approximately 1 to 3 cm in most patients. After negative aspiration, an incremental bolus of local anesthetic (typically 5–15 mL) is administered under dynamic ultrasound visualization to confirm proper placement of local anesthetic.

## SIDE EFFECTS AND COMPLICATIONS

Nerve damage or neuritis can occur secondary to needle trauma or pharmacologic toxicity but is uncommon and usually self-limited. Local anesthetic toxicity as a result of intravascular injection should be guarded against by careful aspiration and incremental injection. The phrenic nerve is frequently blocked because of its anatomic proximity on the anterior surface of the anterior scalene muscle, which may result in subjective shortness of breath in a healthy patient. The risk of pneumothorax is low when the needle is correctly placed at the C5 or C6 level because of the distance from the dome of the pleura. Blockade of the vagus, recurrent laryngeal, and cervical sympathetic nerves, as well as epidural and intrathecal injection, have been reported during this block. Reports of catastrophic nerve damage resulting from cord injection or high-dose spinal injections

underscore that *performing this block in a heavily sedated or anesthetized patient is advised against.*

## Supraclavicular Brachial Plexus Block

Because of the compact arrangement of the trunks/divisions of the brachial plexus at the level of the first rib, the supraclavicular approach is extremely efficient with relatively small volumes of local anesthetic, resulting in rapid and profound neural blockade. The supraclavicular approach provides excellent surgical anesthesia for the elbow, forearm, and hand (Table 94.1).

### TECHNIQUE

The trunks/divisions of the brachial plexus are compactly arranged cephaloposterior and around the subclavian artery at the level of the first rib, inferior to the clavicle at approximately its midpoint (Fig. 94.4). The use of ultrasound for the supraclavicular block allows the practitioner to visualize the brachial plexus structures to be blocked, as well as the subclavian artery and pleura, just above and below the first rib, respectively. The patient is positioned in the supine position with the head turned toward the contralateral shoulder and the arm adducted and stretched as far as possible toward the ipsilateral knee. The ultrasound probe is placed just cephalad and parallel to the clavicle. The probe is moved medially and laterally until the plexus is viewed just lateral to the subclavian artery. The needle is advanced in plane, lateral to medial, toward the plexus. After negative aspiration, 20 to 40 mL of local anesthetic agent is injected around the plexus; spread around the neural structures can be seen on the ultrasound (Fig. 94.5).

### SIDE EFFECTS AND COMPLICATIONS

The major complication associated with supraclavicular blockade is pneumothorax, which usually presents in the postoperative period. The incidence ranges from 0.5% to 6%, decreasing with the experience of the practitioner. Blockade of the phrenic (50%–60%), recurrent laryngeal, and cervical sympathetic nerves is a minor inconvenience requiring often only reassurance in a healthy patient. Nerve damage is uncommon and usually transient. Practitioners may wish to be mindful of high injection pressures and also consider limiting bolus volumes of local anesthesia, as pressure ischemia has been reported. Intravascular injection is largely preventable by careful technique, including the use of test doses, aspiration, and incremental injection.

## Infraclavicular Brachial Plexus Block

Although deeper than the supraclavicular approach, the compact arrangement of the brachial plexus cords near and around the axillary artery inferior and caudal to the clavicle provides an efficient single-injection block with a fast onset, as well as an ideal location for a continuous catheter. The infraclavicular approach provides surgical anesthesia for the elbow, forearm, and hand (Table 94.1).

### TECHNIQUE

The cords of the brachial plexus inferior to the clavicle are compactly arranged adjacent to the axillary artery (proximal) and as the nerves course distally with orientation around the axillary artery.

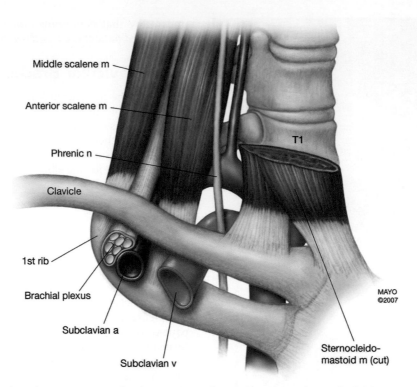

**Fig. 94.4**   Supraclavicular anatomy. (Used with permission of Mayo Foundation for Medical Education and Research.)

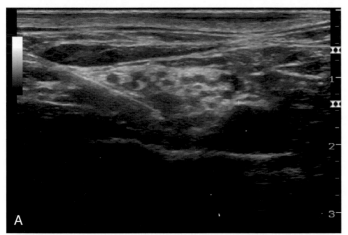

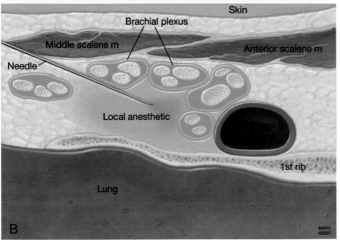

**Fig. 94.5**   Ultrasound-guided supraclavicular block. **A,** Ultrasound image showing injection of local anesthetic around neural structures. **B,** Corresponding anatomy. (Used with permission of Mayo Foundation for Medical Education and Research.)

The use of ultrasound guidance for the infraclavicular block allows the practitioner to visualize the brachial plexus structures to be anesthetized, as well as the axillary artery and vein (Fig. 94.6). The patient is positioned in the supine position with the head turned away from the side to be blocked and the arm abducted if possible, to displace the clavicle and improve imaging. The ultrasound probe is placed just caudal to the lateral third of the clavicle in a long-axis orientation. The probe is moved medially and laterally until the axillary artery is easily viewed under the pectoralis minor. The needle is advanced in plane, cranial to caudal, to the location between the posterior cord and the axillary artery (6 o'clock position). After negative aspiration, typically 30 to 40 mL of local anesthetic agent is often needed for primary anesthesia.

## SIDE EFFECTS AND COMPLICATIONS

Although rare, the major complications associated with infraclavicular blockade are pneumothorax, phrenic nerve blockade, and nerve damage. Intravascular injection is largely preventable by careful technique, including the use of a test dose, aspiration, and incremental injection.

## Axillary Brachial Plexus Block

The axillary approach to the brachial plexus is used because of its ease of performance, safety, and reliability, particularly for hand and forearm surgery (see Table 94.1). A variety of approaches to the axillary block have been described, including elicitation of paresthesias, transarterial injection, sheath blocks, the use of a nerve stimulator, and the use of ultrasound guidance. In experienced hands, all approaches to the axillary block seem to result in a reasonable success rate; however, given there is considerable anatomic variation from individual to individual, the use of ultrasound may provide advantages to the other, more traditional approaches for practitioners infrequently using this technique.

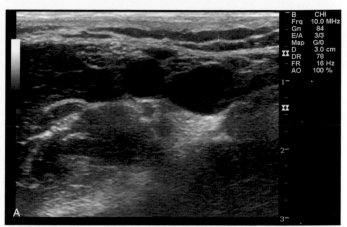

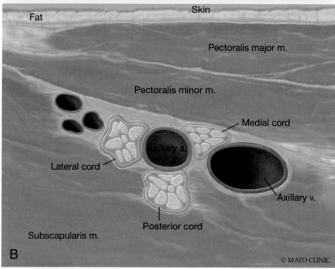

**Fig. 94.6** Ultrasound-guided infraclavicular block. **A,** Ultrasound image **B,** Corresponding anatomy. (Used with permission of Mayo Foundation for Medical Education and Research, all rights reserved.)

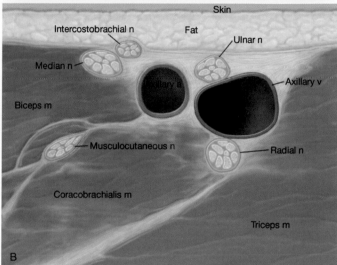

**Fig. 94.7** Ultrasound-guided axillary block. **A,** Ultrasound image. **B,** Corresponding anatomy. (Used with permission of Mayo Foundation for Medical Education and Research, all rights reserved.)

## TECHNIQUE

For all approaches to the axillary block, the patient is positioned supine with the arm to be anesthetized abducted at right angles with the body and the elbow flexed to 90 degrees to allow access to the neurovascular bundle within the axilla. The axillary artery is palpated as close to the axillary crease as possible, and a line is drawn tracing the course of the artery distally.

The ultrasound approach to the axillary block involves visualizing the axillary artery and surrounding distinct neural structures at various positions relative to the artery. The block requires several needle redirections to adequately deposit local anesthetic agent. The ultrasound probe is placed just distal and parallel to the axillary crease at a point that best identifies the artery in proximity to the median, ulnar, and radial nerves (Fig. 94.7). The needle is advanced in an in-plane approach to individually block each nerve (total local anesthetic volume of typically 30–50 mL for primary anesthesia). Alternatively, a perivascular approach to depositing local anesthesia posterior to the axillary artery (6 o'clock position) and anteromedial to the artery has been suggested to be equally efficacious to the perineural approach. Further consideration for upper arm analgesia (e.g., tourniquet-related pain or axillary fistula formation) requires additional separate injections in order to block the cutaneous innervation of the musculocutaneous nerve, medial brachial cutaneous nerve, and intercostobrachial nerve. The musculocutaneous nerve can be identified by scanning further laterally within the coracobrachialis muscle, whereas the medial brachial cutaneous nerve (branch of medial cord) and the intercostobrachial nerve (T2), which provide cutaneous sensation to the anteromedial and posteromedial portion of the upper arm, lie in a separate more superficial plane away from the brachial plexus between the latissimus dorsi muscle and subcutaneous tissue.

## SIDE EFFECTS AND COMPLICATIONS

Because of the large volumes of local anesthetic often recommended for axillary blocks, the proximity of large blood vessels and the popularity of "immobile" needle techniques, local anesthetic toxicity from rapid uptake or intravascular injection may be a higher risk with this technique, compared with other approaches to the brachial plexus. Frequent aspiration combined with incremental injection is an important feature of any method used for a brachial plexus block. Hematoma, sometimes with associated vascular compromise of the upper extremity, and infection are rare but reported complications.

## SUGGESTED READINGS

El-Boghdadly, K., Chin, K. J., & Chan, V. W. (2017). Phrenic nerve palsy and regional anesthesia for shoulder surgery: Anatomic, physiologic, and clinical considerations. *Anesthesiology, 127,* 173–191.

Franco, C. D., & Williams, J. M. (2016). Ultrasound-guided interscalene block: Reevaluation of the "stoplight" sign and clinical implications. *Regional Anesthesia & Pain Medicine, 41,* 452–459.

Magazzeni, P., Jochum, D., Iohom, G., Mekler, G., Albuisson, E., & Bouaziz, H. (2018). Ultrasound-guided selective versus conventional block of the medial brachial cutaneous and the intercostobrachial nerves: A randomized clinical trial. *Regional Anesthesia & Pain Medicine, 43,* 832–837.

McCartney, C. J., Lin, L., & Shastri, U. (2010). Evidence basis for the use of ultrasound for upper-extremity blocks. *Regional Anesthesia & Pain Medicine, 35,* S10–S15.

Neal, J. M., Brull, R., Horn, J. L., Liu, S. S., McCartney, C. J., Perlas, A., et al. (2016). The second American Society of Regional Anesthesia and Pain Medicine evidence-based medicine assessment of ultrasound-guided regional anesthesia: Executive summary. *Regional Anesthesia & Pain Medicine, 41,* 181–194.

Panchamia, J. K., Amundson, A. W., Jacob, A. K., Sviggum, H. P., Nguyen, N. T. V., Sanchez-Sotelo, J., et al. (2019). A 3-arm randomized clinical trial comparing interscalene blockade techniques with local infiltration analgesia for total shoulder arthroplasty. *Journal of Shoulder and Elbow Surgery, 28,* e325–e338.

Sehmbi, H., Johnson, M., & Dhir, S. (2019). Ultrasound-guided subomohyoid suprascapular nerve block and phrenic nerve involvement: A cadaveric dye study. *Regional Anesthesia & Pain Medicine, 44,* 561–564.

Tran, D. Q., Elgueta, M. F., Aliste, J., & Finlayson, R. J. (2017). Diaphragm-sparing nerve blocks for shoulder surgery. *Regional Anesthesia & Pain Medicine, 42,* 32–38.

# 95

# Peripheral Nerve Blocks of the Posterior Trunk

ALBERTO E. ARDON, MD, MPH  |  ROY A. GREENGRASS, MD, FRCP

## Introduction

The use of peripheral nerve blocks for surgery of the chest and abdomen has increased in recent years. Advantages of the use of these techniques include the ability to perform unilateral blockade and therefore decreased risk of sympathectomy. Peripheral nerve blocks of the posterior trunk can be performed in either single or multiple injections or catheter-based fashion, allowing for continuous infusion of local anesthetics if needed.

## Paravertebral Block

### RELEVANT ANATOMY

The paravertebral space is a wedge-shaped anatomic compartment adjacent to the vertebral bodies. The space is defined anterolaterally by the parietal pleura, posteriorly by the superior costotransverse ligament (thoracic levels), medially by the vertebra and intervertebral foramina, and superiorly and inferiorly by the ribs (Fig. 95.1). The paravertebral space contains the spinal nerve root, which branches into dorsal and ventral rami; sympathetic nerve fibers; and intercostal vessels.

### CLINICAL INDICATIONS

Paravertebral blockade (PVB) can provide anesthesia and analgesia for a number of procedures, including breast surgery, herniorrhaphy, thoracotomy/thoracoscopy, and abdominal wall surgery. Additionally, PVB can be useful in patients with multiple rib fractures and associated spinal trauma, in which placement of a thoracic epidural catheter is contraindicated. In this situation, PVB can decrease or eliminate the need for opioid analgesia, which facilitates continuous neurologic assessment.

### REVIEW OF TECHNIQUE

With the patient in the seated position, the spinous process of each level is identified, and a mark is placed at the most superior aspect. The needle insertion point is marked approximately 2.5 cm lateral from the midline. In the thoracic spine, these marks overlie the transverse process (TP) of the immediately caudal vertebra.

#### Landmark Technique

With aseptic technique, a skin wheal is placed at each mark. A 22-gauge Tuohy needle is inserted perpendicular to the skin, with the goal of contacting TP (2–6 cm, depending on body habitus of the patient). As a safety measure, the needle is grasped at a point from its tip that is equal to the estimated depth from the skin to the TP. The needle is inserted to this predicted depth; if TP is not identified, then the needle is redirected in a cephalad-caudad arc. Advancement of no more than 1 cm in depth with each needle redirection

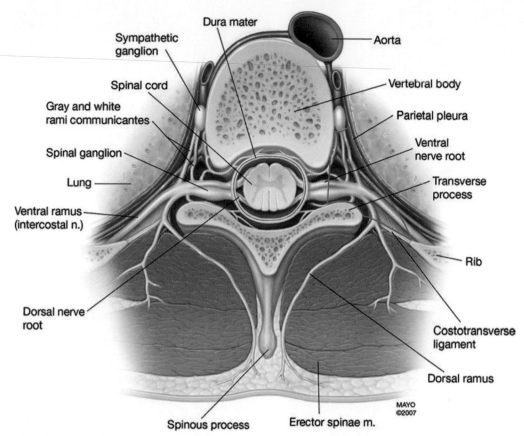

**Fig. 95.1** Cross-section of spine showing location of spinal nerve roots in relation to transverse process. Paravertebral space is highlighted in *blue*. (Courtesy Mayo Clinic.)

is allowed. Once TP is contacted, the needle is withdrawn to subcutaneous tissue and angled in a caudal direction, then slowly advanced with the purpose of entering the paravertebral space at an approximate depth of 1 to 1.5 cm past initial contact with TP. A loss of resistance or "pop" may be appreciated as the needle traverses the superior costotransverse ligament. Once in the paravertebral space, after negative aspiration, 2 to 5 mL of local anesthetic is incrementally injected at each level.

### Ultrasound-Guided Technique

With aseptic technique, an ultrasound probe is positioned in a sagittal orientation 2.5 cm lateral from the midline. The probe can be moved laterally if needed, with rib visualization as the lateral limit for transverse probe movement. With this probe positioning, the paravertebral space can be visualized immediately caudal to the TP, with pleura denoting the anterior border of the space (Fig. 95.2). A 22-gauge Tuohy needle is inserted in a caudal-cranial or cranial-caudal fashion until the tip enters the paravertebral space (Fig. 95.3). After negative aspiration, 2 to 5 mL of local anesthetic is injected. Traditionally, displacement of pleura in a downward direction has been associated with successful performance of PVB. A transverse or oblique approach to the block can also be used. Continuous catheter PVB techniques use an 18-gauge Tuohy needle. A 20-gauge soft-tipped catheter is recommended for reliable positioning in the paravertebral space.

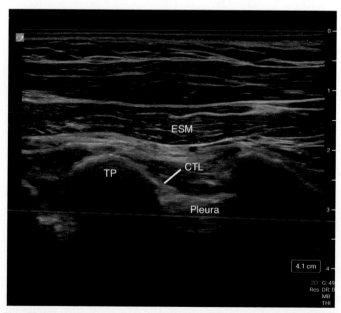

**Fig. 95.2** Sagittal plane view of paravertebral space. Note that this view can be used for either a paravertebral or erector spinae plane block. *CTL*, Costotransverse ligament; *ESM*, erector spinae musculature; *TP*, transverse process.

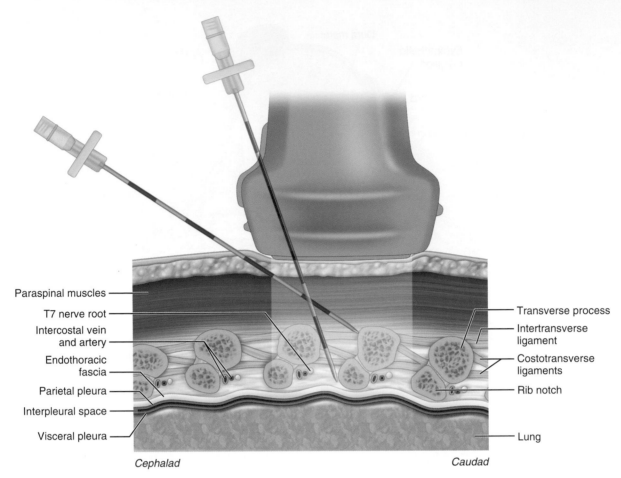

Paraspinal muscles

T7 nerve root

Intercostal vein and artery

Endothoracic fascia

Parietal pleura

Interpleural space

Visceral pleura

Transverse process

Intertransverse ligament

Costotransverse ligaments

Rib notch

Lung

*Cephalad*                    *Caudad*

**Fig. 95.3** Sagittal plane view of ultrasound probe and needle positioning for paravertebral block. (Used with permission of Mayo Foundation for Medical Education and Research, all rights reserved.)

## SIDE EFFECTS AND COMPLICATIONS

Potential complications associated with PVB include vascular puncture and pneumothorax, which are rare with cautious technique. Significant epidural spread may be seen with large-volume blockade.

## Quadratus Lumborum Block

### RELEVANT ANATOMY

The quadratus lumborum (QL) is a posterior abdominal wall muscle that originates from the iliac crest and inserts into the 12th rib and TPs of the first to fourth lumbar vertebrae. The QL lies anterior to the erector spinae muscle group (Fig. 95.4). In the three-layer model of the thoracolumbar fascia, the anterior thoracolumbar fascia lies anterior to the QL and psoas muscles; the middle thoracolumbar fascia lies between the erector spinae and QL; and the posterior thoracolumbar fascia lies posterior to the erector spinae muscle group. The iliohypogastric and ilioinguinal nerves course the ventral surface of the QL. The dorsal rami of the spinal nerves are located on the medial aspect of the middle thoracolumbar fascia posterior to the QL. Although the exact mechanism of action of the QL block remains to be elicited, evidence suggests that local anesthetic spread is not confined to the described fascial planes and to the middle

thoracolumbar fascia intertranse area but also may involve the ipsilateral paravertebral space, somatic nerves, and thoracic sympathetic trunk.

## CLINICAL INDICATIONS

The QL block is a relatively recent technique first described in 2007. QL block has been shown to decrease opioid requirements in renal surgery and in cesarean delivery where intrathecal morphine has not been used. Data on the efficacy of this block for hip surgery is conflicting; considerable heterogeneity exists among the orthopedic studies.

## REVIEW OF TECHNIQUE

The patient is positioned lateral, prone, or in the sitting position. Using sterile technique, a curvilinear ultrasound probe is placed at the level of L2–L4 at the posterior or midaxillary line; both sagittal and horizontal probe positions have been described in the literature. The aponeuroses of the abdominal wall muscles, QL and psoas muscles, and the lumbar TPs should be visualized (Fig. 95.5). A 10- to 15-cm 20-gauge needle is used and advanced in an in-plane fashion. For the anterior QL, the needle is advanced into the plane between the

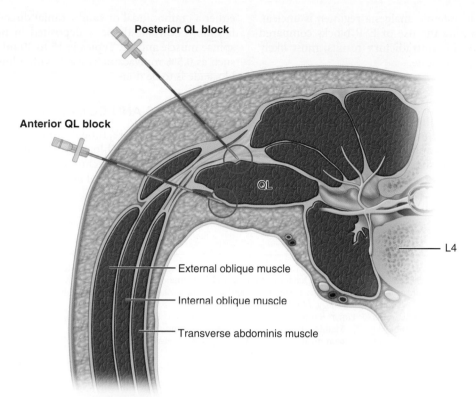

**Fig. 95.4** Transverse plane view showing quadratus lumborum (QL) muscle and needle positioning for anterior QL and posterior QL blocks. (Used with permission of Mayo Foundation for Medical Education and Research, all rights reserved.)

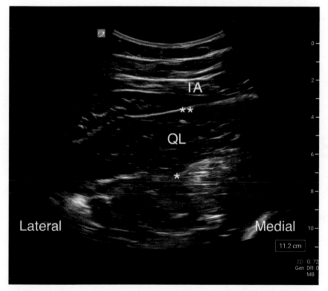

**Fig. 95.5** Transverse-plane ultrasound view of quadratus lumborum (QL). TA, Transversus abdominis muscle; *, endpoint for anterior QL block; **, endpoint for posterior QL block.

psoas and QL muscles. For the posterior QL, the needle is advanced into the plane between the QL and erector spinae muscles. Yet another variation is the lateral QL block, where local anesthetic is deposited between the transversus abdominis aponeurosis and the transversalis fascia. At the target site, 20 to 30 mL of ropivacaine 0.5% or bupivacaine 0.25% is injected. If performing bilateral blockade, consider reducing local anesthetic dosages.

## SIDE EFFECTS AND COMPLICATIONS

Although rare, lower extremity weakness can occur after any QL block. As with any large volume block, local anesthetic systemic toxicity is a potential risk. Despite ultrasound guidance, injury to renal structures remains a potential complication, particularly when performing an anterior QL block. Because the QL block is considered a deep block, care should be taken to follow the American Society of Regional Anesthesia and Pain Medicine guidelines for nerve blockade in the anticoagulated patient to minimize the risk of hematoma.

## Erector Spinae Block

### RELEVANT ANATOMY

The erector spinae muscle group consists of the iliocostalis, longissimus, and spinalis muscles, which extend from the skull to the pelvis along the posterolateral aspect of the spine bilaterally. This muscle group lies directly superficial to the TPs. The erector spinae (ESP) block involves injection of local anesthetic into the fascial plane that lies between the erector spinae muscle and TP (Fig. 95.2). The mechanism of action of the ESP block, though not yet conclusive, is theorized to be anesthetization of the dorsal and ventral rami of the spinal nerves at the involved levels.

### CLINICAL INDICATIONS

The ESP block was first described in 2016. Studies have explored its use in thoracic surgery, breast surgery, and laparoscopic cholecystectomy, with favorable results compared with no blockade. However, the efficacy of ESP block in the presence of a robust multimodal systemic analgesia regimen is unclear. Likewise, studies examining the use of ESP blocks compared with PVB have resulted in contradictory results, most likely because of variations in technique.

## REVIEW OF TECHNIQUE

The patient is positioned in either the sitting or lateral decubitus position. Using sterile technique, an ultrasound probe is placed in a sagittal orientation approximately 3 cm lateral to the midline. The subcutaneous tissue, erector spinae muscle group, and TP are identified. A 21- or 22-gauge needle is introduced in either a craniocaudal or caudocranial direction, in an in-plane fashion. Local anesthetic is deposited in between the erector spinae muscle and TP. Typically 15 to 30 mL of local anesthetic such as 0.5% ropivacaine is used, with a lower dose if bilateral blockade is to be done.

## SIDE EFFECTS AND COMPLICATIONS

The available literature, though limited, suggests that the complication rate after ESP blockade appears to be low. As with any peripheral nerve block technique, the anesthesiologist should be aware of the risk of local anesthetic systemic toxicity.

## SUGGESTED READINGS

Ardon, A. E., Lee, J., Franco, C. D., Riutort, K. T., & Greengrass, R. A. (2020). Paravertebral block: Anatomy and relevant safety issues. *Korean Journal of Anesthesiology, 73*, 394–400.

Chin, K. J., & El-Boghdadly, K. (2021). Mechanisms of action of the erector spinae plane (ESP) block: A narrative review. *Canadian Journal of Anaesthesia, 68*, 387–408.

Elsharkawy, H., El-Boghdadly, K., & Barrington, M. (2019). Quadratus lumborum block: Anatomical concepts, mechanisms, and techniques. *Anesthesiology, 130*, 322–335.

Hojer Karlsen, A. P., Geisler, A., Petersen, P. L., Mathiesen, O., & Dahl, J. B. (2015). Postoperative pain treatment after total hip arthroplasty: A systematic review. *Pain, 156*, 8–30.

Jones, M. R., Hadley, G. R., Kaye, A. D., Lirk, P., & Urman, R. D. (2017). Paravertebral blocks for same-day breast surgery. *Current Pain and Headache Reports, 21*, 35.

# 96

# Peripheral Nerve Blocks of the Anterior Trunk

NIGEL GILLESPIE, MD   |   ALBERTO E. ARDON, MD, MPH

## Introduction

Although neuraxial blockade remains the gold standard for achieving postoperative analgesia of the anterior chest and abdomen, contraindications such as anticoagulation may preclude the use of these techniques. In situations where neuraxial blockade is not feasible, peripheral nerve block options are available. These techniques can provide analgesia of the chest and abdominal wall, producing relief from incisional pain. Both single injection and continuous infusion techniques can be used. Every needle technique and injection of local anesthetic (LA) carries the following basic risks: bleeding, infection, tissue injury, nerve injury, vascular injury, intravascular injection, and LA systemic toxicity.

## Interpectoral, Pectoserratus, and Serratus Anterior Plane Blocks

### NOMENCLATURE

The interpectoral plane (IPP) block has been referred to as Pecs, PECS, PECs, or simply the pectoral nerve block in the literature. For the purposes of this chapter, we will refer to it as the IPP. The IPP had previously been classified as a PECS I block; the pectoserratus plane (PSP) block had previously been labeled as PECS II. The superficial and deep serratus anterior plane (SAP) blocks are associated conceptually with the IPP and PSP blocks but are independent of these techniques.

## RELEVANT ANATOMY

The anterior and lateral chest wall receives sensory innervation from the brachial plexus via the lateral and medial pectoral nerves and from the ventral rami of thoracic spinal nerve roots (T2–T6), which become intercostal nerves with lateral and the anterior cutaneous branches. Additionally, the intercostobrachial branches from the T2 and T3 nerve roots can contribute to anterolateral chest wall sensation approaching the axilla, and the superficial cervical plexus can also contribute to the superior chest wall innervation.

The lateral and medial pectoral nerves reliably pass between the fascial layers of the pectoralis major and pectoralis minor muscle. The thoracoacromial artery or its pectoral branch is also in close relation to these structures. Injection in the plane between the pectoralis major and minor is referred to as an IPP block (previously PECS I block; see Fig. 96.1). Just lateral to the midclavicular line, the serratus anterior muscle lies deep to the pectoralis minor. The lateral cutaneous branches of the dorsal rami that innervate this area course between the fascial layers of the pectoralis minor and serratus anterior muscle. Injection in this plane is labeled as a PSP block (previously PECS II block). Further lateral, in the midaxillary line, the serratus anterior muscle lies deep to the latissimus dorsi muscle and superficial to the ribs. The lateral cutaneous branches of the dorsal rami and the intercostobrachial nerve can be found between the fascial layers of latissimus and serratus, as well as the thoracodorsal artery and nerve and the long thoracic nerve. Injection in this plane is called the superficial SAP block.

## CLINICAL APPLICATIONS

IPP, PSP, and SAP blocks can provide effective analgesia for breast and lateral chest wall surgery by relieving both incisional and muscular pain. There is some evidence to suggest SAP blocks may be helpful in rib fractures. We suggest 15 to 20 mL of long-acting, low-concentration LA per injection while staying within the maximum total dose guidelines to minimize risk of LA toxicity.

## REVIEW OF TECHNIQUE

With the patient in the supine position, a linear high-frequency ultrasound (US) probe is placed in a sagittal orientation below the clavicle at the midclavicular line. Needling and injection should be performed using sterile or aseptic technique.

### Interpectoral Block

The pectoralis major and minor muscles are visualized (see Fig. 96.2). The probe can be adjusted slightly cranial and lateral as needed to visualize the thoracoacromial artery or its pectoral branch in this fascial layer. Nerve structures may also be visualized in this plane. Color Doppler can be helpful in identifying the thoracodorsal artery if it is not readily visible with probe adjustment. The needle is then advanced from cranial to caudal using an in-plane technique (or from anterior to posterior using an out-of-plane technique) until the tip terminates in the fascial layer between the pectoralis major and pectoralis minor. After negative aspiration, LA is injected with resultant separation of these two muscles.

### Pectoserratus Block

The US probe is placed below the clavicle in a sagittal orientation just lateral to the midclavicular line. The pectoralis major, pectoralis minor, and serratus anterior muscles are visualized. The probe can be adjusted laterally as needed. The needle is advanced to the fascial layer between the pectoralis minor and serratus anterior muscles. After negative aspiration, LA is injected with resultant separation of the fascial layer. An IPP block can be performed concurrently, as described earlier.

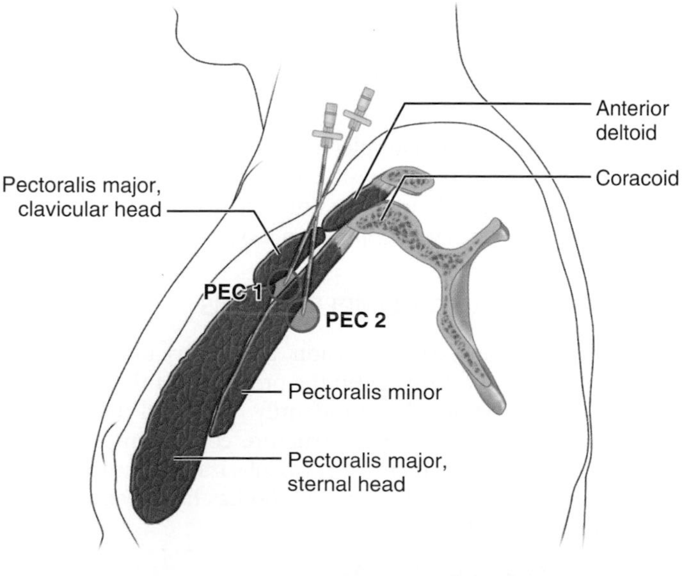

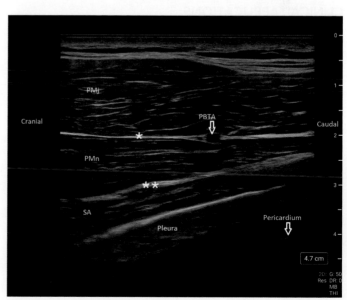

**Fig. 96.1** Illustration of thoracic wall in sagittal plane. Needle tips indicate end points for PECS I (now referred to as interpectoral plane block) and PECS II (now referred to as pectoserratus plane block) blocks, respectively. (Used with permission of Mayo Foundation for Medical Education and Research, all rights reserved.)

**Fig. 96.2** Parasagittal view of anterior chest wall for pectoralis plane block. *PBTA*, Pectoral branch of the thoracoacromial artery; *PMj*, Pectoralis major muscle; *PMn*, pectoralis minor muscle; *SA*, serratus anterior muscle; *, needle end point for interpectoral plane block; **, needle end point for pectoserratus plane block.

## Superficial Serratus Anterior Plane Block

The US probe is placed in a sagittal orientation approaching the midaxillary line at the level of the fourth to sixth ribs. The latissimus dorsi and serratus anterior muscles are visualized in addition to the ribs. Color Doppler can be helpful in identifying the thoracodorsal artery if it is not readily visible with probe adjustment. The needle is advanced from cranial to caudal using an in-plane technique (or from anterior to posterior using an out-of-plane technique) until the tip terminates in the fascial layer between latissimus dorsi and serratus anterior. Injection on the surface of the rib just inferior to the serratus anterior results in a deep SAP block. After negative aspiration, LA is injected.

## SIDE EFFECTS AND COMPLICATIONS

Pneumothorax and scapular winging due to long thoracic nerve blockade are possible, albeit rare, complications of this block.

## Parasternal Intercostal Plane Block

### RELEVANT ANATOMY

The anterior cutaneous branches of the intercostal nerves provide sensation to the anterior ribs, sternum, and anterior cutaneous region of the chest (T2–T6) and reliably are found deep to the internal intercostal muscle and superficial to the transversus thoracis muscle just lateral to the sternum. The internal thoracic artery and vein are also found in this plane. The transversus thoracis fascia is contiguous with the fascia of the innermost intercostal muscle. The anterior cutaneous branches of the intercostal nerves continue superficially through the external intercostal muscles and can be found deep to the pectoralis major. Parasternal injection between the internal intercostal muscle and transversus thoracis muscle is called a deep parasternal intercostal plane (PIP) block. Parasternal injection between the pectoralis major and external intercostal muscle is called a superficial PIP block.

### CLINICAL APPLICATIONS

These blocks provide effective chest wall analgesia for surgery requiring sternotomy. There is some evidence to suggest they facilitate earlier postoperative extubation. We suggest 15 to 20 mL of long-acting, low-concentration LA per injection while staying within the maximum total dose guidelines to minimize risk of LA toxicity. For superficial PIP blocks multiple injections per side may be necessary for complete analgesic coverage. We suggest no more than 5 mL of long-acting, low-concentration anesthetic per injection site while staying within the maximum total dose guidelines.

### REVIEW OF TECHNIQUE

Bowel perforation and rectus sheath hematoma are possible complications of this blocka linear high-frequency US probe is used to acquire images. Needling and injection should be performed using sterile or aseptic technique.

#### Superficial Parasternal Intercostal Plane

The probe is placed in the sagittal orientation just lateral to the sternum at the level of the targeted intercostal space (T2–T6) (see Fig. 96.3a). Once the ribs are seen in cross section and the intercostal space is identified, the needle is advanced in plane

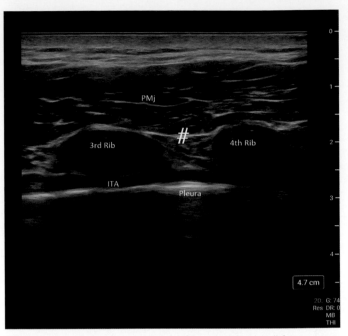

**Fig. 96.3a** Initial parasagittal view of anterior chest wall for parasternal intercostal plane (PIP) block. *ITA,* Internal thoracic artery; *PMj,* pectoralis major muscle; *#,* needle end point for superficial PIP block.

until the tip terminates between the pectoralis major muscle and the external intercostal muscle. After negative aspiration, LA is injected. Alternatively, the superior border of the rib just deep to the pectoralis major can be used as the target for the needle tip termination with confirmed spread of LA beneath the pectoralis muscle.

#### Deep Parasternal Intercostal Plane

The probe is placed in the sagittal orientation just lateral to the sternum at the level of the third and fourth ribs (see Fig. 96.3a). Once the ribs are seen in cross section and the intercostal space is identified, the probe is then rotated over the intercostal space to the transverse orientation. Small adjustments are made until the internal thoracic artery is visible between the layers of the inner intercostal muscle and the transversus thoracis muscle (see Fig. 96.3b). Color Doppler can be helpful in identifying the artery if it is not readily visible with probe adjustment. The needle is then advanced in plane until the tip terminates in this fascial layer. After negative aspiration, LA is injected.

### SIDE EFFECTS AND COMPLICATIONS

Pneumothorax, pericardial effusion, and ventricular puncture are possible complications given the proximity of the heart and lungs. Care should be taken to identify and avoid the internal thoracic artery. Injury to this structure could compromise a primary graft target in planned revascularization surgeries and could be catastrophic for a patient who has had revascularization with this vessel.

## Rectus Sheath Block

### RELEVANT ANATOMY

The ventral rami of the T6/7–T12 nerve roots give rise to the anterior and lateral cutaneous branches of nerves that provide

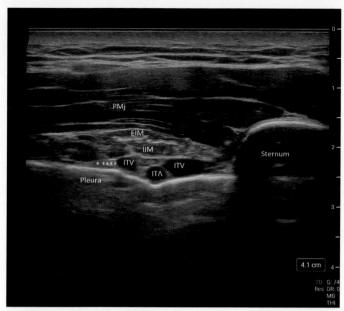

**Fig. 96.3b** Transverse view of anterior chest wall for parasternal intercostal plane (PIP) block. *EIM*, External intercostal muscle; *IIM*, internal intercostal muscle; *ITA*, internal thoracic artery; *ITV*, internal thoracic vein; *PMj*, pectoralis major muscle; *****, needle end point for deep PIP block.

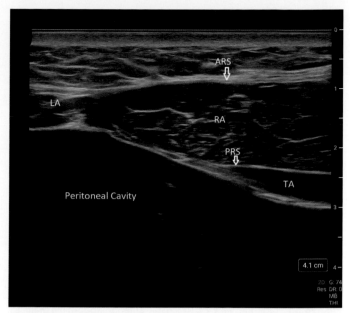

**Fig. 96.4** Transverse view of anterior abdominal wall for rectus sheath block. *ARS*, Anterior rectus sheath; *LA*, linea alba; *PRS*, posterior rectus sheath; *RA*, rectus abdominis muscle; *TA*, transversus abdominis muscle. Arrow indicates needle end point.

sensory innervation to the anterior abdominal wall. The rectus abdominis muscle extends from pubis to sternum and is enveloped by an anterior and posterior sheath above the level of the arcuate line. The posterior rectus sheath contains the anterior cutaneous nerves and the superior and inferior epigastric vessels.

## CLINICAL APPLICATIONS

The rectus sheath block provides cutaneous and some superficial abdominal wall muscle analgesia for surgery requiring a midline incision. There is some limited evidence to suggest it has analgesic utility in laparoscopic surgery as well. We suggest 15 to 20 mL of low-concentration LA per injection while staying within the maximum total dose guidelines to minimize risk of LA toxicity.

## REVIEW OF TECHNIQUE

The patient is placed in the supine position and a linear high-frequency US probe is used to acquire images. Needling and injection should be performed using sterile or aseptic technique.

The US probe is placed in the transverse orientation in the midline just above the umbilicus. The linea alba should be visible. The probe is moved laterally until the rectus abdominis muscle is visualized. The anterior rectus sheath should be visible superficial to the muscle; the posterior rectus sheath will lie deep to the muscle (see Fig. 96.4). The inferior epigastric vessels may be visible in this plane. The needle is advanced anterior to posterior, either in or out of plane, until the tip terminates in the posterior rectus sheath. After negative aspiration, LA is injected.

## SIDE EFFECTS AND COMPLICATIONS

Bowel perforation and rectus sheath hematoma are possible complications of this block.

## Transversus Abdominis Plane Block

### RELEVANT ANATOMY

The lateral abdominal wall has three major muscles: external oblique, internal oblique, and transversus abdominis. The fascial layer between the internal oblique muscle and the transversus abdominis muscle contains the lateral cutaneous and anterior cutaneous branches of the intercostal nerves (T6/7–T12) that provide sensation to the anterior abdominal wall. The peritoneal cavity lies deep to the transversus abdominis muscle. Analgesic distribution of the transversus abdominis plane (TAP) block will depend on the site of injection given the broad area of coverage. A more superior and anterior injection site such as subcostal may provide better superior and anterior analgesic coverage. Likewise, a more lateral and inferior injection site may provide better lateral and inferior abdominal wall analgesia.

### CLINICAL APPLICATIONS

The TAP block provides cutaneous and some superficial abdominal wall muscle analgesia. There is some evidence it can decrease postoperative opioid use after a variety of abdominal surgeries. However, some evidence suggests the TAP block provides minimal to no analgesic benefit in laparoscopic surgery and is likely equivalent to multimodal analgesia. We suggest 15 to 20 mL of low-concentration, long-acting LA bilaterally while staying within the maximum total dose guidelines to minimize risk of LA toxicity.

### REVIEW OF TECHNIQUE

The patient is placed in the supine position and a linear high-frequency US probe is used to acquire images. In the presence of a larger body habitus, a curvilinear probe may be more effective for visualizing the muscular layers. Needling and injection should be performed using sterile or aseptic technique.

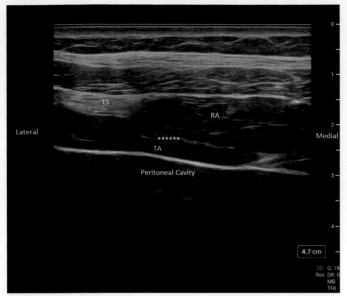

**Fig. 96.5a** Oblique view of subcostal anterior abdominal wall. *LS,* Linea semilunaris; *RA,* rectus abdominis muscle; *TA,* transversus abdominis muscle; \*\*\*\*\*\*, needle end point for subcostal TAP block.

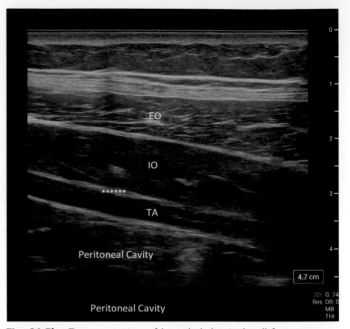

**Fig. 96.5b** Transverse view of lateral abdominal wall for transversus abdominis (TAP) block. *EO,* External oblique muscle; *IO,* internal oblique muscle; *TA,* transversus abdominis muscle; \*\*\*\*\*\*, needle end point for midaxillary TAP block.

### Subcostal Approach

The probe is placed in the transverse orientation underneath the xiphoid process. The rectus muscles and linea alba are visualized. The probe is then moved laterally and in an oblique fashion to remain parallel to and underneath the costal margin. As the anterior and posterior rectus sheaths converge into the linea semilunaris, the external oblique, internal oblique, and transversus abdominis muscles become visible (see Fig. 96.5a: US of subcostal TAP). The needle is advanced from anterior to posterior, either in plane or out of plane, until the tip terminates in the fascial layer between the internal oblique and transversus abdominis. After negative aspiration, LA is injected.

### Midaxillary Approach

The probe is placed in the transverse orientation on the lateral abdomen along the anterior axillary line. The external oblique, internal oblique, and transversus abdominis muscles are visualized (see Fig. 96.5b). The needle is advanced from anterior to posterior, either in plane or out of plane, until the tip terminates in the fascial layer between the internal oblique and transversus abdominis muscles. After negative aspiration, LA is injected.

## SIDE EFFECTS AND COMPLICATIONS

Critically, the TAP block provides no visceral analgesia. Possible complications of this block include bowel perforation.

## Ilioinguinal/Iliohypogastric Nerve Block

### RELEVANT ANATOMY

The ilioinguinal and iliohypogastric nerves are part of the lumbar plexus and originate from the T12 and L1 nerve roots. They pass through the fascial layer between internal oblique and transversus abdominis near the anterior superior iliac spine (ASIS) and are near the deep circumflex branch of the external iliac artery. These nerves provide cutaneous sensation to the hypogastric region, inguinal crease, upper middle thigh, and the base of the genitalia.

## CLINICAL APPLICATIONS

Ilioinguinal and iliohypogastric blocks can provide analgesia for inguinal surgeries and abdominal surgeries that use a subumbilical incision. We suggest 15 to 20 mL of LA per injection while staying within the maximum total dose guidelines to minimize risk of LA toxicity.

## REVIEW OF TECHNIQUE

The patient is placed in the supine position and a linear high-frequency ultrasound probe is used to acquire images. Depending on the patient's body habitus, a curvilinear probe may be more effective for visualizing the muscular layers. Needling and injection should be performed using sterile or aseptic technique.

The probe is placed in a transverse orientation in the lower abdomen with the lateral edge of the probe just medial to ASIS. The probe is moved slightly obliquely toward the umbilicus and adjusted slightly inferiorly until the ilioinguinal and iliohypogastric nerves are seen in the fascial layer between the internal oblique and transversus abdominis muscles. However, one should be aware that these nerves may be difficult to visualize. The needle is advanced from anterior to posterior, either in plane or out of plane, until the tip terminates in the fascial layer between the internal oblique and transversus abdominis. After negative aspiration, 15 to 20 mL of LA is injected.

## SIDE EFFECTS AND COMPLICATIONS

Bowel perforation and urinary retention are potential complications of ilioinguinal and iliohypogastric nerve blocks.

## SUGGESTED READINGS

Chin, K. J., McDonnell, J., Carvalho, B., Sharkey, A., Pawa, A., & Gadsden, J. (2017). Essentials of our current understanding: Abdominal wall blocks. *Regional Anesthesia and Pain Medicine, 42*, 133–183.

Chin, K. J., Versyck, B., & Pawa, A. (2021). Ultrasound-guided fascial plane blocks of the chest wall:

A state-of-the-art review. *Anaesthesia, 76*, 110–126.

Chong, M., Berbenetz, N., Kumar, K., & Lin, C. (2019). The serratus plane block for postoperative analgesia in breast and thoracic surgery: A systematic review and meta-analysis. *Regional Anesthesia and Pain Medicine, 44*, 1066–1074.

Ma, N., Duncan, J., Scarfe, A., Schuhmann, S., & Cameron, A. L. (2017). Clinical safety and effectiveness of transversus abdominis plane (TAP) block in post-operative analgesia: A systematic review and meta-analysis. *Journal of Anesthesia, 31*, 431–452.

# Lower Extremity Peripheral Nerve Blocks

CATHERINE WANJIRU NJATHI-ORI, MD | SANDRA L. KOPP, MD

## Clinical Applications

Peripheral nerve blockade (PNB) of the lower extremity provides selective anesthesia and/or analgesia for procedures from the hip down to the foot. Improving analgesia allows for earlier mobilization and discharge in addition to overall reduction in health care costs.

## Complications

Most PNB share common block-related complications, including inadvertent intravascular injection leading to systemic local anesthesia toxicity (LAST), hematoma formation, infection, neural injury, and "block-specific" complications. Contemporary practice of PNB is primarily completed via ultrasound (US) guidance, although knowledge of nerve stimulator (NS) localization techniques can be invaluable when practicing in locations with limited resources. Additionally, combining NS with US can be helpful in localizing neural targets when visualization with US is poor.

## Posterior Lumbar Plexus Block (Psoas Compartment Block)

First introduced as an alternative to 3-in-1 nerve block, the psoas compartment block (PCB) is an advanced, deep block with similar periprocedural anticoagulation implications as neuraxial procedures. US-guided PCB or alternative blocks have replaced classic NS-guided psoas blocks. Because of the greater depth, proximity to the neuraxial structure, and potential risk to retroperitoneal structures, psoas block requires advanced regional anesthesia training.

### CLINICAL APPLICATIONS

The PCB facilitates complete blockade of the lumbar plexus with a single injection, providing analgesia to the hip and upper thigh. When combined with a sciatic nerve (SN) block, complete anesthesia of the lower extremity may be achieved. The PCB is most used to provide postoperative analgesia for major hip or knee operations.

### RELEVANT ANATOMY

The lumbar plexus, formed from the ventral rami of L1 through L4 with some contributions from T12 and L5 branches, lies anterior to the transverse processes of the lumbar vertebrae and descends vertically with the psoas muscle. The main lumbar plexus nerves are femoral (L2–L4), obturator (L2–L4), lateral femoral cutaneous (L2–L3), iliohypogastric (L1), ilioinguinal (L1), and genitofemoral (L1–L2) (Fig. 97.1). The lumbar plexus provides sensory innervation to the anterior thigh, the medial aspect of the lower leg via the saphenous nerve (distal branch of the femoral nerve [FN]), and the majority of the femur, ischium, and ilium.

### Technique

The patient is positioned laterally (operative side up), with the hips flexed and perpendicular to the horizontal plane. Although there are various approaches to US-guided PCB, because of tissue depth, a curved transducer (5–2 MHz) is typically required. Key sonoanatomic landmarks at the L4 level are skin and subcutaneous tissues, the quadratus lumborum (superficial), the erector spinae (deep and posterior), and the psoas muscle (deep

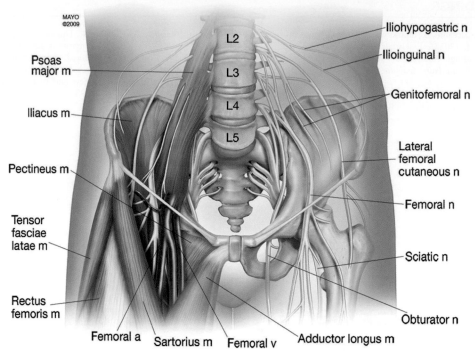

**Fig. 97.1** Anatomy of the lumbar plexus. Used with permission of Mayo Foundation for Medical Education and Research, all rights reserved.

and anterior). Ideally, the target is just lateral to the intervertebral foramen and posterior to the psoas muscle. Using a curvilinear transducer (5–2 MHz) placed parallel to the iliac crest, cephalad and medial scanning is used to identify the transverse process (TP) at L4, the quadratus lumborum (superficial to TP), the erector spinae (deep and posterior), and the psoas muscle (deep and anterior). Using an in-plane approach, the needle is inserted parallel to the intercrestal line, 3 to 4 cm lateral to the midline. The target is posterior to the psoas muscle at the L3 level. Caution to avoid direct trauma to the L3 nerve root or adjacent vasculature is warranted.

## SIDE EFFECTS AND COMPLICATIONS

Due to proximity to the neuraxis, intrathecal injection or epidural spread are potential complications. Factors contributing to epidural spread (incidence 1.8%–16%) include extreme medial needle direction, large local anesthetic (LA) volumes, and spinal deformities. The lumbar plexus is in a deep, highly vascularized location, increasing risk of hemorrhagic complications. Adherence to American Society for Regional Anesthesia and Pain Medicine anticoagulation guidelines may reduce this risk. Given the associated risks, PCB should not be performed under a general anesthetic.

## Femoral Nerve Block

### CLINICAL APPLICATIONS

The femoral nerve block (FNB) is most commonly used for analgesia during knee procedures and can be combined with an SN block for complete analgesia of the lower extremity. The significant quadriceps motor weakness after an FNB has decreased the popularity of this block.

## RELEVANT ANATOMY

Derived from L2 to L4 posterior divisions and forming within the psoas major muscle, the FN is the largest lumbar plexus–derived nerve. Emerging laterally and descending in the groove between the psoas and iliacus muscles, the nerve enters the thigh lateral to the femoral artery. Distal to the inguinal ligament, the FN divides into anterior and posterior branches. The FN supplies sensorimotor innervation to the anterior thigh muscles (quadriceps and sartorius) and skin between the inguinal ligament and the knee. The saphenous nerve, a terminal branch, provides sensory innervation medially below the knee down to the medial malleolus (Fig. 97.2).

## TECHNIQUE

US-guided technique using a high-frequency linear transducer is the preferred method of completing FNB. With the patient supine and the inguinal triangle region exposed, the transducer is placed longitudinally, scanning lateral to medial at the inguinal crease. Ideal sonoanatomy reveals the FN as a honeycombed, often oval-shaped structure immediately lateral to a single femoral artery. An out-of-plane or in-plane approach may be used. With an in-plane approach, the needle is inserted in a lateral to medial direction. The appropriate needle tip location is deep to the fascia iliaca but superficial to the iliacus muscle. A catheter may be placed above or below the nerve for a continuous infusion. Complementary use of both US and NS has the potential to improve nerve detection and may reduce likelihood for intraneural injection with current 0.4 mA or greater. After negative aspiration, 10 to 30 mL of LA solution is injected incrementally.

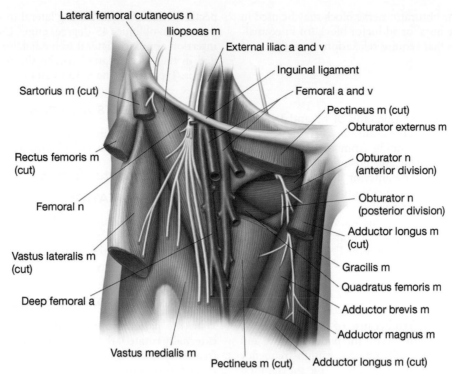

**Fig. 97.2** Neurovascular and muscular anatomy of the femoral region. (Used with permission of Mayo Foundation for Medical Education and Research, all rights reserved.)

## ADVERSE EFFECTS AND COMPLICATIONS

The proximity of the femoral vasculature increases hematoma and intravascular injection risks. Caution is warranted when performing FNB in patients who have undergone femoral vascular grafts because of the increased risk of bleeding due to distorted anatomy.

## Fascia Iliaca Nerve Block

### CLINICAL APPLICATIONS

The fascia iliaca block (FIB), covering both femoral and lateral femoral cutaneous distributions, is an alternative to the psoas block and can be a rescue block when other lower extremity blocks have failed. Increasingly, FIB has become a popular block to treat pain after hip fracture, aiding positioning for neuraxial anesthesia for surgical repair. Needle insertion site is more lateral to the femoral neurovascular structures compared with the femoral block, making FIB potentially safer in heavily sedated, anesthetized patients or patients who may have already received a regional block.

### ANATOMY AND TECHNIQUE

There are two approaches to the FIB: infrainguinal, or classic, versus suprainguinal approach. Both require a high-frequency linear transducer (13–6 MHz) typically held longitudinally. For the *infrainguinal or classic* approach, with the patient supine, the inguinal region is scanned lateral to medial along the inguinal crease until femoral neurovascular structures with the fascia iliaca immediately superficial are identified. The groin is then scanned more laterally tracing out the fascia iliaca superficial to the iliopsoas muscle and medial to the sartorius muscle. The ideal needle insertion point would be deep to the sartorius muscle but superficial to the iliopsoas muscle. For the *suprainguinal* approach, the fascia iliaca and the iliopsoas muscle are identified and traced out laterally. The groin is scanned more lateral and cephalad until immediately above the inguinal crease. Ideal sonoanatomy reveals the sartorius muscle lateral and superficial to the fascia iliaca, and the iliacus muscle deep but superficial to the anterior superior iliac spine. The lateral edge of the internal oblique muscle (IOM) should be medial and slightly superficial to the fascia iliaca. The deep circumflex iliac artery and vein can be identified via color Doppler deep to the IOM. The needle approach can be in plane or out of plane, although the in-plane approach is often preferred for better needle trajectory and LA deposit visualization. The FIB relies on spread; thus larger volumes (30–40 mL) of local anesthesia are required. A catheter may be placed for continuous infusion.

### ADVERSE EFFECTS AND COMPLICATIONS

With the infrainguinal or classic approach, the femoral neurovascular structures are more medial to the insertion site; thus risk of neurovascular injury may be reduced. For the suprainguinal approach, caution is warranted because of the proximity to the deep circumflex iliac artery and vein and the potential for intraabdominal injury. For both approaches, caution is warranted in patients with distorted anatomy due to previous surgery, radiation, or scarring.

## Obturator Nerve Block

### CLINICAL APPLICATIONS

Because the obturator nerve is primarily a motor nerve, it usually requires combination with another lower extremity PNB for desired coverage. The obturator nerve block may be used in combination with the femoral or adductor block for knee analgesia or any procedures that require relaxation or analgesia of the adductor muscles.

## RELEVANT ANATOMY

Derived primarily from the anterior rami of L3 and L4, with variable contributions from L2, the obturator nerve lies deep in the obturator canal after descending from the medial psoas muscle border, forming anterior and posterior branches as it exits the obturator foramen. The anterior branch supplies an articular branch to the anterior adductor muscles and a variable cutaneous branch to the lower medial thigh. The posterior branch supplies the deep adductor muscles, with a variable articular branch to the knee. An accessory obturator nerve branch arising from L3 to L4 and traveling with the FN to innervate the hip may be observed.

## TECHNIQUE

US-guided technique is preferred because of the proximity to femoral neurovascular structures. With the patient supine and the thigh abducted and externally rotated, a high-frequency linear transducer is placed longitudinally along the femoral crease with the needle insertion point medial to the femoral vein. Local anesthesia is deposited along the fascial planes of the adductor brevis and magnus muscles (posterior branch) and the fascial plane between the pectineus and adductor brevis muscles (anterior branch). The anterior branch is typically more superficial to the posterior branch. Typically, 10 to 15 mL of LA solution is injected. Caution to avoid intramuscular injection is warranted.

## ADVERSE EFFECTS AND COMPLICATIONS

The obturator canal contains vascular and neural structures, increasing the potential risk of intravascular injection or nerve damage.

## Pericapsular Nerve Group Block

### CLINICAL APPLICATION

The pericapsular nerve group (PENG) block aims to provide analgesia to the hip by targeting the femoral, obturator, and accessory obturator nerves as these three nerves provide main innervation to the anterior hip. The PENG block may be used as an alternative peripheral nerve blockade for hip procedures while reducing risk of muscle weakness.

### RELEVANT ANATOMY

The femoral and accessory obturator nerve branches course between the anterior inferior iliac spine and the iliopubic eminence, and the obturator nerve courses proximal to the inferomedial acetabulum to innervate the anterior hip capsule.

### TECHNIQUE

With the patient supine, a curvilinear transducer (2–5 MHz) is typically used to identify the iliopsoas muscle, FN, and

pectineus muscle by scanning lateral to medial with the transducer at an oblique (45-degree) angle. Using an in-plane needle insertion approach, lateral to medial, local anesthesia is deposited in the fascial plane between the psoas tendon and pubic ramus. Typical volume is 15 to 20 mL.

## ADVERSE EFFECTS AND COMPLICATIONS

Potential complications include injury to neurovascular structures in addition to the risk of myonecrosis.

## Adductor Canal Block

### CLINICAL APPLICATIONS

The adductor canal block (ACB) is an alternative to the FNB for postoperative pain management during knee procedures. The main benefit of the ACB is the ability to provide analgesia to the knee while decreasing quadriceps weakness.

### RELEVANT ANATOMY AND TECHNIQUE

With the patient supine and the leg abducted and slightly externally rotated, the thigh is scanned typically using a high-frequency linear transducer held transversely along the thigh. Ideal sonoanatomy reveals the sartorius muscle superficially (muscle width changes as one scans proximal to distal along the thigh), the vastus medialis laterally, and the adductor longus medially. Lining the "roof" of the canal is the vastoadductor membrane (VAM), and the superficial femoral artery (SFA) forms a focal point of all three muscles (Fig. 97.3). With the needle approach either in plane or out of plane, local anesthesia deposition must occur deep to the VAM for a successful block. The neural structures, though not always visualized, are lateral to the SFA. Although the saphenous nerve is the main target, the medial vastus and medial femoral cutaneous nerves are likely covered depending on the injection site. Combining NS with US if using an in-plane needle approach may aid in identifying the primary motor nerve to the vastus medialis. Typical volumes are 10 to 15 mL of local anesthesia. Intramuscular spread of LA should be avoided.

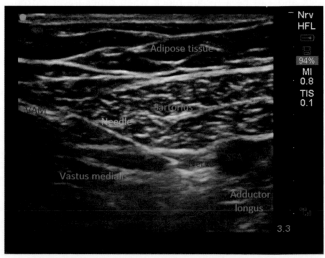

**Fig. 97.3** Ultrasound-guided adductor canal block.

## ADVERSE EFFECTS AND COMPLICATIONS

Complications unique to the ACB include myotoxicity or myonecrosis, and vascular injuries leading to SFA pseudoaneurysm. Neural injury to the nerves could range from saphenous distribution (terminal) to higher branches leading to thigh muscle weakness. Any unexpected thigh weakness should prompt evaluation to rule out myotoxicity or necrosis versus nerve injury.

# Sciatic Nerve Block

## CLINICAL APPLICATIONS

The SN block can be used alone or combined with other lower extremity PNB for analgesia or anesthesia for many procedures below the thigh, such as complex knee procedures and below- or above-knee amputations.

## ANATOMY

Derived from L4 to S3 lumbosacral plexus nerve roots, the SN exits the pelvis with the posterior femoral cutaneous nerve through the sacrosciatic foramen beneath the piriformis muscle, coursing between the greater trochanter of the femur and the ischial tuberosity. As it begins its descent down the posterior thigh toward the popliteal fossa, the SN becomes superficial at the lower border of the gluteus maximus muscle. The SN supplies sensation to the largest area of the lower extremity, including the posterior thigh and everything below the knee, with the exception of a thin medial strip supplied by the saphenous nerve.

## TECHNIQUE

Although the US technique is the most preferred method, sonoanatomy may prove challenging in patients with obesity. In such cases, a combination of US and NS techniques may be warranted. With the US technique, a subgluteal approach is preferred, as the nerve is more superficial. The patient is positioned prone, semiprone, or lateral decubitus. A low-frequency curvilinear transducer is typically used, but in a thin patient a high-frequency linear transducer may suffice. With the transducer placed transversely along the gluteal fold, the SN can be identified as a flat, hyperechoic honeycombed structure medial to the greater trochanter, lateral to the hyperechoic border of the ischial tuberosity, and deep to the gluteus maximus muscle. The needle approach may be in plane or out of plane. If using the combined US-NS technique, tibial (plantar flexion, foot inversion) or common peroneal (dorsiflexion, foot eversion) NS response would confirm appropriate placement. Typical local anesthesia injectate is 25 to 30 mL. A catheter may be placed for a continuous infusion.

## ADVERSE EFFECTS AND COMPLICATIONS

SN block may be technically challenging and uncomfortable for the patient. A lower concentration or volume may be warranted given the SN's risk for ischemia due to poor vascularity. Intramuscular injection should be avoided.

# Popliteal Block

## CLINICAL APPLICATIONS

Popliteal block provides distal leg, ankle, and foot analgesia either as a single injection or a continuous infusion. A saphenous nerve block is typically required if medial leg coverage is desired.

## ANATOMY

The SN diverges into the tibial and common peroneal nerves proximal to the popliteal crease. The tibial nerve continues straight through the popliteal fossa, whereas the peroneal branch lies along the lateral border of the biceps femoris muscle and then wraps laterally around the head of the fibula. The nerves are lateral and superficial to the popliteal artery. The popliteal fossa is bound by semimembranous and semitendinosus muscles medially and the biceps femoris muscle laterally. In patients with greater tissue depth, the common peroneal and tibial nerve may need to be blocked individually for easier block placement.

## TECHNIQUE

Patient positioning may be supine, semiprone, or prone. Similar to the SN, although US-guided technique is preferred, combined US and NS may be warranted in challenging cases. Dorsiflexion/eversion for common peroneal and plantar flexion/inversion for tibial nerve with NS indicates proper nerve identification. A high-frequency linear transducer (13–6 MHz) is typically used, although occasionally a low-frequency curvilinear probe (2–6 MHz) may be required for larger patients. Scanning at the popliteal fossa reveals the tibial nerve immediately superficial to the popliteal vein and artery, respectively, although typically the vein is occluded due to transducer pressure. Scanning more proximally would reveal the common peroneal nerve more laterally but deep to the bicep femoris. Ideal block placement is typically more proximal at the bifurcation of the distal sciatic before the branching of the common peroneal and the tibial nerve occurs. In patients with obesity, this confluence may be too deep, necessitating blocking the nerves separately. Typical LA is 25 to 30 mL.

## ADVERSE EFFECTS AND COMPLICATIONS

Adverse effects and complications associated with a popliteal block are like those associated with a SN block. Caution is warranted to avoid direct injury to the popliteal artery, which may lead to formation of a pseudoaneurysm.

## SUGGESTED READINGS

Aliste, J., Layera, S., Bravo, D., Jara, Á., Muñoz, G., & Barrientos, C., et al. (2021). Randomized comparison between pericapsular nerve group (PENG) block and suprainguinal fascia iliaca block for total hip arthroplasty. *Regional Anesthesia and Pain Medicine, 46,* 874–878.

Gautier, P. E., Hadzic, A., Lecog, J. P., Brichant, J. F., Kuroda, M. M., & Vandepitte, C. (2016). Distribution of injectate and sensory-motor blockade after adductor canal block. *Anesthesia and Analgesia, 122,* 279–282.

Giron-Arango, L., Peng, P. W. H., Chin, K. J., Brull, R., & Perlas, A. (2018). Pericapsular Nerve Group (PENG) block for hip fracture. *Regional Anesthesia and Pain Medicine, 43,* 859–863.

Gray, A. T. (2013). *Atlas of Ultrasound-Guided Regional Anesthesia* (2nd ed.). Philadelphia: Elsevier Inc.

Hebl, J. R., & Lennon, R. L. (2010). *Mayo Clinic Atlas of Regional Anesthesia and Ultrasound-Guided Nerve Blockade.* Rochester, MN: Mayo Clinic Scientific Press.

Karmakar, M. K., Li, J. W., Kwok, W. H., & Hadzic, A. (2015). Ultrasound-guided lumbar plexus block using a transverse scan through the lumbar intertransverse space: A prospective case series. *Regional Anesthesia and Pain Medicine, 40,* 75–81.

Kuang, M. J., Ma, J. X., Fu, L., He, W. W., Zhao, J., & Ma, X. L. (2017). Is adductor canal block better than femoral nerve block in primary total knee arthroplasty? A GRADE analysis of the evidence through a systematic review and meta-analysis. *Journal of Arthroplasty, 17,* 30421–30427.

Njathi, C. W., Johnson, R. L., Laughlin, R. S., Schroeder, D. R., Jacob, A. K., & Kopp, S. L. (2017). Complications after continuous posterior lumbar plexus blockade for total hip arthroplasty: A retrospective cohort study. *Regional Anesthesia and Pain Medicine, 42,* 446–450.

# 98

# Peripheral Nerve Blocks at the Ankle

ADAM D. NIESEN, MD

Anesthesia distal to the ankle is accomplished by depositing local anesthetic adjacent to the five major nerves that innervate the foot. Specifically, these nerves are the tibial, deep fibular (peroneal), superficial fibular (peroneal), sural, and saphenous nerves. The tibial nerve is the largest of the five nerves and provides the greatest distribution of innervation to the foot. The ankle block is relatively easy to learn using landmarks, nerve stimulation, ultrasound, or a combination of these techniques. As with any regional procedure, a good understanding of the relevant anatomy is essential. Ankle blocks are effective for nearly any surgical procedure of the foot. Major complications are rare.

Neuroanatomy of the foot can vary from patient to patient; therefore the following descriptions should serve as a general guide. As with many nerve structures, the five nerves of the ankle block reside near vascular structures. The tibial nerve supplies the sole of the foot and plantar portions of the toes. It maintains a close relationship to the posterior tibial artery, typically lying posterior or deep to the artery and anteromedial to the Achilles tendon. Furthermore, the tibial nerve is located deep to the flexor retinaculum, which must be penetrated for a successful block (Fig. 98.1). The deep fibular nerve courses midway between the malleoli before assuming a position between the anterior tibial tendon and the extensor hallucis longus tendon beneath the extensor retinaculum at the dorsum of the foot. It is closely associated with the deep fibular (dorsalis pedis) artery in this location, innervates the short extensors of the toes, and provides skin sensation to the interdigital cleft between the great and second toes. With the patient dorsiflexing the foot, the tendons of the anterior tibial and extensor hallucis longus muscles can be readily identified at a level just above a line connecting the malleoli. The pulsation of the anterior tibial (dorsalis pedis) artery will often be felt. The nerve is deep to the extensor retinaculum and usually lateral to the artery. The superficial fibular nerve supplies cutaneous sensation to the dorsum of the foot and toes (except between the great and second toes). The saphenous nerve is anterior to the medial malleolus near the great saphenous vein and supplies cutaneous innervation to the anteromedial side of the lower leg and medial foot midway to the toes. The sural nerve is a superficial nerve that provides cutaneous sensation to the lower posterolateral ankle, lateral foot, and fifth toe. It is located adjacent to the small saphenous vein, posterior to the lateral malleolus.

## Technique

Typically, the patient is in the supine position with the procedural leg elevated on a padded support. An ankle block can be quite painful; thus adequate sedation will improve patient experience.

### FIELD BLOCK/NERVE STIMULATOR BLOCK

The block is started by injecting a small amount of local anesthetic agent medial to the Achilles tendon at the level of the upper border of the medial malleolus. A 3-cm to 5-cm 25G needle is directed at right angles to the tibia. The needle tip is

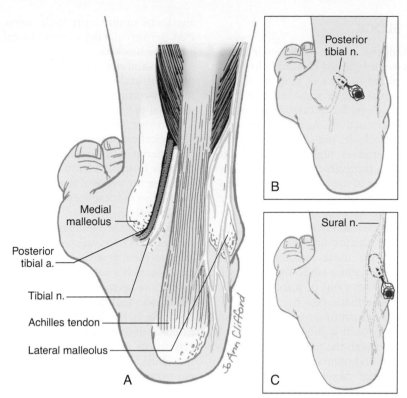

**Fig. 98.1** **A**, Anatomic landmarks for block of the tibial and sural nerves at the ankle. **B**, Tibial nerve: method of needle placement for block at the ankle. **C**, Sural nerve: method of needle placement for block at the ankle. (From Miller RD, ed. Nerve block at the ankle. In: Miller RD, ed. *Miller's Anesthesia.* 9th ed. Elsevier, 2020:1450–1479.)

slowly advanced until a paresthesia is elicited or bone is contacted. At this point, 5 to 7 mL of local anesthetic agent without epinephrine is injected near the posterior aspect of the tibia, with an equal volume of local anesthetic injected during withdrawal of the needle to the skin surface if a paresthesia is not elicited. The tibial nerve is the only nerve of the ankle block that will produce a reliable motor response to stimulation. If a nerve stimulator is used, a 5-cm 22G insulated needle is advanced in a similar course to that described for field block until a response of plantar flexion of the toes is elicited. Then a similar volume of 5 to 7 mL of local anesthetic is injected. When performing an ankle block, it is advisable to perform the tibial nerve block first, as it provides innervation to most of the deep structures of the foot, and onset of anesthesia may be delayed because of its comparatively large size.

Then the deep fibular, superficial fibular, and saphenous nerves can all be blocked using a single injection site. A 3-cm to 5-cm 25G needle is inserted perpendicular to the skin, as depicted in Fig. 98.2. A loss of resistance will often be felt during passage through the extensor retinaculum, at which time 3 to 5 mL of local anesthetic agent is injected. Blockade of the superficial fibular nerve can be achieved by injecting local anesthetic agent subcutaneously laterally from the site of injection of the deep fibular nerve toward the superior aspect of the lateral malleolus using 5 to 10 mL of solution; then the saphenous nerve is blocked with 3 to 5 mL of local anesthetic agent injected subcutaneously medially from the site of injection of the deep fibular nerve toward the saphenous vein.

Sural nerve blockade is accomplished by infiltrating 5 to 10 mL of local anesthetic agent solution posterior to the lateral malleolus to the Achilles tendon at the level of the upper border of the lateral malleolus.

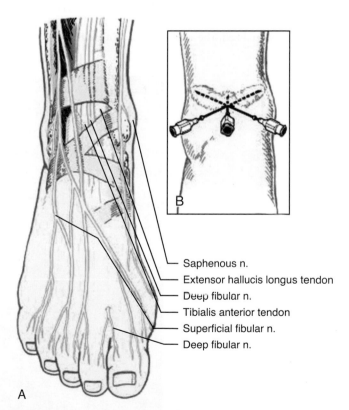

**Fig. 98.2** **A**, Anatomic landmarks for block of the deep fibular (peroneal), superficial fibular (peroneal), and saphenous nerves at the ankle. **B**, Method of needle placement for block of the deep fibular (peroneal), superficial fibular (peroneal), and saphenous nerves through a single needle entry site. (From Miller RD: Nerve block at the ankle. In Miller RD, ed. *Miller's Anesthesia.* 9th ed. Elsevier; 2020:1450–1479.)

## ULTRASOUND-GUIDED BLOCK

The superficial positions of all five nerves of the ankle block make them amenable to ultrasound-guided blockade. However, not all nerves are easily visualized because of their small size. Other complicating factors, such as edema of the lower extremity, may create challenging conditions for ultrasound visualization of the desired neurovascular anatomy. As the largest nerve of the five involved in ankle blockade, the tibial nerve is the easiest to identify with ultrasound. A high-frequency linear ultrasound probe is placed in a transverse orientation in the space between the posterior border of the medial malleolus and Achilles tendon. The posterior tibial artery is identified, with the hyperechoic posterior tibial nerve typically immediately posterior or deep to the artery. Adjacent tendon structures may mimic the appearance of the nerve. If this occurs, the practitioner should slide the ultrasound probe more proximally, as the tendons will transition to muscle bellies while the nerve will maintain its appearance. An in-plane or out-of-plane needle approach is used to deposit local anesthetic near the tibial nerve, depending on nerve position and surrounding anatomy. If an anterior to posterior in-plane approach is chosen, care must be taken to allow sufficient space between the malleolus and ultrasound probe for needle insertion and redirection.

Ultrasound-guided deep fibular nerve blockade involves placement of a high-frequency linear ultrasound probe in a transverse position over the anterior ankle. After the deep fibular artery is identified, the nerve may be visualized as a hyperechoic structure lateral to the artery; however, it may not be easily seen in all patients because of its small size. Typically, an out-of-plane approach is used to deposit local anesthetic. If the nerve is visualized, the aim should be to deliver the local anesthetic in proximity to the nerve. If the nerve is not visualized, perivascular deposition of local anesthetic will also achieve adequate blockade.

The sural nerve is usually associated with the small saphenous vein at the ankle. Both structures are quite superficial, and the easy compressibility of the vein requires the application of minimal pressure with the ultrasound probe in comparison to other nerve blocks. Application of a tourniquet may aid the identification of the small saphenous vein, which indicates the sural nerve is nearby. Like the deep fibular nerve, if the sural nerve is formally identified, local anesthetic should be deposited near the nerve; if the nerve is not identifiable, perivascular deposition of local anesthetic around the small saphenous vein is appropriate.

Although the saphenous and superficial fibular nerves may occasionally be visualized with ultrasound, both are quite difficult to identify at the level of the ankle. The superficial fibular nerve branches substantially above the level of the ankle. Scanning more proximally (10–15 cm) on the lateral aspect of the leg allows identification of the nerve in a position amenable to blockade. In this location, the nerve lies at the confluence of the extensor digitorum longus and peroneus brevis muscles, with a prominent groove appearing between the muscles leading to the fibula. Fig. 98.3 demonstrates ultrasound imaging for the neurovascular structures of the posterior tibial, deep fibular, sural, and superficial fibular nerves.

Although complications resulting from ankle blockade are rare, cases of prolonged paresthesia and local anesthetic toxicity have been reported. Use of epinephrine-containing local anesthetic agents when performing an ankle block is controversial; however, epinephrine should be avoided in patients with peripheral vascular disease or other causes of distal circulatory compromise.

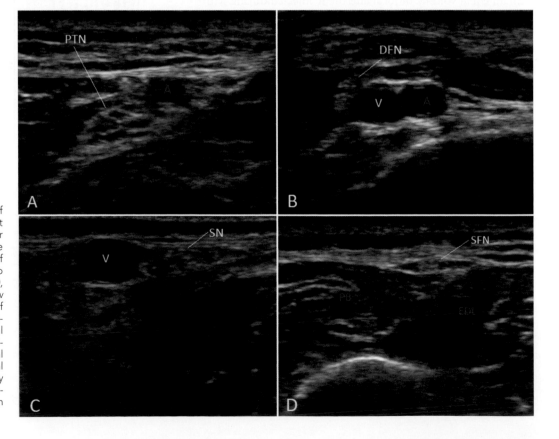

**Fig. 98.3** Ultrasound images of the ankle block. **A**, Medial aspect of the ankle showing the posterior tibial artery (*red A*) and tibial nerve (*yellow PTN*). **B**, Anterior surface of the ankle demonstrating the deep fibular artery (*red A*), vein (*blue V*), and deep fibular nerve (*yellow DFN*). **C**, Posterolateral aspect of the ankle illustrating the small saphenous vein (*blue V*) and the sural nerve (*yellow SN*). **D**, Lateral surface of the leg in a more proximal position revealing the superficial fibular nerve (*yellow SFN*) closely associated with the peroneus brevis (*red PB*) and extensor digitorum longus (*red EDL*) muscles.

## SUGGESTED READINGS

Gray, A. T. (2010). *Atlas of Ultrasound-Guided Regional Anesthesia* (2nd ed.). Philadelphia: Saunders Elsevier.

Hadzic, A. (2011). *Hadzic's peripheral nerve blocks and anatomy for ultrasound-guided regional anesthesia* (2nd ed.). New York: McGraw-Hill.

Miller, R. D. (2020). *Miller's Anesthesia* (9th ed.). Philadelphia: Elsevier.

Vandepitte, C., Lopez, A. M., Van Boxstael, S., & Jalil, H. (2021). *Ultrasound-Guided Ankle Nerve Block*. Retrieved from https://www.nysora.com/regional-anesthesia-for-specific-surgical-procedures/lower-extremity-regional-anesthesia-for-specific-surgical-procedures/foot-and-anckle/ultrasound-guided-ankle-block/. Accessed December, 2021.

# 99

# Perioperative Antifibrinolytic Medication Use

ALLAN M. KLOMPAS, MB, BCh, BAO  |  REBECCA L. JOHNSON, MD

## Introduction

Tissue injury, including surgery, damages endothelium resulting in the exposure of collagen and release of tissue factor initiating complex hemostatic processes, including activation of the clotting cascade, to promote clot formation and prevent excessive blood loss. Additionally, anticoagulant factors and activation of the fibrinolytic cascade promote clot regulation and contain the clot to the damaged site. To achieve this, circulating liver-derived plasminogen, along with endothelium-derived tissue plasminogen activator (tPA), bind to formed and forming clots at lysine residues, where it is converted to its active form plasmin. Once active, plasmin enzymatically cleaves fibrin to induce clot breakdown and limit clot propagation. Tranexamic acid (TXA) is a synthetic derivative of the amino acid lysine. By acting as an alternative lysine site, TXA competitively inhibits the activation of plasminogen to plasmin, which thwarts the breakdown of fibrin and promotes clot stability (Fig. 99.1). TXA has also been proposed to have anti-inflammatory properties in some settings. Although not inherently procoagulant, TXA allows fibrin clots to mature and stabilize, contributing to ongoing hemostasis. Simply, TXA prevents the breakdown of clots *that have already formed* without directly contributing to clot formation or interrupting ongoing coagulation.

Excessive bleeding is a common concern in nearly every surgical discipline. Countless efforts have been employed to mitigate this, including advances in surgical techniques such as minimally invasive approaches, use of tourniquets, deliberately induced or passive hypotension, medical optimization, topical hemostatic agents, and antifibrinolytic medication use as means to reduce blood transfusion.

In an effort to control peripartum and obstetric bleeding, antifibrinolytic medications were synthesized in the 1960s. ε-Aminocaproic acid (EACA) was the first of its kind but was quickly superseded by TXA, which was found to be 27 times more potent, as well as the introduction of a non–lysine-based serine protease inhibitor, aprotinin. Numerous studies over the ensuing decades found antifibrinolytics being employed to reduce blood loss and prevent transfusions in cardiac surgery, trauma, obstetrics and gynecology, neurosurgery, orthopedic surgery, organ transplantation, and gastrointestinal (GI)/hepatobiliary surgeries. Although use has been widespread, caution remains over concerns that antifibrinolytics may tip the hemostatic balance toward pathologic clot and contribute to venous or arterial thromboses, particularly in areas that already have elevated perioperative risk, such as in orthopedic surgery and obstetrics. This chapter will highlight the key evidence supporting antifibrinolytic use with a focus on the most widely studied agent, TXA, across multiple perioperative settings.

## Routes, Dosage, and Side Effects

The most commonly used routes include oral, intravenous (IV), and topical administration or combination thereof.

Topical applications of TXA have mostly been studied in orthopedic and cardiac surgery; this approach has generally been perceived as equivalent to IV use in these settings. In a

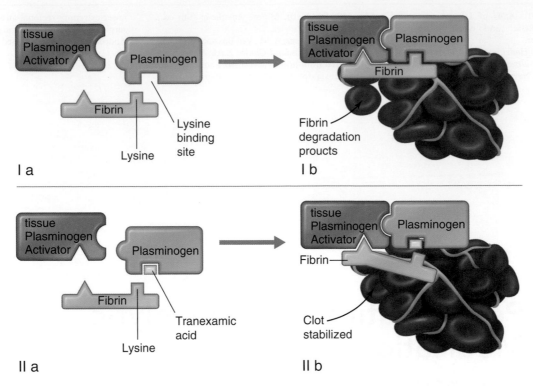

**Fig. 99.1** Fibrinolysis pathway (panel Ia → Ib); competitive inhibition in presence of tranexamic acid (panel IIa → II b) mechanism of action of tranexamic acid. (Used with permission of Mayo Foundation for Medical Education and Research, all rights reserved.)

metaanalysis of six trials and 679 patients, Wang and colleagues studied topical versus IV administration of TXA in primary total knee arthroplasty and found no statistically significant differences in drain output, blood loss, hemoglobin change, or transfusions regardless of method of delivering TXA; however, all routes of TXA administration were found more effective than placebo. Similarly, in a metaanalysis of intrapericardial use in cardiac surgery, Habbab and colleagues demonstrated that TXA use decreased postoperative bleeding and trended to a decrease in transfusion requirements. Despite these findings, IV use is by far the most common route of administration selected by many centers to ensure medication adherence.

Although a wide range of doses have been used across contexts and routes, local pharmacy guidelines should be consulted prior to clinical use. TXA duration of action is approximately 3 h, with a half-life between 2 and 11 h, depending on renal function. It has been advised to reduce the dose or extend the dosing interval of TXA during repeat administration for patients with renal insufficiency, malnutrition/low weight, or in those with seizure histories; however, no formal adjustments to guidelines for simple intraoperative administration have reached consensus. Also based on TXA pharmacokinetics, postoperative anticoagulation regimens for deep venous thrombosis (DVT) prevention do not need to be adjusted based upon administration of TXA.

It is generally agreed that only a small percentage of TXA injected intravenously reaches the target location to inhibit local tissue fibrinolysis and stabilize the clot; therefore it may be that IV administration decreases external blood loss but not hidden blood loss. Further, it is still unknown whether topical or intraarticular administration results in lower systemic absorption and therefore fewer adverse effects or lower potential for thromboembolic complications.

## Usage and Efficacy

Decades of research on antifibrinolytics have amassed data across nearly every procedural arena, with TXA receiving the most attention of the three. Although the discussion that follows is not exhaustive, it will highlight some of the most significant findings across disciplines with a central focus on TXA.

### CARDIOVASCULAR SURGERY

Because of the risk of significant perioperative bleeding, much of the foundational work on the efficacy of antifibrinolytics occurred in cardiac surgery, with their use being considered standard of care by the mid-1990s. Because of its powerful effects on hemostasis, aprotinin use was widespread until a hallmark study in 2006 directly compared EACA, aprotinin, and TXA and suggested that aprotinin was associated with higher rates of end organ dysfunction. At the same time, a case-control study found that aprotinin and TXA had similar efficacy but that aprotinin was associated with increased renal dysfunction. The BART trial from 2008, which randomized 2331 high-risk cardiac surgical patients to aprotinin, TXA, or EACA, also provided compelling evidence to shift contemporary practice toward TXA use. Despite a modest improvement in efficacy over its peers, aprotinin was associated with a higher mortality (6% vs. approx. 4%). Although study results were highly controversial, they were extremely impactful and aprotinin was withdrawn from the market.

Since the shift away from aprotinin toward TXA and EACA, there have been numerous studies supporting the efficacy of antifibrinolytics in cardiac surgery, such as a recent metaanalysis showing its efficacy in coronary artery revascularization without increasing the risk of thrombotic complications. The recent ATACAS study from 2017 evaluated the use of aspirin and TXA in 4631 patients undergoing coronary artery revascularization. TXA was associated with a lower risk of bleeding and did not increase the risk of death or thrombotic complications at 30 days; however, it was associated with a higher risk of postoperative seizures. Together, the data for antifibrinolytic use in cardiac surgery has garnered a class I, level A recommendation on multiple guidelines and is now generally considered the standard of care.

## TRAUMA

Antifibrinolytic use in trauma has gained significant attention in recent years after the landmark CRASH-2 trial, which compared TXA use to placebo in over 20,000 patients suffering acute trauma. This randomized controlled trial (RCT) demonstrated a significant improvement in all-cause mortality in the TXA group (14.5% vs. 16.0%) with the relative risk (RR) of death due to bleeding of 0.85 (95% CI, 0.76–0.96). Subsequent analysis suggested that this mortality benefit only occurred when TXA was given within the first 3 h of injury and actually increased the risk of death due to bleeding when given after 3 h. A recent metaanalysis incorporating five clinical trials found that administration of TXA in the emergency department was associated with decreased mortality in severe trauma and improved functional status.

Although TXA use in trauma become widespread after CRASH-2, questions remained over its efficacy and safety in the setting of head injuries. In a subsequent trial published in 2019, the CRASH-3 trial randomized 12,737 patients to either TXA or placebo after traumatic brain injury (TBI). In those treated within 3 h, the risk of head injury–related death was decreased in the TXA group without increasing the risk of vascular occlusive events or seizures. Conversely, a 2020 RCT comparing early prehospital administration of TXA versus placebo in TBI did not demonstrate significant improvements in a 6-month neurologic outcome. Similarly, the 2020 STAMP trial evaluated prehospital TXA versus placebo in trauma at risk of significant hemorrhage. Although there was no difference in 30-day mortality or thrombotic complications, there was a dramatic improvement in 30-day mortality in patients with severe shock (18.5% vs. 35.5%; improvement of 17%; 95% CI, −25.8 to −8.1%).

Following this evidence, the European Society of Intensive Care Medicine released a practice guideline in late 2021 issuing a *strong* recommendation for the early use of TXA (<3 h) in critically ill patients with bleeding or suspected bleeding due to trauma and a *conditional* recommendation for its use in critically ill patients with acute TBI and bleeding due to trauma.

## OBSTETRICS AND GYNECOLOGY

As the initial impetus for the development of antifibrinolytic medications, it is unsurprising that antifibrinolytics have a long history of use in the management of gynecologic bleeding. As an example, TXA has been used for as an oral therapy for menorrhagia for over 40 years.

What is surprising, however, is how long it took to demonstrate the same robust usage in the management of postpartum hemorrhage (PPH), which continues to be a significant contributor of maternal morbidity and mortality globally. Part of the hesitation for use comes from the "prothrombotic" state of pregnancy and concerns for propagating pathologic thrombus.

Early studies on TXA use to prevent PPH demonstrated efficacy but suffered from methodological issues and a large variation in the dosage, which limited its impact in clinical practice. In 2017, the WOMAN trial randomized 20,060 women with clinical PPH after vaginal or cesarean delivery to either TXA or placebo. This study was unique in that it occurred in 21 countries, including many developing or underresourced centers. Although the effect size on bleeding-related death was modest favoring the TXA group (1.5% in TXA vs. 1.9% in placebo; 95% CI, 0.65–1.00), the WOMAN trial reiterated the need for early use (<3 h) from bleeding onset. Importantly, in this presumed high-risk population, there was no increase in expected adverse events including thromboembolism. Similarly, the 2021 TRAAP2 trial randomized 4551 women undergoing cesarean delivery to either TXA or placebo who were also receiving prophylactic uterotonic agents and reported a modest reduction in estimated blood loss greater than 1 L or receipt of red blood cell transfusion within 2 days of delivery. Also, there were no differences in thromboembolic events reported between groups. A recent metaanalysis on prophylactic TXA for prevention of PPH in cesarean delivery, which included 10,659 women in 36 studies, concluded that TXA use is effective in lowering postpartum blood loss, transfusion requirements, supplemental uterotonic requirements, and hemoglobin drop.

Altogether, these studies have resulted in the World Health Organization recommending the early use (<3 h) of TXA after vaginal or cesarean delivery with clinical evidence of PPH. Despite its apparent efficacy and safety profile, questions remain about its cost-effectiveness that limit the widespread implementation for routine use outside of the rare case of a parturient expected to have a large volume blood loss.

## NEUROSURGERY

Although most surgical specialties have been most concerned about TXA's theoretical risk of pathologic thromboses, there have been decades of controversy surrounding TXA use in neurosurgery relating to its effects on bleeding, seizures, and possible stroke risk.

In 2018, the TICH-2 trial randomized 2325 patients with intracerebral hemorrhage to either TXA or placebo. Study findings indicated no difference in functional status at

90 days; however, there was a decrease in early mortality and serious adverse events. The recent 2020 STOP-AUST trial randomized 100 patients with intracerebral hemorrhage to TXA versus placebo failed to demonstrate evidence that TXA halts hemorrhage growth or induces thromboembolic complications. Similarly, the 2021 ULTRA trial randomized 955 with subarachnoid hemorrhage to TXA with usual care or usual care alone and did not demonstrate a difference in clinical outcome at 6 months, rebleeding, or other serious adverse effects. As of late 2021, in a metaanalysis performed for TXA in spontaneous intracranial hemorrhage, TXA seems effective in reducing hematoma expansion but does not affect neurologic function, infections, craniotomy, or thromboembolic effects.

Similarly, other areas of neurosurgery have had conflicting results. In brain tumor surgery, an assessment of several small studies concluded that TXA reduced the volume of blood loss but did not affect the need for blood transfusion, whereas in multilevel spine surgery it was found TXA is effective at reducing blood loss and the need for transfusions. Although there seems to be support in TBI, the same robust evidence does not support its use in operative neurosurgery and extracranial surgery based on equivocal effects on outcome scores.

Altogether, antifibrinolytic use seems to have support primarily in TBI and spine surgery but remains less robust for most other areas of neurosurgery.

## GASTROINTESTINAL AND HEPATOBILIARY

Although most attention has been on the intraoperative use of antifibrinolytics, the use of TXA in medical bleeding has recently gained interest. One of the most influential, the HALT-IT trial randomized 12,009 patients with upper or lower GI bleeding to either TXA or placebo. There was no difference in bleeding-related deaths, myocardial infarction (MI), or stroke; however, there was an increased risk of venous thromboembolism in the TXA group (RR 1.85; 95% CI, 1.15–2.98). A subsequent metaanalysis in TXA for GI bleeding from late 2021 included five trials with both IV and oral administration. Study findings indicated that high-dose IV TXA did not improve mortality or bleeding outcome but was associated with increased adverse events including DVT, pulmonary embolism (PE), and seizures. Altogether, there is currently insufficient evidence to support TXA use in GI bleeding.

## ORTHOPEDIC SURGERY

In 2014, Huang and colleagues published a metaanalysis of 46 RCTs involving 2925 patients. These authors found that the use of TXA reduced total blood loss, the number of blood transfusions by almost 1 unit per patient; this data left authors to conclude a significant reduction in transfusion requirements (RR, 0.51; 95% CI, 0.46–0.56) with no additional increase in the risks of DVT in this sample (RR, 1.11; 95% CI, 0.69–1.79). Further, although a higher preoperative hemoglobin level may obviate the need for TXA for blood loss prevention, researchers at the Mayo Clinic provided evidence to support routine TXA use in all total joint arthroplasty patients. In a retrospective investigation of more than 2000 primary total joint arthroplasty patients, transfusion universally decreased with TXA use (in fact, the group with the largest *relative* decrease in transfusion rates was the group with preoperative hemoglobin levels >15 g/dL). Whiting and colleagues further showed that hospital length of stay may also be significantly reduced among patients given TXA. Together, this data has led to a *strong* recommendation for TXA use in total joint arthroplasty in a multidisciplinary guideline by Fillingham and colleagues published in 2019.

## Complications and Safety

Concern for serious complications centers around a theoretical increased risk of thromboembolic events due to the reduction in clot breakdown. Surgeons and anesthesiologists alike hesitate to provide TXA particularly in those patients with a history of coronary artery disease, history of thromboembolic events, and chronic renal insufficiency. However, it remains unknown if these assumed risks warrant a relative contraindication to TXA administration in these subpopulations of patients presenting for total joint replacement inherently at higher risk of perioperative thromboembolism. Certainly, a counterargument may be made that TXA actually reduces the incidence of thromboembolic events by permitting clot formation where it is needed while preventing upregulation of the entire coagulation cascade. Further, patients with comorbidities benefit greatly from avoidance of transfusion. These latter arguments appear to have some emerging evidentiary basis supporting more widespread TXA use.

As highlighted earlier, the highly favorable safety profiles of TXA in both the CRASH-2 and WOMAN trials including over 40,000 patients at high risk of thrombotic complications have been influential in assuaging clinicians of its overall safety. In a recent metaanalysis in JAMA, the safety of IV TXA was assessed by analyzing 216 studies including over 125,000 patients. Importantly, they found no difference in the risk of thromboembolic complications (2.1% in TXA vs. 2.0% in placebo), which included venous thrombosis, PE, myocardial ischemia or infarction, and cerebral ischemia or infarction.

The other primary concern over TXA use relates to its association with seizures. Because of its chemical similarities with inhibitory neurotransmitters and its ability to disrupt γ-aminobutyric acid type A activity, it has long been known that high doses of TXA can precipitate seizures. A recent metaanalysis on the safety of TXA including 234 studies and over 100,000 patients found that although overall there was not an increased risk of seizures, this risk increased when the daily dose was greater than 2 g/day (RR 3.05; 95% CI, 1.01–9.2), which increased in proportion to total dose. From this, we would recommend using the lowest acceptable dose and consider dose adjustment or omission in those with an elevated risk of seizure.

Other serious complications have been reported but are rare (generalized urticaria, angioedema, itching). One patient showed a positive response to an intradermal challenge test with TXA. Another case report detailed epidermal necrolysis in a liver failure patient and a case report of anaphylaxis. Minor side effects, as with any medication are reported, and may be related to dosing and drug levels.

## HIGH-RISK CASES

In addition to the perioperative risk of thrombosis resulting from the procedure, many patients undergoing major surgery are at high risk of thromboembolic complications due to intrinsic coagulation abnormalities, withholding chronic anticoagulation, advanced age, and mobility restrictions. In this context, a high-risk patient is one in whom cardiovascular occlusive events would appear to pose specific and increased risk. "High risk" would be defined as American Society of Anesthesiologists III–IV patients with histories of hypercoagulable states, DVT, PE, stroke, and MI requiring revascularization.

In addition to its efficacy and safety in known high-risk groups such as coronary artery bypass grafting, obstetrics, and major trauma, this has also been specifically addressed in orthopedic surgery. A 2021 report by Poeran and colleagues evaluated over 100,000 hip and knee arthroplasty patients with high-risk medical comorbidities including hypercoagulable patients, those with history of seizures, cerebrovascular accidents, atrial fibrillation, and renal dysfunction. Compared with those without high-risk comorbidities that received TXA, there was a demonstrable decrease in blood transfusion requirements without differences in complication rates, including thromboembolic, strokes, MIs, or seizures. Providers may wish to consider withholding TXA in some high-risk scenarios on a case-by-case basis, albeit across multiple surgical specialties, it appears the risk:benefit ratio for most patients will favor the use of TXA to reduce the risk of excessive bleeding and decrease transfusion requirements.

## Summary

- TXA is a lysine analog with antifibrinolytic activity, *not* a procoagulant.
- There is evidence of reduced bleeding and blood transfusions in many clinical settings (cardiac surgery, trauma, obstetrics and gynecology, spine surgery, and orthopedic surgery).
- Ongoing research is required before recommending routine use in intracranial neurosurgery, GI hemorrhage, and other forms of nonsurgical bleeding.
- Ideal routes and doses are still being investigated, but 80% to 100% inhibition of fibrinolysis occurs at 10 mcg/kg.
- Large trauma and orthopedic investigations show a trend toward *lower* vaso-occlusive events and reduced 30–day mortality.
- Limiting hyperactivity of coagulation cascade (stabilizing fibrin clot) may actually reduce venous thromboembolism risk.
- Specific comorbidity risks remain unknown, but generally, TXA use is associated with low complication rates even in high-risk groups where avoidance of blood transfusion is equally beneficial.

## SUGGESTED READINGS

Shakur, H., Roberts, I., Bautista, R., Caballero, J., Coats, T., Dewan, Y., et al. (2010). Effects of tranexamic acid on death, vascular occlusive events, and blood transfusion in trauma patients with significant haemorrhage (CRASH-2): A randomized, placebo-controlled trial. *Lancet, 76*, 23–32.

Fillingham, Y. A., Ramkumar, D. B., Jevsevar, D. S., Yates, A. J., Bini, S. A., Clarke, H. D., et al. (2019). Tranexamic acid in total joint arthroplasty: The endorsed clinical practice guides of the American Association of Hip and Knee Surgeons, American Society of Regional Anesthesia and Pain Medicine, American Academy of Orthopaedic Surgeons, Hip Society, and Knee Society. *Regional Anesthesia and Pain Medicine, 44*, 7–11.

HALT-IT Trial Collaborators. (2020). Effects of a high-dose 24-h infusion of tranexamic acid on death and thromboembolic events in patients with acute gastrointestinal bleeding (HALT-IT): An international randomized, double-blind, placebo-controlled trial. *Lancet, 395*, 1927–1936.

Hong, Pan, Liu, Ruikang, Rai, Saroj, Liu, JiaJia, Ding, Yuhong, & Li, Jin (2022). Does tranexamic acid reduce the blood loss in various surgeries? An umbrella review of state-of-the-art meta-analysis. *Front Pharmacol, 13*, 887386. doi:10.3389/fphar.2022.887386. 35662737.

Poeran, J., Chan, J. J., Zubizarreta, N., Mazumdar, M., Galatz, L. M., & Moucha, C. S. (2021). Safety of tranexamic acid in hip and knee arthroplasty in high-risk patients. *Anesthesiology, 135*, 57–68.

Taeuber, I., Weibel, S., Herrmann, E., Neef, V., Schlesinger, T., Kranke, P., et al. (2021). Association of intravenous tranexamic acid with thromboembolic events and mortality: A systematic review, meta-analysis, and meta-regression. *JAMA Surgery, 156*, e210884.

WOMAN Trial Collaborators. (2017). Effect of early tranexamic acid administration on mortality, hysterectomy, and other morbidities in women with post-partum haemorrhage (WOMAN): An international, randomized, double-blind, placebo-controlled trial. *Lancet, 389*, 2105–2116.

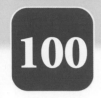

# Basics of Ultrasound-Guided Regional Anesthesia

DAVID OLSEN, MD

## Introduction

Ultrasound imaging has become ubiquitous within anesthesia. From intravenous access to intraoperative monitoring, ultrasonic imaging is routinely used in the perioperative setting. Arguably, no area of anesthesia has seen more growth in the use of ultrasound than regional anesthesia. Ultrasound imaging is noninvasive, free of ionizing radiation, and allows the practitioner to directly visualize the neurovascular structures, the advancement of the block needle, and the deposition of local anesthetic at the target site.

Ultrasound was first used in medicine in 1947 and introduced into regional anesthesia in 1978. Advancements in ultrasound technology in the 1990s created an explosion of interest in ultrasound-guided regional anesthesia. Ultrasound imaging allows for the teaching of neuroanatomy, improves block onset time and success rate, has reduced the number of needle passes, and allows for new approaches to neurovascular structures.

Competency in the use of ultrasound for regional anesthesia requires an understanding of the physics of the ultrasonic transducer to better appreciate both the capabilities and limitations of the device.

## Ultrasound Imaging Physics

Ultrasound imaging is produced by an ultrasonic transducer, usually located in a handheld probe, and a signal-processing unit. The transducer is an electromechanical device that uses a piezoelectric element to convert electrical signals into vibratory longitudinal mechanical sound (pressure) waves in the ultrasonic frequency range, a frequency above the threshold of human hearing (20 kHz). For medical imaging, a 2 to 15 MHz frequency is commonly used. The transducer, shown in Fig. 100.1, both transmits and receives ultrasonic sound waves, converting the reflected mechanical waves into electrical signals that are processed into a medical image.

The ultrasonic pressure waves traverse human soft tissue at approximately 1540 m/s with the speed of propagation dependent on the *acoustic impedance* (Z), or opposition to flow, of the different tissue types. Acoustic impedance is related to both the stiffness and density of the tissue. Ultrasonic waves are partially reflected to the transducer at a *Z-interface*, the plane between tissues with different acoustic impedances. Each reflected wave is termed an *echo*, and the greater the difference in acoustic impedances at the Z-interface, the more the wave will be reflected and the stronger the echo (Fig. 100.1). By measuring the time from transmission to reception of the echo, the signal processor can calculate the depth of each Z-interface and generate an ultrasonic image where the brightness at each depth is related to the amount of signal returned to the probe. This type of ultrasound imaging is termed *B-mode*, or brightness mode

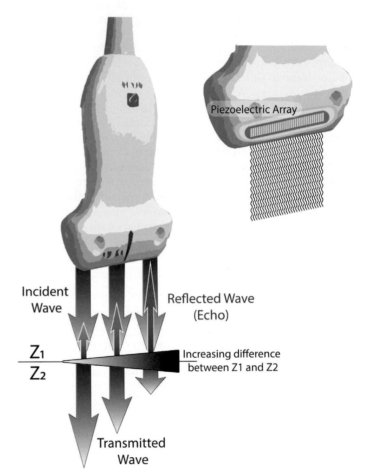

**Fig. 100.1 Ultrasound Probe.** The ultrasound probe transmits an array of mechanical vibrations from the piezoelectric elements. These vibrations hit a tissue interface, the Z-interface, between tissues with different acoustic impedance (Z). Some of the energy is reflected back as an echo in the reflected wave, and the remainder is transmitted to deeper tissues. The greater the difference in acoustic impedance, the stronger the reflected wave and the smaller the transmitted wave. For example, the left arrow with the small echo could represent the interface between water (Z = 1.5) and muscle (Z = 1.7), whereas the right arrow with a large echo could represent the interface between muscle and bone (Z = 6.5).

imaging, and is the imaging modality commonly used in regional anesthesia.

The amount of signal returned to the probe depends partially on the *angle of incidence* between the Z-interface and the direction of propagation. As the angle of incidence increases, less energy is reflected to the transducer, and the structure is less easily visualized.

An important consideration of ultrasound imaging is the relationship of imaging frequency, resolution, and depth. As the frequency increases, the *resolution* (ability to distinguish adjacent objects) of the image increases; however, the imaging depth or penetration decreases. Penetration decreases with frequency because high-frequency waveforms are more easily scattered by the tissue. Scattering results in insufficient signal returning to the probe from deeper depths to generate an image.

Because regional anesthesia imaging relies on high-resolution (high-quality) imaging, most ultrasound-guided blocks use high-frequency probes at shallow depths. For example, high-frequency probes (10–18 MHz) can be used for an interscalene block because the depth of imaging is only 1 to 2 cm, giving a very high-resolution image. Contrast this with neuraxial imaging, which at around 6 to 10 cm requires the use of low frequency (1–5 MHz) probes to penetrate these depths and will generate a much lower resolution image.

## ULTRASOUND EQUIPMENT

Ultrasonic probes are available in several different shapes and sizes to match the surface contours of the anatomic site of interest. Most probes are either linear or curvilinear. Within the head of the probe, the piezoelectric array is made up of many tiny crystal elements. Each element can emit and detect the reflected waveform independently. This type of ultrasound is called a *phased array*. Using advanced computer algorithms and variable waveform timing, these zones can "steer" the ultrasonic beam in different directions. By taking multiple images and averaging the results, called *spatial compound imaging*, the signal-to-noise ratio can be improved. In addition to frequency, discussed earlier, other parameters of the ultrasound machine include *gain*, an adjustment of the intensity or brightness of the image at a given depth, and *focus*, whereby adjusting the timing of the waveform generation more ultrasound energy can be delivered to a given depth of tissue, increasing the image quality at that depth. Most modern ultrasound machines will have preset options to optimize internal parameters to the study of interest.

Ultrasonic gel is applied between the probe and the skin to eliminate air, which rapidly attenuates (decreases) the ultrasound waveform, and to reduce the Z-interface at the skin surface, which improves propagation of the waveform into the tissue.

Needle characteristics are important for ultrasonic regional anesthesia. The larger the diameter of the needle, the easier it is to image with ultrasound. Some manufacturers include notches on the shaft of the needle to improve the angle of incidence and reflect more ultrasonic energy back to the transducer, improving visualization of the needle with steep approach angles.

As many regional techniques rely on the periarterial location of nerve structures, imaging blood flow is important to both identify and avoid vascular structures. Color Doppler ultrasound imaging works on the principle of the *Doppler effect*, the change in frequency of the echo when a sound wave hits a moving object. As the ultrasound wave is incident on a moving red blood cell, the cell will reflect the wave back at a different frequency proportional to the velocity of the cell. By measuring this change in frequency, the direction and speed of the blood can be estimated.

## TISSUE ULTRASOUND CHARACTERISTICS

Each tissue will transmit, absorb, or reflect the sound waves differently depending on the *echodensity* of the tissue. Tissues that conduct sound waves well, called *echolucent* or *anechoic*, will appear black on ultrasound and typically have high water content, such as cerebrospinal or blood. Conversely, those tissues that conduct sound poorly are termed *hyperechoic* and will reflect most of the energy back to the transducer and appear bright. Tendons, bone, and fascial planes are hyperechoic. Muscle and fat tissue reflects less sound; these are *hypoechoic* and are typically outlined by their respective hyperechoic fascial planes.

Some tissues exhibit *anisotropy*, a change in echogenicity when imaged from a different axes or orientation. This property can be useful to distinguish a neuronal structure, which has moderate anisotropy, from tendons, which are highly anisotropic as shown in Fig. 100.2.

When imaging neurovascular structures for regional anesthesia, it is important to understand the typical imaging characteristics of peripheral nerves. Proximal nerves (brachial plexus), with their tightly packed axonal bundles, appear hypoechoic or dark on ultrasound imaging. Distal nerves (axillary, femoral, radial), with more connective tissue and fewer axons, appear hyperechoic or "honeycombed" (Fig. 100.3).

## ULTRASOUND IMAGING ARTIFACTS

Understanding the errors in the representative ultrasound image, called *artifacts*, is important to improve safety and block success. Some common artifacts seen in ultrasound imaging include reverberation, refraction, acoustic enhancement, and

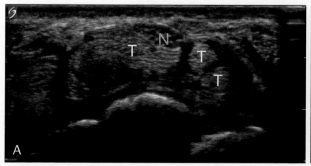
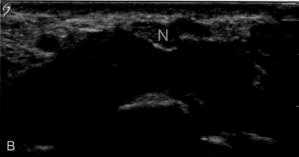

**Fig. 100.2 Anisotropy.** Both tendons and nerves exhibit *anisotropy*, a change in echogenicity when imaged from a different axes or orientation. A slight tilt of the ultrasound probe (about 2 degrees) between (A) and (B) of an image at the wrist shows a dramatic change in echogenicity of the tendons *(T)* while highlighting the median nerve *(N)*.

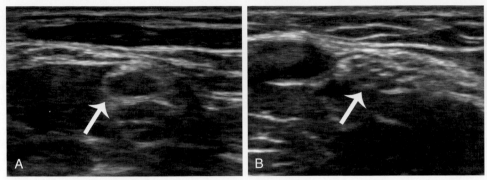

**Fig. 100.3 Nerve Characteristics.** The nerves in the proximal brachial plexus (A) appear hypoechoic secondary to their tightly bound axonal bundles, whereas the more distal median nerve (B) appears hyperechoic or "honeycombed" because it has more connective tissue and fewer axons.

acoustic shadowing. *Reverberation* occurs when the waveform bounces back and forth between two parallel Z-interfaces (such as the shaft of a hollow needle) causing multiple delayed signals to return to the probe. The signal processor assumes that an echo returns after a single reflection and interprets these delayed echoes as deeper structures because it takes longer for a reverberated wave to return to the transducer (Fig. 100.4*A*). Similarly, *mirror artifacts* occur when a strong smooth reflector reflects the waveform to an overlying tissue. It thus acts like a deep transmitter below the object and causes a secondary signal to appear.

*Refraction* artifact is caused by the ultrasound beam changing direction at the interface of two tissues with different propagation speeds. This can cause the needle to appear "bent" on the display similar to how a straw can appear bent in a glass of water. A similar artifact, termed a "bayonet" or velocity artifact, occurs because the speed of sound is not constant but varies with the tissue. If the sound velocity slows above part of the

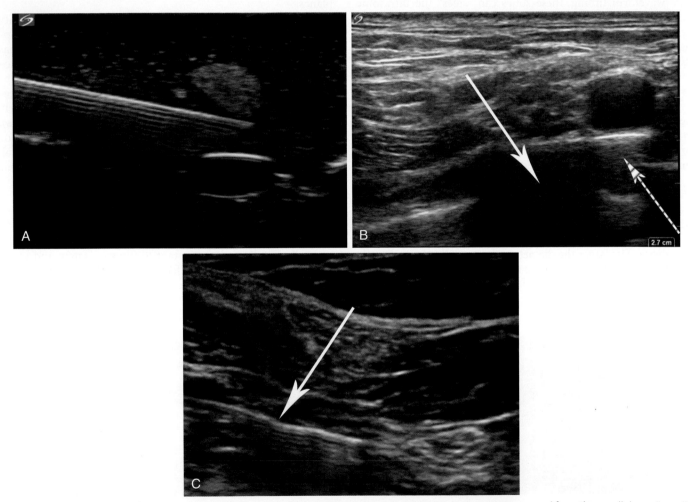

**Fig. 100.4 Ultrasound Artifacts.** Common artifacts include (A) Reverberation, secondary to multiple echoes returned from the parallel needle walls; (B) Acoustic shadowing *(solid arrow)* below the first rib in the supraclavicular view and acoustic enhancement *(striped arrow)* below the artery; and (C) "bayonet artifact," which makes the needle appear wavy or bent in the popliteal view secondary to errors in velocity estimation.

needle, the echo will take longer to return, and the signal processor, which assumes constant sound velocity, will display the needle part deeper in the image (Fig. 100.4C).

As the ultrasound wave travels through the tissue, it becomes attenuated or weakened secondary to scattering and absorption of the wave. The ultrasound display compensates for this attenuation by amplifying later echoes, termed *time gain compensation*, to make the display brightness uniform. When the beam passes through tissues with low attenuation (fluid), more energy is returned from deeper structures than anticipated and these deeper structures appear brighter. This is called *acoustic enhancement* and is particularly important in regional anesthesia as it can create the false appearance of nerves below vessels. The converse, *acoustic shadowing*, occurs with structures deep to tissues with high attenuation. In this case there will be shadowing and loss of signal, such as occurs below bones, as shown in Fig. 100.4B.

The orientation of the needle is important and can be inserted into the tissue "in plane" or "out of plane" with respect to the ultrasound transducer. In-plane imaging allows for the entire shaft of the needle to be visualized during needle insertion. Out-of-plane imaging will only reflect a cross-section of the needle shaft. With in-plane imaging, the angle of incidence between the needle and the probe will determine the ability to visualize the needle shaft. Shallow angles reflect more ultrasonic energy to the probe and improve visualization, whereas steep angles give poor visualization as most of the echo is reflected away from the probe. Needle approaches that maintain a shallow angle can improve block success.

## Ultrasound Safety

Ultrasound imaging for regional anesthesia is considered safe. Concerns for localized tissue heating or mechanical stress from ultrasound waves have not been shown with the duration or energies used for regional anesthesia. Regarding safety, it is important for the operator to realize that only the narrow window of tissue below the probe is visualized at a given time. A needle passed away from or oblique to this imaging plane can cause damage to structures not visualized in the ultrasound beam, including vessels, nerves, or lung parenchyma. Furthermore, direct visualization does not prevent all intravascular injection. Always identify the needle tip before advancing a needle near critical structures and direct the needle toward the tangent rather than the center of the target nerve.

Ultrasound guidance has been shown to reduce the risk of local anesthetic systemic toxicity, intravascular injection, and both hemidiaphragmatic paresis and pneumothorax with supraclavicular blocks. However, the use of ultrasound to reduce peripheral nerve injury remains unclear. Ultimately, all the benefits of using ultrasound in regional anesthesia require a competent and well-trained practitioner.

## SUGGESTED READINGS

Baad, M., Lu, Z. F., Reiser, I., & Paushter, D. (2017). Clinical significance of US artifacts. *Radiographics, 37,* 1408–1423.

Barrington, M. J., & Uda, Y. (2018). Did ultrasound fulfill the promise of safety in regional anesthesia? *Current Opinion in Anaesthesiology, 31,* 649–655.

Gray, A. T. (2019). *Atlas of Ultrasound-Guided Regional Anesthesia* (3rd ed.). Philadelphia: Elsevier.

Liu, S. S. (2016). Evidence basis for ultrasound-guided block characteristics onset, quality, and duration. *Regional Anesthesia and Pain Medicine, 41,* 205–220.

Neal, J. M., Brull, R., Horn, J. L., Liu, S. S., McCartney, C. J., Perlas, A., et al. (2016). The Second American Society of regional anesthesia and pain medicine evidence-based medicine assessment of ultrasound-guided regional anesthesia: Executive summary. *Regional Anesthesia and Pain Medicine, 41,* 181–194.

Xu, D., De Meirsman, S., & Schreurs, R. (2022). Optimizing an ultrasound image. In A. Hadzic (Ed.), *Hadzic's peripheral nerve blocks and anatomy for ultrasound-guided regional anesthesia* (3rd ed.). New York: McGraw Hill.

# Speciality Anesthesia: Neuroanesthesia

# Cerebral Protection

BENJAMIN FREDRICK GRUENBAUM, MD, PhD  |  SHAUN EVAN GRUENBAUM, MD, PhD

Cerebral ischemia results when the metabolic demands of the cerebral tissue exceed substrate (primarily $O_2$) delivery. Ischemia can be categorized as either global, which reflects a complete interruption of substrate delivery to the entire brain (e.g., after cardiac arrest), or focal, which reflects an interruption of substrate delivery to a defined region of the brain (e.g., after embolic cerebral arterial occlusion). Cerebral neuroprotective strategies include any modality that prolongs the ischemic tolerance of brain tissue and reduces neuronal injury that results from ischemia.

The traditional concept of cerebral metabolism is illustrated in Fig. 101.1. Cerebral metabolism includes a functional component and a cellular integrity component. The functional component comprises 60% of neuronal $O_2$ utilization. This component is responsible for generating action potentials and can be quantified by electroencephalogram assessment. The cellular integrity component consists of the remaining 40% of $O_2$ utilization for protein synthesis and other activities that maintain cellular integrity.

Anesthetic agents and hypothermia decrease the functional component of cerebral metabolism, reducing $O_2$ consumption by up to 60%. Hypothermia can further reduce $O_2$ utilization by decreasing the metabolic requirements for cellular integrity maintenance. In this simple $O_2$ supply–metabolic demand paradigm, cerebral neuroprotection can be achieved in ischemic conditions by optimizing the cerebral perfusion pressure (CPP) and $O_2$ delivery, whereas cerebral metabolism is reduced with the use of anesthetic agents and hypothermia.

The process of cerebral ischemia includes an initial ischemic event, followed by a secondary cascade of events that continues long after the initial event has resolved, which results in neuronal loss (Fig. 101.2). Excitotoxicity reflects a cascade of glutamate-mediated reactions that results in neuronal apoptosis (i.e., protease-mediated programmed cell death) shortly after the onset of neuronal ischemia. Apoptosis and inflammation are initiated by the ischemic event and continue to contribute to neuron loss for several days. Therefore it might be possible to limit ischemic damage by invoking cerebral protective therapies before, during, or after an ischemic event (Table 101.1). The currently available evidence that supports the use of cerebral neuroprotective strategies is derived primarily from animal models and limited clinical studies. Currently, conclusive evidence for the neuroprotective effects of anesthetic agents is lacking.

## Regulation of Physiologic Parameters

### TEMPERATURE

Hyperthermia should be avoided after an ischemic insult because it results in increased cerebral metabolism and subsequently worsens neurologic injury. Hypothermia, by contrast, reduces both the functional and cellular integrity components of cerebral metabolism. Profound hypothermia ($<14°C$) induces electrocerebral silence (ECS) in 80% of patients, allowing for 30 min of hypothermic circulatory arrest (HCA) without significant neuronal sequelae. In 20% to 80% of patients, deep hypothermia ($14.1°C–20°C$) induces ECS that is

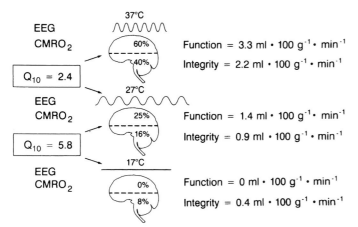

**Fig. 101.1** Theoretical interaction of temperature, brain function, cerebral metabolic $O_2$ consumption (CMRO_2), and calculated $Q_{10}$ value. $Q_{10}$ is defined as the ratio of metabolic rates at two temperatures separated by 10°C. In reducing temperature from 37°C to 27°C, function is maintained and both of the energy-consuming processes (i.e., function and integrity) are presumed to be affected equally, with a reduction in CMRo_2 of slightly more than 50%, thus generating a $Q_{10}$ value of about 2.4. With a further 10°C reduction in temperature to 17°C, function is abolished, resulting in a steep decrease in CMRo_2 such that the calculated $Q_{10}$ value is 5.0 or greater. At this point, the total $O_2$ consumed by the brain is reduced to less than 8% of the normothermic value of $O_2$. EEG, Electroencephalogram. (Reprinted, with permission, from Michenfelder JD, ed. Anesthesia and the Brain. Churchill Livingstone; 1988:14.)

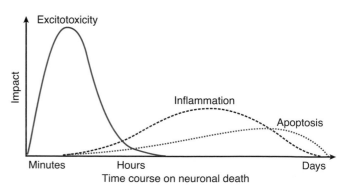

**Fig. 101.2** Time course of neuronal death after cerebral ischemia. Excitotoxicity rapidly leads to neuronal necrosis. Inflammation and neuronal apoptosis contribute to ongoing cell death for a period that extends from several days to weeks. (From Patel P. Cerebral ischemia and intraoperative brain protection. In: Gupta AK, Gelb AW, eds. Essentials of Neuroanesthesia and Neurointensive Care. WB Saunders; 2008:36–48.)

| TABLE 101.1 Evidence-Based Status of Plausible Interventions to Reduce Perioperative Ischemic Brain Injury | | | | | | |
|---|---|---|---|---|---|---|
| | EFFICACY IN EXPERIMENTAL ANIMALS | | EFFICACY IN HUMANS | | SUSTAINED PROTECTION IN | |
| Intervention | Preischemic | Postischemic | Preischemic | Postischemic | Animals | Humans |
| **HYPOTHERMIA** | | | | | | |
| Mild | ++ | ++ | ± | ++* | ++ | ++ |
| Moderate | − − − | − − − | − − | − − | − − − | |
| Hyperventilation | − − | − − | − − | − − | − − | − − |
| Normoglycemia | ++ | − − | + | ++ | ++ | − − |
| Hyperbaric $O_2$ | ++ | − − | − − | ± | − − | − − |
| Barbiturates | ++ | − | + | ++ | ++ | − − |
| Propofol | ++ | + | − | − − | − − | − |
| Etomidate | − − − | − − | − − | − − | − − | − − |
| $N_2O$ | − | − − | − − | − − | − − | − − |
| Isoflurane | ++ | − − | − − | − − | ++ | − − |
| Sevoflurane | | − − | − − | − − | ++ | − − |
| Desflurane | ++ | − − | − − | − − | − − | − − |
| Lidocaine | ++ | − − | + | − − | − − | − − |
| Ketamine | ++ | − − | − − | − − | − − | − − |
| Glucocorticoids | − − − | − − | − − | − − | − − | − − |

*Out-of-hospital ventricular fibrillation cardiac arrest.

++, Supported by evidence from repeated physiologically controlled studies in animals/randomized, prospective, adequately powered clinical trials; +, consistent suggestion by case series/retrospective or prospective trials with small sample sizes or data extrapolated from other paradigms; ±, inconsistent findings in clinical trials, may be dependent on characteristics of insult; −, well-defined absence of benefit; − −, absence of evidence in physiologically controlled studies in animals/randomized, prospective adequately powered clinical trials; − − −, evidence of potential harm.
(Adapted, with permission, from Fukuda S, Warner DS. Cerebral protection. *Br J Anaesth.* 2007;99:10–17.)

proportional to the level of hypothermia and allows for 20 to 30 min of HCA. Moderate hypothermia (20.1°C–28°C) allows for 10 to 20 min of HCA. Mild hypothermia (28.1°C–34°C) provides minimal ECS and resumption of metabolic activity. Studies in adults who have survived out-of-hospital cardiac arrest and in neonates with asphyxia have shown that mild hypothermia (32°C–35°C) has beneficial cerebral neuroprotective effects. The temperature goals in current therapeutic hypothermia protocols are 33°C to 36°C, for which studies have demonstrated similar neurologic outcomes compared with lower temperature goals.

Recently, animal studies and small clinical trials have provided some promising results that support the use of therapeutic hypothermia after ischemic stroke and traumatic brain injury (TBI). Larger clinical trials, however, have failed to demonstrate any neurologic or mortality benefit when therapeutic hypothermia is used. Therefore therapeutic hypothermia is currently not recommended as a neuroprotective strategy for these conditions.

## CEREBRAL PERFUSION PRESSURE

Mathematically, the CPP equals the mean arterial pressure minus the intracranial pressure (CPP = MAP − ICP). Under normal conditions, cerebral blood flow (CBF) autoregulates over a range of CPP from 50 to 150 mm Hg. The autoregulation curve is shifted to the right in patients with chronic hypertension. Studies of CBF in patients with TBI have demonstrated that the CPP goal should be in the range of 60 to 70 mm Hg if clinically feasible. Hypotension can decrease CBF and worsen ischemia.

## CO$_2$ TENSION

$CO_2$ is a known potent cerebral vasodilator, and hyperventilation results in hypocapnia and cerebral vascular vasoconstriction. Profound hypocapnia can result in decreased CBF and worsened neurologic outcome after TBI and other acute ischemic events.

## OXYGENATION

Restoration of $O_2$ delivery to ischemic tissues should theoretically resolve the deleterious effects of ischemia. However, supraphysiologic concentrations of $O_2$ in the cerebral tissue can result in the formation of reactive $O_2$ species, which paradoxically leads to worsened neurologic outcomes.

## GLUCOSE METABOLISM

During ischemic conditions, glucose undergoes anaerobic metabolism that results in intracellular acidosis and poor neurologic outcomes. Frequent glucose monitoring is recommended in patients at risk for developing cerebral ischemia, with the goal of achieving euglycemia. Hypoglycemia and hyperglycemia should be avoided.

## Anesthetic Agents

Some anesthetic agents have demonstrated neuroprotective effects. However, much of the research on the neuroprotective effects of these drugs after an ischemic event lacks the necessary standardization of dosage, frequency, and risk factors. This introduction aims to provide an overview of several commonly used anesthetic agents and highlights the need for further studies that evaluate their proposed neuroprotective effects.

## BARBITURATES

Historically, barbiturates have been considered the gold standard for providing neuroprotection when administered prior to a focal ischemic event. The neuroprotective properties of barbiturates are supported by a single human study in patients undergoing cardiopulmonary bypass, and corroborative evidence in other clinical trials is currently lacking. Historically, it has been argued that the underlying mechanism of barbiturate-mediated cerebral neuroprotection in laboratory animals reflected a dose-dependent reduction in the cerebral metabolic rate. However, subsequent studies have demonstrated that barbiturate doses that result in electroencephalographic isoelectricity or burst suppression are equally neuroprotective, suggesting additional neuroprotective mechanisms. Undesirable effects of high-dose barbiturates, such as cardiovascular instability and delayed emergence and neurologic assessment, should always be considered when barbiturates to achieve neuroprotection.

## DEXMEDETOMIDINE

Alpha-2 adrenoceptor agonists are often administered for their sedative and analgesic effects. Dexmedetomidine has been found to decrease the inflammatory response and neuroendocrine release during neurologic surgery. These effects are thought to be in part due to decreased heart rate and blood pressure. A recent metaanalysis has shown that the use of dexmedetomidine also reduces the surge of TNF-alpha and IL-6, which are known for their inflammatory and neurodegenerative effects during the acute phases of brain ischemia. Dexmedetomidine also suppresses serum-specific enolase (NSE) and S100-beta, neurobiochemical markers secreted by neurons during ischemic conditions. S100-beta worsens inflammatory responses and contributes to neuronal toxicity. Other studies have suggested that dexmedetomidine may decrease cortisol and glucose release, leading to improved neurologic outcomes after cerebral ischemia. Additionally, dexmedetomidine was found to facilitate hemodynamic stability, decrease elevation in intracranial pressure, and inhibit inflammatory and neuroendocrine responses resulting from an ischemic insult. Studies addressing optimal dosing regimens and times of administration are currently lacking.

## PROPOFOL

Laboratory studies in animal models of ischemia have suggested that propofol has neuroprotective effects; however, this has not yet been confirmed in human studies.

## REMIFENTANIL

Studies have failed to demonstrate neuroprotective effects of intraoperative remifentanil administration in patients after ischemic stroke.

## MANNITOL

There is currently little evidence to suggest that mannitol provides neuroprotection in human studies.

## HYPERTONIC SALINE

Hypertonic saline has not been established as an effective neuroprotective strategy after cerebral ischemia.

## INHALATION ANESTHETIC AGENTS

Commonly used volatile anesthetics produce significant and reversible electroencephalographic suppression at clinical doses. Animal studies have demonstrated potent neuroprotective effects of volatile anesthetics in the setting of focal and transient global ischemia; however, conclusive human data are currently lacking.

## LIDOCAINE

In typical antiarrhythmic doses, lidocaine may inhibit neuronal apoptosis. Supratherapeutic (i.e., toxic) doses are necessary to achieve a reduction in cerebral metabolism.

## ETOMIDATE

Etomidate decreases cerebral metabolism in a manner similar to that observed by barbiturates, although the data supporting its neuroprotective effects are less convincing than for barbiturates. The lack of observed neuroprotective effects with etomidate may be due to its inhibition of nitric oxide production, which subsequently decreases CBF.

## Conclusion

Pharmacologic and physiologic modalities that protect the nervous system from the cascade of delirious events that follow an ischemic insult are important to consider. Current neuroprotective strategies include a few promising interventions; however, most strategies are speculative or have not yet been supported by clinical data. Box 101.1 provides a basic evidence-based framework for using neuroprotective strategies after an ischemic insult.

---

**BOX 101.1  CONSIDERATIONS WHEN ANTICIPATING OR MANAGING A PERIOPERATIVE ISCHEMIC INSULT**

Ensure the absence of hyperthermia
Manage blood glucose concentration with insulin to induce normoglycemia
Optimize oxyhemoglobin saturation*
Establish normocapnia
Consider the use of inhalation anesthetic agents if the operation is prolonged[†]
Resist the use of glucocorticoids
Consider the use of postoperative sustained induced moderate hypothermia if global ischemia is present[‡]

---

*Increasing concern has arisen that hypoxemia may be adverse in global ischemia.
[†]Not tested by clinical trials in the perioperative environment but supported by consistent efficacy when used in out-of-hospital ventricular fibrillation cardiac arrest.
[‡]No evidence of efficacy; preclinical evidence of adverse effect in global ischemia.
(Adapted, with permission, from Fukuda S, Warner DS. Cerebral protection. *Br J Anaesth.* 2007;99:10–17.)

## SUGGESTED READINGS

Badenes, R., Gruenbaum, S., & Bilotta, F. (2015). Cerebral protection during neurosurgery and stroke. *Current Opinion in Anaesthesiology, 28*(5), 532–536.

Jiang, L., Hu, M., Lu, Y., Cao, Y., Chang, Y., & Dai, Z. (2017). The protective effects of dexmedetomidine on ischemic brain injury: A meta-analysis. *Journal of Clinical Anesthesia, 40,* 25–32.

Powers, W. J., Rabinstein, A. A., Ackerman, T., Adeoye, O. M., Bambakidis, N. C., Becker, K., et al. (2019).

Guidelines for the early management of patients with acute ischemic stroke: 2019 Update to the 2018 guidelines for the early management of acute ischemic stroke: A guideline for professionals from the American Heart Association/American Stroke Association. *Stroke, 50*(12), e344–e418.

Stocchetti, N., Taccone, F. S., Citerio, G., Pepe, P. E., Le Roux, P. D., Oddo, M., et al. (2015). Neuroprotection in acute brain injury: An up-to-date review. *Critical Care, 19*(1), 186.

Urits, I., Jones, M. R., Orhurhu, V., Sikorsky, A., Seifert, D., Flores, C., et al. (2019). A comprehensive update of current anesthesia perspectives on therapeutic hypothermia. *Advances in Therapy, 36,* 2223–2232.

Zwerus, R., & Absalom, A. (2015). Update on anesthetic neuroprotection. *Current Opinion in Anaesthesiology, 28*(4), 424–430.

# 102

# Increased Intracranial Pressure

BENJAMIN FREDRICK GRUENBAUM, MD, PhD   |   SHAUN EVAN GRUENBAUM, MD, PhD

Intracranial pressure (ICP) refers to the pressure within the intracranial vault. The intracranial vault consists of three volume compartments: brain parenchyma, cerebrospinal fluid (CSF), and blood. Intracranial hypertension is defined as ICP above 20 mm Hg that persists for more than 5 minutes. Without immediate treatment, increased intracranial pressure can lead to cerebral ischemia, herniation, and death.

## Brain

The brain parenchyma is composed of cellular elements as well as intracellular and interstitial water. The average adult brain weighs between 1350 and 1450 g and accounts for approximately 90% of the intracranial volume. This compartment can expand through tumor growth or cytotoxic cerebral edema.

## Cerebrospinal Fluid

The CSF occupies approximately 5% of the intracranial volume (i.e., approx. 75 mL, of which approximately 25 mL is confined to the ventricles). The rate of CSF production is about 0.35 mL/min in the normal adult, or about 580 mL per 24 h. Expansion of this compartment can occur in the presence of obstructive or communicating hydrocephalus.

## Blood

Intracranial blood accounts for the remaining 5% of the intracranial volume. The cerebral blood volume (CBV) is 3 to 7 mL/100 g brain weight. Elevation of the head decreases both CBV and ICP. Expansion of the blood compartment can result from cerebral hemorrhage or dilation of resistance or capacitance vessels (e.g., vasogenic cerebral edema). This compartment is most responsive to acute therapeutic intervention. With few exceptions (e.g., cerebral vasospasm), profound hypotension results in increased cerebral blood flow (CBF) and parallel increases in CBV and ICP.

## Intracranial Elastance

Historically, the intracranial pressure-volume relationship has been termed *compliance* in the medical literature. Compliance is defined as a unit change in volume (e.g., intracranial volume) divided by a unit change in pressure (e.g., ICP). This relationship can be mathematically defined as $\Delta V/\Delta P$. However, another common way to consider this relationship is presented in Fig. 102.1; the figure also depicts elastance, which is mathematically the reciprocal of compliance.

Elastance is mathematically defined as $\Delta P/\Delta V$. Under normal physiologic conditions, small volume increases in any one of the three intracranial compartments results in little or no change in ICP. The compensatory mechanisms that initially protect against an elevation in ICP include (a) translocation of intracranial CSF through the foramen magnum to the subarachnoid space surrounding the spinal cord, (b) increased CSF absorption through the arachnoid granulations, and (c) translocation of blood out of the intracranial vault. Once these mechanisms are exhausted, significant increases in ICP can result from small increases in intracranial volume (see Fig. 102.1). Under these conditions, intracranial elastance is increased and intracranial compliance is decreased.

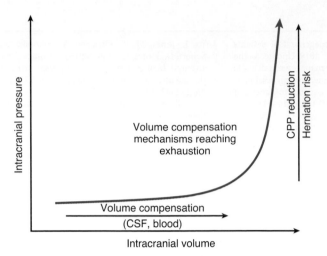

**Fig. 102.1** Idealized intracranial pressure-volume curve. The horizontal segment depicts maintenance of intracranial pressure (ICP) via physiologic compensatory mechanisms that respond to expanding intracranial volume (e.g., tumor, hematoma). Once these compensatory mechanisms are exhausted, elastance is increased, and small changes in intracranial volume result in large changes in ICP. *CPP,* Cerebral perfusion pressure; *CSF,* cerebrospinal fluid. (From Drummond JC, Patel PM. Neurosurgical anesthesia. In: Miller RD, ed. *Miller's Anesthesia.* Churchill Livingstone Elsevier; 2009:2045–2087.)

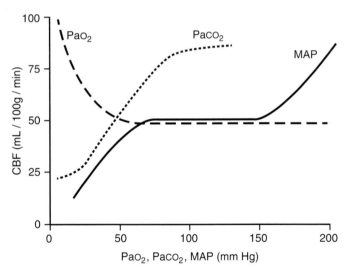

**Fig. 102.2** Effects of $PaO_2$, $PaCO_2$, and mean arterial pressure on cerebral blood flow. *CBF,* Cerebral blood flow; *MAP,* mean arterial pressure.

## Anesthetic Considerations

The goals of managing a patient with intracranial hypertension include the prevention of cerebral ischemia and subsequent brain herniation.

### RESPIRATORY

$PaCO_2$ is the single most potent physiologic determinant of CBF (Fig. 102.2) and CBV. At a $PaCO_2$ between 20 and 80 mm Hg, CBF decreases 1 mL/100 g brain weight/min and CBV decreases 0.05 mL/100 g brain weight for each 1-mm Hg decrease in $PaCO_2$. Decreasing $PaCO_2$ to 25 to 28 mm Hg should provide near-maximal reductions in ICP. This effect lasts up to 24 h without adversely affecting acid-base or electrolyte status or decreasing cerebral $O_2$ delivery (i.e., resulting from combined cerebral vasoconstriction and leftward shift in the oxyhemoglobin dissociation curve). Accordingly, in the setting of severe traumatic brain injury (TBI), the Brain Trauma Foundation advises that aggressive hyperventilation (i.e., $PaCO_2$ ≤25 mm Hg) is contraindicated because extreme $PaCO_2$ reductions can result in iatrogenic brain injury.

Hypoxia ($PaO_2$ <50 mm Hg) increases CBF and ICP. Application of positive end-expiratory pressure can decrease the venous effluent from the cranium and exacerbate intracranial hypertension.

Similarly, coughing against a closed glottis (i.e., during the Valsalva maneuver) significantly increases the ICP. Lidocaine, esmolol, or opioids can be administered to prevent cough-associated ICP increases during intubation.

### CARDIOVASCULAR

Mean arterial pressure (MAP) is an important determinant of the cerebral perfusion pressure, or CPP (i.e., CPP = MAP − ICP or CVP, whichever is higher). The blood-brain barrier and autoregulatory mechanisms can be disrupted at the site of cerebral ischemic, traumatic, hemorrhagic, or osmolar insults. CBF is thought to be passively dependent on CPP in these regions. Before the dura is opened, hypertensive episodes should be preemptively avoided by deepening the anesthetic depth and administering antihypertensive drugs that do not dilate cerebral vessels (e.g., esmolol, labetalol, metoprolol). With respect to CPP, the critical threshold for ischemia is approximately 50 to 60 mm Hg. Maintaining CPP that approaches 60 to 70 mm Hg is advisable in the setting of TBI. Routine use of vasopressors and intravenously administered fluids to maintain CPP greater than 70 mm Hg is not advised.

### FLUIDS

Intravenous fluid administration should not be limited at the expense of hemodynamic instability. Osmolar, not oncotic, pressure is the primary determinant of fluid shifts within the brain. Therefore maintaining intravascular isovolemia with a near-isoosmolar solution (e.g., normal saline, or lactated Ringer solution) is safe and beneficial to achieve end organ preservation. The use of hypo-osmolar glucose-containing fluids (e.g., $D_5W$) is avoided because these solutions can result in cerebral edema, increased ICP, and hyperglycemia, which can further worsen ischemic neurologic injury.

Hypertonic saline is currently the treatment of choice for reducing intracranial hypertension after TBI, which has been shown in recent studies to reduce ICP at a faster rate compared with mannitol, opioids, barbiturates, and propofol. However, this finding has not translated to a reduction in morbidity or mortality, and other studies have failed to demonstrate that hypertonic saline is significantly advantageous over alternative ICP reduction strategies.

Both osmotic (e.g., mannitol) and loop diuretics (e.g., furosemide) reduce the parenchymal fluid compartment and decrease CSF formation.

## Metabolic Considerations

Evidence supports the use of mild hypothermia for neuroprotection after acute coronary syndromes, and there is much interest in the use of hypothermia to reduce tissue damage after central nervous system injury. Hypothermia reduces ICP by decreasing cerebral metabolism by approximately 6% per 1°C reduction in temperature. Conversely, hyperthermia can worsen postischemic neurologic outcome.

Therapeutic hypothermia can be effective at preventing intracranial hypertension when initiated immediately after a brain insult, but it has also been shown to be effective in reducing ICP after the onset of intracranial hypertension. Despite convincing animal studies on the effects of hypothermia on neurologic outcomes after an ischemic brain insult, large multicenter clinical trials have yielded inconsistent and variable results. Currently, the Brain Trauma Foundation does not include therapeutic hypothermia in its most recent clinical guidelines for TBI intervention.

## MUSCULOSKELETAL

To facilitate tracheal intubation and maintain neuromuscular blockade, the use of nondepolarizing neuromuscular blocking agents such as rocuronium, vecuronium, or cisatracurium is recommended. Atracurium can release histamine and should be avoided. In the pathologic brain, pancuronium and gallamine can induce systemic and intracranial hypertension.

Succinylcholine may transiently increase ICP, possibly by increasing muscle afferent activity, but the clinical significance of this increased ICP is likely negligible.

## SPECIFIC ANESTHETIC AGENTS

All commonly used inhalation anesthetic agents are cerebral vasodilators that cause dose-dependent increases in CBF, CBV, and ICP in normocapnic patients. These effects are similar in isoflurane, sevoflurane, and desflurane at clinical doses. The cerebral vasodilation observed with volatile agents can be mitigated by the concomitant use of hyperventilation. There is a lack of clinical evidence to suggest that nitrous oxide has any effect on neurologic deficits, total hospital stay, or hospital cost in neurosurgical patients.

With the exception of ketamine, which has a spectrum of neuroprotective and detrimental cerebral effects, all intravenously administered anesthetic agents cause some degree of reduction in cerebral metabolism, CBF, and ICP (assuming ventilation is not reduced).

## Postoperative Care

A rapid and smooth emergence from general anesthesia minimizes the hemodynamic effects on ICP and helps facilitate a comprehensive neurologic assessment prior to discharge from the operative suite.

### SUGGESTED READINGS

Alnemari, A. M., Krafcik, B. M., Mansour, T. R., & Gaudin, D. (2017). A comparison of pharmacologic therapeutic agents used for the reduction of intracranial pressure after traumatic brain injury. *World Neurosurg, 106*, 509–528.

Carney, N., Totten, A. M., O'Reilly, C., Ullman, J. S., Hawryluk, G. W., Bell, M. J., et al. (2017). Guidelines for the management of severe traumatic brain injury, fourth edition. *Neurosurgery, 80*(1), 6–15.

Chen, H., Song, Z., & Dennis, J. A. (2020). Hypertonic saline versus other intracranial pressure-lowering agents for people with acute traumatic brain injury. *Cochrane Database of Systematic Reviews, 17*(1), 1.

De-Lima-Oliveira, M., Salinet, A. S. M., Nogueira, R. C., de Azevedo, D. S., Paiva, W. S., Teixeira, M. J., et al. (2018). Intracranial hypertension and cerebral autoregulation: A systematic review and meta-analysis. *World Neurosurg, 113*, 110–124.

Farrell, D., & Bendo, A. A. (2018). Perioperative management of severe traumatic brain injury: What is new? *Current Anesthesiology Reports, 8*, 279–289.

Gruenbaum, S. E., Zlotnik, A., Gruenbaum, B. F., Hersey, D., & Bilotta, F. (2016). Pharmacologic neuroprotection for functional outcomes after traumatic brain injury: A systematic review of the clinical literature. *CNS Drugs, 30*(9), 791–806.

# 103

# Functional Neurosurgery

LINDSAY ROYCE HUNTER GUEVARA, MD | JEFFREY J. PASTERNAK, MS, MD

Functional neurosurgery is a broad term applied to a variety of neurosurgical procedures performed to treat conditions in which the function of the brain is abnormal, typically in the context of normal gross structure and anatomy. These conditions include movement disorders, psychiatric diseases, pain disorders, cervical dystonia, and epilepsy. Some of these procedures can be used to treat a broad range of disease states. The major challenge during functional neurosurgical procedures is to accurately and safely identify the abnormal regions of brain tissue. This identification is accomplished either via neurologic assessment in an awake or minimally sedated patient or through the use of radiographically guided or electrophysiologically guided techniques.

## Deep Brain Stimulation

Deep brain stimulation (DBS) involves the implantation of electrodes into select regions of the brain, allowing for electrical stimulation of the area to modulate brain activity. This results in attenuation, if not elimination, of the symptoms and signs of a number of disease states. Indications for DBS are summarized in Table 103.1. The specific site of electrode implantation depends on the disorder for which the patient requires treatment, as illustrated in Fig. 103.1. DBS is believed to modulate abnormal neuronal function, either by acting directly on neuronal action potentials or altering neurotransmitter release. Use of DBS has generally replaced ablative procedures as DBS is less invasive and is reversible.

| TABLE 103.1 | Disease States and Potential Anatomic Targets for Deep Brain Stimulation | |
|---|---|
| **Disease** | **Potential Targets for Deep Brain Stimulation** |
| Parkinson's disease and essential tremor | Subthalamic nucleus |
| | Globus pallidus |
| Dystonia | Globus pallidus |
| Cerebellar tremor from multiple sclerosis | Thalamic ventral intermediate nucleus |
| Pantothenate kinase–associated neurodegeneration | Globus pallidus |
| Medical refractory depression | Subgenual cingulate region |
| Tourette's syndrome | Anterior limb of the internal capsule |
| | Thalamic centromedian-parafascicular complex |
| Obsessive-compulsive disorder | Nucleus accumbens |
| | Anterior limb of the internal capsule |
| Central pain syndromes | Motor cortex |
| | Peri-aqueductal gray matter |
| | Peri-ventricular gray matter |
| | Thalamus |
| Medically refractory epilepsy | Anterior nucleus of the thalamus |
| | Centromedian nucleus of the thalamus |
| | Subthalamic nucleus |
| Cluster headaches | Posterior hypothalamus |
| Obesity | Lateral hypothalamus |
| | Ventromedial hypothalamus |
| | Nucleus accumbens |

Modified with permission from Siddiqui MS, Ellis TL, Tatter SB, Okun MS. Deep brain stimulation: treating neurological and psychiatric disorders by modulating brain activity. *Neurorehabilitation.* 2008;23:105–113.

DBS implantation is typically conducted via frame-based stereotactic techniques. A stereotactic head frame is applied, after which the patient undergoes imaging to localize the deep brain target relative to the stereotactic head frame. With the patient in a semiseated position, the electrode is advanced through a burr hole in the cranium to the target location. Implantation of the electrode into the exact target nucleus may be facilitated by single-neuron recordings and by the resolution of symptoms upon stimulation in patients receiving sedation. In patients having general anesthesia, placement of electrodes is assisted by the use of stereotactic coordinates. After electrode implantation, wires are tunneled under the skin to reach a generator, which is typically implanted in the pectoral region.

Monitored anesthesia care is typically used to facilitate lead placement. Monitored anesthesia care allows for the use of both single-neuron microelectrode recordings and awake neurologic assessment as supplements to the use of coordinates derived from imaging relative to the stereotactic head frame to correctly identify the target location within the brain. Deep brain targets can be identified by their characteristic signature of neuronal discharges on single-neuron microelectrode recordings. Additionally, during monitored anesthesia care, attenuation of signs and symptoms of the patient's disease can be observed when the correct target is identified and electrically stimulated. Sedatives are administered to keep the patient "comfortable" but not so sedated that the surgeon cannot intraoperatively assess neurologic status and optimize the efficacy of electrode placement. Typically, $\gamma$-aminobutyric acid (GABA)-ergic sedatives are avoided because they can interfere with the reliability of single-neuron microelectrode recordings, whereas opioids and dexmedetomidine appear to have much less of a suppressive effect. A means to rapidly secure the airway (i.e., laryngeal mask airway, video laryngoscope, fiberoptic bronchoscope) should be readily available given the potential challenges with airway management with a patient in a stereotactic head frame. Tunneling of electrode leads and implantation of the pulse generator are usually performed with general anesthesia after removal of the stereotactic head frame.

In patients not able to tolerate the procedure with sedation, such as children, implantation of a DBS electrode can be conducted with general anesthesia. Drugs used to maintain general anesthesia can significantly affect the ability to identify and monitor single-neuron microelectrode recordings. Further, intraprocedural attenuation of signs and symptoms to confirm successful target acquisition is not possible during general anesthesia. In these situations, proper placement of the depth electrode is then dependent only on imaging data referenced to the stereotactic head frame.

Clinically significant venous air embolism has been reported, and precordial Doppler sonography monitoring should be considered. Of note, electrical impedance from precordial Doppler sonography may impair neuronal electrical recording and may require termination during recording of neuronal activity.

## Cervical Denervation for Dystonia

Dystonias are a group of disorders in which inappropriate and sustained muscle contractions lead to twisting movements and abnormal postures. For patients in whom conservative treatments have failed, cervical denervation to treat cervical dystonia (i.e., torticollis) or DBS may be options.

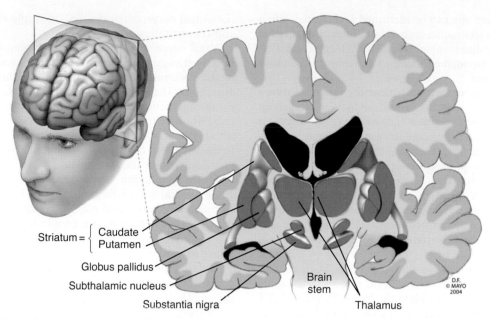

**Fig. 103.1**  The basal ganglia are primary targets for the treatment of a variety of disorders via deep brain stimulation. (Used with permission of Mayo Foundation for Medical Education and Research, all rights reserved.)

Cervical denervation involves identifying and transecting the nerves supplying the affected muscles in the neck. This procedure is conducted with general anesthesia with the patient in the prone or sitting position. In either case, the surgeon will directly stimulate nerves with an electric current to identify specific muscular innervation; hence the use of neuromuscular blocking drugs is contraindicated during this step of the procedure. In patients undergoing cervical denervation in the sitting position, monitors for venous air embolism (i.e., transesophageal echocardiography, precordial Doppler sonography) should be used.

## Epilepsy Surgery

Epilepsy, or recurrent seizure disorder, affects 50 million people worldwide and occurs in all age groups. Surgical treatment is usually considered for patients with seizures that are refractory of optimized pharmacotherapy or for those unable to tolerate the side effects of pharmacotherapy. There are two major types of epilepsy surgery: (1) resective and (2) nonresective procedures.

### RESECTIVE PROCEDURES

The goal of resective procedures is to remove an epileptogenic focus, an abnormal region of brain that is thought to initiate seizures. Because many epileptogenic foci amenable to surgery are located in the anterior temporal lobe, resection of lesions in this region is common, accounting for 75% of resective procedures. Perioperative identification of the epileptogenic focus is usually based on history and physical examination, brain imaging, and electroencephalography-based techniques.

In some patients, craniotomy is performed to facilitate the placement of depth electrodes or cortical electrode grids. Seizure focus resection could be performed during this same procedure if the focus can be identified via the electrodes. The monitoring technique used intraoperatively to identify the focus is called electrocorticography and is similar to electroencephalography except that electrode recordings are obtained directly from the brain instead of via surface electrodes on the scalp. In cases in which electrocorticography is employed intraoperatively, anesthetic drugs that suppress epileptiform activity should be avoided or minimized during mapping. These drugs include halogenated inhalational anesthetics, sedative and anesthetic doses of barbiturates and propofol, and benzodiazepines. Nitrous oxide, opioids, and dexmedetomidine may be used to maintain sedation or general anesthesia during this period. Additionally, low-dose methohexital (0.3–1 mg/kg), etomidate (0.1–0.3 mg/kg), remifentanil (4 μg/kg), or alfentanil (50 μg/kg) may be administered as a bolus to enhance epileptiform activity generated by the seizure focus. Patients requiring intraoperative electrocorticography should be counseled preoperatively on the increased risk of intraoperative awareness.

If an epileptogenic focus is not identified during the procedure where grids or depth electrodes were placed, the patient can be allowed to awaken from anesthesia and monitored in an epilepsy monitoring unit. The patients are then monitored for clinical seizure activity that can be correlated with simultaneous recordings from the depth electrodes and grid, facilitating the identification of a possible epileptogenic focus. If a focus is found, the patient can be brought back to the operating room for electrode removal and resection.

Stereoelectroencephalography (SEEG) is increasingly being use to identify epileptogenic foci. Instead of performing a craniotomy to allow for electrode placement, during a SEEG procedure electrodes are stereotactically placed via burr holes in the cranium to allow for identification of the seizure focus, and the patient is later monitored in an epilepsy-monitoring unit. The advantage of the SEEG technique is avoiding the need for a craniotomy in a patient for whom either a specific focus cannot be identified or where one can be identified and treated with a less invasive ablative technique, such as laser interstitial thermal therapy (LITT). The disadvantage of the SEEG technique is that ablation cannot be performed during the same procedure as electrode implantation.

In patients undergoing resection near the language center located in the temporal lobe, the procedure may be carried out with local anesthesia and sedation (i.e., awake craniotomy) allowing for intraoperative language assessment. Given the possibility of an intraprocedural seizure, the clinician should be prepared with airway equipment to secure an airway in a situation with limited airway access. Termination of a seizure should be accomplished with drugs that cause minimal respiratory depression in the setting of an unsecured airway such as with small doses of midazolam or propofol. Additionally, the surgeon may irrigate the brain surface with cold saline solution in an effort to terminate a seizure.

For patients in whom a seizure focus has been reliably identified via either SEEG or magnetic resonance imaging (MRI), LITT may be used to ablate the focus. During a LITT procedure, the patient is placed in a stereotactic head frame and then imaged to identify the coordinates of the epileptogenic focus relative to the head frame. Through a burr hole, a fiberoptic laser probe is placed into the epileptogenic focus. The laser is then used to ablate the focus, typically with MRI guidance such that MRI-derived tissue temperature estimates can be used to guide ablation of the focus and to minimize injury to surrounding normal brain parenchyma. LITT procedures are performed with general anesthesia and can also be used to ablate other types of intracranial lesions, such as brain tumors.

## NONRESECTIVE PROCEDURES

For patients who continue to have frequent seizures despite resective treatment or are deemed not to be candidates for resective options, other nonresective surgical procedures may be considered. Nonresective procedures are generally palliative and employed as a means to achieve a reduction in seizure frequency, as opposed to achieving a cure of epilepsy. These procedures include electrical stimulation techniques (i.e., vagal nerve, cortical, DBS), multiple subpial transection, and corpus callosotomy.

Vagal nerve stimulation involves placement of an electrode in the left vagal nerve sheath in the neck and a pulse generator in the pectoral region; it is typically performed with general anesthesia. The left vagus nerve is the preferred target because parasympathetic innervation of the heart is predominantly derived from the right vagus nerve. The exact mechanism by which vagal nerve stimulation results in a reduction in seizure frequency is not currently understood. The most common side effects are cough and hoarseness.

Other stimulation techniques used for seizure control include cortical stimulation and DBS. The major advantage of stimulation-based techniques for epilepsy control is reversibility, such that if patients are unable to tolerate side effects or experience no benefit, the device can be removed with minimal injury to brain tissue.

The treatment goal of the multiple subpial transsection or corpus callosotomy is to limit seizure spread to the adjacent cortex. These techniques are typically performed with general anesthesia.

## Focused Ultrasound

Transcranial focused ultrasound (FUS) uses high-intensity ultrasound waves to target specific areas of the brain to treat movement, psychiatric, and some pain disorders. The major advantage of FUS is avoidance of a surgical incision.

During a FUS procedure, a stereotactic head frame is placed and the brain is subsequently imaged to determine the coordinates of the lesion relative to the head frame. The patient's head and head frame are placed in a special ultrasound-generating device, and then all are placed in an MRI scanner. MRI-derived tissue temperature estimates can be used to guide ultrasonic ablation of the lesion and to minimize injury to surrounding normal brain parenchyma.

FUS is typically performed with patients receiving minimal or no sedation unless they are unable to tolerate the procedure due to factors such as claustrophobia. Common complications include headache and nausea and vomiting. Intracranial hemorrhage is a potential risk of FUS.

## SUGGESTED READINGS

Cardinale, F., Rizzi, M., Vignanti, E., Cossu, M., Castana, L., d'Orio, P., et al. (2019). Stereoelectroencephalography: Retrospective analysis of 742 procedures in a single center. *Brain, 142*, 2688–2704.

Chui, J., Manninen, P., Valiante, T., & Venkatraghavan, L. (2013). The anesthetic considerations of intraoperative electrocorticography during epilepsy surgery. *Anesthesia and Analgesia, 117*, 479–486.

Dinsmore, M., & Venkatraghavan, L. (2021). Anesthesia for deep brain stimulation: An update. *Current Opinion in Anaesthesiology, 34*, 563–568.

Dunn, L. K., Durieux, M. E., Elias, W. J., Nemergut, E. C., & Naik, B. I. (2018). Innovations in functional neurosurgery and anesthetic implications. *Journal of Neurosurgical Anesthesiology, 30*, 18–25.

Meng, Y., Hynynen, K., & Lipsman, N. (2021). Applications of focused ultrasound in the brain: From thermoablation to drug delivery. *Nature, 17*, 7–22.

Prince, E., Hakimian, S., Ko, A. L., Ojemann, J. G., Kim, M. S., & Miller, J. W. (2017). Laser interstitial thermal therapy for epilepsy. *Current Neurology and Neuroscience Reports, 17*, 63.

# Anesthesia for Awake Intracranial Surgery

PATRICK B. BOLTON, MD

## Introduction

Anesthesia for awake intracranial surgery poses many unique challenges to the anesthesiologist. Some of those challenges include obtaining a fine balance of analgesia, sedation, and hemodynamic stability while avoiding anxiety or oversedation in an awake patient during critical parts of the operation. Airway management is of utmost importance because these patients are in pinions, with limited mobility and access to the airway. The success of the procedure is dependent on many factors such as appropriate patient selection, communication between the surgical staff and the anesthesia team, and appropriate intraoperative management of these patients.

Although awake craniotomies in the modern era have been performed for more than 50 years, its application has been constantly evolving. In this chapter, we explore the indications for awake intracranial surgery, the evidence in favor of awake versus asleep craniotomy, the importance of patient selection, the general steps of the procedure, anesthetic management, and potential intraoperative complications.

## Indications for Awake Craniotomy

The indications for awake craniotomy have expanded over the years. As early as the 1950s, intraoperative surface electrocorticography was used to guide surgical excision of epileptic foci. These procedures were performed with an awake patient to minimize the effect anesthetic agents had on the cortical recordings. However, with the advancement in imaging techniques, the use of intraoperative electrocorticography for localizing epileptic foci has decreased. Surgical excision of neoplastic lesions or vascular malformations near eloquent cortical tissue that control speech, language, or movement are currently the most frequent indications for awake craniotomy. These procedures require patient participation during the cortical mapping phase of the operation, which will delineate the individual's functional brain topography and safe surgical resection boundaries. This allows the surgeon to remove as much of the lesion as possible but avoid removal of functional tissue. Lesions in the frontal lobe are most commonly considered for awake resection as the primary motor cortex (Brodmann area 4), the primary sensory cortex (Brodmann areas 3,1,2), and the language centers (Broca's area in the inferior frontal lobe of the dominant hemisphere) are part of the frontal lobe. Wernicke's area in the posterior temporal lobe contains motor neurons involved in the comprehension of speech and preservation of this area is a known indication for an awake procedure (Fig. 104.1). Awake surgery for direct arterial bypass for Moyamoya disease has been described with the benefit being frequent and robust neurologic examinations and avoidance of hypotension.

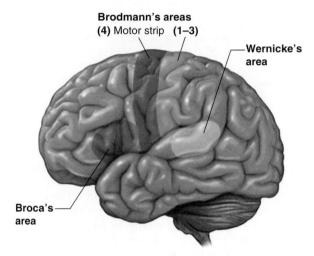

**Fig. 104.1** Topographic illustration of eloquent brain regions an awake craniotomy hopes to preserve: Broca's area (speech), Wernicke's area (language comprehension), and primary motor cortex (planning and execution of movements).

## Awake Craniotomy Versus General Anesthesia

Awake craniotomy for functional cortical mapping facilitates maximum tumor resection and minimizes neurologic damage. This approach results in fewer postoperative neurologic deficits and higher total resection of lesions in the eloquent brain areas versus patients undergoing a general anesthetic and surgical guidance with functional imaging. Many studies also demonstrate earlier hospital discharge, shorter intensive care unit stays, less resource utilization, and higher patient satisfaction. Postoperative nausea and vomiting and the need for analgesic medications are less frequent in patients undergoing awake craniotomy compared with patients undergoing a general anesthetic. Protocols for awake craniotomy using monitored anesthesia care with a scalp block and no airway instrumentation have been dubbed "enhanced recovery after neurosurgery" (ERANS).

## Preoperative Assessment and Patient Selection

Essential to the success of an awake craniotomy is patient selection and preparation. Building rapport with the patient is extremely important and should ideally be done in a preoperative clinic well in advance of the procedure. The discussion should include a general description of what to expect during the entire procedure, and topics such as positioning, awareness, cooperation, and participation should be reviewed in detail. The importance of good rapport and alleviating the patient's

| TABLE 104.1 | Considerations for Patient Selection for Awake Craniotomy |
|---|---|

**COOPERATION**
- Age
- Mental maturity
- Psychiatric disorders (anxiety, schizophrenia, claustrophobia)
- Pain disorders
- Movement disorders

**AIRWAY**
- Ease of mask ventilation, insertion of laryngeal mask airway, and intubation
- Prior intubation history
- Risk of upper airway obstruction (obesity, obstructive sleep apnea)

**SURGICAL**
- Hemorrhagic risk
- Size of tumor
- Hemodynamic stability

anxiety is of utmost importance, because having a cooperative patient in an unfamiliar and stressful environment is crucial to the success of an awake craniotomy.

Patient selection should be based not only on airway assessment and patient comorbidities but also on the risks of sedation failure and the patient's ability to cooperate during the procedure (Table 104.1). Risk factors for sedation failure include psychiatric disorders, anxiety, and chronic pain disorders, history of alcohol or drug abuse, and low tolerance to pain. Absolute contraindications to awake craniotomy include patient refusal, language barrier, altered mental status, and inability to cooperate. Obesity, gastroesophageal reflux disease, and chronic cough may be relative contraindications depending on the severity of the condition. Given that the patient is rigidly fixed in pinions and is being intermittently sedated, preoperative airway evaluation is essential. A plan to emergently secure the airway must be in place, and the equipment to do so must be readily available. Other factors that should be taken into consideration are tumor size, hemorrhagic risk, and hemodynamic instability during the procedure. Overall, a thorough individualized preoperative assessment is necessary to identify appropriate candidates for awake craniotomy.

## Anesthetic Management

Effective analgesia of the cranial skin and soft tissues is essential for the success of an awake craniotomy, and a scalp block can be performed in an alert or sedated patient. The block technique involves infiltration of a long-acting and short-acting local anesthetic mixture with epinephrine around six superficial nerves (four branches of the trigeminal nerve and two branches from C2 and C3) on both sides of the head. The blocks are performed using superficial anatomic landmarks, although ultrasound-guided blocks of the occipital nerves have been described. The supraorbital and supratrochlear nerves innervate the anterior region of the scalp; the auriculotemporal and zygomaticotemporal nerves innervate the lateral portion; and the greater and lesser occipital nerves innervate the posterior region. The great auricular nerve can also be included in the block bilaterally if the planned surgical incision is in proximity to the posterior ear or mastoid bone. It is also advisable to block the three sites of contact before Mayfield pinion application with 3 to 5 mL of the local anesthetic mixture.

Repeat infiltrations may be necessary if the patient identifies areas of discomfort during the awake portion of the case.

The auriculotemporal nerve runs with the superficial temporal artery, and appropriate precautions should be taken not to inject into the artery. In addition, the facial nerve and branches run inferior to the auriculotemporal nerve, and it can be inadvertently blocked, resulting in temporary facial paralysis. Postoperative facial paralysis after an awake neurosurgical procedure confounds the postoperative neurologic examination. To minimize inferior spread of the local anesthetic unintentionally blocking the facial nerve, the auriculotemporal nerve block is best done 1 cm above the tragus. However, if a pterional incision is used, injecting too superiorly near the incision may expose the skin and subcutaneous tissue to copious amounts of irrigation during burr-hole placement. This can dilute the local anesthetic and shorten its effect. Depending on the location, the dura mater is innervated by branches of the trigeminal nerve, C1 to C3 cervical nerves, and cranial nerves IX and X. Thus for intraoperative analgesia, innervation to the dura must be directly blocked with local anesthetic under direct vision by the surgeon (Fig. 104.2).

Augmenting the scalp block are various anesthetic methods that include monitored anesthesia care (MAC), asleep-awake-asleep (AAA), and asleep-awake (AA) technique. It is important to note that none of these methods has proven superior. Whichever anesthetic method is used, the goal is rapid and smooth transition of anesthetic depth and stable cerebral and cardiovascular hemodynamics. Like all intracranial procedures, avoidance of hypercapnia and hypoxemia is desirable, as well as maintenance of adequate cerebral perfusion pressure.

## Monitored Anesthesia Care

With MAC (sometimes called sedation only), the patient is sedated before the placement of the scalp block, and it is continued until the mapping and neuropsychological testing phase. The goal is preservation of spontaneous ventilation and rapid emergence for accurate brain mapping. The advantages of MAC are the

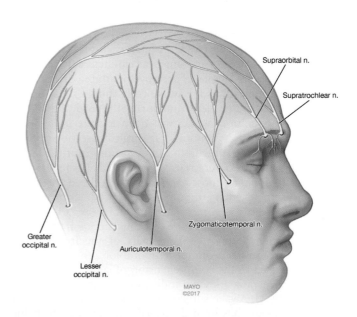

**Fig. 104.2**  Illustration of the six peripheral nerves targeted in a scalp block.

preservation of responses to verbal stimulation and light tactile stimulation and the avoidance of general anesthesia and airway instrumentation. The first phase of the procedure (head pinning, craniotomy, opening of dura) is extremely stimulating, and a dense scalp block allows for lighter sedation during times that sedation is required. Short-acting, easily titratable agents such as propofol, remifentanil, or dexmedetomidine are preferred to provide rapid shifts through the various phases of sedation necessary for the procedure. These drugs, at levels used for sedation, also do not interfere with the electrophysiological mapping signals or increase the risk of nausea and vomiting. Once the testing phase is complete, the sedation is restarted and usually continued through lesion resection and closure.

## Asleep-Awake-Asleep Method

In this method, the patient undergoes general anesthesia with either a laryngeal mask airway (LMA) or endotracheal tube (ETT) until the brain is exposed. The patient is then awakened, and the LMA or ETT is removed to allow for functional cortical mapping and neurologic assessment. After the lesion is removed, general anesthesia is induced again, and an LMA or ETT is reinserted until surgery is completed. Advantages of this method include a secure airway with control of ventilation and patient comfort during the initial stages of the procedure. AAA avoids oversedation in an uninstrumented airway and its consequences of apnea, hypoxemia, hypercapnia, and increases in cerebral mass. It also avoids undersedation and its consequences of hypertension, tachycardia, and psychological distress. The disadvantages of this technique involve instrumentation of the airway. Removal of the LMA or ETT may cause coughing, which can result in upward herniation of the brain through the craniotomy. Reinsertion of the airway device may be difficult in a patient with a fixed head position under surgical drapes, and there may be residual airway irritation and edema after the initial airway manipulation.

## Asleep-Awake Method

In this method, the patient undergoes general anesthesia up until the brain is exposed and patient participation is required. After the patient has emerged from anesthesia and the LMA or ETT is removed, the patient remains awake for cortical mapping and tumor resection and is then sedated for the remainder of the procedure. The benefit of this method over AAA is risk avoidance of airway instrumentation "under the drapes," and it allows the opportunity for remapping toward the end of the procedure, if needed. If inhalation agents are used during the asleep portion, there is a risk for nausea and vomiting and diminished cortical signals.

## Intraoperative Complications

Intraoperative complications are common and include respiratory depression, seizure, loss of patient cooperation, nausea and vomiting, air embolism, cerebral edema, airway obstruction, and leaking LMA (Table 104.2). By report, 6.4% of patients fail to complete mapping because of the onset of seizures, loss of patient cooperation, or development of mixed dysphagia. Although rare and usually focal in nature, intraoperative seizures can be treated with ice-cold saline applied to the brain and/or medications such as propofol and benzodiazepines. Loss of patient cooperation can usually be prevented by careful patient selection, establishment of rapport, and satisfactory titration of intravenous hypnotic and/or analgesic agents. AAA cases have been reported to have more frequent occurrences of desaturation, hypertension, hypotension, tachycardia, and hypercapnia. The possibility of airway fire should always be considered and discussed during the time-out, as these procedures can present an elevated fire risk given the presence of an uncontained oxygen source (nasal cannula/facemask) under a canopy of drapes with fuel (skin prep sanitizer) and an ignition source present (electrocautery).

## Summary

Awake craniotomy with cortical mapping allows for more precise neurosurgical resection of a lesion near language or motor pathways. To increase the success of the procedure, meticulous attention to patient selection and patient education is crucial. Placement of a scalp block and proper titration of anesthetic agents facilitate patient comfort, surgical conditions, neuropsychological testing conditions, and safety. Although no technique is superior over another (MAC, AAA, or AA), it is important to understand the advantages and disadvantages of each technique to adequately anticipate and manage their respective complications.

| TABLE 104.2 | Intraoperative Complications in Awake Intracranial Surgery |
|---|---|

- Oxyhemoglobin desaturations
- Hypoventilation
- Hypercapnia
- Increased brain swelling
- Hypertension
- Hypotension
- Tachycardia
- Agitation/uncooperativeness
- Movement
- Venous embolism
- Seizure

## SUGGESTED READINGS

Andersen, J., & Olsen, K. (2010). Anesthesia for awake craniotomy is safe and well-tolerated. *Danish Medical Bulletin*, 57(10), A4194.

Aoun, R. J. N., Sattur, M. G., Krishna, C., Gupta, A., Welz, M. E., Nanney, A. D., III, et al. (2017). Awake surgery for brain vascular malformations and Moyamoya disease. *World Neurosurgery*, 105, 659–671.

Erickson, K. M., & Cole, D. J. (2012). Anesthetic considerations for awake craniotomy for epilepsy and functional neurosurgery. *Anesthesiology Clinics*, 30, 241–268.

Gupta, D. K., Chandra, P. S., Ojha, B. K., Sharma, B. S., Mahapatra, A. K., & Mehta, V. S. (2007). Awake craniotomy versus surgery under general anesthesia for resection of intrinsic lesions of eloquent cortex – A prospective randomised study. *Clinical Neurology and Neurosurgery*, 109, 335–343.

Osborn, I., & Sebeo, J. (2010). Scalp block during craniotomy: A classic technique revisited. *Journal of Neurosurgical Anesthesiology*, 22(3), 187–194.

Pacquin-Lanthier, G., Subramaniam, S., Leong, K. W., Daniels, A., Singh, K., Takami, H., et al. (2021). Risk Factors and Characteristics of Intraoperative Seizures During Awake Craniotomy: A Retrospective Cohort Study of 562 Consecutive Patients With a Space-occupying Brain Lesion. *Journal of Neurosurgical Anesthesiology*, 35(2), 1–7. doi:10.1097/ANA.0000000000000798.

Piccioni, F., & Fanzio, M. (2008). Management of anesthesia in awake craniotomy. *Minerva Anestesiologica*, 74(7–8), 393–408.

Sacko, O., Lauwers-Cances, V., Brauge, D., Sesay, M., Brenner, A., & Roux, F. E. (2011). Awake craniotomy vs surgery under general anesthesia for resection of supratentorial lesions. *Neurosurgery*, 68, 1192–1198, discussion 1198–1199.

# Cerebral Circulation

JASON M. WOODBURY, MD

The brain is highly perfused, receiving approximately 15% to 20% of cardiac output. The cerebral arterial circulation is supplied by the paired internal carotid arteries (80% of total cerebral flow) and the paired vertebral arteries (20% of total cerebral flow), which communicate through a series of anastomoses at the circle of Willis (cerebral arterial circle), a ring of vessels located in the suprasellar cistern at the base of the brain (Fig. 105.1). The circle of Willis connects the anterior and posterior cerebral circulation, providing collateral perfusion throughout the brain. Anatomic variations within the circle of Willis are common.

## Anterior Circulation

In adults, the common carotid artery bifurcates into the external carotid and internal carotid arteries between the third and fifth cervical vertebrae. Before coursing superiorly, the internal carotid artery dilates to form the carotid sinus, an innervated baroreceptor critical for blood pressure regulation. The internal

carotid artery ascends within the carotid sheath and enters the cranium through the carotid canal in the temporal bone, where it courses anteromedially before exiting above the foramen lacerum and eventually pierces the dural layers of the cavernous sinus. The *carotid siphon* refers to the S-shaped course of the artery within the sinus. Before joining the circle of Willis, the internal carotid artery gives rise to the ophthalmic artery (which subsequently gives rise to the central artery of the retina) and the superior hypophyseal artery. The terminal segment gives rise to the anterior choroidal and posterior communicating arteries before bifurcating into the anterior and middle cerebral arteries. The anterior cerebral arteries connect via the anterior communicating artery just superior to the optic chiasm to supply the midline components of the frontal lobes and the superior medial portions of the parietal lobes (Fig. 105.2). The middle cerebral arteries supply the lateral cerebral hemispheres, including the lateral frontal and parietal lobes and the superior temporal lobes, underlying insular lobes, and portions of the internal capsule and basal ganglia. The middle cerebral artery also perfuses Broca's and Wernicke's areas.

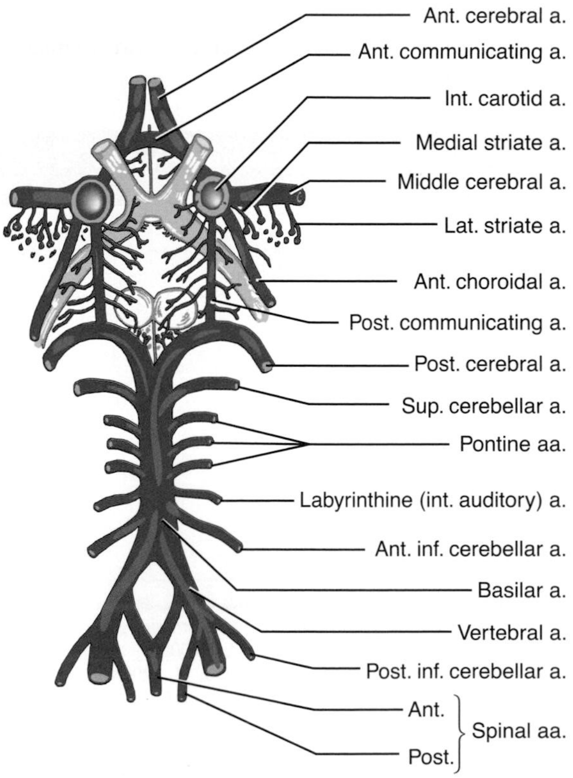

## Posterior Circulation

The bilateral vertebral arteries arise from the subclavian arteries and ascend through the transverse processes of C6 to C1 before entering the skull through the foramen magnum. Branches of the vertebral arteries form the single anterior spinal artery and the paired posterior inferior cerebellar arteries. The paired posterior spinal arteries may arise from the vertebral artery itself or originate from the posterior inferior cerebellar artery. On the inferior surface of the brainstem, the vertebral arteries join to form the singular basilar artery. As the basilar artery courses along the pons toward the circle of Willis, it gives off branches that include the anterior inferior cerebellar arteries, the pontine arteries, the superior cerebellar arteries, and finally the posterior cerebral arteries. The anastomotic connection to the anterior circulation of the brain occurs via the posterior communicating arteries. This vertebrobasilar arterial system supplies the midbrain, pons, medulla, cerebellum, a portion of the thalamus, and the posterior cerebrum, including the occipital, inferior, and medial temporal lobes.

## Meningeal Arteries

The arterial blood supply to the dura originates as branches extending from the external carotid artery. The anterior meningeal artery supplies the dura of the anterior cranial fossa, and the posterior meningeal artery supplies the dura of the posterior cranial fossa. The middle meningeal artery is a large branch of the maxillary artery that enters the foramen spinosum to supply the majority of the dura, including the calvarial aspect.

**Fig. 105.1** Diagram of the arterial supply to the brainstem and the constituents of the circle of Willis. *Ant.*, Anterior; *inf.*, inferior; *Int.*, internal; *Lat.*, lateral; *Post.*, posterior; *Sup.*, superior. (Reprinted, with permission, from Pansky B. *Review of Gross Anatomy.* 5th ed. Macmillan; 1984.)

Labels in figure:
- Ant. cerebral a.
- Ant. communicating a.
- Int. carotid a.
- Medial striate a.
- Middle cerebral a.
- Lat. striate a.
- Ant. choroidal a.
- Post. communicating a.
- Post. cerebral a.
- Sup. cerebellar a.
- Pontine aa.
- Labyrinthine (int. auditory) a.
- Ant. inf. cerebellar a.
- Basilar a.
- Vertebral a.
- Post. inf. cerebellar a.
- Ant. } Spinal aa.
- Post. }

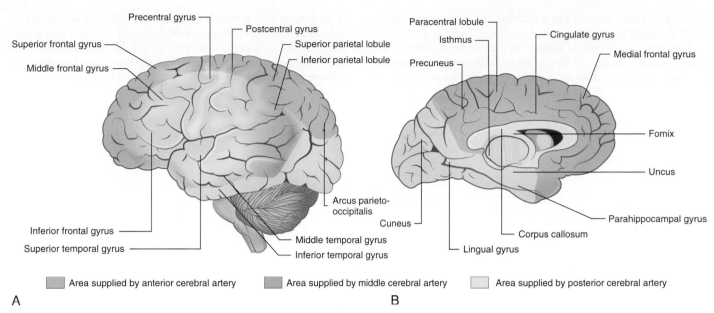

**Fig. 105.2**  Distribution of the cerebral arterial supply, shown on the (**A**) lateral and (**B**) medial surfaces of the left cerebral hemisphere. (Reprinted, with permission, from Standring S. Vascular supply and drainage of the brain. In: Standring S, ed. *Gray's Anatomy: The Anatomical Basis of Clinical Practice*. 41st ed. Elsevier; 2016:280–290.)

The anterior branch of the middle meningeal artery runs just behind the pterion (a weak portion of the skull at the junction of the frontal, parietal, temporal, and sphenoid bones), where it is vulnerable to trauma and resulting epidural hemorrhage.

## Venous Drainage of the Head

The venous structure of the brain consists of dura-lined sinuses and thin-walled, valveless veins. After draining the scalp, veins on the surface of the skull connect via emissary veins to the intracerebral venous sinuses and can serve as a conduit to spread infection. Diploic veins are endothelium-lined canals draining the skull. The four main diploic veins on each side of the skull are identified by the anatomic region that they drain: frontal, anterior temporal, posterior temporal, and occipital. The superior, middle, and inferior superficial cerebral veins and their connections, which drain into the superior sagittal sinus, drain the external portion of the brain parenchyma. The internal cerebral veins drain the deeper cerebral parenchyma. There are also superior and inferior cerebellar veins that drain the cerebellum. Dural venous sinuses are located between the endosteal and meningeal layers of the dura mater, where they receive blood from the brain, meninges, skull, and scalp, along with cerebrospinal fluid from arachnoid granulations. Venous drainage from the brain ultimately empties into the superior vena cava via the internal jugular veins.

## Clinical Considerations

Strokes are classified as either hemorrhagic or ischemic. A patient with a suspected stroke should be imaged using noncontrast CT, which will reliably distinguish between an acute intracranial hemorrhage and ischemia. Hemorrhagic strokes are further categorized by the location of bleeding within the intracranial vault.

Intraparenchymal (or intracerebral) hemorrhage is bleeding that occurs within the brain proper and may result from arteriovenous malformation rupture, trauma, or bleeding from a brain tumor, or it may occur spontaneously. Arterial anastomoses are numerous on the surface of the brain but relatively rare within the brain parenchyma. Occlusion or rupture of an intraparenchymal artery will likely cause more damage than a similar occlusion or rupture on the surface of the brain due to lack of collateral circulation.

Subarachnoid hemorrhage classically presents as a thunderclap headache described as the "worst headache" of the patient's life and typically presents after head trauma or aneurysm rupture. Head imaging will reveal subarachnoid blood, often within the region of the cerebral arterial circle, as this area has a strong association with aneurysm formation and rupture. These hemorrhages may, however, occur in any region of the brain.

Epidural hematomas are most commonly caused by traumatic disruption of meningeal arteries that are located between the dura mater and the periosteum of the cranial bones. Imaging typically shows a biconvex collection of blood between the dura and the skull. Patients with head injuries resulting in epidural hematomas characteristically present with a lucid interval after the initial trauma, followed by progressive waning of consciousness as intracranial pressure rises due to hematoma expansion.

A subdural hematoma results from venous bleeding and is associated with a more insidious presentation of symptoms, with headache or altered mental status progressively evolving and fluctuating over several days. Blood collects between the dura and the arachnoid, characteristically resulting from tearing of subdural bridging veins. On brain imaging this appears acutely as a homogeneous, crescent-shaped fluid collection with diffuse extraaxial spread over the affected hemisphere. Subdural hematomas are associated with high morbidity and mortality.

Cavernous sinus thrombosis is a life-threatening condition in which sinus, dental, or facial infection spreads intracranially, leading to clot formation within the sinus. There are no valves in the dural venous sinuses or within the diploic, emissary, or meningeal veins, resulting in a channel for infection to spread from the scalp to the intracranial vault.

Other vascular cerebral anomalies include venous angiomas, cavernous angiomas, capillary telangiectasias, and arteriovenous fistulae. Moyamoya disease is characterized by the development of an intertwined network of collateral capillaries secondary to progressive stenosis of intracerebral arterial vessels. Cranial imaging shows a characteristic "puff of smoke" appearance, from which the disease gets its Japanese name. Moyamoya patients are at increased risk for developing intracranial aneurysms.

## SUGGESTED READINGS

Cipolla, M. J. (2016). *The cerebral circulation* (2nd ed.). San Rafael, CA: Morgan & Claypool Life Sciences.

Donnelly, J., Budohoski, K. P., Smielewski, P., & Czosnyka, M. (2016). Regulation of the cerebral circulation: Bedside assessment and clinical implications. *Critical Care, 20*(1), 129.

Hunter Guevara, L. R., & Pasternak, J. J. (2022). Diseases affecting the brain. In R. L. Hines, S. B. Jones (Eds.), *Stoelting's anesthesia and co-existing disease* (8th ed., pp. 273–308). Philadelphia, PA: Elsevier Saunders.

Standring, S. (2021). Vascular supply and drainage of the brain. In S. Standring (Ed.), *Gray's anatomy: The anatomical basis of clinical practice* (42nd ed., pp. 415–424). Amsterdam: Elsevier.

# 106

# Management of Cerebral Aneurysms

JUAN G. RIPOLL, MD    |    ARNOLEY S. ABCEJO, MD

## Epidemiology and Risk Factors

The prevalence of intracranial aneurysms in the United States is estimated at 4% to 6% in the general population. The global incidence of aneurysmal subarachnoid hemorrhage (aSAH) ranges from 2 to 16 cases per 100,000 persons per year. However, the incidence of aSAH may be underestimated, as death from this condition often occurs before hospital admission.

The risk of hemorrhage from unruptured aneurysms is estimated at 1% to 2% per year. The 1-year risk of rupture in known unruptured aneurysms after growth detection may be 1 out of 25. The incidence of aSAH is increased among adults 50 years and older, females (1.24 times greater risk than men), and nonwhites (especially Hispanics and African Americans). Moreover, the incidence of this clinical condition is nearly twice as high in low- and middle-income countries as in high-income countries. Modifiable risk factors for aSAH include smoking, hypertension, use of sympathomimetic drugs (e.g., cocaine), and alcohol abuse. The risk of aSAH also increases with a previous history of aSAH, large cerebral aneurysms (>7 mm), if the aneurysm is located within the posterior circulation, has an irregular anatomic shape, or coincides with vasculopathic genetic conditions (e.g., Ehlers-Danlos syndrome).

## Aneurysm Rupture

When an aneurysm ruptures, blood flows into the subarachnoid space. Signs of meningismus often occur as blood from the rupture spreads. The classic presenting complaint is sudden onset of severe headache typically described as "the worst headache of my life." Additional symptoms include nausea, vomiting, seizures, photophobia, nuchal rigidity, altered mental status, focal or global neurologic deficits, and coma.

The severity of the rupture is categorized using the Hunt-Hess classification system and the Fisher scale. Clinicians often use these methods interchangeably to assess the severity of an aSAH. The Hunt-Hess classification system employs a 5-grade scoring scale (Table 106.1A). Grades 1 and 2 are associated with increasing headache, grades 3 and 4 are associated with increasing neurologic deficits, and grade 5 signifies deep coma. Higher grades are associated with progressively worse outcomes.

The Fisher scale provides an index of vasospasm risk based on the hemorrhage pattern seen on the initial head computed tomography (CT) scan (Table 106.1B). This scale employs a 4-grade scoring scale ranging from no blood (grade 1) to intraventricular or intracerebral clots with diffuse or no subarachnoid blood (grade 4). Typically, higher grades predict delayed cerebral ischemia.

| TABLE 106.1 | Classification Systems for Patients With Subarachnoid Hemorrhage |
|---|---|

**1. HUNT-HESS CLASSIFICATION SYSTEM**

| Grade | Clinical Description |
|---|---|
| 0 | Unruptured aneurysm |
| 1 | Asymptomatic or minimal headache and slight nuchal rigidity |
| 2 | Moderate to severe headache, nuchal rigidity, but no neurologic deficit other than cranial palsy |
| 3 | Drowsiness, confusion, or mild focal deficit |
| 4 | Stupor, mild or severe hemiparesis, possible early decerebrate rigidity, vegetative disturbance |
| 5 | Deep coma, decerebrate rigidity, moribund appearance |

**2. FISHER SCALE**

| Grade | Head CT Findings |
|---|---|
| 1 | No blood detected |
| 2 | Diffuse thin layer of subarachnoid blood (vertical layers <1 mm thick) |
| 3 | Localized clot or thick layer of subarachnoid blood (vertical layers ≥1 mm thick) |
| 4 | Intracerebral or intraventricular blood with diffuse or no subarachnoid blood |

*CT,* Computed tomography.

| TABLE 106.2 | Complications of Aneurysmal Subarachnoid Hemorrhage |
|---|---|

| | Complication(s) |
|---|---|
| Neurologic | Seizures<br>Rebleeding<br>Vasospasm<br>Hydrocephalus<br>Delayed cerebral ischemia<br>Cerebral salt wasting syndrome<br>SIADH |
| Cardiovascular | Conduction abnormalities (including life-threatening arrythmias)<br>Takotsubo cardiomyopathy<br>Myocardial ischemia<br>Elevated troponins |
| Pulmonary | Cardiac-induced pulmonary edema<br>Neurogenic pulmonary edema<br>Acute respiratory distress syndrome<br>Aspiration pneumonia |
| Hematologic | Anemia, thrombocytopenia, leukocytosis |
| Others | Hyponatremia, hypokalemia, hypocalcemia, hypomagnesemia, hyperglycemia |

*SIADH,* Syndrome of inappropriate secretion of antidiuretic hormone.

Head CT and magnetic resonance imaging are sensitive diagnostic tools. Lumbar puncture frequently confirms a clinical suspicion of aSAH among patients with negative or inconclusive head imaging and no overt signs of increased intracranial pressure (ICP). Nevertheless, the presence of bilirubin in the cerebrospinal fluid (CSF) resulting from breakdown of hemoglobin (xanthochromia) is only detectable 12 hours after the initial presentation. A CT angiogram is another useful tool to identify the aneurysm and guide therapeutic interventions. More recently, three-dimensional digital subtraction angiography has been used to provide a more detailed reconstruction of the vascular anatomy prior to neurointerventional procedures.

## POSTOPERATIVE COMPLICATIONS

Major causes of morbidity and death include rebleeding, cerebral vasospasm, and obstructive hydrocephalus (Table 106.2).

### Rebleeding

Aneurysm rebleeding is associated with high postoperative morbidity and mortality. The incidence of rebleeding is estimated at 4% to 14% within the first 24 hours. Risk factors associated with this clinical condition include systolic blood pressure greater than 160 mm Hg, delayed treatment, worse neurologic status on admission, larger aneurysm size, and loss of consciousness. Preventable strategies include a strict control of the systolic blood pressure (<160 mm Hg) while avoiding systemic hypotension and prompt reversal of anticoagulation.

### Vasospasm

Vasospasm is a particularly devastating complication of aSAH. The exact mechanism of vasospasm is unknown but is most likely related to hemoglobin products irritating cerebral arteries. If vasospasm is left untreated, permanent neurologic damage from ischemia is likely to occur. This clinical condition usually manifests about 72 hours after the aneurysm rupture, and the risk peaks between 4 to 14 days after the initial bleed.

Cerebral vasospasm is diagnosed clinically based on changes in neurologic status. Transcranial Doppler ultrasonography allows definitive diagnosis and prophylactic monitoring of vasospasm. In addition to the measurement of absolute velocities, the Lindegaard ratio (middle cerebral artery velocity compared with external carotid artery velocity) is also commonly used to assess the risk of vasospasm. Cerebral artery velocities greater than 120 cm/sec and Lindegaard ratios of 3 and above are highly suggestive of ongoing vasospasm.

Nimodipine is the standard drug used to prevent vasospasm. It has been shown to improve the neurologic outcomes after aSAH and reduce the risk of delayed cerebral ischemia (Table 106.3). However, nimodipine does not relieve the vasospasm of the main vessel. Therefore the demonstrated therapeutic effect of nimodipine in improved neurologic outcome does not result from direct treatment of vasospasm. Studied mechanisms responsible for the effectiveness of this therapy include reduction of calcium-dependent excitotoxicity, diminished platelet aggregation, and vasodilation of smaller arteries (not visualized on angiograms).

Optimal supportive management includes (1) preventing hypotension (allowing the blood pressure to remain elevated if it encourages good neurologic exam), (2) preventing hypovolemia, and (3) treatment with nimodipine. Specifically, "Triple H therapy" (hypertension, hydration, and hemodilution), once thought to be the gold standard of care, has been disproven and may be harmful. Patients refractory to these interventions may be candidates for endovascular intervention including angioplasty or intraarterial injection of vasodilators (i.e., verapamil).

| TABLE 106.3 | Management of Cerebral Aneurysms | |
|---|---|---|
| | **ANEURYSM CATEGORY** | |
| **Management Aspect** | **Nonruptured** | **Ruptured** |
| Monitoring | Standard | Standard plus ICP |
| Brain protection | No | Probable |
| Vasospasm | No | Most likely |
| Surgical treatment | Elective | Emergent |
| Surgical treatment vs. endovascular coil placement | Location dependent | Location dependent |
| Nimodipine | No | Yes |
| Outcomes | Good | Depends on Hunt-Hess classification and Fisher scale |

*ICP*, Intracranial pressure.

### Obstructive Hydrocephalus

Hydrocephalus is a serious complication and carries a high risk of morbidity and mortality after aSAH. It results from the accumulation of blood in the cerebral cisterns that ultimately occlude the arachnoid granulations, thus preventing the reabsorption of CSF. The incidence ranges from 20% to 30% and occurs in about one-fifth of patients within the first 3 to 4 days and in 10% to 20% of patients after 2 weeks after aSAH. Timely diagnosis and rapid restoration of cerebral perfusion by the placement of an external ventricular drain are paramount to improve the patient's neurologic deterioration, particularly in the acute setting.

Additional complications after aSAH include cardiopulmonary perturbations resulting from an intense sympathetic discharge. Although some electrocardiographic changes are benign, new electrocardiographic changes after aSAH may indicate myocardial damage. Takotsubo cardiomyopathy (apical stunning) may be seen after aSAH. When echocardiographic changes coincide with hemodynamic collapse, invasive monitoring may be indicated. If coronary intervention is required, percutaneous endovascular therapy may be preferred given the need to avoid anticoagulation. Moreover, pulmonary edema is a common sequela after aSAH secondary to the sympathetic surge.

Hyponatremia is common after aSAH. Reduced serum sodium levels can occur due to cerebral salt-wasting syndrome or syndrome of inappropriate antidiuretic hormone secretion (SIADH). The former results from secretion of atrial natriuretic hormone from the brain, causing a clinical triad of hyponatremia, hypovolemia, and high urine sodium concentration. These patients frequently require fluid resuscitation. SIADH results from inappropriate release of antidiuretic hormone and subsequent excessive free-water retention. In contrast with cerebral salt-wasting syndrome, hypervolemia and euvolemia are hallmarks of SIADH. Treatment includes fluid restriction, which may be difficult in the setting of vasospasm, because of the need to avoid hypovolemia. Administration of hypertonic saline should be considered in this setting.

## TREATMENT OPTIONS

The mainstay of aSAH treatment is a timely obliteration of the ruptured aneurysm by surgery or endovascular intervention. Moreover, patients with aSAH should be transferred promptly to specialized high-volume centers with the availability of multidisciplinary teams and expertise in the management of neurocritically ill patients to improve patient outcomes.

## Surgical Treatment Versus Endovascular Interventions

Previously, patients with a diagnosis of aSAH were observed for 10 to 14 days for resolution of vasospasm and cerebral edema. However, the incidence of rebleeding with resultant morbidity and mortality was unacceptably high. Current management of patients with cerebral aneurysms focuses on early endovascular or open surgical intervention. Endovascular repair involves coil embolization or pipeline diversion of the cerebral aneurysm resulting in thrombosis and obliteration of the dilated arterial sac. Open aneurysm repair through a craniotomy involves direct clipping of the neck of the aneurysm.

Multiple factors influence the decision to select endovascular or open surgical therapy. These include the location of the aneurysm (posterior vs. anterior circulation), the anatomy of the dilated vessel, the durability of the repair, the recurrence rate of the aneurysm, and the previous experience of the surgical team. Each approach has advantages and disadvantages. In the International Subarachnoid Aneurysm Trial, endovascular coiling was more likely to result in survival at 1 year, and the survival benefit persisted for more than 7 years. However, the incidence of late rebleeding was higher with endovascular coiling, and the rate of complete aneurysm obliteration was higher after surgical clipping. Currently, the American Heart Association and American Stroke Association recommend endovascular coiling as the preferred method for aSAH if amenable to both clipping and coiling.

## Anesthetic Management

General anesthesia is the preferred method for surgical clipping and endovascular coiling of cerebral aneurysms. Endotracheal intubation is usually indicated among patients with aSAH for airway protection. Indeed, 30% of patients develop pulmonary edema as a short-term complication of an aSAH.

### INTRAOPERATIVE MONITORING

The use of standard American Society of Anesthesiologists monitors and direct arterial blood pressure monitoring are indicated. Direct arterial blood pressure monitoring facilitates tight blood pressure control and expedites intraoperative arterial blood gas analyses. Placement of a central venous catheter may be considered based on the patient's comorbid conditions. If hydrocephalus is present, the neurosurgeon may elect to place a ventriculostomy to monitoring ICP and facilitate CSF drainage. Brain swelling can also be decreased with intravenously administered mannitol.

Cerebral function can be monitored using evoked potentials (brainstem auditory, somatosensory, and motor). Total intravenous anesthesia is recommended when evoked potentials are assessed, as volatile anesthetics interfere with evoked potential monitoring (especially motor) more than intravenous anesthetics such as remifentanil and propofol do.

## ANESTHETIC GOALS

The primary anesthetic goal among patients with unruptured cerebral aneurysms or aSAH is optimization of metabolic and hemodynamic conditions to promote good neurologic outcome. The aim for induction of anesthesia is to prevent excessive exacerbations in hypertension during laryngoscopy, which can lead to a sudden increase in the transmural pressure of the aneurysmal sac. Anesthesia may be induced with propofol and analgesia maintained with an opioid such as fentanyl. An inhalational agent such as isoflurane may also be used. It may become necessary to avoid an anesthesia level that exceeds 1 MAC (minimum alveolar concentration) of an inhalation agent to avoid uncoupling, cerebral vasodilation, and subsequent increases in ICP. If the brain is extremely edematous, use of a total intravenous anesthetic technique should be considered.

Controlled hypotension was previously used to decrease intraoperative bleeding. Now, most surgeons prefer to maintain the blood pressure at baseline to ensure sufficient cerebral perfusion pressure. Temporary clipping of the main feeder vessel to the aneurysm is sometimes required. In this case relative hypotension may be required to reduce blood flow to the aneurysmal sac before clipping. Less commonly, intravenous adenosine may be administered to transiently interrupt blood flow. It may be necessary to temporarily increase the patient's blood pressure to improve collateral circulation once the aneurysm is clipped. After the temporary clip is removed, any dramatic increase in blood pressure that could lead to bleeding should be avoided.

In general, hypotonic fluids (i.e., dextrose or lactated Ringer solution) should be avoided in patients undergoing cerebral aneurysm repair, as they can worsen underlying hyponatremia and/or cerebral edema. Normal saline is the typical fluid of choice, as it is isotonic. Hypertonic fluids (1.5% or 3% saline) may be indicated to correct hyponatremia in select cases.

Avoiding hyperglycemia (blood glucose >180 mg/dL) and fever during periods when the brain is at risk for developing ischemic injury are the only techniques for which there is definitive evidence for brain protection in humans. Despite this, many physicians use barbiturates or propofol to achieve burst suppression (4–6 bursts/min) during critical periods of aneurysm repair. The Intraoperative Hypothermia for Aneurysm Surgery Trial did not show any benefit of mild hypothermia (to 33°C) during aneurysm repair. Therapeutic hypothermia is generally reserved for cases that require complex cerebrovascular bypass procedures or long temporary clip ligation.

## ANESTHETIC MANAGEMENT OF ENDOVASCULAR PROCEDURES FOR INTRACRANIAL ANEURYSMS

Endovascular techniques are used to treat both ruptured and unruptured aneurysms. Although monitored anesthesia care has been used as a primary anesthetic, most anesthesiologists prefer the use of general anesthesia with paralysis to prevent complications related to patient's movement (i.e., dissection, aneurysm rupture). Neurointerventional procedures are commonly performed in interventional radiology suites. Therefore in addition to the standard anesthesia setup, the anesthesia provider must be mindful of some additional concerns that are specific to these cases.

### Before the Case

Before the procedure, the anesthesiologist must set up the operating room acknowledging the expected motion of the fluoroscopy machine, as well as the position of the neurointerventionalist and the surgical team in the room. The addition of extensions to the breathing circuit and to the intravenous and intraarterial access must be also considered. The anesthesia provider is also responsible for ensuring the availability of protective lead aprons and/or screen for the anesthesia team and should secure the breathing circuit is away from the field to limit the risk of imaging interference and poor image quality. In addition to the standard drugs used in anesthesia, infusions of vasopressors (phenylephrine, norepinephrine, and vasopressin) as well as blood pressure–reducing agents (clevidipine and nicardipine) must be readily available. Last, in the event of an undesired aneurysm rupture, protamine should be accessible for immediate heparin reversal.

### During the Case

Intraoperatively, there are some specific concerns related to endovascular procedures. Patients are commonly heparinized, and an activated clotting time goal should be discussed with the proceduralist before starting the case. Also, the administration of antiplatelet agents is not uncommon, and an orogastric or nasogastric tube should be placed after intubation but before heparin administration. In the event of an aneurysm rupture, protamine must be administered to reverse the anticoagulation, and if thromboembolism is detected prior or during coiling, the use of an antiplatelet agent (abciximab, glycoprotein IIb/IIIa inhibitor) is highly recommended.

Intraarterial verapamil may be administered locally by the proceduralist for cerebral vasospasm treatment. Although given focally to promote targeted cerebral vasodilation, systemic hypotension may be seen especially with repeated doses.

## GOALS FOR EMERGENCE FROM ANESTHESIA AND DISPOSITION OF CARE

Emergence is an important phase of the anesthetic management of patients treated with endovascular procedures, clipping via craniotomy, or a combination of both techniques. Ideally, the goals for emergence include avoiding hypertension and limiting cough or straining. Also, the anesthesiologist must facilitate a rapid emergence to allow a brief neurologic examination by the proceduralist before leaving the operating room.

After neurointerventional procedures for aneurysm repair, patients should be admitted to the neurointensive care or monitored unit. Indeed, these patients require precise blood pressure control and monitoring, serial neurologic examinations to facilitate prompt recognition of postoperative neurologic changes, optimal postoperative nausea and vomiting treatment, and an individualized pain management strategy.

## Recovery

Regardless of whether the patient has undergone endovascular coiling or surgical clipping, smooth emergence from general anesthesia facilitates early postoperative neurologic examination. Patients with a Hunt-Hess grade 3 or 4 aneurysm may benefit from continued postoperative airway and sedative management, as well as ICP monitoring with a ventriculostomy or a Camino intracranial device. Patients can be monitored with transcranial Doppler ultrasonography if vasospasm is suspected, and therapy can be initiated if vasospasm becomes evident. Repeat CT scan or angiography may also be considered.

## SUGGESTED READINGS

Connolly, E. S., Jr., Rabinstein, A. A., Carhuapoma, J. R., Derdeyn, C. P., Dion, J., Higashida, R. T., et al. (2012). Guidelines for the management of aneurysmal subarachnoid hemorrhage: A guideline for healthcare professionals from the American Heart Association/American Stroke Association. *Stroke, 43,* 1711–1737.

Datar, S., & Rabinstein, A. A. (2017). Postinterventional critical care management of aneurysmal subarachnoid hemorrhage. *Current Opinion in Critical Care, 23,* 87–93.

Diringer, M. N., Bleck, T. P., Claude Hemphill, J., III, Menon, D., Shutter, L., Vespa, P., et al. (2011). Critical care management of patients following aneurysmal subarachnoid hemorrhage: Recommendations from the Neurocritical Care Society's Multidisciplinary Consensus Conference. *Neurocritical Care, 15,* 211–240.

Lawton, M. T., & Vates, G. E. (2017). Subarachnoid hemorrhage. *New England Journal of Medicine, 377,* 257–266.

Macdonald, R. L., & Schweizer, T. A. (2017). Spontaneous subarachnoid haemorrhage. *Lancet, 389,* 655.

Maher, M., Schweizer, T. A., & Macdonald, R. L. (2020). Treatment of spontaneous subarachnoid hemorrhage: Guidelines and gaps. *Stroke, 51,* 1326–1332.

Molyneux, A. J., Kerr, R. S., Yu, L. M., Clarke, M., Sneade, M., Yarnold, J. A., et al. (2005). International subarachnoid aneurysm trial (ISAT) of neurosurgical clipping versus endovascular coiling in 2143 patients with ruptured intracranial aneurysms: A randomised comparison of effects on survival, dependency, seizures, rebleeding, subgroups, and aneurysm occlusion. *Lancet, 366,* 809–817.

Sharma, D. (2020). Perioperative management of aneurysmal subarachnoid hemorrhage. *Anesthesiology, 133,* 1283–1305.

Steiner, T., Juvela, S., Unterberg, A., Jung, C., Forsting, M., Rinkel, G., et al. (2013). European Stroke Organization guidelines for the management of intracranial aneurysms and subarachnoid haemorrhage. *Cerebrovascular Diseases, 35,* 93–112.

Van der Kamp, L. T., Rinkel, G. J. E., Verbaan, D., van den Berg, R., Vandertop, W. P., Murayama, Y., et al. (2021). Risk of rupture after intracranial aneurysm growth. *JAMA Neurology, 78,* 1228–1235.

# 107

# Anesthesia for Pituitary Surgery

JEFFREY J. PASTERNAK, MS, MD

The pituitary gland is located inferior to the hypothalamus within the sella turcica (Fig. 107.1). Despite its small size, the pituitary gland plays a crucial role in human physiology. It consists of two functionally separate regions: (1) the anterior pituitary, or adenohypophysis; and (2) the posterior pituitary, or neurohypophysis. The pituitary gland secretes a variety of hormones that either directly affect other tissues or regulate the release of other hormones. Pituitary tumors are a common cause of primary pituitary dysfunction and can manifest by hypersecretion or hyposecretion of hormones or by invasion of the structures surrounding the sella turcica. Other disorders that can affect the function of the pituitary gland include but are not limited to infection, inflammation, infarction, or hemorrhage.

## Adenohypophysis

The adenohypophysis secretes an array of hormones under the regulation of the hypothalamus. Releasing and inhibiting factors are secreted into a capillary network within the hypothalamus (Table 107.1). Via portal vessels, these compounds then enter a second capillary network within the adenohypophysis, where they either enhance or inhibit secretion of adenohypophyseal hormones (Fig. 107.2). Further secretion of hormones by the anterior pituitary is then regulated via feedback control of hypothalamic and adenohypophyseal secretion in response to concentrations of hormones secreted by the pituitary gland or other target organs. Given the complex interactions among the hypothalamus, anterior pituitary, target endocrine glands, and end organs, disease or dysregulation at any point within these pathways can cause dysfunction of one or more hormone axes.

## Cushing Disease

Adrenocorticotropic hormone (ACTH) acts on adrenal cortex to increase cortisol production. In patients with Cushing disease, excessive production of ACTH by an ACTH-producing pituitary adenoma results in hypercortisolemia. Cortisol has a broad range of physiologic effects, including increased gluconeogenesis, reduced systemic glucose utilization, protein

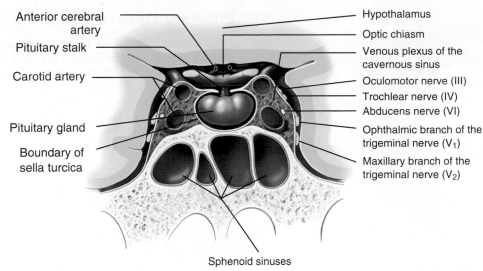

**Fig. 107.1**  Coronal section of the sella turcica depicting the anatomic relationships among the pituitary gland, cranial nerves, carotid arteries, and cavernous and sphenoid sinuses.

| TABLE 107.1 | **Hypothalamic Hormones and Adenohypophyseal Responses** | | |
|---|---|---|---|
| **Hypothalamic Hormone** | **Pituitary Cell Target** | **Pituitary Response** | **Overall Effect** |
| CRH | Corticotrophs | ↑ production of ACTH | ↑ production of cortisol by the adrenal gland |
| TRH | Thyrotrophs | ↑ production of TSH | ↑ production of $T_3$ and $T_4$ by the thyroid gland |
| GnRH | Gonadotrophs | ↑ production of FSH and LH | Regulates estrogen, progesterone, testosterone, and inhibin production by gonads |
| GHRH | Somatotrophs | ↑ production of GH | ↑ production of IGF |
| Somatostatin | Somatotrophs | ↓ production of GH | ↓ production of IGF |
| PRF | Lactotrophs | ↑ production of prolactin | Promotes lactation |
| Dopamine | Lactotrophs | ↓ production of prolactin | Inhibits lactation |

*ACTH*, Adrenocorticotropic hormone; *CRH*, corticotropin-releasing hormone; *FSH*, follicle-stimulating hormone; *GH*, growth hormone; *GHRH*, growth hormone–releasing hormone; *GnRH*, gonadotropin-releasing hormone; *IGF*, insulin-like growth factor; *LH*, luteinizing hormone; *PRF*, prolactin-releasing factor; $T_3$, triiodothyronine; $T_4$, thyroxine; *TRH*, thyroid-releasing hormone; *TSH*, thyroid-stimulating hormone.

catabolism, increased lipolysis, increased gastric acid production, bone reabsorption, and immune suppression. Clinical manifestations include hyperglycemia, skeletal muscle weakness, "moon facies," "buffalo hump," osteoporosis, poor wound healing, and increased infection rate. Perioperative concerns include possible difficulty with airway management, aberrant serum electrolyte or glucose concentrations, muscle weakness, and difficulty positioning due to osteoporosis or body habitus.

## Acromegaly

Acromegaly results from excessive secretion of growth hormone by the adenohypophysis. Growth hormone exerts its effect either directly on target cells or via stimulating hepatic secretion of insulin-like growth factor, also known as somatomedin C. Together, excessive growth hormone and insulin-like growth factor production result in inappropriately increased protein synthesis, gluconeogenesis, lipolysis, chondrocyte proliferation, bone mineralization, and muscle sarcomeric hyperplasia. This results in organomegaly and overgrowth of bones, muscles, and connective tissues.

The effects of these changes on the respiratory and cardiac systems are of primary concern during the perioperative period. Specifically, hypertrophy of facial bones, tongue, airway soft tissues, and glottic structures render the patient susceptible to developing obstructive sleep apnea. Additionally, difficulties with mask fit, bag-mask ventilation, and direct laryngoscopy can occur. Mandibular hypertrophy increases the distance between the lips and vocal cord. Vocal cord dysfunction, secondary to stretching of the recurrent laryngeal nerve, and impaired mobility of the cricoarytenoid joints can further affect airway management. Videolaryngoscopic or awake fiberoptic intubations are prudent options when managing the airway. Intubation may be performed after the induction of anesthesia, but difficulty with mask ventilation and laryngoscopy by any means should be anticipated, and backup equipment should be readily available. Costal cartilage hypertrophy can lead to restrictive pulmonary physiology.

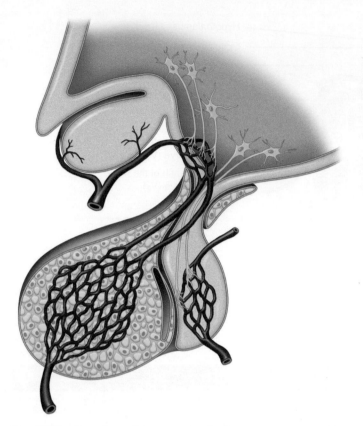

**Fig. 107.2** Physiology of the pituitary gland. Hormones secreted by the hypothalamus reach the adenohypophysis via the portal vessel. These hypothalamic hormones enter a second capillary network and act upon adenohypophyseal cells, thus regulating the secretion of hormones by the adenohypophysis. The neurohypophysis contains axons of neurons located in the supraoptic and paraventricular nuclei of the hypothalamus. When stimulated, these neurons secrete either oxytocin or vasopressin into the capillary network of the neurohypophysis.

Cardiovascular manifestations of acromegaly include hypertension, cardiac hypertrophy, left ventricular diastolic dysfunction (generally with preserved systolic function at rest until late in the course of the disease), and arrhythmias. Coronary artery insufficiency can occur and is related to increased $O_2$ demand from a hypertrophic heart and reduced coronary blood flow due to increased cardiac filling pressures that occur with diastolic dysfunction. Despite beliefs to the contrary, hypertrophy of the transverse carpal ligament does not increase the risk of ischemic complications of the hand with cannulation of the radial artery.

## Hyperprolactinemia

Signs and symptoms of increased prolactin production are more concrete in women (i.e., galactorrhea, amenorrhea, infertility) than in men (e.g., decreased libido, erectile dysfunction). As such, prolactin-secreting tumors tend to be larger and more invasive in men at the time of surgery because of delayed diagnosis. Although the manifestations of hyperprolactinemia cause no overt concerns for anesthesia, medications used to pharmacologically manage increased serum prolactin concentration (e.g., bromocriptine or cabergoline) can be associated with nausea, orthostatic hypotension, and cardiac valvular dysfunction.

## Pituitary Hyperthyroidism

Pituitary hyperthyroidism results from excessive production of thyroid-stimulating hormone (TSH) that causes increased tri-iodothyronine ($T_3$) and thyroxine ($T_4$) production (both are important metabolic regulators). These tumors are rare, and thus many patients undergo treatment for other causes of hyperthyroidism (e.g., Graves disease) prior to detection of the pituitary disease, thereby delaying the diagnosis. Such interventions include radioactive thyroid ablation or thyroidectomy that lead to decreased thyroid hormone production and loss of negative feedback on secretion of TSH, which, in turn, can enhance tumor growth. Delayed diagnosis and tumor growth increase the likelihood of encroachment on surrounding structures (e.g., the cavernous sinus), which places the patient at increased risk for developing intraoperative bleeding and iatrogenic central nervous system injury during the resection. Patients may also be hyperthyroid, hypothyroid, or euthyroid at the time of surgery. Unless visual loss is acutely threatened, patients should be rendered physiologically euthyroid, using medical treatment, prior to surgery.

## Hypopituitarism

Hypopituitarism is the condition where the production of one or more pituitary hormones is inadequate to meet physiologic demands. Hypopituitarism can result from compression of the normal gland by pituitary tumors and can also occur after pituitary surgery. Other causes include infection, inflammation, trauma, apoplexy (where pituitary hemorrhage occurs typically at the site of a preexisting pituitary tumor), or Sheehan syndrome (where pituitary infarction occurs in the setting of severe systemic hypotension during obstetric hemorrhage). Signs and symptoms may be nonspecific and depend on the extent of hormone deficiencies. In acute pituitary failure, decreases in serum ACTH and subsequent cortisol concentrations occur quickly because of their short half-lives. As such, signs and symptoms of acute pituitary failure include acute hyponatremia, profound hypotension, and shock. Treatment with corticosteroids is critical, especially to facilitate vascular responsiveness to endogenous and exogenous catecholamines that may be used to treat hypotension. In those with chronic hypopituitarism, growth hormone and ACTH deficiencies are most common with deficiencies of TSH, prolactin, and hormones produced by the neurohypophysis (i.e., oxytocin and vasopressin) being less common. Patients with chronic hypopituitarism will likely require perioperative corticosteroid supplementation.

## Neurohypophysis

Unlike the adenohypophysis, which contains hormone-secreting cells, the neurohypophysis contains distal axons of peptidergic neurons with cell bodies located in the hypothalamus. These neurons synthesize and secrete either oxytocin or vasopressin (i.e., antidiuretic hormone), which are released into the systemic circulation via capillaries located in the neurohypophysis (see Fig. 107.2).

Oxytocin is best known for modulating labor and delivery and release of breast milk. Vasopressin is one of the principal hormones regulating water balance. Normally, the strongest stimulus for vasopressin secretion is increased serum osmolality mediated via hypothalamic osmoreceptors. Vasopressin increases water reabsorption by the kidney and causes systemic arteriolar constriction.

The most common manifestation of the syndrome of inappropriate antidiuretic hormone secretion (SIADH) is hyponatremia. SIADH is usually asymptomatic if the syndrome is mild; however, seizures and coma can occur if the serum sodium concentration acutely decreases below 120 mEq/L. In the setting of chronic SIADH, adaptive mechanisms minimize symptoms despite very low serum sodium concentrations. Treatment usually involves fluid restriction for mild cases and otherwise slow ($<1$–$2$ mEq$\cdot$L$^{-1}$$\cdot$h$^{-1}$) correction of hyponatremia with hypertonic saline, as rapid correction can potentially cause central pontine myelinolysis.

Diabetes insipidus (DI) refers to inappropriate production of hypotonic urine due to either inadequate production of vasopressin (i.e., central DI) or renal unresponsiveness to vasopressin (i.e., nephrogenic DI). Initial treatment should focus on replenishing intravascular volume (which may require use of 0.9% saline in patients with severe hypovolemia, despite hypernatremia) and correcting hypernatremia. Additionally, for central DI, vasopressin or a synthetic analog (i.e., 1-desamino-8-D-arginine vasopressin) may be administered.

## Management of Patients Having Pituitary Surgery

The most common indication for pituitary surgery is tumor resection. Tumors derived from secretory cells are typically smaller at the time of diagnosis and often present with endocrinopathies, whereas nonsecreting tumors are usually larger at diagnosis and manifest due to compression or invasion of surrounding structures.

The pituitary gland is most commonly approached transnasally via the sphenoid sinus, whereas craniotomy is usually reserved for patients with large and invasive tumors. The preoperative evaluation should focus on the physiologic and anesthetic implications of any endocrinopathy, any preexisting neurologic deficits should be noted, and the risk of intraoperative bleeding or surgical disruption of adjacent structures (i.e., cavernous sinus, optic chiasm) should be considered.

For transnasal operations, the hypopharynx may be packed with moistened gauze after orotracheal intubation to minimize gastric accumulation of blood. Otherwise, it may be prudent to place an orogastric tube to remove blood that may have accumulated in the stomach as intragastric blood may be a trigger for emesis. The surgeon may request placement of a lumbar cerebrospinal fluid (CSF) drain. This will allow injection of air into the CSF, slightly increasing CSF volume and thus displacing a tumor inferiorly, or withdrawal of CSF, displacing a tumor superiorly within the sella turcica. Alternative, a lumbar drain may be placed if the surgeon anticipates significant dural disruption during surgery. The lumbar drain will allow CSF to exit via the drain instead of via the dural deficit, allowing the dural deficit a better opportunity to close, thus minimizing risk for chronic CSF leakage via the dural deficit. N$_2$O should be used with care in patients in whom air was injected into the lumbar CSF drain. Local anesthetics containing epinephrine may be injected into the nasal mucosa, with or without application of topical cocaine, to reduce bleeding. This intervention may induce transient but significant hypertension. A motionless patient is critical during transsphenoidal pituitary surgery given the proximity of the surgical site to the cavernous sinuses that contain the carotid arteries and a venous plexus (Fig. 107.1).

Common complications after surgery include nausea and vomiting, CSF leak, hypopituitarism, or disorders of water balance related to altered secretion of vasopressin by the neurohypophysis. Other complications include infection or injury to neural (i.e., optic chiasm, cranial nerves contained within the cavernous sinus) or vascular (i.e., carotid artery) structures. Increases in airway pressure should be avoided in patients with recent pituitary surgery via the transsphenoidal approach to minimize risk for entrainment of intracranial air. This includes use of continuous positive airway pressure devices in patients with obstructive sleep apnea or positive pressure mask ventilation. In the event that positive pressure mask ventilation is emergently required, a laryngeal mask airway or tracheal intubation should be considered to avoid the need for positive pressure mask ventilation.

## SUGGESTED READINGS

Esfahani, K., & Dunn, L. K. (2021). Anesthetic management during transsphenoidal pituitary surgery. *Current Opinion in Anaesthesiology, 34*, 575–581.

Krings, J. G., Kallogjeri, D., Wineland, A., Nepple, K. G., Piccirillo, J. F., & Getz, A. E. (2015). Complications following primary and revision transsphenoidal surgeries for pituitary tumors. *The Laryngoscope, 125*, 311–317.

Lee, H. C., Kim, M. K., Kim, Y. H., & Park, H. P. (2019). Radiographic predictors of difficult laryngoscopy in acromegaly patients. *Journal of Neurosurgical Anesthesiology, 31*, 50–56.

Liu, M. M., Reidy, A. B., Saatee, S., & Collard, C. D. (2017). Perioperative steroid management: Approaches based on current evidence. *Anesthesiology, 127*, 166–172.

Nemergut, E. C., & Zuo, Z. (2006). Airway management in patients with pituitary disease: A review of 746 patients. *Journal of Neurosurgical Anesthesiology, 18*, 73–77.

Pasternak, J. J. (2010). The pituitary gland. In M. F. M. James (Ed.), *Anaesthesia for patients with endocrine disease* (pp. 15–46). New York: Oxford University Press.

# 108

# Anesthesia for the Sitting Position

THOMAS J. CHRISTIANSON, MD | ROBERT M. CRAFT, MD

The sitting position is used in neurosurgery for posterior approaches to the cervical spinal and for procedures involving the posterior cranial fossa. Alternative positions for these procedures include supine with the head turned to the side, park bench, and the prone position. Properly positioned, a surgical patient in the sitting position case is actually in a modified recumbent position (Fig. 108.1). In addition to applications for neurosurgery, the sitting position, "beach chair," is often used in orthopedic surgery, particularly for shoulder surgery. The extent to which a patient is upright for shoulder surgery varies, but often these patients are positioned more upright than are neurosurgical patients. The lateral position is an alternative position for shoulder surgery.

Patients undergoing cervical spine surgery require careful preoperative evaluation for decreased cervical range of motion, cervical instability, or position-related neurologic symptoms. Any of these situations may require additional steps for airway management. Patients with posterior fossa tumors should be approached with the knowledge that brainstem structures may be adversely affected by compression or direct surgical insult and that obstructive hydrocephalus may result in elevated intracranial pressure.

Right-to-left intracardiac shunt should be considered an absolute contraindication to surgery in the sitting position.

Relative contraindications to the sitting position are listed in Box 108.1.

Catastrophic complications of the sitting position, especially during orthopedic procedures, have resulted in devastating complications from inadequate cerebral perfusion or inadequate cervical spinal cord perfusion. Recognition of the potential for this severe complication has focused attention on the importance of maintenance of adequate perfusion while in the sitting position. Cerebral autoregulation in normal adults occurs between mean arterial pressures (MAPs) of 70 to 150 mm Hg. It is essential to consider the difference between arterial blood pressure at the site of measurement and blood pressure at the brain in any position in which these values may differ. In the sitting position the gradient between the brachial MAP and the MAP at the circle of Willis (CoW) is approximately 25 mm Hg. Neurosurgical patients often have arterial lines allowing for placement of the transducer at the level of the external auditory canal (correlates to the CoW). Most patients undergoing shoulder surgery do not have arterial lines, so consideration of this gradient is important. Note that even larger gradients may occur if a lower extremity blood pressure cuff is used. Recall the MAP changes by 7.5 mm Hg for every 10 cm of height difference.

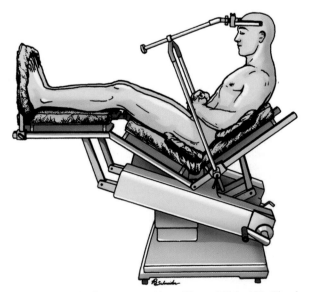

**Fig. 108.1** Standard sitting position. (From Milde LN. The head-elevated positions. In: Martin JT, Warner MA, eds. *Positioning in Anesthesia and Surgery.* 3rd ed. WB Saunders: 1997:71–93.)

## BOX 108.1 RELATIVE CONTRAINDICATIONS TO THE USE OF THE SITTING POSITION

Cerebral ischemia when the patient is upright and awake
LA pressure (PAOP) < RA pressure
Platypnea-orthodeoxia*
Preoperative demonstration of patent foramen ovale or right-to-left shunt
Hypotension†
Extremes of age
Ventriculoatrial shunt in place and open

*Platypnea-orthodeoxia is a condition in which there is a right-to-left shunting of the blood at the atrial level only with assumption of the upright position.
†Usually due to decreased intravascular volume; note that if the patient were to have a cardiac arrest in this position, chest compressions would be ineffective.
*LA,* Left atrial; *PCOP,* pulmonary artery occlusion pressure; *RA,* right atrial.
Reprinted with permission from Black S, Cucchiara RF. Tumor surgery. In: Cucchiara RF, Michenfelder JD, eds. *Clinical Neuroanesthesia.* 2nd ed. Churchill Livingstone; 1998:343–365.

> **BOX 108.2   ADVANTAGES TO THE SITTING POSITION FOR SURGERY**
>
> ↓ Blood loss
> ↑ Surgical exposure with less tissue retraction
> ↑ Access to the tracheal tube, extremities, and chest
> ↓ Facial swelling
> ↓ Intracranial pressure by ↑ drainage of both venous blood and cerebrospinal fluid

> **BOX 108.3   COMPLICATIONS ASSOCIATED WITH THE USE OF THE SITTING POSITION FOR SURGERY**
>
> Cerebral ischemia
> Circulatory instability
> Cranial nerve dysfunction
> Impaired venous drainage
> Paradoxical air embolism
> Peripheral nerve injury
> Postoperative central apnea
> Quadriplegia
> Subdural hematoma
> Tension pneumocephalus
> Venous air embolism

## Advantages of the Sitting Position

Advantages of the sitting position are listed in Box 108.2.

## Complications of the Sitting Position (Box 108.3)

### VENOUS AIR EMBOLISM AND PARADOXICAL AIR EMBOLISM

Although most often feared as a complication of the sitting position, venous air embolism (VAE) occurs in a variety of other settings including cesarean section, laparoscopy, orthopedic surgery, and prostate surgery. A large study demonstrated that although the incidence of VAE is greater in sitting patients than in horizontal patients (45% vs. 12%), no difference was noted in morbidity or mortality. Clinically significant VAE appears to occur more frequently in suboccipital craniotomies performed in the sitting position than in sitting cervical spine surgeries. Paradoxical air embolism (PAE) occurs when air crosses from the venous circulation to the arterial circulation, usually through a patent foramen ovale. A patent foramen ovale is present in approximately 27% of adults. Some authors have recommended routine screening for patent foramen ovale using echocardiography during a Valsalva maneuver prior to using the sitting position. VAE and PAE are further discussed in Chapter 109.

### TENSION PNEUMOCEPHALUS

Although there is a near 100% frequency of pneumocephalus in sitting position craniotomies, symptomatic pneumocephalus is uncommon. Cerebrospinal fluid is more likely to drain through the wound in sitting patients with cortical atrophy, allowing the entrapment of air (inverted Coke bottle phenomenon). The effect of nitrous oxide on the frequency and severity of pneumocephalus has not been confirmed.

### CIRCULATORY INSTABILITY

Anesthesia in the sitting position is associated with decreases in MAP, systolic blood pressure, stroke volume index, cardiac index, and pulmonary capillary wedge pressure. Heart rate, systemic vascular resistance, and pulmonary vascular resistance often increase.

A large retrospective comparison failed to show a difference in the incidence of hypotension between sitting and horizontal patients. Recommendations for minimizing the hemodynamic changes of the sitting position include preoperative hydration, compression stockings, slow positional change, and maintenance of appropriate degrees of hip and knee flexion. Hypotension and bradycardia, attributed to the Bezold-Jarisch reflex, is reported in shoulder surgery when regional anesthesia, with or without general anesthesia, is combined with the beach chair position.

### IMPAIRED VENOUS DRAINAGE

Venous drainage may be compromised by extreme neck flexion resulting in significant tongue and airway swelling. Limiting head flexion to allow at least 1 inch between the mandible and the sternum is often recommended to avoid compromising venous drainage.

### POSTOPERATIVE CENTRAL APNEA

Potential causes of postoperative central apnea include brainstem hematoma and surgical damage to the respiratory centers. Careful avoidance and treatment of postoperative hypertension are indicated to help decrease the incidence of hematoma formation.

### CRANIAL NERVE DYSFUNCTION

Cranial nerves V, VII, IX, X, XI, and XII may be involved. Postoperative airway protection may be impaired by dysfunction of cranial nerve IX, X, or XII.

### QUADRIPLEGIA

Mechanical compression of the spinal cord and ischemia resulting from stretching of the spinal cord blood vessels secondary to neck flexion are proposed mechanisms for reported cases of quadriplegia. Preventive measures include preoperative examination of the cervical range of motion and radiographic determination of cervical canal dimensions, as well as prompt intraoperative treatment of hypotension and limitation of neck flexion.

### PERIPHERAL NERVE INJURY

Common postoperative neuropathies involve the sciatic nerve and its division, the common peroneal nerve. Careful positioning, to avoid extreme hip or knee flexion, and padding of pressure points are recommended to limit the occurrence peripheral neuropathies.

## CEREBRAL ISCHEMIA

Devastating complications of cerebral ischemia have been attributed to inadequate perfusion in the sitting position. Most reports have been during orthopedic shoulder surgery. Please see the earlier discussion of blood pressure differences between cerebral, upper extremity, and lower extremity locations in the sitting position. Plans for deliberate hypotension during surgery in the sitting position should be viewed with great caution and with consideration for this complication.

## MONITORING

Frequently used monitoring techniques for patients undergoing surgery in the sitting position include electrocardiography (ECG), pulse oximetry, direct arterial pressure monitoring (transduced at the level of the external auditory canal), expired gas analysis, right atrial catheter, precordial Doppler, and transesophageal echocardiography (TEE). Electrophysiologic monitoring and employing modalities such as brainstem auditory evoked response (BAER), somatosensory evoked potential (SSEP), and electromyography (EMG) can provide additional information.

The cardiopulmonary system may be assessed with ECG, pulse oximetry, arterial line, central venous line, and perhaps TEE. The brainstem can be evaluated for signs of surgical trespass with BAER or SSEP monitoring. The ECG may also provide evidence of surgical transgression with potential warning signs including tachycardia, bradycardia, and ectopic beats.

Evidence of cranial nerve stimulation may be revealed through examination of the ECG, arterial line, EMG, and BAER. Manipulation of cranial nerve V results in hypertension and bradycardia, whereas manipulation of cranial nerve X results in hypotension and bradycardia. Mechanical stimulation of cranial nerves V, VII, and XI may be detected with EMG monitoring of the corresponding muscle groups. Cranial nerve VIII can be monitored with BAER.

TEE is the most sensitive intraoperative monitor for VAE and also offers the advantage of direct visualization of air in the left heart (PAE). Precordial Doppler is a sensitive and simple monitor. The classic physical finding of a "mill-wheel" murmur is an insensitive sign of VAE.

## CHOICE OF ANESTHETICS

Anesthetic concerns that may influence the choice of anesthetic agents include maintenance of cardiovascular stability, the risk of air embolism, possible increased intracranial pressure, and the desire for rapid emergence to allow for prompt postoperative neurological evaluation. No specific anesthetic technique is universally recommended. Many clinicians favor sevoflurane, low-dose opioids, and nondepolarizing neuromuscular blocking agents (or higher-dose volatile anesthetics without neuromuscular blockade in cases where EMG monitoring is used). Combinations of volatile anesthetics, nitrous oxide, and short-acting opioids allow for easily controlled anesthetic depth, stable hemodynamic parameters, and rapid emergence. The use of nitrous oxide is tempered by the knowledge of its effects on intracranial pressure and VAE. Total intravenous anesthesia, using propofol and opioid infusions, is a well-accepted technique especially when neurophysiologic monitoring is employed.

## SUGGESTED READINGS

Bapteste, L., Carrillon, R., Javelier, S., Guyotat, J., Desgranges, F. P., Lehot, J. J., et al. (2020). Pulse pressure variations and plethysmographic variability index measured at ear are able to predict fluid responsiveness in the sitting position for neurosurgery. *Journal of Neurosurgical Anesthesiology, 32*(3), 263–267.

Drummond, J. C. (2013). A beach chair, comfortably positioned atop an iceberg. *Anesthesia and Analgesia, 116,* 1204–1206.

Himes, B. T., Mallory, G. W., Abcejo, A. S., Pasternak, J., Atkinson, J. L. D., Meyer, F. B., et al. (2017). Contemporary analysis of the intraoperative and perioperative complications of neurosurgical procedures performed in the sitting position. *Journal of Neurosurgery, 127,* 182–188.

Rains, D. D., Rooke, A. R., & Wahl, C. J. (2011). Pathomechanisms and complications related to patient positioning and anesthesia during shoulder arthroscopy. *Arthroscopy: The Journal of Arthroscopic and Related Surgery, 27,* 532–541.

Tufegdzic, B., Lamperti, M., Siyam, A., & Roser, F. (2021). Air-embolism in the semi-sitting position for craniotomy: A narrative review with emphasis on a single centers experience. *Clinical Neurology and Neurosurgery, 209,* 106904. doi:10.1016/j.clineuro.2021.106904.

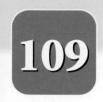

# 109

# Physiology and Treatment of Venous Air Embolism

BENJAMIN FREDRICK GRUENBAUM, MD, PhD | SHAUN EVAN GRUENBAUM, MD, PhD

## Etiology

A venous air embolism (VAE) can result when an open, noncollapsible vein is exposed to air or gas, and a pressure gradient favors air entrainment into the circulation rather than bleeding. VAE typically occurs when the operative site is above the level of the heart, but it can also occur when noncollapsible veins are open in an operative field in which gas has been insufflated under pressure.

## Prevalence

VAE has been reported in several types of surgical procedures in which the operative site is above the level of the heart. VAE can also occur when gas is used for insufflation or to cool surgical instruments, resulting from the inadvertent injection of gas into a cavity, joint, or directly into the vasculature. VAE has been reported in most types of neurosurgical procedures, with the highest incidence (76%) observed during posterior fossa craniotomy (Table 109.1).

| TABLE 109.1 Operative Incidence of Venous Air Embolism | |
|---|---|
| **Procedure** | **Reported Frequency of VAE, %** |
| **NEUROSURGICAL** | |
| Sitting posterior fossa craniotomy | 45–55 |
| Posterior fossa procedures | 76 |
| Cervical laminectomy | 23–25 |
| Transsphenoidal pituitary resection | 12 |
| Craniosynostosis | 85 |
| Lumbar spine procedures | 1–2 |
| Intracranial electrode placement for movement disorder | * |
| **OB/GYN** | |
| Cesarean section | 11–44 |
| Hysteroscopy, laser endometrial ablation | * |
| **ORTHOPEDIC** | |
| Total hip replacement | Up to 65 |
| Intramedullary femur nailing, irrigation of pelvic fractures, removal of bone cyst, arthroscopy | * |
| **GENERAL SURGERY** | |
| Laparoscopy, laser tumor resection, instillation of liquid nitrogen, insertion of peritoneovenous shunt, hepatic resection, GI endoscopy, venovenous bypass during liver transplantation | * |
| **PLASTIC SURGERY** | |
| Removal of tissue expander | * |
| **TRAUMA** | |
| Head and neck trauma, penetrating lung trauma | * |
| **DENTAL** | |
| Dental implant procedures | * |
| **UROLOGIC** | |
| Prostatectomy | * |
| Interventional radiology | |
| ERCP | * |
| **ICU** | |
| Mechanical ventilation, central line placement and removal | * |

*Case reports.
*ERCP*, Endoscopic retrograde cholangiopancreatography; *GI*, gastrointestinal; *ICU*, intensive care unit; *OB/GYN*, obstetrics and gynecology; *VAE*, venous air embolism.

## Pathophysiology

The amount of air and rate of air entrapment are the most important factors that determine the systemic and hemodynamic effects that result from VAE. Rarely, a massive VAE can create an "air lock" in the right ventricle (RV), resulting in RV outflow obstruction, RV failure, and cardiovascular collapse. More commonly, VAE reflects a slow entrainment of air into the venous system, right side of the heart, and pulmonary vasculature, which increases the pulmonary vascular resistance via two mechanisms: mechanical obstruction of small arteries and arterioles, and release of endogenous vasoactive agents that cause pulmonary vasoconstriction. RV afterload, pulmonary artery pressure, and central venous pressure increase as the RV function worsens. As VAE progresses, hypotension ensues as cardiac output decreases. Acute respiratory distress syndrome can develop after a large VAE.

Paradoxical air embolism (PAE) or arterial air embolism can also occur when air passes from the right to the left side of the heart through an intracardiac shunt or through the pulmonary vasculature. In the setting of PAE, serious complications can result from coronary and cerebral artery obstruction. Known complications of PAE include arrhythmias, myocardial ischemia, and focal neurologic deficits.

## Morbidity and Mortality

The risk of morbidity and mortality from VAE is low in procedures in which precautions are taken to reduce the risk of significant VAE and when VAE is rapidly diagnosed, communicated with the surgical team, and treated. However, complete cardiovascular collapse and death from VAE can occur, particularly during procedures in which VAE is thought to be unlikely. In these procedures, the diagnosis and treatment of VAE is often delayed, resulting in further entrapment of air and worsening hemodynamic instability. For example, reported cases of VAE during spine operations are associated with a near 50% mortality rate, when the diagnosis is typically made late in the clinical course and in the presence of severe hemodynamic instability.

## Diagnosis

The most sensitive monitors for VAE are transesophageal echocardiography (TEE) and precordial Doppler, followed by expired nitrogen, end-tidal CO$_2$, pulmonary artery pressure, central venous pressure, right atrial (RA) catheter, and esophageal stethoscope (Fig. 109.1).

The precordial Doppler is often used in the perioperative setting for the diagnosis of VAE because it is highly sensitive, relatively inexpensive, easy to use, and noninvasive. The Doppler probe should be placed at the fourth or fifth intercostal space at the right sternal border and moved until the maximal heart tones are heard (Fig. 109.2). Injection of agitated saline via a central or large-bore free-running peripheral intravenous catheter assists in verifying proper placement. A characteristic sound ("mill-wheel murmur") of turbulent flow is heard when air enters the right heart chambers.

TEE is a sensitive monitor for VAE that detects localized air in the cardiac chambers. Although TEE may be slightly more sensitive than the precordial Doppler, there are disadvantages to its use: (1) TEE requires more experience to place properly and interpret; (2) it carries a potential risk of esophageal injury or

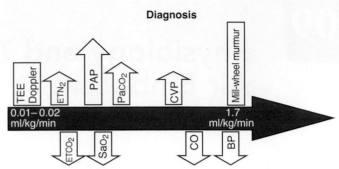

**Fig. 109.1** Changes in detection parameters for venous air embolism with increasing volumes of air. Data are aggregated from human and animal studies. The mill-wheel murmur is the characteristic sound of turbulent flow heard on Doppler when the agitated saline (air) enters the right heart chambers. *BP,* Blood pressure; *CO,* cardiac output; *CVP,* central venous pressure; *ETCO$_2$,* end-tidal carbon dioxide; *ETN$_2$,* end-tidal nitrogen; *PaCO$_2$,* partial pressure of carbon dioxide; *PAP,* pulmonary artery pressure; *SaO$_2$,* arterial oxygen saturation; *TEE,* transesophageal echocardiography.

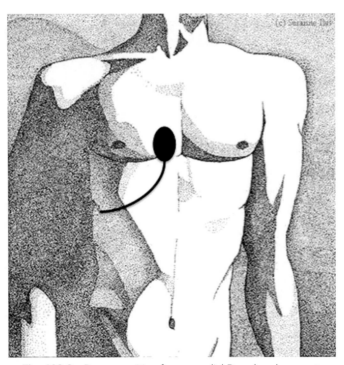

**Fig. 109.2** Proper position for precordial Doppler placement.

airway compression (if neck flexion is required for surgical positioning); (3) the image must be continuously watched (unlike the Doppler, which is an audible monitor); and (4) its high sensitivity can make it difficult to differentiate clinically insignificant microemboli from clinically significant VAE. However, recent advancements in automated VAE detection with TEE have yielded promising results.

A multiorifice central venous catheter can be used for the aspiration of air from the RA during massive VAE. Proper placement of the RA catheter high in the RA is necessary to optimize the surface area of the orifices that make contact with the entrapped air. Correct catheter placement can be confirmed by three methods: (1) recording of the electrocardiogram via the RA catheter and identification of large negative P waves when the catheter tip is high in the RA; (2) transducing pressure recordings obtained when the catheter enters the RV and is pulled back; or (3) chest radiograph.

## Treatment

Successful treatment of VAE relies on its rapid diagnosis, which is necessary to prevent any further entrapment of air into the open vessel, and to support and optimize the cardiac output. Flooding the surgical field with saline prevents any further air entry in the circulation. The application of manual jugular venous compression for about 15 seconds will frequently raise the venous pressure at the operative site during craniotomy sufficiently to allow the vessel to back-bleed and be identified.

If $N_2O$ is being used, it should be immediately discontinued because its low solubility will facilitate its diffusion into the VAE, thereby increasing its size and hemodynamic effects. The administration of vasopressors and isotonic fluids will increase the preload and cardiac output and will aid in pushing the VAE through the heart and peripheral pulmonary circulation. Aspiration of air from the RA catheter should be attempted, although its effectiveness in this setting has been questioned. To decrease VAE, some authors have recommended the use of positive end-expiratory pressure (PEEP) to increase central venous pressure and cerebral venous pressure, but most studies have demonstrated that the use of PEEP is ineffective. Also, with the use of PEEP, increased right-sided heart pressures can increase the risk of PAE.

In the presence of VAE-related cardiovascular collapse, it is generally recommended that the patient be immediately placed in the Durant position (left lateral decubitus position) or Trendelenburg position (head down, except when there is a risk of intracranial hypertension) to relieve RV outflow obstruction. Some studies, however, have suggested that repositioning does not offer any significant benefit. As addressed earlier, the most important prognostic indicators for VAE is its rapid diagnosis, prevention of further air entrainment, and cardiovascular/hemodynamic support.

Similarly, the initial treatment of PAE should aim to prevent further air entrapment. If myocardial ischemia develops, the use of positive inotropic agents such as epinephrine is recommended to maintain adequate blood pressure and increase ventricular contractility, which can assist in dissolving the emboli. If symptomatic cerebral ischemia occurs, hyperbaric $O_2$ therapy should be considered as soon as the patient can be safely transported into a hyperbaric chamber.

## Anesthetic Considerations

When VAE or PAE develop, there are some conditions that can increase the risk of significant morbidity. In the presence of these risk factors, efforts should be focused on decreasing the likelihood of the occurrence of VAE. For example, although controversial, the use of $N_2O$ in procedures that carry a risk for VAE is generally contraindicated in high-risk patients or in high-risk surgeries. However, animal and human data suggest that if $N_2O$ is discontinued when VAE is rapidly diagnosed with precordial Doppler, the risk of significant VAE-associated morbidity is not increased. When sensitive diagnostic monitors for VAE are used, $N_2O$ can be used safely in procedures that carry an increased risk for VAE. In the event of VAE, $N_2O$ should be immediately discontinued. If the use of sensitive diagnostic monitors are not available, $N_2O$ should generally be avoided.

## SUGGESTED READINGS

Brull, S. J., & Prielipp, R. C. (2017). Vascular air embolism: A silent hazard to patient safety. *Journal of Critical Care, 42*, 255–263.

Lee, C. C., Wu, A., & Li, M. (2020). Venous air embolism during neurosurgery. In A. Brambrink, J. Kirsch (Eds.), *Essentials of neurosurgical anesthesia & critical care* (pp. 287–291). Champlain: Springer.

McCarthy, C. J., Behravesh, S., Naidu, S. G., & Oklu, R. (2016). Air embolism: Practical tips for prevention and treatment. *Journal of Clinical Medicine, 5*(11), 93.

McCarthy, C. J., Behravesh, S., Naidu, S. G., & Oklu, R. (2017). Air embolism: Diagnosis, clinical management and outcomes. *Diagnostics, 7*(1), 5.

Rau, T. R., Plaschke, K., Weigand, M. A., Maier, C., & Schramm, C. (2021). Automatic detection of venous air embolism using transesophageal echocardiography in patients undergoing neurological surgery in the semi-sitting position: A pilot study. *Journal of Clinical Monitoring and Computing, 35*(5), 1103–1109.

Schlimp, C. J., Bothma, P. A., & Brodbeck, A. E. (2014). Cerebral venous air embolism: What is it and do we know how to deal with it properly? *JAMA Neurology, 71*(2), 243.

# 110

# Perioperative Implications of Caring for Patients With Epilepsy

BENJAMIN FREDRICK GRUENBAUM, MD, PhD | SHAUN EVAN GRUENBAUM, MD, PhD

Epilepsy is one of the most common neurologic disorders globally and can affect both children and adults of all races and economic status. Approximately 3.5 million people in the United States suffer from a seizure disorder, which are characterized in accordance with their clinical presentation and electroencephalographic (EEG) features.

Anecdotal observations and case reports suggest that anesthesia and surgery are associated with an increased risk of perioperative seizure activity (frequency and duration). Proposed etiologic factors include missing one or more doses of the patient's antiepileptic drugs (AEDs) on the day of surgery; pathophysiological conditions such as hypoglycemia, hyponatremia, hyperpyrexia, environmental factors such as sleep deprivation, fatigue, stress, and excessive alcohol consumption; and exposure to proconvulsant medications. Anesthetics implicated in triggering seizure activity include inhalational anesthetic agents; local anesthetic (LA) agents (e.g., lidocaine, bupivacaine); opioids (e.g., fentanyl, alfentanil, sufentanil, meperidine); and some sedative-hypnotic medications (e.g., etomidate, ketamine, methohexital). Because these drugs are commonly used in patients undergoing general anesthesia, their effects in patients with seizure disorders must be fully understood.

In addition to the increased risk of perioperative seizure activity, patients with epilepsy have a greater risk of postoperative morbidity including stroke, myocardial infarction, and traumatic brain injury. Therefore, anesthesia providers must approach the perioperative care of epilepsy patients presenting for neurological or nonneurological surgery with an understanding of these associated risks.

## Perioperative Seizure Frequency

Studies have suggested that the frequency of perioperative seizures in epilepsy patients during either regional or general anesthesia is higher than in the general population but is considerably variable. Approximately 2% to 6% of epilepsy patients can experience postoperative seizures that, based on the temporal relationship, are thought to be unlikely directly related to the anesthetic management. Evidence from recent investigations demonstrates that, although many regional and general anesthetic medications have proconvulsant properties, the risk of perioperative seizures is mostly related to the patient's underlying seizure history (i.e., baseline frequency) and the requirement of multiple AEDs. Although it is difficult to establish a rate of perioperative seizure activity in the general population (i.e., in nonepileptic patients), some patients have been shown to experience nonepileptic seizures while under anesthesia.

## Effect of Anesthetics on Epilepsy

### INHALED ANESTHETIC AGENTS

Inhaled anesthetic agents have both proconvulsant and anticonvulsant properties. At low doses, these inhaled anesthetic agents have the potential to induce EEG-identified epileptiform activity in individuals with or without a history of seizures. Although the mechanism of action has yet to be fully elucidated, these changes likely result from preferential inhibition of inhibitory central nervous system neurotransmission. As a result, excitatory neurotransmission freely occurs in cortical and subcortical brain regions. In contrast, with escalating doses of the inhaled agents, the EEG progresses through a continuum of increased beta activity followed by burst suppression and, eventually, isoelectricity. Accordingly, inhaled anesthetic agents can be used to facilitate cortical mapping during epilepsy surgery or, at higher doses, to terminate status epilepticus in patients whose seizures are refractory to conventional therapy.

### OPIOIDS

It is well established that opioids can induce epileptiform activity in both laboratory animals and humans. Opioid-induced epileptiform activity may be used to localize the epileptogenic zone activity in patients undergoing epilepsy surgery. Alfentanil, sufentanil, and remifentanil (i.e., short-acting opioids) can be used to initiate epileptiform loci during intraoperative electrocorticography (ECoG) at the time of focal cortical resection. The cause of opioid-induced limbic system seizures has not yet been fully determined. Proposed mechanisms include selective activation of limbic opioid receptors, augmented release of excitatory amino acids (like glutamate), facilitation of coupling between excitatory postsynaptic potentials and somatic spike-generating sites, and suppression of inhibitory interneurons (i.e., the disinhibition hypothesis). According to the disinhibition hypothesis, opioids indirectly excite limbic system structures by inhibiting neighboring $\gamma$-aminobutyric acid (GABA)–secreting inhibitory interneurons.

### LOCAL ANESTHETIC AGENTS

LA toxicity is a potential risk for patients with and without epilepsy undergoing regional anesthesia, particularly during procedures that require a large dose of LA agents such as epidural, caudal, or peripheral nerve blocks. Systemic LA toxicity presents as a spectrum of neurologic symptoms and signs that worsen as plasma drug concentrations rise. A preexisting epilepsy diagnosis does not appear to increase the likelihood of LA-induced seizures in patients undergoing regional anesthesia.

## BENZODIAZEPINES

Intraoperative cortical mapping and ECoG are important tools to identify, treat, and prevent seizure activity. Benzodiazepines profoundly suppress seizures due to their potent GABA agonist effects and therefore should be used with caution in patients undergoing procedures to identify epileptogenic foci. Clinical discretion and counseling with the patient care team are recommended in order to avoid the suppression of epileptic activity in these cases.

## Effect of Antiepileptic Drugs on Perioperative Patient Care

There is little evidence to suggest that additional seizure prophylaxis with AEDs is beneficial for patients in the postoperative period. However, these drugs are often administered in patients undergoing surgery for other indications, and it is therefore prudent to understand the interactions between AEDs and commonly used anesthetics.

The most relevant interaction between AEDs and anesthetic agents pertains to the use of nondepolarizing neuromuscular blocking agents (NMBAs) in patients chronically taking phenytoin, carbamazepine, and phenobarbital. This patient population may require a larger initial bolus dose of an NMBA to induce muscle relaxation, and more frequent dosing is often necessary to maintain a steady-state plasma concentration. Although the cause is not fully understood, the larger initial dose is partially attributable to increased plasma concentrations of $\alpha$1-acid glycoprotein (AAG), which is an inducible plasma protein responsible for binding basic drugs such as NMBAs. In the setting of chronic AED use, AAG synthesis increases, thereby decreasing the quantity of free (i.e., unbound and pharmacologically active) NMBA available to interact with nicotinic receptors at the neuromuscular junction. More frequent dosing may also be required, as AEDs induce the hepatic enzyme activity that metabolically inactivates NMBA activity.

By contrast, the bolus and infusions doses of propofol necessary to maintain a patient on AEDs at a bispectral index of 30 to 50 are significantly lower than in controls. Moreover, the time to emergence in patients taking AEDs is significantly longer than for those not taking AEDs. The interaction of propofol and AEDs is thought to be due to hepatic enzyme inhibition of the cytochrome P450 pathways CYP2B6, CYP2C9, and CYP2C19, which metabolize drugs like valproic acid, carbamazepine, phenytoin, and phenobarbital.

Studies have further observed that AED use can also result in significant hematologic perturbations. For example, chronic use of valproate can result in a dose-dependent thrombocytopenia, as well as hepatotoxicity as reflected by abnormal liver function tests including $\gamma$-glutamyl transpeptidase, alkaline phosphatase, and alanine aminotransferase. These alterations are often asymptomatic, transient, and are thought to be clinically insignificant.

## SUGGESTED READINGS

Benish, S. M., Cascino, G. D., Warner, M. E., Worrell, G. A., & Wass, C. T. (2010). Effect of general anesthesia in patients with epilepsy: A population-based study. *Epilepsy and Behavior, 17,* 87–89.

Chang, H. C., Liao, C. C., Chang, C. C., Huang, S. Y., Yeh, C. C., Hu, C. J., et al. (2018). Risks of epilepsy in surgical patients undergoing general or neuraxial anaesthesia. *Anaesthesia, 73*(3), 323–331.

Couch, C. G., Menendez, M. E., & Barnes, C. L. (2017). Perioperative risk in patients with epilepsy undergoing total joint arthroplasty. *Journal of Arthroplasty, 32*(2), 537–540.

Niesen, A. D., Jacob, A. K., Aho, L. E., Botten, E. J., Nase, K. E., Nelson, J. M., et al. (2010). Perioperative seizures in patients with a history of a seizure disorder. *Anesthesia and Analgesia, 111,* 729–735.

Orihara, A., Hara, K., Hara, S., Shimizu, K., Inaji, M., Hashimoto, S., et al. (2020). Effects of sevoflurane anesthesia on intraoperative high-frequency oscillations in patients with temporal lobe epilepsy. *Seizure, 82,* 44–49.

Ouchi, K., & Sugiyama, K. (2015). Required propofol dose for anesthesia and time to emerge are affected by the use of antiepileptics: prospective cohort study. *BMC Anesthesiology, 15,* 34.

Shetty, A., Pardeshi, S., Shah, V. M., & Kulkarni, A. (2016). Anesthesia considerations in epilepsy surgery. *International Journal of Surgery, 36,* 454–459.

Turnbull, D., Singatullina, N., & Reilly, C. A. (2016). Systematic appraisal of neurosurgical seizure prophylaxis. *Journal of Neurosurgical Anesthesiology, 28,* 233–249.

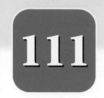

# 111

# Effects of Anesthetic Agents and Sedation Medications on Electroencephalograms

R. DORIS WANG, MD

## Normal Electroencephalogram

The electroencephalogram (EEG) is a continuous depiction of the summation of excitatory and inhibitory postsynaptic potentials from pyramidal neurons of the cerebral cortex. In addition, the EEG also reflects the state of deeper brain structures due to the rich interconnections between cortical and subcortical structures such as the thalamus, hippocampus, and brainstem. The disruption of these neuronal signal connections is thought to reduce the capacity of information integration and thus decrease the level of consciousness. Raw EEG tracings contain several identifiable rhythms, which are defined by the frequency. The five commonly recognized patterns of human EEG oscillations and their characteristics are listed in Table 111.1, and the four categories of frequencies that are the most clinically relevant appear in Figure 111.1. In general, there is an inverse relationship between EEG frequency and amplitude. The frequency and amplitude of the EEG become slower as the level of arousal diminishes. In infancy, low-frequency oscillations tend to dominate until around age 8, when the alpha rhythm becomes the predominate oscillation. In healthy elderly patients, the frequency of alpha oscillation can become slower with increasing age but remains above 8 Hz. Compared to younger patients, EEG amplitudes tend to be smaller in elderly patients. Some awake patients may have pathological slowing of the EEG due to underlying system or central nervous system pathology.

## EEG PARAMETERS FOR THE ASSESSMENT OF CHANGES ASSOCIATED WITH ANESTHESIA AND SEDATION

Changes in intraoperative EEG reflect the effects of a combination of different types of medications, anesthetic agents, levels of

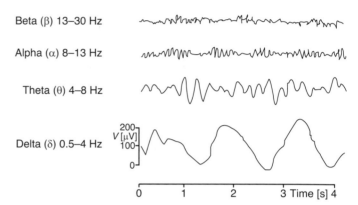

**Fig. 111.1** Clinically relevant electroencephalographic frequencies. (Constant I, Sabourdin N. The EEG signals: a window on the cortical brain activity. *Pediatric Anesthesia.* 2012;22:539–552.)

anesthesia, a patient's underlying physiological state, and the level of surgical stimulation. A general pattern of EEG progression from sedation to general anesthesia state is seen in Figure 111.2. The strength of EEG activity is described by the amplitude or power for a particular frequency band and can be presented as a compressed spectral array or spectrogram for rapid review of the EEG trend. Coherence, a metric in the study of rhythmic neuronal interaction, is a measure of similarity between two EEG oscillation recordings from different brain regions. Under general anesthesia, particularly with γ-aminobutyric acid type A (GABA_A) receptor–mediated agents, the normal posterior dominant alpha oscillation disappears and a frontal alpha coherent oscillation emerges. This spatial shift is called anteriorization of alpha oscillation. The coherent frontal alpha oscillations are thought to reduce the capacity of the thalamocortical network to coordinate exogenous inputs and communicate with the cortical neurons. Lower frontal alpha band power under anesthesia has been found to associate with higher propensity for burst suppression independent of age and other factors. In general, EEG signals become more regular with increasing anesthesia depth and are associated with a decrease in entropy. The burst suppression EEG pattern, an independent predictor of postoperative delirium, is characterized by alternating periods of high amplitude activity (burst) and relatively low amplitude activity (suppression) and represents a very deep state of general anesthesia.

The relationship between anesthetic agents and EEG patterns has been extensively studied. In particular, the GABA_A-mediated and *N*-methyl-D-aspartate (NMDA) receptor–mediated anesthetic agents appear to have distinct EEG patterns, particularly during the maintenance phase of anesthesia.

| TABLE 111.1 | Categories of the Most Clinically Relevant Electroencephalographic Frequencies | |
| --- | --- | --- |
| **Wave Pattern** | **Frequency Range (Hz)** | **Level of Consciousness** |
| Delta | <4 | Ischemia<br>Slow-wave sleep |
| Theta | 4–8 | Drowsiness (also first stage of sleep) |
| Alpha | 8–12 | Relaxed but alert |
| Beta | 12–30 | Highly alert and focused |
| Gamma | 30–80 | Learning, formation of working memory |

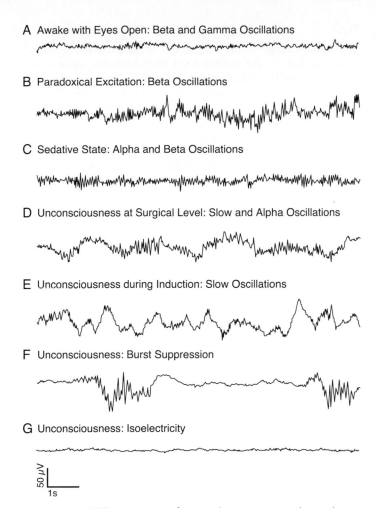

A Awake with Eyes Open: Beta and Gamma Oscillations

B Paradoxical Excitation: Beta Oscillations

C Sedative State: Alpha and Beta Oscillations

D Unconsciousness at Surgical Level: Slow and Alpha Oscillations

E Unconsciousness during Induction: Slow Oscillations

F Unconsciousness: Burst Suppression

G Unconsciousness: Isoelectricity

50 μV
1s

**Fig. 111.2** EEG progression from sedation to general anesthesia. (Purdon PL, et al. Clinical electroencephalography for anesthesiologists. *Anesthesiologist.* 2015;123:937–960.)

## GABAERGIC ANESTHETICS

Isoflurane, sevoflurane, thiopental, and propofol produce anesthesia by potentiating inhibitory $GABA_A$ receptors. Although each agent has its own characteristic EEG changes due to interaction with different subunits of GABA receptors, the EEG waveforms undergo similar changes as the concentration of administered anesthetic increases. The change in the EEG signature of $GABA_A$ receptor–mediated anesthetic agents from light sedation to the state of unconsciousness includes the appearance of spatially coherent frontal alpha oscillations in most patients and a general progression from small amplitude and high-frequency oscillation to larger amplitude and lower-frequency oscillations.

### Propofol

Propofol enhances $GABA_A$ receptor–mediated inhibition in the neocortex, thalamus, and brainstem. During slow induction of anesthesia with propofol infusion, raw EEG shows small and high-frequency activity (paradoxical excitation) during light sedation. At loss of consciousness (LOC), the EEG may continue to be small in amplitude and fast in frequency but slower than during awake state. As overall EEG frequency slows, amplitude becomes larger and alpha oscillations become coherent in the frontal region. Further increases in propofol concentration

lead to diminishing of alpha activity, whereas theta and delta oscillation becomes dominant. Eventually, the burst suppression pattern emerges. Rapid induction of general anesthesia with a large dose of propofol bolus is associated with the appearance of delta waves followed by coherent alpha and delta oscillations and high-amplitude incoherent slow wave (0.1–1 Hz) oscillations. Compared to volatile anesthetics, propofol induced burst suppression has lower amplitudes and a strong oscillatory component around 10 Hz.

## Inhalation Anesthetic Agents

The EEG pattern of different inhalational agents are similar. At minimum alveolar concentration (MAC) level of anesthesia, the EEG pattern is characterized by coherent alpha, slow-delta, and theta oscillations. With EEG progression from sedation to general anesthesia with sevoflurane, there is augmentation of beta power, which persists despite loss of responsiveness. Alpha, theta, and delta power remain unchanged, and frontal alpha oscillation does not consistently emerge at the LOC. Frontal alpha oscillation intensifies at greater sevoflurane concentrations.

The alpha and delta oscillations observed with sub-MAC level of inhalational agents resemble those of propofol. However, unlike propofol, a distinct theta coherence oscillation is observed with increasing sevoflurane end tidal concentrations at MAC level and above. As with propofol, burst suppression can occur with surgical depth–inhalation anesthesia. Sevoflurane-induced burst appears to have the lowest entropy and is indicative of a more regular signal pattern compared to isoflurane and propofol.

A burst suppression pattern usually occurs with isoflurane concentrations of greater than 2% in $O_2$ or 1.5% in 70% $N_2O$. For desflurane, burst suppression occurs at a MAC of at least 1.25. Substitution of $N_2O$ for 0.42 MAC desflurane reduces the degree of EEG suppression relative to the equipotent administration of desflurane and $O_2$.

Epileptiform activities are often observed with rapid inhalational induction with 7% to 8% sevoflurane and during steady state anesthesia with greater than 1.5 MAC of sevoflurane in both adult and pediatric patients. Rapid inhalational induction, hyperventilation particularly in adult patients, and female sex are associated with higher incidence of epileptiform activities on EEG. These EEG spikes can appear in a background of slow delta waves or during burst suppression.

## BARBITURATES

Barbiturates are also $GABA_A$ receptor–mediated anesthetic agents. When comparing thiopental and propofol for rapid sequence induction in pregnant patients, thiopental is associated with an increase in spectral entropy, which signifies a lighter state of anesthesia compared to propofol.

Barbiturate-induced burst suppression therapy is associated with more systemic hypotension and recovery compared to propofol. Thiopental, though widely use throughout Europe, is no longer available for use in the United States.

## ETOMIDATE

Etomidate exerts its actions through potentiation of the $GABA_A$ receptor containing β2 and β3 subunits. The β2 subunit is associated with a sedative effect, whereas the β3 subunit is responsible for anesthetic properties. As with propofol and thiopental, burst suppression is seen with administration of high-dose etomidate. The frontal EEG signature of etomidate-induced LOC is associated with increases in delta-wave, alpha-wave, and theta-wave coherence. Coherence of the theta oscillation pattern has been indicated in interference in hippocampal interactions with the prefrontal cortex, another significant memory-associated pathway.

## BENZODIAZEPINES

Benzodiazepines also exert their sedation and axolysis effects through interaction with the $GABA_A$ receptors. Benzodiazepines are associated with increased delta activity in the bilateral frontotemporal and temporal-occipital regions and decreased alpha activity in the frontal, temporal, and occipital regions. At high doses, benzodiazepines produce frontally dominant delta and theta activity. However, burst suppression cannot be achieved with benzodiazepines alone. Comparison of light sedation under midazolam versus propofol revealed a more integrated network in the beta frequency band with midazolam.

## NMDA RECEPTOR ANTAGONISTS

### Ketamine

Ketamine induces general anesthesia by inhibiting NMDA receptor–mediated interactions leading to excitatory activity in the neocortex, hippocampus, and limbic system. In healthy volunteers with multichanneled EEG monitors, ketamine administration is associated with local resting-state synchrony within the gamma and theta bands and an increase in gamma and theta band long-range oscillatory coupling. Frontal EEG changes associated with administration of induction dose of ketamine include a "gamma burst" pattern with alternation of slow delta and gamma oscillations, an increase in theta oscillations, and a decrease in alpha and beta oscillations. For these reasons, EEG indices tracking the suppression of high-frequency EEG activity and the activation of low-frequency oscillations (as triggered by the GABAergic-mediated anesthetics) do not correlate well with NMDA receptor–mediated sedatives.

### $N_2O$

The initial change in EEG with $N_2O$ is the progressive loss of alpha rhythm. As the patient loses consciousness, alpha waves disappear. Fast frontal oscillatory activity ($>30$ Hz) is observed with inspired $N_2O$ concentrations greater than 50%. The fast activity is especially prominent in frontal regions. Theta waves increase in frequency and amplitude, particularly in the temporal region. Addition of $N_2O$ to volatile anesthetics has an additive effect for increasing anesthetic depth to surgical stimulation but may not have an additional effect on suppression of EEG activity.

## OPIOIDS

Opioids generally induce a slowing of the spontaneous EEG and an increase in the delta band. However, high-dose opioids do not result in a burst-suppression pattern.

### Dexmedetomidine

Dexmedetomidine alters arousal primarily through its actions on presynaptic $\alpha_2$ adrenergic receptors on neurons projecting from the locus ceruleus. EEG with full scalp electrodes revealed dexmedetomidine-induced sedation is associated with increased slow delta power in the frontal and occipital regions, increased occipital theta power, increased frontocentral spindle waves, and decreased beta power. Clinically, the EEG signature of the dexmedetomidine-induced sedation state is slow delta oscillations and episodic sleep spindles (12–16 Hz) in the frontal electrodes. These spindles resemble the EEG pattern of the early stage of sleep, which is a state of unconsciousness that is less profound than non–rapid eye movement stage III or slow-wave sleep. With increasing infusion rates, the spindles disappear, and the amplitude of the slow delta oscillations increases.

### Other

Scopolamine, a centrally acting anticholinergic agent, is known to cause cognitive impairments. Scopolamine is associated with reduced corticocortical coherence in the fast oscillations and the shift of coherence toward the slow delta range.

## SUGGESTED READINGS

Bombardieri, A. M., Wildes, T. S., Stevens, T., Wolfson, M., Steinhorn, R., Ben Abdallah, A., et al. (2020). Practical training of anesthesia clinicians in electroencephalogram-based determination of hypnotic depth of general anesthesia. *Anesthesia and Analgesia, 130*(3), 777–786.

Bowyer, S. (2016). Coherence a measure of the brain networks: Past and present. *Neuropsychiatric Electrophysiology, 2*, 1–12.

Kreuzer, M. (2017). EEG based monitoring of general anesthesia: Taking the next steps. *Front Comput Neurosci, 11*, 56. Retrieved from https://doi.org/10.3389/fncom.2017.00056.

Marchant, N., Sanders, R., Sleigh, J., Vanhaudenhuyse, A., Bruno, M. A., Brichant, J. F., et al. (2014). How electroencephalography serves the anesthesiologist. *Clinical EEG and Neuroscience, 45*(1), 22–32.

Purdon, P. L., Pavone, K. J., Akeju, O., Smith, A. C., Sampson, A. L., Lee, J., et al. (2015). The ageing brain: Age-dependent changes in the electroencephalogram during propofol and sevoflurane general anesthesia. *British Journal of Anaesthesia, 115*, i46–i57.

Purdon, P. L., Sampson, A., Pavone, K., & Brown, E. N. (2015). Clinical electroencephalography for anesthesiologists. Part I: Background and basic signatures. *Anesthesiology, 123*(4), 937–960.

# 112 Carotid Endarterectomy

DAVID M. BURIC, MD

Carotid artery stenosis can be treated surgically by performing a carotid endarterectomy (CEA) or endovascularly by placing a carotid stent. The discussion in this chapter will be limited to anesthetic considerations for CEA. CEA is indicated for symptomatic patients (i.e., those who present with transient ischemic attacks of visual loss [amaurosis fugax], paresthesia, unsteadiness, and speech problems) or permanent sequelae because of cerebral infarction with greater than 70% stenosis of one or both carotid arteries. Current evidence supports early operation in these patients, ideally within 2 weeks of the patient's most recent neurologic symptoms. Results of previous randomized controlled studies have shown a 17% reduction in the occurrence of ipsilateral stroke at 2 years with CEA compared with medical management alone. Only marginal benefit has been shown in symptomatic patients with 50% to 69% stenosis. For asymptomatic patients with stenosis, current research supports medical management alone. However, new research is underway to evaluate whether medical management alone or medical management with carotid revascularization (CEA vs. stenting) is the safest and most effective treatment for the prevention of stroke in asymptomatic patients.

## Preoperative Evaluation

Patients with known carotid artery disease should undergo a thorough preoperative evaluation with a focus on cardiovascular comorbidities and functional status. CEA surgery is considered intermediate risk for perioperative cardiac events, with myocardial ischemia being the most common cause of perioperative death. Because of this increased risk, evaluation by a cardiologist before surgery should be considered for those individuals with active cardiac disease (acute myocardial ischemia [<1 week], severe valvular disease, arrhythmias, or decompensated congestive heart failure) or two or more risk factors with unknown functional status.

## Carotid Endarterectomy Procedure

General and regional anesthesia are equally effective for CEA. An international, multicenter randomized trial comparing outcomes in patients who received general anesthesia with those who received local anesthesia for CEA showed no differences between groups in rates of perioperative morbidity and mortality, quality of life, and long-term stroke-free survival.

Key aspects of the surgery involve making an incision in the neck and placing a carotid clamp proximal and distal to the diseased portion of the vessel to allow dissection of the plaque from the artery in a bloodless field. Some surgeons also place a shunt to reroute blood around the clamped vessel. Not all surgeons routinely place shunts because of the risk of thromboembolic events; instead, some first evaluate the patient's need for a

shunt by assessing the adequacy of cerebral blood flow and oxygenation. Several monitoring options exist, each with theoretical and practical advantages and limitations. A more detailed discussion of intraoperative neurologic monitoring follows.

## PHYSIOLOGIC EFFECTS

CEA causes physiologic changes related to temporary obstruction of the blood flow through the carotid artery. Surgical technique requires temporary total occlusion of the carotid artery, thereby rendering the ipsilateral hemisphere dependent solely on collateral blood flow from the vertebral arteries and the contralateral carotid artery through the circle of Willis (Fig. 112.1), which is complete in only 42% to 47% of people. During CEA surgery, an incomplete circle of Willis predisposes approximately one-sixth of individuals to cerebral ischemia during carotid clamping or transient closure of the carotid

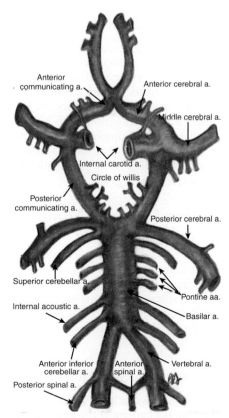

**Fig. 112.1** Blood supply of the circle of Willis. During cross-clamping of the internal carotid artery, blood supply to the ipsilateral cerebral hemisphere is from the contralateral internal carotid artery and from the basilar artery through the circle of Willis. (Image © Brooke Albright-Trainer, MD.)

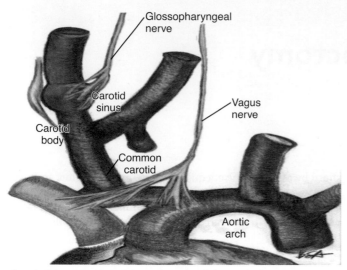

**Fig. 112.2** Anatomy of the right side of the neck showing the common carotid artery, demonstrating the relationship of the carotid body to the carotid sinus at the origin of the internal carotid artery. (Image © Brooke Albright-Trainer, MD.)

artery. In those patients with coexisting contralateral internal carotid artery occlusion, the risk of cerebral ischemia rises more than threefold. Some institutions use preoperative cerebral angiograms to assess collateral flow, to predict the need for additional cerebral protection or monitoring, and to determine the need for intraluminal shunting during the procedure.

## POTENTIAL ADVERSE EVENTS

Complications of CEA surgery include new neurologic deficits attributed primarily to thromboembolic events that occur intraoperatively, cerebral hyperperfusion syndrome resulting from excess blood flow to the brain because of impaired autoregulation, and poor control of blood pressure postoperatively because of carotid sinus dysfunction, with hypertension more common than hypotension. Compensatory hyperventilation in response to hypoxemia may be abolished because of disruption of the carotid bodies at the level of the carotid bifurcation if a bilateral CEA is performed (Fig. 112.2).

# Techniques for Cerebral Monitoring

Ensuring adequate cerebral blood flow to the ipsilateral brain during clamping of the carotid artery is a critical aspect of CEA surgery. Some clinicians use cerebral monitoring in an effort to decrease the incidence of perioperative stroke by monitoring for thromboemboli, intraoperative hypoperfusion, and postoperative hyperperfusion syndrome. However, not all clinicians use cerebral monitoring because of concerns over actual benefit and associated high costs.

## EVALUATING THE AWAKE PATIENT

The most sensitive and specific cerebral monitor is neurologic assessment of the awake patient. If the patient and surgeon are comfortable performing the operation while the patient is awake, verbal communication and frequent examination of strength using contralateral handgrip can be used to assess level of consciousness, motor function, and cerebral perfusion.

Assessment is best performed every 2 to 5 minutes. Adequate anesthesia for CEA in the awake patient is provided by regional blockade of the superficial and deep cervical plexus. Awake monitoring may not be feasible in extremely anxious or claustrophobic patients or in patients with cardiopulmonary disease who are unable to lie flat because of dyspnea, those who experience coughing spells, or those who are otherwise unable to remain still. Another potential disadvantage to performing CEA in awake patients is the anesthesia provider's inability to maintain control of the patient's airway, especially if cerebral blood flow is compromised: if the patient loses consciousness, emergency intervention to protect the airway is required. It is also possible that the duration of the regional anesthetic may not be sufficient for the surgical procedure.

## ELECTROENCEPHALOGRAPHY

Electroencephalography (EEG) is the most reliable cerebral monitor for detecting cerebral ischemia in anesthetized patients. A standard 16-channel EEG monitor uses 20 scalp electrodes, with eight channels for each hemisphere, covering the parasagittal and temporal brain regions. EEG changes, which are apparent within seconds of changes in cerebral blood flow, are defined as ipsilateral or bilateral increased theta or delta activity, suppression of alpha or beta activity of more than 50%, or both. EEG changes occur in about 20% of patients during carotid occlusion and are indicative of potentially serious ischemia. Data show a strong correlation between persistent EEG changes of 10 minutes or longer and postoperative neurologic deficit; however, not all changes in electrical activity are specific for life-threatening cerebral ischemia. Nonetheless, because of the strong correlation, most surgeons consider changes in EEG activity an indication for immediate shunt placement.

Disadvantages of EEG monitoring are the need for continuous observation by a highly trained technician, the inability to detect subcortical ischemia, and the decreased predictive value of EEG in the patients with preexisting neurologic deficits. Physiologic changes in temperature, $Paco_2$, depth of anesthesia, and anesthetic technique can also affect EEG monitoring reliability.

## SOMATOSENSORY EVOKED POTENTIALS

Monitoring of somatosensory evoked potentials (SSEPs) involves electrically stimulating a peripheral or cranial nerve and comparing the latency and amplitude of the stimulation to baseline values. Latency is the time from the application of the stimulus to the peak onset of the response. The amplitude is the voltage of the recorded response. A decrease in amplitude of 50% or more from baseline or an increase in latency of more than 10% is considered clinically significant and, if the cause is uncorrected, can be associated with new postoperative neurologic deficits.

Monitoring of EEG and SSEPs has similar sensitivity and specificity for detecting cerebral ischemia. SSEP monitoring offers some potential advantage over a 16-channel EEG in that it is technically easier to perform and interpret and provides information specific to the sensory cortex, an area supplied by the middle cerebral artery, which is at risk during cross-clamping of the carotid artery. SSEPs may also detect ischemia in subcortical structures better than EEG can. However, like EEG, SSEP monitoring requires the presence of trained technicians.

## CAROTID STUMP PRESSURE

Systolic pressure beyond the carotid clamp can be measured by placing either a needle or an intraluminal Fogarty balloon catheter in the distal carotid artery. Some studies have suggested that a carotid artery stump pressure of at least 40 mm Hg systolic may be considered an equally reliable but more cost-effective method than EEG to predict the need for carotid shunting during CEA under general anesthesia; however, other research using stump-pressure measurements of less than 40 mm Hg as an indication for selective shunt placement (compared with routine shunt placement) showed no difference in stroke rate when either stump pressure or EEG was used. Measured stump pressures may not always correlate with cerebral perfusion pressure or accurately predict cerebral ischemia because the threshold for ischemia may vary considerably among patients. In some patients, stump pressures of 40 mm Hg may be high enough to ensure adequate cerebral blood flow, whereas in others, particularly chronic hypertensives and patients with cerebral vascular disease, higher pressures may be required.

## TRANSCRANIAL DOPPLER ULTRASOUND

Transcranial Doppler ultrasound uses the thin petrous temporal bone as an acoustic window for detecting Doppler signals and ultrasound visualization of the middle cerebral artery. Unlike other cerebral monitors, transcranial Doppler ultrasound can measure blood flow velocities and detect embolic signals in real time. Because most perioperative neurologic events are embolic or thrombotic in nature, the transcranial Doppler ultrasound can prove to be a very useful monitor when performed by a trained technologist. Three transcranial Doppler ultrasound variables are predictors of stroke after CEA: the occurrence of emboli during dissection or wound closure, a greater than 90% decrease in middle cerebral artery peak systolic velocity when the cross-clamp is applied, and a 100% or greater increase in the pulsatility index of the Doppler signal at clamp release. One limitation related to the use of transcranial Doppler ultrasound is that the location of the probe is relatively near the surgical site, which may hinder observance of the monitor by the operator and may require continual readjustment of the monitor.

## Other Considerations

Dissection of the atheromatous plaque at the level of the carotid bifurcation can disrupt carotid sinus baroreceptor function and lead to direct and indirect hemodynamic effects. Normally functioning carotid sinus baroreceptors sense arterial wall stretch, sending afferent input to the vasomotor center in the medulla via the glossopharyngeal nerve. In response, efferent impulses transmitted via the vagus nerve result in decreased sympathetic output, increased parasympathetic output, bradycardia, and hypotension. Patients with coronary artery disease, increased age, or a low ejection fraction are at greatest risk of developing severe symptoms during manipulation of the carotid sinus. Discontinuation of the sinus stimulation attenuates the signs; however, if they persist, 1 to 2 mL of a local anesthetic agent injected into the area of the carotid bifurcation blocks the impulse propagation. In certain situations, it may be necessary to intravenously administer atropine, fluid boluses, or vasopressors when manipulation of the sinus causes profound hypotension or bradycardia.

After removal of atheromatous plaques in patients who have intact functioning of the carotid sinus, postoperative hypotension may occur because of hyperactivity of the newly exposed carotid sinus to the perceived increased blood pressure. Hypersensitivity of the carotid sinus after CEA can eventually lead to carotid sinus syndrome, which is characterized by nausea, vomiting, dizziness, syncope, severe hypotension, and asystole. Treatment may require a pacemaker, glossopharyngeal nerve block or ablation, or surgical denervation of the glossopharyngeal nerve at the level of the carotid bifurcation. More commonly, removal of the plaque may result in denervation of the baroreceptor nerve fibers within the arterial wall, leading to sympathomimetic electrocardiographic changes and hypertension.

## SUGGESTED READINGS

Aburahma, A. F., Stone, P. A., Hass, S. M., Dean, L. S., Habib, J., Keiffer, T., et al. (2010). Prospective randomized trial of routine versus selective shunting in carotid endarterectomy based on stump pressure. *Journal of Vascular Surgery, 51*, 1133–1138.

Apinis, A., Sankalp, S., & Leff, J. (2014). Intraoperative management of carotid endarterectomy. *Anesthesiology Clinics, 32*, 677–698.

Bozzani, A., Arici, V., Ticozzelli, G., Pregnolato, S., Boschini, S., Fellegara, R., et al. (2022). Intraoperative cerebral monitoring during carotid surgery: A narrative review. *Vascular Surgery, 78*, 36–44. doi:10.1016/j.avsg.2021.06.044.

Jovic, M., Unic-Stojanovic, D., Isenovic, E., Manfredi, R., Cekic, O., Ilijevski, N., et al. (2015). Anesthetics and cerebral protection in patients undergoing carotid endarterectomy. *Journal of Cardiothoracic and Vascular Anesthesia, 29*, 178–184.

Manninen, H., Mäkinen, K., & Vanninen, R. (2009). How often does an incomplete circle of willis predispose to cerebral ischemia during closure of carotid artery? Postmortem and clinical imaging studies. *Acta Neurochirurgica, 151*, 1099–1105.

Toorop, R. J., Scheltinga, M. R., Moll, F. L., & Bleys, R. L. (2009). Anatomy of the carotid sinus nerve and surgical implications in carotid sinus syndrome. *Journal of Vascular Surgery, 50*, 177–182.

Unic-Stojanovic, D., Babic, S., & Neskovic, V. (2013). General versus regional anesthesia for carotid endarterectomy. *Journal of Cardiothoracic and Vascular Anesthesia, 27*, 1379–1383.

# 113

# Management of Acute Spinal Cord Injury

ASHLEY V. WONG GROSSMAN, MD | TIMOTHY R. LONG, MD

## Pathophysiologic Factors

Spinal cord injury can result in hemorrhage, cord edema, and potentially catastrophic neurogenic shock. Because the area surrounding the spinal cord at C1–C2 is anatomically larger, injuries at this level are less likely to damage the spinal cord compared with injuries at the C3 vertebrae and lower. Injuries to the C1 and C2 vertebrae have a high mortality rate, often due to associated injuries such as traumatic brain or airway injury. Patients who survive the initial injury have a good chance of retaining neurologic function.

Spinal cord lesions are not always static. For example, a spinal cord lesion may involve an enlarging hematoma, which leads to increased edema and progressive ischemia of the spinal cord. Spinal cord injury may also be incomplete, such as in Brown-Séquard syndrome, in which the damage is located in half of the spinal cord, resulting in ipsilateral paralysis and loss of proprioception and contralateral loss of pain and temperature sensation.

## Respiratory Considerations

Lesions above T7 may adversely affect respiratory function because of the involvement of intercostal muscles, accessory muscles of respiration, and diaphragmatic function. As a result, vital capacity, expiratory reserve volume, and forced expiratory volume may decrease.

Neurons exiting the spinal cord at C3, C4, and C5 provide innervation of the diaphragm. Spinal cord injury at C3 or C4 therefore results in paralysis of the diaphragm and respiratory distress. If the injury is not recognized and treated immediately, patients with lesions that paralyze the diaphragm asphyxiate. Conversely, lesions at C5 may result in only partial diaphragmatic paralysis. Lesions below C5 enable patients to maintain ventilation as innervation of the diaphragm remains intact. However, these patients may have some respiratory compromise due to intercostal and accessory muscle dysfunction. These patients frequently present with sternal retraction, paradoxical breathing, compromised cough, and inability to clear secretions.

Anterolateral lesions at C2 through C4 may result in Ondine curse or central hypoventilation syndrome. Patients with traumatic spinal cord injury with associated neurologic deficits have an increased risk of developing deep venous thrombosis (DVT) and pulmonary embolic events. Other pulmonary disorders associated with spinal cord injury include neurogenic pulmonary edema, aspiration pneumonia, and acute respiratory distress syndrome.

## Gastrointestinal Considerations

Many patients with spinal cord injury subsequently develop paralytic ileus that results in gastric distention, further impinging diaphragmatic excursion. This results in decreased functional residual capacity and more rapid desaturation after periods of apnea. Gastric distention and delayed gastric emptying place these patients at increased risk of aspiration during induction of anesthesia.

## Cardiovascular Considerations

After spinal cord injury, blood pressure and heart rate may transiently increase due to increased catecholamine release from the adrenal glands. This sympathetic surge is often short-lived and followed by parasympathetic dominance, which manifests as bradycardia, sinus node pauses, sick sinus syndrome, supraventricular arrhythmias, ventricular ectopy, and possible ST-segment changes.

Neurogenic shock is a complication that occurs with injury to the sympathetic chain from T1–L2, most commonly with injuries at T6 and above. This results in loss of sympathetic input and parasympathetic predominance, mediated through the vagus nerve. Neurogenic shock manifests as hypotension and bradycardia. Hypothermia is another common finding, with peripheral vasodilation initially presenting with warm and flushed skin that subsequently leads to rapid heat loss. Neurogenic shock often lasts 1 to 6 weeks.

Autonomic dysreflexia is a chronic complication of spinal cord injuries at T6 and above that can occur at any time after injury but is more common in the first months after injury. This phenomenon is characterized by hypertension and bradycardia in response to stimuli below the level of injury, most commonly bladder distention. This stimulus results in sympathetic discharge that causes hypertension above the level of injury and a reactive parasympathetic response that causes bradycardia. Hypertensive crisis as a result of autonomic dysreflexia can be life-threatening but often resolves with treatment of the underlying stimuli.

## Metabolic Considerations

Patients with a spinal cord injury between T1 and L2 with disruption of the sympathetic nervous system lose the ability to thermoregulate. Hypothermia can lead to peripheral and coronary vasoconstriction, resulting in metabolic acidosis and myocardial ischemia, respectively. Conversely, patients with spinal cord lesions above C7 have an inability to sweat, which can manifest as hyperthermia. In patients with long-standing paralysis from spinal cord injury, bone reabsorption can lead to hypercalcemia, which can increase the risk of arrhythmias and cause decreased response to nondepolarizing neuromuscular blocking agents. Patients with impaired ventilatory drive can present with respiratory acidosis, with or without a compensatory metabolic alkalosis.

# Anesthetic Management

## PREOPERATIVE MANAGEMENT

Airway management mandates stabilization of the neck while intubating the trachea in an expeditious manner. Chest physiotherapy, DVT prophylaxis (beginning 2–3 days after the injury to avoid hemorrhage at the site of injury), decompression of the stomach, administration of stress-related ulcer prophylaxis, and monitoring effective ventilation and oxygenation are important considerations in the preoperative setting.

## PHARMACOLOGY

Succinylcholine may be used for airway management after acute spinal cord injury. However, these patients develop progressive muscle denervation, which begins as early as 48 to 72 hours after injury. The denervation injury is associated with proliferation of extrajunctional acetylcholine receptors. After the acute phase of injury, succinylcholine should be avoided, as these patients can have an exaggerated hyperkalemic response resulting in ventricular fibrillation and cardiac arrest. The use of a nondepolarizing muscle relaxant is preferred in these patients. Rocuronium can be used as an alternative for rapid sequence induction, particularly considering the availability of sugammadex for rapid reversal of muscle relaxation induced by rocuronium if necessary.

The use of corticosteroids, such as methylprednisolone (30 mg/kg bolus followed by 5.4 $mg \cdot kg^{-1} \cdot h^{-1}$ for 24–48 hours), may be associated with a small but statistically significant improvement in outcome—assuming that the spinal cord is not completely transected—if therapy is started within 8 hours of injury. Use is controversial but may be considered when clinically appropriate.

## AIRWAY MANAGEMENT

Patients with cervical spine fractures are considered to have difficult airways. The primary goal of care is to maintain cervical stability and to oxygenate, ventilate, and protect the airway by placing an endotracheal tube in a timely manner. Choice of airway technique should be dictated by the clinical conditions and urgency.

Direct laryngoscopy provides for a fast, widely available, and well-known method of intubation. However, it requires increased movement of the mouth and cervical spine and may be technically complicated by the cervical stabilization technique (i.e., rigid collar vs. inline stabilization). Availability and familiarity with a variety of airway adjuncts is advantageous for this patient population.

Indirect video laryngoscopy may allow for less cervical spine movement during intubation and provide a better view of the larynx when compared with direct laryngoscopy. However, use may be limited by provider experience and availability. Blood, secretions, or other foreign matter in the airway may impair visualization of the glottic opening with this technique.

Awake intubation is associated with less cervical spine movement and the ability to conduct a neurologic assessment before and after intubation. However, use is heavily dependent on urgency, availability, provider experience, and patient cooperation. In addition, without proper topical anesthesia to the airway, patients may cough or gag, resulting in further neurologic insult. Supraglottic airway devices may be a useful adjunct in the difficult airway but are associated with increased cervical spine movement and increased risk of aspiration. Nasal intubation should be avoided in patients with basilar skull fractures, raccoon eyes, Battle sign, Le Fort fractures, or any evidence of cerebrospinal fluid leak.

## CARDIOVASCULAR CONSIDERATIONS

Acute lesions above T6 can be associated with neurogenic shock. Restoration of an adequate perfusion pressure is critical to prevent extension of the neurologic deficit. Though fluid resuscitation is the preferred initial choice for blood pressure support, these patients often require vasopressors because of the lack of sympathetic tone. Prompt treatment of neurogenic shock with intravascular fluids and vasoactive agents to maintain a mean arterial pressure (MAP) of 85 to 90 mm Hg for 5 to 7 days may improve neurologic outcome.

Hemodynamic instability from spinal shock usually stabilizes after 10 to 14 days. However, patients with lesions at T6 or above are at risk for developing autonomic dysreflexia in the perioperative period, presenting as hypertension in response to a stimulus below the level of spinal cord injury. Despite lack of sensation below the site of injury, adequate anesthesia is required for procedures below this level to prevent this complication. In addition to adequate depth of anesthesia to avoid noxious stimuli, emptying of the bladder and bowels and invasive blood pressure monitoring are often required.

In summary, the goals in the treatment of patients with spinal cord injuries include the following:

- Maintain an adequate airway while minimizing spine movement.
- Treat neurogenic shock promptly and maintain MAP of 85 to 90 mm Hg.
- Consider starting corticosteroid treatment within 8 hours of injury, if clinically appropriate.
- Treat other multisystem involvement, including respiratory insufficiency, electrolyte abnormalities, and temperature fluctuation, and assess other multiorgan–multisystem trauma.
- Avoid succinylcholine beyond the acute phase of injury.

## SUGGESTED READINGS

Austin, N., Krishnamoorthy, V., & Dagal, A. (2014). Airway management in cervical spine injury. *International Journal of Critical Illness and Injury Science, 4*, 50–56.

Hurlbert, J., Hadley, M., Walters, B., Aarabi, B., Dhall, S. S., Gelb, D. E., et al. (2013). Pharmacological therapy for acute spinal cord injury. *Neurosurgery, 72*, 93–105.

Petsas, A., & Drake, J. (2015). Perioperative management of patients with a chronic spinal cord injury. *BJA Education, 15*(3), 123–130.

Rao, S., & Treggiari, M. M. (2021). Anesthesia for acute spinal cord injury. *Anesthesiology Clinics, 39*(1), 127–138.

Rogers, W. K., & Todd, M. (2016). Acute spinal cord injury. *Best Practice and Research. Clinical Anaesthesiology, 30*(1), 27–39.

Ryken, T., Hurlbert, J., Hadley, M., Aarabi, B., Dhall, S. S., Gelb, D. E., et al. (2013). The acute cardiopulmonary management of patients with cervical spinal cord injuries. *Neurosurgery, 72*, 84–92.

# Anesthesia for Adult Complex Spine Surgery

PATRICK B. BOLTON, MD

Complex spine surgery (e.g., scoliosis correction) is a technically demanding neurosurgical or orthopedic subspecialty. The anesthesia management is similarly complex because cases to correct severe spinal deformities are often long, are associated with significant blood loss, and are performed on an increasingly elderly population with significant comorbidities. In addition, anesthetic techniques must consider the various modes of intraoperative neurologic monitoring (IONM) and plan for the possibility of an intraoperative Stagnara wake-up test.

## Epidemiology

In older adults, most cases of scoliotic deformity are from progressive asymmetric disc degeneration and facet degeneration, but some may originate from untreated idiopathic juvenile scoliosis that persisted into adulthood. The prevalence of adult spinal deformity (ASD) in the general population is increasing as the elderly population in the United States increases. One estimate reported an adult scoliosis prevalence of 68% in a population aged 60 years or older.

## Preoperative Evaluation

Severe and/or extensive spinal deformities may negatively affect airway management, cardiovascular function, respiratory function, and neuromuscular function. Preoperative assessment should include careful airway assessment. Advanced spinal rotational deformities may cause restrictive lung physiology, hypoxia, and pulmonary hypertension. Thus, preoperative pulmonary function tests should be considered. Secondary cardiovascular effects of immobility and poor functional status should be considered in patients with pain-related restricted activity. The

patient's preoperative neurological deficits should be documented in the anesthesia note and compared with baseline IONM readings before positioning prone. Knowledge of baseline neurological strength is important should an intraoperative wake-up test be required. The anesthesiologist should also review the risks of prone positioning during the preoperative interview.

## Surgery

The goal of the surgery is to correct sagittal (kyphosis and lordosis) and coronal (scoliosis) spinal imbalances that cause symptomatic neural compression and pain. Spinal balance is a broad term that describes the ability to maintain the head correctly over the pelvis, which enables energy-efficient motion. As normal spine-to-hip angles deviate from progressive degeneration, patient-reported disability scores increase and quality-of-life measures decrease. Surgical restoration of lumbar lordosis, reduction of thoracic kyphosis, and correction of rotational asymmetry result in greater quality-of-life outcome scores than nonoperative management.

ASD correction may be a long, multiphase operation that involves a large surgical exposure (thorax to sacrum), removal of the posterior spinal elements, focal neurologic decompressions, pedicle screw placement, titanium rod placement, placement of bone fusion material, and closure. To reduce kyphosis or enhance lordosis, the surgeon may also perform an osteotomy at one or more levels (Fig. 114.1). An osteotomy is the removal of strategic spine material that increases the ability of the surgeon to reshape the spine toward its natural curvatures. The procedure is technically challenging and is associated with significantly increased blood loss and potential injury to the surrounding dura and nerves (Fig. 114.1).

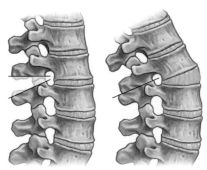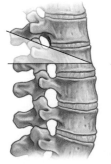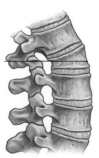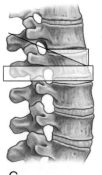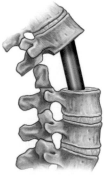

A         B         C

**Fig. 114.1** **A,** A Smith-Peterson osteotomy, where just posterior elements are removed. **B,** Pedicle subtraction osteotomy, where a wedge is cut into the vertebral body. **C,** Vertebral column resection, where the entire vertebral body is removed. Bone graft is applied to the resulting gap.

Several structures anterolateral to the spine can be inadvertently injured during surgery. It is important that the anesthesiologist is aware of the potential sudden complications that can occur while decompressing or instrumenting the spine. During decompression, the thorax, peritoneum, and retroperitoneum can be unintentionally breached, resulting in bleeding, spillage of viscous contents, or pneumothorax. During osteotomy creation, the dura and neural elements are at risk of injury from retraction and from their proximity to the bone being cut. Noticeable dural tears are repaired intraoperatively. Unrecognized dural injury may result in slow but large-volume cerebrospinal fluid (CSF) losses. Postoperatively, excessive loss of CSF can cause venous cerebellar or cerebral parenchymal hemorrhage from an overrelaxed brain once upright posture is initiated. Misplaced pedicle screws have the potential to injure a variety of important structures. Depending on the vertebral level (thoracic through lumbar), pedicle screws that are advanced too far anterior can breach the vertebral periosteum and enter the aorta, vena cava, or iliac vessels. Anterior violations can also injure small segmental arteries that supply the anterior spinal cord. Screws with a medial trajectory can pierce the nerve root or spinal cord, and those placed too lateral can enter the chest or retroperitoneal space (Figure 114.2). The increasing use of navigation-guided and robotic pedicle screw placement reduces the incidence of misplaced spinal hardware. Given the presence of epidural veins and open osseous cuts in the spine, air embolism or fat embolism may also occur.

## Blood Loss and Management Strategies

Blood loss in ASD surgery may be significant because of the length and depth of the exposure, the removal of significant amounts of bone, injury to epidural veins, placement of several pedicle screws, and dilution or consumption of coagulation

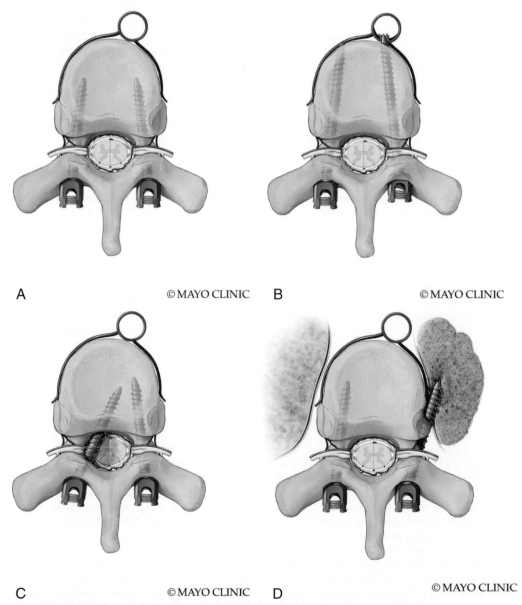

A    ©MAYO CLINIC    B    ©MAYO CLINIC

C    ©MAYO CLINIC    D    ©MAYO CLINIC

**Fig. 114.2**  Bottom-up axial view of T9 vertebral body with properly placed and malpositioned pedicle screws. **A,** Appropriately placed pedicle screws. **B,** Anterior perforation of pedicle screws with injury to segmental artery and aorta. **C,** Medial pedicle screw violation with injury to nerve root and spinal cord. **D,** Lateral breach of pedicle with pleural and parenchymal lung injury resulting in pneumothorax. (Used with permission of Mayo Foundation for Medical Education and Research, all rights reserved.)

factors. Barring injury to a large blood vessel, the rate of blood loss in ASD surgery is low to moderate, but it may continue over many hours. One study assessed a mean operative time for ASD surgery of 7.1 hours. If osteotomies are performed, the rate of blood loss can increase significantly. By one analysis, the incidence of major blood loss in ASD surgeries with osteotomies is greater than 4 L in 24% of procedures and another showed the range to be 0.2 to 12.2 L. Patients with low bone mineral density are at higher risk for bleeding, presumably from thinned periosteum and wider vascular channels.

Antifibrinolytics, including tranexamic acid and epsilon-aminocaproic acid infusions, can be used to decrease blood loss and blood product administration. Both are lysine analogues that competitively block the binding site for plasminogen and plasmin and prevent the degradation of fibrin clots. Their benefit in reducing blood loss in orthopedic and cardiac surgery is well established, and the data suggesting the same benefit without an increase in thromboembolic events in spine surgery is growing. The data are inconsistent in establishing one compound as superior to the other.

There is no consensus about blood product replacement trigger values or transfusion strategies in ASD surgeries. This, coupled with the difficulty in estimating blood loss and the time lag in obtaining intraoperative laboratory measurements, contributes to a lack of standardized resuscitation guidelines. Many anesthesiologists follow blood replacement strategies (i.e., 1:1 packed red blood cells to fresh frozen plasma) used in trauma resuscitations. Obtaining a baseline fibrinogen and following it throughout the case helps guide the need for cryoprecipitate transfusion. Rotational thromboelastometry (ROTEM), a rapid viscoelastometric method for testing whole blood hemostasis, has been shown to reduce intraoperative blood loss and reduce transfusion requirements by early identification of hypofibrinogenemia and resulting coagulopathy. Although ROTEM shows promise as a method to guide transfusion, it is not routinely used outside of large institutional centers. Red blood cell salvage techniques are an attractive method to reduce allogenic red blood cell transfusion, but the data supporting this practice in ASD surgery are conflicting. Because the resuscitation needs in ASD cases are often large, adequate intravenous access for blood product administration and vasopressor infusion is essential.

## Intraoperative Neuromonitoring

IONM uses electrophysiological methods (continuous or intermittent) to monitor the integrity of neurological pathways. The most common modalities employed in ASD cases are somatosensory evoked potentials (SSEPs), "free-running" and "triggered" electromyography (EMG), and transcranial evoked potentials (TcMEPs). In general, SSEPs monitor the integrity of the posterior spinal cord by stimulating peripheral nerves on the extremities and recording the responses cortically. TcMEPs intermittently evaluate anterior spinal cord function by stimulating the motor cortex and recording at distal muscle groups. Free-running EMG detects nerve root irritation by continually monitoring the activity of specific skeletal muscle groups. Skeletal muscle responses are produced with nonelectric stimuli such as nerve traction or ischemia. Triggered EMG is used to detect the proper placement of pedicle screws by stimulating pedicle screw heads with an increasing current. If the screw trajectory is proper and well surrounded by bone, the threshold

for muscle response is high. If the screw has been placed too medial near the spinal canal, the threshold for muscle response is low and the screw must be repositioned.

Warning criteria for SSEPs are 50% loss of baseline amplitude or 10% prolongation of the latency, whereas TcMEP warning criteria are less clear but involve increased threshold response and/or decreased response magnitude. IONM measurements that have decreased from baseline require the anesthesiologist to evaluate and normalize the following potential physiologic contributors:

1. Hypothermia
2. Hypotension
3. Anemia
4. Hypoxia
5. Hypocapnia
6. Nerve compression

The Stagnara wake-up test can be employed if needed to evaluate extremity strength/function during the procedure. Waking up a patient with a large open wound is typically only done if the IONM suggests a significant deterioration of spinal cord function that is not responsive to standard IONM troubleshooting and surgical corrective measures (i.e., lessening spinal distraction). Though modern electrophysiologic monitoring has lessened the need to perform a wake-up test, some surgeons still ask for it as secondary confirmation. When working with surgeons who are known to rely on wake-up tests, patients should be counseled preoperatively about the possibility of intraoperative awareness and recall.

Placement of a soft bite block, optimally placed to prevent molar occlusion, is essential when TcMEPs are being monitored. Without it, jaw muscle movement from transcranial stimulation can injure lingual, buccal, and dental tissues. Prolonged prone positioning can also cause significant dependent edema of the tongue, increasing the likelihood of lingual injury during TcMEP stimulation.

Operating room staff should be aware that 1-cm subdermal needle electrodes are used as stimulating conduits and detectors for TcMEPs, SSEPs, and EMG. In some instances, more than 50 needle electrodes in a single patient may be required to obtain high-fidelity recordings. All staff, not just the IONM technologist, who have contact with the patient are at risk of needlestick exposure.

## Anesthesia

The challenge for ASD cases is to provide an adequate and stable anesthetic during dynamic physiologic disruptions while constrained by the need to consider the effects of anesthetics on IONM. Although some advocate for a total intravenous anesthesia technique in the setting of IONM, others feel that prolonged infusions of propofol prolong wake-up times and that precision intravenous dosing is lost given the large fluid volume exchanges that occur in these cases. Some anesthesiologists prefer to add small concentrations of halogenated gas to the anesthetic regimen to reduce the amount of propofol infused and ensure amnesia.

Halogenated gases, though known to have a negative, dose-dependent effect on TcMEP, have been shown to allow reliable signals at 0.5 minimum alveolar concentration and below. Thus, balanced combinations of low-dose anesthetic gas, propofol, opioid infusions, and perhaps ketamine administration are preferred by many anesthesiologists. Propofol boluses as

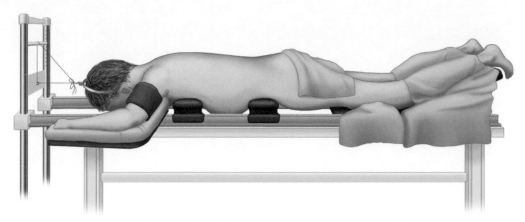

**Fig. 114.3** Illustration of prone positioning on a Jackson table with the head suspended with Gardner-Wells tongs. The face is free of pressure and the abdomen hangs free as the body is supported by pads at the thorax and pelvis. Despite meticulous padding, injuries can occur at pressure points.

little as 0.5 mg/kg and high-dose infusions (150 mcg/kg/min) have also been shown to impair TcMEP signals. Dexmedetomidine is generally thought to not significantly degrade TcMEPs at infusion doses of 0.5 mcg/kg/h or less. All anesthetic gases and intravenous hypnotics exert a negative effect on TcMEPs over time, despite the dose. This phenomenon is called *anesthetic fade.*

If a Stagnara wake-up test is indicated, all anesthetics are typically stopped, and the patient is allowed to "wake up" sufficiently to follow simple commands to move the extremities. Once the surgeon has confirmed the presence of retained extremity strength or new neurological weakness, anesthesia can be reinduced quickly with a bolus of hypnotic. It is advisable that an antihypertensive be administered or available during the execution of the wake-up test, as the pain from an open wound and psychological distress can raise blood pressures dramatically. Airway security is a key consideration during wake-up tests.

## Positioning

Many ASD cases are performed on a Jackson table, which provides support inferiorly and laterally at the thorax and pelvis and allows the abdomen to hang free (Fig. 114.3). This table design, compared with older rigid-framed tables, increases abdominal compliance, which increases end-organ perfusion and venous return, reduces vertebral venous pressure, and facilitates ventilation. The table can accommodate a cradle-type head holder or Gardner-Wells tongs, which suspend the head with the support of control pins screwed to the skull, thus keeping the eyes and face free of pressure. The tables are made of radiolucent carbon fiber, which supports patient weights of up to 500 pounds and facilitates intraoperative imaging. Although these advances in table design solve many problems, myocutaneous pressure wounds at the sites of support remain common after exceptionally long cases, and compartment syndrome of the lower extremities has been described. Brachial plexus injuries can occur, especially if the arms are abducted greater than 90 degrees and the more distal nerves can be injured by brachial artery compression or direct nerve compression or stretch. When IONM is used for the surgical aspect of the case, obtaining supine baseline measurements can help identify positional error and nerve compression after turning prone.

Permanent vision loss after spine surgery has been attributed to periorbital pressure, blood loss anemia, and hypotension—factors that make ASD surgery high-risk for this rare ophthalmologic complication.

Cardiac arrest while prone is a scenario that must be planned for by the surgical team. There is no consensus on how to manage a prone cardiac arrest. Depending on the stage of the procedure, advanced cardiac life support protocols may best be employed while remaining prone because turning a patient with ongoing blood loss, an unstable spine, and protruding instrumentation supine may not be feasible.

## SUGGESTED READINGS

Buhl, L., Bastos, A. B., Pollard, R. J., Arle, J. E., Thomas, G. P., Song, Y., et al. (2021). Neurophysiologic intraoperative monitoring for spine surgery: A practical guide from past to present. *Journal of Intensive Care Medicine*, *36*, 1237–1249.

DePasse, J. M., Palumbo, M., Haque, M., Eberson, C. P., & Daniels, A. H. (2015). Complications associated with prone positioning in elective spinal surgery. *World Journal of Orthopedics*, *6*, 351–359.

Naik, B. I., Pajewski, T. N., Bogdonoff, D. L., Zuo, Z., Clark, P., Terkawi, A. S., et al. (2015). Rotational thromboelastometry-guided blood product management in major spine surgery. *Journal of Neurosurgery Spine*, *23*, 239–249.

Norton, R. P., Bianco, K., Lafage, V., Schwab, F. J., & International Spine Study Group Foundation. (2013). Complications and intercenter variability of three-column resection osteotomies for spinal deformity surgery: A retrospective review of 423 patients. *Evidence-Based Spine-Care Journal*, *4*(2), 157–159.

Sloan, T. B., Tolekis, J. R., Tolekis, S. C., & Koht, A. (2015). Intraoperative neurophysiological monitoring during spine surgery with total intravenous anesthesia or balanced anesthesia with 3% desflurane. *Journal of Clinical Monitoring and Computing*, *29*, 77–85.

Smith, J. S., Klineberg, E., Lafage, V., Shaffrey, C. I., Schwab, F., Lafage, R., et al. (2016). Prospective multicenter assessment of perioperative and minimum 2-year postoperative complication rates associated with adult spinal deformity surgery. *Journal of Neurosurgery Spine*, *25*(1), 1–14.

Smith, J. S., Shaffrey, C. I., Lafage, V., Schwab, F., Scheer, J. K., Protopsaltis, T., et al. (2015). Comparison of best versus worst clinical outcomes for adult spinal deformity surgery: A retrospective review of a prospectively collected, multicenter database with 2-year follow-up. *Journal of Neurosurgery Spine*, *23*, 349–359.

Soroceanu, A., Oren, J. H., Smith, J. S., Hostin, R., Shaffrey, C. I., Mundis, G. M., et al. (2016). Effect of antifibrinolytic therapy on complications, thromboembolic events, blood product utilization and fusion in adult spinal deformity surgery. *Spine*, *41*, E879–E886.

# Specialty Anesthesia: Cardiac

# Coronary Circulation and the Myocardial Conduction System

ARCHER KILBOURNE MARTIN, MD  |  HARISH RAMAKRISHNA, MD, FACC, FESC, FASE

## Coronary Circulation

The right and left main coronary arteries arise from ostia (small openings) located behind the right and left aortic valve cusps toward the more cephalad portion of the sinus of Valsalva (Fig. 115.1). The third aortic cusp is the posterior, or noncoronary, cusp. The left main coronary artery travels anteriorly and leftward from the left coronary sinus and, after a 2- to 10-mm course between the pulmonary trunk and the left atrium, divides into the left anterior descending (LAD) and left circumflex arteries. Occasionally, a diagonal branch is also present.

The LAD artery, or left interventricular coronary, is a direct continuation of the left main coronary artery, traveling anterior and caudad and descending in the anterior interventricular groove. This artery terminates in the inferior aspect of the cardiac apex. Branches of this artery include (1) the first diagonal, (2) the first septal perforator, (3) the right ventricular branches (variable), (4) three to five additional septal perforators, and (5) two to six additional diagonal branches. The LAD supplies blood to most of the ventricular septum (the anterior two-thirds); the anterior, lateral, and apical walls of the left ventricle; most of the right and left bundle branches; and the anterolateral papillary muscle of the left ventricle. It can provide collateral vessels to the anterior right ventricle via the circle of Vieussens, to the ventricular septum via septal perforators, and to the posterior descending artery territory via the distal LAD artery or a diagonal branch.

The left circumflex artery travels posteriorly around the heart in the left atrioventricular (AV) sulcus. In 85% to 90% of individuals, it terminates near the obtuse margin of the left ventricle; in the remaining 10% to 15%, it continues around to the crux of the heart to become the posterior descending artery. The coronary artery (left circumflex vs. right coronary) that leads to the posterior descending artery determines coronary dominance. Branches include (1) a branch to the sino-atrial (SA) node in 40% to 50% of individuals, (2) a left atrial circumflex branch, (3) an anterolateral marginal branch, (4) a distal circumflex artery, (5) posterolateral marginal branches, and (6) the posterior descending artery, as noted. This artery provides blood to the left atrium, the posterior and lateral left ventricle, the anterolateral papillary muscle of the left ventricle, and the SA node, as noted earlier. If it continues as the posterior descending artery (in 10%–15% of hearts), it also supplies blood to the AV node, the proximal bundle branches, the remainder of the inferoposterior left ventricle, the posterior interventricular septum, and the posteromedial papillary muscle of the left ventricle.

The right coronary artery (RCA) passes forward to emerge between the pulmonary trunk and the right atrium, and then it descends in the right AV sulcus. In most hearts, once it reaches the apex, the RCA continues traveling in the posterior AV sulcus around the posterior of the heart to terminate as a left ventricular branch or to anastomose with the left circumflex artery. Branches include (1) the conus artery, (2) the artery to the SA node (in 50%–60% of hearts), (3) anterior right ventricular branches, (4) right atrial branches, (5) an acute marginal branch, (6) an artery to the AV node and proximal bundle branches, (7) the posterior descending artery (in 85%–90% of hearts), and (8) terminal branches to the left atrium and left ventricle. The RCA supplies blood to the SA node (as noted earlier), the right ventricle, the crista supraventricularis, and the right atrium. If it provides the posterior descending artery, it also supplies blood to those areas discussed previously. The RCA provides collaterals to the LAD artery via the conus artery and septal perforators.

The coronary venous system consists of three primary systems: (1) the coronary sinus, (2) the anterior right ventricular veins, and (3) the thebesian veins (Fig. 115.2). The coronary sinus is located in the posterior AV groove and receives blood from the great, middle, and small cardiac veins; the posterior veins of the left ventricle; and the left oblique atrial vein (oblique vein of Marshall). The coronary sinus drains blood primarily from the left ventricle and opens into the right atrium. The two to three anterior right ventricular veins originate in and drain blood from the right ventricular wall. These veins enter the right atrium directly or enter into a small collecting vein at the base of the right atrium. The thebesian veins are tiny venous outlets that drain directly into the cardiac chambers, primarily the right atrium and right ventricle.

## Myocardial Conduction System

The conducting system of the heart is composed of specially differentiated cardiac muscle fibers that are responsible for initiating and maintaining normal cardiac rhythm and for ensuring proper coordination between atrial and ventricular contraction. This system comprises the SA node, the AV node, the bundle of His, the right and left branch bundles, and the Purkinje fibers.

The SA node is a horseshoe-shaped structure located in the upper part of the sulcus terminalis of the right atrium (Fig. 115.3). It extends through the atrial wall from the epicardium to the endocardium. SA nodal fibers have a higher intrinsic rate of depolarization than do any other cardiac muscle fibers and act as the pacemaker of the heart. Three internodal pathways facilitate the conduction of impulses between the SA and AV nodes: the anterior (Bachmann bundle), middle, and posterior internodal tracts. The AV node lies in the medial floor of the right atrium at the base of the atrial septum above the orifice of the coronary sinus. The bundle of His begins at the anterior aspect of the AV node and penetrates through the central fibrous body. Here, the bundle of His divides into the

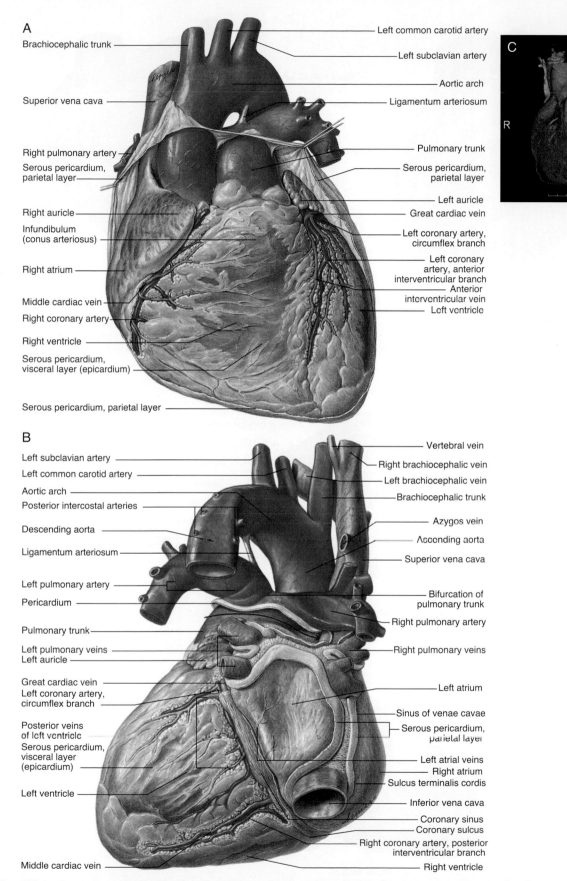

**A**

Brachiocephalic trunk

Superior vena cava

Right pulmonary artery
Serous pericardium, parietal layer

Right auricle
Infundibulum (conus arteriosus)

Right atrium

Middle cardiac vein
Right coronary artery

Right ventricle
Serous pericardium, visceral layer (epicardium)

Serous pericardium, parietal layer

Left common carotid artery
Left subclavian artery
Aortic arch
Ligamentum arteriosum

Pulmonary trunk
Serous pericardium, parietal layer

Left auricle
Great cardiac vein
Left coronary artery, circumflex branch
Left coronary artery, anterior interventricular branch
Anterior interventricular vein
Left ventricle

C    H

R                L

F

**B**

Left subclavian artery
Left common carotid artery
Aortic arch
Posterior intercostal arteries
Descending aorta
Ligamentum arteriosum

Left pulmonary artery
Pericardium

Pulmonary trunk

Left pulmonary veins
Left auricle

Great cardiac vein
Left coronary artery, circumflex branch

Posterior veins of left ventricle
Serous pericardium, visceral layer (epicardium)

Left ventricle

Middle cardiac vein

Vertebral vein
Right brachiocephalic vein
Left brachiocephalic vein
Brachiocephalic trunk

Azygos vein
Ascending aorta
Superior vena cava

Bifurcation of pulmonary trunk
Right pulmonary artery

Right pulmonary veins

Left atrium

Sinus of venae cavae
Serous pericardium, parietal layer

Left atrial veins
Right atrium
Sulcus terminalis cordis
Inferior vena cava
Coronary sinus
Coronary sulcus
Right coronary artery, posterior interventricular branch
Right ventricle

**Fig. 115.1** Coronary arterial distribution. **A,** Anterior view. The right and circumflex coronary arteries travel in the atrioventricular sulcus, adjacent to the tricuspid and mitral valves, respectively. The left anterior descending and posterior descending coronary arteries travel in the interventricular sulcus and demarcate the plane of the ventricular septum. **B,** Posteroinferior view showing right dominance. **C,** Coronary CT depicting heart and great vessels. (From Standring S. The heart and great vessels. In: *Gray's Anatomy.* Churchill Livingstone; 2008:chap 56.)

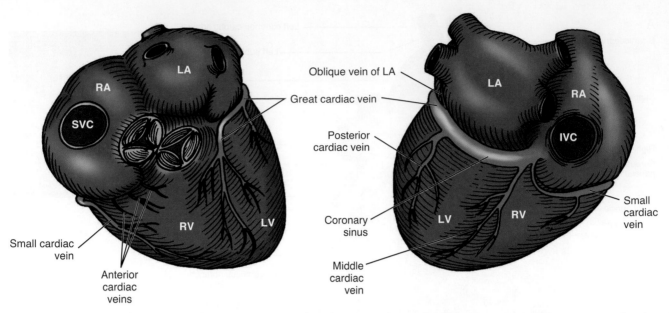

**Fig. 115.2** Coronary veins. The anterior cardiac veins empty into the right atrium, whereas the other major epicardial coronary veins drain into the coronary sinus. *IVC*, Inferior vena cava; *LA*, left atrium; *LV*, left ventricle; *RA*, right atrium; *RV*, right ventricle; *SVC*, superior vena cava. (Adapted from Williams PL, ed. The anatomical basis of medicine and surgery. In: *Gray's Anatomy*. 38th ed. Churchill Livingstone; 1995.)

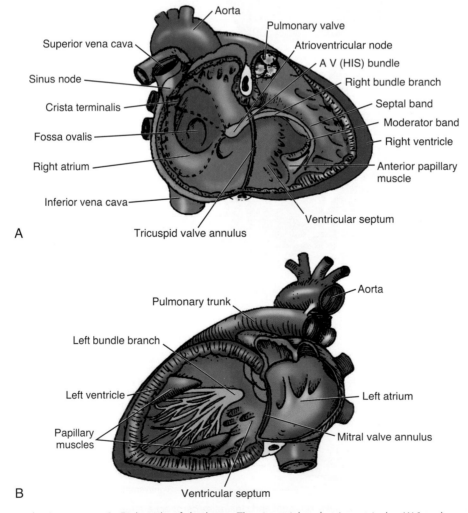

**Fig. 115.3** Cardiac conduction system. **A,** Right side of the heart. The sinoatrial and atrioventricular *(AV)* nodes are both right atrial structures. **B,** Left side of the heart. The left bundle branch forms a broad sheet that does not divide into distinct anterior and posterior fascicles.(Adapted from Williams PL, ed. The anatomical basis of medicine and surgery. In: *Gray's Anatomy*. 38th ed. Churchill Livingstone; 1995.)

left and right branch bundles. The division straddles the upper border of the muscular ventricular septum, and the bundles run superficially down either side of the septum. About midway to the apex, the left bundle divides into the anterior superior and posterior inferior fascicles. These fascicles continue to the base of the papillary muscles of the left ventricle, where they form plexuses of Purkinje fibers that distribute to all portions of the left ventricular myocardium. The right branch bundle continues to the anterior papillary muscle of the right ventricle, where it forms a plexus of Purkinje fibers that distribute to all portions of the right ventricular myocardium.

## SUGGESTED READINGS

Malouf, J. F., Maleszewsk, J. J., Tajik, A. J., & Seward, J. B. (2017). Functional anatomy of the heart. In V. Fuster, R. A. Harrington, J. Narula, & Z. J. Eapen (Eds.), *Hurst's the heart* (14th ed.). New York: McGraw-Hill.

Murphy, J. G., & Wright, R. S. (2012). Applied anatomy of the heart and great vessels. In J. G. Murphy, & M. A. Lloyd (Eds.), *Mayo clinic cardiology concise textbook* (4th ed., pp. 20–43). Oxford University Press.

Standring, S. (2021). The heart and great vessels. In *Gray's anatomy: The anatomical basis of clinical practice* (42nd ed.). Elsevier.

# 116

# Transesophageal Echocardiography: Anatomic Considerations

KENT H. REHFELDT, MD, FACC, FASE  |  WESLEY L. ALLEN, MD

Echocardiography typically uses ultrasound frequencies of 2 million to 10 million hertz (or 2–10 MHz), which is well above the audible range of humans (20–20,000 Hz). Sound waves are absorbed, reflected, and scattered to varying degrees by passage through human tissue. Reflected echoes are produced at boundaries between two inhomogeneous media (e.g., blood-soft tissue interface). More homogeneous tissues result in greater ultrasound scattering and less reflection.

Modern transesophageal echocardiography (TEE) probes possess multiplane imaging capability. That is, the imaging plane of the transducer at the distal tip of the probe can be electronically rotated between 0 degrees (horizontal or transverse plane) and 180 degrees. The image obtained at 180 degrees represents a right-left mirror image of the view obtained at 0 degrees. These multiplane probes use linear phased array imaging technology, and sequential activation of 64 to 128 piezoelectric crystals generates 2D triangular, or "pie-shaped," sectors. Newer matrix-array probes incorporate 2500 piezoelectric crystals at the probe tip, arranged in a square grid that has 50 elements per side. Matrix-array probes are capable of generating 3D images. Sequential activation of piezoelectric crystals in both azimuthal and elevational planes yields voxels that combine to form the 3D image. Matrix-array probes are also capable of generating standard 2D images with 0- to 180-degree multiplane rotation. The simultaneous display of two orthogonal 2D images also represents a function of the matrix-array probe.

## Transesophageal Echocardiography Safety

Numerous complications have been attributed to TEE use, including vocal cord paresis, dysphagia or odynophagia, inadvertent manipulation of the tracheal tube, bronchospasm, arrhythmias, and vascular compression during flexion of the probe tip, particularly in infants. Minor, often subclinical trauma to the hypopharynx is not an uncommon finding after probe insertion. In fact, hypopharyngeal hematoma or laceration may occur in nearly one-fourth of adult patients after typical blind insertion of the TEE probe, although specific treatment of these injuries is almost never needed. Probe insertion with direct visualization with laryngoscopy probably reduces the rate of hypopharyngeal injury. More serious complications, such as esophageal perforation, although fortunately rare, may occur more often than previously believed. Studies of TEE-related esophageal perforation are frequently retrospective and may be complicated by missing data. Nonetheless, the reported frequency of esophageal tear or perforation as a result of

TEE use typically ranges in the literature from 0.1 to 1 per 1000 TEE insertions. Serious TEE-related injury probably occurs more commonly in the operative setting compared with studies performed in a clinic environment. This may relate to longer and repeated examinations performed in patients unable to communicate discomfort while under general anesthesia. It is important to realize that TEE-related esophageal perforation that occurs in conjunction with cardiac surgery may first manifest several days after surgery and may present with nonspecific symptoms and signs, including dyspnea, pleural effusion on chest x-ray, and subcutaneous emphysema. A high index of suspicion is required for early diagnosis.

## Anatomic Correlations

Irrespective of the reason for the TEE study, a comprehensive examination is recommended for every patient, preferably before a specific question or application of TEE is addressed. It is beyond the scope of this brief description to detail all of the anatomic views obtainable with TEE, and the reader is referred to other reviews of the subject.

### INTRAOPERATIVE IMAGE ORIENTATION

The transducer location and the near field (vertex) of the image sector are at the top of the display, and far field at the bottom. At a multiplane angle of 0 degrees (horizontal or transverse plane), with the imaging plane directed anteriorly from the esophagus through the heart, the patient's right side appears on the left of the image display.

The advent of 3D imaging has allowed users to crop and rotate data sets to produce images of variable size that can be viewed from any perspective. Although standard 3D display formats are not defined, some image projections are commonplace. For example, 3D images of the mitral valve are often shown from a left atrial perspective with the aortic valve at the top of the image and the left atrial appendage at the left side ("surgeon's view"). In addition to the area of interest, the inclusion of other recognizable structures in 3D displays aids in viewer orientation.

### BASIC PROBE MOVEMENTS

To generate the desired images, manipulation of the TEE probe is required in addition to changing the multiplane angle (Fig. 116.1). Probe movement is determined by the spatial relationships of the anatomic structures. The multiplane angle allows for cross-sectional imaging of a central image. The basic probe movements include insertion and withdrawal of the probe within the esophagus or stomach. Anteflexion and retroflexion of the probe tip are controlled with the large wheel on the probe and result in cephalad and caudad angulation of the imaging plane, respectively. Left-side and right-side flexion can be achieved by manipulating the smaller wheel on the probe, which causes deflection of the probe tip within a coronal plane. *Rotation* of the probe refers to clockwise or counterclockwise spinning of the probe shaft.

## Standard Views

The American Society of Echocardiography and the Society of Cardiovascular Anesthesiologists task force recommended

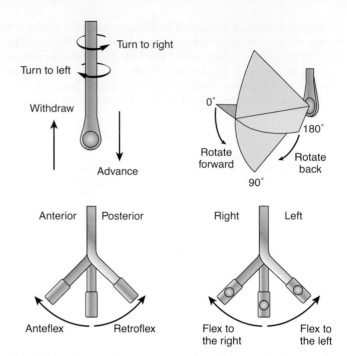

**Fig. 116.1** Basic probe movements, including anteflexion, retroflexion, side flexion, and withdrawal and advancement of the probe, are demonstrated. (From Kahn RA, Shernan SK, Konstadt SN. Intraoperative echocardiography. In: Kaplan JA, ed. *Kaplan's Cardiac Anesthesia*. 5th ed. Saunders Elsevier; 2006:451.)

views that make up the standard intraoperative TEE examination are shown, along with the associated icon depicting a typical multiplane angle at which the image may be generated, in Fig. 116.2. It is important to remember that additional "off-axis" or nonstandard views may be required to adequately examine specific findings in any given patient. Further, the multiplane angles suggested by the images should be considered a rough guide; the precise multiplane angle at which a given structure is best imaged varies among patients. A complete description of the probe maneuvers necessary to obtain these views is beyond the scope of this chapter. Readers are referred to the task force consensus statement.

When studying the images that make up a comprehensive multiplane intraoperative TEE examination, several tips may prove helpful. First, in the majority of midesophageal (ME) images, the structure closest to the probe (i.e., the chamber at the apex of the image) is the left atrium. The only exception is when the probe is withdrawn above the left atrium and resides directly behind the great vessels. In this superior position, the probe is nearest the right pulmonary artery, which can be seen in the long-axis (LAX) view, along with the pulmonary artery bifurcation in the ME ascending aortic short-axis (SAX) view. Increasing the multiplane angle by approximately 90 degrees yields the ME ascending aortic LAX view, in which the right pulmonary artery is seen in the SAX view. These two views demonstrate the orthogonal relationship between the ascending aorta and the right pulmonary artery. (The aortic and pulmonary valves also have a near-orthogonal relationship.) Second, the transgastric (TG) LAX views are most useful for placing a Doppler cursor in near-parallel alignment with the left ventricular outflow tract and aortic root. In this position, the aortic valve or left ventricular outflow tract velocity may be

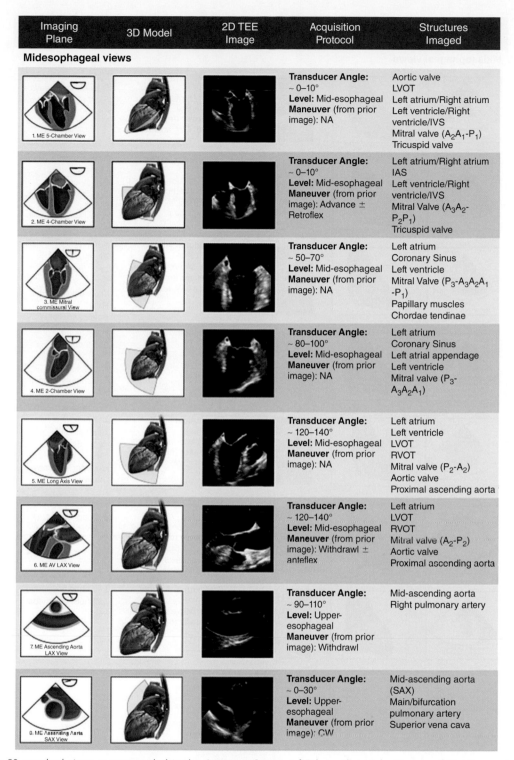

| Imaging Plane | 3D Model | 2D TEE Image | Acquisition Protocol | Structures Imaged |
|---|---|---|---|---|
| **Midesophageal views** | | | | |
| 1. ME 5-Chamber View | | | **Transducer Angle:** ~ 0–10° **Level:** Mid-esophageal **Maneuver** (from prior image): NA | Aortic valve LVOT Left atrium/Right atrium Left ventricle/Right ventricle/IVS Mitral valve ($A_2A_1$-$P_1$) Tricuspid valve |
| 2. ME 4-Chamber View | | | **Transducer Angle:** ~ 0–10° **Level:** Mid-esophageal **Maneuver** (from prior image): Advance ± Retroflex | Left atrium/Right atrium IAS Left ventricle/Right ventricle/IVS Mitral Valve ($A_3A_2$-$P_2P_1$) Tricuspid valve |
| 3. ME Mitral commissural View | | | **Transducer Angle:** ~ 50–70° **Level:** Mid-esophageal **Maneuver** (from prior image): NA | Left atrium Coronary Sinus Left ventricle Mitral Valve ($P_3$-$A_3A_2A_1$-$P_1$) Papillary muscles Chordae tendinae |
| 4. ME 2-Chamber View | | | **Transducer Angle:** ~ 80–100° **Level:** Mid-esophageal **Maneuver** (from prior image): NA | Left atrium Coronary Sinus Left atrial appendage Left ventricle Mitral valve ($P_3$-$A_3A_2A_1$) |
| 5. ME Long Axis View | | | **Transducer Angle:** ~ 120–140° **Level:** Mid-esophageal **Maneuver** (from prior image): NA | Left atrium Left ventricle LVOT RVOT Mitral valve ($P_2$-$A_2$) Aortic valve Proximal ascending aorta |
| 6. ME AV LAX View | | | **Transducer Angle:** ~ 120–140° **Level:** Mid-esophageal **Maneuver** (from prior image): Withdrawl ± anteflex | Left atrium LVOT RVOT Mitral valve ($A_2$-$P_2$) Aortic valve Proximal ascending aorta |
| 7. ME Ascending Aorta LAX View | | | **Transducer Angle:** ~ 90–110° **Level:** Upper-esophageal **Maneuver** (from prior image): Withdrawl | Mid-ascending aorta Right pulmonary artery |
| 8. ME Ascending Aorta SAX View | | | **Transducer Angle:** ~ 0–30° **Level:** Upper-esophageal **Maneuver** (from prior image): CW | Mid-ascending aorta (SAX) Main/bifurcation pulmonary artery Superior vena cava |

**Fig. 116.2** These 28 standard views recommended in the American Society of Echocardiography/Society of Cardiovascular Anesthesiologists guidelines make up the minimum comprehensive intraoperative transesophageal echocardiography exam. (From Hahn RT, Abraham T, Adams MS, et al. Guidelines for performing a comprehensive transesophageal echocardiographic examination: recommendations from the American Society of Echocardiography and the Society of Cardiovascular Anesthesiologists. *J Am Soc Echocardiogr.* 2013;26:921–964. Used by permission.)

*Continued*

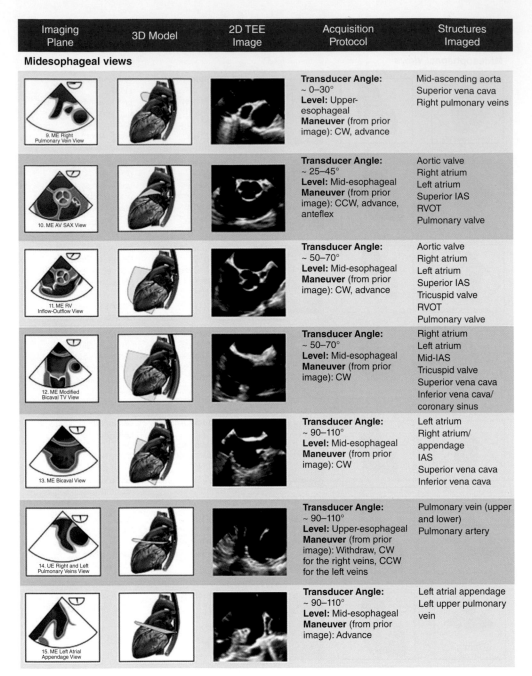

| Imaging Plane | 3D Model | 2D TEE Image | Acquisition Protocol | Structures Imaged |
|---|---|---|---|---|
| **Midesophageal views** | | | | |
| 9. ME Right Pulmonary Vein View | | | **Transducer Angle:** ~ 0–30° **Level:** Upper-esophageal **Maneuver** (from prior image): CW, advance | Mid-ascending aorta Superior vena cava Right pulmonary veins |
| 10. ME AV SAX View | | | **Transducer Angle:** ~ 25–45° **Level:** Mid-esophageal **Maneuver** (from prior image): CCW, advance, anteflex | Aortic valve Right atrium Left atrium Superior IAS RVOT Pulmonary valve |
| 11. ME RV Inflow-Outflow View | | | **Transducer Angle:** ~ 50–70° **Level:** Mid-esophageal **Maneuver** (from prior image): CW, advance | Aortic valve Right atrium Left atrium Superior IAS Tricuspid valve RVOT Pulmonary valve |
| 12. ME Modified Bicaval TV View | | | **Transducer Angle:** ~ 50–70° **Level:** Mid-esophageal **Maneuver** (from prior image): CW | Right atrium Left atrium Mid-IAS Tricuspid valve Superior vena cava Inferior vena cava/coronary sinus |
| 13. ME Bicaval View | | | **Transducer Angle:** ~ 90–110° **Level:** Mid-esophageal **Maneuver** (from prior image): CW | Left atrium Right atrium/appendage IAS Superior vena cava Inferior vena cava |
| 14. UE Right and Left Pulmonary Veins View | | | **Transducer Angle:** ~ 90–110° **Level:** Upper-esophageal **Maneuver** (from prior image): Withdraw, CW for the right veins, CCW for the left veins | Pulmonary vein (upper and lower) Pulmonary artery |
| 15. ME Left Atrial Appendage View | | | **Transducer Angle:** ~ 90–110° **Level:** Mid-esophageal **Maneuver** (from prior image): Advance | Left atrial appendage Left upper pulmonary vein |

**Fig. 116.2, cont'd**

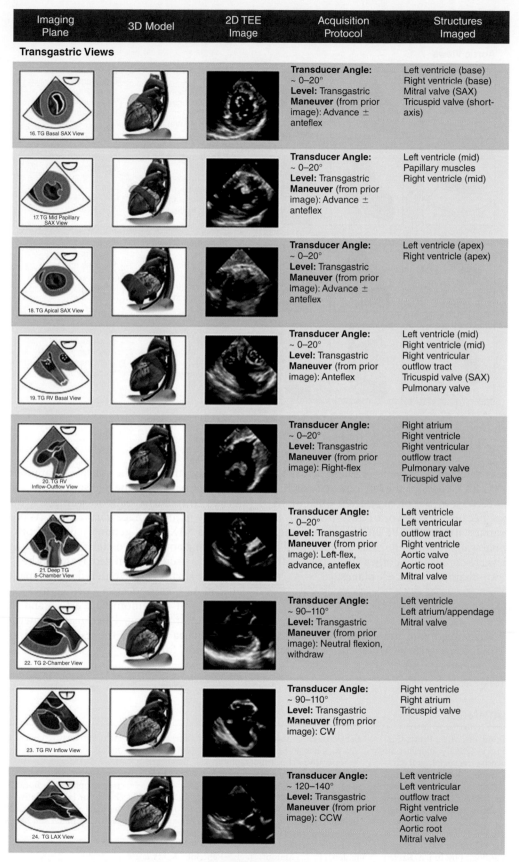

| Imaging Plane | 3D Model | 2D TEE Image | Acquisition Protocol | Structures Imaged |
|---|---|---|---|---|
| **Transgastric Views** | | | | |
| 16. TG Basal SAX View | | | **Transducer Angle:** ~ 0–20° **Level:** Transgastric **Maneuver** (from prior image): Advance ± anteflex | Left ventricle (base) Right ventricle (base) Mitral valve (SAX) Tricuspid valve (short-axis) |
| 17. TG Mid Papillary SAX View | | | **Transducer Angle:** ~ 0–20° **Level:** Transgastric **Maneuver** (from prior image): Advance ± anteflex | Left ventricle (mid) Papillary muscles Right ventricle (mid) |
| 18. TG Apical SAX View | | | **Transducer Angle:** ~ 0–20° **Level:** Transgastric **Maneuver** (from prior Image): Advance ± anteflex | Left ventricle (apex) Right ventricle (apex) |
| 19. TG RV Basal View | | | **Transducer Angle:** ~ 0–20° **Level:** Transgastric **Maneuver** (from prior image): Anteflex | Left ventricle (mid) Right ventricle (mid) Right ventricular outflow tract Tricuspid valve (SAX) Pulmonary valve |
| 20. TG RV Inflow-Outflow View | | | **Transducer Angle:** ~ 0–20° **Level:** Transgastric **Maneuver** (from prior image): Right-flex | Right atrium Right ventricle Right ventricular outflow tract Pulmonary valve Tricuspid valve |
| 21. Deep TG 5-Chamber View | | | **Transducer Angle:** ~ 0–20° **Level:** Transgastric **Maneuver** (from prior image): Left-flex, advance, anteflex | Left ventricle Left ventricular outflow tract Right ventricle Aortic valve Aortic root Mitral valve |
| 22. TG 2-Chamber View | | | **Transducer Angle:** ~ 90–110° **Level:** Transgastric **Maneuver** (from prior image): Neutral flexion, withdraw | Left ventricle Left atrium/appendage Mitral valve |
| 23. TG RV Inflow View | | | **Transducer Angle:** ~ 90–110° **Level:** Transgastric **Maneuver** (from prior image): CW | Right ventricle Right atrium Tricuspid valve |
| 24. TG LAX View | | | **Transducer Angle:** ~ 120–140° **Level:** Transgastric **Maneuver** (from prior image): CCW | Left ventricle Left ventricular outflow tract Right ventricle Aortic valve Aortic root Mitral valve |

**Fig. 116.2, cont'd**

*Continued*

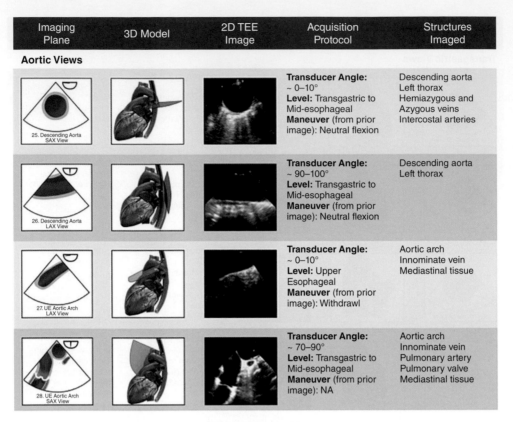

| Imaging Plane | 3D Model | 2D TEE Image | Acquisition Protocol | Structures Imaged |
|---|---|---|---|---|
| **Aortic Views** | | | | |
| 25. Descending Aorta SAX View | | | **Transducer Angle:** ~ 0–10° **Level:** Transgastric to Mid-esophageal **Maneuver** (from prior image): Neutral flexion | Descending aorta Left thorax Hemiazygous and Azygous veins Intercostal arteries |
| 26. Descending Aorta LAX View | | | **Transducer Angle:** ~ 90–100° **Level:** Transgastric to Mid-esophageal **Maneuver** (from prior image): Neutral flexion | Descending aorta Left thorax |
| 27. UE Aortic Arch LAX View | | | **Transducer Angle:** ~ 0–10° **Level:** Upper Esophageal **Maneuver** (from prior image): Withdrawl | Aortic arch Innominate vein Mediastinal tissue |
| 28. UE Aortic Arch SAX View | | | **Transducer Angle:** ~ 70–90° **Level:** Transgastric to Mid-esophageal **Maneuver** (from prior image): NA | Aortic arch Innominate vein Pulmonary artery Pulmonary valve Mediastinal tissue |

**Fig. 116.2, cont'd**

measured and used to calculate a pressure gradient across the aortic valve. Third, TG SAX views of the left ventricle, such as the TG midpapillary SAX views, are often selected when monitoring for ischemia because the myocardium perfused by the three major coronary arteries can be visualized in a single image. Ideally, regional wall motion abnormalities identified in the TG mid-SAX view are confirmed in other views, such as the ME four-chamber, two-chamber, and LAX planes.

## THORACIC AORTA

Thorough intraoperative imaging of the thoracic aorta is important to detect conditions, such as severe atherosclerosis, that may modify the surgical approach (aortic cross-clamping) or inform the decision to place mechanical support devices (intraaortic balloon pump). A number of standard views are used to image various aspects of the thoracic aorta. LAX and SAX views generally image both the ascending and descending aorta. The distal aortic arch and subclavian artery orifice are usually visualized as the probe is withdrawn slowly while the aorta is kept centered in the image. Occasionally, the left common carotid artery orifice may be seen. In contrast, the origin of the innominate artery and the distal ascending aorta are rarely imaged because of interposition of the air-filled trachea between the esophagus and aorta, creating a "blind spot" for TEE.

## SUGGESTED READINGS

Hahn, R. T., Abraham, T., Adams, M. S., Bruce, C. J., Glas, K. E., Lang, R. M., et al. (2013). Guidelines for performing a comprehensive transesophageal echocardiographic examination: Recommendations from the American Society of Echocardiography and the Society of Cardiovascular Anesthesiologists. *Journal of the American Society of Echocardiography, 26,* 921–964.

Kahn, R. A., Maus, T., Salgo, I., Weiner, M.M., & Shernan, S.K., et al. (2017). Basic intraoperative transesophageal echocardiography. In J. A. Kaplan (Ed.), *Kaplan's cardiac anesthesia* (7th ed., pp. 427–504). Philadelphia: Elsevier.

Michelena, H. I., Abel, M. D., Suri, R. M., Freeman, W. K., Click, R. L., Sundt, T. M., et al. (2010). Intraoperative echocardiography in valvular heart disease: An evidence-based appraisal. *Mayo Clinic Proceedings, 85,* 646–655.

Piercy, M., McNichol, L., Dinh, D. T., Story, D. A., & Smith, J. A. (2009). Major complications related to the use of transesophageal echocardiography in cardiac surgery. *Journal of Cardiothoracic and Vascular Anesthesia, 23,* 62–65.

Thaden, J. J., Malouf, J. F., Rehfeldt, K. H., Ashikhmina, E., Bagameri, G., Enriquez-Sarano, M., et al. (2020). Adult intraoperative echocardiography:

A comprehensive review of current practice. *Journal of the American Society of Echocardiography, 33,* 735–755.

Vegas, A., & Meineri, M. (2010). Three-dimensional transesophageal echocardiography is a major advance for intraoperative clinical management of patients undergoing cardiac surgery: A core review. *Anesthesia and Analgesia, 110,* 1548–1573.

# Detection and Treatment of Perioperative Acute Coronary Syndromes

RYAN C. CRANER, MD

Significant advances in anesthesia safety have been made over the past 50 years that allow more patients to undergo operations that prolong and improve the quality of life. Because of these advances, it has been estimated that more than 300 million noncardiac surgical procedures are completed each year worldwide. Thankfully, death while in the operating room is rare; however, the true incidence of perioperative mortality is difficult to capture because definitions vary among reporting bodies. It is estimated that the 30-day mortality rate of adult patients who undergo noncardiac surgery is 1% to 3%. If perioperative death were considered as its own category in the annual mortality tables from the Centers for Disease Control and Prevention, it would represent the third leading cause of death in the United States. Cardiac complications, including myocardial ischemia, are a leading cause of perioperative mortality.

## Monitoring for Myocardial Injury and Infarction

*Myocardial infarction* (MI) is defined as myocardial cell death as a result of prolonged ischemia and is classified into various types, depending on the etiology of the ischemic event. Type 1 MI (Fig. 117.1) is caused by atherosclerotic plaque rupture, with resulting intraluminal thrombus. This is the characteristic acute coronary syndrome (ACS). Type 2 MI is the most common type of MI encountered in clinical settings and occurs when myocardial necrosis occurs as a result of supply/demand mismatch. Type 3 MI is characterized by patients who succumb prior to any elevation in troponin. Types 4 and 5 are related to coronary revascularization procedures like percutaneous coronary intervention (PCI) or coronary artery bypass grafting.

Myocardial injury often initially presents with the usual ischemic symptoms, including chest discomfort, nausea, weakness, and dyspnea. In extreme cases, ventricular arrhythmia or cardiac arrest may be the first manifestation. In addition, the characteristic symptoms of myocardial ischemia may be vague or absent in the postoperative patient because of the effects of analgesia and residual anesthesia. In one trial, only 34% of patients who had perioperative MI after noncardiac surgery had ischemic symptoms, possibly as a result of receiving perioperative analgesics.

In patients where an ACS is suspected, initial stratification of ACS is traditionally based on characteristic ECG findings. These include ST-segment elevation MI (STEMI), non–ST-segment elevation MI (NSTEMI), and unstable angina pectoris. Early in the course of NSTEMI, distinguishing between NSTEMI and prolonged unstable angina may be difficult. The latter is diagnosed if cardiac enzyme markers do not become abnormal; fortunately, the initial management is similar.

The pathogenesis of perioperative ACS is similar to that of spontaneously developing myocardial ischemia and infarction. In many cases plaque rupture or erosion leads to the formation of a partially or totally occlusive intracoronary thrombus (type 1), most often at the site of a preexisting nonstenotic plaque. In cases without plaque rupture, increased $O_2$ demand as a result of catecholamine release from surgical stress and a hypercoagulable state secondary to the surgical procedure cause ischemia (type 2). Total coronary occlusion most often leads to STEMI, whereas subtotal occlusion is most commonly associated with non–ST-segment elevation coronary syndromes. However, many factors, including the degree of preexistent collateral vessels, level of $O_2$ demand, and coronary vasomotion, create exceptions to this generalization. Intraoperative detection of ACS is enhanced by appropriate monitoring of high-risk patients. Electrocardiography is an integral part of intraoperative monitoring and the diagnostic workup and stratification of patients with MI. However, its diagnostic utility is limited in the setting of conduction defects and ventricularly paced rhythms and in situations when the chest is inaccessible during thoracic or upper abdominal procedures. Intraoperative ST-segment changes are associated with myocardial injury; however, the sensitivity is much lower than that of echocardiography evaluation of regional and global left ventricular function. Intraoperative use of transesophageal echocardiography requires specialized equipment and personnel who are comfortable with interpreting the transesophageal echocardiography images, which may limit its widespread use. Another possible modality for intraoperative monitoring for myocardial ischemia is trend monitoring of pulmonary artery occlusion pressure.

Postoperative monitoring modalities include continuous electrocardiogram (ECG) monitoring and serum measurement of cardiac enzyme markers of necrosis, usually troponin T or I. These markers, troponin T and I, are more sensitive and specific for myocardial injury than other markers, such as creatine kinase-MB. Although elevation of troponin is sensitive for necrosis, mild elevations may occur with tachycardia (including rapid atrial fibrillation), pulmonary embolism, cardiac contusions, cardiac pacing, stress cardiomyopathy (apical ballooning syndrome), acute neurologic disease, and critical illness (e.g., respiratory or renal failure) and thus do not alone define MI. A recent multinational trial evaluated serum troponin levels during the first 3 perioperative days and found that

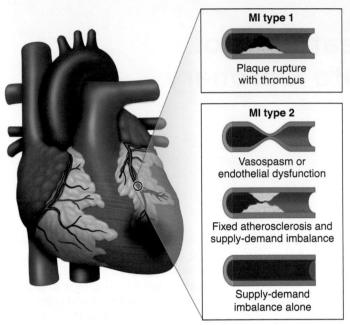

**Fig. 117.1** Differentiation between myocardial infarction (*MI*) types 1 and 2 according to the condition of the coronary arteries.

an "abnormally" elevated troponin level was an independent predictor of 30-day mortality, irrespective of ischemic symptoms. This phenomenon, known as *myocardial injury after noncardiac surgery* (MINS), had prognostic relevance as the 30-day mortality rate was 9.8% among patients who had MINS as opposed to 1.1% among patients who did not (odds ratio, 10.07; 95% confidence interval, 7.84–12.94). Currently, there are no clear strategies to prevent or treat MINS, but postoperative troponin measurements should be considered in patients who are considered to be at high risk for cardiovascular complications.

## Treatment of Acute Coronary Syndrome

A general approach to the management of ACS is shown in Fig. 117.2. Urgent cardiology consultation is warranted when ACS is suspected. Necessary adjustments in anesthetic and fluid management should be made to optimize key components of the patient's physiology. These include oxygenation, intravascular fluid volume, and hemoglobin concentrations.

Because the underlying problem in ACS is often platelet-rich thrombus, pharmacotherapy includes the administration of antiplatelet and antithrombotic agents. These agents greatly increase the risk of bleeding in the perioperative setting and, thus, must be used cautiously. When the risk of postoperative hemorrhage is low, aspirin should be administered immediately, and the use of intravenously administered unfractionated heparin should be considered. Low-molecular-weight (LMW) heparin has been shown to be more effective than unfractionated heparin in treating ACS; however, the effects of LMW heparin are more difficult to monitor with commonly available tests and are more difficult to reverse quickly. The use of the potent intravenously administered glycoprotein IIb/IIIa platelet antagonists is generally contraindicated in the setting of ongoing or recent surgery because of the high risk of hemorrhagic complications.

The treatment approach then diverges based on ECG findings. Patients with ST-segment elevation or new left bundle branch block will be considered separately from those with ST-segment depression or nonspecific ECG changes (see Fig. 117.2).

## ST-Segment Elevation Myocardial Infarction

ST-segment elevation is a highly specific finding indicative of acute MI. Such patients typically have occlusion of an epicardial coronary artery and are candidates for urgent reperfusion therapy, which is most beneficial if achieved early but is of some

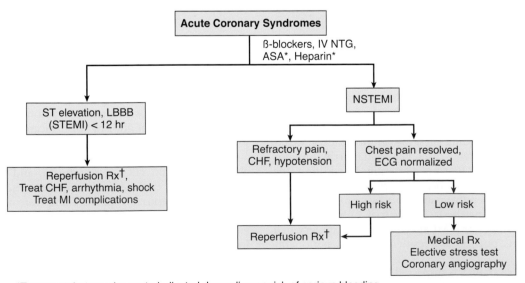

*Treatment that may be contraindicated depending on risk of serious bleeding

†Usually with percutaneous coronary intervention (thrombolysis contraindications)

**Fig. 117.2** Therapy and decision-making for patients with acute coronary syndromes. Reperfusion therapy includes angioplasty, thrombolysis, or both. *ASA,* Aspirin; *CHF,* congestive heart failure; *ECG,* electrocardiogram; *IV,* intravenously administered; *LBBB,* left bundle branch block; *MI,* myocardial infarction; *NSTEMI,* non–ST-segment elevation MI; *NTG,* nitroglycerin; *Rx,* therapy; *STEMI,* ST-segment elevation MI.

value up to 12 hours after onset of the event. Although thrombolytic therapy is contraindicated in the immediate postoperative setting, many postoperative patients may tolerate aspirin and intravenously administered heparin with acceptable bleeding risk. Ongoing assessment of the patient to evaluate and treat for heart failure includes use of an afterload-reducing agent, such as nitroglycerin (if no hypotension or recent use of phosphodiesterase inhibitors). If hypertension persists, β-blockers, such as metoprolol, may be administered. Ultimately, cardiology consultation should be obtained and determination made if the patient is a candidate for angiography and potential PCI where needed. If cardiac catheterization services are not available, emergent patient transfer to a center that provides PCI may be necessary.

## Non–ST-Segment Elevation Acute Coronary Syndrome

Non–ST-segment elevation ACS most commonly results from an incompletely occlusive coronary thrombus. Patients may present with chest pain or, more commonly, have elevated cardiac enzyme markers postoperatively. Medical therapy includes aspirin, intravenous or sublingual nitrates, lipid-lowering agents, and antithrombotic agents. Antiischemic therapy should also be initiated if no evidence of shock is present, and a short-acting intravenous β-adrenergic receptor blocking agent may be used.

Patients who are at high risk for subsequent morbidity and mortality include those with persistent ST-segment depression; elevated cardiac serum markers, such as troponin or creatine kinase-MB; and hemodynamic instability, including hypotension, shock, pulmonary edema, right-sided heart failure, and frequent ventricular arrhythmia. These high-risk patients and those with refractory ischemic pain should be considered for coronary angiography and reperfusion therapy. The same caveats regarding assessment of bleeding risk and the use of potent platelet and thrombin inhibitors apply. For other patients who are minimally symptomatic and hemodynamically stable, urgent angiography is not necessary as long as the patient's condition remains stable. ECG monitoring with serial assessment of cardiac enzyme markers is appropriate. The use of coronary computed tomography angiography may also be useful to identify patients that may not benefit from invasive angiography. Further investigation can be delayed until later in the patient's convalescence and usually includes stress imaging, angiography as indicated, or both. Guidelines for the management of preoperative risk stratification and acute MI and for the use of PCI are available.

Complications of MI include congestive heart failure, ventricular arrhythmia, cardiogenic shock, and cardiac arrest. Patients must be diligently monitored for these conditions, and the complications must be corrected with appropriate pharmacologic measures. In the setting of cardiogenic shock, placement of an intraaortic balloon pump or other percutaneous left ventricular support device may be considered (Impella [ABIOMED, Danvers, MA], TandemHeart [LivaNova, London, UK]). Angiotensin-converting enzyme inhibitors, aspirin, β-adrenergic receptor blocking agents, and appropriate lipid-lowering therapy are indicated over the long term.

## Special Situations

For patients who are allergic to aspirin, clopidogrel may be substituted. Heparin-induced thrombocytopenia typically does not occur during the first 5 days of therapy unless recent earlier exposure to heparin has occurred. Patients with this disorder usually have an antibody to the heparin-platelet factor 4 complex. A direct-acting thrombin inhibitor that is structurally and functionally unrelated to heparin, such as bivalirudin or argatroban, may be substituted for heparin in this circumstance.

The use of β-adrenergic receptor blocking agents is contraindicated in patients with second-degree or greater atrioventricular block, shock, cardiogenic pulmonary edema, severe heart failure, or severe asthma, but these drugs should not be withheld in patients with diabetes mellitus. The use of calcium channel blockers is indicated for rate control of rapid atrial fibrillation, which may accompany or precipitate ACS in some patients. For patients with refractory ventricular tachycardia or ventricular fibrillation, the current drug of choice is intravenous amiodarone, although other antiarrythmics may also be used.

For patients with an anterior wall MI, pump failure is the most serious complication and is a strong indication for reperfusion therapy and inotropic and left ventricular support. For those with an inferior wall MI, complications such as papillary muscle dysfunction or rupture and hemodynamically significant right ventricular MI are more common. The use of surface or transesophageal echocardiography allows rapid and accurate differentiation of these disorders.

In any patient in the postanesthesia care unit who has sudden hemodynamic collapse, a diagnosis of ACS must be considered. The differential diagnosis should also include pulmonary embolus, aortic dissection, pneumothorax, cardiac tamponade, and sepsis.

## SUGGESTED READINGS

Amsterdam, E. A., Wenger, N. K., Brindis, R. G., Casey, D. E., Jr., Ganiats, T. G., Holmes, D. R., Jr., et al. (2014). 2014 AHA/ACC Guideline for the management of patients with non-ST-elevation acute coronary syndromes: A report of the American College of Cardiology/American Heart Association Task Force on Practice Guidelines. *Journal of the American College of Cardiology, 64*(24), e139–e228.

Botto, F., Alonso-Coello, P., Chan, M. T., Villar, J. C., Xavier, D., Srinathan, S., et al. (2014). Myocardial injury after noncardiac surgery: A large, international, prospective cohort study establishing diagnostic criteria, characteristics, predictors, and 30-day outcomes. *Anesthesiology, 120*(3), 564–578.

Devereaux, P. J., Xavier, D., Pogue, J., Guyatt, G., Sigamani, A., Garutti, I., et al. (2011). Characteristics and short-term prognosis of perioperative myocardial infarction in patients undergoing noncardiac surgery: A cohort study. *Annals of Internal Medicine, 154*(8), 523–528.

Kunkel, K. J., Lemor, A., Mahmood, S., Villablanca, P., & Ramakrishna, H. (2022). 2021 Update for the diagnosis and management of acute coronary syndromes for the perioperative clinician. *Journal of Cardiothoracic and Vascular Anesthesia, 36*(8), 2767–2779. doi:10.1053/j.jvca.2021.07.032.

Tabit, C. E., & Nathan, S. (Winter 2021). Management of perioperative acute coronary syndromes

by mechanism: A practical approach. *International Anesthesiology Clinics, 59*(1), 61–65. doi:10.1097/AIA.0000000000000310.

Thygesen, K., Alpert, J. S., Jaffe, A. S., Chaitman, B. R., Bax, J. J., Morrow, D. A., et al. (2018). Fourth universal definition of myocardial infarction 2018. *Journal of the American College of Cardiology, 72*(18), 2231–2264. Retrieved from https://www.jacc.org/doi/full/10.1016/j.jacc.2018.08.1038.

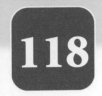

# Heart Failure: Classification, Compensation, and Treatment

CHRISTOPHER A. THUNBERG, MD

Heart failure (HF) is a clinical syndrome in which cardiac output does not satisfy the body's metabolic needs. Patients may present with fatigue, dyspnea, and reduced exercise capacity. Some HF patients have volume overload with pulmonary edema, congestion of visceral organs, and peripheral fluid accumulation; in these patients the term *congestive heart failure* is often used.

## Types of Heart Failure

Many HF patients have left ventricular (LV) dysfunction that precedes the onset of HF symptoms. LV dysfunction can be divided into systolic and diastolic categories. LV ejection fraction (EF) is an echocardiographic measure of systolic function used to classify and monitor HF. The term *HF with reduced EF* (HF*r*EF) describes patients with HF and EF less than or equal to 40%. It is important to recognize that diastolic dysfunction can cause HF at any degree of LV systolic function. Because of this, clinicians use the term *HF with preserved EF* (HF*p*EF) for patients with HF and EF greater than 40%. HF*p*EF constitutes approximately 50% of all HF.

HF is a clinical syndrome with many etiologies (Table 118.1). Disorders that target any part of the heart (pericardium, myocardium, endocardium, cardiac valves, coronary arteries) or great vessels may result in HF.

## Classification of Heart Failure

The New York Heart Association classification system (Table 118.2) is symptom based, whereas the American College of Cardiology Foundation/American Heart Association (ACCF/AHA) classification emphasizes disease progression (Table 118.3). Clinicians managing HF patients use the ACCF/AHA staging system to target appropriate therapy for their patients.

## Compensatory Mechanisms in Heart Failure

HF results in a reduction in cardiac output (CO) and decreased organ perfusion. As CO falls, the body activates compensatory neurohormonal systems (Table 118.4) that promote vasoconstriction and vascular volume expansion. According to the *Frank-Starling mechanism*, an increase in LV end-diastolic pressure (LVEDP) leads to an increase in CO due to augmented myocardial stretch. Over time, neurohormonal activation puts the LV under hemodynamic stress (volume overload, pressure overload, tachycardia) that results in pathologic remodeling (dilation, hypertrophy, fibrosis). As remodeling progresses, it takes ever-increasing LVEDP to maintain CO, setting up a cycle of worsening HF.

| TABLE 118.1 | Etiologies of Heart Failure |
| --- | --- |
| **Etiology** | **Comments** |
| Hypertension | Associated with diastolic dysfunction and HFpEF |
| Coronary artery disease | Major cause of HFrEF |
| Valvular heart disease | Results in volume or pressure overload |
| Dilated cardiomyopathy | Myocardial disorders characterized by ventricular dilation and reduced contractility |
| Familial cardiomyopathy | Idiopathic dilated cardiomyopathy arising in closely related family members |
| Endocrine/metabolic | Obesity, diabetes mellitus, thyroid disease |
| Toxic | Alcohol, cocaine, ephedra, amphetamines, heavy metals |
| Tachycardia induced | LV myocardial dysfunction due to tachyarrhythmia or ventricular pacing at high rates |
| Myocarditis/inflammatory | Systemic lupus erythematosus, AIDS, Chagas disease |
| Peripartum | LV dysfunction arising late in pregnancy or soon after birth |
| Amyloidosis | Deposition of insoluble proteins (fibrils) in heart tissue |
| Sarcoidosis | Infiltration of cardiac tissue with inflammatory cells |
| Stress (takotsubo) | Acute, reversible LV dysfunction due to severe physical or emotional stress |
| Hemochromatosis | Iron overload |

*HFpEF*, Heart failure with preserved ejection fraction; *HFrEF*, heart failure with reduced ejection fraction; *LV*, left ventricular.

| TABLE 118.2 | New York Heart Association Functional Classification of Heart Failure | |
|---|---|---|
| **Class** | **Description** | |
| I | No limitation—symptoms of heart failure only at activity levels that would limit most normal individuals | |
| II | Slight limitation—symptoms with ordinary levels of exertion | |
| III | Marked limitation—symptoms with less than normal levels of exertion | |
| IV | Symptoms at rest—very poor prognosis | |

| TABLE 118.3 | American College of Cardiology Foundation/American Heart Association Stages of Heart Failure | |
|---|---|---|
| **Stage** | **Description** | **Clinical Correlation/Presentation** |
| A | High risk for developing HF but without structural heart disease or symptoms of HF | Hypertension, lipid disorders, diabetes, coronary artery disease, obesity, family history of cardiomyopathy |
| B | Structural heart disease but without signs of symptoms of HF | Previous myocardial infarction, left ventricular dysfunction, asymptomatic valvular heart disease |
| C | Structural heart disease with prior or current symptoms of HF | Dyspnea and fatigue, impaired exercise capacity |
| D | Refractory end-stage HF | Marked symptoms at rest despite maximal medical therapy |

*HF*, Heart failure.

| TABLE 118.4 | Neurohormonal Systems Activated in Patients With Heart Failure | |
|---|---|---|
| **System** | **Actions** | |
| Sympathetic nervous system | Vasoconstriction Increased inotropy Increased chronotropy | |
| Renin-angiotensin-aldosterone system | Vasoconstriction Sodium retention | |
| Antidiuretic hormone (vasopressin) | Vasoconstriction Water retention | |
| Endothelin | Vasoconstriction | |

## Biomarkers in Heart Failure

B-type natriuretic peptides (BNPs) are produced by cardiac myocytes in response to myocardial stretch. BNPs counteract the neurohormonal systems described in Table 118.4 by stimulating vasodilation and excretion of water and sodium. Clinicians use assays to detect BNP and NT-proBNP (N-terminal pro-B-type natriuretic peptide) to diagnose HF, monitor severity, and gauge patient response to HF therapy. Concentrations of cardiac troponin (troponins I and T) are also increased in HF, suggesting myocyte injury or necrosis, and may have prognostic significance.

## Treatment of Heart Failure

Modern HF treatments are multidisciplinary, guideline driven, and conform to the patient's ACCF/AHA staging status.

## STAGE A

Medical therapy for stage A (high risk for HF but without structural heart disease) is directed at controlling hypertension and dyslipidemia to avoid the development of HF. Diuretics, β-blockers, angiotensin-converting enzyme (ACE) inhibitors, and angiotensin receptor blockers (ARBs) are effective treatments for high blood pressure, whereas statins may be given for dyslipidemia. Other conditions, such as obesity, diabetes mellitus, and tobacco use, should be controlled or avoided.

## STAGE B

Patients in stage B are asymptomatic but have evidence of structural heart disease. Therapy is tailored to the patient's condition. Those with a history of myocardial infarction should receive ACE inhibitors (or ARBs), β-blockers, and statins to reduce mortality and prevent progression to symptomatic HF. Patients with a reduced EF should receive ACE inhibitors and β-blockers to prevent progression to HF. In patients with other structural abnormalities (such as LV hypertrophy), ACE inhibitors/ARBs and β-blockers are indicated. Coronary revascularization and valvular surgery should be done as appropriate.

## STAGE C

Patients in stage C have prior or current symptoms of HF and are at risk of repeated hospitalization. A sodium-restricted diet may reduce symptoms of congestion. Treatment of sleep disorders (obstructive sleep apnea) and enrollment in cardiac rehabilitation may improve functional status.

As in stages A and B, pharmacologic therapy continues to rely on ACE inhibitors/ARBs and β-blockers. In addition, loop diuretics may be added for patients with volume overload. Vasodilator therapy with hydralazine and isosorbide dinitrate is recommended in Black patients. Aldosterone antagonists (spironolactone, eplerenone) and angiotensin receptor–neprilysin inhibitor (ARNI) have been shown to reduce mortality and hospitalization. ARNI refers to the combination of valsartan, an ARB, with sacubitril, an inhibitor of the enzyme neprilysin, which degrades natriuretic peptides. Ivabradine, an inhibitor of the $I_f$ current in the sinoatrial node, slows heart rate without lowering blood pressure and is indicated to reduce heart rate in patients with HFrEF who do not tolerate up-titration of β-blockers. Sodium-glucose cotransporter-2 inhibitors (such as dapagliflozin) are used for glycemic control in type 2 diabetes mellitus and have benefit in patients with HFrEF through reduction of preload and afterload. Dapagliflozin has been shown to reduce HF mortality and hospitalization in patients with and without diabetes.

Placement of an implantable cardioverter-defibrillator is recommended in patients with ischemic heart disease and reduced EF to prevent lethal ventricular tachyarrhythmias, and cardiac resynchronization therapy with a biventricular pacemaker is recommended for patients with low EF and left bundle branch block to improve LV function. As in stage B, consideration of coronary revascularization and valvular repair is appropriate.

## STAGE D

Stage D is marked by advanced, refractory HF. At this stage, patients may not tolerate β-blockers and ACE inhibitors/ARBs due to hypotension. Dietary sodium, fluid restriction, and diuretics may be required to manage volume overload. Treatment of refractory volume overload is possible with ultrafiltration, a form of renal replacement therapy. Intravenous inotropic support with adrenergic agonists (dopamine, dobutamine) and phosphodiesterase inhibitors (milrinone) can be used to stabilize the patients with low CO. If hypotension is absent, infusions of vasodilators, such as nitroglycerin, nitroprusside, and nesiritide (human BNP), can reduce preload and afterload on the failing heart. Insertion of an intraaortic balloon pump will temporarily augment CO and coronary artery perfusion. Mechanical circulatory support (MCS) refers to placement of a ventricular assist device. Percutaneously inserted assist devices serve as short-term MCS for cardiogenic shock. Surgical implantation of a left ventricular assist device provides durable MCS permanently (destination therapy) or until cardiac transplantation is feasible (bridge-to-transplant). Cardiac transplantation is the ultimate solution for HF with a 5-year survival around 70% but requires lifetime therapy with antirejection drugs.

## SUGGESTED READINGS

Kemp, C. D., & Conte, J. V. (2012). The pathophysiology of heart failure. *Cardiovascular Pathology*, 21, 365–371.

Maddox, T. M., Januzzi, J. L., Allen, L. A., Breathett, K., Butler, J., Davis, L. L., et al. (2021). 2021 update to the 2017 ACC expert consensus decision pathway for optimization of heart failure treatment: Answers to 10 pivotal issues about heart failure with reduced ejection fraction: A report of the American College of Cardiology Solution Set Oversight Committee. *Journal of the American College of Cardiology*, 77(6), 772–810.

Yancy, C. W., Jessup, M., Bozkurt, B., Butler, J., Casey, D. E., Jr., Drazner, M. H., et al. (2013). 2013 ACCF/AHA guideline for the management of heart failure: A report of the American College of Cardiology Foundation/American Heart Association task force on practice guidelines. *Journal of the American College of Cardiology*, 62, e147–e239.

Yancy, C. W., Jessup, M., Bozkurt, B., Butler, J., Casey, D. E., Jr., Colvin, M. M., et al. (2017). 2017 ACC/AHA/HFSA focused update of the 2013 ACCF/AHA guideline for the management of heart failure: A report of the American College of Cardiology/American Heart Association task force on clinical practice guidelines and the Heart Failure Society of America. *Journal of the American College of Cardiology*, 70(6), 776–803.

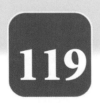

# 119

# Right Heart Failure, Tricuspid and Pulmonary Valve Pathology

WESLEY L. ALLEN, MD

## The Right Ventricle

Compared with the left ventricle (LV), the right ventricle (RV) is a physiologic low-pressure, high-volume system with different geometry, design, and structure. Although previously disregarded as only a passive channel to the LV, more recent investigations have shown the independent importance of right ventricular performance and management to patients' exercise tolerance, outcomes, procedural success, and long-term mortality rates. Clinical symptoms of right-sided heart dysfunction include hypotension, peripheral edema, abdominal pain caused by hepatic congestion, chest pain, syncope, dyspnea, and shock.

## Anatomy

The RV lies anteromedial in relation to the LV and can be divided into three segments: inflow (smooth muscle), trabeculated apical region, and outflow. The inflow extends from the tricuspid valve to the heavily trabeculated RV wall before transitioning to the RV outflow tract. A remnant of the bulbus cordis, the outflow tract contains the infundibulum and the pulmonic valve. It is smooth and nontrabeculated and has different fiber orientation and coronary blood supply compared with the RV inflow portion. The systolic and diastolic performance of the RV and LV are intrinsically linked via the shared interventricular septum, creating interventricular dependence.

Unique to the RV (and used for identification of ventricular "sided-ness" in congenital heart disease) are the tricuspid valve, with three associated papillary muscles, and the moderator band. The tricuspid valve is trileaflet, with a distinctive septal leaflet in addition to the posterior and anterior leaflets (vs. the anterior/posterior bileaflet mitral valve). The moderator band is a horizontal muscular band of tissue in the apex that separates the inflow and outflow tracts and connects the shared ventricular septum to the anterior papillary muscle. It contains part of the right bundle branch of the atrioventricular bundle and acts primarily as a conduction pathway to the anterior papillary muscle and free wall.

## Electrocardiography of the Right Ventricle

The RV is represented on the standard 12-lead electrocardiogram (ECG) by precordial leads V1, V2, and II, III, and aVF for the free wall and inferior walls, respectively. Right ventricular hypertrophy will present with an R wave of greater than 1 in V1 and repolarization abnormalities (T-wave inversion with ST-segment depression) in II, III, aVF, and V1 to V3. Injury to the right atrioventricular bundle can cause a right bundle branch block that traditionally presents with prolonged QRS, a large R wave in leads V1 or V2, and a broad, deep S wave in lead V5 or V6. Conduction abnormalities can also be of mechanical origin from guidewires or catheters (e.g., central venous catheters, pulmonary artery catheters, right-sided heart catheter procedures) entering the RV. This mostly causes right bundle branch block, with the incidence of complete heart block secondary to pulmonary artery catheters varying from 3% to 12% in the literature. Although consensus is lacking, some studies note up to a nearly fivefold increased incidence of complete heart block in patients with a preexisting left bundle branch block.

Diagnosis of RV myocardial ischemia or infarction (RVMI), however, may be difficult using the standard 12-lead ECG. Originally designed with a focus on the LV, the precordial leads V1 and V2 fail to represent the RV free wall in its entirety. Up to 50% of inferior wall infarctions (ECG leads II, III, aVF) will have concomitant right ventricular wall injury that may not be represented in leads V1 and V2, increasing the risk of mortality 2.6-fold. ST-segment elevation in the V4 lead (V4R) of a "right-sided" ECG is highly sensitive and specific for identification of RVMI and is associated with decreased right ventricular ejection fraction and increased in-hospital mortality. Hemodynamically, hypotension and shock will be seen without evidence of pulmonary congestion in acute RVMI (as can be seen with LV failure).

Further, hypotension and shock in RVMI may have a delayed presentation, with greater onsets after hospital admission compared with LV failure (preadmission/presenting symptom predominance), and thus can be missed on initial evaluation.

## Coronary Perfusion

Right ventricular perfusion occurs during both systole and diastole under normal physiologic conditions, as opposed to the LV. This is a result of coronary driving pressure exceeding RV wall tension and chamber pressure during systole. As wall tension or systolic chamber pressure increases, as with acute or chronic increases in afterload, the RV assumes a systolic dominant perfusion pattern that is more congruent with that of the LV.

The right coronary artery is responsible for perfusing the RV free wall and the inferior third of the basal midventricular septum (Fig. 119.1). It also perfuses the sinoatrial node and the atrioventricular node in 60% and 80% to 90% of patients, respectively. As a result, injury or ischemia to right coronary blood flow can have significant effects not only on right ventricular performance but also on left ventricular function, the conduction system, and atrioventricular synchrony.

## Design and Function

The RV is a crescent-shaped chamber (vs. the circular or bullet shape of its counterpart) that extends to near, but does not share, the cardiac apex in normal physiologic conditions. Compared with the LV, the muscle wall is more heavily trabeculated and thinner, with increased compliance. Although the stroke volume is equal to that of the LV in the absence of shunts or valvular disease, because of the increased end-systolic and end-diastolic chamber volumes, the RV ejection fraction is slightly lower, with a normal range of 40% to 60%. The RV has one-third to one-fourth the muscle mass of the LV, and under normal conditions it performs one-fourth to one-sixth the stroke work (adjusted to body surface area). The RV free wall contains subepicardial circumferential and subendocardial longitudinal contraction fibers, but it lacks the helical fiber layer of the LV that accounts for most of the ejection. This helical muscle layer component of the RV is restricted to the ventricular septum. During septal contraction, the helical fibers thicken, creating longitudinal strain throughout the RV. This longitudinal shortening accounts for roughly 40% or more of the RV systolic ejection. Thus RV performance is significantly dependent on interventricular septum function and is the basis for interventricular dependence.

## Preload

The Frank-Starling curve applies differently for the RV compared with the LV. The LV increases contractility with increasing volume because of optimum stretch of the myofibrils. This "stretch" occurs uniformly throughout the left ventricular wall as the chamber radially expands equidistant from the center, increasing regional contractility homogeneously. During low-pressure environments, RV chamber expansion secondary to increasing volume is uneven, with a greater increase in the septal/free chamber wall diameter. In this scenario, the Frank-Starling mechanism plays a lesser role. As the chamber pressure rises, the RV becomes more cylindrical, with uniform dimension expansion, thus increasing the Frank-Starling contribution.

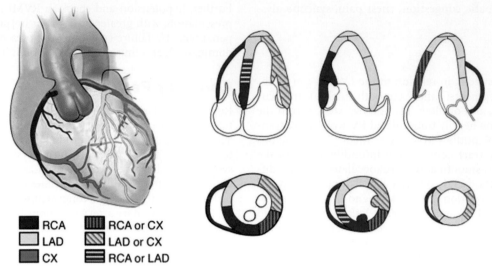

**Fig. 119.1  Coronary blood flow distribution.** *CX,* Circumflex artery; *LAD,* left anterior descending artery; *RCA,* right coronary artery. (Reproduced from Lang R, et al. Recommendations for cardiac chamber quantification by echocardiography in adults: an update from the American Society of Echocardiography and the European Association of Cardiovascular Imaging. *J Am Soc Echocardiogr.* 2015;28(1):1–39.e14. Copyright 2015 with permission from Elsevier.)

## Afterload

RV afterload is multifactorial, with pulmonary artery resistance, left atrial pressure, and left ventricular cardiac output all contributing (Table 119.1). In the setting of rising afterload, the RV has a more substantial decline in stroke volume compared with the LV (Fig. 119.2). This can best be explained by LaPlace's law and wall stress (Table 119.2). The reduced capacity of the RV to contract against a load is secondary to increased wall tension in the setting of decreased wall thickness and increasing radius (which occurs during normal contraction). Understanding this relationship and the components of afterload is important for proper management and maintenance of RV performance.

## Evaluation of the Right Ventricle

Advancements in RV performance evaluation techniques through imaging and hemodynamic assessments have grown. Hemodynamic assessments have shown predictive value as the Pulmonary Artery Pulsatility Index is a sensitive predictor for RV failure. Imaging includes cardiac computed tomography, cardiac magnetic resonance imaging (MRI), and echocardiography. Evaluation of the RV via echocardiography should include wall thickness, chamber size, and interventricular septum positioning in systole and diastole and systolic function. Because of the unique shape of the RV and the inability to capture its entirety in a single plane, systolic performance traditionally was mostly

| TABLE 119.1 | Factors That Increase Right Ventricular Afterload | | |
|---|---|---|---|
| **Pulmonary Vascular Resistance** | **Increased Left Atrial Pressure** | **Cardiac Output** |
| **PHYSIOLOGIC:** acidosis, hypothermia, hypoxia | **VALVULAR:** mitral regurgitation, mitral valve stenosis, aortic valve insufficiency | Decreased left ventricular contractility |
| **VENTILATION:** atelectasis, hypercapnia, extreme high/low lung volume | **MYOCARDIAL DYSFUNCTION:** left ventricular diastolic dysfunction, left ventricular systolic dysfunction | – |
| **MEDICATIONS:** $\alpha_1$-agonists, methylene blue, protamine, high-dose vasopressin, serotonin | **CONDUCTION SYSTEM:** atrioventricular dyssynchrony atrial fibrillation | – |
| **INFLAMMATORY:** endothelin–1, tumor necrosis factor-α, histamine, thromboxane $A_2$, arachidonic acid, sepsis | – | – |
| **SPECIAL CIRCUMSTANCES:** Stenotic pulmonary vein anastomosis after heart or lung transplant Pulmonary embolism | – | – |

$$\text{Pulmonary vascular resistance} \left(\text{dyne.s.cm}^{-5}\right) = \frac{80^* \left(\text{Mean Pulmonary Arterial Pressure} - \text{Pulmonary Capillary Wedge Pressure}\right)}{\text{Cardiac Output}}$$

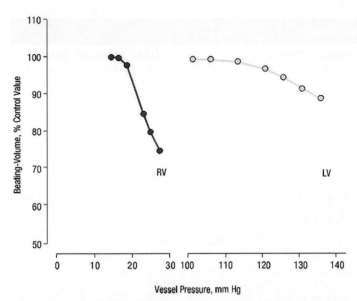

**Fig. 119.2 Stroke volume: afterload relationship of the right (RV) and left ventricles (LV).** In comparison with the LV, the RV is less able to compensate for an acute increase in afterload. Note the substantial decrease in RV ejection fraction in response to an increase in afterload. (Reproduced from Wiedemann HP, Matthay RA. Cor pulmonale. In: Braunwald E, ed. *Heart Disease*. 5th ed. Philadelphia: W.B. Saunders; 1997: 1606. Copyright 1997, with permission from Elsevier.)

| TABLE 119.2 | Chamber Pressure or Afterload Described by LaPlace's Law and Wall Stress |
|---|---|
| LaPlace's law | $P = \dfrac{T}{r}$ $\qquad$ $p = \dfrac{\sigma * h}{r}$ |
| Wall stress | $\sigma = \dfrac{T}{h}$ |

where $P$ = chamber pressure or afterload; $T$ = wall tension; $r$ = chamber radius; $\sigma$ = wall stress; $T$ = tension; $h$ = wall thickness.

qualitative with modest predictive values, with the best measure being the degree of longitudinal shortening. New advancements in 3D echocardiography have shown 3D RV ejection fraction to be more reliable, with similar accuracy and reproducibility to MRI assessments. Myocardial speckle tracking and strain measurements are also evolving as reliable measures. Despite the overall larger chamber size and volume, the normal relative RV cavity size in a standard midesophageal four-chamber view is two-thirds or less of the LV and does not extend to the apex (Fig. 119.3). This is because the beam cuts through the shorter diameter of the crescent-shaped RV (compared with the circular or ellipsoid LV). Dysfunction in chronic disease, as seen in pulmonary hypertension, chronic tricuspid regurgitation, or chronic left-sided heart pathology, begins with chamber dilation with maintained systolic function. RV dilation is described as RV diastolic size of greater than two-thirds of the LV and/or ventricular sharing of the apex (Fig. 119.4). With time, the systolic performance progressively declines.

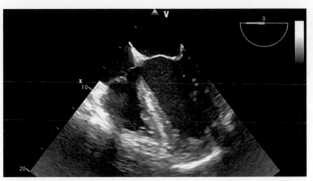

**Fig. 119.3 Midesophageal four-chamber view showing normal right ventricular size/dimension.** The normal right ventricle (RV) is significantly smaller than the left ventricle (LV) (less than two-thirds in size). Additionally, with normal RV morphology, the apex of the heart is composed of the LV and septum (apical involvement is not shared by the RV). With progressive RV failure, these features change so that as the RV increases in size, apical involvement of the RV develops.

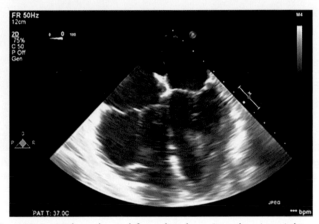

**Fig. 119.4 Midesophageal four-chamber view showing right ventricular failure.** The right ventricle (RV) is dilated (more than two-thirds the size of the left ventricle). Also note that there is apical involvement because of the change in morphology of the RV.

## Management of Right Ventricular Dysfunction

Right ventricular dysfunction is multifactorial, and management should target the specific underlying pathology. RV perfusion deficits, RV volume overload, RV pressure overload secondary to elevated pulmonary vascular resistance or left-sided pathology (i.e., LV failure, severe mitral regurgitation) (see Table 119.1), and direct myocardial or physiologic depressants all effect RV contractility (Table 119.3).

Direct $\beta_1$-agonist is the first-line treatment for impairment of RV contractility not resultant from compromised perfusion. $\beta_1$-agonism vasodilates the arterial beds while simultaneously increasing contractility. Dobutamine infusion is recommended for stable or mild dysfunction, and epinephrine infusion or bolus for severe compromise or rescue therapy. Dopamine is less favorable than dobutamine or epinephrine because it is associated with tachycardia and lower relative reduction in pulmonary vascular resistance. Milrinone, although considered ionotropic, only has a mild effect on contractility, and its main benefits occur through afterload reduction.

| TABLE 119.3 | Etiologies of Direct Right Ventricular Myocardial Depression | | | |
|---|---|---|---|---|
| **PHYSIOLOGIC:** | **INFLAMMATORY:** | **CORONARY PERFUSION:** | | **VOLUME/STARLING CURVE:** |
| acidosis, hypothermia, hypocalcemia, hypophosphatemia | histamine tumor necrosis factor-$\alpha$, interleukin–1, interleukin–6 (sepsis), inflammatory mediators released in cardiopulmonary bypass | $O_2$ demand mismatch, acute ischemia, insufficient protection in cardiopulmonary bypass, air into right coronary artery during open heart procedures | | acute increase in right ventricular end-diastolic volume (sarcomeres stretched beyond optimal length) |

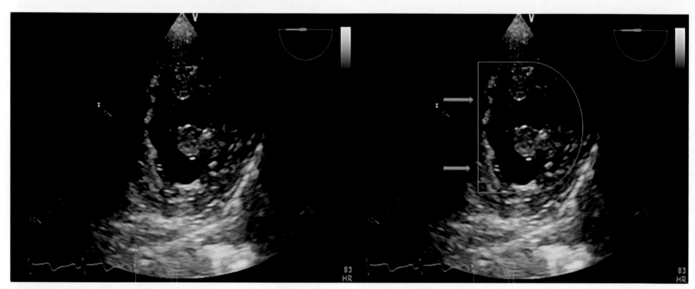

**Fig. 119.5**   **Diastolic septal flattening seen in right ventricle (RV) volume overload.** The *arrows* show flattening of the interventricular septum secondary to right ventricular filling pressures exceeding left ventricular filling pressures during diastole. This conformational change from a circular left ventricle (LV) to a D-shaped LV is the hallmark sign of RV volume overload.

Because of interventricular dependence, RV dysfunction can have dramatic effects on LV function, and vice versa. Evaluation of the interventricular septum in diastole and systole can be diagnostic of the pathologic state. Pressure overload physiology will cause septal shifting into the LV during systole when the maximal chamber pressure is generated. Volume overload physiology causes septal shifting into the LV during diastole when the ventricle fills (Fig. 119.5).

Treatment of primary pulmonary pressure overload with normal RV contractility should be directed at afterload reduction. This can be accomplished by reducing pulmonary vascular resistance via improving ventilation and correcting hypoxia, hypothermia, hypercarbia, and acidosis. Direct pulmonary vasodilator medications, such as prostaglandin $E_1$ agonists, inhaled nitric oxide, sildenafil, and inhaled or intravenous milrinone infusion, are all effective therapies for decreasing pulmonary vascular resistance and improving right ventricular performance. For acute collapse secondary to pulmonary artery spasms (e.g., in protamine administration), rapid and effective treatment is 30 to 50 μg/kg intravenous milrinone bolus. The most common side effect of the intravenous medications, however, is a concomitant decrease in systemic vascular resistance. This is generally absent with inhaled therapy. Once there is evidence of RV systolic dysfunction, $\beta_1$-agonists should be first-line therapy to maintain RV EF and prevent rises in RV end-systolic volume and volume overload while vasodilator/afterload therapy is initiated.

Goal-directed therapy for volume overload should aim at decreasing preload. Venodilators, such as nitroglycerin, have preferential venous over arterial dilation, increasing venous capacitance and decreasing preload to a greater extent than decreasing systemic vascular resistance. For acute collapse or severe compromise, rapid maneuvers for decreasing preload include placing the patient in the reverse Trendelenburg position and providing direct volume aspiration from a central venous catheter if present.

In the setting of systemic vasodilatory hypotension with elevated pulmonary vascular resistance, the management goal is to augment the systemic vascular resistance to maintain myocardial oxygen delivery, minimize hyperdynamic LV outflow obstruction, and maximize right ventricular ejection fraction without exacerbating pulmonary vascular resistance. Because vasopressors have varying pharmacodynamic effects in the pulmonary and systemic vascular systems, understanding the specific interactions and relationships of individual vasopressors with these vascular beds and their effects on RV ejection fraction is paramount (Table 119.4).

Although oversimplified, understanding the physiology behind RV design, function, pathologic states, and directed therapy is vital. Right ventricular afterload, preload, and

| TABLE 119.4 | Effects of Medication on Systemic Vascular Resistance, Pulmonary Vascular Resistance, Right Ventricular Ejection Fraction, and Heart Rate | | |
|---|---|---|---|
| **Medication** | **SVR vs. PVR** | **Right Ventricular Ejection Fraction** | **Heart Rate** |
| Vasopressin infusion (low dose) | SVR > PVR (minimal effect) | No change | No change vs. ↓ |
| Vasopressin (bolus) | SVR ≥ PVR | Mild ↓ vs.no change | No change vs. ↓ |
| Phenylephrine (pure α₁ agonists) | SVR < PVR | ↓ | ↓ |
| Norepinephrine | SVR ≥ PVR | No change | ↑ (minimal effect) |
| Epinephrine | SVR > PVR | ↑↑ (≥25%) | ↑ |

*PVR,* Pulmonary vascular resistance; *SVR,* systemic vascular resistance.

myocardial perfusion are intrinsically linked and are targets during management. For example, an acute increase in RV afterload can quickly lead to RV compromise that progresses to failure. Initially, the RV cannot contract against an increased afterload. The reduced RV ejection fraction leads to increased RV end-diastolic volume. As the RV acutely dilates, the sarcomeres stretch beyond optimal length and contraction further decreases. Myocardial perfusion declines during acute dilation because of increased wall tension and chamber pressure. As myocardial perfusion declines, contractility progressively worsens. This progression illustrates the interconnection of afterload, preload, and myocardial perfusion and why the RV decline accelerates in failure. Although it may be counterintuitive in the setting of systemic hypotension, nitroglycerin administration to decrease preload and RV end-diastolic volume improves sarcomere length and the position on the Starling curve. Reduction in RV end-diastolic pressure and wall tension improves perfusion. This, coupled with β₁-agonism, improves RV ejection fraction and left ventricular filling. Vasopressin or norepinephrine administration can be used to augment SVR without impairing RV ejection fraction to improve coronary perfusion. This will also reduce left ventricular outflow tract obstruction commonly seen in the setting of a hyperdynamic underfilled LV. In summary, systemic hypotension secondary to RV failure is a result of inadequate filling of the LV and decreased cardiac output. Therefore therapy should be directed at maximizing RV ejection fraction to optimize LV filling.

## Tricuspid Valve

The tricuspid valve is the largest of the cardiac valves, with a valve area of 4 to 6 cm². It is trileaflet, with septal, anterior, and posterior leaflets, and its annulus is more apically displaced in relation to the plane of the mitral valve annulus in the atrioventricular groove. Three papillary muscles arise from the septal, anterior, and posterior walls and are named respectively.

## Tricuspid Regurgitation

Tricuspid regurgitation can be an acquired or a congenital pathology secondary to a predominant leaflet problem or a predominant annulus problem. Most commonly, tricuspid regurgitation is acquired secondary to annular dilation with normal leaflet function and is classified as *functional*. Other causes of acquired tricuspid regurgitation secondary to

leaflet pathology include rheumatic heart disease, carcinoid syndrome, radiation therapy, endocarditis, medications (fenfluramine/phentermine, methysergide), leaflet restriction from pacemaker wires, and inadvertent damage secondary to right-sided heart biopsy, among others. Trauma, tumors (myxoma), and right ventricular infarction can also cause valvular incompetence. Patients may experience fatigue or decreased exercise tolerance in addition to peripheral edema, decreased appetite, ascites, and atrial fibrillation because of right atrial enlargement.

Tricuspid regurgitation is evaluated by color flow Doppler with echocardiography and graded (mild, moderate, severe), most commonly based on regurgitant jet size, area, orifice diameter, jet density, and hepatic vein flow. Severe tricuspid regurgitation can cause end organ damage by decreasing organ perfusion pressures from increased venous congestion. The liver is an organ commonly affected, because severe tricuspid regurgitation can lead to hepatic congestion and injury. Tricuspid regurgitation also causes right atrial and ventricular dilation over time secondary to elevated inflow volumes. Isolated surgical correction of tricuspid regurgitation is traditionally reserved for severe asymptomatic or symptomatic regurgitation. Surgical correction at the time of left-sided valve surgery is recommended for mild tricuspid regurgitation or greater with annular dilation of more than 4 cm on echocardiography or moderate tricuspid regurgitation or greater with or without annular dilation. The valve can be openly repaired with ring annuloplasty or replaced with a prosthetic valve. Current endovascular repair techniques are being evaluated but are not yet approved by the U.S. Food and Drug Administration. The therapeutic intervention is determined by the etiology of the regurgitation, leaflet integrity, and annular dimension.

## Tricuspid Stenosis

Tricuspid stenosis is much less frequent than regurgitation, with the vast majority of cases secondary to rheumatic fever. Other causes include systemic lupus erythematosus, carcinoid syndrome, right atrial myxoma, congenital malformation, metastatic tumor, and radiation. Tricuspid stenosis evaluated by echocardiography with color flow Doppler is traditionally characterized by high velocity and turbulent flow. The evaluation of severity is similar to that for other stenotic lesions by jet velocity (higher stenosis grade causes higher jet velocity), mean gradient, calculated valve area, and pressure half-time.

Tricuspid valve replacement is reserved for symptomatic patients or asymptomatic patients with a severely stenotic lesion.

## Pulmonic Valve

The pulmonic valve is a trileaflet semilunar valve with anterior, right, and left leaflets, respectively, positioned between the right ventricular outflow tract (composed of the right ventricular free wall, infundibulum, and ventricular septum) and the pulmonary artery. It is the most anterior valve in the chest, and as a result, it is best evaluated via transthoracic echocardiography as opposed to transesophageal echocardiography.

## Pulmonic Regurgitation

Parameters evaluating the severity of pulmonic regurgitation are less validated than those for other valves. The most common etiology of pulmonic valve regurgitation is pulmonary hypertension. Less common causes include endocarditis, carcinoid syndrome, and rheumatic fever. Physical examination findings show a decrescendo diastolic murmur at the left sternal border in the second intercostal space. The clinical consequence of significant pulmonic regurgitation is right ventricular enlargement secondary to chronically increased volume to the RV. Although it is usually asymptomatic, severe disease can present with symptoms of right-sided heart failure.

## Pulmonic Stenosis

Pulmonic stenosis is most commonly of congenital origin as a component of tetralogy of Fallot, and it primarily affects children. Adult etiology is rare and most often secondary to carcinoid syndrome. Physical examination findings are significant for a harsh crescendo-decrescendo systolic murmur at the left sternal border of the second intercostal space, best heard with the patient leaning forward. Symptoms of syncope, angina and/or dyspnea, or heart failure may appear. Intervention is usually reserved for symptomatic patients or asymptomatic patients with severe grading, with or without chamber dilation.

## SUGGESTED READINGS

Addetia, K., Muraru, D., Badano, L. P., & Lang, R. M. (2019). New directions in right ventricular assessment using 3-dimensional echocardiography. *JAMA Cardiology, 4*(9), 936–944.

Buckberg, G., & Hoffman, J. (2014). Right ventricular architecture responsible for mechanical performance: Unifying role of ventricular septum. *Journal of Thoracic and Cardiovascular Surgery, 148*(6), 3166–3171.

Kawel-Boehm, N., Maceira, A., Valsangiacomo-Buechel, E. R., Vogel-Claussen, J., Turkbey, E. B.,

Williams, R., et al. (2015). Normal values for cardiovascular magnetic resonance in adults and children. *Journal of Cardiovascular Magnetic Resonance, 17,* 29.

Lang, R. M., Badano, L. P., Mor-Avi, V., Afilalo, J., Armstrong, A., Ernande, L., et al. (2015). Recommendations for cardiac chamber quantification by echocardiography in adults: An update from the American Society of Echocardiography and the European Association of Cardiovascular Imaging. *Journal of the American Society of Echocardiography, 28*(1), 1–39.e14.

Naeije, R., & Badagliacca, R. (2017). The overloaded right heart and ventricular interdependence. *Cardiovascular Research, 113,* 1474–1485.

Sanz, J., Sánchez-Quintana, D., Bossone, E., Bogaard, H. J., & Naeije, R. (2019). Anatomy, function, and dysfunction of the right ventricle: JACC state-of-the-art review. *Journal of the American College of Cardiology, 73*(12), 1463–1482.

# 120

# Management of End-Stage Heart Failure: Heart Transplantation Versus Ventricular Assist Device

ADAM J. MILAM, MD, PhD

*Heart failure* is defined as insufficient cardiac output to meet the metabolic requirements of the tissues at normal cardiac filling pressures. Heart failure can be systolic (impaired contractility with impaired ejection fraction) or diastolic (decreased relaxation and compliance). *Cardiogenic shock* is defined as sustained hypotension and tissue hypoperfusion. With heart failure, there is activation of the compensatory neurohormone system (renin-angiotensin-aldosterone system and release of natriuretic peptides, angiotensin II, norepinephrine, and endothelin) resulting in fluid retention, peripheral vasoconstriction, downregulation of β-adrenergic receptors, and ventricular remodeling. Eventually, left ventricular (LV) failure leads to pulmonary hypertension and right ventricular (RV) failure.

Echocardiography is used to assess ventricular function, identify structural and functional cardiac abnormalities and status, and guide therapy. The American Heart Association classification defines four stages of heart failure, A through D, where stage D is end-stage heart failure (Fig. 120.1). Coronary artery disease is the most common cause of both systolic and diastolic failure. Other causes include dilated nonischemic, restrictive, hypertrophic, and stress-induced cardiomyopathy. The most common cause of death in patients with heart failure is ventricular dysrhythmia.

Patients with coronary artery or valvular heart disease should have medical therapy optimized and, depending on the anatomy, revascularization performed or valves repaired or replaced as appropriate. In patients with an ejection fraction of less than 30%, placement of an implantable cardioverter defibrillator (ICD), pacemaker resynchronization therapy, or both is recommended. Routine anticoagulation is not recommended. Surgical treatment options include placement of an intraaortic balloon pump, ventricular assist device (VAD), total artificial heart (TAH), or orthotopic heart transplantation; each treatment option has specific indications and contraindications.

Clinical indications for the use of a mechanical device before multisystem organ failure occurs include myocardial infarction, failed percutaneous coronary intervention, acute viral myocarditis, peripartum cardiomyopathy, cardiac contusion, postcardiotomy shock, chronic cardiomyopathy with acute decompensation,

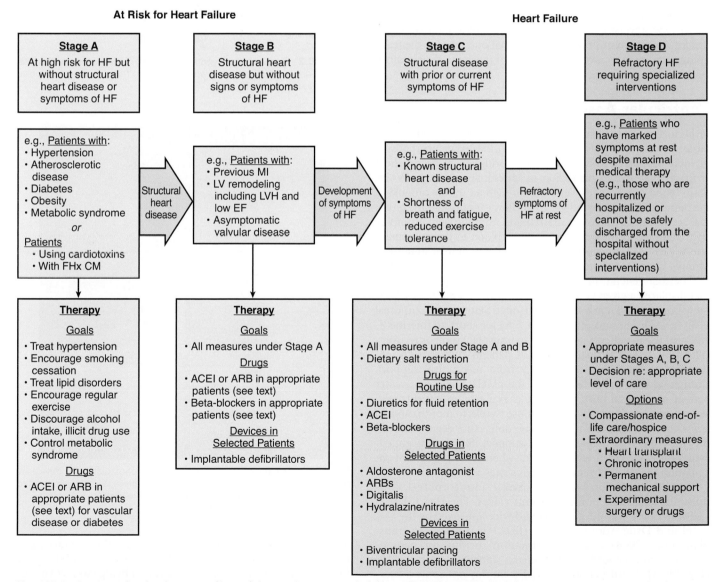

**Fig. 120.1** Stages in the development of heart failure and recommended therapy by stage. *ACEI,* Angiotensin-converting enzyme inhibitor; *ARB,* angiotensin II receptor blocker; *EF,* ejection fraction; *FHx CM,* family history of cardiomyopathy; *HF,* heart failure; *LV,* left ventricular; *LVH,* left ventricular hypertrophy; *MI,* myocardial infarction. (Modified from Jessup M, Abraham WT, Casey DE, et al. 2009 focused update: ACCF/AHA Guidelines for the Diagnosis and Management of Heart Failure in Adults: a report of the American College of Cardiology Foundation/American Heart Association Task Force on Practice Guidelines: developed in collaboration with the International Society for Heart and Lung Transplantation. *Circulation.* 2009;119:1977–2016. © 2013 American Heart Association, Inc. All rights reserved.)

and intractable ventricular dysrhythmia. Early intervention improves survival.

Since 2005, the Interagency Registry for Mechanically Assisted Circulatory Support (INTERMACS) has collected clinical data relevant to patients requiring mechanical circulatory support devices for end-stage heart failure in North America. According to INTERMACS, nearly 28,000 adult patients received a durable MCS from 2010 to 2019; 93.6% of these patients had an isolated left VAD (LVAD) implantation, 0.1% had an isolated right VAD (RVAD) implantation, 3.8% had BiVAD (RVAD and LVAD) implantation, and 1.6% of patients had a TAH implanted. INTERMACS data reflect an overall increase in the use of LVADs for destination therapy: from 2010 to 2014, 42.7% of LVADs were implanted for destination therapy compared with 56.1% for 2015 to 2019. The International Society for Heart and Lung Transplantation Mechanically Assisted Circulatory Support (IMACS) registry includes data from the INTERMACS registry and several other databases worldwide. Its first annual report was published in 2016 and includes data from 31 countries and 5942 patients. Data collection and analysis of patient demographics, survival, device type, adverse events, competing outcomes, and risk factors will improve current practices and overall outcomes as the technology continues to evolve and the use of mechanical circulatory assist devices continues to expand.

## Ventricular Assist Devices

VADs to support the left or right ventricle, or both, are either pulsatile or continuous flow (most common), located paracorporeally or intracorporeally, and are used as a bridge to recovery (short term), a bridge to transplantation, or as destination therapy. LVADs drain blood from the left ventricle through an inflow cannula to the pump and return blood via an outflow cannula into the proximal aorta. Similarly, RVADs drain blood from the right atrium or right ventricle to the pump and return blood to the pulmonary artery. The VAD system consists of an inflow cannula, an outflow cannula, a pump, a tunneled driveline, and an electrical controller.

The first-generation VADs used pulsatile pumps with valves that displaced a given volume of blood with every beat. One pulsatile pump is still marketed in the United States, a paracorporeal VAD (pVAD; Thoratec, Pleasanton, CA) for short, to intermediate-term use in patients as a bridge to transplantation or recovery (Fig. 120.2). Approximately 10% of patients recover sufficient function to be weaned completely from mechanical support. Compared with previous devices, the pVAD allows for greater patient mobility (a portable device is available for patients who leave the hospital) and longer-term use (weeks to months and, in a few cases, years). The pVAD is the only assist device that can provide longer-term biventricular support. Short-term anticoagulation is provided with heparin, whereas long-term anticoagulation requires warfarin and sometimes aspirin.

Second-generation VADs are smaller, intracorporeal, nonpulsatile, axial flow pumps without valves. The HeartMate II (Thoratec) is a second-generation device approved by the U.S. Food and Drug Administration (FDA) as a bridge to transplantation (2008) and for destination therapy for patients who are not candidates for heart transplantation (2010) (Fig. 120.3). Third-generation VADs employ noncontact bearings using a combination of magnetically and hydrodynamically suspended impellers. The third-generation devices are the HeartWare VAD system (HVAD; HeartWare International, Framingham, MA), approved in 2012 by the FDA as a bridge

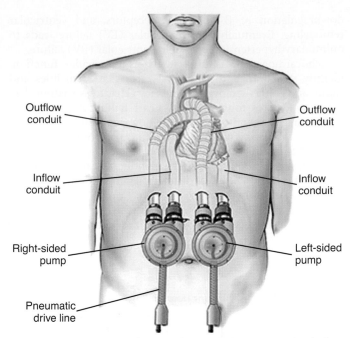

**Fig. 120.2** Paracorporeal ventricular assist device—a pulsatile first-generation device. (Reprinted with permission from Thoratec Corporation, Pleasanton, CA.)

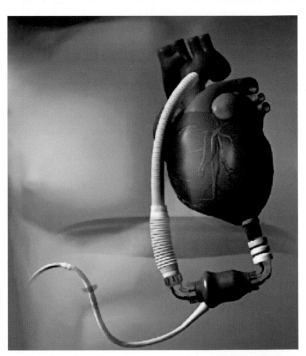

**Fig. 120.3** HeartMate II, an intracorporeal ventricular assist device—a second-generation, continuous-flow ventricular assist device. (Reprinted with permission from Thoratec Corporation, Pleasanton, CA.)

to transplantation and in 2017 for destination therapy; and the HeartMate III (Thoratec; [Fig. 120.4]), approved by the FDA in 2017 for short-term support as a bridge to recovery or transplantation and in 2018 for destination therapy. The HVAD was recalled in 2021 for an increased risk of adverse neurologic events. The timing of implantation is important; the Randomized Evaluation of Mechanical Assistance for the

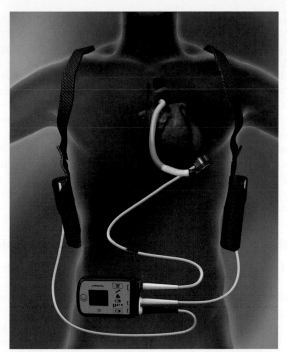

**Fig. 120.4** HeartMate 3 Left Ventricular Assist System (LVAS)—a third-generation, continuous-flow ventricular assist device. (HeartMate 3 is a trademark of Abbott or its related companies. Reproduced with permission of Abbott, © 2021. All rights reserved.)

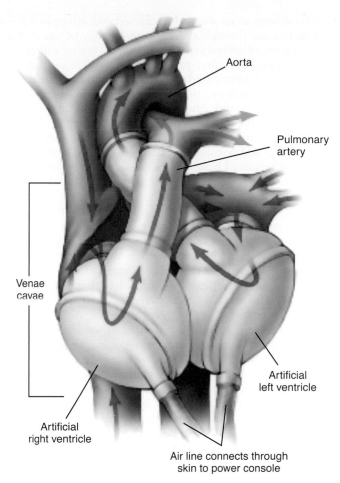

**Fig. 120.5** Total artificial heart. (Reprinted with permission from SynCardia, Tucson, AZ.)

Treatment of Congestive Heart Failure (REMATCH) trial demonstrated that patients had better outcomes when the device implanted sooner rather than later (before organ dysfunction developed, e.g., kidney failure). The long-term survival rate was approximately 80% at 1 year and more than 50% at 2 years after device implantation in this study.

## Total Artificial Heart

TAH provides biventricular support for patients with end-stage heart failure. SynCardia (Tucson, AZ) produces two TAHs, consisting of two independent pulsatile devices (ventricles) each with two mechanical valves, two tunneled drivelines, and an external controller. When implanting the TAH, the native ventricles are excised, cuffs are placed at the position of the atrioventricular valve, and outflow grafts are attached to the ascending aorta and main pulmonary artery. The pulsatile devices are attached to the cuffs (at the tricuspid and mitral valve position) and then the great arteries. The FDA approved the 75-mL TAH (Fig. 120.5) as a bridge to transplant in 2004 and the 50-mL TAH in 2020. There is currently a clinical trial to evaluate the 75-mL TAH for destination therapy.

## Anesthetic Considerations for Patients With End-Stage Heart Failure Who Require Implantation of a Ventricular Assist Device or Total Artificial Heart

### PREOPERATIVE CONSIDERATIONS

The preparation of patients requiring VAD and TAH implantation in addition to heart transplantation is similar to that required for other patients undergoing cardiac surgical procedures involving cardiopulmonary bypass (CPB). However, patients who are receiving VADs, TAHs, or heart transplants are at greater risk for right heart failure, hemorrhage, systolic dysfunction, ventricular dysrhythmias, and sudden death before CPB.

A thorough preoperative evaluation should include an extensive review of the patient's cardiac, pulmonary, renal, and metabolic history; a thorough examination of the patient; and a complete assessment of all laboratory results and imaging studies. All previously implanted devices, such as pacemakers and ICDs, should be interrogated. Packed red blood cells (cytomegalovirus free), fresh frozen plasma, cryoprecipitate, and platelets must be available in the blood bank because these patients often receive anticoagulant therapy, have chronic anemia, and are at high risk for perioperative bleeding, especially if they have had a previous sternotomy.

### Intraoperative Management

#### PATIENTS RECEIVING A VENTRICULAR ASSIST DEVICE

In addition to standard American Society of Anesthesiologists monitoring devices, these patients should have a cannula placed in a radial, brachial, or femoral artery before induction of anesthesia for continuous measurement of arterial blood pressure.

Central venous access should be achieved with either an 8.5F or a 9F introducer through which a catheter may be inserted for measurement of central venous, pulmonary artery, and/or pulmonary artery occlusion pressure, and cardiac output. The pharmacologic agents used for induction and maintenance of anesthesia are similar to those used for any other patient with severe cardiomyopathy. After tracheal intubation, a transesophageal echocardiography (TEE) probe should be inserted. Patients with preexisting coagulopathy require baseline coagulation studies and possibly thromboelastography. Defibrillation pads must be placed before deactivation of defibrillation therapy. Pacemakers must be interrogated, and appropriate changes must be made.

Before CPB, a TEE examination must be performed to assess RV function, evaluate for valvular abnormalities (especially tricuspid regurgitation, mitral stenosis, and aortic insufficiency [AI]), identify shunts (patent foramen ovale or septal defects), and identify thrombi in the atria or ventricles. RV failure is a common occurrence after LVAD implantation; therefore careful interrogation of the RV is necessary (e.g., tricuspid regurgitation, RV dilatation). The LVAD will create negative pressure at the tip of the cannula in the left ventricle; therefore it is important to repair a shunt to prevent paradoxical embolism of air bubbles and thrombi, as well as to shunt desaturated blood from the right side of the heart to the left. If the patient has AI, the LVAD may create a flow loop, in which blood flowing from the device into the aortic root is drawn back through the incompetent aortic valve, into the device, and back into the root, resulting in insufficient flow to vital organs. Severe AI requires aortic valve repair, replacement, or closure (with sutures), whereas mild to moderate AI may be managed medically and with adjustments in pump parameters. Significant pulmonary valve stenosis and moderate or severe mitral valve stenosis must be addressed to ensure adequate inflow to the LVAD. Aortic valve stenosis is not generally a concern with LVAD implantation; however, mechanical aortic valves must be replaced with a bioprosthetic valve as reduced flow through the aortic valve increases the risk for thromboembolic events. Removing cardiac thrombi is critical to avoid their entry into the pump. Intraoperative TEE findings should be discussed with the surgeon to decide whether deficits should be corrected surgically. Midesophageal four- or two-chamber TEE views help identify the ventriculostomy site for the inflow cannula and the presence of intracardiac air (see American Society of Echocardiography guidelines for echocardiography during management of LVAD patients). Because of the severity of the cardiomyopathy, any reduction in preload, heart rate, or contractility before CPB may produce sudden cardiovascular collapse. Vasoactive agents, such as phenylephrine, ephedrine, epinephrine, norepinephrine, vasopressin, and milrinone, may be required to maintain hemodynamic stability.

The primary cause of failure to wean from CPB is inadequate LV preload. This may be a result of decreased intravascular volume, vasodilation, or RV failure—most commonly secondary to pulmonary hypertension. Therapeutic options to improve LV preload include intravascular volume replacement, vasoconstrictor therapy (vasopressin, norepinephrine, phenylephrine), appropriate inotropic support in the case of RV failure (milrinone, epinephrine, dobutamine), and/or primary pulmonary vasodilator therapy (nitric oxide, prostaglandins). After implantation of the device, TEE is used to assess RV function, valve pathology, shunts, inflow and outflow to the LVAD, and LV preload. The inflow cannula of the device at the LV apex

should be directed toward the mitral valve. The outflow graft is anastomosed to the ascending aorta. Hemodynamic assessment guides the management of the VAD including the pump speed. Low pump speeds may result in a dilated LV, increased LV pressure, increased mitral regurgitation, and pulmonary artery and central venous pressures, whereas high speeds may cause increased AI and suction events (reduced preload causing negative pressure in the LV). Familiarity with the VAD parameters is necessary (i.e., pump speed, pump flow, pump power, and pulsatility index). Once the patient is weaned from CPB, the most common causes of hypotension are decreased intravascular volume, decreased systemic vascular resistance (e.g., vasoplegia), and right-sided heart failure, which must be appropriately treated.

## PATIENTS RECEIVING A TOTAL ARTIFICIAL HEART

A TAH may be an option for patients with biventricular failure when VADs do not provide sufficient support and when confounding factors make heart transplantation unlikely or contraindicated. The anesthetic management for patients undergoing TAH implantation is similar to that previously described. However, because the native ventricles are excised, no benefit is gained from the use of inotropes for the treatment of hypotension. Fluid administration is required to increase intravascular volume and therefore venous return, and vasopressors are used to increase systemic vascular resistance. Again, nitric oxide and prostaglandins may be required to treat pulmonary hypertension. A pulmonary artery catheter, if present, must be removed because it will interfere with the mechanical valves. After anastomosis of the artificial ventricles to the native atria, the mechanical ventricles must be primed. The patient is placed in the Trendelenburg position, and with the use of TEE, the de-airing of the artificial heat is monitored, and the venae cavae and pulmonary veins are inspected for compression. Once the mechanical ventricles are functioning and the hemodynamics are satisfactory, the patient is weaned from CPB, and bleeding is controlled. Familiarity with the TAH parameters (e.g., rate, filling volume, ejection pressures) is necessary for management of these patients. Of note, compression of the venae cavae and pulmonary veins can occur when the chest is closed, with significant bleeding, and in patients with smaller thoracic cavities. TEE is used to assess for compression of these vessels during and after chest closure.

## Postoperative Management

Complications of all devices include bleeding, thromboembolism, infection, hemolysis, device malfunction, and multiorgan failure. The management of the patient with an LVAD or a BiVAD is similar to the management of patients who have had a cardiac surgical procedure with CPB: postoperative bleeding and hemodynamics must be carefully monitored and stabilized, and the patient must be weaned from mechanical ventilation. The possibility of RV dysfunction must be considered in a patient with only an LVAD, if hypotension develops. Once the patient leaves the intensive care unit, the most likely cause of hypotension is decreased preload secondary to decreased intravascular volume.

As the number of patients with VAD implanted continues to increase along with the improved survival, more patients are presenting for noncardiac surgery. For unknown reasons, but probably related to the nonpulsatile blood flow with the second- and third-generation devices, approximately 40% to 50% of these patients will have gastrointestinal bleeding secondary to arteriovenous malformations that form in the walls of the gastrointestinal tract. Therefore these patients often require upper or lower gastrointestinal endoscopy procedures with sedation. For such procedures, noninvasive blood pressure monitoring is usually adequate when there is a palpable radial pulse present. If a pressure reading is attainable with the automated noninvasive blood pressure monitor, the mean cuff pressure is used. Alternatively, Doppler can be used to approximate the mean systemic pressure. The Doppler probe is placed over the brachial artery, distal to a manual blood pressure cuff, and the mean systemic blood pressure is the opening pressure reading (mm Hg) determined by auscultation. For patients requiring general anesthesia, most providers prefer an arterial line for blood pressure monitoring; TEE and central line placement may be necessary when there is significant blood loss, with positioning changes (e.g., prone position), or with increased intraabdominal or intrathoracic pressures (e.g., in laparoscopic and thoracoscopic procedures). Anticoagulation should be managed in consultation with the multidisciplinary team; factors include the urgency of the surgery (elective vs. emergent), the risk of bleeding, and the specific patient risk for thrombosis. Vasoconstrictors are the drug of choice to counteract vasodilation. Dysrhythmia is the most common complication. Appropriate perioperative pacemaker and ICD management is important, and half of patients are observed in the intensive care unit afterward.

## Considerations for Patients for Heart Transplantation

Patients with end-stage heart disease being evaluated for heart transplantation are carefully screened. The patient must be compliant with treatment, without substance abuse (including alcohol), have an adequate support system, be free of cancer, and have a body mass index of less than 38. Severe irreversible pulmonary hypertension is an absolute contraindication to heart transplantation (pulmonary vascular resistance >6 Wood units or >480 dynes·sec$^{-1}$·cm$^{-5}$).

When the United Network for Organ Sharing is notified that a patient has been declared brain dead and the organs are available for transplantation, potential recipients are identified by matching the donor heart with potential recipients, based on the severity of the recipient's disease, through human leukocyte antigen typing, ABO blood group compatibility, and body size. Once the best recipient is identified, the transplant center is notified. If the transplant team and the patient agree, the candidate is posted for transplantation.

Heart transplantation cases always have emergency priority. Donor heart ischemic time should optimally be kept at less than 4 hours. Sterile technique is imperative because the patient will be immunosuppressed and at high risk for infection. Immunosuppression protocols vary; commonly, methylprednisolone is administered intraoperatively. Other immunosuppressant agents may be used, depending on the preferences of the institution's transplant service.

RV failure secondary to pulmonary hypertension is the most common cause of failure to wean from CPB after heart transplantation. Preventing hypoxia and hypercarbia is essential, and the use of pulmonary vasodilators (prostaglandin E$_1$, nitric oxide, milrinone) and inotropes (epinephrine, dobutamine, milrinone) to support the right ventricle may be necessary. Norepinephrine and vasopressin may be needed to maintain systemic vascular resistance. Heart transplantation leads to denervation of the donor heart; only direct-acting β-adrenergic agents or pacing will increase the heart rate. In the early postoperative period, patients are at risk for hyperacute and acute rejection, pulmonary and systemic hypertension, cardiac dysrhythmia, respiratory failure, renal failure, and infection.

Allograft coronary artery disease is the major limiting factor to long-term survival after heart transplantation. This is diffuse disease that involves the vessels circumferentially. Cyclosporine and corticosteroids are the mainstays of long-term immunosuppression and may cause nephrotoxicity, hypertension, and malignant neoplastic disease. The survival rates for transplantation approach 90% for the first year and 75% at the seventh year.

## Conclusion

Management of patients with end-stage heart failure is constantly evolving with the introduction of new technology and devices. The perioperative management of this patient population is complex and requires a multidisciplinary approach. Challenges during the perioperative period include RV failure, coagulopathy, dysrhythmias, systemic inflammatory response syndromes, vasoplegia, and multiorgan failure. As patients with heart failure, a transplanted heart, or a heart with an implanted VAD are presenting for noncardiac surgery with increasing frequency, it is important that all providers understand the pathophysiology of end-stage heart failure, as well as the device and perioperative management of this complex patient population.

## SUGGESTED READINGS

Dalia, A. A., Cronin, B., Stone, M., Turner, K., Hargrave, J., Vidal Melo, M. F., et al. (2018). Anesthetic management of patients with continuous-flow left ventricular assist devices undergoing noncardiac surgery: An update for anesthesiologists. *Journal of Cardiothoracic and Vascular Anesthesia, 32,* 1001–1012.

Kirklin, J. K., Cantor, R., Mohacsi, P., Gummert, J., De By, T., Hannan, M. M., et al. (2016). First annual IMACS report: A global International Society for Heart and Lung Transplantation Registry for Mechanical Circulatory Support. *Journal of Heart and Lung Transplantation, 35,* 407–412.

Molina, E. J., Shah, P., Kiernan, M. S., Cornwell, W. K., III, Copeland, H., Takeda, K., et al. (2021). The Society of Thoracic Surgeons Intermacs 2020 Annual Report. *Annals of Thoracic and Cardiovascular Surgery, 111,* 778–792.

Sladen, R. N. (2017). New innovations of circulatory support with ventricular assist device and extracorporeal membrane oxygenation therapy. *Anesthesia and Analgesia, 124*(4), 1071–1086.

Slininger, K. A., Haddadin, A. S., & Mangi, A. A. (2013). Perioperative management of patients with left ventricular assist devices undergoing non-cardiac surgery. *Journal of Cardiothoracic and Vascular Anesthesia, 27,* 752–759.

Stainbeck, R. F., Estep, J. D., Agler, D. A., Birks, E. J., Bremer, M., Hung, J., et al. (2015). Echocardiography in the management of patients with left ventricular assist devices: Recommendations from the American Society of Echocardiography. *Journal of the American Society of Echocardiography, 28,* 853–909.

Stone, M., Hinchey, J., Sattler, C., & Evans, A. (2016). Trends in the management of patients with left ventricular assist devices presenting for noncardiac surgery: A ten-year institutional experience. *Seminars in Cardiothoracic and Vascular Anesthesia, 20*(3), 197–204.

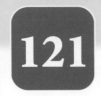

# Coronary Artery Stents

AMY G. VOET, DO, MS, BS | JAMES A. GIACALONE, PhD, MS, BS

Coronary artery stents were first developed in the 1980s and are now placed in most percutaneous coronary interventions (PCIs). Interventional cardiologists have a wide choice of stents for implantation. The choices range from a bare metal stent (BMS) or a drug-eluting stent (DES), both of which are widely used in contemporary practice, to new types of stent, such as a DES with novel coatings, a DES with biodegradable polymers, a DES that is polymer free, biodegradable stents, dedicated bifurcation stents, and self-expanding stents. A number of types of DES are currently undergoing study or are available outside of the United States.

Ulrich Sigwart placed the first stent in 1986. This BMS proved to be effective as a rescue device for patients who were in imminent danger of vessel closure, and it reduced the number of patients undergoing emergency coronary artery bypass grafting. However, the risk of subacute thrombotic coronary occlusion hindered the further development of these stents. Coronary artery stenting finally became widely accepted in 1994 after evidence showed that stenting was safe with the use of dual antiplatelet therapy (DAPT; typically, aspirin and a platelet P2Y12 inhibitor). By 1999, the placement of coronary artery stents made up more than 80% of PCIs. The risk of subacute thrombosis remained, and the new iatrogenic problem of in-stent neointimal hyperplasia developed, which resulted in 20% to 30% restenosis rates, stimulating the development of the DES. The risk of stent thrombosis after the placement of either a BMS or a DES can be reduced by implementation of DAPT, consisting of a P2Y12 inhibitor in combination with aspirin therapy (Table 121.1).

Stent thrombosis has surfaced as the major safety concern after the placement of coronary artery stents. A review of published data showed little difference between DES and BMS in terms of risk of acute and subacute (early stent thrombosis), or late stent thrombosis. However, the risk of very late stent thrombosis with a DES is much higher than with a BMS (0.6%–0.7% vs. 0%–0.2%, respectively). The data also indicate that the risk of stent thrombosis is higher in patients treated

with a DES for off-label use compared with patients treated for on-label use. The exact mechanism remains unclear, but several factors have been implicated. Some risk factors associated with early or late stent thrombosis include early cessation of DAPT, clopidogrel unresponsiveness, complexity of lesions, multistent implantation, small lesion diameter, and lesions longer than 28 to 30 mm. Risk factors associated with very late stent thrombosis include renal failure and previous brachytherapy. Other complications of PCI include hemorrhage, myocardial infarction (MI), stroke, and contrast-induced nephropathy (Table 121.2). Compared with first-generation

| TABLE 121.1 | Definitions |
| --- | --- |
| **Bare metal stent (BMS):** Non–drug-coated vascular stent composed of various metal alloys deployed into a coronary artery or vascular conduit to restore the luminal integrity of the vessel | |
| **Drug-eluting stent (DES):** Drug-coated stent deployed into a coronary artery or vascular conduit to restore the luminal integrity of the vessel and designed to release the coating into the vessel wall to prevent neointimal growth and restenosis | |
| **Acute stent thrombosis:** Stent thrombosis occurring in less than 24 hours | |
| **Subacute stent thrombosis:** Stent thrombosis occurring in less than 30 days | |
| **Late stent thrombosis:** Stent thrombosis occurring in 30 days to 1 year | |
| **Very late stent thrombosis:** Stent thrombosis occurring more than 1 year after implantation | |
| **Aspirin effect:** Aspirin irreversibly acetylates platelet cyclooxygenase–1, preventing formation of thromboxane $A_2$ and thus stimulation of platelet aggregation | |
| **P2Y12 inhibitor:** A class of pharmacologic agents that irreversibly bind to the platelet P2Y12 receptor, inhibiting platelet activation through adenosine diphosphate (ADP) and limiting ADP-mediated conversion of glycoprotein IIb-IIIa to its active form | |

| TABLE 121.2 | Risk Factors for Stent Thrombosis | | | |
| --- | --- | --- | --- | --- |
| **Lesion-Specific Factors** | **Patient Risk Factors** | | **Procedural Factors** | **Device Factors** |
| Bifurcation stenting | Renal failure | | Inadequate stent expansion | Hypersensitivity to drug coating/polymer |
| Ostial stenting | Diabetes mellitus | | Incomplete stent apposition | Incomplete endothelialization |
| Lesion/stent length | Left ventricular impairment (ejection fraction 40%) | | Stent deployment in necrotic lumen | First-generation drug-eluting stent |
| Vessel/stent diameter | Prior brachytherapy | | | |
| Multiple stents/vessels | Prior subacute stent thrombosis | | | |
| Left main artery stent | Premature cessation of dual antiplatelet therapy | | | |
| Bypass graft stent | Clopidogrel unresponsiveness | | | |
| Calcification of vessel | Acute coronary syndrome presentation | | | |

stents, newer-generation DES have an improved safety profile and a lower risk of stent thrombosis.

Hemorrhage that results in hemodynamic instability or transfusion therapy arises in approximately 0.5% to 4% of patients who have undergone PCI and is dependent on several factors, including patient characteristics, the specifics of the procedure, and patient-specific pharmacologic variables. These factors include, but are not limited to, age and sex, location of the femoral arteriotomy, and the level of antithrombotic therapy. The risk of stroke is relatively low (<0.2%), whereas MI complicates 5% to 38% of PCIs, with the rate depending on the definition used for MI. New Q-wave appearance has an incidence of 1%, whereas any elevation of creatine kinase–MB occurs in up to 38% of patients. Contrast-induced nephropathy is also dependent on multiple variables, including age, presence of congestive heart failure, preexisting renal failure, previous exposure to contrast agents, and presence of peripheral vascular disease, and is seen in approximately 5% to 6% patients.

## Recommendations

The American College of Cardiology/American Heart Association (ACC/AHA) guidelines were updated in 2016. The 2016 ACC/AHA guideline focused on duration of dual antiplatelet therapy in patients with coronary artery disease. In December 2021, an update for the ACC/AHA/SCAI Guideline for Coronary Artery Revascularization: A Report of the American College of Cardiology/American Heart Association Joint Committee on Clinical Practice Guidelines was published. This contained an update with recommendations for DAPT after PCI. The caveat was that the new recommendations are to be used as a supplemental guide to the 2016 DAPT recommendations given the limitations of the studies, as well as the multiplicity of antiplatelet regimens now available. The primary studies used for the new recommendations came from the STOPDAPT-2 trial, the SMART-CHOICE trial, and the TICO trial. These trials had many limitations. The patient population tended to have a low ischemic risk, few had an ST-segment elevation MI, and there were underrepresented racial and ethnic groups.

The recommendations for DAPT after PCI have been broken down into stable ischemic heart disease (SIHD) and acute coronary syndrome (ACS), as well as patient risk for ischemia. The risk of bleeding is also a consideration that is addressed in the recommendations (Fig. 121.1). For a patient with SIHD who is receiving a DES, there is class I evidence to use a P2Y12 inhibitor for at least 6 months. There is now class IIa evidence that discontinuation of aspirin after 1 to 3 months with continuation of P2Y12 inhibitor monotherapy is reasonable to reduce overt bleeding risk. If there is high risk of overt bleeding, there is class IIb evidence to discontinue P2Y12 inhibitors. If there is not a high risk of bleeding and there is no significant overt bleeding on DAPT, there is class IIb evidence to suggest continuing DAPT for longer than 6 months. SIHD with BMS has class I evidence to continue a P2Y12 inhibitor for at least 1 month. If there is not a high risk of bleeding and there is no overt bleeding, there is class IIb evidence to continue for longer than 1 month. For ACS, whether there is BMS or DES, there is class I evidence to continue the P2Y12 inhibitor for 12 months. There is now class IIa evidence that it may be reasonable to discontinue aspirin after 1 to 3 months and continue DAPT as monotherapy. If there is no significant risk of bleeding and there is no overt bleeding, there is class IIb evidence to continue DAPT for longer than 12 months. If there is a high risk of bleeding, there is class IIb evidence to suggest discontinuing DAPT after 6 months. No optimal duration of prolonged DAPT has been established past 12 months. A DAPT risk score has been developed by Yeh and colleagues that may be helpful in guiding prolonged use of DAPT for longer than 1 year. A score of 2 or greater indicates that the benefit of prolonged DAPT outweighs the risk. A score of less than 2 indicates that the risk may outweigh the benefit (Table 121.3).

The guidelines state that there is class III evidence of harm for a patient treated with PCI involving a DES and DAPT for less than 1 to 3 months who is facing elective noncardiac surgery; thus surgery should be delayed. For patients treated for 3 to 6 months, when the risk of delaying surgery is greater than the risk of stent thrombosis, there is class IIb evidence to discontinue DAPT and proceed with surgery. If it has been longer than 6 months since DES implantation, there is class I evidence to proceed with surgery. If it has been less than 30 days since BMS implantation, there is class III evidence of harm; thus surgery should be delayed. If it has been 30 days or more since implantation, there is class I evidence to proceed with surgery. If the operation cannot be delayed, it may need to be performed while the patient is receiving dual therapy or aspirin alone because surgery itself causes a prothrombotic state. If the P2Y12 inhibitor must be withheld, it should optimally be held for 5 days or less preoperatively for patients with DES, who are at higher risk for thrombosis. After the procedure, platelet P2Y12 inhibitor therapy should be restarted as soon as possible. Maximizing the success of the operation requires collaboration among the cardiologist, surgeon, and anesthesiologist and sufficient lead time (2 weeks) before the procedure to allow for implementation of perioperative, intraoperative, and postoperative plans. Although this collaboration can be logistically challenging, it is an essential component of high-quality, safe perioperative care. Discussion with the patient about treatment options is also necessary for the patient to make an informed decision. The operation should be performed at a facility with the ability to perform emergency PCI or cardiac surgery. Stent thrombosis typically presents as acute MI, cardiogenic shock, and sudden death; thus immediate thrombus retrieval is essential. Finally, it is imperative to educate patients about the risks of early discontinuation of DAPT and to clearly encourage compliance with the prescribed regimen. It is important to seek the most recent ACC/AHA guidance in this complex area of practice.

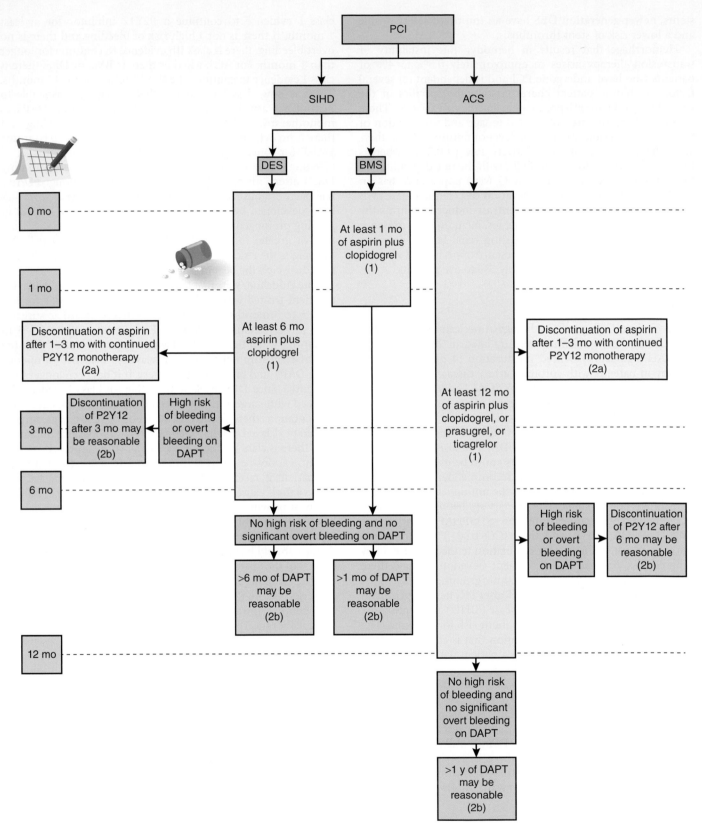

**Fig. 121.1** **Treatment algorithm for duration of P2Y12 inhibitor therapy in patients treated with percutaneous coronary intervention** *(PCI).* Colors correspond to Class of Recommendation in Table 121.1. *Arrows* at the bottom of the figure denote that the optimal duration of prolonged dual antiplatelet therapy *(DAPT)* is not established. Clopidogrel is the only currently used P2Y12 inhibitor studied in patients with stable ischemic heart disease *(SIHD)* undergoing PCI. Aspirin therapy is almost always continued indefinitely in patients with coronary artery disease. "High risk of bleeding" denotes those who have or develop a high risk of bleeding (e.g., treatment with oral anticoagulant therapy) or are at increased risk of severe bleeding complication (e.g., major intracranial surgery). *ACS,* acute coronary syndrome; *BMS,* bare metal stent; *DES,* drug-eluting stent. (From Lawton JS, Tamis-Holland JE, Bangalore S, et al. 2021 ACC/AHA/SCAI Guideline for Coronary Artery Revascularization: A Report of the American College of Cardiology/American Heart Association Joint Committee on Clinical Practice Guidelines. Circulation. 2022;145:e18–e114.)

| TABLE 121.3 | Clinical Prediction Score to Stratify Individual Risk of Benefit Versus Harm With Continuation of Dual Antiplatelet Therapy Beyond 1 Year After Percutaneous Coronary Intervention | |
| --- | --- | --- |
| **Variable** | | **Points** |
| Age ≥75 years | | −2 |
| Age 65 to <75 years | | −1 |
| Age <65 years | | 0 |
| Current smoker | | 1 |
| Diabetes mellitus | | 1 |
| MI at presentation | | 1 |
| Prior PCI or MI | | 1 |
| Stent diameter <3 mm | | 1 |
| Paclitaxel-eluting stint | | 1 |
| CHF or LVEF <30% | | 2 |
| Saphenous vein graft PCI | | 2 |

*CHF,* Congestive heart failure; *LVEF,* left ventricular ejection fraction; *MI,* myocardial infarction; *PCI,* percutaneous coronary intervention.

## SUGGESTED READINGS

Hahn, J. Y., Song, Y. B., Oh, J. H., Chun, W. J., Park, Y. H., Jang, W. J., et al. (2019). Effect of P2Y12 inhibitor monotherapy vs dual antiplatelet therapy on cardiovascular events in patients undergoing percutaneous coronary intervention: The SMART-CHOICE randomized clinical trial. *JAMA, 321,* 2428–2437.

Kim, B. K., Hong, S. J., Cho, Y. H., Yun, K. H., Kim, Y. H., Suh, Y., et al. (2020). Effect of ticagrelor monotherapy vs ticagrelor with aspirin on major bleeding and cardiovascular events in patients with acute coronary syndrome: The TICO randomized clinical trial. *JAMA, 323,* 2407–2416.

Lawton, J. S., Tamis-Holland, J. E., Bangalore, S., Bates, E. R., Beckie, T. M., Bischoff, J. M., et al. (2022). 2021 ACC/AHA/SCAI Guideline for coronary artery revascularization: A Report of the American College of Cardiology/American Heart Association Joint Committee on Clinical Practice Guidelines. *Circulation, 145,* e18–e114.

Levine, Glen N., et al. (2016). Chair of ACC/AHA Task Force. 2016 ACC/AHA guideline focused on duration of dual antiplatelet therapy in patients with coronary artery disease. *Journal of the American College of Cardiology, 68*(10), 1082-1115.

Savonitto, S., D'Urbano, M., Caracciolo, M., Barlocco, F., Mariani, G., Nichelatti, M., et al. (2010). Urgent surgery in patients with a recently implanted coronary drug-eluting stent: A phase II study of "bridging" antiplatelet therapy with tirofiban during temporary withdrawal of clopidogrel. *British Journal of Anaesthesia, 104,* 285–291.

Watanabe, H., Domei, T., Morimoto, T., Natsuaki, M., Shiomi, H., Toyota, T., et al. (2019). Effect of 1-month dual antiplatelet therapy followed by clopidogrel vs 12-month dual antiplatelet therapy on cardiovascular and bleeding events in patients receiving PCI: The STOPDAPT-2 randomized clinical trial. *JAMA, 321,* 2414–2427.

Yeh, R. W., Secemsky, E., Kereiakes, D. J., Normand, S. L., Gershlick, A. H., Cohen, D. J., et al. (2016). Development and validation of a prediction rule for benefit and harm of dual antiplatelet therapy beyond one year after percutaneous coronary intervention: An analysis from the randomized Dual Antiplatelet Therapy Study. *JAMA, 315*(16), 1735–1749.

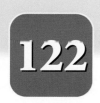

# 122

# Cardiopulmonary Bypass

EDUARDO S. RODRIGUES, MD  |  ARCHER KILBOURNE MARTIN, MD

## Basic Cardiopulmonary Bypass Structure

When centrally cannulated, a right atrial or bicaval cannulae (superior venous cannula [SVC] and inferior venous cannula [IVC]) are the sources for venous blood return into the venous reservoir. For peripheral cannulation, femoral and internal jugular veins provide alternative sites for venous cannulation; this approach is frequent during minimally invasive cardiac surgery. The deoxygenated blood exits the reservoir, traveling to a pump (roller or centrifugal), where it is pumped through an oxygenator (typically hollow fiber) and an integrated heat exchanger. $Pao_2$ is determined by the $Fio_2$ of the fresh gas flow passing countercurrently through the hollow fibers for hollow-fiber oxygenators, whereas the total gas flow rate determines $Paco_2$ through the oxygenator (sweep speed). The pressurized oxygenated blood typically passes through an arterial line filter before entering the arterial cannula (centrally placed in the proximal aorta or alternative peripheral sites). The pressure in the cardiopulmonary bypass (CPB) arterial line is directly measured and managed by the perfusionist, with general perfusion guidelines recommending avoidance of arterial line pressures above 300 mm Hg. Standard adult arterial cannula sizes range from 18F to 22F, with the larger cannulae allowing higher flow rates with lower line pressure levels. Additional features of the CPB circuit include several monitors of line pressures, flow, temperature and oxygenation, a cardioplegia delivery system, and a means for cardiotomy suctioning and ventricular venting.

## Control of Systemic Oxygenation During Cardiopulmonary Bypass

The factors that control systemic oxygenation during non-CPB conditions also control oxygenation during CPB. Oxygen requirements are most profoundly affected by body temperature, whereas $O_2$ delivery ($\dot{D}o_2$) is determined by pump flow and hematocrit.

## Basic Relationships

Arterial $O_2$ content $\left(CaO_2\right)$

$$= 1.34 \,(\text{hemoglobin}) \left(O_2\text{sat}\%\right) + 0.003 \left(PaO_2\right)$$

Arteriovenous $O_2$ content difference $\left(CaO_2 - C\overline{v}o_2\right)$

$$= CaO_2 - C\overline{v}o_2$$

Systemic $\dot{D}o_2 = \text{cardiac output or CPB pump flow}$

$$\times \, CaO_2 \text{ Systemic } O_2 \text{ consumption } \left(\dot{V}o_2\right)$$

$$= \text{cardiac output} \times \left(CaO_2 - C\overline{v}o_2\right)$$

The temperature coefficient ($Q_{10}$) describes the ratio of metabolic rates at two temperatures separated by 10°C. In humans, the $Q_{10}$ is approximately 2 (i.e., when a patient's temperature increases from 27°C to 37°C, the metabolic rate doubles). Conversely, every 10°C decrease in body temperature decreases the by approximately 50%.

## General Practice of Cardiopulmonary Bypass

Although cardiopulmonary bypass can occur with either pulsatile or nonpulsatile flow, the latter method of perfusion predominates. There are no relevant differences in clinical outcomes when pulsatile flow is compared with nonpulsatile flow. Nonpulsatile flow (2.0–2.5 $L \cdot min^{-1} \cdot m^{-2}$) is based on the cardiac index under anesthesia in non-CPB conditions. The flow rate may also be expressed as $mL \cdot kg^{-1} \cdot min^{-1}$. The most recent

literature suggests that mild to moderate hypothermia close to the normal range (i.e., 28°C–35°C) reduces the incidence of low cardiac output syndromes post-CPB without an attendant increase in neurologic complications.

Moderate normovolemic hemodilution should be maintained. The literature, comprising primarily retrospective data, suggests that increased complication rates (neurologic, cardiovascular, and renal) occur when the hematocrit is less than 20% to 23%. However, other data suggest that addressing this anemia with transfusion of red blood cells may worsen outcomes. It is likely that CPB-related anemia is a function of the prebypass period and therefore is primarily a marker of greater comorbidity instead of being an independent determinant of adverse outcome.

There isn't consensus in the literature regarding the ideal mean arterial pressure (MAP) during CPB. Even with moderate hypothermia, cerebral autoregulation begins to fail below a cerebral perfusion pressure of 50 to 55 mm Hg. A recent study suggests that tailoring MAP to a patient's specific autoregulation may improve neurologic outcomes, as they found that the product of duration and magnitude of MAP below autoregulatory limits was associated with perioperative risk of stroke in cardiac surgery. In patients with a history of hypertension or peripheral vascular disease, keeping the MAP at 70 mm Hg or higher reduces the incidence of adverse cardiac and neurologic outcomes. It is the author's preference to maintain the MAP during CPB within 20% of preoperative mean blood pressure, respecting the patient's baseline cerebral autoregulation. A very practical way to calculate the goal MAP during CPB is to use the patient's age as a goal for MAP in patients older than 60 years.

## Cardiopulmonary Bypass Hemodynamics and Hemodilution

Under non-CPB conditions, moderate hemodilution decreases $Cao_2$ but may not decrease $\dot{D}o_2$ because hemodilution is associated with increases in cardiac output. However, during CPB, pump flow is typically less than the cardiac output that would be seen with equivalent hemodilution under non-CPB conditions, resulting in a decrease in whole body $\dot{D}o_2$ during CPB that is approximately equivalent to the degree of hemodilution. Additionally, in the absence of increases in compensatory flow, MAP during CPB is typically reduced secondary to lower blood viscosity associated with hemodilution that subsequently reduces systemic vascular resistance (SVR).

## Effect of Temperature Change on Systemic Oxygenation

Hypothermia to 27°C reduces systemic $O_2$ requirements by approximately 60%. Because $O_2$ demand decreases so dramatically with hypothermia, adequate oxygenation can be maintained with reduced flow, greater degrees of hemodilution, or a combination thereof. However, during early and late CPB, when patients approximate normothermia, the margin between systemic $O_2$ supply and demand is narrowed. A beneficial effect of hypothermia is that the associated increases in SVR may offset the reductions in SVR associated with hemodilution alone.

## Effect of Anesthetic Depth on Systemic Oxygenation

Anesthetic depth has less influence than does hypothermia on $\dot{V}o_2$ during CPB. However, anesthetic depth is of greater relative importance at body temperatures greater than 32°C. Plasma levels of anesthetic agents decrease with the onset of CPB secondary to dilution from an increased circulatory volume. Therefore intravenous infusion techniques or inhalation agents integrated into the circuit structure during CPB help ensure adequate anesthesia.

## Monitoring the Adequacy of Perfusion During Cardiopulmonary Bypass

### SYSTEMIC $O_2$ SATURATION

Mixed venous $O_2$ saturation ($S\bar{v}o_2$) reflects venous $O_2$ content (i.e., the amount of $O_2$ left in the venous blood after systemic $O_2$ requirements are met). Although $S\bar{v}o_2$ does not measure either $\dot{V}o_2$ or $\dot{D}o_2$, it does provide an index of the adequacy of their matching. As such, $S\bar{v}o_2$ monitoring conveys extremely valuable information on the interaction among systemic $O_2$ requirements, pump flow, arterial $O_2$ content, hematocrit level, and temperature. $S\bar{v}o_2$ greater than 65% generally indicates a satisfactory margin of safety for systemic oxygenation. A higher saturation is indicated during hypothermia, given that hypothermia increases the $O_2$ affinity of hemoglobin.

Inline hemoglobin or hematocrit monitors are available and are usually coupled to the detector. Temperature monitoring is performed in three areas: the venous line (reflecting the adequacy of whole-body cooling or warming), the arterial inflow line, and the heat exchanger, where the temperature should not exceed 38.5°C. Optional arterial inflow line monitoring devices are available to monitor gases ($Pao_2$, pH, $Paco_2$, base deficit, and temperature).

## Difficulties in Maintaining Systemic Oxygenation During Cardiopulmonary Bypass

During stable hypothermia, systemic oxygenation is easy to maintain, but the transitions to and from hypothermia can be a problem. Initiation of CPB is associated with nearly instantaneous hemodilution and decreased SVR. In the absence of increased flow, hypotension commonly occurs until cooling is initiated, SVR is increased pharmacologically, or volume resuscitation occurs. During rewarming from CPB, SVR and MAP will fall as vasodilation occurs and blood viscosity decreases. This occurs at a time when systemic $O_2$ demand may double (27°C–37°C).

## Cardioplegia

Cardioplegia with a high-$K^+$ solution results in depolarization and cardiac arrest. This induces electromechanical silence and reduces myocardial $O_2$ demand by more than 80%. The use of cardioplegia is indicated when the aortic cross-clamp is in place because there is no coronary blood flow at this time. Cardioplegia may consist of an oxygenated blood–high-$K^+$ mixture (blood cardioplegia) or a high-$K^+$ solution alone (crystalloid cardioplegia). Cardioplegia is usually given intermittently into the aorta proximal to the cross-clamp (antegrade) or directly into the coronary ostia. Retrograde cardioplegia via the coronary sinus is also used, particularly in aortic regurgitant lesions or in the presence of severe coronary artery disease. Left ventricular hypertrophy and coronary artery disease make myocardial protection more difficult to achieve and may require the perfusion team to deliver higher amounts of cardioplegia than normal in order to achieve electromechanical silence.

## SUGGESTED READINGS

Engelman, R., Baker, R. A., Likosky, D. S., Grigore, A., Dickinson, T. A., Shore-Lesserson, L., et al. (2015). The Society of Thoracic Surgeons, The Society of Cardiovascular Anesthesiologists, and the American Society of ExtraCorporeal Technology: Clinical Practice Guidelines for Cardiopulmonary Bypass – Temperature Management During Cardiopulmonary Bypass. *Journal of Extra-Corporeal Technology, 47*(3), 145–154.

Gravlee, G. P., Davis, R. F., Hammon, J., & Kussman, B. (2016). *Cardiopulmonary bypass and mechanical support: Principles and practice* (4th ed.). Philadelphia: Wolters Kluwer.

Grocott, H. P., Stafford-Smith, M., & Mora-Mangano, C. T. (2017). Cardiopulmonary bypass management and organ protection. In J. A. Kaplan (Ed.), *Cardiac anesthesia for cardiac and non-cardiac surgery* (7th ed., Vol. 31, pp. 1111–1161). Philadelphia: Elsevier.

Hori, D., Nomura, Y., Ono, M., Joshi, B., Mandal, K., Cameron, D., et al. (2017). Optimal blood pressure during cardiopulmonary bypass defined by cerebral autoregulation monitoring. *Journal of Thoracic and Cardiovascular Surgery, 154*(5), 1590–1598.e2.

Murphy, G. S., Hessel, E. A., & Groom, R. C. (2009). Optimal perfusion during cardiopulmonary

bypass: An evidence-based approach. *Anesthesia and Analgesia, 108,* 1394–1417.

Sarwar, M., Searles, B. E., Stone, M. E., & Shore-Lesserson, L. (2020). Anesthesia for cardiac surgical procedures. In R. D. Miller (Ed.), *Anesthesia* (9th ed., pp. 1717–1814). Philadelphia: Saunders.

Wahba, A., Milojevic, M., Boer, C., De Somer, F. M. J. J., Gudbjartsson, T., van den Goor, J., et al. (2020). 2019 EACTS/EACTA/EBCP guidelines on cardiopulmonary bypass in adult cardiac surgery. *European Journal of Cardio-Thoracic Surgery, 57*(2), 210–251.

# 123

# Evaluation of the Coagulation System

PATRICK O. MCCONVILLE, MD, FASA | ROBERT M. CRAFT, MD

Classically, the coagulation system has been described in terms of the extrinsic and intrinsic pathways for the secondary phase of hemostasis, ultimately arriving in a common pathway for hemostasis (Fig. 123.1). However, this description is inadequate, as the pathways are linked from the beginning of the process. More recently, coagulation systems are described as a three-part process: the initiation phase, the amplification phase, and the propagation phase. This three-stage process contains multiple complex interactions with platelets, the endothelium, and coagulation factors.

## Preoperative Assessment

Current evidence does not support the routine use of screening tests in the perioperative period in patients without risk factors for coagulopathy. A thorough history and physical with emphasis on family history of bleeding disorders, perioperative bleeding in the past, liver disease, and medication review is a sufficient screening tool in most patients.

## Common Point-of-Care Tests of Coagulation

Point-of-care (POC) tests have continued to increase in the perioperative period because of the expanding spectrum of available tests, the ease of running the tests, and the ability to obtain rapid results. Although in vitro coagulation tests including the prothrombin time (PT) and the activated partial thromboplastin time (aPTT) provide information on initial thrombin formation in plasma, several POC tests evaluate the ability of whole blood to generate clot. A variety of tests may be used to assess the coagulation system perioperatively depending on the clinical scenario.

### VISCOELASTIC MEASUREMENT OF COAGULATION

Viscoelastic measures of coagulation include thromboelastography, rotational thromboelastography, and the Sonoclot analyzer (Sienco Inc, Boulder, CO). These whole-blood tests measure the time from early fibrin strand generation to clot fibrinolysis. Coagulation is measured and displayed graphically in Figs. 123.2 and 123.3, and the variables and common abnormalities are shown. These viscoelastic POC tests are helpful in providing information for goal-directed therapy in the setting of major blood loss, disseminated intravascular coagulation (DIC), or other unknown coagulopathies. Some studies have shown that transfusion protocols triggered by thromboelastography compared with conventional coagulation tests modestly reduced the transfusion of red blood cells, platelets, and plasma in cardiac surgery. The Society of Cardiovascular Anesthesiologists 2019 guidelines for management of hemostasis in patients

in Enhanced Recovery After Cardiac Surgery (ERACS) protocols include the use of viscoelastic coagulation tests to guide transfusion therapy. There is insufficient evidence, however, showing improved clinically relevant outcome in trauma surgery and postpartum hemorrhage patients. Viscoelastic coagulation tests are limited in their ability to detect coagulopathies caused by hypothermia or hyperthermia, abnormalities in pH, calcium ion concentration, or hematocrit.

## Functional Measurement of Anticoagulation

### ACTIVATED CLOTTING TIME

Activated clotting time (ACT) is widely used to measure the adequacy of heparin-induced anticoagulation for cardiac catheterization and extracorporeal circuit use, such as cardiopulmonary bypass (CPB) and extracorporeal oxygenation. Although it is used commonly because of its simplicity and low cost, the ACT has poor reproducibility and is prolonged in hypothermia, hemodilution, thrombocytopenia, and platelet dysfunction.

### HEPARIN CONCENTRATION MEASUREMENT

Protamine titration is the most common method for assessing heparin concentration in the perioperative period. Protamine titration is capable of measuring heparin concentrations because every 1–1.5 mg of protamine will neutralize 100 units of heparin (1 mg). Thus, if a blood sample is divided and analyzed with several doses of protamine, the portion with the closest heparin and protamine concentrations will clot the most rapidly. The approximate heparin dose to obtain a specific plasma heparin concentration can be determined, as well as the amount of protamine needed to reverse a specific heparin concentration. Advantages of the protamine titration method include relative resistance to the effects of hypothermia and hemodilution, as well as sensitivity at low heparin concentrations. POC monitors currently in use, such as Hepcon HMS (Medtronic Blood Management, Parker, CO), use automated measurement techniques.

### PLATELET FUNCTION MONITORING

Although platelet dysfunction can be detected using viscoelastic POC tests, specificity and sensitivity are limited. CPB, DIC, and multiple platelet-altering medications can alter both platelet quantity and quality in the perioperative period. POC platelet function tests have been created to determine the effects of antiplatelet medications on platelet function. These can be used to guide antiplatelet therapy or to determine the degree of a perioperative patient's platelet dysfunction.

## Blood Coagulation: Pathways of Activation

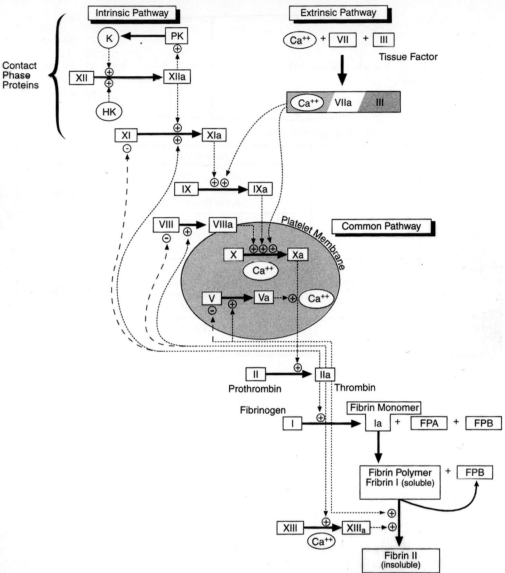

**Fig. 123.1** Activation of proteins leading to blood coagulation. A positive feedback system (amplification) magnifies initial pathway reactions. A negative feedback system (inhibition) serves as a countervailing force and limits coagulation. *Dotted arrows* and + signs indicate facilitation of the process; *dashed arrows* and − signs indicate inhibition of the process. The intrinsic pathway is initiated by the action of kallikrein *(K)* and high-molecular-weight kininogen *(HK)* and prekallikrein *(PK)* cofactors on factor XII. Fibrinopeptide A *(FPA)* and fibrinopeptide B *(FPB)* are two peptides that are released when the fibrin monomer is formed. (From Carvalho ACA. Hemostasis and thrombosis. In: Schiffman FJ, ed. *Hematologic Pathophysiology*. Lippincott-Raven; 1998:161–243.)

Some of the POC platelet function analyzers include the PFA-100 (Platelet Function Analyzer; Dade International Inc. Deerfield, IL), Plateletworks (Helena Laboratories, Beaumont, TX), Multiplate (Roche Diagnostics GmbH, Basel, Switzerland), and VerifyNow (Accumetrics, San Diego, CA). PFA-100 uses whole blood pulled with a vacuum through a membrane containing various platelet activators, simulating vascular injury, and can be used to identify platelet dysfunction from various congenital disorders or medications. The Plateletworks test measures platelet aggregation in the presence and absence of adenosine diphosphate or collagen, which correlates with optical platelet aggregometry. Multiplate simulates platelet aggregation with various agonists, thereby measuring the ability of

platelet response to stimulation. VerifyNow is an additional POC platelet aggregation test that can detect thienopyridine, glycoprotein 11b-111a antagonists, and aspirin-induced antiplatelet effects.

## COAGULATION TESTS

Table 123.1 summarizes the most common preoperative coagulation studies. In vitro coagulation POC coagulation tests include aPTT, PT, and the international normalized ratio (INR). These tests are widely available and can help guide treatment for patients on warfarin therapy. They provide information on initial thrombin formation in plasma.

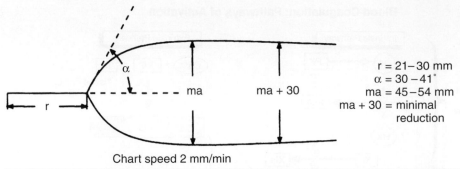

Chart speed 2 mm/min

$$r = 21 - 30 \text{ mm}$$
$$\alpha = 30 - 41°$$
$$ma = 45 - 54 \text{ mm}$$
$$ma + 30 = \text{minimal reduction}$$

| Variable | Measures | Abnormality | | Example |
|---|---|---|---|---|
| r<br>reaction<br>time | thromboplastin<br>generation via the<br>intrinsic pathway | ↑ r | Factor deficiency<br>Heparin<br>Severe thrombocytopenia | Factor deficiency 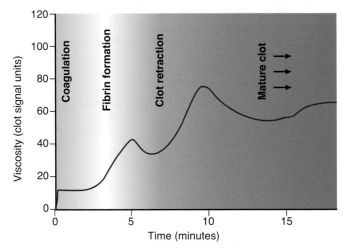 |
| α<br>angle of<br>divergence | rate of clot<br>formation | ↓ α | Hypofibrinogenemia<br>Thrombocytopenia<br>Thrombocytopathy | Hypofibrinogenemia |
| ma<br>maximum<br>amplitude | maximum clot<br>strength/elasticity | ↓ ma | Thrombocytopenia<br>Thrombocytopathy<br>Hypofibrinogenemia<br>Factor XIII deficiency | Thrombocytopenia |
| ma + 30 | clot retraction<br>after 30 minutes | ↓ ma + 30 | Fibrinolysis | Fibrinolysis |

**Fig. 123.2**  Typical thromboelastograph pattern and variables measured, normal values, and examples of abnormal tracings.

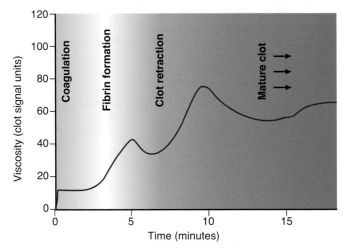

**Fig. 123.3**  As the blood sample clots, a variety of hemostasis-related mechanical changes occur that alter the signal value of the clot. A typical Sonoclot signature is shown (Sienco Inc, Arvada, CO).

| TABLE 123.1 | Common Preoperative Studies to Assess Coagulation Status | |
|---|---|---|
| Test | Measured Aspect | Comments |
| PT | Extrinsic pathway and common pathway | PT is prolonged if any of factors VII, X, V, II, and I are deficient, abnormal, or inhibited. <br><br> The coagulant activity of these factors must be <30% of normal and the fibrinogen concentration must be <100 mg/dL for PT to be prolonged. <br><br> PT may be used as a screening test for patients receiving oral anti-coagulant therapy. <br><br> PT may be used to assess the synthetic function of the liver. |
| aPTT | Intrinsic pathway and common pathway | The aPTT is prolonged when any of factors XII, XI, IX, VIII, X, V, II, and I are deficient, abnormal, or inhibited. <br><br> The coagulant activity of these factors must be <30% of normal and the fibrinogen concentration must be <100 mg/dL for PT to be prolonged. <br><br> The aPTT is prolonged by heparin therapy. <br><br> The aPTT is prolonged in those with hemophilia and usually in those with von Willebrand disease. |
| Fibrinogen | Fibrinogen level and common pathway | Levels <100 mg/dL may be associated with inability to form a clot and severe bleeding. |
| Platelet count | Quantitative platelet assessment | Platelet count does not provide information on platelet function. <br><br> Thrombocytopenia is defined as a platelet count <150,000/μL. <br><br> Bleeding during surgery may be severe in patients with platelet counts of 40,000–70,000/μL. <br><br> Spontaneous bleeding is unlikely to occur if the platelet count is >10,000–20,000/μL. |
| Bleeding time | Platelet function assessed by evaluating the time for a platelet plug to form after vascular injury | Bleeding time is prolonged in patients with platelet dysfunction (e.g., those receiving aspirin therapy or those with uremia). <br><br> Because of the techniques used for the test, reproducibility is poor and results are imprecise. <br><br> Bleeding time is not useful for routine screening. |
| Platelet aggregometry | Ability of platelets to aggregate after exposure to adenosine diphosphate, epinephrine, collagen, or ristocetin | Only qualitative results (clot retraction vs. no clot retraction) are reported. <br><br> Quantitative results are difficult to obtain. |

*aPTT,* Activated partial thromboplastin time; *PT,* prothrombin time.

## SUGGESTED READINGS

Bolliger, D., & Tanaka, K. A. (2013). Roles of thromb-elastography and thromboelastometry for patient blood management in cardiac surgery. *Transfusion Medicine Reviews, 27,* 213–220.

Bolliger, D., & Tanaka, K. A. (2017). Point-of-care testing in cardiac surgery. *Seminars in Thrombosis and Hemostasis, 43,* 386–396.

Karkouti, K., McCluskey, S. A., Callum, J., Freedman, J., Selby, R., Timoumi, T., et al. (2015). Evaluation of a novel transfusion algorithm employing point-of-care coagulation assays in cardiac surgery, retrospective cohort study with inter-rupted Time-Series Analysis. *Anesthesiology, 122,* 560–570.

Keyl, C., Bashota, A., Beyersdorf, F., & Trenk, D. (2022). Rotational thromboelastometry and con-ventional coagulation tests in patients undergoing major cardiac or aortic surgery: A retrospective single-center cohort study. *Journal of Thrombosis and Thrombolysis, 53,* 149–157.

Nath, S. S., Pandey, C. K., & Kumar, S. (2022). Clinical application of viscoelastic point-of-care tests of coagulation-shifting paradigms. *Annals of Cardiac Anaesthesia, 25,* 1–10.

Panigrahi, A. K., & Liu, L. L. (2020). Patient blood management: Coagulation. In M. A. Gropper (Ed.), *Miller's anesthesia* (9th ed., pp. 1579–1602). Philadelphia, PA: Elsevier.

Patel, P. A., Henderson, R. A., Jr., Bolliger, D., Erdoes, G., & Mazzeffi, M. A. (2021). The year in coagulation: Selected highlights from 2020. *Journal of Cardiotho-racic and Vascular Anesthesia, 35,* 2260–2272.

Rafael, J., Mazer, C. D., Subramani, S., Schroeder, A., Abdalla, M., Ferreira, R., et al. (2019). Society of Cardiovascular Anesthesiologists Clinical Prac-tice Improvement Advisory for management of perioperative bleeding and hemostasis in cardiac surgery patients. *Anesthesia and Analgesia, 129,* 1209–1221.

Terwindt, L. E., Karlas, A. A., Eberl, S., Wijnberge, M., Driessen, A. H. G., Veelo, D. P., et al. (2019). Patient blood management in the cardiac surgical setting: An updated overview. *Transfusion and Apheresis Science, 58,* 397–407.

# Anticoagulation and Reversal for Cardiopulmonary Bypass

BRIAN S. DONAHUE, MD, PhD

## Heparin

Heparin anticoagulation and reversal by protamine constitute the mainstay of cardiopulmonary bypass (CPB) management. Heparin is a glycosaminoglycan, or mucopolysaccharide, composed of alternating D-glucuronic N-acetyl-D-glucosamine acid residues. Commercial heparin is a mixture of these polysaccharides, having molecular weights in the range of 5000 to 30,000 Da (5–35 saccharide units). Heparin has one of the highest negative charge-to-size ratios of any known biologic compound. Heparan sulfate is a related biologic compound that has fewer sulfate groups than heparin and, therefore, has less potency. Heparin inhibits coagulation by serving as a catalyst: antithrombin III (AT) binds to its surface, inducing a conformational change in AT, making its active site more accessible to any of several proteases involved in the intrinsic and common coagulation pathways (thrombin [IIa], factor Xa, factor XIa, factor XIIa, and factor IXa). However, the anticoagulant effects of heparin are primarily mediated by the inhibition of thrombin and factor Xa that occurs when thrombin and factor Xa are bound by AT. Once these covalent bonds are established, the heparin moiety is released and available to bind to another molecule of AT.

Heparin has many other effects on coagulation independent of AT. There is some evidence that heparin can activate plasmin, contributing to fibrinolysis during cardiac surgery. Heparin binds platelets and can induce some aggregation, but the physiologic results of this interaction are not well understood, especially in cardiac surgery. Heparin also induces the release of tissue factor pathway inhibitor from endothelium, independent of AT. Fragments of tissue factor pathway inhibitor persist in circulation after protamine reversal and may contribute to post-CPB coagulopathy.

Heparin use is complex because not all molecules in a preparation of heparin have similar biologic activity or have any biologic activity at all. The ability of a specific heparin molecule to bind and activate AT is dependent on it having a critical pentasaccharide sequence, which is present in only about a third of all heparin molecules in a commercial preparation. Longer chains (>18 saccharides) are needed for the resulting heparin-AT complex to inhibit thrombin, whereas the critical pentasaccharide sequence alone is sufficient to inhibit factor Xa. Therefore a major drawback to the clinical of use of heparin is the variability in heparin response. In addition to polysaccharide chain length and composition, numerous other factors account for variability in response, such as availability of AT, availability of heparin cofactor II, and nonspecific heparin binding to plasma proteins, lipoproteins, macrophages, and endothelium. There is some evidence that heparin can activate plasmin, contributing to fibrinolysis during cardiac surgery. Heparin does bind platelets, but the physiologic results of this interaction are not well understood.

## Administration and Monitoring of Heparin During Cardiopulmonary Bypass

Heparin for CPB is administered intravenously as a bolus dose of 300 to 400 units/kg. Traditionally, the extent of inhibition of coagulation has been monitored using the whole-blood activated clotting time (ACT). With this technique, the patient's blood is mixed in a test tube with an activator (e.g., diatomite or kaolin), and the time until clot forms is recorded as the ACT. Although practice varies markedly, most surgical teams require an ACT of 350 to 450 seconds before they will allow initiation of CPB. The ACT is widely used because it has several advantages: the prolongation of the ACT is generally linear with the heparin level, and the test is widely available, is inexpensive, is easy to perform, and has stood the test of time.

The use of ACT has many drawbacks: there is wide variability not only between tests of blood run on different instruments but also between aliquots of the same blood run on the same instrument. In addition, numerous factors associated with cardiac surgery affect the ACT, such as hypothermia, thrombin inhibitors, protamine, and antiphospholipid antibodies. Hemodilution decreases availability of contact factors (factors XII and XI, kallikrein, high-molecular-weight kininogen), common pathway factors (factors X and V, prothrombin), and fibrinogen, thus prolonging ACT through multiple mechanisms. Coagulation factor reactions typically occur on platelet surfaces, hence low platelet count and presence of antiplatelet drugs can also prolong ACT.

Other methods of anticoagulation monitoring include high-dose thrombin time, or measurement of heparin levels by either protamine titration or the heparin concentration test. Protamine titration involves combining patient blood with measured amounts of protamine in several channels and determining the channel to first show production of a clot. Because the protamine titration method relies on the first channel to show a clot, and not the time to generate clot, the method is independent of factor levels and platelet count or function. The heparin concentration test has been compared with the ACT in efforts to arrive at the most optimal evidence-based management. In a few randomized trials the heparin concentration test, compared with the ACT, was found to be associated with greater suppression of the coagulation pathway, decreased perioperative transfusion requirements, and greater total heparin dosing. Overall, a 2006 best evidence review of point-of-care coagulation testing during CPB concluded that using the heparin-concentration test results in higher heparin and lower protamine dosing, with possible sparing of coagulation system activation and decreased transfusion requirements. Because of variability in patient response to heparin, however, the same heparin levels do not necessarily imply the same anticoagulant effect across a patient population.

Thromboelastography (TEG) is a method of assessing the coagulation system that provides information about factor levels, fibrinogen, platelet function, and fibrinolysis. Its use in cardiac surgery is limited to assessment of the post-CPB state when bleeding is present and the specific cause is unclear. As a monitoring method for CPB anticoagulation, TEG has not been formally validated or standardized, as have methods that involve ACT or heparin assay.

In response to wide practice variability involving the dosing of heparin for CPB, monitoring of its anticoagulant effect, and reversing its effect, the literature was reviewed in 2018 by a Task Force consisting of members from the Society of Thoracic Surgeons (STS), the Society of Cardiovascular Anesthesiologists (SCA), and the American Society of Extracorporeal Technology (AmSECT). The Task Force then issued practice guidelines for anticoagulation management during CPB, with assessment of the level of evidence supporting each recommendation. Measurement of a whole-blood clotting time received a class I recommendation, whereas class IIa recommendations were issued for establishing anticoagulation prior to CPB and maintaining ACT above 480 seconds. Use of a heparin-response formula, as opposed to weight-based dosing, and heparin concentration monitoring received class IIb recommendations because outcomes data regarding the efficacy of such practices were inconsistent.

## Problems Associated With the Use of Heparin

### HEPARIN-INDUCED THROMBOCYTOPENIA

The occasional patient with heparin-induced thrombocytopenia (HIT) presents a challenge to the cardiac surgical team. Heparin-induced thrombocytopenia is classified into two subtypes. HIT I describes a non–immune-mediated reaction to heparin therapy associated with a transient decline in platelet count within 72 hours of exposure to heparin. It is thought to be due to heparin's nonspecific binding and proaggregatory effects on platelets, and it typically resolves after 4 days of discontinuation of heparin. It is not associated with thrombosis.

HIT II is caused by immunoglobulin G antibodies that bind to heparin–platelet factor (PF) 4 complexes on platelets, thus activating the platelets and leading to microaggregate formation, thrombocytopenia, and vascular thrombosis (usually arterial). A positive serotonin-release assay, where donor platelets activate and release serotonin in response to patient serum and heparin, can confirm the diagnosis. HIT II is likely when (1) platelet count drops by 50% from preheparin counts, (2) platelet count improves when heparin is discontinued, and (3) other causes of thrombocytopenia have been excluded. Even without thrombocytopenia, the very presence of antibodies directed against heparin-PF4 complexes is a risk factor for the occurrence of major adverse events in patients with cardiovascular disease.

For cardiac surgery, patients with active HIT can be managed in several ways. Postponing elective surgery until platelet count is restored, and then performing CPB with an alternative anticoagulant, is one option. This approach received a class IIa recommendation from the 2018 STS/SCA/AmSECT Task Force in their recently published guidelines. Plasmapheresis before surgery to effectively reduce antibody levels may be considered. If plasmapheresis is not available or an emergency arises that does not allow time to perform plasmapheresis, then alternate anticoagulants are indicated to safely anticoagulate the patient regardless of platelet count. The use of bivalirudin received a class IIa recommendation from the 2018 Task Force, whereas other approaches, such as plasmapheresis, other anticoagulants, and antiplatelet agents, received class IIb recommendations.

### HEPARIN RESISTANCE

Up to 20% of patients have heparin resistance (i.e., an inadequate response to an acceptable dose of heparin [as measured via the ACT]). Frequently, the cause is AT deficiency, which can be congenital, or acquired secondary to nephrotic syndrome, liver disease, malnutrition, and previous heparin treatment. AT supplementation typically restores heparin sensitivity for many but not all patients with heparin resistance caused by AT deficiency, indicating an AT-independent mechanism for heparin resistance. Nitroglycerin, elevated factor VIII levels, and nonspecific binding of heparin to various plasma proteins account for some known causes of AT-independent heparin resistance.

When heparin resistance is encountered clinically, surgical teams generally supplement with additional heparin or with administration of AT in the form of either plasma or AT preparations. The use of additional heparin is often effective but may be limited by a ceiling effect; additional heparin is unlikely to produce a further increase in ACT when levels are higher than 4.0 U/mL. Because of lack of sufficient outcome data for the use of plasma in this setting, plasma for this specific indication has been recommended by the FDA only if AT concentrates are not available.

### NONHEMORRHAGIC SIDE EFFECTS

As many as 80% of patients receiving heparin will have a transient increase in aminotransferase levels. Approximately 5% to 10% of patients who have received heparin will develop hyperkalemia secondary to heparin-induced aldosterone suppression. The hyperkalemia may appear hours to days after the infusion of heparin.

## Problems Associated With Heparin Manufacture

In 2007, lots of heparin were removed from the market because several syringes were found to be contaminated with *Serratia marcescens*. In 2008, Baxter withdrew all of its heparin from the market after more than 80 deaths were associated with its use. The heparin, imported from China, had a contaminant: oversulfated derivatives of chondroitin sulfate, a shellfish-derived supplement.

In 2009, the U.S. Food and Drug Administration notified physicians of a new reference standard to measure the potency of heparin to bring the U.S. Pharmacopeia unit dose in compliance with the World Health Organization international standard unit dose. This change resulted in an approximately 10% reduction in the potency of the heparin sold in the United States.

## Heparin Alternatives for Cardiopulmonary Bypass

Although heparin-induced thrombocytopenia and heparin resistance have typically fueled the search for other anticoagulants, they are not the only drawbacks to the use of heparin for CPB. Despite the lack of obvious clot formation during heparin-managed CPB, activation of the coagulation system still occurs, resulting in some degree of thrombin formation and coagulation factor consumption. Thrombin formation during CPB also occurs in patients with complete factor XII or factor XI deficiencies, indicating that activation of the extrinsic (tissue factor) pathway plays some role in the activation of coagulation during CPB, and heparin alone is insufficient to completely attenuate the coagulation process. Thrombin activation during CPB has been shown to be directly related to postoperative bleeding.

Alternatives to heparin in CPB include direct thrombin inhibitors, such as lepirudin and bivalirudin; danaparoid and other heparinoids; and ancrod. Because a specific reversal agent, such as protamine, is lacking for all these agents, bivalirudin is the most used heparin alternative because it has the shortest duration of action. The ACT is typically not sensitive enough to the effects of thrombin antagonists to be useful during CPB; therefore a similar test, the ecarin clotting time, has been developed. In medical institutions in which the ecarin clotting time is not available, success has been reported with the use of a modified ACT.

Bivalirudin inhibits plasma thrombin, as well as clot-bound thrombin and thrombin-dependent platelet activation, through its inhibition of PAR-1 cleavage. For these reasons, bivalirudin may provide improved early vein graft patency when used for coronary bypass operations. In two open-label safety trials of bivalirudin in patients with heparin-induced thrombocytopenia who were undergoing either on-pump or off-pump cardiac procedures, the authors reported procedural success rates equivalent to those from cases in which heparin was used. Investigators of the EVOLUTION-ON study—a randomized, open-label, multicenter trial comparing heparin and bivalirudin—reported similar procedural success rates and hemostatic outcomes in patients undergoing either on-pump and off-pump cardiac operations. Koster and colleagues reported acceptable hemostatic results with the use of bivalirudin as an anticoagulant in a series of 141 patients undergoing on-pump or off-pump operations. Bivalirudin dosing consists of a 1-mg/kg loading dose with infusion at 2.5 mg/kg/hr. Some authors have reported supplementing the CPB prime with 50 mg; others report additional bolus doses of 0.1 to 0.5 mg/kg as needed throughout CPB.

## Reversal of Heparin After Cardiopulmonary Bypass

Protamine is a polyanionic peptide that binds rapidly and noncovalently to circulating heparin to inactivate the anticoagulant effect. Although protamine is the chief heparin-reversal agent used in clinical practice, other agents—such as heparinase and PF4—have been used.

Accurate dosing of protamine for heparin reversal is important for reestablishing hemostasis after CPB. Protamine reversal of the heparin effect can be performed by fixed dose, ACT-guided dosing, or dosing based on heparin level. Fixed-dose protamine administration is generally the simplest and relies on the assumption that 1 mg protamine neutralizes 100 units of heparin. Protamine is then administered according to the previously administered heparin doses. However, without accounting for heparin consumption over time, this method can result in excessive protamine administration. Excess free protamine impairs postoperative platelet function, increases ACT, and may contribute to coagulopathy after CPB. ACT-guided dosing involves generating heparin-ACT response curves, which yield estimates of the quantity of remaining heparin in circulation; this therefore results in more accurate protamine dosing. Likewise, heparin concentration-based protamine dosing relies on measurements of heparin levels at the conclusion of CPB. The 2018 Task Force provided a class IIa recommendation for calculation of a precise protamine dose based on titration of circulating heparin, because consistent evidence exists that this practice reduces bleeding and transfusion.

Protamine administration has been associated with a range of systemic cardiovascular reactions, such as vasodilation, pulmonary hypertension, bronchospasm, anaphylaxis, myocardial depression, and circulatory collapse. These reactions may range from mild and clinically inconsequential to severe and ultimately fatal. The immunologic mechanism responsible for protamine reactions is complex and probably involves release of anaphylatoxins and eicosanoids, complement activation, histamine, and preformed antiprotamine or antiprotamine-heparin complex antibodies. Fish or shellfish allergy, prior use of NPH insulin, and previous vasectomy have been classically taught as risk factors for protamine reactions, although the evidence supporting these associations is weak or anecdotal. Previous exposure to protamine appears to increase the incidence of protamine-induced pulmonary vasoconstriction, whereas preoperative aspirin use seems to decrease it. Treatment of protamine reactions is generally supportive and aimed at restoring normal hemodynamics. The use of inhaled nitric oxide to manage pulmonary hypertension and right-sided heart failure associated with protamine has been reported.

## SUGGESTED READINGS

Erdoes, G., Ortmann, E., DeArroyabe, B. M. L., Reid, C., & Koster, A. (2020). Role of bivalirudin for anticoagulation in adult perioperative cardiothoracic practice. *Journal of Cardiothoracic and Vascular Anesthesia, 34*, 2207–2214.

Finley, A., & Greenberg, C. (2013). Review article: Heparin sensitivity and resistance: Management during cardiopulmonary bypass. *Anesthesia and Analgesia, 116*, 1210–1222.

Hessel, E. A. (2019). What's new in cardiopulmonary bypass. *Journal of Cardiothoracic and Vascular Anesthesia, 33*(8), 2296–2326.

Koster A, Buz S, Krabatsch T, et al. Bivalirudin anticoagulation during cardiac surgery: a single-center experience in 141 patients. *Perfusion* 2009; 24: 7–11.

Lander, H., Zammert, M., & FitzGerald, D. (2016). Anticoagulation management during cross-clamping and bypass. *Best Practice and Research. Clinical Anaesthesiology, 30*, 359–370.

McNair, E., Marcoux, J. A., Bally, C., Gamble, J., & Thomson, D. (2016). Bivalirudin as an adjunctive anticoagulant to heparin in the treatment of heparin resistance during cardiopulmonary bypass-assisted cardiac surgery. *Perfusion, 31*, 189–199.

Salter, B. S., Weiner, M. M., Trinh, M. A., Heller, J., Evans, A. S., Adams, D. H., et al. (2016). Heparin-induced thrombocytopenia: A comprehensive clinical review. *Journal of the American College of Cardiology, 67*(21), 2519–2532.

Shore-Lesserson, L., Baker, R. A., Ferraris, V., Greilich, P. E., Fitzgerald, D., Roman, P., et al. (2018). STS/SCA/AmSECT Clinical Practice Guidelines: Anticoagulation during Cardiopulmonary Bypass. *Journal of Extra-Corporeal Technology, 50*, 5–18.

Sniecinski, R. M., & Levy, J. H. (2015). Anticoagulation management associated with extracorporeal circulation. *Best Practice and Research. Clinical Anaesthesiology, 29*, 189–202.

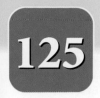

# 125

# Aortic Stenosis

MARTIN L. DE RUYTER, MD, MS, FASA

## Clinical Features

Aortic valve stenosis (AS) is the second most common valvular lesion in the United States and presents in about 5% of the population at age 65 years and increases in prevalence with advancing age. In a population study of subjects from Europe and North America in patients over 75 years of age, the observed prevalence of AS was 1 in 8, yet AS was rare in patients less than 65 years of age. The three major etiologies of AS are (1) rheumatic aortic valve disease, which usually occurs in conjunction with mitral valve abnormalities after rheumatic fever and which in developing countries remains the leading cause of AS; (2) calcification or degeneration in a previously normal tricuspid aortic valve; and (3) a congenital malformation (e.g., bicuspid valve) that becomes stenotic over decades. Medical management has limitations, and aortic valve replacement (AVR) is the definitive treatment of AS. Surgical aortic valve replacement (SAVR), the one-time standard, is increasingly giving way to transcatheter aortic valve replacement (TAVR).

In the United States, calcific stenosis of a tricuspid aortic valve or a congenital bicuspid aortic valve that later calcifies are the more common causes of AS. The risk factors for calcific degenerative AS are similar to those for atherosclerosis (e.g., older age, male sex, hypertension, tobacco smoking, diabetes, hyperlipidemia with evidence of inflammation at the site of disease). Renal failure has also been associated as a risk factor. In patients over the age of 70 years who undergo surgical replacement, 60% have a degenerative tricuspid aortic valve.

It is estimated that between 0.5% and 2% of the population has a bicuspid aortic valve, yet these congenitally abnormal valves account for nearly half of the aortic valves that are surgically treated. Bicuspid aortic valves are thought to be inherited as an autosomal-dominant trait with variable penetrance. Flow through a bicuspid aortic valve is turbulent, creating abnormal pressures on the leaflets, which incites an inflammatory component. This results in a thickening of the leaflets and eventual stenosis. In a recent metanalysis of patients with bicuspid aortic valve, 12% to 37% develop moderate to severe AS (Fig. 125.1).

Eighty percent of patients with symptomatic AS are men, approximately 50% will have coronary artery disease, and most of these patients will be at least 70 years of age. Severe aortic stenosis is observed in 3.4% of adults older than 75 years. In a study of 5201 men and women over the age of 65 years, 26% had aortic sclerosis (a thickening of the valve without hemodynamic sequelae), and 2% had AS. The prevalence of aortic sclerosis increased with age: 20% in patients aged 65 to 75 years, 35% in those aged 75 to 85 years, and 48% in patients older than 85 years. AS rates were 1.3%, 2.4%, and 4% in these age groups, respectively.

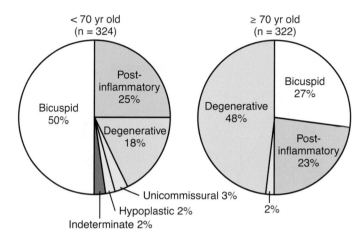

Fig. 125.1   Distribution of aortic valve disease based on age. (Adapted from Fuster V, O'Rourke RA, Walsh RA, Poole-Wilson P. *Hurst's The Heart.* 13th ed. Chapter 76. Available at http://www.accessmedicine.com.)

## Natural History

The typical natural history of AS consists of a prolonged asymptomatic period. This is followed by a gradual onset of symptoms manifest in the fifth to seventh decades of life. Stages have been proposed by the American College of Cardiology/American Heart Association to acknowledge and describe the continuum of AS: stage A includes those at risk of developing AS; stage B includes mild to moderate AS; stage C includes severe AS without symptoms and normal left ventricular function (ejection fraction [EF] >50%); and stage D includes severe AS with symptoms and/or reduced EF (<50%). Stage D is further subdivided into three categories based on gradient, flow across the aortic valve, and EF. Patients with AS are at increased risk of sudden death (likely from cardiac arrhythmia due to ischemia from mismatching of $O_2$ supply and demand). Aortic sclerosis is not an uncommon finding in patients older than 65 years, but about 16% of patients with sclerosis develop AS within 7 years. Patients with aortic sclerosis are asymptomatic, but once the pressure gradient across the valve increases, exertional dyspnea, angina, and syncope—the cardinal symptoms of AS—can appear within 5 years. The typical time frames from the onset of symptoms until death are 4.5 years for patients with angina, 2.6 years for patients with syncope, 2 years for patients with dyspnea, and 1 year for patients with congestive heart failure, with the latter being the cause of death in one-half to two-thirds of patients with untreated AS (Fig. 125.2).

The mortality rate is approximately 25% per year among symptomatic patients, with three-quarters whose AS is untreated dying within 3 years of the onset of symptoms (Fig. 125.3). Asymptomatic patients, on the other hand, even those with severe disease, have a more favorable outlook (risk of death <1% per year).

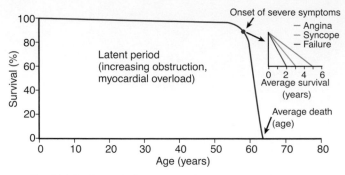

**Fig. 125.2** Survival of patients with aortic stenosis over time.

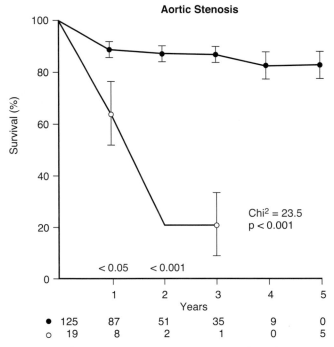

**Fig. 125.3** Effect of medical intervention on mortality risk in patients with aortic stenosis. (Adapted from Fuster V, O'Rourke RA, Walsh RA, Poole-Wilson P. *Hurst's The Heart*. 13th ed. Chapter 76. Available at: http://www.accessmedicine.com.)

Patients with AS due to a bicuspid aortic valve tend to be younger than 70 years. In these patients, AS is less likely associated with coronary artery disease but more associated with aortic root dilatation.

## Anatomic Considerations

The internal cross-sectional area of a normal aortic valve during systole is 3 to 4 cm²; significant hemodynamic obstruction does not occur until the valve area is less than 1.5 cm². Based upon measurements of valve area, peak blood flow velocity across the valve, mean pressure gradient, and effective orifice area, the degree of AS is categorized as mild, moderate, or severe. These measurements are typically assessed with echocardiography (Table 125.1). The measurement of pressure gradients is accurate less than 50% of the time because the pressure gradient is flow dependent. Measuring the valve area is the most reliable method of assessing severity of AS because it depends less on ventricular contractility than do pressure gradients, but measuring valve area using two-dimensional echocardiography has several factors that may limit

| TABLE 125.1 | Aortic Stenosis: Measurements and Severity of Disease | | | |
|---|---|---|---|---|
| | **CLINICAL STATUS/DISEASE SEVERITY** | | | |
| **Stenotic Lesion Characteristic** | **Normal** | **Mild** | **Moderate** | **Severe** |
| Valve area (cm²) | 3.0–4.0 | >1.5 | 1.0–1.5 | <1.0 |
| AoVmax (m/sec) | <1.5 | 2.5–3.0 | 3.0–4.0 | >4.0 |
| MPG (mm Hg) | 0 | <20 | 20–40 | >40 |
| EOA (cm²) | 3.0–4.0 | >1.5 | 1.0–1.5 | <1.0 |

*AoVmax,* Peak blood flow velocity across the valve; *EOA,* effective orifice area; *MPG,* mean pressure gradient.

its usefulness, including the difficulty in obtaining the correct short-axis view, the presence of calcifications that create shadowing on the image, and the inability with a "pinhole" valve to identify the orifice during systole. Therefore the effective valve area or the effective orifice area is calculated using the equation:

$$\text{Aortic Valve Area} = \frac{(\text{LVOT}_{\text{Area}} \times \text{LVOT}_{\text{VTI}})}{\text{Aortic Valve}_{\text{VTI}}}$$

where LVOT is the left ventricular outflow tract and VTI is the velocity time integral.

## Valve Replacement

AS is a disease of the elderly, and as the population ages, it is anticipated that more patients will need intervention. In a recent Norwegian study, the prevalence of AS was 1.3% in those aged 60 to 69 years, 3.9% in those aged 70 to 79, and 9.8% in those aged 80 to 89. In the United States, aging baby boomers are accounting for major shifts in the population. Based on US Census data, in 2019 the population aged 65 years or older was 40 million (16.5%). The population in this age group is estimated to be 77 million (20%) by 2034 and 94.7 million (33%) by 2060, thus suggesting a strong demand for AVR in the future.

The timing of the AVR operation is based on the type, duration, and severity of symptoms and the degree of valve narrowing. At present, each year approximately 80,000 to 85,000 AVRs are performed in the United States, and these numbers are increasing annually. SAVR, namely bioprosthetic (tissue) valves and mechanical valves, have been the traditional approach to replace a diseased valve. Valve selection depends on balancing the risks associated with the use of chronic anticoagulation, the likelihood of structural failure of a bioprosthetic valve (hence the need for subsequent replacement), and the patient's expected longevity and functional status. An 11-year follow-up study of patients who were randomly assigned to receive either a bioprosthetic valve or a mechanical valve found no difference in survival rates between the two groups. Structural valve failure was observed in the bioprosthetic group, but this was offset by increased bleeding complications in the patients who were anticoagulated because they had a mechanical valve. In general, 10-year survival rate after AVR is approximately 67%.

Enthusiasm for noninvasive percutaneous transluminal aortic valvuloplasty quickly abated after clinical experience. Postoperative improvements in pressure gradients across the valve and in symptoms were often only temporary, and overall mortality rates did not improve. Today this approach is mostly abandoned.

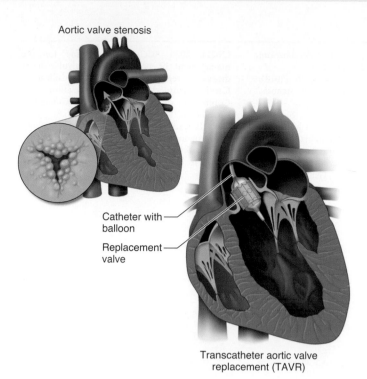

Aortic valve stenosis

Catheter with balloon

Replacement valve

Transcatheter aortic valve replacement (TAVR)

**Fig. 125.4** Transcatheter aortic valve replacement (TAVR).

TAVR was introduced in 2011 and consists of placing a prosthetic aortic valve typically via a transfemoral arterial approach (other approaches described include transapical, aortic, and subclavian) (Fig. 125.4). TAVR was initially offered to AS patients considered to be too high-risk for SAVR. This expanded to include intermediate-risk patients, with high-quality randomized controlled trials supporting its use in this population as well.

A review of the Transcatheter Valve Therapy Registry and the Society of Thoracic Surgeons National Database compared outcomes for more than 9000 propensity-matched intermediate- and high-risk patients who underwent either TAVR or SAVR. This review found TAVR patients had a lower incidence of in-hospital mortality and were more often discharged home. After 1 year, results were similar with regard to rates of death, stroke, and days alive and out of hospital. In 2019, the TAVR volume (72,991) exceeded all forms of SAVR (57,626), and TAVR received U.S. Food and Drug Administration approval for patients of low-risk for AVR. It is projected that the TAVR volume will exceed 130,000 by 2026.

## Concomitant Diseases

Patients with AS often have additional medical problems, including coronary artery disease, with asymptomatic patients having an incidence of coronary artery disease of up to 33%. Heyde syndrome, which occurs in the elderly, includes AS, acquired coagulopathy, and anemia due to bleeding from intestinal angiodysplasia. In patients with a bicuspid aortic valve, aortic root dilatation is not uncommon, and these patients undergo routine surveillance for possible intervention.

## Anesthetic Considerations for Aortic Valve Replacement

For the surgical, sternotomy approach to AVR, many clinicians previously preferred using an opioid-based technique when anesthetizing patients. Compared with inhalational anesthetic agents, opioids preserve systemic vascular resistance (SVR) and left ventricular contractility. However, many of the concerns with regard to inhalational anesthetic agents are of little clinical consequence. In practice, most clinicians use a combination of an opioid and either an inhalational agent or an intravenously administered hypnotic to produce optimal hemodynamics and early weaning from mechanical ventilation and tracheal extubation in the intensive care unit (ICU).

In addition to routine monitors recommended by the American Society of Anesthesiologists, arterial catheter and transesophageal echocardiography are commonly used. Pulmonary artery catheters may be placed, as the intensivist may use this monitor for guiding postoperative management. Echocardiography permits assessment of preload, left ventricular function, valve gradients, and prosthetic valve function and provides real-time information to the surgical team. Arrhythmias and hypotension should be treated aggressively. Anesthetic goals are summarized in Box 125.1.

For TAVR procedures, approaches with either a balanced general anesthetic with an endotracheal tube or deep sedation with local anesthetic infiltration of the insertion site have been used. In either approach, an arterial line and transesophageal echocardiography are common. A recent metaanalysis compared local anesthesia/sedation versus general anesthesia in patients undergoing TAVR and found that the local anesthesia/sedation approach was associated with a lower 30-day mortality and shorter procedure time, ICU length of stay, hospital length of stay, and reduced need of inotropic support. Of note, it is not uncommon for patients to have transient, temporary heart block after TAVR and, although most resolve, it has been reported that 27% of patients may need a permanent pacemaker within 30 days after the procedure.

## Anesthesia for Patients With Aortic Stenosis Undergoing Noncardiac Surgery

Patients with AS who undergo noncardiac surgery are at an increased risk of developing perioperative myocardial infarction, congestive heart failure, and arrhythmia. An adequate history for symptoms should be obtained and appropriate diagnostic testing should be performed before patients with AS undergo elective procedures. Anesthetic goals for noncardiac surgery are like those for AVR (see Box 125.1). Given the potential for deleterious effects of reduced SVR and subsequent reduced coronary perfusion, central neuraxial anesthesia (e.g., spinal or epidural) is relatively contraindicated.

---

**BOX 125.1 ANESTHETIC GOALS FOR AORTIC VALVE REPLACEMENT**

Avoid hypotension
Maintain sinus rhythm, avoiding both bradycardia and tachycardia
Optimize intravascular volume to maintain venous return and left ventricular filling
Avoid sudden increases or decreases in systemic vascular resistance
Identify and treat myocardial ischemia

## SUGGESTED READINGS

Acona, R., & Pinzt, S. (2020). Epidemiology of aortic valve stenosis and aortic valve incompetence: Is the prevalence similar in different parts of the World? *Journal of Cardiology Practice, 18,* 1–8.

Brennan, J. M., Thomas, L., Cohen, D. J., Shahian, D., Wang, A., Mack, M. J., et al. (2017). Transcatheter versus surgical aortic valve replacement. *Journal of the American College of Cardiology, 70,* 439–450.

Carroll, J. D., Mack, M. J., Vemulapalli, S., Herrmann, H. C., Gleason, T. G., Hanzel, G., et al. (2020). STS-ASS TVT registry of transcatheter aortic valve replacement. *Journal of the American College of Cardiology, 76*(2), 2492–2516.

Kanwar, A., Thaden, J., & Nkomo, V. (2018). Management of patients with aortic valve stenosis. *Mayo Clinic Proceedings, 93*(4), 488–508.

Masri, A., Syensson, L. G., Griffin, B. T., & Desai, M. Y. (2017). Contemporary natural history of bicuspid aortic valve disease: A systematic review. *Heart, 103,* 1323–1330.

Otto, C. M., Nishimura, R. A., Bonow, R. O., Carabello, B. A., Erwin, J. P., III, Gentile, F., et al. (2021). 2020 ACC/AHA guideline for the management of patients with valvular heart disease: A report of the American College of Cardiology/American Heart Association Joint Committee on Clinical Practice Guidelines. *Circulation, 143,* e72–e227.

Pellikka, P. A. (2022). Natural history, epidemiology, and prognosis of aortic stenosis. In C. M. Otto & S. B. Yeon (Eds.), *UpToDate.* Waltham, MA: UpToDate. Accessed April, 2023.

# 126

# Mitral Regurgitation

ADAM J. MILAM, MD, PhD  |  SHAWN MALAN, MD

## Anatomy of the Mitral Valve

Although the approach to the repair of an incompetent mitral valve (MV) is constantly evolving, successful anesthetic management of a patient with mitral regurgitation (MR) undergoing surgical correction is predicated on a clear understanding of the anatomy and physiology of the MV (Fig. 126.1). The MV, so named because it resembles a bishop's miter, is composed of a fibrous annulus and anterior and posterior leaflets—the combined area of the two leaflets is more than twice the area of the annulus. The two leaflets are connected to the anterolateral and posteromedial papillary muscles by primary, secondary, and tertiary chordae tendineae. Primary chordae connect the papillary muscle to the tips of the mitral leaflets, secondary chordae connect the papillary muscle to the leaflet body, and tertiary chordae connect the basal region of the posterior valve leaflet to the ventricular free wall. The anterior leaflet attaches to approximately one-third of the annulus, and the ratio of its height to its base is greater than that of the posterior leaflet, which in turn attaches to the other two-thirds of the annulus. The two leaflets are connected at the sides of the annulus to form the anterolateral and posteromedial commissures. The posterior MV has three components, the P1, P2, and P3 segments, which are often referred to as *scallops.* Likewise, the anterior leaflet of the MV is composed of the corresponding segments known as the A1, A2, and A3 segments based on their proximity to the posterior leaflet scallops (Fig. 126.2). The P1 and A1 segments are attached at the anterolateral commissure, whereas the A3 and P3 segments adjoin at the posteromedial commissure.

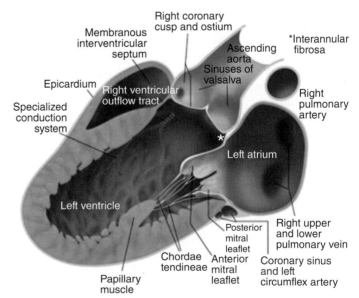

**Fig. 126.1** Normal mitral valve anatomy. An anatomic illustration oriented similar to an echocardiographic parasternal long-axis view in diastole shows normal mitral valve anatomy, including the mitral annulus, anterior and posterior mitral leaflets, mitral chords, and papillary muscles. The medial papillary muscle is shown for reference, although slight medial angulation typically is needed to visualize this structure in the long-axis view. (From Narang A, Puthumana J, Thomas JD. Diagnostic evaluation of mitral regurgitation. In: C. Otto, ed. *Valvular Heart Disease: A Companion to Braunwald's Heart Disease.* 5th ed. Elsevier; 2020:289–310, fig. 15.1.)

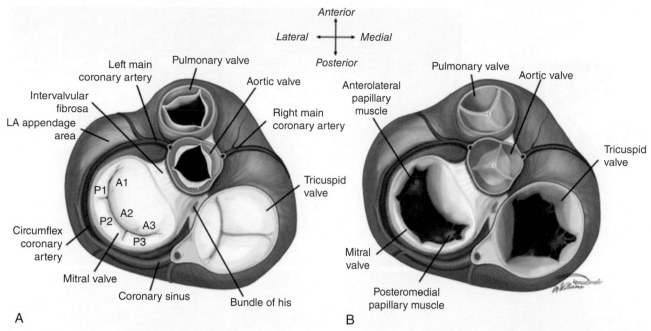

**Fig. 126.2** Anatomic relationships of the mitral valve (MV). The base of the heart is shown in an anatomic orientation from the left atrial *(LA)* aspect. The relationship of the MV and adjacent cardiac structures is demonstrated. **A,** Systole. The posterior leaflet of the MV has two natural clefts. The clefts divide the posterior leaflet into three segments that (using the Carpentier nomenclature) are called P1, P2, and P3. Although there are no natural clefts in the anterior leaflet, its corresponding segments are called A1, A2, and A3. For purposes of echocardiographic orientation, it is useful to observe that P1 is adjacent to the LA appendage and P3 is adjacent to the tricuspid valve. **B,** Diastole. The anterolateral and posteromedial papillary muscles support the anterior and posterior leaflets symmetrically. The anterolateral muscle supports A1/P1 and the anterolateral half of A2/P2; the posteromedial muscle supports A3/P3 and the posteromedial half of A2/P2. (From Drake DH, Zimmerman KG, Sidebotham DA. Transesophageal echocardiography for surgical repair of mitral regurgitation. In: Otto C, ed. *The Practice of Clinical Echocardiography.* 5th ed. Elsevier; 2017:343–373, fig. 25.1.)

Three-dimensional echocardiography has significantly improved the evaluation of the MV and the anatomic derangements that are causing MR. In the past, the mitral annulus was believed to be a fixed cartilaginous structure to which the anterior and posterior leaflets were attached. It is now recognized that the annulus undergoes significant conformational changes throughout the cardiac cycle. During systole, the annulus "contracts," or narrows, allowing the edges of the anterior and posterior leaflets to coapt, thereby preventing regurgitation of blood into the atrium during ventricular systole. The opposite occurs during diastole: the annulus "widens," increasing the cross-sectional area of the MV orifice, thereby facilitating inflow into the left ventricle (LV) during diastole.

## Classification Mitral Regurgitation

Incompetence of the MV resulting in regurgitation of blood from the LV into the left atrium (LA) during systole is a common physiologic finding (Fig. 126.3). MR is classified as organic (primary), when there is an abnormality of the MV apparatus (i.e., myxomatous changes, endocarditis); or functional (secondary), when the MV apparatus is normal but changes to the LV (from ischemic or dilated cardiomyopathy) cause displacement of the papillary muscles or poor coaptation of the MV leaflets. MR can also be classified by chronicity: acute, chronic compensated, or chronic decompensated. Last, MR can be classified based on the severity of the MR: mild, moderate, or severe based on qualitative (e.g., color Doppler jet area, MV morphology) and quantitative measurements (e.g., regurgitant volume, effective regurgitant orifice area). In the developed world, MR most commonly occurs as a result of degeneration of the mitral

leaflets, and its prevalence increases with age. In lower-income countries, rheumatic heart disease is the most common cause of MR. Other causes of MR include endocarditis, congenital clefts, papillary muscle rupture, systolic anterior motion (SAM) of the anterior mitral leaflet, and annular dilation.

## Natural History of Mitral Regurgitation

Acute MR is usually quite symptomatic and requires surgical intervention. Acute MR (as might be caused by rupture of a chorda tendinea) leads to a large volume of blood being ejected retrograde into the LA during LV systole because LA pressure is lower than aortic root pressure. In turn, increased LA blood volume leads to an increased LA pressure, which is ultimately transmitted retrograde into the pulmonary vasculature. As a result, pulmonary artery pressure, pulmonary artery occlusion pressure (PAOP), and pulmonary capillary wedge pressure acutely increase. As described by Starling, the increase in end capillary hydrostatic pressure leads to transudation of fluid into the alveoli, which is manifested clinically by dyspnea, orthopnea, paroxysmal nocturnal dyspnea, rales (as can be heard on auscultation of the lungs), and pulmonary edema (as can be seen on chest radiograph).

In patients in whom incompetence of the valve develops over time (chronic regurgitation, i.e., changes because of senescence), the volume of blood that regurgitates into the LA is initially small; therefore cardiac output can be maintained by an equivalent increase in LV end-diastolic volume (LVEDV), and stroke volume ejected into the aorta remains unaffected. The regurgitant volume in the LA is not large enough to increase PAOP and end capillary hydrostatic pressure. Consequently, there is no transudation of fluid into the alveoli. However, as the regurgitant volume increases,

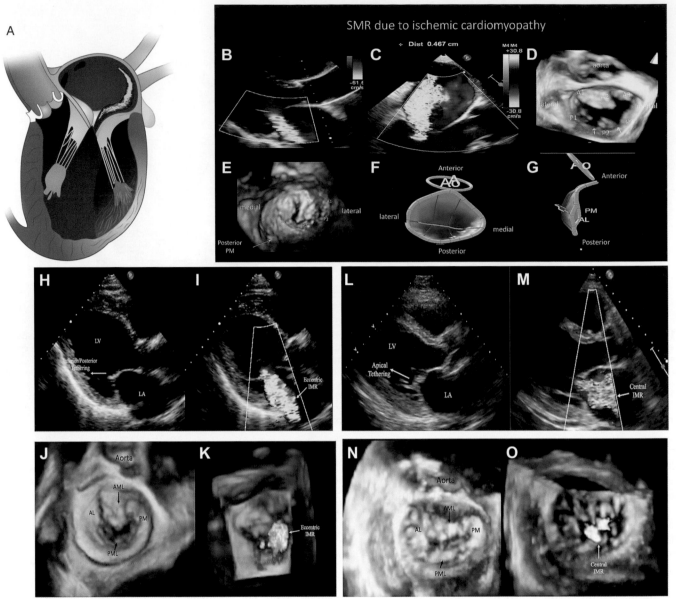

**Fig. 126.3** **A,** Carpentier type IIIB represents restricted leaflet motion in systole. **B–G,** Multimodality echocardiographic imaging for ischemic mitral regurgitation *(IMR)*. Transthoracic echocardiography parasternal long-axis view **(B)** and transesophageal echocardiography (TEE) left ventricular outflow tract view **(C)** show eccentric jet of MR due to asymmetric tethering. **D,** 3D TEE (en face view from left atrium) shows marked indentations between P2–P3 and P2–P1 *(white arrow)* due to left ventricular remodeling. **E,** 3D TEE (en face view from left ventricle) shows an apical and posterior secondary displacement of posterior papillary muscle *(white arrow)*. **F–G,** Reconstruction and model of the mitral valve (MV) shows the malcoaptation of mitral leaflets due to a tethering of the posterior valve. **H–K,** Asymmetric pattern of MV tethering on 2D and 3D echocardiography in the inferior/posterior direction *(yellow arrow)* results in posteriorly directed eccentric IMR. **L–O,** Symmetric pattern of MV tethering on 2D and 3D echocardiography. Note central IMR jet. *AL,* Anterolateral; *AML,* anterior mitral leaflet; *LA,* left atrium; *LV,* left ventricle; *PM,* posteromedial; *PML,* posterior mitral leaflet; *SMR,* secondary mitral regurgitation. (From Nappi F, Singh SSA, Padala M., et al. The choice of treatment in ischemic mitral regurgitation with reduced left ventricular function. *Ann Thorac Surg.* 2019;108(6):1901–1912, fig. 1.)

the LV hypertrophies to reduce the wall stress that accompanies the rise in total stroke volume (total stroke volume equals LA regurgitant volume plus stroke volume into the aorta). Over time, as the valve becomes more incompetent, the increasing volume of regurgitation into the LA dilates the LA while maintaining a relatively "normal" LA pressure. These compensatory changes allow cardiac output to be maintained and minimizes the effects of increasing regurgitant volume on the pulmonary vasculature. The compensatory phase of MR may last for many years but eventually will manifest by LV dysfunction, the hallmark of decompensated MR. It is not completely clear why or when a patient transitions from

the compensated to the decompensated phase of MR, but, as mentioned previously, it is important to intervene surgically before the patient's condition decompensates. Once LV dysfunction develops, it is difficult if not impossible to reverse, and life expectancy is considerably reduced.

Chronic compensated MR transitions to decompensated chronic MR when the LV begins to dilate to accommodate the LVEDV necessary to accommodate both the LA regurgitant fraction and the stroke volume ejected to the aorta (i.e., the total volume ejected from the LV). As the LV dilates, the cardiomyocytes are no longer able to contract adequately to compensate, which leads to signs and symptoms of volume overload. Furthermore, cardiac stroke volume begins to decrease. The reduced stroke volume decreases cardiac output, and LV end-systolic volume subsequently increases. A vicious cycle ensues: an increase in end-systolic volume in the LV increases LVEDV, LA pressure, and PAOP. As the PAOP increases, alveoli begin to fill with fluid, leading to the symptoms and signs of pulmonary edema and congestive heart failure. Mild MR is associated with few, if any, complications. However, severe MR may lead to the development of a variety of sequelae (Box 126.1).

## Concomitant Disease

As was discussed earlier, the clinical manifestations of MR are caused by dilation of the LA. This dilatation can lead to atrial fibrillation (with increased risk for thromboembolic events), an increased LA pressure manifested by pulmonary hypertension, and heart failure. Although these sequelae of MR can initially be managed medically, as soon as there is any evidence of end-diastolic enlargement of the LV, surgical correction of the MV incompetence should be considered to thwart the progression of the sequelae.

MR, per se, does not lead to coronary artery disease (CAD). However, CAD can lead to MR in two ways: myocardial ischemia and infarction can lead to necrosis and rupture of a papillary muscle (most commonly the posteromedial papillary muscle with its single blood supply), resulting in the acute onset of severe MR. Likewise, CAD resulting in regional wall motion abnormalities can lead to papillary dysfunction and annular architectural changes, both of which contribute to MR (i.e., secondary or functional MR). Nevertheless, the principal etiology of MR in high-income countries is senescence of the MV leaflets and accompanying MV apparatus. Because the incidence of CAD likewise increases with age, older patients often present for treatment of CAD and are found to have some degree of MR. If the MR is caused by ischemia (e.g., as a result of regional wall motion abnormalities such as hypokinesis or akinesis in the subvalvular LV), the management can be challenging because none of the options for correcting these abnormalities is ideal. In such patients, depending on a variety of factors, the surgeon may choose to replace the valve rather than attempt to repair it because the success rate of repair in patients with MR caused by ischemia is much lower than the rate in patients with MR because of degenerative changes.

## Surgical Correction of Mitral Regurgitation

Acute MR generally requires immediate surgical intervention. However, the management of chronic regurgitation of the MV is controversial; patients who are symptomatic or who have a decreased ejection fraction (EF) are at increased risk of developing complications and are usually considered candidates for surgery.

Asymptomatic patients with LV systolic dysfunction (EF ≤60%, LV end-systolic diameter ≥40 mm), as well as new-onset atrial fibrillation and pulmonary hypertension, should also be recommended for surgery treatment. Surgical repair or replacement of the MV not only relieves symptoms but has increasingly been shown to improve long-term outcomes, with reductions in morbidity and mortality. Patients who have MR and a decreased EF, an increased LVEDV (i.e., dilated LV), chronic atrial fibrillation, or pulmonary hypertension have better long-term outcomes when the valve incompetence is surgically corrected earlier in the course of the disease. Fortunately, the success of valve repair (compared with replacement) and the low morbidity and mortality rates associated with surgical intervention favor early elective surgery. To prevent progression to worsening disease and subsequent increase in morbidity and mortality rates, current efforts focus on identifying patients with asymptomatic MV disease whose long-term outcome may be favorably affected if their MR is corrected at an early stage.

Dr. Alain Carpentier revolutionized the treatment of MR when, more than 30 years ago, he published his experience with repairing the MV as opposed to replacing it. His findings, and those of others, have led to MV repair being the preferred technique for correcting MR. Approximately 50,000 patients have MV repair annually in the United States. The most common technique to repair the valve is annuloplasty, with or without surgical correction of any defects in the leaflets themselves, or repair of dysfunctional chordae tendineae or reattachment of a ruptured chorda tendinea (Fig. 126.4).

The goal of annuloplasty is to implant a "device" (commonly referred to as a *ring*) onto the annulus to restore its structural integrity and function. The cardiac surgeon has multiple options from which to choose when selecting a ring to perform the annuloplasty: the plastic rings can be complete 360-degree rings or incomplete rings; rigid, semirigid, or flexible; adjustable or nonadjustable; and flat or saddle-shaped. The goal is to restore the annulus in such a way that the anterior and posterior leaflets coapt during ventricular systole. If there is redundancy or prolapse of one of the components of the valve leaflets, then the redundant tissue can be resected, or alternately, if there is incompetence between subcomponents of the leaflets (e.g., between P2 and P3), such an area of the valve can be plicated. If there is incompetence of the valve leaflets because of abnormalities of the chordae, the surgeon can shorten them or reattach them if they are ruptured. Increasingly, in as many as 20% of institutions, MV repair is being performed with minimally invasive techniques that involve a right minithoracotomy (or ministernotomy) with or without robotic assistance.

As the field has advanced, interventional cardiologists are using a variety of new devices to repair incompetent valves in the cardiac catheterization suite using percutaneous techniques (Figs. 126.5 and 126.6). This technology is important for patients who are not surgical candidates. The efficacy of percutaneous repair has been demonstrated in patients with MR who underwent repair using the MitraClip (Abbott Laboratories, Santa Clara, CA). The MitraClip uses the principles of an Alfieri stitch (introduced by Dr. Ottavio Alfieri in 1991), relying on a functional repair versus the anatomic repair (e.g., annuloplasty). The Alfieri stitch is an edge-to-edge repair with the application of a suture at the site of regurgitation; similarly, the MitraClip is a device that is attached to the MV at the site of regurgitation creating a double orifice MV. At 12 months after MitraClip repair, MV function and LV EF had improved. In addition, compared with a control group, the MitraClip cohort

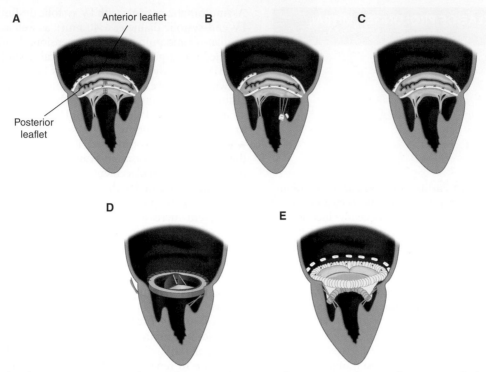

**Fig. 126.4** Surgical techniques in primary mitral regurgitation. **A,** Posterior prolapse repair with triangular resection. **B,** Anterior prolapse repair with artificial chords. **C,** Commissural prolapse repair with commissuroplasty. Almost all repairs include an annuloplasty ring. Chordal sparing mitral valve replacement using **(D)** a mechanical prosthetic valve and **(E)** a tissue prosthetic valve. (From El Sabbagh A, Reddy YN, Nishimura RA. Mitral valve regurgitation in the contemporary era: insights into diagnosis, management, and future directions. *JACC Cardiovasc Imaging.* 2018;11(4):628–643, fig. 4.)

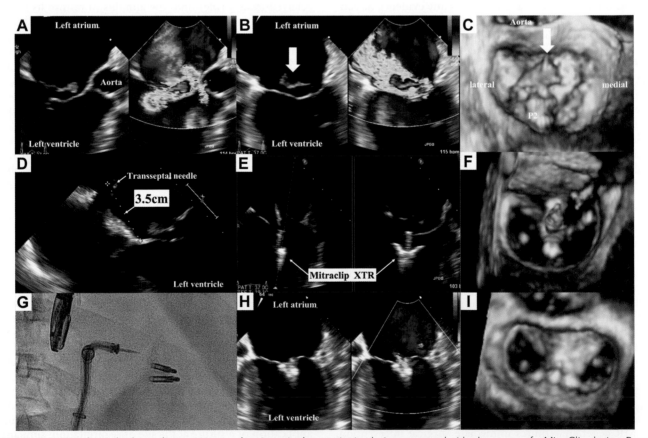

**Fig. 126.5** Transesophageal echocardiogram images showing mitral regurgitation being corrected with placement of a MitraClip device. Preprocedural images of the mitral valve include **(A)** midesophageal (ME) long-axis view, **(B)** ME bicommissural view, and **(C)** a 3D image. **D,** The torn papillary muscle is seen *(white arrow).* Also labeled is the 3.5-cm septal puncture height. X-plane views **(E)** and 3D image **(F)** of implantation of first MitraClip XTR device. **G,** Fluoroscopic image after implantation of two clips. Postrepair views include the ME bicommissural view **(H)** and a 3D image **(I).** (From Komatsu I, Cohen EA, Cohen GN, Czarnecki A. Transcatheter mitral valve edge-to-edge repair with the new MitraClip XTR system for acute mitral regurgitation caused by papillary muscle rupture. *Can J Cardiol.* 2019;35(11):1604-e5, fig. 1.)

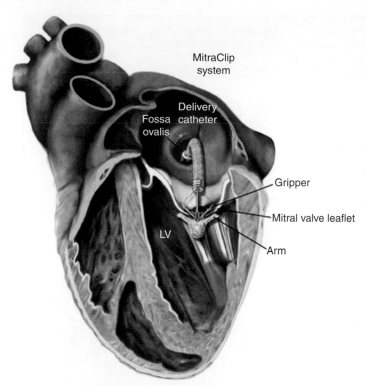

**Fig. 126.6** The MitraClip leaflet edge-to-edge repair system. This device (Abbott Vascular) creates a bridge between the P2 and A2 segments of the mitral valve similar to that created in the Alfieri stitch operation. The clip delivery system is advanced across the atrial septum and through the mitral valve in the open position before the leaflets are grasped. *LV*, Left ventricle. (From Salcedo EE, Quaife RA, Kim MS, et al. Transcatheter mitral valve repair: role of echocardiography in patient selection, procedural guidance, and evaluation of outcomes. In: Otto CM, ed. *The Practice of Clinical Echocardiography*. 5th ed. Elsevier; 2017:376, fig. 20.2.)

demonstrated greater reduction in diastolic and systolic LV dimensions and volumes, LV mass, and peak wall stress.

## Anesthetic Considerations in the Patient With Mitral Regurgitation

Understanding the nature and etiology of the patient's MR is critical to formulating an anesthetic plan for patients undergoing MV procedures. During the preoperative visit, in addition to the customary history and physical examination conducted on all patients about to undergo an anesthetic, the anesthesiologist must determine the etiology of the MR. Although senescence of the MV is the most common cause of MR, patients may also have MR as a consequence of rheumatic fever, ischemic cardiomyopathy, or other, less common causes. The anesthesiologist must also determine whether the patient has mild symptomatic chronic MR or acute regurgitation imposed on chronic MR. Any concomitant disease processes must be elucidated and medical therapies (e.g., the use of anticoagulants or β-adrenergic receptor blocking agents) must be considered.

In the operating room, the monitoring requirements and management of patients undergoing a midline sternotomy and atriotomy are the same as for other patients having cardiopulmonary bypass. Minimally invasive techniques may require special considerations and should be discussed with the surgeon and cardiologist. Often, minimally invasive approaches to MV repair require lung isolation, groin cannulation, and in some cases the placement of a bypass cannula in the superior vena cava. In addition, surgeons may request that a coronary sinus catheter be placed via the jugular vein cannula site for retrograde perfusion.

The priorities for managing patients with MR include maintaining or decreasing systemic vascular resistance during induction and maintenance of anesthesia, as any increase in systemic vascular resistance will decrease LV output into the aorta, along with a corresponding increase in the severity of MR. Equal emphasis should be placed on maintaining normal sinus rhythm or slight tachycardia; a higher heart rate will decrease filling volumes and may reduce regurgitant volume and fraction.

Intraoperative transesophageal echocardiography (TEE) is an integral part of the MV repair process. After induction of anesthesia and tracheal intubation, an orogastric tube should be inserted, the stomach suctioned (in this case, primarily to remove air), the gastric tube removed, and, unless the patient has a condition in which the use of TEE is absolutely contraindicated, an echocardiographic probe should be inserted into the esophagus. A preprocedural intraoperative examination using TEE should be performed, noting the patient's systemic blood pressure and central venous pressure (or pulmonary artery pressure, if available). TEE is used to describe the anatomy of the MV, the cause and severity of MR, and to evaluate for any concomitant disease. Real-time 3D has added additional utility to the diagnostic capacity of echocardiography and is an especially important tool for transcatheter MV repair (Fig. 126.3).

This baseline examination is important because it provides the surgeon with valuable information about the nature and etiology of the MR and can help direct the repair or replacement. Dr. Carpentier also developed a classification system to succinctly communicate the cause of MR that can help guide the decision to replace or repair a diseased valve (Fig. 126.7). MR with normal leaflet mobility (e.g., perforation, congenital cleft, annular dilation) is classified as type I MR. Type II MR is characterized by degeneration leading to excessive leaflet motion (i.e., leaflet flail or prolapse). Restricted leaflet movement is the hallmark of type III MR (i.e., rheumatic disease, ischemia, or LV dilation), which is further divided into types IIIA (restricted mobility during systole and diastole) and IIIB (restricted mobility during systole).

Hemodynamic conditions should be noted during the echocardiographic examination with the goal of reproducing similar hemodynamics that a patient exhibits while not under general anesthesia. The reduction of systemic vascular resistance that often accompanies the maintenance of a general anesthetic can significantly alter the severity of MR and may not highlight all areas of regurgitation. Volume loading, the use of vasopressors, or a combination thereof may be necessary to reproduce preoperative hemodynamic values and are commonly performed during the preprocedural TEE.

Before complete separation from cardiopulmonary bypass, a second, postprocedural echocardiographic examination should be performed to assess the adequacy of the repair or replacement, to identify any concerns about the repair or replacement, and to identify any complications. One common concern (incidence 2%–16%) after a MV repair with annuloplasty is that of SAM of the MV and the LV outflow tract obstruction that it may, in turn, create. The preprocedural intraoperative TEE may also help identify patients at high risk of developing SAM after repair (e.g., small LV, long anterior MV leaflet) and help surgeons modify their repair to reduce the likelihood of SAM. Often, with mild SAM, medical management, including volume loading, heart rate control, and increasing system

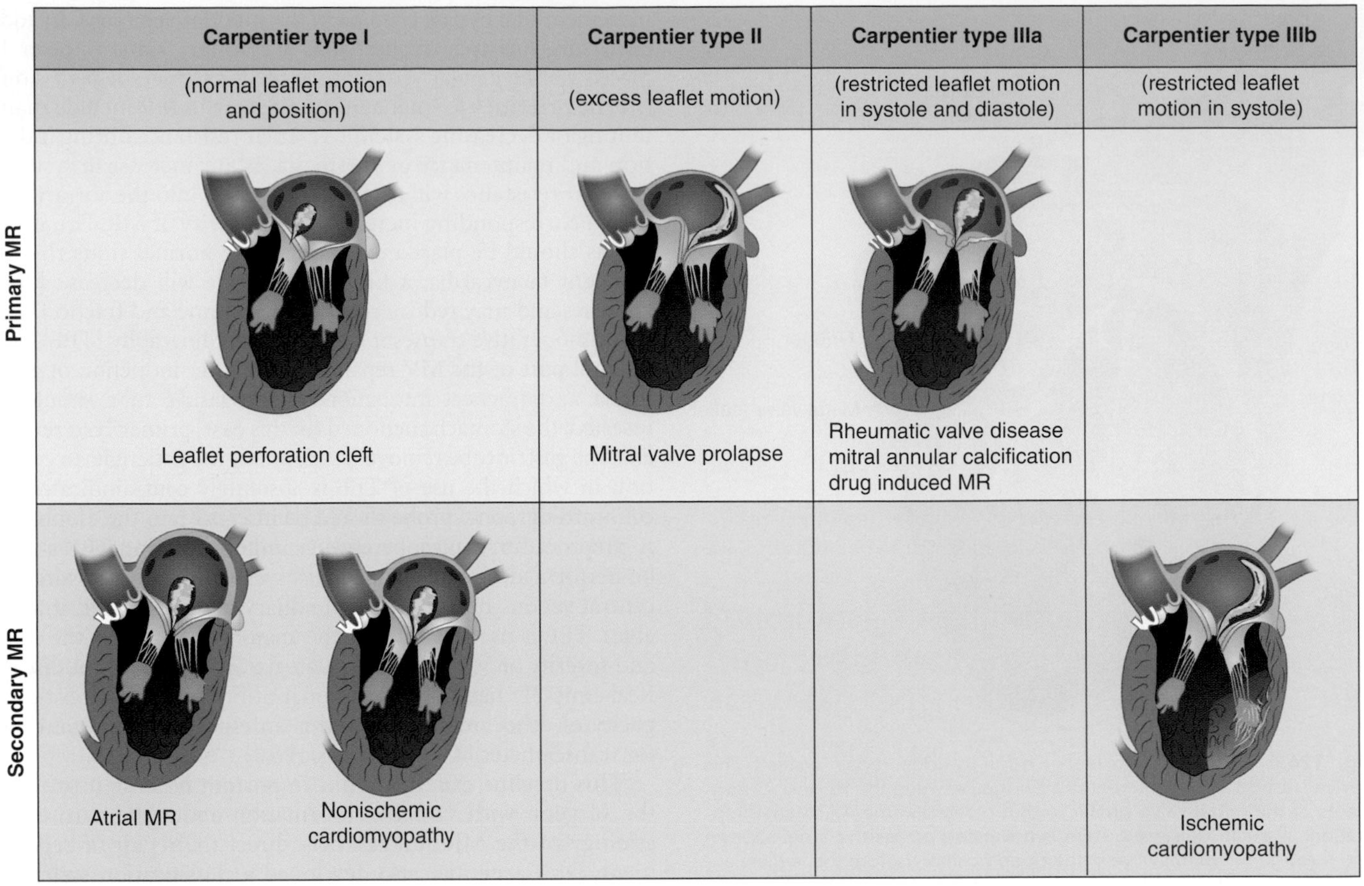

| | Carpentier type I | Carpentier type II | Carpentier type IIIa | Carpentier type IIIb |
|---|---|---|---|---|
| | (normal leaflet motion and position) | (excess leaflet motion) | (restricted leaflet motion in systole and diastole) | (restricted leaflet motion in systole) |
| **Primary MR** | Leaflet perforation cleft | Mitral valve prolapse | Rheumatic valve disease mitral annular calcification drug induced MR | |
| **Secondary MR** | Atrial MR    Nonischemic cardiomyopathy | | | Ischemic cardiomyopathy |

**Fig. 126.7** Classification of the etiology of mitral regurgitation *(MR)*. Primary and secondary MR groupings with their respective Carpentier functional classification. Carpentier type I represents normal leaflet motion and position. Carpentier type II represents excess leaflet motion. Carpentier type IIIA represents restricted leaflet motion in systole and diastole. Carpentier type IIIB represents restricted leaflet motion in systole. (From El Sabbagh A, Reddy YN, Nishimura RA. Mitral valve regurgitation in the contemporary era: insights into diagnosis, management, and future directions. *JACC Cardiovasc Imaging.* 2018;11(4):628–643, cent. illus.)

vascular resistance may resolve the obstruction of the LV outflow tract. However, if obstruction of the LV outflow tract persists despite these maneuvers, the MV repair may need to be revised, often by using a larger-size annuloplasty and, at times, using an Alfieri repair to reduce leaflet excursion during diastole.

Once the repair or replacement is determined to be successful, separation from cardiopulmonary bypass may ensue, anticoagulation (heparinization) can be reversed, the heart and vessels can be decannulated, and the patient managed as any other patient would be who has undergone cardiopulmonary bypass.

## SUGGESTED READINGS

Ashikhmina, E., Schaff, H. V., Daly, R. C., Stulak, J. M., Greason, K. L., Michelena, H. I., et al. (2021). Risk factors and progression of systolic anterior motion after mitral valve repair. *Journal of Thoracic and Cardiovascular Surgery, 162,* 567–577.

Bax, J. J., Debonnaire, P., Lancellotti, P., Ajmone Marsan, N., Tops, L. F., Min, J. K., et al. (2019). Transcatheter interventions for mitral regurgitation: Multimodality imaging for patient selection and procedural guidance. *JACC Cardiovascular Imaging, 12,* 2029–2048.

Essayagh, B., Mantovani, F., Benfari, G., Maalouf, J. F., Mankad, S., Thapa, P., et al. (2022). Mitral annular disjunction of degenerative mitral regurgitation: Three-dimensional evaluation and implications for mitral repair. *Journal of the American Society of Echocardiography, 35*(2), 165–175.

Grayburn, P. A., & Thomas, J. D. (2021). Basic principles of the echocardiographic evaluation of mitral regurgitation. *JACC Cardiovascular Imaging, 14,* 843–853.

Kampaktsis, P. N., Lebehn, M., & Wu, I. Y. (2021). Mitral regurgitation in 2020: The 2020 focused update of the 2017 American College of Cardiology Expert Consensus Decision Pathway on the management of mitral regurgitation. *Journal of Cardiothoracic and Vascular Anesthesia, 35,* 1678–1690.

Lawrie, G. M. (2020). Surgical treatment of mitral regurgitation. *Current Opinion in Cardiology, 35,* 491–499.

Otto, C. M., Nishimura, R. A., Bonow, R. O., et al. (2021). 2020 ACC/AHA guideline for the Management of Patients with Valvular Heart Disease: A report of the American College of Cardiology/American Heart Association Joint Committee on Clinical Practice Guidelines. *Journal of the American College of Cardiology, 77*(4), e25–e197. Erratum in: J Am Coll Cardiol. 2021;77(4):509. Erratum in: J Am Coll Cardiol. 2021;77(9):1275.

Silbiger, J. J., Lee, S., Christia, P., & Perk, G. (2019). Mechanisms, pathophysiology, and diagnostic imaging of left ventricular outflow tract obstruction following mitral valve surgery and transcatheter mitral valve replacement. *Echocardiography (Mount Kisco, N.Y.), 36,* 1165–1172.

Sweeney, J., Dutta, T., Sharma, M., Kabra, N., Ranjan, P., Goldberg, J., et al. (2022). Variations in mitral valve leaflet and scallop anatomy on three-dimensional transesophageal echocardiography. *Journal of the American Society of Echocardiography, 35,* 77–85.

Virk, S. A., Tian, D. H., Sriravindrarajah, A., Dunn, D., Wolfenden, H. D., Suri, R. M., et al. (2017). Mitral valve surgery and coronary artery bypass grafting for moderate-to-severe ischemic mitral regurgitation: Meta-analysis of clinical and echocardiographic outcomes. *Journal of Thoracic and Cardiovascular Surgery, 154*(1), 127–136.

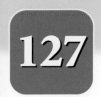

# 127

# Percutaneous Approaches to Valvular Disease: Transcatheter Aortic Valve Replacement and Transcatheter Mitral Valve Repair

RYAN C. CRANER, MD  |  BRANTLEY D. GAITAN, MD  |  RICARDO WEIS, MD

Valvular heart disease accounts for a significant portion of cardiac surgical procedures. Aortic stenosis (AS) is the most common valvular heart disease worldwide. Calcific AS is thought to be a disease of the elderly and increases in prevalence with age, occurring in 2.5% of patients 75 years old and up to 8.1% at 85 years. In the United States, mitral regurgitation (MR) is the most frequently encountered valvular lesion, although this includes patients diagnosed but not necessarily requiring surgical correction. Like calcific AS, degenerative mitral valve disease is seen with increasing frequency in the aging population, affecting more than 6% of patients 65 years and older. When severe AS or MR becomes symptomatic or left ventricular (LV) systolic dysfunction develops, surgery is recommended and the prognosis is poor if left untreated, with a 2-year mortality approaching 50%. However, patients diagnosed with severe valvular disease often have comorbidities that increase their risk for open surgical intervention.

## Treatment Options for Aortic Stenosis and Mitral Regurgitation

Surgical aortic valve replacement (SAVR) has long been the gold standard for treatment of calcific AS. The first reported open SAVR was performed in 1960 using a porcine valve xenograft. Early surgical experience for mitral valve disease was around the same time, with the first open repair for regurgitation performed in the late 1950s and the development of the first commercially available artificial mitral valve in the 1960s. The decades since have seen advances in surgical techniques, perfusion technology, and anesthetic practices, which have allowed open heart surgery to be performed with relative safely for most patients. Despite these advances, many patients with valvular disease are not surgical candidates because of comorbid conditions.

Operative risk associated with cardiac surgery in the elderly can be as high as 10% and increases with associated comorbidities such as LV dysfunction and chronic renal disease. In fact, in the 1980s, patients over the age of 70 were disqualified from candidacy for open surgical repair, which motivated the search for less invasive options. In 2002, Cribier and colleagues described the first percutaneous placement of a prosthetic aortic valve, which was soon followed by feasibility trials restricted to compassionate use. The early success of transcatheter aortic valve replacement (TAVR) and continued technologic advances ultimately led to development of the SAPIEN valve (Edwards Lifesciences, Irvine, CA) and the CoreValve (Medtronic, Inc., Minneapolis, MN). In 2014, the first generation valves (SAPIEN

XT and CoreValve System) were both U.S. Food and Drug Administration (FDA) approved for use in high-risk patients, and in 2017 the FDA expanded the indication for use of the newer generation valves (SAPIEN 3 and CoreValve Evolut R System) to include treatment of patients with severe AS at intermediate risk for surgery.

Surgical intervention has also historically been the preferred definitive treatment for severe degenerative MR. This has evolved to mitral repair being preferred when possible (rather than replacement) because of superior outcomes and lower risk. As with degenerative AS, a large percentage of patients with degenerative MR are not surgical candidates because of comorbidities. Alfieri originally described an edge-to-edge open mitral valve repair (MVR) technique in the 1990s, where a suture is placed to attach the redundant mitral leaflets together, creating two effective orifices between the leaflets and therefore reducing the regurgitant fraction. Percutaneous MVR is based on the Alfieri technique because it involves the placement of a clip rather than suture to attach the two mitral leaflets to each other and effectively decrease regurgitation. Early experience with this device led to the first randomized trial comparing a transcatheter mitral repair device (MitraClip, Abbott Vascular, Santa Clara, CA) with standard MVR, showing the MitraClip to be effective and safe in high-risk patients who are poor operative candidates. MitraClip was subsequently FDA approved in 2013 for use in patients who meet prohibitive risk criteria. With further experience its indications may be eventually be expanded (i.e., for patients with functional MR).

## Patient Selection

Candidacy for percutaneous intervention for valvular disease should be determined through a multidisciplinary team. Management of severe valvular heart disease and appropriate selection of patients for TAVR/transcatheter aortic valve implantation (TAVI) or transcatheter mitral valve repair (TMVR) requires a focused heart valve team that includes cardiologists, structural valve interventional cardiologists, cardiovascular imaging specialists (echocardiographers), cardiac surgeons, and cardiac anesthesiologists.

As noted earlier, the population of AS patients considered for TAVR has expanded with FDA approval of intermediate risk patients. This is now reflected in the American College of Cardiology/American Heart Association (ACC/AHA) guidelines for the management of patients with valvular heart disease as well. The 2014 guidelines recommended TAVR to be considered in AS patients with prohibitive or high risk for SAVR, with predicted survival post-TAVR greater than 12 months. These were updated in 2017 to recommend TAVR to be considered in both intermediate and high surgical risk patients with symptomatic AS.

Regarding patients with MR considered for TMVR, the ACC/AHA guidelines remained unchanged with the 2017 update. Current recommendation is to consider TMVR for patients with chronic severe primary MR who are severely symptomatic and have prohibitive or high surgical risk, have favorable anatomy for the procedure, and reasonable life expectancy.

TAVR/TAVI and TMVR are contraindicated in patients who cannot tolerate procedural anticoagulation or a postprocedural antiplatelet regimen, have active endocarditis or other ongoing infection, or intracardiac, inferior vena cava, or femoral venous thrombus. Preexisting mechanical heart valves may prevent use of percutaneous valve systems, although there has been success with some valve-in-valve techniques for AS. Sensitivity to contrast media (if severe or not amenable to pretreatment) may preclude placement of the devices. Use of the devices is also contraindicated if there is an allergy to any components of the revalving system (e.g., titanium or nickel).

## Devices and Insertion Techniques

There are currently two types of valves approved by the FDA for TAVR. Both SAPIEN (SAPIEN XT and SAPIEN 3; Edwards Lifesciences) and CoreValve (CoreValve and Evolut R; Medtronic, Inc.) are bioprosthetic aortic valves on metal alloy frames that are deployed within the native aortic valve (Figs. 127.1 and 127.2). The differences in valve design and in the valve delivery systems will affect which valve is most appropriate for use (Table 127.1). Additional patient factors that are considered include patient size, annulus size, distance from annulus to coronary vessels within the coronary sinus, and presence of

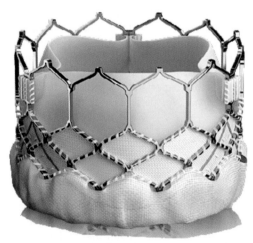

**Fig. 127.1** SAPIEN is a trileaflet valve that is deployed within the native calcified aortic valve after it has been opened with balloon dilation. Low-profile access (smaller diameter delivery system) allows the valve to be delivered through smaller or diseased vessels, and it can be delivered through multiple approaches so it may be used in patients whose anatomy or vascular disease might otherwise prohibit transcatheter aortic valve replacement. The newer generation SAPIEN 3 has lower-profile delivery catheters (14F), improvements in valve frame design and composition (cobalt alloy), and an outer skirt to reduce paravalvular leak. (From Edwards Lifesciences LLC, Irvine, CA. Edwards, Edwards Lifesciences, Edwards SAPIEN, SAPIEN, SAPIEN XT, and SAPIEN 3 are trademarks of Edwards Lifesciences Corporation.)

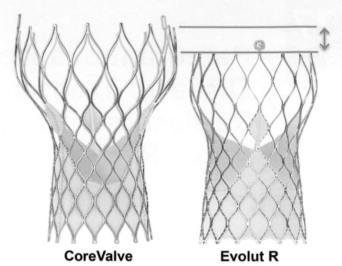

**CoreValve**      **Evolut R**

**Fig. 127.2** CoreValve is a trileaflet valve prosthesis with a self-expanding nitinol frame that displaces the native aortic valve (does not require balloon dilation) and seats in a supraannular position. The newer-generation CoreValve Evolut R can be repositioned and recaptured, and its largest-size valve (CoreValve Evolut R 34 mm) expanded options to patients with larger (26–30 mm) native aortic valves who previously were unable to receive a transcatheter aortic valve implantation. (From Popma JJ et al. Early clinical outcomes after transcatheter aortic valve replacement using a novel self-expanding bioprosthesis in patients with severe aortic stenosis who are suboptimal for surgery. *JACC.* 2017;10(3):fig. 1.)

| TABLE 127.1 | SAPIEN and CoreValve | |
|---|---|---|
| | **Edwards SAPIEN** | **Medtronic CoreValve** |
| Leaflet design | Trileaflet | Trileaflet |
| Leaflet material | Bovine pericardial | Porcine pericardial |
| Frame material | Stainless steel (SAPIEN XT) | Nickel-titanium alloy (Nitinol) |
| | Cobalt alloy (SAPIEN 3) | |
| Deployment mechanism | Balloon dilation | Self-expanding |
| Valve sizing | 20, 23, 26, 29 mm | 23, 26, 29, 34* mm |
| Design | Low valve frame height / Outer skirt to reduce paravalvular leak | Supraannular |
| Delivery profile | 14 or 16F† | 14F, <1/5 inch‡ |
| Approach | Transfemoral / Transaxillary / Transapical / Transaortic | Transfemoral / Transaxillary / Transsubclavian |

*34 mm is indicated for annulus size up to 30 mm.
†14F for 20, 23, 26 mm and 16F for 29 mm.
‡Vessel indication of 5.0 mm in Evolut 23, 26, and 29; others require vessels >5.5 mm.

peripheral vascular disease or vascular anatomy, which may preclude a transfemoral approach.

The MitraClip device is currently the only device approved by the FDA for TAMR. The clip is cobalt-chromium and has a polyester cover designed to promote tissue growth. Like the TAVR devices, the MitraClip has a specialized delivery system

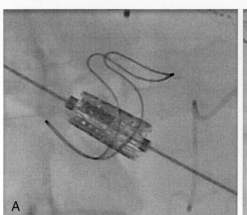
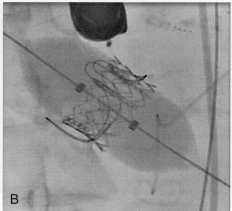
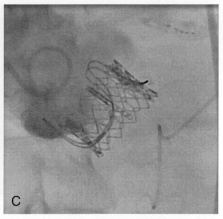

**Fig. 127.3**  **A,** Fluoroscopic images during positioning of the aortic valve prosthesis during a valve-in-valve transcatheter aortic valve replacement (SAPIEN). The wire frame and prosthetic sewing ring of the previously placed aortic valve are visible. **B,** During rapid ventricular pacing, balloon expansion within the aortic valve annulus is performed and the valve deployed. **C,** Aortography demonstrates a successful placement of a competent prosthetic valve. (From Webb JG et al. Transcatheter valve-in-valve implantation for failed bioprosthetic heart valves. *Circulation.* 2010;121:1848–1857.)

that allows the clip to be threaded into its intracardiac position via transfemoral approach (into the left atrium through a transseptal puncture). The delivery system is larger (24F) than the TAVR systems because it requires a more sophisticated, highly steerable catheter that can be manipulated for accurate placement of the clip on the mitral leaflets. The controls are on the proximal end of the delivery system and allow for real-time positioning and repositioning of the clip(s).

Percutaneous valve procedures are routinely performed in the hybrid operating room or the catheterization laboratory. Fluoroscopy and echocardiography (more often transesophageal echocardiography [TEE]) are used throughout the procedures to guide placement of the devices, determine successful placement, and monitor for potential complications. TAVR procedures are performed with a team of cardiac surgeons and interventional cardiologists, with a perfusionist readily available should there be a need for emergent conversion to cardiopulmonary bypass. In contrast, TAMR is usually performed by an interventional cardiologist, without cardiopulmonary bypass capabilities readily available. Vascular access is obtained first, usually via the femoral artery, although a transcarotid approach has been utilized for those with significant femoro/iliac arterial disease. Transaortic or transapical approaches for TAVR require more invasive access (ministernotomy or minianterior thoracotomy).

After vascular access is obtained, TAVR/TAVI involves positioning of a guidewire across the diseased aortic valve. The compressed valve is then threaded into position over the guidewire and deployed within the native valve. Position of the wire and the compressed valve are confirmed with fluoroscopy and echocardiography (TEE if under general anesthesia, transthoracic if under monitored anesthesia care [MAC]). The SAPIEN valve requires balloon dilation of the calcified native valve; rapid ventricular pacing is used during this phase and results in severe aortic insufficiency immediately after dilation until the prosthesis is deployed. The CoreValve is self-expanding and does not require dilation before being deployed. Fluoroscopy and echocardiography are used continuously before and during deployment to ensure accurate placement (Fig. 127.3). When successful deployment is confirmed, the delivery system is removed and the vascular access site repaired.

For MitraClip procedures, a right heart catheterization is performed to document baseline pressures. Next, under guidance of

fluoroscopy and echocardiography, a transseptal puncture is performed and the 24F guide catheter is introduced. The steerable catheter with the open clip is advanced across the septal puncture into the left atrium (Fig. 127.4A). The clip is positioned over the mitral valve with the arms open toward the left ventricle, so the leaflets can be grasped by the clip when it is closed (Fig. 127.4B; see also corresponding TEE loop Video 127.1) TEE is used to assess leaflet capture and to evaluate for residual MR and/or presence of mitral stenosis (MS) after the clip is placed. The clip can be reopened and repositioned if needed, and additional clips can also be placed (Fig. 127.5; see also corresponding TEE loop Videos 127.2–127.4).

## Anesthetic Management

### TRANSCATHETER AORTIC VALVE REPLACEMENT/ TRANSCATHETER AORTIC VALVE IMPLANTATION

The anesthetic technique for TAVR depends on patient comorbidities and planned procedural approach. Both general anesthesia and MAC have been used with success. General anesthesia offers several advantages including control of airway and ventilation, blunted sympathetic response and its effect on hemodynamic control, and ease of use of TEE. Controlled ventilation facilitates breath holding and reduces the likelihood of patient movement during valve placement. General anesthesia (GA) may also be preferred for patients who may not tolerate the supine position for the duration of the procedure (e.g., obstructive sleep apnea [OSA], morbid obesity, claustrophobia, back pain). Disadvantages to GA include difficult airway management, delayed emergence, myocardial depressant effects of anesthetics, and potential hemodynamic disturbances on induction and emergence. Because of the required surgical exposure, transapical and transaortic approaches for TAVR require GA with an endotracheal tube.

GA is often accomplished with standard induction agents and maintained with inhalational agents. Invasive monitoring is usually required, with placement of pulmonary artery catheter often at the discretion of the anesthesiologist. If extubation at the end of the case is planned, the anesthetic should be tailored accordingly. Disposition of the patient varies based on patient condition and local practice.

MAC is being used more frequently for elective TAVR placement. Transfemoral or transaxillary approaches can be

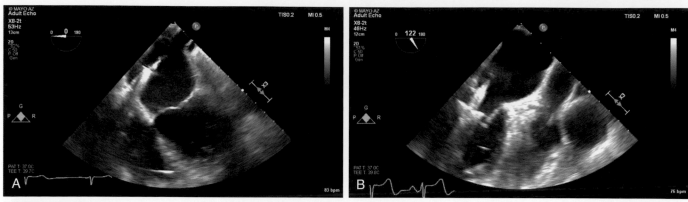

**Fig. 127.4**   Two-dimensional transesophageal echocardiography images during transcatheter mitral valve repair procedure. **A,** The delivery catheter has been threaded into the left atrium through the transseptal puncture. **B,** The MitraClip device is positioned at the tip of the steering catheter before placement.

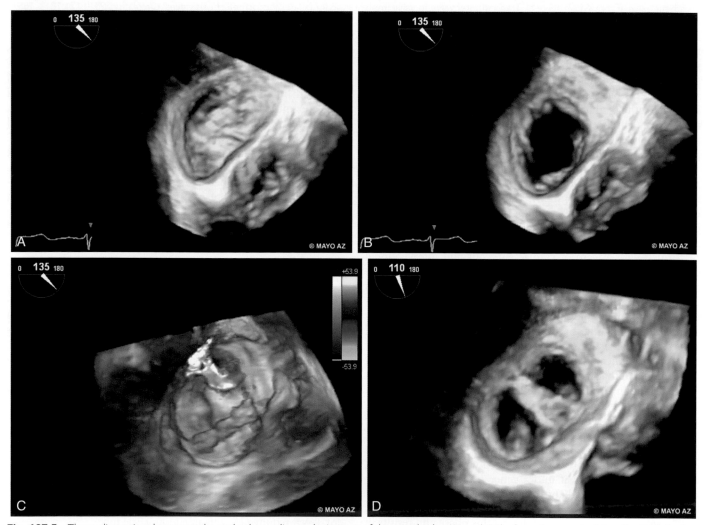

**Fig. 127.5**   Three-dimensional transesophageal echocardiography images of the mitral valve **(A)** and **(B)** before placement of the clip. **C,** Color flow demonstrating the regurgitant jet through mitral valve before placement of the clip. **D,** After placement of the clip.

performed with MAC, but this requires patient cooperation and suitability (e.g., OSA or morbid obesity may prevent this technique). Infusions or boluses of dexmedetomidine, propofol, remifentanil, or ketamine (in combination or as monotherapy) have been used for MAC. TAVR under MAC can be performed without central venous access in appropriate patients; these patients have an arterial line and two large-bore intravenous lines. Many institutions performing TAVR under MAC allow for the patients to be discharged from the postanesthesia care unit to a non–intensive care (non-ICU) setting. Advantages of MAC are shorter procedural time, ability to monitor mental status and therefore cerebral perfusion, shorter (or no) ICU stay, shorter hospital length of stay, and lower in-hospital mortality. Disadvantages include inability to use TEE (most MAC cases use transthoracic), difficulty providing advanced airway management (because of C-arm of fluoroscopy and other equipment), and possible lower procedural success rate (determined by rate of paravalvular leak and requirement for permanent pacemaker after the procedure). Lower procedural success rates with MAC could be caused by transthoracic versus TEE imaging or by patient movement during critical portions of the procedure.

Regardless of anesthetic technique or valve being used, vasoactive and inotropic medications should be readily available. Before deployment of the valve, heparin is administered and monitored with activated clotting time with a goal of greater than 250 seconds. The most critical portion of the procedure is during valve deployment because any movement may interfere with successful valve deployment. Thus ventilation is often held during this portion for patients under GA, and depth of sedation is usually increased for patients under MAC. Hemodynamic support should be provided if needed throughout rapid ventricular pacing (RVP) and deployment of the valve, because a mean arterial pressure of less than 75 before RVP can be associated with prolonged hypotension. When RVP is terminated, the systemic blood pressure typically recovers as normal loading conditions and cardiac output are restored. There can be transient ST segment changes or wall motion abnormalities because of the demand ischemia.

Complications can include malposition of the valve; the CoreValve can be retrieved and repositioned, whereas the SAPIEN cannot. SAPIEN malposition may require a second valve to be placed within the first prosthesis (valve-in-valve). Both valve malposition and folding of the native calcified leaflets can potentially occlude the coronary arteries, so continued vigilance and preparedness for intervention is paramount. Postprocedural arrhythmias can occur; the CoreValve is associated with a higher rate of atrioventricular block than SAPIEN. Vascular injuries are possible in all transvascular approaches (i.e., transfemoral and transaxillary/subclavian), and there is potential risk of cardiac tamponade or lung injury during transapical TAVR.

## TRANSCATHETER MITRAL VALVE REPAIR

GA with endotracheal intubation is the prevalent anesthetic technique used in these procedures because it facilitates the intraoperative prolonged use of TEE, allows to control the ventilation and breath holding, and ensures that the patient does not move during the case. Deep sedation is a less commonly used method.

Hemodynamic monitoring is achieved with electrocardiography, pulse oximetry, TEE, and discretionary use of invasive arterial blood pressure and central venous pressure. At the time of transseptal puncture, heparin is administered. Breath holding is needed during critical steps, such as during difficult grasping attempts or when a second or third clip is being advanced from left atrium to the left ventricle. Vasopressor agents may be necessary, and TEE may also be used to assess location and severity of residual MR and to guide clip placement.

Complications can include rare clip malposition, partial clip detachment, or clip embolization. Vascular injury and bleeding complications are unusual but more commonly encountered versus TAVR/TAVI procedures because of the larger size of the delivery system.

Visit Elsevier eBooks+ (https://eBooks.Health.Elsevier.com) for videos.

## SUGGESTED READINGS

Chung, M., & Vazquez, R. (2020). Non-operating room anesthesia. In M. A. Gropper (Ed.), *Miller's anesthesia* (9th ed., pp. 2284–2312). Philadelphia: Elsevier.

Gaemperli, O., & Corti, R. (2012). MitraClip for the treatment of mitral regurgitation. *Cardiovascular Medicine*, *15*(10), 276–286.

Guarracino, F., Baldassarri, R., Ferro, B., Giannini, C., Bertini, P., Petronio, A. S., et al. (2014). Transesophageal echocardiography during MitraClip® procedure. *Anesthesia and Analgesia*, *118*(6), 1188–1196.

Hyman, M. C., Vemulapalli, S., Szeto, W. Y., Stebbins, A., Patel, P. A., Matsouaka, R. A., et al. (2017). Conscious sedation versus general anesthesia for transcatheter aortic valve replacement: Insights from the National Cardiovascular Data Registry Society of Thoracic Surgeons/American College of Cardiology Transcatheter Valve Therapy Registry. *Circulation*, *136*(22), 2132–2140.

Kothandan, H., Vui, K. H., Khung, K. Y., & Nian, C. H. (2014). Anesthesia management for MitraClip device implantation. *Annals of Cardiac Anaesthesia*, *17*(2), 132.

Nishimura, R. A. , Otto, C, Bonow, R, Carabello, B, & Erwin, J, et al. (2018). 2017 focused update of the 2014 ACC/AHA guideline for the management of patients with valvular heart disease. *Circulation*, *137*(9), 1–59.

Otto, C. M., Nishimura, R. A., Bonow, R. O., Carabello, B. A., Erwin, J. P., III, Gentile, F., et al. (2021). 2020 ACC/AHA guideline for the management of patients with valvular heart disease: A report of the American College of Cardiology/American Heart Association Joint Committee of Clinical Practice Guidelines. *Circulation*, *143*(5), e72–e227.

Patzelt, J., Ulrich, M., Magunia, H., Sauter, R., Droppa, M., Jorbenadze, R., et al. (2017). Comparison of deep sedation with general anesthesia in patients undergoing percutaneous mitral valve repair. *Journal of the American Heart Association*, *6*(12), e007485.

Thourani, V. H., Kodali, S., Makkar, R. R., Herrmann, H. C., Williams, M., Babaliaros, V., et al. (2016). Transcatheter aortic valve replacement versus surgical valve replacement in intermediate-risk patients: A propensity score analysis. *Lancet*, *387*(10034), 2218–2225.

Zakhary, W., & Ender, J. K. (2018). Procedures in the hybrid operating room. In J. A. Kaplan, B. Cronin, T. Maus (Eds.), *Kaplan's essentials of cardiac anesthesia* (2nd ed., pp. 534–550). Philadelphia: Elsevier.

Zakhary, W., & Ender, J. K. (2017). Procedures in the hybrid operating room. In J. A. Kaplan, J. T. G. Augoustides, G. R. Manecke, T. Maus, D. L. Reich (Eds.), *Kaplan's cardiac anesthesia* (7th ed., pp. 1022–1041). Philadelphia: Elsevier.

# 128

# Pacemakers

TARRAH FOLLEY, MD | CHELSEA CAMBA ALFAFARA, MD

## Overview

The prevalence of cardiac arrhythmias in the United States is increasing each year. The most common of these arrythmias are atrial fibrillation (AF) and atrial flutter (AFL). Many of these patients will have cardiac implantable electronic devices (CIEDs) placed to treat conduction problems, arrhythmias, and ventricular dysfunction associated with cardiac arrhythmias. The number of implanted devices continues to rise dramatically, with more than three million people in the United States estimated to have a conventional pacemaker and more 300,000 estimated to have an implantable cardioverter-defibrillator (ICD) with pacing capabilities. It is important that anesthesia personnel have an understanding of these devices and the anesthetic implications and potential complications for both initial placement and generator changes. Additionally, with the increasing incidence of patients presenting with CIEDs for other surgical procedures, it is essential for anesthesia care providers to have a comprehensive understanding of CIEDs and their function during the perioperative period, as one of the primary issues facing the care team remains that of electromagnetic interference (EMI).

Although technologic improvements have revolutionized pacemaker function, improved outcomes, and diminished issues such as EMI, there remain both short- and long-term complications associated with transvenous CIEDs. Pacemakers consist of two components: a pulse generator, which provides an electrical impulse; and one or more electrodes or leads, which are usually placed transvenously to deliver the electrical impulse from the pulse generator to the myocardium. The generator is usually placed in a subcutaneous or subpectoral pocket on the side where the leads are threaded through the venous system into the heart, where they are attached to the endocardium. Immediate (short-term) complications are related to the placement of the device and include pneumothorax, lead dislodgement, vascular injury, and cardiac perforation. Long-term complications include central venous thrombosis and obstruction, tricuspid valve injury, lead failures, lead endocarditis, and pocket infections. Newer nontransvenous CIED devices mitigate these risks to a degree and include both leadless pacemakers and subcutaneous defibrillators with extravascular leads.

## Generic Codes of Pacemakers

Developed originally by the International Conference on Heart Disease and subsequently modified by the North American Society of Pacing and Electrophysiology/British Pacing and Electrophysiology Group (NASPE/BPEG) alliance, the NASPE/BPEG code consists of five letters of the alphabet that describe the five programmable functions of the pacing system (Box 128.1). The first letter of the code indicates the chamber

---

### BOX 128.1  NORTH AMERICAN SOCIETY OF PACING AND ELECTROPHYSIOLOGY/BRITISH PACING AND ELECTROPHYSIOLOGY GROUP (NASPE/BPEG) GENERIC PACEMAKER CODES

Position 1 (chamber paced): V, A, D, S, O*
Position 2 (chamber sensed): V, A, D, S, O*
Position 3 (mode of response): T, I, D, O†
Position 4 (programmability, rate modulation): P, M, C, R, O‡
Position 5 (multisite pacing): V, A, D, O§

*V, Ventricular; A, atrial; D, dual chamber (i.e., ventricle and atrium); S, single chamber (i.e., ventricle or atrium); O, none.
†T, Triggered; I, inhibited; D, dual chamber (atrial triggered and ventricular inhibited); O, none.
‡P, Programmable (rate and/or output); M, multiprogrammable; C, communicating; R, rate modulated; O, none.
§V, Ventricular; A, atrial; D, dual; O, none.

---

being paced; the second letter, the chamber being sensed; and the third letter, the response to sensing (I and T indicate inhibited or triggered responses, respectively). An R in the fourth position indicates that the pacemaker incorporates a sensor to detect a physical index, like increased vibration, or a physiologic index, like increased lead impedance to modulate the heart rate independently. The fifth letter position was previously assigned to an antitachycardia arrhythmia function, such as rapid pacing or shocks, but more recently it is used to describe the presence of multisite pacing options. Usually, a V indicates multisite pacing in the ventricles. However, letters in the fifth position are uncommonly used. Table 128.1 summarizes commonly used configurations.

## Preoperative Evaluation/Preparation

Preoperative evaluation of the patient and the pacemaker is an important aspect of the anesthetic management of a patient with a permanent pacemaker who is undergoing surgery. Recommendations are well detailed in the American Society of Anesthesiologists (ASA) Practice Advisory on Perioperative Management (2020). Preoperative evaluation consists of four steps: (1) identifying patients with a CIED; (2) determining the CIED type, manufacturer, and primary indication for placement; (3) determining whether a patient is pacing-dependent; and (4) determining the device's current settings and if it is functioning properly (either by the most recent interrogation report or interrogating the device directly).

Identification of patients with CIEDs can be obtained through a detailed patient history, physical examination, and testing such as a chest x-ray and electrocardiogram. Once the device manufacturer has been identified, they can be consulted

| TABLE 128.1 | Common Permanent Pacemaker Modes | | |
|---|---|---|---|
| Pacing Mode | Indication | Function | Perioperative Management |
| VVI | Bradycardia without the need for preserved AV conduction | Demand ventricular pacing | Magnet use may be helpful and converts to asynchronous pacing, usually at 72 beats/min |
| VVIR | Bradycardia without the need for preserved AV conduction; chronotropic incompetence | Allows a somewhat physiologic response to exercise | Pacemaker may sense perioperative changes (e.g., temperature, respiratory rate) as related to exercise or unpredictable response to magnet placement; suggest postoperative interrogation |
| DDD | Bradycardia when AV synchrony can be preserved | Provides more physiologic response; maintains AV concordance | Unpredictable response to magnet placement; suggest postoperative interrogation |
| DDDR | Patients requiring physiologic response of heart rate (i.e., chronotropic incompetence) | Provides increased physiologic response to exercise; maintains AV concordance | Pacemaker may sense perioperative changes (e.g., temperature, respiratory rate) as related to exercise or unpredictable response to magnet placement; suggest postoperative interrogation |

AV, Atrioventricular.

for detailed information regarding a patient's CIED. Most manufacturers maintain a 24 hours per day, 7 days per week technical support hotline. Operative information necessary for the CIED team would include the location of surgery, proximity to the pacemaker, and the likelihood of EMI during the procedure.

After establishing the presence, type, and function of the device, the determination is made whether the patient is CIED dependent for antibradycardiac function. A discussion between the CIED team and the anesthesiologist can then facilitate management in the operating room, including (1) leaving the pacemaker as is, (2) reprogramming to an asynchronous mode, (3) disabling rate-responsive functions, (4) suspending antiarrhythmic functions for devices with this capability, and (5) assessing the need for alternative pacing methods.

If the patient also has an ICD, one should consider disabling it before induction of anesthesia for surgical procedures that will use electrocautery superior to the umbilicus.

## Effect of a Magnet on Pacemaker Function

Magnets are used in the operating room to protect the pacemaker-dependent patient from the effects of EMI. Magnets most commonly affect a magnetic reed switch that switches the on-and-off circuitry within the device. Newer pacemaker models may have similar alternative technology using a Hall-effect sensor, giant magnetosensitive resistors, or telemetry coils. In general, a magnet placed over a pacemaker pulse generator triggers an asynchronous pacing mode at a fixed rate. However, the response varies with the model and the manufacturer and may be in the form of no apparent change in rate or rhythm, brief asynchronous pacing, continuous or transient loss of pacing, or asynchronous pacing without rate response. Thus it is advisable to have the pacemaker interrogated by a qualified technician and to consult with the manufacturer to determine the exact behavior of the CIED with magnet application. The routine use of a magnet during surgery is not without risk and at times may result in undesirable outcomes. Switching to asynchronous pacing may trigger atrioventricular dyssynchrony, which may cause myocardial ischemia, hypoxia, or electrolyte imbalance in selected patients. Some new-generation pacemakers are relatively immune to magnet application, and placement of a magnet may not convert a pacemaker to an asynchronous mode. Constant

magnet application over the pacemaker may alter its programming, leading to either inhibited or triggered pacing, or may cause continuous or transient loss of pacing. Magnets placed over programmable pacemakers, in the presence of EMI, have been known to reprogram the pulse generator. This change may not be evident until after the magnet is removed. A further problem with magnetic application is the variability of response between devices because there is no universal standard between device manufacturers.

## Intraoperative Management

Intraoperative monitoring should be based on the patient's underlying disease and the type of operation to be performed. ASA standards for patient monitoring should be applied. The presence of a pacemaker should not affect the choice of anesthetic agent; both intravenous and inhalation agent–based techniques can be used because they do not alter the current and voltage thresholds of the pacemaker. Skeletal myopotentials, electroconvulsive therapy (ECT), succinylcholine fasciculation, myoclonic movements, and direct muscle stimulation can inappropriately inhibit or trigger pacemaker stimulation, depending on the programmed pacing modes. Case reports have indicated that myoclonus associated with the use of etomidate and ketamine may affect pacemaker function. In patients with rate-responsive pacemakers, the rate-responsive mode should be deactivated before surgery. If this is not possible, the mode of rate response must be known so that conditions causing changes in paced heart rate can be avoided. For example, shivering and fasciculations should be avoided if the pacemaker is "activity" rate responsive, ventilation (respiratory rate and tidal volume) should be controlled if the pacemaker is "minute ventilation" rate responsive, and temperature must be kept constant in "temperature" rate-responsive pacemakers.

## Electromagnetic Interference

Among the various sources of EMI, electrocautery is the most important. Electrocautery involves the use of radiofrequency currents of 300 to 500 kHz to cut or coagulate tissue during surgical procedures. Fatal arrhythmias and deaths have been reported with the use of electrocautery leading to failure of pacemakers. Between 1984 and 1997, the U.S. Food and Drug

Administration was notified of 456 adverse events with the use of pulse generators—255 from electrocautery—with a significant number of device failures. The most common CIED interaction with EMI is oversensing, which occurs most commonly when the electric current used with electrocautery is mistaken for cardiac conduction. This results in possible inhibition of pacing output, which can be fatal in those who are pacemaker-dependent. Other effects may include mode switching or alteration in rate responsiveness. Less common are reports of pacemaker resetting, pulse generator damage, and lead tissue interface damage. The following measures may decrease the possibility of adverse effects caused by electrocautery:

- Bipolar cautery should be used as much as possible because it causes less EMI.
- If unipolar cautery is planned superior to the umbilicus, reprogram the device to asynchronous pacing mode in pacing-dependent patients. If the device has ICD capabilities, suspend antitachycardia functioning in a monitored environment.
- Position the electrosurgical return electrode (pad) such that the current pathway does not pass through or near the CIED generator or leads. The pad should be placed close to the operative site and as far away as possible from the site of the pacemaker, usually on the patient's thigh. In cases where the thigh is not accessible, the electrosurgical return electrode can be placed on the posterior superior aspect of the shoulder contralateral to the generator position.
- Electrocautery should not be used within 15 cm of a pacemaker.
- The use of electrocautery should be limited to 1-s bursts in every 10 s to prevent asystole.
- During the use of cautery, the magnet should not be placed on the pulse generator because it may cause pacemaker malfunction. Ask for a pause in EMI use before placement.
- Drugs such as isoproterenol and atropine should be available.
- If defibrillation is required in a patient with a pacemaker, paddles should be positioned as far away as possible from the pacemaker generator. If possible, the paddles should be placed anterior to posterior.
- The lead from nerve stimulators should not overlay the generator.
- The device should always be rechecked after the operation if electrocautery was used during the procedure.
- For certain patients with unipolar sensing configuration of their device, switching to bipolar configuration sensing, if possible, can reduce oversensing as well.

## Magnetic Resonance Imaging

Traditionally, magnetic resonance imaging (MRI) has been contraindicated for people with CIED even when it may be the most appropriate diagnostic imaging method for the patient's medical condition. With the increasing number of placements of CIEDs and the likelihood of patients requiring MRIs during their lifetime, attention is being directed to improve access for patients with CIEDs to this diagnostic modality.

Over the past 20 years, the design of CIEDs has improved their shielding and reduced the ability of EMI to interfere with normal pacemaker functioning in general. Manufacturers continue to work on "MRI-conditional" devices and may hopefully make "MRI-safe" devices at some point in the future.

Recent controlled studies examining pacemaker function during and after MRI have shown encouraging results, primarily in non–pacemaker-dependent patients. Given these results, many institutions have developed protocols that coordinate care between their respective radiology and cardiology departments to allow for specific patients with pacemakers to have MRIs. These examinations are done under controlled and monitored conditions.

## Special Situations

There are other specialized procedural areas where the anesthesia care team will encounter CIED patients. Each of these requires an understanding of the energy sources and their proximity to the device and leads. These include cardioversion, catheter ablations, lithotripsy, therapeutic radiation, ECT therapy, and implantable stimulation devices. Appropriate management of the device after a thorough discussion with the implanting/procedural physicians and the manufacturers should mitigate any potential problems with CIEDs and anesthetic care in these areas.

## Summary

Patients with implanted pacemakers can be managed safely for surgery and other nonsurgical procedures, but to do so requires a thorough understanding of the indication for and the programming of the pacemaker. Anesthetic management should be planned preoperatively according to the patient's medical status, and a plan for the intraoperative device management should be made with the patient's or the institution's CIED team. Precautions should be taken to minimize EMI while using electrocautery. The magnet should not be placed over the pacemaker in the operating room while electrocautery is in use. Rate-responsive pacemakers should have the rate-responsive mode disabled before the operation begins. Provision of temporary pacing should be available in the operating room to deal with pacemaker malfunction (Table 128.2).

## Acknowledgement

Our sincere thanks to Dan Sorajja, MD, for his guidance in preparing this chapter.

| TABLE 128.2 | **Pacemaker Malfunctions: Mechanisms and Potential Causes** | |
|---|---|---|
| **Malfunction** | **Description/Manifestation** | **Potential Causes** |
| Failure to output | No pacing artifact is present despite an indication to pace | Battery failure<br>Lead fracture<br>Fractured lead insulation<br>Oversensing (inhibiting pacer output)<br>Poor lead connection at the takeoff from the pacer<br>"Cross-talk" (i.e., a phenomenon occurring when atrial output is sensed by a ventricular lead in a dual-chamber pacer) |
| Failure to capture | Pacing artifact is not followed by an atrial or a ventricular complex | Lead fracture<br>Lead dislodgement<br>Fracture lead insulation<br>Elevated pacing threshold<br>Myocardial infarction at the lead tip<br>Drugs (e.g., flecainide)<br>Metabolic abnormalities (e.g., hyperkalemia, acidosis, alkalosis)<br>Cardiac perforation<br>Poor lead connection at the takeoff from the generator<br>Improper amplitude or pulse width settings |
| Oversensing* | A pacer senses noncardiac electrical activity and is inhibited, resulting in a heart rate lower than the present rate | Muscle activity, particularly of the diaphragm or pectoralis muscles<br>Electromagnetic interference<br>Fractured lead insulation |
| Undersensing[†] | A pacer misses intrinsic depolarization and paces despite intrinsic activity, resulting in the pacemaker's operating in an asynchronous mode | Poor lead positioning<br>Lead dislodgement<br>Magnet application<br>Low battery<br>Myocardial infarction |
| Pacemaker-mediated tachycardia* | A PVC occurs in a patient with a dual-chamber pacemaker | If a PVC is transmitted in a retrograde manner through the AV node, it may in turn depolarize the atria. The depolarization is detected by the atrial sensor, which then stimulates the ventricular leads to fire, thereby creating an endless loop. Although the maximum rate is limited by the programmed upper limit of the pacemaker, ischemia may develop in susceptible patients. |
| Runaway pacemaker | A malfunction of the pacemaker generator resulting in life-threatening rapid tachycardia (up to 200 beats/min) | Battery failure<br>External damage to the generator |
| Pacemaker syndrome | Patient feels worse after pacemaker placement and presents with progressively worsening CHF | Loss of AV synchrony, whereby the pathway is reversed and now has a ventricular origin |
| Twiddler syndrome[‡] | Chest radiograph reveals twisting, coiling, fracture, dislodgement, or migration of the leads | Patient persistently disturbs or manipulates the generator, resulting in malfunction |
| Cardiac monitor pseudomalfunction[§] | Cardiac monitor reports incorrect heart rate | No malfunction is present; the monitor inappropriately interprets pacing artifacts |
| Pacemaker pseudomalfunction[¶] | Pacing system appears to malfunction | No malfunction is present; the "malfunction" is a normal programmed pacer function, primarily caused by new algorithms that preserve intrinsic conduction and more physiologic pacing |
| R on T phenomenon | Superimposition of an ectopic beat on the T wave of a preceding beat, increasing the risk of sustained ventricular tachyarrhythmias | Asynchronous pacing<br>Sensing malfunction |

*This condition is diagnosable and treatable with magnet application.
[†]Management is similar to that for other types of failures.
[‡]Requires surgical correction and patient counseling and education.
[§]Clinicians faced with this issue should first palpate the patient's pulse and correlate this finding with the results of a pulse oximeter plethysmogram to verify the findings on the cardiac monitor. New monitors have settings to adapt for patients with pacemakers and provide more accurate heart rates.
[¶]Correction may involve changing the programming or changing the device.
*AV,* Atrioventricular; *CHF,* congestive heart failure; *PVC,* premature ventricular contraction.

## SUGGESTED READINGS

Cody, J., Graul, T., Holliday, S., Streckenbach, S., Hussain, N., Dalia, A. A., et al. (2021). Nontransvenous cardiovascular implantable electronic device technology: A review for the anesthesiologist. *Journal of Cardiothoracic and Vascular Anesthesia, 35,* 2784–2791.

Liaquat, M. T., Ahmed, I., & Alzahrani, T. (2023). Pacemaker malfunction. In *StatPearls* [Internet]. Treasure Island, FL: StatPearls Publishing.

# Implantable Cardioverter-Defibrillators

TARRAH FOLLEY, MD | CHELSEA CAMBA ALFAFARA, MD

## Overview

Approximately 380,000 Americans die each year from sudden cardiac arrest. Many of these individuals were taking antiarrhythmic drugs, but drugs alone are not sufficient to prevent ventricular tachycardia and fibrillation. The implantable cardioverter-defibrillator (ICD) has revolutionized the treatment of patients at risk for experiencing sudden cardiac death caused by these ventricular tachyarrhythmias. The superiority of the ICD device over antiarrhythmic therapy has been confirmed in several randomized trials for both secondary and primary prevention of sudden cardiac death in patients with ischemic and nonischemic substrates. The indications of ICD placement are numerous, including survivors of cardiac arrest with ventricular arrythmias and those with ischemic and nonischemic heart failure with reduced ejection fraction of 35% or less. The number of ICD implants continues to increase, with the United States leading the world in both total number and rate (434 new implants per 1 million people). In 2009 alone, based on industry statistics, 133,262 ICDs were implanted in the United States. ICD technology has progressed exponentially since its introduction by Michel Mirowski and colleagues in the early 1980s.

## The Implantable Cardioverter Defibrillator System

The ICD system comprises a microprocessor/pulse generator, a battery, and a conducting lead system. The lead system is required for sensing, pacing, and the delivery of therapy. Early devices were true "shock boxes," capable of detecting a tachycardia and delivering a shock without the ability to pace. The pulse generators for these earlier devices were large enough that they had to be placed abdominally. Defibrillation was delivered via two epicardial patches positioned anteriorly and posteriorly. However, more recent years have seen advancements in lead and generator technology and the development of biphasic defibrillation electric impulses, the latter of which lowered the energy requirements necessary for successful defibrillation. The creation of a bipolar lead combining pacing and sensing capabilities with a high-voltage electrode coil allowed for nonthoracotomy system implants, which reduced surgical morbidity and mortality rates. The leads were positioned transvenously via the subclavian vein and fixed to the inside of the right ventricle. In current practice, transvenous system generators are relatively small—the smallest commercially available devices today are about the size of a stopwatch, approximately $7 \times 5 \times 1$ cm, and weigh 30 to 40 g—allowing for subcutaneous pectoral implantation and simplification of the implantation process.

The ICD generator houses the batteries, high-voltage capacitors, and microprocessors necessary to process any sensed intrinsic cardiac electrical activity. In essence, the generator is a minicomputer within a hermetically sealed titanium box, which can store an electric charge that can be delivered, "shocking" the atria and ventricles back to a sinus rhythm. Typically, ICDs deliver no more than six shocks per event, although some can deliver as many as 18. Within an event, each successive therapy must be at equal or greater energy than the previous attempt. Once a shock is delivered, no further antitachycardia pacing can take place.

Typical ICDs contain lithium silver vanadium oxide cells that store between 2 and 7 volts. The high voltages necessary for defibrillation are generated with the aid of high-voltage capacitors that can generate 700 to 800 volts of defibrillation energy in less than 10 s.

Current devices allow extensive programmability for tiered antitachycardia pacing, tiered high-voltage therapies, bradycardia pacing, supraventricular tachycardia discrimination algorithms, and detailed diagnostics of tachycardic and bradycardic episodes. They also allow physicians to conduct completely noninvasive programmed stimulation. The most recent iterations provide dedicated dual-chamber and antitachycardia pacing and options for atrial defibrillation. Diagnostic functions, including stored electrocardiograms, allow for verification of shock appropriateness. Device battery longevity has also increased; early devices lasted 2 years or less, whereas newer lithium silver vanadium batteries now last up to 9 years.

The U.S. Food and Drug Administration approved the subcutaneous implantable cardioverter-defibrillator (S-ICD) in 2012. This device is implanted in the subcutaneous tissue over the left chest wall with the lead tunneled over the rib cage and along the sternum. It performs basic biphasic defibrillation to terminate lethal arrhythmias. Although it provides a brief period of postshock pacing, it is not meant for patients who require antibradycardiac therapy or cardiac resynchronization therapy. The S-ICD compared favorably to the transvenous system in the Subcutaneous versus Transvenous Arrhythmia Recognition Testing (START) trial and in the ongoing EF-FORTLESS (Evaluation of Factors Impacting Clinical Outcome and Cost Effectiveness of the S-ICD) trial. Preliminary evidence comparing myocardial injury after shock delivery from the two systems favors the S-ICD despite the higher Joules delivered.

## Implantable Cardioverter Defibrillator Placement

Transvenous placement is performed by cardiologists, usually in the left or right infraclavicular area with the leads tunneled transvenously while the patient receives intravenous sedation under monitored anesthesia care (MAC). A deeper level of sedation or general anesthesia is briefly provided to the patient for the discomfort that occurs when the unit is tested (i.e., discharged) and an electric shock is delivered to the patient.

Defibrillation can lead to prolonged periods of asystole that can result in significant myocardial and cerebral ischemia. Enough time should be allowed between tests to ensure reperfusion and restoration of hemodynamic stability. The anesthesia provider must monitor the duration and frequency of testing and ischemic periods. Vasoactive drugs are often used to stabilize these patients during and immediately after the testing period. Minimum monitoring includes standard American Society of Anesthesiologists (ASA) monitors and continuous arterial pressure measurement, usually through an arterial cannula placed by the cardiologist.

## Implantable Cardioverter Defibrillator Functioning as a Pacemaker

ICDs also have the capability to function as pacemakers. An ICD with a built-in capability for pacing will begin pacing when the RR interval (longer RR interval equates to slower heart rates) is greater than previously set limits. Beginning around 1993, most ICDs incorporated backup VVI pacing to protect the patient from the common occurrence of postshock bradycardia. Because many ICDs are programmed to address tachyarrhythmias only, there are occasions where bradytherapy support is required. If a patient with an ICD requires temporary pacing, increasing the lower rate limit of the ICD is preferred. In patients in whom there is only a single chamber RV lead, the pacing from the RV lead can result in AV dyssynchrony or right ventricular–left ventricular dyssynchrony, and it may not be tolerated. In such cases, right atrial pacing may be preferable and can be accomplished by placement of a temporary right atrial lead. Of note, with placement of a magnet over an ICD, the tachytherapy functions will be inactivated, removing the risk of inappropriate and appropriate shock therapy, but the pacing function will remain intact.

## Electromagnetic Interference and Implantable Cardioverter Defibrillators

The ability of ICDs to function is dependent on their ability to sense intrinsic cardiac electrical activity. Hermetic shielding, filtering, interference rejection circuits, and bipolar sensing have safeguarded ICDs (and pacemakers) against the effects of common electromagnetic sources. However, exposure to electromagnetic interference (EMI) may still result in oversensing, asynchronous pacing, ventricular inhibition, and spurious ICD discharges. EMI may also lead to loss of output, increased pacing thresholds, and decreased R-wave amplitude. Common sources of EMI include cellular phones, electronic article surveillance (antitheft) devices, and metal detectors. Occupational sources of EMI include high-voltage power lines, electrical transformers, and arc welding. Interference of concern to anesthesia providers can occur during procedures, such as magnetic resonance imaging, electrocautery, spinal cord stimulators, transcutaneous electrical nerve stimulator units, radiofrequency catheter ablation, therapeutic diathermy, and lithotripsy.

## Inappropriate Implantable Cardioverter Defibrillator Shocks

One of the risks associated with an ICD is that of inappropriate ICD shocks, which can occur from EMI or noise, as mentioned previously, or from detection of other arrhythmias. An inappropriate ICD shock is one that is not precipitated by accurate detection of a malignant ventricular arrhythmia, ventricular tachycardia, or ventricular fibrillation. Typically, inappropriate ICD shocks result when atrial arrhythmias, such as atrial fibrillation, atrial tachycardia, or atrial flutter, accelerate the ventricular rate beyond the set detection heart rate for delivery of ICD shock therapy. Analysis of the MADIT II trial data revealed that 11.5% of the patients with an ICD received inappropriate ICD shocks and that 31.2% of all ICD shocks were deemed inappropriate. Inappropriate ICD shocks caused by arrhythmias were attributed to atrial fibrillation (44%), supraventricular tachycardia (36%), and abnormal sensing (20%). Patients with inappropriate shocks had greater all-cause mortality rate (hazard ratio, 2.29; $P = .025$).

## Implantable Cardioverter Defibrillator Magnets

As with pacemakers, ICDs can be altered by magnets. In general, magnet application to an ICD will result in its antitachycardia therapies being disabled, and the pacing mode will continue unaffected. The switch from "on" to "off" and back most commonly relates to a magnetic reed switch built into the ICD. Newer ICD models may incorporate a Hall-effect sensor, giant magnetosensitive resistor, or telemetry coil, instead of the reed switch, to have similar effect for the switch in programming. The magnetic field effect is proportional to the magnet strength and inversely proportional to the distance of the magnet from the ICD. Therefore in obese patients, sometimes more than one magnet may be required to initiate the switch in programming. Regular functioning of the ICD is restored by removing the magnet. Interrogating the device by a trained technician or calling the manufacturer remain the most reliable ways to determine magnet responsiveness.

## Preoperative Evaluation

ICDs should have the antitachycardia therapy disabled before induction of anesthesia and commencement of the procedure if electrocautery is to be used above the umbilicus. As with pacing devices, monopolar electrosurgical cautery has been reported to "confuse" an ICD into delivering inappropriate therapy. Also, many ICDs have no noise reversion behavior, so electrosurgical cautery–induced ventricular oversensing might cause nonpacing in a patient who depends on an ICD for pacing. For those undergoing anesthesia with ICDs disabled as opposed to with a magnet, anesthesia providers should consider attaching defibrillator pads prior to the induction of anesthesia and should be prepared to quickly provide external defibrillation as long as the device remains disabled.

## Intraoperative Management

No special monitoring or anesthetic technique is required for the patient with an ICD. However, the Heart Rhythm Society and ASA have developed guidelines and recommendations for how the patient with an ICD coming to the operating room for an elective procedure (Box 129.1) or an emergent procedure (Box 129.2) should be managed. For surgeries below the umbilicus, there is minimal need to reprogram an ICD or place a magnet on the ICD because the risk of an adverse event is small. There have, however, been case reports of inadvertent firing

## BOX 129.1   GENERAL PRINCIPLES OF IMPLANTABLE CARDIOVERTER-DEFIBRILLATOR MANAGEMENT

The perioperative management of ICDs must be individualized to the patient, the type of ICD, and the procedure being performed.

An ICD team is defined as the physicians and physician extenders who monitor the ICD function of the patient.

The anesthesia team should communicate the type of procedure and likely risk of EMI with the ICD team.

The ICD team should communicate with the anesthesia team to deliver a prescription for the perioperative management of patients with ICDs:
1. Manufacturer and model
2. Indication for device
3. What is the response of this device to magnet placement?
4. Will ICD detection resume automatically with removal of the magnet?

*Note:* Inactivation of ICD detection is not a universal requirement for all procedures.

*EMI,* Electromagnetic interference; *ICD,* implantable cardioverter-defibrillator.

Modified from Practice advisory for the perioperative management of patients with cardiac implantable electronic devices: pacemakers and implantable cardioverter-defibrillators 2020: an updated report by the American Society of Anesthesiologists Task Force on Perioperative Management of Patients with Cardiac Implantable Electronic Devices. *Anesthesiology.* 2020;132:225–252.

## BOX 129.2   APPROACH TO EMERGENT/URGENT PROCEDURES

**IDENTIFY THE DEVICE TYPE, MANUFACTURER, AND INDICATION FOR PLACEMENT:**

Obtain the manufacturer's identification card from the patient or other source.

Review the medical record.

Obtain and review the most recent CIED interrogation report.

Refer to supplemental resources (e.g., manufacturer's databases, CIED clinic records).

Order a chest x-ray if no other data are available.

**DETERMINE WHETHER THE PATIENT IS PACING DEPENDENT:**

From the focused history and medical record, assess for one or more of the following indicators:

Bradycardia that caused syncope or other symptoms resulting in CIED implantation

Successful atrioventricular nodal ablation resulting in CIED implantation

A CIED interrogation showing no evidence of spontaneous ventricular activity when the CIED's pacing function is temporarily programed to a nontracking mode (i.e., ventricular-only pacing and sensing) at the lowest programmable rate

**DETERMINE THE CARDIAC IMPLANTABLE ELECTRONIC DEVICE'S CURRENT SETTING**

Reinterrogate the CIED if there is any question of proper function.

*CIED,* Cardiac implantable electronic device.

Modified from Practice advisory for the perioperative management of patients with cardiac implantable electronic devices: pacemakers and implantable cardioverter-defibrillators 2020: an updated report by the American Society of Anesthesiologists Task Force on Perioperative Management of Patients with Cardiac Implantable Electronic Devices. *Anesthesiology.* 2020;132:225–252.

## BOX 129.3   PROBLEMS THAT CAN OCCUR DURING PROCEDURES IN PATIENTS WITH IMPLANTABLE CARDIOVERTER-DEFIBRILLATORS

Bipolar electrosurgery does not cause EMI unless it is applied directly to an ICD.

EMI from monopolar electrosurgery is the most common problem incurred during surgical procedures.

ICDs with antitachycardia function may be inhibited or may falsely detect arrhythmias when exposed to EMI.

Pulse generator damage from electrosurgery can occur but is uncommon.

Impedance-based rate-responsive systems may go to upper rate behavior with electrosurgery exposure.

Risk mitigation strategies can be effective.

Position the electrosurgical unit's dispersive electrode so that the current pathway does not pass through or near the CIED generator and leads.

Avoid proximity of the electrosurgical unit's electrical current to the generator or leads.

Use intermittent and irregular bursts of monopolar electrosurgery at the lowest feasible energy levels.

Use bipolar electrosurgery.

Use ultrasonic (harmonic) scalpel.

Radiofrequency ablation can cause all of the interactions that monopolar electrosurgery can cause but may have a more significant risk profile because of the prolonged exposure to current.

TENS units can result in EMI.

*CIED,* Cardiac implantable electronic device; *EMI,* electromagnetic interference; *ICD,* implantable cardioverter-defibrillator; *TENS,* transcutaneous electrical nerve stimulation.

Modified from Practice advisory for the perioperative management of patients with cardiac implantable electronic devices: pacemakers and implantable cardioverter-defibrillators 2020: an updated report by the American Society of Anesthesiologists Task Force on Perioperative Management of Patients with Cardiac Implantable Electronic Devices. *Anesthesiology.* 2020;132:225–252.

when the return electrode for monopolar electrocautery was placed on the contralateral lower extremity. Care should be taken to evaluate the return electrode placement and presumed discharge pathway before deciding on ICD management for surgery. Magnets can be used, but the provider must know what the response will be for the specific ICD. Electrocardiographic monitoring and the ability to deliver prompt external cardioversion or defibrillation must be present if the ICD is being disabled, regardless of whether the device is used for pacing or whether the patient is pacemaker dependent (Box 129.3). Should external defibrillation become necessary, device manufacturers recommend using the lowest possible energy, placing the paddles perpendicular to the path of the implanted leads, and keeping the paddles away from the implanted generator—the same as with a standard pacemaker device. The guidelines outline when and how the ICD must be reinterrogated and re-enabled postoperatively (Box 129.4).

## Complications

Implantation of an ICD has an intraoperative and perioperative risk of approximately 1% to 3%, including a death rate of 1% or less, perforation and cardiac tamponade of 1% or less, and acute lead dysfunction. Postimplantation pocket infection is a major complication, which generally requires the removal of the complete system. It is reported to occur in 1% to 2% of patients. Infection risk seems to be a little higher at the time of battery or lead replacement than at the time of initial implantation. Lead dislodgement can occur shortly after implantation or at any time thereafter. In patients in whom the lead is completely dislodged, monitoring and timely removal of the lead are mandatory to avoid mechanically induced arrhythmias. Lead dysfunction from insulation breakage or insulation erosion is most frequently preceded by inappropriate ICD discharge caused by electrical noise on the rate electrocardiogram. It usually displays high, frequent, irregular signals with pseudo-RR intervals at the resolution boundary of the device. Some newer devices provide a counter for these specific signals to detect the problems early and avoid inappropriate discharges.

## Acknowledgement

Our sincere thanks to Dan Sorajja, MD, for his guidance in preparing this chapter.

### SUGGESTED READINGS

Al-Khatib, A. M., Friedman, P., & Ellenbogen, K. (2016). Defibrillators, selecting the right device for the right patient. *Circulation, 134,* 1390–1404.

Ammannaya, G. K. K. (2020). Implantable cardioverter defibrillators: The past, present and future. *Archives of Medical Sciences Atherosclerotic diseases, 5,* e163–e170.

Cronin, B., & Essandoh, M. K. (2018). Update on cardiovascular implantable electronic devices for anesthesiologists. *Journal of Cardiothoracic and Vascular Anesthesia, 32,* 1871–1884.

Essandoh, M. K., Mark, G. E., Aasbo, J. D., Joyner, C. A., Sharma, S., Decena, B. F., et al. (2018). Anesthesia for subcutaneous implantable cardioverter-defibrillator implantation: Perspectives from the clinical experience of a U.S. panel of physicians. *Pacing and Clinical Electrophysiology, 41,* 807–816.

Practice advisory for the perioperative management of patients with cardiac implantable electronic devices: Pacemakers and implantable cardioverter-defibrillators 2020: An updated report by the American Society of Anesthesiologists Task Force on perioperative management of patients with cardiac implantable electronic devices. (2020). *Anesthesiology, 132,* 223–252.

Schulman, P. M., Treggiari, M. M., Yanez, N. D., Henrikson, C. A., Jessel, P. M., Dewland, T. A., et al. (2019). Electromagnetic interference with protocolized electrosurgery dispersive electrode positioning in patients with implantable cardioverter defibrillators. *Anesthesiology, 130,* 530–540.

Virani, S. S., Alonso, A., Benjamin, E. J., Bittencourt, M. S., Callaway, C. W., Carson, A. P., et al., (2020). Heart disease and stroke statistics–2020 update: A report from the American Heart Association. American Heart Association Council on Epidemiology and Prevention Statistics Committee and Stroke Statistics Subcommittee. *Circulation, 141*(9), e139–e596.

# 130

# Intra-Aortic Balloon Pump

EDUARDO S. RODRIGUES, MD

## Equipment

Historically, the adult intra-aortic balloon pump (IABP) consisted of an 8.5-F to 12-F catheter, the distal 30 cm of which was covered with a polyurethane balloon. With the advancement in technology, 7-F catheters and 25-mL to 50-mL balloons are most used today; the size of the balloon depends on the patient's height (Fig. 130.1). The pediatric catheter is 4.5-F to 7-F with a 2.5-mL to 12-mL balloon.

The catheter is inserted into the common femoral artery percutaneously by the Seldinger technique or an open surgical procedure. It is then threaded proximally so that the balloon lies

## Sizing Guidelines*

| Arrow® IAB catheters | 30 cc | 40 cc | 50 cc |
|---|---|---|---|
| Height (feet/inches) | 4'10"–5'4" | 5'4"–6' | > 5'8" |
| Height (centimeters) | 147–162 cm | 162–182 cm | > 173 cm |
| Body surface area | < 1.8 m² | > 1.8 m² | > 1.8 m² |

*Refer to IFU

**Fig. 130.1** Arrow® Intra-Aortic 50 cc Balloon Catheters With New Sizing Guidelines. Meeting your patients' counterpulsation needs. Image courtesy of Teleflex Incorporated. © 2023 Teleflex Incorporated. All rights reserved.

high in the descending thoracic aorta, approximately 2 cm distal to the origin of the left subclavian artery.

The catheter is connected to a drive console that has a pneumatic pump that uses helium to inflate the balloon rapidly and, just as quickly, deflate the balloon after a brief period. Balloon cycling is triggered either from the electrocardiogram R wave, inflating with diastole and deflating with the onset of systole (Fig. 130.2), or from the aortic pressure waveform. It should be adjusted to inflate when the dicrotic notch occurs in the pressure cycle (Fig. 130.3). The balloon can be set to trigger with every beat, every other beat, or some other pattern.

## Hemodynamic Effects

With balloon deflation at the onset of systole, the peak aortic systolic pressure falls 10% to 15% (systolic unloading) and inflates immediately with the appearance of the dicrotic notch. Balloon inflation can increase intra-aortic diastolic pressure by approximately 70%. The cardiac index increases 10% to 15%, whereas the pulmonary artery occlusion pressure falls by a similar amount. Coronary blood flow increases as a result of increased diastolic pressure and consequent coronary perfusion pressure (mean diastolic pressure minus left ventricular end-diastolic pressure).

As the balloon deflates, a decrease occurs in the pressure in the aorta in proximity to the balloon, reducing the systemic vascular resistance (SVR), which in turn reduces myocardial oxygen ($O_2$) demand and results in a shift of the Starling curve to the right. These effects can last up to 48 to 72 h after initiation of balloon counterpulsation.

## Counterpulsation Adjustment

For proper IABP adjustment, the device is set up to a 1:2 ratio so the unassisted cardiac cycle can be compared with the assisted cycle.

## INFLATION

The balloon should inflate at the onset of diastole, evident by the dicrotic notch in the arterial waveform; inflation should occur just before the dicrotic notch. The balloon should occlude 85% to 90% of the lumen of the aorta. If the balloon inflates too soon, earlier than the dicrotic notch, early closure of the aortic valve will result, causing a decrease in stroke volume, an increase in left ventricular end-diastolic volume (preload), and a consequent increase in myocardial oxygen consumption ($MVO_2$). Late inflation will cause suboptimal increases in coronary perfusion and no significant decrease in $MVO_2$.

## DEFLATION

Counterpulsation is a diastolic event. The balloon should deflate at the end of diastole before the initiation of systole. The assisted diastolic pressure should be lower than the unassisted diastolic pressure, and the assisted systolic pressure should be lower than the unassisted systolic pressure. Late deflation will increase left ventricular afterload, increasing myocardial oxygen consumption and preload. Early deflation will create suboptimal results similar to late inflation.

Suboptimal results can also be caused by improper occlusion of the aorta due to a highly compliant aorta (low SVR) or suboptimal filling of the balloon due to size, improper positioning (too low in the aorta), or kinking of the helium gas line.

## Indications

The IABP is used primarily to manage acute cardiac failure refractory to pharmacologic intervention. Most commonly, it is used for low-output states associated with acute coronary syndromes and after cardiopulmonary bypass (CPB). The pump

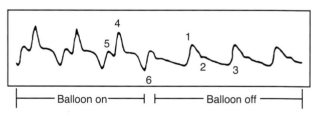

**Fig. 130.3** Arterial pressure tracing (balloon on 1:1 and balloon off). Note diastolic peak (4) balloon augmentation and systolic peak (1), dicrotic notch (2), diastolic low (3), diastolic peak (4), systolic peak (5), and end-diastolic dip (6). (Modified from Gray JR, Faust RJ. Intraaortic balloon counterpulsation and ventricular assist devices. In: Tarhan S, ed. *Cardiovascular Anesthesia and Postoperative Care*. 2nd ed. Year Book Medical; 1989:513.)

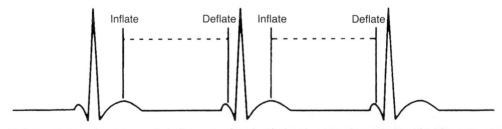

**Fig. 130.2** Inflation/deflation timing of an intra-aortic balloon correlated with the electrocardiogram. (Modified from Gray JR, Faust RJ. Intraaortic balloon counterpulsation and ventricular assist devices. In: Tarhan S, ed. *Cardiovascular Anesthesia and Postoperative Care*. 2nd ed. Year Book Medical; 1989:513.)

can also be placed preoperatively when the surgical stress is anticipated to exceed the functional capacity of a diseased heart. In high-risk coronary artery bypass grafting operations, the elective preoperative placement of an intra-aortic balloon and initiation of counterpulsation can improve the patient's prognosis. In recent years, the IABP has also found use as a temporary bridge to cardiac transplantation, placement of a left ventricular assist device, or placement of a total artificial heart.

Approximately 3% to 4% of patients undergoing CPB need IABP support. If the patient is not hypovolemic and the heart rhythm is suitable for IABP use, the criteria listed in Box 130.1 can be used to determine the appropriate initiation of IABP support.

## Contraindications

The classic contraindications to the use of intra-aortic counterpulsation are severe aortic insufficiency, severe peripheral vascular disease, thrombocytopenia (platelet count $<50,000$), contraindication to anticoagulation, acute stroke, and active bleeding.

## Weaning From Intra-Aortic Balloon Pump Support

After resolution of the problem for which the intra-aortic balloon was placed, patients have traditionally been weaned from IABP support by a gradual reduction in augmentation rate (1:1, then 1:2, then 1:3, etc.). Most hemodynamic changes occur during the transition from full support to partial support, from 1:1 to 1:2 augmentation. To institute a more gradual reduction in circulatory assist and reduce the risk of thrombus formation around a static balloon, an alternate weaning approach is to maintain a 1:1 counterpulsation rate but gradually reduce the degree of balloon inflation and consequent hemodynamic support.

## Complications

Previously reported complication rates with the use of IABP were 5% to 27%, but more recent reviews suggest a complication rate around 3% to 4%. Placement of a large catheter in the common femoral artery can occlude the artery, which is manifested by a loss of distal pulses; the aortotomy site can bleed, or the insertion site can become infected. The relative frequency of each of these complications varies widely among reports, and the literature is inconsistent as to the effect of chronic placement on complication rates. Nevertheless, it may be reasonable to expect up to a 9% incidence of bleeding or vascular compromise in these patients. These complications may readily become life-threatening.

## Outcome

Clinicians have evaluated immediate and long-term prognosis after IABP support to identify reliable determinants of survival but have made their assessments using nonrandomized groups. The primary determinant of survival after using an IABP is an early recovery (within 24 h) of cardiac function with the maintenance of vital organ perfusion. Conversely, inotropes, direct current cardioversion, chronic left ventricular failure, and the functional severity of the patient's heart disease have been associated with poor outcomes.

Theoretically, the predicted improvement in the O$_2$ demand-supply ratio offered by IABP support can benefit patients with acute cardiac decompensation. Nevertheless, it has been a challenge to demonstrate long-term benefits as multiple studies have not shown significant change in survival with the use of this ingenious device.

## SUGGESTED READINGS

Deppe, A. C., Weber, C., & Liakopoulos, O. J. (2017). Preoperative intra-aortic balloon pump use in high-risk patients prior to coronary artery bypass graft surgery decreases the risk for morbidity and mortality: A meta-analysis of 9,212 patients. *Journal of Cardiac Surgery, 32*(3), 177–185.

Dhruva, S. S., Ross, J. S., Mortazavi, B. J., Hurley, N. C., Krumholz, H. M., Curtis, J. P., et al. (2020). Association of use of an intravascular microaxial left ventricular assist device vs intra-aortic balloon pump with in-hospital mortality and major bleeding among patients with acute myocardial infarction complicated by cardiogenic shock. *JAMA, 323*(8), 734–745.

Rossini, R., Valente, S., Colivicchi, F., Baldi, C., Caldarola, P., Chiappetta, D., et al. (2021). ANMCO POSITION PAPER: Role of intra-aortic balloon pump in patients with acute advanced heart failure and cardiogenic shock. *European Heart Journal Supplements, 23*(Suppl. C), C204–C220. doi:10.1093/eurheartj/suab074.

Vieira, J. L., Ventura, H. O., & Mehra, M. R. (2020). Mechanical circulatory support devices in advanced heart failure: 2020 and beyond. *Progress in Cardiovascular Diseases, 63,* 630–639.

Yang, F., Wang, J., Hou, D., Xing, J., Liu, F., Xing, Z. C., et al. (2016). Preoperative intra-aortic balloon pump improves the clinical outcomes of off-pump coronary artery bypass grafting in left ventricular dysfunction patients. *Scientific Reports, 6,* 27645. doi:10.1038/srep27645.

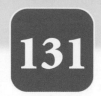

# 131 Extracorporeal Membrane Oxygenation

JUAN G. RIPOLL, MD | SURAJ M. YALAMURI, MD

Extracorporeal membrane oxygenation (ECMO) is a form of mechanical cardiopulmonary life support that allows partial and temporary bypass of the heart and lungs. ECMO is mainly used for short-term carbon dioxide removal, oxygenation, and improvement in perfusion. Based on its configuration, it can provide primary pulmonary support (for respiratory failure) or combined cardiopulmonary support (for cardiogenic shock). Its ability to augment both the cardiac and pulmonary function renders this technology unique among the currently available extracorporeal system devices.

## Basic Principles of Extracorporeal Membrane Oxygenation

### THE EXTRACORPOREAL MEMBRANE OXYGENATION CIRCUIT

The basic ECMO circuit requires a semipermeable membrane oxygenator (used for gas exchange: carbon dioxide elimination and oxygen uptake), blood pump (centrifugal or roller), gas blender/mixer, drainage and return cannulae, conduit tubing, heat exchanger, and the console.

In a typical configuration, the circuit drains deoxygenated blood from the venous system via the drainage/inflow cannula and pumps it through a semipermeable membrane oxygenator. The semipermeable membrane provides an interface for the

blood and fresh gas, known as *sweep gas*, in the oxygenator. Sweep gas flow can be anywhere between 21% to 100% oxygen, and the fraction of oxygen is controlled by a mixture of air and oxygen. The fraction of oxygen used depends on how much oxygenation is being provided through the ECMO circuit. Blood passing through the oxygenator is decarboxylated and oxygenated and then returned to the patient via the outflow/return cannula (Fig. 131.1).

In general, the main determinants of blood oxygenation for a given ECMO device include the fraction of oxygen delivered through the oxygenator, the blood flow through the circuit, and the contribution of the native lungs. Conversely, the major determinants of carbon dioxide removal are the rate of gas flow through the oxygenator (sweep gas flow rate) and, to a lesser degree, the total blood flow rate. Total blood flow rate contributes more toward oxygenation as opposed to decarboxylation given the intrinsic properties of the two gases.

There are two basic types of configurations in ECMO: venoarterial (VA) and venovenous (VV). The differences between both types of ECMO support are presented in Table 131.1.

VA-ECMO is very similar to standard cardiopulmonary bypass because it allows circulatory and pulmonary support. Some of the main differences between VA-ECMO and CPB include the lack of a venous reservoir, cardioplegia delivery systems, and an open blood-to-air interface. Based on the position of the arterial cannula, it can be classified as central (cannula in the aorta) or

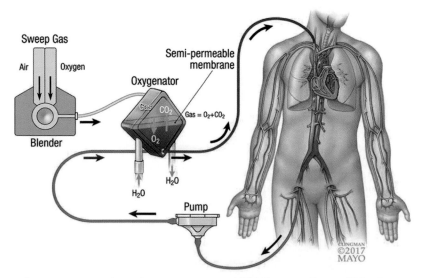

**Fig. 131.1** Basic components of an extracorporeal membrane oxygenation (ECMO) circuit. Types of ECMO: venovenous and venoarterial. (Used with permission of Mayo Foundation for Medical Education and Research, all rights reserved.)

| TABLE 131.1 | Major Differences Between Venoarterial and Venovenous ECMO | |
|---|---|---|
| **Venoarterial (VA) ECMO** | **Venovenous (VV) ECMO** | |
| Requires arterial cannulation | Requires only venous cannulation | |
| Most of the native pulmonary blood flow is circumvented | Native pulmonary blood flow is maintained | |
| Provides both cardiac and pulmonary support | Only provides pulmonary support | |

*ECMO,* Extracorporeal membrane oxygenation.

peripheral (cannula in peripheral artery). Drainage cannulas placed via central access or peripheral access both typically drain from the right atrium. Central VA-ECMO configuration requires a sternotomy or thoracotomy to position the inflow and outflow cannula in the right atrium and aorta, respectively. Minimally invasive approaches to cannulation, such as direct aortic cannulation through the second intercostal space, is achievable but not routinely employed. The femoral artery is the most accessible and most frequently used vessel for peripheral VA-ECMO; additional cannulation sites such as the subclavian artery and axillary artery might also be used. The peripheral configuration of VA-ECMO is presented in Fig. 131.2.

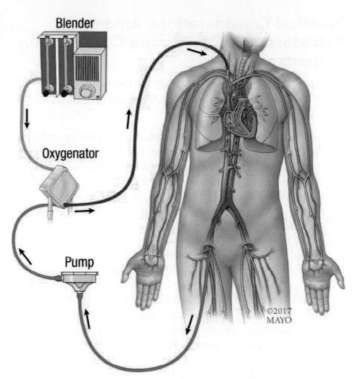

**Fig. 131.3** Double venous cannulation technique for venovenous–extracorporeal membrane oxygenation configuration. The femoral (extending into the junction of inferior vena cava and right atrium) cannula drains deoxygenated blood *(purple)* from the central venous circulation. Subsequently, the oxygenated blood is reinfused *(red)* to the patient via the internal jugular vein (extending into the junction of superior vena cava and right atrium) return cannula. This cannulation technique is also called the *femoroatrial* or *cavoatrial* approach. (Used with permission of Mayo Foundation for Medical Education and Research, all rights reserved.)

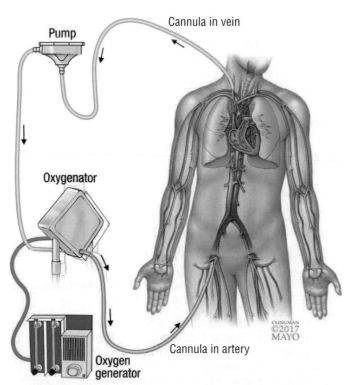

**Fig. 131.2** Peripheral (femoral) venoarterial–extracorporeal membrane oxygenation configuration. The drainage cannula is positioned in the right internal jugular vein with poorly oxygenated blood flowing *(blue)* to the oxygenator. The blood is reinfused oxygenated *(pink)* to the patient via a femoral arterial cannula. (Used with permission of Mayo Foundation for Medical Education and Research, all rights reserved.)

VV-ECMO provides partial or complete pulmonary support. It is therefore commonly indicated among patients with adequate native cardiac function and isolated respiratory failure. Under this configuration, deoxygenated blood is drained from the central venous system and oxygenated blood is returned to the right side of the heart, typically in the right atrium. Among adult patients, there are several cannula configurations for VV-ECMO. The most used has been the double-venous cannulation. Within this configuration, the blood is extracted from the hepatic inferior vena cava with a cannula placed from the common femoral vein, and oxygenated blood is returned to the patient via the femoral vein or right internal jugular vein (Fig. 131.3). Additionally, a single venous cannulation technique is also possible. Utilizing a dual-lumen cannula (Crescent Jugular Dual Lumen Catheter [MC3 Cardiopulmonary, Dexter, MI]), the blood is drained from both vena cavae and reinfused directly into the right atrium directed at the tricuspid valve. Advantages of this technique include less recirculation if the cannula is properly positioned and one-site cannulation. Although strictly not VV-ECMO, as it provides right ventricular support, the ProtekDuo dual lumen cannula (CardiacAssist, Inc., Pittsburgh, PA) is another option. Placed via the right internal jugular vein, the cannula drains the blood from the superior vena cava/right atrial junction and allows for bypass of the right ventricle with reinfusion of the oxygenated blood in the main pulmonary artery.

# Practical Considerations Among Extracorporeal Membrane Oxygenation Patients

## OPTIMIZING GAS EXCHANGE WITHIN THE EXTRACORPOREAL MEMBRANE OXYGENATION CIRCUIT

The initial ECMO settings are commonly titrated according to the hemodynamics and respiratory needs of each patient. There are three variables that are commonly manipulated to achieve the desirable levels of oxygenation and carbon dioxide removal in ECMO patients: (1) blood flow; (2) fraction of oxygen in the sweep gas; and (3) sweep gas flow rate.

### Blood Flow

The blood flow among patients under ECMO is dependent on the revolutions per minute (RPM) of the pump, the afterload, and the preload. The centrifugal pump is preload dependent and afterload sensitive. Mechanical factors such as the oxygenator or circuit clots might reduce the blood flow for a given RPM by increasing the resistance throughout the ECMO circuit. Similarly, clinical conditions that reduce the preload or increase the afterload (e.g., tension pneumothorax, systemic hypertension, cardiac tamponade, hypovolemia) also compromise the blood flow through the ECMO circuit.

### Fraction of Oxygen in the Sweep Gas

As depicted in Fig. 131.1, the ECMO oxygenator contains a gas blender that allows the mixing of oxygen and air. This property allows for a thorough regulation of the oxygen concentration in the circuit. Notably, an increase in the fraction of oxygen is reflected as an increase in the partial pressure of oxygen in the blood.

### Sweep Gas (Fresh Gas) Flow Rate

The interaction between the sweep gas (fresh gas) and the venous blood of the ECMO system translates into carbon dioxide removal and blood oxygenation. An increase in the sweep gas flow rate translates into increased carbon dioxide removal from the venous blood of the ECMO circuit.

## MECHANICAL VENTILATION

The current strategies of lung protective ventilation among critically ill patients also apply to patients on ECMO. Indeed, a low tidal volume strategy has been correlated with reduction of ventilator-induced lung injury causing a significant reduction in mortality in ECMO patients. A tidal volume of 6 mL/kg predicted body weight and plateau pressure less than or equal to 30 cm $H_2O$ should be targeted in this setting.

The use of ECMO allows lower airway pressure and tidal volumes in patients whose gas exchange could otherwise be maintained only at the expense of mechanical ventilation. Therefore some groups advocate for the use of "ultra-lung-protective" ventilation with the use of lower tidal volumes (3–4 mL/kg) and airway pressures (e.g., <25 cm $H_2O$). The rationale is that despite conventional lung-protective mechanical ventilation strategies, lung injury may still ensue. However, lowering tidal volumes may result in respiratory acidosis with detrimental effects for a patient's recovery. At this point, a concomitant increase in sweep gas flow must be provided in order to counteract the resulting respiratory acidosis. The use of extracorporeal carbon dioxide removal ($ECCO_2R$), a form of

extracorporeal gas exchange, has been proposed as a solution for respiratory acidosis during ultralung protective ventilation when a patient is not on ECMO. Unfortunately, despite showing promise as a feasible strategy in patients with acute hypoxemic respiratory failure due to acute respiratory stress syndrome (ARDS) (SUPER-NOVA trial, 2019), it failed to demonstrate a significant reduction in 90-day mortality (REST trial, 2021).

## ANTICOAGULATION

Anticoagulation among patients under ECMO represents a challenge for the intensivist. The main goal is to achieve an optimal balance between mitigating the risk of bleeding while avoiding a life-threatening thrombosis. The goal of anticoagulation in ECMO is to prevent contact phase activation and subsequent thrombin generation.

Traditionally, unfractionated heparin has been used for anticoagulation in ECMO. It is easily reversible, cheap, widely available, and has a rapid onset of action. Current tests used to assess the efficacy of the anticoagulation under heparin include the activated clotting time (ACT) (goal: 180–220 s), the heparin concentration (goal: 0.3–0.7 U/mL), the thromboelastogram, the activated partial thromboplastin time (aPTT) (goal: 1.5–2.5 times the control), and the antifactor Xa functional assay.

Bivalirudin, a direct thrombin inhibitor, has demonstrated safety and feasibility as an alternative agent for patients on ECMO compared with heparin-based systemic anticoagulation. More importantly, it has shown improvement in hospital survival compared with unfractionated heparin. As a result, bivalirudin is now used in some centers in the world as a first-line agent for systemic anticoagulation in adult and pediatric patients on ECMO. Advantages of bivalirudin include a short half-life (25 min) with clearance mainly by proteolytic cleavage and the fact that it does not trigger immune or non–immune-mediated thrombocytopenia. Despite the lack of a reversal agent, bivalirudin can be removed by hemodialysis. Efficacy of the anticoagulation is monitored with the aPTT (goal: 1.5–2.5 times baseline).

# Indications

Medical providers need to be aware of three basic ECMO principles before considering this form of extracorporeal support. First, ECMO is a short-term form of pulmonary and/or cardiac support that is considered if the primary pathology of the patient is potentially reversible in nature. Second, if it is used as rescue therapy or bridge to transplantation, it should only be used when conventional therapy has failed. Third, ECMO requires a 24-hour multidisciplinary team readily available.

## INDICATIONS FOR EXTRACORPOREAL MEMBRANE OXYGENATION IN CARDIAC FAILURE

ECMO remains a useful alternative for the management of patients undergoing cardiac failure. Typically, it is used among individuals with refractory shock displaying a cardiac index below 2 L/min/m², hypotension (systolic blood pressure <90 mm Hg), lactic acidosis despite adequate volume resuscitation, optimal inotropic support, and/or failure in other forms of invasive mechanical circulatory support (i.e., intraaortic balloon pump or Impella). The most common indications of VA-ECMO for cardiac failure are the inability to wean from cardiopulmonary bypass after cardiac surgery or heart transplantation; nonischemic cardiogenic shock (e.g., myocarditis); bridge to long-term therapy (e.g., ventricular-assisted devices or heart transplantation); recovery from severe cardiogenic shock (acute myocardial infarction, drug toxicity/overdose, acute anaphylaxis, sepsis-induced myocardial depression, pulmonary embolism, trauma to myocardium or major vessels, and recurrent dysrhythmias such as ventricular tachycardia/fibrillation); periprocedural support among high-risk patients undergoing percutaneous cardiac interventions; and in selected patients who develop out-hospital or in-hospital cardiac arrest, also known as *extracorporeal cardiopulmonary resuscitation* (ECPR).

### Extracorporeal Cardiopulmonary Resuscitation

It is well known that patients with longer cardiopulmonary resuscitation (CPR) times (30–40 min) due to refractory cardiac arrest despite adequate advanced cardiac life support (ACLS) display a very poor prognosis. Over the last 5 years, multiple observational studies have suggested an increase survival among patients who develop out-of-hospital refractory cardiac arrest who failed initial management and were treated with peripheral VA-ECMO. A recent phase 2, single-center, safety and efficacy randomized clinical trial (ARREST trial, 2020) further reinforced the survival benefit and improvement in functional status in patients who developed out-of-hospital refractory cardiac arrest unresponsive to initial ACLS treatment and required ECMO compared with those patients who only received standard ACLS resuscitation.

### INDICATIONS FOR EXTRACORPOREAL MEMBRANE OXYGENATION IN RESPIRATORY FAILURE

ECMO is indicated among patients with life-threatening but potentially reversible respiratory failure. Either VA-ECMO or VV-ECMO can be used as rescue therapy among patients with acute respiratory failure as a bridge to recovery or lung transplantation. Currently, the most common indications of VV-ECMO in the setting of respiratory failure include ARDS, bridge to lung transplantation, primary graft failure after lung transplantation, extracorporeal assistance needed to ensure lung rest (e.g., pulmonary contusion, airway obstruction), and status asthmaticus.

Based on the Extracorporeal Life Support Organization guidelines, VV-ECMO should be considered in patients with hypoxic respiratory failure when the mortality risk is 50% or greater and is indicated when the mortality risk is 80% or greater. A 50% mortality risk translates into a partial pressure of oxygen in arterial blood ($Pao_2$)/fraction of inspired oxygen ($Fio_2$) ratio less than 150 on $Fio_2$ >90 % with a Murray Score of 2 to 3. Meanwhile, an 80% mortality risk is defined by a ($Pao_2$)/($Fio_2$) ratio less than 100 on $Fio_2$ >90 % and/or Murray Score of 3 to 4 despite optimal care for 6 hours or less. Additional indications include severe hypercapnia on mechanical ventilation despite high plateau airway pressure (>30 cm of $H_2O$), severe air leaks, sudden and potentially reversible causes of respiratory or cardiovascular collapse, and the need for intubation in patients listed for a lung transplant. Accepted flow rates on VV-ECMO are to capture at least 60% of the patient's native cardiac output to achieve oxygen saturation of 90%.

### LANDMARK STUDIES

The Conventional Ventilatory Support Versus Extracorporeal Membrane Oxygenation for Severe Acute Respiratory Failure (CESAR, 2009) trial randomly assigned patients with severe acute respiratory failure to either undergo continued conventional management or to be referred to an ECMO center. This landmark study concluded that patients with severe but potentially reversible respiratory failure should be referred to an ECMO center early in the course of their disease to improve survival. Furthermore, the ECMO to Rescue Lung Injury in Severe ARDS (EOLIA, 2018) trial revealed that patients with severe ARDS who fail to respond to conventional treatment (lung protective ventilation strategies, prone ventilation, neuromuscular blockade, and inhaled pulmonary vasodilators) should be managed with ECMO early in the course of the disease (<2 days after onset) to improve survival, instead of a rescue/late treatment (>6 days).

## Outcomes

Overall, there are three possible clinical outcomes among patients under ECMO support. The first is a full recovery of the pulmonary and cardiac dysfunction followed by weaning from the extracorporeal support, also known as *bridge to recovery.* The second is an irreversible respiratory and cardiac failure with ECMO dependence, leading to transplantation or bridge to long-term mechanical circulatory devices (e.g., ventricular assist devices), also named as *bridge to transplant* or *bridge to bridge*, respectively. Third, a permanent neurologic injury or lack of recovery might ensue, requiring withdrawal of ECMO support.

## Contraindications

An elderly population, immunodeficiency caused by an underlying disease (e.g., malignancy), pharmacologic immune suppression, and severe peripheral vascular disease are among the most common relative contraindications of ECMO. Although there are specific contraindications based on modality of ECMO and sites of cannulation, it is important to remember that any terminal condition resulting in a life expectancy of <6 weeks should be viewed as a contraindication to provide a resource intensive medical therapy such as ECMO.

Absolute contraindications for ECMO include multiorgan failure, inability to tolerate anticoagulation therapy, end-stage renal or liver disease, prolonged CPR (>1 h), and refusal by the surrogate decision maker. Severe aortic valve regurgitation and unrepaired aortic dissection are also included in this category when considering VA-ECMO, especially peripheral VA-ECMO where retrograde flow is established. During VA-ECMO the ventricular end-diastolic pressure can be excessively increased, resulting in overdistention of the left ventricle, thus altering the oxygenation of the myocardium and worsening the patient's heart failure. Therefore in severe left ventricular systolic failure, LV venting should be considered. Recent trials have shown improved survival with left ventricular venting with an Impella, termed ECPELLA, as opposed to nonventing.

## Complications

Complications among patients under ECMO are common and are associated with an increased risk of morbidity and mortality. Typically, these complications are the result of the underlying patient's comorbidities leading to the ECMO therapy or by the circuit itself (e.g., anticoagulation, surgical insertion). In the following section, we revisit the most common complications documented in patients under ECMO.

## HEMORRHAGE

Hemorrhage is the most common complication in patients under ECMO, with an incidence varying between 10% to 30%. The risk of bleeding is elevated because of platelet dysfunction, clotting factor hemodilution, and systemic anticoagulation. Hemorrhage might occur at the cannula site, at the surgical site, or into the site of a prior invasive surgical intervention. Pulmonary, abdominal, retroperitoneal, and intrathoracic bleeding might also occur.

## COMPLICATIONS DERIVED FROM THE EXTRACORPOREAL MEMBRANE OXYGENATION CIRCUIT

There are two critical and devastating complications intrinsic to the circuit that require prompt clamping and immediate discontinuation of ECMO support: massive blood loss secondary to disconnections or tubing rupture, and gas embolism (incidence <2% in adults). Gas embolism is more frequent with centrifugal pumps because of the ability to cause cavitation in setting of repeated suck-downs. This is generated between the interface of the blood vessel walls and the drainage cannula, eventually leading to loss of preload at the pump head. Repeated, rapid stopping and restarting the pump results in extremely elevated negative pressures that cause cavitation. The resulting air entrapment within this section of the circuit has the potential to cause a massive gas embolism. Other ECMO circuit complications include blood clots, loss of circuit flow (most likely secondary to hypovolemia), and primary failure of the circuit components.

Thrombus formation represents a devastating complication of ECMO. Major thrombus formation can cause oxygenator failures, systemic and pulmonary emboli, and severe consumption coagulopathy. Its effect is more prominent among patients receiving VA-ECMO than VV-ECMO, as result of the direct communication with the arterial systemic circulation. Anticoagulation to target a specific functional coagulation target and a thorough observation of the circuit for clot formation represent successful strategies to prevent systemic thromboembolism in ECMO patients. Avoidance of low blood flow states is also helpful.

## HEPARIN-INDUCED THROMBOCYTOPENIA

Because of continuous and prolonged heparin exposure, heparin-induced thrombocytopenia (HIT) might arise among patients under ECMO. Immediately after the diagnosis, heparin should be discontinued and replaced by a nonheparin anticoagulant such as bivalirudin or argatroban. In patients with severe HIT with associated thrombotic complications, plasma exchange and/or intravenous immune globulin administration should also be considered.

## OTHER COMPLICATIONS

Intracranial hemorrhage, seizures, and ischemic stroke are the most common neurologic complications among patients under ECMO. Intracerebral hemorrhage is a fatal complication and represents a significant risk for morbidity and mortality in ECMO patients, with a reported incidence ranging between 1.6% to 18.9%. Intracranial hemorrhage and ischemic stroke arise because of systemic heparinization, coagulopathy, systemic hypertension, and critical illness–induced thrombocytopenia. Infections and worsening sepsis might occur among patients under ECMO as the circuit represents a large intravascular foreign body. During the first 24 hours, an oliguric phase is frequently identified as the ECMO circuit induces an acute inflammatory reaction. If this condition is untreated, the capillary leak and intravascular volume depletion lead to acute tubular necrosis. Renal failure secondary to acute tubular necrosis requiring hemodialysis has been reported in up to 13% of ECMO patients. Hypoxemia, hemodynamic instability, and local complications derived from the peripheral insertion site might also occur (e.g., leg ischemia).

# Challenges and Future Directions

ECMO has continued to increase in use since 2009, primarily because adult patients with acute hypoxic respiratory failure from influenza showed positive results in large trials when ECMO was used as rescue therapy. Additionally, due to the growing evidence highlighting the survival benefits of ECPR, the need for structured multidisciplinary ECMO teams with experts allowed to respond timely to out-of-hospital cardiac arrests cannot be overstated. At a state level, the geographic allocation and timely delivery of this therapy remains a significant challenge, particularly in rural areas.

In the future, new technologies will improve the safety and simplicity of the ECMO components (pumps, oxygenators, and surface coatings). The oxygenators will be smaller, more portable, and the care of the ECMO patient will most likely not be in the intensive care unit but in an ambulatory or a step-down unit of the hospital. Improvements in cannula design and cannulation methods, including hybrid schemes, will also become available. Moreover, improvement in surface coating components might reduce the thrombogenicity of the ECMO cannulas, thus limiting the need for continuous anticoagulation and ultimately reducing the incidence of bleeding complications. Last, although the use of ECCO$_2$R, a form of "respiratory dialysis" and low-flow AV-ECMO, is growing in popularity for patients with hypercapnic respiratory failure, additional data is needed to confirm its benefits.

# Conclusions

Current advances in extracorporeal oxygenation technology have led to widespread usage of ECMO among patients with cardiac, respiratory, or mixed cardiopulmonary failure. Scientific innovations made over the past decade are primarily responsible for the increased use of this technology in critically ill patients. Although the practice is gaining wide acceptance across the medical field, there are still numerous unresolved challenges and issues. Additional research studies in conjunction with more clinical experience are required to capitalize the benefits of ECMO while avoiding iatrogenic harms.

## SUGGESTED READINGS

Abrams, D., Schmidt, M., Pham, T., Beitler, J. R., Fan, E., Goligher, E. C., et al. (2020). Mechanical ventilation for acute respiratory distress syndrome during extracorporeal life support: Research and practice. *American Journal of Respiratory and Critical Care Medicine, 201*, 514–525.

Combes, A., Fanelli, V., Pham, T., Ranieri, V. M., & European Society of Intensive Care Medicine Trials Group and the "Strategy of Ultra-Protective lung ventilation with Extracorporeal CO2 Removal for New-Onset moderate to severe ARDS" (SUPERNOVA) investigators. (2019). Feasibility and safety of extracorporeal CO2 removal to enhance protective ventilation in acute respiratory distress syndrome: the SUPERNOVA study. *Intensive Care Medicine, 45*, 592–600.

Combes, A., Hajage, D., Capellier, G., Demoule, A., Lavoué, S., Guervilly, C., et al. (2018). Extracorporeal membrane oxygenation for severe acute respiratory distress syndrome. *New England Journal of Medicine, 378*, 1965–1975.

Kuhl, T., Michels, G., Pfister, R., Wendt, S., Langebartels, G., & Wahlers, T. (2015). Comparison of the avalon dual-lumen cannula with conventional cannulation technique for venovenous extracorporeal membrane oxygenation. *Thoracic and Cardiovascular Surgeon, 63*, 653–662.

McNamee, J. J., Gillies, M. A., Barrett, N. A., Perkins, G. D., Tunnicliffe, W., Young, D., et al. (2021). Effect of lower tidal volume ventilation facilitated by extracorporeal carbon dioxide removal vs standard care ventilation on 90-day mortality in patients with acute hypoxemic respiratory failure: The REST Randomized Clinical Trial. *JAMA, 326*, 1013–1023.

Patel, S. M., Lipinski, J., Al-Kindi, S. G., Patel, T., Saric, P., Li, J., et al. (2019). Simultaneous venoarterial extracorporeal membrane oxygenation and percutaneous left ventricular decompression therapy with impella is associated with improved outcomes in refractory cardiogenic shock. *ASAIO Journal, 65*, 21–28.

Seelhammer, T. G., Bohman, J. K., Schulte, P. J., Hanson, A. C., & Aganga, D. O. (2021). Comparison of bivalirudin versus heparin for maintenance systemic anticoagulation during adult and pediatric extracorporeal membrane oxygenation. *Critical Care Medicine, 49*, 1481–1492.

Yannopoulos, D., Bartos, J., Raveendran, G., Walser, E., Connett, J., Murray, T. A., et al. (2020). Advanced reperfusion strategies for patients with out-of-hospital cardiac arrest and refractory ventricular fibrillation (ARREST): A phase 2, single centre, open-label, randomised controlled trial. *Lancet, 396*, 1807–1816.

# Specialty Anesthesia: Thoracic

# Intraoperative Bronchospasm: Etiology and Treatment

LINDSAY ROYCE HUNTER GUEVARA, MD

## Introduction

Bronchoconstriction, a reflex spasm of airway smooth muscle, is a common and potentially devastating occurrence during anesthesia. Signs of bronchospasm include wheezing and prolonged expiration. For a patient who is intubated and mechanically ventilated, early signs of airway obstruction or bronchospasm may be an increase in peak airway pressure, a decrease in tidal volume, or a decrease in the slope of the expiratory carbon dioxide curve. Persistent and severe airway obstruction may be followed by oxygen ($O_2$) desaturation, hypercapnia, and hypotension secondary to increased intrathoracic pressure from decreased expiratory flow and air trapping.

Resting bronchial tone is regulated primarily by the parasympathetic nervous system via vagal nerve fibers and muscarinic acetylcholine receptors. Bronchoconstriction can either be centrally mediated via the parasympathetic nervous system or caused by local airway irritation. Most (80%) of the resistance to flow in airways occurs in the large central airways, leaving 20% of airway resistance from the peripheral bronchioles. Thus, large changes in the caliber of small airways may result in small changes in resistance, making the small airways a clinically silent area. The obstruction can be extrinsic to the airway, intrinsic (within the airway wall), or within the lumen (Box 132.1).

## Differential Diagnosis for Bronchospasm

### REACTIVE AIRWAY DISEASE

Wheezing may indicate the presence of underlying obstructive lung disease—asthma or chronic obstructive pulmonary disease (COPD), including emphysema and chronic bronchitis.

### Asthma

Asthma, a reactive airway disease, is manifested by chronic airway inflammation, hyperreactive airways, and reversible airway obstruction. The immunologic component to asthma is well recognized and includes immunoglobulin E antibody fixed to mast cells and basophils, which release immune mediators in response to challenge with specific antigens. Numerous factors—including exercise, cold air, allergens, respiratory infections, emotional factors, β-adrenergic blockade, and the use of a prostaglandin inhibitor such as aspirin—may override the baseline bronchial tone, provoking an attack in patients with bronchospastic disease. Cross-sensitivity between aspirin and other nonsteroidal antiinflammatory drugs is common and should be considered as a cause for bronchospasm, especially in patients with the triad of asthma, nasal polyps, and aspirin-induced asthma.

### Chronic Obstructive Pulmonary Disease (Additional Information in Chapter 21)

COPD differs from asthma in that airflow obstruction is not completely reversible because the mechanism is primarily destruction of lung parenchyma. Pulmonary infections are common and can increase the risk of bronchospasm in a patient. For patients who are having an exacerbation of their COPD, management principles include bronchodilator therapy (β-adrenergic agonists and anticholinergic agents), glucocorticoids, and antibiotics (in patients who display signs and symptoms of a moderate to severe exacerbation or are at increased risk of a bacterial infection).

---

### BOX 132.1 CAUSES OF VENTILATORY OBSTRUCTION

**AIRWAY DISEASE**

- Asthma
- Bronchitis
- Chronic obstructive pulmonary disease
- Cystic fibrosis
- Tumors of the larynx or pharynx
- Foreign body
- Bronchiectasis
- Tracheomalacia
- Laryngeal edema or infection

**BRONCHOCONSTRICTION DURING ANESTHESIA**

- Airway manipulation
- Tracheal intubation
- Bronchial intubation
- Carinal pressure from the tracheal tube
- Light anesthesia
- Secretions in large airways
- Aspiration of stomach contents
- Infection, pneumonia
- Pulmonary edema
- Pulmonary or amniotic fluid embolus
- Pneumothorax
- Allergens
- Anaphylaxis, anaphylactoid reactions
- Drug reactions from histamine release, antagonism
- Carcinoid tumors

**MECHANICAL OBSTRUCTION**

- Kinked tracheal tube
- Secretions in tracheal tube
- Obstructed tracheal tube
- High intraabdominal pressure (laparoscopy)

---

## PERIOPERATIVE MEDICATIONS

Histamine release may occur with administration of anesthetic drugs, including mivacurium, atracurium, meperidine, morphine, and vancomycin. When administered rapidly or in large doses (as occurs during induction and subsequent airway manipulation), these drugs are more likely to increase the risk of bronchoconstriction. The muscarinic action of cholinesterase inhibitors used for reversal of a neuromuscular blocker may precipitate bronchospasm. In these situations, experience suggests using larger than usual doses of atropine ($>1.0$ mg) or glycopyrrolate ($>0.5$ mg) can minimize potential bronchospasm in patients who are actively wheezing.

The use of $\beta_2$-adrenergic receptor antagonists (labetalol, esmolol) may increase the risk of bronchoconstriction. Although they have been used without untoward effect in the treatment of hypertension in patients with stable COPD, the American College of Chest Physicians recommends that these agents be used with extreme caution, if at all, in patients with reactive airway disease.

The use of methohexital is associated with wheezing if other drugs are not used to blunt the effect or if adequate depth of anesthesia is not achieved before airway manipulation. The use of either propofol or ketamine offers advantages in patients with a history of bronchospasm or reactive airway disease. Propofol reduces airway resistance in patients with asthma and COPD by relaxing airway smooth muscle. Ketamine helps protect against irritant reflexes, although it increases secretions from salivary and tracheobronchial mucous glands (which can be prevented by administering a small dose of an anticholinergic medication). Ketamine also stimulates the sympathetic system by preventing the reuptake of catecholamines and attenuates vagal reflexes, leading to smooth muscle relaxation.

Inhalation anesthetic agents can be used to deepen the level of anesthesia before airway manipulation and surgical stimulation or when bronchospasm is mild. In true bronchospasm, the administration of inhalation anesthetic agents will depress airway reactivity and bronchoconstriction by blunting parasympathetic constrictive reflexes and directly relaxing bronchiolar smooth muscle. Sevoflurane has the most significant bronchodilation of the currently used volatile anesthetics, in contrast with desflurane, which can increase airway resistance, especially in smokers.

Sugammadex has also been implicated as a cause of bronchospasm, especially with use of desflurane for maintenance of general anesthesia with reversal of rocuronium neuromuscular blockade. The etiology of the bronchospasm is thought to be related to sugammadex-rocuronium complexes combined with the airway irritation caused by desflurane.

## ANAPHYLACTIC/ANAPHYLACTOID REACTIONS (ADDITIONAL INFORMATION IN CHAPTER 228)

Wheezing and bronchospasm may occur during an anaphylactic or anaphylactoid reaction. Antibiotic drugs, neuromuscular blockers, blood products, or intravenously administered contrast agents may be the trigger, with an initial manifestation of wheezing accompanied by hypotension, periorbital and airway edema, urticaria, tachycardia, and arrhythmias.

## ASPIRATION

Aspiration of gastric contents, which can occur during induction of, maintenance of, or emergence from anesthesia, can cause an inflammatory response in the airways causing bronchospasm. Wheezing and rhonchi can be auscultated.

## CARCINOID SYNDROME (ADDITIONAL INFORMATION IN CHAPTER 161)

Hormonally symptomatic carcinoid tumors (carcinoid syndrome) secrete a variety of active compounds (e.g., serotonin, prostaglandins, vasoactive peptides) into the systemic circulation, which can trigger bronchospasm. This symptom frequently accompanies other acute manifestations of the carcinoid syndrome, such as hypotension/hypertension, diarrhea, and flushing. Increased sympathetic activity can trigger carcinoid tumor hormone release, so conventional treatment for bronchospasm (with catecholamines like albuterol and epinephrine) may actually worsen a carcinoid crisis. Octreotide (a somatostatin analog) stabilizes carcinoid tumor membranes and can decrease the likelihood of tumor hormone release. Patients should be prepared preoperatively with octreotide, and additional octreotide should be immediately available to treat carcinoid crisis. Additional anesthetic care involves avoiding histamine-releasing agents (see earlier) and indirect- or direct-acting catecholamines, and extremes of blood pressure to decrease carcinoid tumor release.

# Perioperative Evaluation, Planning, and Bronchospasm Management

## HISTORY

Obtaining a thorough history of reactive airway disease is important for perioperative planning and prevention of bronchospasm. In a patient with a diagnosis of chronic airway disease, an understanding of their bronchodilator use, as well as their hospitalization and endotracheal intubation history, can be helpful in determining the severity and control of their disease. A history of recent upper respiratory infection (within 4 weeks, especially in patients with obstructive airway disease); recent smoking, cough, dyspnea, or fever; intolerance to cold air, dust, or smoke; and prior intolerance of general anesthesia with tracheal intubation are all pertinent in predicting intraoperative wheezing.

## PHYSICAL EXAMINATION

Wheezes are typically described as high-pitched notes that most often occur during expiration. An awake patient may additionally present with tachypnea and cough. Of note, it may be difficult to determine the severity of airway obstruction in a patient with bronchospastic disease based on the presence or absence of wheezing. A finding of wheezing on preoperative examination may suggest the need for further optimization before induction of anesthesia or that the patient may benefit from a regional anesthetic technique, if appropriate.

## PREMEDICATION

After identifying patients at risk for intraoperative bronchospasm, pharmacologic management includes the use of bronchodilators and antiinflammatory drugs. Prevention should also be directed toward the cause of bronchospasm. $\beta_2$-Adrenergic receptor agonists, such as the short-acting albuterol, can work within minutes. Longer-acting $\beta_2$-adrenergic receptor agonists, such as salmeterol, are more helpful in the control of chronic bronchospastic disease. Adequate anxiolysis additionally plays a role in prevention of bronchospasm. Antimuscarinic drugs—such as atropine, ipratropium, and glycopyrrolate—have been used to prevent bronchoconstriction. However, these medications are nonselective and, at low doses, may block the beneficial effects of $M_2$ more than $M_1$ and $M_3$, thereby worsening bronchoconstriction. At higher doses, antimuscarinic drugs block all three receptors, resulting in bronchodilation.

## INDUCTION OF ANESTHESIA

For patients that are at higher risk for bronchospasm, consideration should be given to using a regional anesthetic technique with limitation of airway manipulation, if possible. Additionally, an intravenous induction is recommended over an inhalation induction. During induction of general anesthesia, the goal is to establish adequate anesthetic depth and avoid stimulation of airway reflexes. Consideration should be given to the use of an inhaled bronchodilator immediately before induction. Lidocaine (1–2 mg/kg), administered topically or intravenously (1–3 min before intubation), may be helpful in preventing bronchoconstriction during airway manipulation. As described previously, propofol and ketamine can reduce airway resistance. Opioids can also help by depressing airway reflexes, keeping in mind that morphine can stimulate histamine release.

## AIRWAY MANIPULATION

Although wheezing can occur throughout the perioperative period, it more commonly occurs during airway manipulation because of reflex bronchoconstriction. Wheezing can be a sign of airway irritation from stimulation of the cholinergic system and subsequent bronchiolar constriction, which occurs when intubation is undertaken in a hyperreactive airway or if the depth of anesthesia is inadequate at the time of intubation. If appropriate for the patient and procedure, use of mask ventilation or placement of a laryngeal mask airway can reduce the risk of bronchospasm.

## CRISIS MANAGEMENT

When intraoperative bronchospasm occurs and causes $O_2$ desaturation or inadequate ventilation, the following must occur almost simultaneously: administration of 100% $O_2$, deepening of anesthesia, cessation of stimulation or surgery, and calling for help. Next, hand ventilation and evaluation of breath sounds over the chest and central epigastrium should be performed. These actions will isolate the patient from the anesthesia machine and exclude esophageal or bronchial intubation as potential causes of desaturation or inadequate ventilation. The position of the endotracheal tube should be examined for potential carinal stimulation with slow withdrawal of the tube, if needed. If, while passing a suction catheter down the tracheal tube, the anesthesia provider encounters an obstruction, the tracheal tube may be misplaced, kinked, or blocked.

A $\beta_2$-adrenergic receptor agonist (e.g., 4–8 puffs of albuterol initially followed by 2 puffs every 10 min) should be administered via the tracheal tube, timed with patient inhalation, through a connector into the tracheal tube. Ipratropium (6 puffs, followed by 2 puffs every 10 min) can also be given in this manner. Dosage of these inhaled medications can be adjusted to effect if administered via a breathing circuit. Once the initial assessment has been completed, corticosteroids (e.g., methylprednisolone 1–2 mg/kg) can be given, if appropriate, with the understanding that their onset of action may be delayed.

For severe bronchospasm that does not resolve with these interventions, intravenously administered epinephrine (1 mcg/kg bolus followed by 10–25 mcg·kg$^{-1}$·min$^{-1}$ titrated to vital signs and response) can be used for its bronchodilating effects. Increasing the time for expiration and changing from an anesthesia machine ventilator to a higher-performance intensive care unit ventilator with consideration for stopping the operation as quickly as possible may be necessary. The administration of inhaled anesthetic agents increases anesthetic depth. However, delivery of inhaled medications may be difficult or impossible in patients with acute bronchospasm because of ventilation/perfusion mismatch. There is also some evidence to suggest that the use of heliox is beneficial in severe cases of obstruction by decreasing airway resistance. Aminophylline and theophylline have less of a role in treating acute bronchospasm compared with $\beta_2$-adrenergic receptor agonists.

## POSTOPERATIVE MANAGEMENT OF A PATIENT WITH INTRAOPERATIVE BRONCHOSPASM

Extubating a wheezing patient can present additional hazards. Although deep extubation will likely reduce bronchospasm, it exposes the patient to residual anesthetic effects, including ventilation/perfusion mismatch, hypercapnia, narcosis, and aspiration of gastric contents.

## SUGGESTED READINGS

Bayable, S. D., Melesse, D. Y., Lema, G. F., & Ahmed, S. A. (2021). Perioperative management of patients with asthma during elective surgery: A systematic review. *Annals of Medicine and Surgery, 70*, 102847.

Chandler, D., Mosieri, C., Kallurkar, A., Pham, A. D., Okada, L. K., Kaye, R. J., et al. (2020). Perioperative strategies for the reduction of postoperative pulmonary complications. *Best Practice and Research Clinical Anaesthesiology, 34*(2), 153–166.

Ponsoye, P., Vecellio, L., Espitalier, F., Remerand, F., & Laffon, M. (2019). Pressurized metered-dose inhaler for beta-2 agonist delivery during intraoperative bronchospasm: Comparison of different administration methods. *British Journal of Anaesthesia, 122*(2), e26–e28.

von Ungern-Sternberg, B. S., Sommerfield, D., Slevin, L., Drake-Brockman, T. F. E., Zhang, G., & Hall, G. L. (2019). Effect of albuterol premedication vs placebo on the occurrence of respiratory adverse events in children undergoing tonsillectomies: The REACT Randomized Clinical Trial. *JAMA Pediatrics, 173*(6), 527–533.

# Anesthesia for Bronchoscopy

RYAN CHADHA, MD | J. ROSS RENEW, MD

Bronchoscopy allows direct visualization of the tracheobronchial tree using either a rigid metallic tube with an attached light source (rigid bronchoscope) or a flexible tube with a bundle of optical fibers running through the tube (flexible bronchoscope). Because of its size and rigidity, the rigid bronchoscope is used primarily to examine central airways, where it is used for removing endobronchial tumors, inserting stents to dilate major bronchi, removing foreign bodies, or aspirating blood. The fiber-optic bronchoscope (FOB) provides excellent visualization of, and access to, the tracheobronchial tree and is used in more than 90% of all bronchoscopic procedures. The modern FOB is now used more often, along with laser therapy and stents, to relieve central airway obstruction caused by tumor or airway stenosis especially after lung transplantation.

## Clinical Aspects of Bronchoscopy

The indications for bronchoscopy are outlined in Table 133.1. Concurrent medical problems increase the risks associated with the procedure. Patients with obstructive lung disease have an increased incidence of bronchospasm during bronchoscopy. Similarly, patients with restrictive ventilatory defects (e.g., interstitial lung disease) may have significant hypoxia during the procedure. Patients with lung cancer undergoing bronchoscopy may have other comorbid conditions (e.g., central airway obstruction, superior vena cava obstruction, metastatic lesions [bone, brain, liver], electrolyte imbalance [hyponatremia, hypercalcemia]). Patients with pulmonary hypertension, elevated

| TABLE 133.1 | Indications for Bronchoscopy |
|---|---|
| **Therapeutic** | **Diagnostic** |
| Removal of<br>  Foreign body<br>  Secretions<br>  Control of hemorrhage<br>Treat endobronchial<br>  obstruction with<br>  Thermal lasers<br>  Photodynamic therapy<br>  Brachytherapy<br>Dilate airway with<br>  Rigid scope<br>  Stent<br>  Balloon<br>Close bronchopleural<br>  fistula | Identify source of<br>  Hemorrhage in a patient with<br>    hemoptysis<br>  Unexplained cough<br>Assess<br>  Airway anatomy<br>  Airway function<br>  Tracheobronchial mucosa<br>  Peribronchial structures<br>Brush<br>  Mucosa, lung parenchyma, cytology<br>  Protective brush for quantitative<br>    bacteriologic culture<br>Biopsy<br>  Bronchial wall<br>  Transbronchial lung biopsy<br>  Transbronchial lymph node biopsy<br>Lavage<br>  Qualitative for inflammatory cells,<br>    neutrophils<br>  Quantitative for bacteria |

blood urea nitrogen (>30 mg/dL), chronic renal disease, and aspirin ingestion have an increased risk of postoperative bleeding. Interestingly, patients with recent myocardial infarction, unstable angina, or refractory arrhythmias often undergo bronchoscopy without significant complications.

A preoperative chest radiograph is mandatory; other investigations (e.g., complete blood count, electrolyte panel, coagulation studies) are performed as indicated. Resting pulse oximetry before the procedure is essential in providing baseline information. Pulmonary function testing establishes the presence and severity of either restrictive or obstructive lung disease and the degree of reversibility with treatment. If respiratory failure is suspected or if the patient is on home oxygen ($O_2$), arterial blood gas analysis may be helpful.

## Aims of Anesthesia for Bronchoscopy

The aims of anesthesia depend on the type of bronchoscopy. For FOB, topical upper airway anesthesia and/or sedation is common; however, for rigid bronchoscopy, general anesthesia is typical. For either technique, it is important to suppress patient's cough reflex and the hemodynamic response associated with bronchoscopy.

## Preoperative Preparation

After review of the indication for either FOB or rigid bronchoscopy, a complete history and examination is undertaken. Upper airway difficulties and obstruction of the central airways are noted. After anesthesia and risks are discussed with a fasting (>6 h) patient, an antisialagogue (atropine, 0.4–0.8 mg, or glycopyrrolate, 0.1–0.2 mg) may be administered intramuscularly or intravenously 40 min before the procedure. Aerosolized bronchodilators, $\beta_2$-adrenergic receptor agonists, and anticholinergic agents can be administered to patients with reactive airway disease. Corticosteroids are indicated during an exacerbation of reactive airway disease. The American Heart Association recommends endocarditis prophylaxis for rigid bronchoscopy but not for bronchoscopy using an FOB unless the patient has a prosthetic heart valve, a surgically corrected intracardiac defect, or a history of endocarditis. Depending on the situation, patients on intravenous heparin should have the heparin discontinued 4 to 6 h before the procedure, and platelets should be transfused to maintain platelet levels greater than 50,000/mL. For patients undergoing any type of anesthesia, the American Society of Anesthesiologists guidelines for standard monitoring should be followed.

## Fiber-optic Bronchoscopy

Fiber-optic bronchoscopy is usually performed under local anesthesia using topical local anesthetics or nerve blocks with or without sedation, and with or without the use of an airway. The FOB can be inserted orally or nasally, with patient cooperation being essential. Increasingly, especially in patients undergoing repetitive or interventional FOBs, a supraglottic airway is used.

## Sedation

Without sedation, bronchoscopy is associated with increased cough, increased sense of asphyxiation, and a significant increase in heart rate and blood pressure. Conscious sedation is usually achieved with intravenously administered incremental doses of midazolam (0.5–1.0 mg) or diazepam (1–2 mg). Intravenously administered opioids act synergistically with benzodiazepines to provide sedation and suppress airway reflexes but at the expense of potentiating respiratory depression. Fentanyl, sufentanil, alfentanil, and remifentanil are suitable opioid choices. Propofol can be used as a sedative agent to provide conscious sedation and suppression of cough reflexes; however, significant hypotension and even apnea may result from excess drug administration. Intravenously administered dexmedetomidine has also been used to provide sedation for flexible bronchoscopy with an FOB.

## Upper Airway Anesthesia for Bronchoscopy

The sensory innervation of the upper airway is described in Table 133.2. Local anesthetic agents, administered topically or via peripheral nerve blocks, can be used to anesthetize the upper airway. Two percent lidocaine (liquid or gel) is commonly used for topical airway anesthesia because of its margin of safety, rapid onset, and short duration of action. The maximum safe dose of lidocaine is 4 mg/kg. Toxicity depends on the rate of absorption and the resulting blood levels. Two percent lidocaine sprayed into or 4% viscous lidocaine-soaked pledgets placed in the nares (along with phenylephrine or cocaine to constrict the mucosa vessels) can be used to anesthetize the nasopharynx. Oropharyngeal anesthesia can be achieved by one of several means (Box 133.1). These techniques provide satisfactory anesthesia of the upper airway. If persistent gag reflex prevents bronchoscopy, use of bilateral glossopharyngeal nerve blocks is an option. These blocks should always be performed after superior laryngeal nerve blocks, otherwise significant pharyngeal muscle

---

> **BOX 133.1 METHODS TO ACHIEVE OROPHARYNGEAL ANESTHESIA DURING BRONCHOSCOPY**
>
> Mouth and pharynx—gargle and rinse with 2% viscous lidocaine
> Nebulized 2% lidocaine solution (95% effective when nebulized for 10 min)
> Superior laryngeal nerve blocks
> Transcricothyroid membrane injection
> Topicalization through suction port of the FOB
> Application of 4 mL of EMLA cream to the posterior one-third of the tongue
>
> *EMLA,* Eutectic mixture of local anesthetics (lidocaine and prilocaine); *FOB,* fiber-optic bronchoscope.

---

and tongue relaxation may result, obstructing the airway. Using a tonsillar needle, 3 mL of 2% lidocaine is injected into the midpoint of both posterior tonsillar pillars to a depth of 1 cm. This will effectively block the submucosa pressor receptors at the posterior aspect of the tongue.

## Artificial Airways and Fiber-optic Bronchoscope

For the patient undergoing repeated bronchoscopies (e.g., after lung transplantation), therapeutic procedures (airway stents), or FOB with extensive procedures, artificial airways can be used. Supraglottic airway (SGA) devices may be options in this setting. The principal contraindications for an SGA insertion are anatomic issue precluding placement, a full stomach, or nausea and vomiting (which is a relative contraindication). In these cases, an endotracheal tube is used. If an endotracheal tube is required, a 7.5-ID or larger tracheal tube is necessary to allow passage of an FOB of sufficient size to perform any planned procedures. The decrease in cross-sectional area of the tracheal tube once the FOB is inserted often requires assisted ventilation. A closed system is achieved with a self-sealing rubber diaphragm in the connector to the breathing circuit of the anesthesia machine. As with rigid bronchoscopy, bronchoscopy with an artificial airway can be performed with either a total intravenous technique or an inhalation technique. The topical administration of a local anesthetic agent to the airway before the induction of general anesthesia decreases anesthetic requirements.

## Treatment of Hypoxemia for Bronchoscopy

Hypoxemia during bronchoscopy may occur because of hypoventilation due to excess sedation or upper airway obstruction, ventilation-perfusion mismatch due to pneumothorax secondary to transbronchial biopsy or excessive bleeding, or from the proceduralist performing pulmonary lavage. Pulse oximetry is necessary for monitoring, with a goal of maintaining $O_2$ saturation ($Spo_2$) of at least 90%. Administration of supplemental $O_2$ (4–6 L/min) via nasal prongs or mask may help achieve this goal. The use of transnasal humidified rapid insufflation ventilator exchange (THRIVE) may be helpful to relieve hypoxemia and can provide some ventilatory support. If hypoxia persists, a nasopharyngeal tube should be inserted and $O_2$ administered via this route. If the $Spo_2$ saturation remains

---

| TABLE 133.2 | Sensory Innervation of the Upper Airway |
|---|---|
| **Anatomic Structure** | **Nerve Supply** |
| Nose | Trigeminal V—ophthalmic $V_1$, maxillary $V_2$ |
| **TONGUE** | |
| Anterior | Trigeminal V—lingual $V_3$ |
| Posterior | Glossopharyngeal IX |
| **PHARYNX** | |
| Nasal | Trigeminal V—maxillary branch $V_2$ |
| Oral | Glossopharyngeal IX |
| Larynx | Vagus X—internal laryngeal branch |
| Vocal cords | Vagus X—internal laryngeal branch |
| Trachea | Vagus X—internal laryngeal branch |

below 90%, the next step is to administer $O_2$ via a catheter passed nasally that is placed either above the larynx or in the proximal trachea. If $O_2$ desaturation continues, the bronchoscope should be withdrawn, an arterial blood gas should be measured, the sedation reversed, and an anesthesia bag and mask used to ventilate the patient. In such circumstances, tracheal intubation and ventilation with a high $Fio_2$ may be necessary.

## Rigid Bronchoscopy

An awake intubation should be considered for an anticipated difficult airway. If awake intubation is not feasible, an inhalation induction technique may be an alternative. An intravenous induction technique is used if no airway difficulty is anticipated. Anesthesia can be maintained with either an inhalation or intravenous technique.

Propofol is an ideal choice to maintain anesthesia if a total intravenous anesthetic technique is used because of its rapid onset and offset in addition to its suppression of airway reflexes. The administration of a potent opioid is often necessary because bronchoscopy can increase mean arterial pressure, heart rate, cardiac output, and pulmonary artery occlusion pressure to unacceptable levels. Fentanyl and sufentanil can be administered intermittently, or alfentanil and remifentanil can be given as a continuous infusion after a loading dose.

Neuromuscular blockade, which is often required, can be achieved with the use of a nondepolarizing agent with rapid onset and intermediate duration of action (e.g., rocuronium) or with a succinylcholine infusion. Patients with small cell lung neoplasms may develop Lambert-Eaton syndrome, a neuromuscular disorder that increases the sensitivity of patients who have the syndrome to the effects of both depolarizing and nondepolarizing neuromuscular blocking agents. The introduction of sugammadex has also given clinicians the ability to rapidly restore neuromuscular function after deep levels of aminosteroidal-induced neuromuscular blockade (train-of-four count = 0).

If the duration of the procedure is short, apneic oxygenation with intermittent ventilation may be an option. After induction of anesthesia and neuromuscular blockade, the patient is administered $O_2$ with an $Fio_2$ of 1.0, and then $O_2$ at 6 L/min is insufflated through a catheter passed through the vocal cords to lie just above the main carina. Although it may be possible to maintain $O_2$ saturation, the partial pressure of carbon dioxide in arterial blood tension will increase approximately 4 to 6 mm Hg the first minute and 2 to 4 mm Hg/min thereafter. Intermittent periods of ventilation may be necessary to attenuate the associated respiratory acidosis.

Sealing the open end of a rigid bronchoscope with the attached magnifying glass and attaching the breathing circuit from an anesthesia machine to the side arm of the rigid bronchoscope allows the anesthesia provider to oxygenate and ventilate the patient, with the added benefit of permitting the provider to maintain anesthesia using an inhaled anesthetic agent. When this technique is used for prolonged procedures, hypoxemia and hypercapnia may develop during times that the proximal end of the bronchoscope is open for instrumentation of the airway.

The Sanders jet injector technique, which is now frequently used, makes use of the Venturi principle, in which gas ($Fio_2$ $\geq 0.21$) under high pressure (50 psi) flows through a long metal tube with a small orifice entraining air from the open outlet, maintaining ventilation. This technique works well except in patients with decreased lung compliance in whom ventilation and oxygenation may be difficult to maintain. Because the gas is injected under high pressure, care must be taken to avoid barotrauma.

## Removal of a Foreign Body

The typical patient having a foreign body removed is a young, distressed, nonfasted child who has aspirated. Atropine is typically administered for its vagolytic and antisialagogue effects. Induction is aimed at reducing patient distress, which has the potential to disrupt the foreign body and cause asphyxia. Either systemic ketamine or a gradual inhalation technique with sevoflurane can be used. After induction, the aim is to keep the patient spontaneously breathing to prevent further dislodgement of the foreign body. If neuromuscular blockade is necessary, adequate expiratory time is important to prevent barotrauma from a ball-valve effect of the foreign body. The foreign body usually lodges in the right main bronchus. Adequate oxygenation and ventilation are maintained via the left lung when the foreign body is being removed; however, it may detach from the forceps and obstruct the lumen of the trachea. If the foreign body is not readily retrieved and the patient becomes increasingly hypoxic, the solution is to push the foreign body distally back into the bronchus to relieve the tracheal obstruction. When significant manipulation takes place, postprocedural obstruction because of mucosal edema may occur; therefore corticosteroids are often administered prophylactically.

## Management of Massive Hemoptysis

Massive hemoptysis ($>600$ mL of blood/24 h) is a rare but life-threatening crisis. The immediate therapy involves correcting the hypoxia by placing a tracheal tube (preferably a double-lumen tracheal tube if the bleeding is from either the right or left lung) and administering 100% $O_2$. Intravenous fluid resuscitation is indicated to correct hypovolemia, if present. If the bleeding is from the trachea or proximal main bronchi, the tracheal tube can be withdrawn and replaced with a rigid ventilating bronchoscope to locate the source of bleeding, aspirate blood and clots, instill iced saline and vasoconstrictors, and, if necessary, place a bronchial blocker into the bronchus from which the blood is emanating. A jet ventilation technique would be inappropriate in this situation because dry gas under pressure will cause the blood to solidify, thus exacerbating the obstruction and hypoxemia.

## Bronchoscopy Management of Central Airway Obstruction

Intrinsic processes (tracheomalacia, intraluminal malignancy, and strictures related to lung transplantation or intubation) or extrinsic processes (external compression by tumors) provide challenging cases for therapeutic bronchoscopy. For urgent obstruction relief, laser ablation, electrocautery, argon plasma coagulation, and placement of airway stents (metal, silicone, and hybrid) may be used. Cryotherapy, brachytherapy, and photodynamic therapy provide delayed relief of central airway obstruction. An FOB or a rigid bronchoscope can be used, depending on the planned procedure and skill and experience of the bronchoscopist. With the use of a rigid bronchoscope for relief of an obstruction of the trachea or major bronchi, an inhalation induction technique can be used, with a trial of positive-pressure ventilation used once the patient has been adequately anesthetized. The rigid bronchoscope is then introduced and the patient's nose and mouth packed. Obstruction of the airway because of necrotic tissue and excessive bleeding during treatment of the obstruction, most often with laser therapy, can precipitate hypoxia, requiring cessation of the procedure, administration of 100% $O_2$, and vigorous suction. During laser therapy, it is important to decrease the $Fio_2$ to 0.3 or less to minimize the possibility of airway fire. The anesthesia provider must communicate with the bronchoscopist if unable to maintain an $Spo_2$ of at least 90% with an $Fio_2$ to 0.3 or less; in this situation, the bronchoscopist should stop using the laser until oxygenation is improved and the $Fio_2$ is again decreased to 0.3 or less.

Both lasers and argon plasma coagulation technology involve the use of gas flow, which has the potential to lead to gas embolism, exacerbating hypoxemia and, in some instances, causing cardiac arrest. A review of patients undergoing rigid bronchoscopy under general anesthesia for airway stent placement found a complication incidence of 19.8% and a 30-day mortality rate of 7.8%, which was correlated with the patients' underlying health status and the urgency of the procedure.

## Complications Associated With Bronchoscopy

A mortality rate of less than 0.1%, a rate of major complications of less than 1.5%, and a rate of minor complications of less than 6.5% have been reported with the use of bronchoscopy (Table 133.3). Significantly, 50% of complications are caused by the premedication, the general anesthetic, or the local anesthetic agent used for the procedure. Because rigid bronchoscopy is usually carried out under total intravenous anesthesia, awareness is a recognized complication.

Bronchoscopy-induced hemodynamic changes increase myocardial $O_2$ demand in patients at risk of developing myocardial ischemia. Hypoxemia predisposes the patients to developing cardiac arrhythmias and ST-segment changes, whereas coronary artery disease, per se, does not increase the risk for developing arrhythmias. Hypoxemia and hypercarbia contribute greatly to the cardiovascular complications associated with bronchoscopy. Severe hypoxemia and hypercarbia may also result in seizures, but these are usually associated with local anesthetic toxicity.

| TABLE 133.3 | Complications of Bronchoscopy | |
|---|---|
| **General** | **Local** |
| Hypoxemia<br>  Sedation/anesthesia<br>  Methemoglobinemia<br>Hypercarbia<br>  Sedation/anesthesia<br>  Inadequate ventilation<br>Cardiac arrhythmias<br>Awareness and recall<br>Neurologic—seizures<br>Cardiac arrest and death | Dental and facial trauma<br>Hemorrhage<br>Bronchospasm<br>Pneumothorax<br>Central airway obstruction<br>  Tumor<br>  Blood<br>  Secretions<br>Peripheral airway obstruction<br>  caused by<br>  Asthma<br>  Chronic bronchitis<br>  Emphysema<br>Airway trauma |

## Summary

The anesthesia provider is challenged during a bronchoscopic procedure because the airway is shared with the bronchoscopist. Complications of bronchoscopy, such as hypoxemia and hypercarbia, are common and can result in cardiovascular complications, even cardiopulmonary arrest. Communication, cooperation, vigilance, and attention to detail—especially to $O_2$ saturation and minute ventilation—improve outcomes.

## SUGGESTED READINGS

de Lima, A., Kheir, F., Majid, A., & Pawlowski, J. (2018). Anesthesia for interventional pulmonology procedures: A review of advanced diagnostic and therapeutic bronchoscopy. *Canadian Journal of Anaesthesia*, 65(7), 822–836. doi:10.1007/s12630-018-1121-3.

José, R. J., Shaefi, S., & Navani, N. (2014). Anesthesia for bronchoscopy. *Current Opinion in Anaesthesiology*, 27(4), 453–457.

Londino, A. V., III, & Jagannathan, N. (2019). Anesthesia in diagnostic and therapeutic pediatric bronchoscopy. *Otolaryngologic Clinics of North America*, 52(6), 1037–1048.

# Double-Lumen Tracheal Tubes

EDUARDO S. RODRIGUES, MD

Double-lumen tracheal tubes enable functional separation of the lungs. This separation can prevent spillage or contamination of fluid, blood, and pus from one lung to another and control ventilation distribution. The most common indication for single-lung ventilation is to improve surgical exposure (Table 134.1). Although single-lung ventilation can also be achieved with single-lumen tubes and bronchial blockers, double-lumen tubes have several advantages (Box 134.1).

Lung separation can be lifesaving, but its initiation can produce sudden and substantial impairment of $O_2$ exchange. Other disadvantages, particularly to double-lumen tubes, are that they increase airway resistance and can make clearance of secretions difficult. Relative contraindications must also be considered when contemplating the placement of these tubes (Box 134.2).

## Tube Selection

Double-lumen tubes include Carlens, White, Bryce-Smith, and Robertshaw, which all share standard features: they have two lumina, one terminating in the trachea and the other in the right or left main bronchus; have two cuffs; and are molded to conform to the oropharynx and main bronchus. The Carlens is a left-sided tube with a carinal hook. The White is essentially a right-sided Carlens; the Bryce-Smith lacks a carinal hook and has a slotted cuff on its right-sided version to allow right upper lobe ventilation. More recently, double-lumen tubes include technological adaptations, including bioimpedance for cardiac output monitoring and video assistance for position assistance. These newer devices are prone to increasing cost, more steps, new risk, and provider distraction, and they are not discussed here.

<table>
<tr><td>TABLE 134.1</td><td colspan="2">Indications for Separation of the Two Lungs (Double-Lumen Tube Intubation) or One-Lung Ventilation</td></tr>
<tr><td colspan="2">Absolute Indication</td><td>Relative Indication</td></tr>
<tr><td colspan="2">Isolation of one lung from the other to avoid spillage or contamination because of<br>Infection<br>Massive hemorrhage<br>Bronchopleural fistula<br>Bronchopleural cutaneous fistula<br>Surgical opening of a major conducting airway<br>Lung cyst or bulla<br>Tracheobronchial tree disruption<br>Unilateral bronchopulmonary lavage for pulmonary alveolar proteinosis<br>Video-assisted thoracic surgery<br>Lung transplantation</td><td>Surgical exposure (high priority) for<br>Thoracic aortic aneurysm<br>Pneumonectomy<br>Upper lobectomy<br>Mediastinal exposure<br>Thoracoscopy<br>Surgical exposure (medium [lower] priority) for<br>Middle and lower lobectomies and subsegmental resections<br>Esophageal resection<br>Procedures on the thoracic spine<br>Severe hypoxemia because of unilateral lung disease<br>Minimally invasive heart surgery</td></tr>
</table>

**BOX 134.2 RELATIVE CONTRAINDICATIONS TO THE USE OF A DOUBLE-LUMEN TRACHEAL TUBE**

Presence of a lesion along the pathway of the double-lumen tube
Difficult or impossible conventional direct or videolaryngoscopy vision intubation
Critically ill patients with single-lumen tube in situ who cannot tolerate even a short time without mechanical ventilation
Full stomach or high risk of aspiration (this is more relevant important with less experienced teams)

The Robertshaw DLT is the model widely available for clinical practice as the previously described historic models have been retired. The Robertshaw DLT is made of clear plastic and disposable, with left- and right-sided versions. The distance from the edge of the distal cuff to the lumen is approximately 3 cm (Fig. 134.1). The tubes are available in sizes 41F, 39F, 37F, 35F, 32F, and 28F (Table 134.2). Both cuffs are high-volume, low-pressure type (Fig. 134.2), with the bronchial cuff colored bright blue; this bronchial cuff is also slanted in the right-sided version to improve right upper lobe ventilation. Finally, this version contains a radiopaque line at the end of each lumen to allow for radiographic identification of correct placement.

The left-sided double-lumen tube is easier to position, maintains a good position during surgery, and can be used for most thoracic procedures requiring one-lung ventilation, regardless of the operative side and planned operation. The left-sided double-lumen tube can be used for right thoracotomies requiring right-lung collapse and can also be used for left thoracotomies with left-lung collapse. In left-sided operations, the bronchial portion of the left-sided tube can be withdrawn into the trachea in case of need of left main bronchus clamping and continue to be used for right-lung ventilation through both lumens.

Conversely, the use of the right-sided tube can be more challenging. Most surgeons frown on a right-sided double-lumen tube. To ventilate the right upper lobe, the slot of the bronchial portion of the right-sided tube must be closely opposed to the orifice of the right upper lobe. Because the length of the right main bronchus is shorter and more variable than that of the left main bronchus, right-sided bronchial intubation poses a substantial risk for right upper lobe collapse and hypoventilation. In general, the left main bronchus is approximately 5 cm in

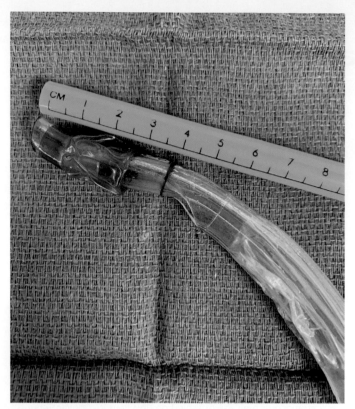

**Fig. 134.1** Left-sided double-lumen tube distal cuff *(blue)* with tip 4 cm from the tracheal lumen. The proximal edge of the blue cuff (3 cm) should be positioned at the carina level.

| TABLE 134.2 | Double Lumen Sizes Chart | |
|---|---|---|
| Tube Size | Internal Diameter (mm) | External Diameter (mm) |
| 28F (left only) | 4.0 | 9.3 |
| 32F (left only) | 4.5 | 10.7 |
| 35F | 5.0 | 11.7 |
| 37F | 5.5 | 12.3 |
| 39F | 6.0 | 13.0 |
| 41F | 6.5 | 13.7 |

French gauge units and internal and external diameter in mm.

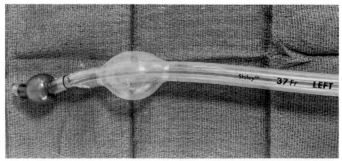

**Fig. 134.2** Left-sided double-lumen tube with both high-volume, low-pressure cuffs inflated for demonstration purposes. The proximal cuff *(transparent)* will be positioned, when deflated, at the tracheal level, and the bronchial cuff *(blue)* will be placed at the left main bronchi with the proximal edge at the level of the carina.

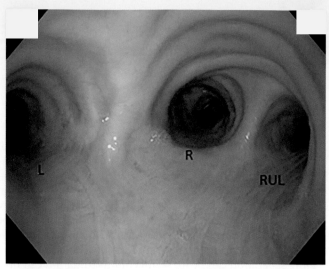

**Fig. 134.3** Fiberoptic bronchoscopy view at the level of the carina, depicting the abnormal takeoff of the right upper lobe (RUL), termed *tracheal bronchus* or *bronchus suis*. The anterior C-shaped cartilaginous rings and the posterior membranous portion of the trachea allow for anterior-posterior orientation. This abnormal connection to the RUL from the trachea rather than the right mainstem bronchus can be found in 0.1% to 3% of the general population.

length until bifurcation of the left upper lobe. On the right side, the upper lobe will depart 2 cm distal to the carina in most patients, but in 10% of patients this could be shorter, and in 3% of patients the right upper lobe departs from the trachea. When the right main bronchi departs from the trachea, also known as *bronchus suis*, it can pose challenges to anatomy identification, and a right-sided tube cannot be used (Fig. 134.3).

The shorter right main bronchus has a small margin of safety on the positioning as small as 1 mm, and dislocation during surgery is more common, making adequate ventilation of the right upper lobe a challenge.

The contraindications to left-sided placement are proximal left main endobronchial lesions, other lesions distorting the left main bronchus, local airway disruption, and previous left-side pneumectomy. Therefore except for these contraindications, a left-sided tube is preferred in the author's institution.

## Double-Lumen Tube Placement Technique

To place the double-lumen tube, the following steps are performed:
- Choose the tube size. There is no consensus in double-lumen tube size selection, but the patient's sex, height, and ethnicity should be considered. For example, females, shorter patients, and those in the Asian population require smaller double-lumen tubes. Using preoperative chest radiographs and computed tomography to measure the patient's trachea and left main bronchus is scientific but not pragmatic and is rarely used in practice. Historically, the largest tube possible was chosen; however, it is well documented that airway trauma and complications are related to the diameter of the endotracheal tube. A 35F tracheal tube is appropriate for most women and a 37F for men. Amar and associates showed that a 35F tube is suitable for most patients and does not increase the risk of hypoxia. Several institutions, including the author's, are migrating to this more pragmatic approach of 35F for females and

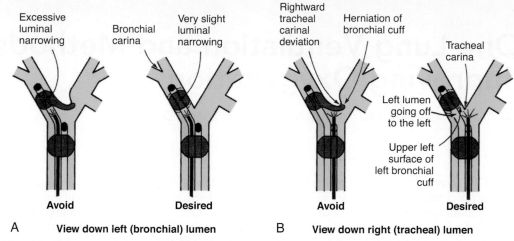

**Fig. 134.4** This schematic diagram depicts the complete fiberoptic bronchoscopy picture of left-sided double-lumen tracheal tubes (both the desired view and the view to be avoided from both of the lumina). **A,** When the bronchoscope is passed down the left lumen of the left-sided tube, the endoscopist should see a very slight left luminal narrowing and a clear straight-ahead view of the bronchial carina off in the distance. Excessive left luminal narrowing should be avoided. **B,** When the bronchoscope is passed down the right lumen of the left-sided tube, the endoscopist should see a clear straight-ahead view of the tracheal carina and the upper surface of the blue left endobronchial cuff just below the tracheal carina. Excessive pressure in the endobronchial cuff, as manifested by tracheal carinal deviation to the right and herniation of the endobronchial cuff over the carina, should be avoided. (Adapted from Benumof JL. *Anesthesia for Thoracic Surgery.* 2nd ed. WB Saunders; 1995.)

37F for males. The amount of airway hygiene required during surgery needs to be considered when selecting the ideal tube size.

- Review the patient's history and examine the patient for conditions that may affect tube choice or require special intubation techniques, like tracheostomy, tracheal stenosis, or need for awake intubation. These conditions are very important and are likely to alter clinical management.
- Check both cuffs for integrity (the bronchial cuff usually requires <3 mL of air); cuffs can be protected at intubation with a tooth guard.
- In most cases, a Macintosh (Mac) blade is used for intubation, as this blade approximates the curvature of the tracheal tube. However, despite our preference for the use of a Mac blade, the Miller blade is also appropriate, and the provider should use the equipment they are more familiar and comfortable with.
- Pass the tip of the tube through the larynx, with the distal curvature concave anteriorly.
- Once the tip is through the larynx, remove the stylet, and rotate the tube 90 degrees toward the correct side: clockwise for a right-sided double-lumen tube and counterclockwise for a left-sided tube.
- A video-laryngoscope can safely and successfully be used in patients with difficult visualization of the vocal cords. It is helpful to have the tube made more malleable in warm saline and have a more pronounced curvature for airway engagement. A continued 360-degree spin facilitates the tube advancement for tube advancement.

- After intubation, the anesthesia provider must use an established routine to verify tube placement. The clinical exam alone, without bronchoscopy, may miss mispositioning 48% of the time and should not be used alone. For this reason, fiberoptic bronchoscopy is routinely used and mandatory to confirm proper positioning (Fig. 134.4).
- Tube position must be reconfirmed after repositioning the patient. Head flexion may cause tube advancement, bronchial placement of the tracheal lumen, or upper lobe obstruction if a right-sided tube is used. Head extension can cause bronchial decannulation. In addition, intraoperative surgical manipulation may displace the tube.
- Most of the complications associated with the placement of double-lumen tracheal tubes (Box 134.3) involve direct tracheobronchial trauma. They can be avoided by checking tube position regularly, selecting an appropriately sized tube, by paying meticulous attention to cuff inflation to avoid high pressures, by means of care in repositioning patients, and by using caution in patients with bronchial wall abnormalities.

---

**BOX 134.3 COMPLICATIONS OF THE USE OF DOUBLE-LUMEN TRACHEAL TUBES, IN ORDER OF FREQUENCY**

Traumatic laryngitis
Tracheobronchial tree trauma and disruption
Suturing of the double-lumen tracheal tube to the intrathoracic structure

## SUGGESTED READINGS

Amar, D., Desiderio, D. P., Heerdt, P. M., Kolker, A. C., Zhang, H., & Thaler, H. T. (2008). Practice patterns in choice of left double-lumen tube size for thoracic surgery. *Anesthesia and analgesia, 106*(2), 379–383.

Falzon, D., Alston, R. P., Coley, E., & Montgomery, K. (2017). Lung isolation for thoracic surgery: From inception to evidence-based. *Journal of Cardiothoracic and Vascular Anesthesia, 31*(2), 678–693.

Hao, D., & Baker, K. (2021). Placement of a double-lumen endotracheal tube. *New England Journal of Medicine, 385*(16), e52.

Joshi, B. L., Lester, L. C., & Grant, M. C. (2018). Placement of the double-lumen endotracheal tube: One size doesn't fit all. *Journal of Cardiothoracic and Vascular Anesthesia, 32*(1), 287–289.

Sunger, P., & Campos, H. (2020). Anesthesia for thoracic surgery. In M. A. Gropper (Ed.), *Miller's anesthesia* (9th ed., pp. 1648–1716). Philadelphia: Elsevier.

# 135

# One-Lung Ventilation and Methods of Improving Oxygenation

SARANG S. KOUSHIK, MD  |  BRANTLEY D. GAITAN, MD

One-lung ventilation (OLV) may be required for optimal exposure for intrathoracic surgical procedures (i.e., cardiac or thoracic). There are multiple indications for OLV, both surgical and nonsurgical, and these are noted in Table 135.1. OLV is achieved through a double-lumen tracheal tube (DLT), through a single-lumen tracheal tube advanced into either the right or left mainstem bronchus, or by advancing a bronchial blocker through a single-lumen tracheal tube into one of the mainstem bronchi.

## Mechanism of Hypoxemia

One of the main considerations in the management of cases requiring OLV is maintenance of oxygenation (i.e., avoidance of hypoxemia that could lead to tissue hypoxia). There is no accepted threshold to define the safest lower limit of oxygenation; however, partial pressure of oxygen ($Pao_2$) greater than 60 mm Hg or oxygenation greater than 90% is generally accepted. Hypoxemia results from ventilation/perfusion (V/Q) mismatching because of both OLV and lateral decubitus positioning used for the majority of these surgical procedures. Several factors can contribute to the development of V/Q mismatching, and consideration of these factors preoperatively can help identify patients who might be at risk for clinically significant hypoxemia.

Lateral decubitus positioning alters the balance of ventilation and perfusion in both lungs compared with normal physiologic conditions (i.e., spontaneous ventilation), as well as the physiologic conditions that exist for the supine patient under anesthesia. These changes are seen even when both lungs are being ventilated (i.e., positioning independently contributes to the development of V/Q mismatching). The dependent lung is compressed by the abdominal contents and by the mediastinum, promoting atelectasis, alveolar collapse, and underventilation of the dependent lung. The nondependent lung is not subject to external compression like the dependent lung; in fact,

it has increased compliance and becomes relatively overventilated, particularly when the corresponding hemithorax is opened. Lateral decubitus positioning also affects distribution of blood flow as a result of gravity, with the dependent lung well perfused and the nondependent lung underperfused. Because of this V/Q mismatching, desaturation and hypoxemia can result with lateral decubitus positioning even when both lungs are being ventilated.

When OLV is initiated, ventilation to the nondependent lung ceases and the dependent lung is the only lung being ventilated. The nondependent lung becomes atelectatic but is still being perfused; thus the V/Q ratio approaches 0, and a transpulmonary shunt is created through the upper lung. Various factors can affect the distribution of blood flow (i.e., hypoxic pulmonary vasoconstriction, addition of positive end-expiratory pressure [PEEP], or continuous positive airway pressure [CPAP]), and the degree of hypoxemia correlates with the degree of the resulting shunt. Interestingly, the physiologic response in ventilation and perfusion as a result of lateral decubitus positioning serve to offset the effect of OLV to a degree, so that patients having OLV in the lateral position will have a better $Pao_2$ than patients having OLV in the supine position.

## Factors Affecting Oxygenation During One-Lung Ventilation

Many factors can affect oxygenation during OLV through changes in ventilation or distribution of pulmonary blood flow. Normally, when part of a lung is not ventilated (e.g., atelectasis, edema), "hypoxic" pulmonary vasoconstriction (HPV) restricts flow to the affected alveoli. Physiologically, this occurs so that blood flow is redistributed to areas of the lung that are being ventilated. When OLV is initiated, HPV quickly develops, and maintenance of oxygenation depends on the effective redistribution of blood flow to the ventilated lung. HPV has a biphasic pattern in response to alveolar hypoxia, with the first plateau being reached around 20 to 30 min and a second plateau phase reaching maximum vasoconstriction at around 2 h. It is of greatest benefit when 30% to 70% of the alveoli in a segment of nonventilated lung either contain a hypoxic gas mixture or are collapsed, as this can decrease the blood flow to the affected area by 50%.

There are many factors that can either blunt or potentiate HPV and therefore affect the physiologic response to V/Q mismatching during OLV (Table 135.2). Anything that increases pulmonary arterial pressure will decrease flow through the dependent lung and increase the shunt through the nondependent lung. Resultant scenarios that worsen hypoxemia include volume overload, elevated left atrial pressure, pulmonary embolism, hypocarbia, or drug-induced vasoconstriction in the

| TABLE 135.1 | Indications for One-Lung Ventilation | |
|---|---|---|
| **Absolute** | | **Relative** |
| Video-assisted thoracoscopy | | Surgery on thoracic aorta or esophagus |
| Protective isolation (infection, hemorrhage) | | Pneumonectomy or lobar resection* |
| Differential ventilation (bronchopleural fistula, cyst, bullae, bronchial disruption) | | |
| Pulmonary alveolar lavage | | |

*If one-lung ventilation is used, the surgical incision can be smaller because the deflation of the nondependent lung enables the surgeon to have better surgical access without a large thoracotomy incision.

| TABLE 135.2 | Factors Affecting HPV Response During One-Lung Ventilation* | |
|---|---|---|
| **Blunt HPV Response** | **Potentiate HPV Response** | |
| COPD | Hypertension | |
| Cirrhosis | Iron deficiency | |
| Sepsis | | |
| Sustained exposure to high altitude | | |
| Metabolic or respiratory alkalosis | Metabolic acidosis (independent of $Pco_2$) | |
| Hypocapnia | Hypercapnia | |
| Hyperventilation | | |
| Hypothermia | Hyperthermia | |
| Trendelenburg position | Lateral decubitus position | |
| Inhalation anesthetic agents (except $N_2O$) Not clinically significant | | |
| Systemic vasodilators (most) (i.e., nitroglycerin, nitroprusside, calcium channel blockers, and many $\beta_2$-receptor agonists) | Retraction of operative lung on surgical field | |

*Blunted response to HPV will worsen hypoxemia during OLV, whereas potentiated/enhanced response to HPV will lessen hypoxemia during OLV.
*COPD*, Chronic obstructive pulmonary disease; *HPV*, hypoxic pulmonary vasoconstriction; $N_2O$, nitrous oxide; *OLV*, one-lung ventilation.

pulmonary vasculature (dopamine, epinephrine, phenylephrine, and other vasoconstrictors preferentially constrict normoxic lung vessels and defeat the HPV mechanism).

Although HPV is responsible for most of the redistribution of blood flow away from the nonventilated lung, manual compression of the nonventilated lung during the surgical procedure may further reduce blood flow to this area.

## Preoperative and Intraoperative Condition of the Dependent Lung

The pulmonary vascular resistance (PVR) of the dependent lung determines the ability of that lung to accept redistributed blood flow from the nondependent lung, so increases in PVR will worsen shunting by distributing more blood flow to the nonventilated lung. Preexisting pulmonary hypertension (i.e., high PVR in the dependent lung) interferes with the ability of HPV to redistribute flow to the dependent lung. As mentioned previously, lateral decubitus positioning will cause increased blood flow to the dependent lung, which can be of benefit during OLV. However, maintaining the patient in the lateral decubitus position for long periods of time may cause a pericapillary transudate in the dependent lung, collapsing alveoli and increasing PVR in the dependent lung. Hyperventilation (high tidal volumes, excessive PEEP) can increase airway pressure and PVR in the ventilated lung, redirecting blood flow into the nondependent lung and worsening the shunt. Clinical conditions that may increase PVR in the dependent lung include atelectasis, low inspired oxygen ($O_2$) tension, hypothermia, hypercapnia, acidosis, and suboptimal pain control.

## Methods to Attenuate Hypoxemia During One-Lung Ventilation

A fraction of inspired oxygen ($Fio_2$) of 1.0 has been associated with $Pao_2$ values between 150 and 250 mm Hg during OLV and can help protect against hypoxemia and promote vasodilation in the dependent lung to accept blood flow redistribution from the hypoxic nondependent lung. Prolonged high $Fio_2$ can lead to absorption atelectasis, $O_2$ toxicity, or lung injury in patients previously treated with bleomycin chemotherapy. The risks and benefits of high $Fio_2$ should be assessed on a case-by-case basis, and application of the lowest $Fio_2$ to maintain satisfactory oxygenation is a reasonable approach to managing most patients. Vigilant control of factors that negatively affect the V/Q ratio (i.e., temperature management, pain control) can affect postoperative morbidity.

Ventilation strategy is usually directed toward preserving oxygenation and decreasing risk of damage to the lung, and this is accomplished with lower tidal volumes and adequate PEEP (which should prevent atelectasis while avoiding overdistention). It is reasonable to initiate OLV using a tidal volume of 4 to 6 mL/kg and PEEP 5 cmH2O, and the rate should be sufficient to maintain the partial pressure of carbon dioxide ($Paco_2$) at 40 mm Hg or less. Because carbon dioxide ($CO_2$) is 20 times more diffusible than $O_2$ in the lung, ventilation through the dependent lung removes sufficient $CO_2$ so that hypercarbia is rarely seen. Any resulting hypercarbia can be rapidly corrected with the cessation of OLV. Lower tidal volumes may lead to increased atelectasis in the dependent lung, and during OLV these have been associated with increased perioperative morbidity through clinically significant hypoxemia and auto PEEP. However, increased airway pressures through overdistention (high tidal volume) or addition of excessive PEEP can impede blood flow to the dependent lung, worsening the shunt fraction. PEEP applied to the dependent lung increases functional residual capacity in that lung and can function to optimize the ventilation-perfusion ratio and attenuate some of the hypoxemia. Therefore it should be either added or increased (if already in use) up to 10 cmH2O, as PEEP higher than this can increase shunting and worsen hypoxia. The optimal value for PEEP remains to be defined and may vary depending on the clinical scenario. Pressure control and volume control ventilation can both be used to accomplish the goals of physiologic tidal volumes and optimal PEEP while minimizing airway pressures. There is no accepted strategy that can be applied to all clinical scenarios, so patient condition, pulmonary mechanics, and underlying physiology must be considered to determine optimal intraoperative management.

Despite these efforts, patients may still develop hypoxemia. The most common causes of hypoxemia during OLV tend to be malposition of the double-lumen tube, inadequate ventilation of the dependent lung with development of atelectasis, and blood or secretions in the airway of the ventilated lung. When hypoxemia occurs, the first priority is correcting it through ensuring an $Fio_2$ of 1.0, delivering recruitment breaths to the dependent lung, and communicating to the surgeon that oxygenation is an issue in case a brief period of reinflation of the operative lung is required. After improving saturation to an acceptable level, the common causes of hypoxemia should be explored with fiberoptic inspection of tube position, removal of blood or secretions, and adjustment of ventilation strategy to include intermittent recruitment maneuvers if needed.

If PEEP is maximized and hypoxemia persists, CPAP at 5 to 10 cmH2O can be applied to the nonventilated lung. This maintains the patency of alveoli that have not already collapsed in the nondependent lung, drawing blood flow from already collapsed alveoli, and allowing some gas exchange to occur in the nondependent lung. CPAP can be effective at lower levels (2–5 cmH$_2$O), which can be particularly important if higher levels are interfering with surgical exposure (i.e., video-assisted thoracoscopic surgery [VATs]); however, the lung must often be briefly reinflated before its application (30 cm H$_2$O for 15 sec).

If neither CPAP nor PEEP improves the hypoxemia, then the anesthesia provider should communicate with the surgeon to advise them of the degree of the patient's desaturation and methods attempted to correct oxygenation. In certain cases, ligation of the pulmonary vessels supplying the lung tissue to be resected can be performed expeditiously to decrease the shunt. If ligation of the pulmonary vasculature is not an option, then the surgeon should pause while the anesthesia provider ventilates both lungs. Adequate CPAP should be applied to the nondependent lung to reexpand that lung and resolve the hypoxic event. If hypoxia progresses, discussion can be had with the surgeon to proceed with intermittent reexpansion and ventilation of the nondependent lung.

## Miscellaneous Causes of Hypoxemia

Endotracheal tube malposition often contributes to the development of hypoxemia. If performing OLV with a DLT, the bronchial lumen can be advanced too distal into the airway, not advanced far enough, or be inadvertently positioned into the incorrect mainstem bronchus. In addition, right-sided DLT can potentially be positioned so that the right upper lobe is not being adequately ventilated. If using a bronchial blocker, this can become malpositioned and obstruct the airway, although this is often accompanied by an increase in airway pressures that allows for detection before pronounced desaturation has occurred.

If surgery is for resection of a tumor, characteristics of the tumor can affect oxygenation intraoperatively. With larger, more centrally located masses, the distribution of blood flow will likely be such that there is already less perfusion of the operative side. In contrast, smaller and/or more peripheral tumors (i.e., metastatic disease) are more likely to develop hypoxemia upon initiation of OLV.

The side of the operation can contribute to hypoxemia. The left lung is smaller than the right, so hypoxemia can be more pronounced in right-sided surgical procedures when oxygenation must be maintained with the smaller left lung in the dependent position.

Other causes include supine positioning (rather than lateral decubitus), atelectasis of the ventilated lung, failure of the operative lung to adequately collapse, bronchospasm, inadequate neuromuscular blockade (coughing), blockage of the tracheal tube lumen by secretions or blood, and failure of the O$_2$ supply or disconnection of the breathing circuit.

### SUGGESTED READINGS

Campos, J. H., & Feider, A. (2018). Hypoxia during one-lung ventilation: A review and update. *Journal of Cardiothoracic and Vascular Anesthesia, 32*(5), 2330–2338.

Campos, J. H., & Peacher, D. (2021). Application of continuous positive airway pressure during video-assisted thoracoscopic surgery. *Current Anesthesiology Reports, 11*(4), 446–456.

de Gama, Abreu M., & Whittenstein, J. (2022). Management of one-lung ventilation: Protective lung ventilation. In E. Cohen (Ed.), *Cohen's comprehensive thoracic anesthesia* (1st ed., pp. 279–292). Elsevier Philadelphia: Elsevier.

Hagerman, A., & Licker, M. (2022). Anesthesia, mechanical ventilation and hypoxic pulmonary vasoconstriction. In E. Cohen (Ed.), *Cohen's comprehensive thoracic anesthesia* (pp. 193–212). Elsevier Philadelphia: Elsevier.

Peel, J. K., Funk, D. J., Slinger, P., Srinathan, S., & Kidane, B. (2020). Positive end expiratory pressure and recruitment maneuvers during one-lung ventilation: A systematic review and meta-analysis. *Journal of Thoracic and Cardiovascular Surgery, 160*(4), 1112–1122.

Peel, J. K., Funk, D. J., Slinger, P., Srinathan, S., & Kidane, B. (2022). Tidal volume during 1-lung ventilation: A systematic review and meta-analysis. *Journal of Thoracic and Cardiovascular Surgery, 163*(4), 1573–1585.e1.

Slinger, P & Campos, JH. (2020) Anesthesia for Thoracic Surgery. In Gropper, MA, Cohen, NH, Eriksson LI, Leslie, K, Wiener-Kronish, JP (Eds.) *Miller's Anesthesia* (9th ed., pp. 1648-1716.e8). Philadelphia: Elsevier.

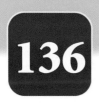

# 136

# Bronchopleural Fistula

THOMAS M. STEWART, MD

A bronchopleural fistula (BPF) is a connection between the bronchi or lung parenchyma and the pleural space. If the fistula communicates with the surface of the chest, it is a bronchopleural cutaneous fistula. Communication between the airways and the pleural space substantially increases the risk of infection and can make ventilation difficult, accounting for the high morbidity associated with this condition. Anesthesia providers may encounter patients with BPFs when these patients present for surgical repair of the fistula or in the intensive care unit when the patients require ventilator management of the condition. In rare cases, a patient may present to the operating room for surgery in which the fistula is an incidental condition.

## Etiology

Common causes of BPF include spontaneous development (usually secondary to underlying pathology or infection) and direct injury (often resulting from trauma, radiation, or surgery.) The mechanism usually involves rupture or erosion of a lung abscess, bronchus, bulla, cyst, suture line, or parenchymal tissue into the pleural space; however, by far the most common modern cause is a complication of thoracic surgery. The incidence of postoperative formation of a BPF has been reported to be 2% to 40% after pulmonary resection. Persistent air leak, expanding pneumothorax, sepsis, empyema, purulent sputum, and respiratory distress may characterize such fistulas. If presenting within the initial 24- to 72-h postoperative period, BPF often indicates insufficient surgical closure of the lung parenchyma or bronchial stump. Postoperative BPF development beyond 72 h may represent failure of the suture line due to ischemia, infection, or necrosis. Predisposing factors include perioperative radiation or chemotherapy, residual neoplasm, age greater than 60 years, infection at the resection site, and an avascular bronchial stump.

Before the movement toward lung-protective ventilation strategies, it was not uncommon to develop BPF in mechanically ventilated patients suffering from acute respiratory distress syndrome (ARDS). Alveolar rupture during mechanical ventilation is thought to be a consequence of both volutrauma from inappropriately high tidal volumes and an elevated transpulmonary pressure gradient.

## Treatment

Treatment of BPFs is highly dependent on the cause and nature of the fistula. In general, attempts are made to reduce the pleural space and seal the fistula by either placing a chest tube or performing pleurodesis. In those patients who are intubated, positive-pressure ventilation management is critical to minimize air leak and give the fistula the best chance of healing while maintaining appropriate gas exchange. If the fistula is large (e.g., disruption of a postpneumonectomy bronchial stump), conservative management is often not effective, and surgical intervention and repair will be necessary.

Treatment of BPFs that result in patients who are mechanically ventilated for ARDS are exceptionally difficult to treat.

Regardless of lung-protective ventilator strategies for ARDS, the increased transpulmonary pressures and high respiratory rates required to adequately ventilate and oxygenate the patient may impede closure of a BPF.

## ANESTHETIC CONSIDERATIONS

The primary clinical concern when caring for patients undergoing surgical repair of BPFs relates to providing adequate alveolar gas exchange during positive-pressure ventilation. The following must be considered:

- Tidal volume is preferentially delivered into the pleural space through the low-resistance fistula.
- Air leak into the pleural space can produce a tension pneumothorax.
- If infection is suspected, healthy lung tissue should be protected from contamination by the affected lung.
- Differences in compliance and gas exchange between healthy lung and diseased lung or diseased lung and the fistula can exacerbate the difficulty in delivering an adequate tidal volume through the fistula.

Tension pneumothorax is prevented or treated by placement of a chest tube. If an empyema or lung abscess is present, drainage under local anesthesia or bronchoscopy should be considered prior to repair of the fistula. Because the use of positive-pressure ventilation may exacerbate difficulties in providing adequate gas exchange, alternative anesthetic techniques—including maintenance of spontaneous ventilation and the use of regional anesthesia (e.g., thoracic epidural anesthesia)—have been used. Unfortunately, most procedures to repair or treat bronchopulmonary fistulas will require general anesthesia and the use of positive-pressure ventilation.

## MECHANICAL VENTILATION

In general, the goal of positive-pressure ventilation in patients with BPFs is to minimize tidal volume loss to the pleura or atmosphere by isolating the fistula (e.g., by using double-lumen tracheal tubes or bronchial blockers). If this is not possible, the goal is to keep airway pressures and tidal volumes to a minimum. In addition, the differing physiology and mechanics of varying regions of diseased and nondiseased lung may require different ventilation strategies for different portions of the lung (Table 136.1). In patients with BPFs, delivering adequate ventilation with conventional mechanical ventilators and single-lumen tracheal tubes may be difficult unless the fistula is small.

| TABLE 136.1 Approaches to Positive-Pressure Ventilation for Reducing Transfistula Gas Flow | | |
|---|---|---|
| **Technique** | **Pro** | **Con** |
| Single-lumen tracheal tube Pressure- or volume-controlled ventilation with increased respiratory rate, low tidal volumes, increased inspiratory time, and minimal, if any, PEEP | Simple to perform | Effective only with very small air leak Difficult to keep airway pressures low enough |
| Timed occlusion of chest tubes during inspiration | Increases pleural pressure during inspiration to decrease transfistula pressure gradient Can be added to other techniques | Requires specialized equipment |

*Continued*

| TABLE 136.1 Approaches to Positive-Pressure Ventilation for Reducing Transfistula Gas Flow—cont'd | | |
|---|---|---|
| **Technique** | **Pro** | **Con** |
| Single-lumen tracheal tube with intubation of contralateral lung | Simple to perform<br>Protects contralateral lung from infection | Underlying pulmonary disease may make one-lung ventilation difficult |
| Double-lumen tracheal tube | Relatively simple to perform<br>Protects contralateral lung from infection<br>Can be positioned with bronchoscope<br>Allows for addition of CPAP with 100% $O_2$ to nonventilated lung | Underlying pulmonary disease may make one-lung ventilation difficult even with the addition of CPAP with 100% $O_2$ |
| Double-lumen tracheal tube with different ventilation of each lung | Protects contralateral lung from infection<br>Can be positioned with bronchoscope<br>Allows for use of optimal ventilatory mode for each lung<br>Can be combined with a bronchial blocker or HFO technique | Complex to perform<br>Still may be difficult to ventilate diseased lung while minimizing tidal volume loss |
| Bronchial blockers | Can provide for highly selective isolation (level of the individual bronchus) of the leak, thereby maximizing amount of lung that can be ventilated<br>Can be combined with other techniques | Requires skillful placement with a bronchoscope<br>Blockers can become dislodged during surgery |
| HFO ventilation | Can be combined with other techniques<br>Airway pressures are decreased<br>Allows for humidification and warming of gases<br>Gas trapping on expiration is decreased<br>Can be used for prolonged ventilation in the ICU | Requires specialized equipment and knowledge |
| High-frequency jet ventilation | Can be combined with other techniques | Requires specialized equipment and knowledge<br>Control of tidal volume and agent delivery may be difficult<br>Warming and humidification may be difficult<br>Ventilation may be complicated by gas trapping |

*CPAP,* Continuous positive airway pressure; *HFO,* high-frequency oscillation; *ICU,* intensive care unit; *PEEP,* positive end-expiratory pressure.

## SUGGESTED READINGS

Alohali, A. F., Abu-Daff, S., Alao, K., & Almaani, M. (2017). Ventilator management of bronchopleural fistula secondary to methicillin-resistant staphylococcus aureus necrotizing pneumonia in a pregnant patient with systemic lupus erythematosus. *Case Reports in Medicine, 2017,* 1492910.

Ha, D. V., & Johnson, D. (2004). High frequency oscillatory ventilation in the management of a high output bronchopleural fistula: A case report. *Canadian Journal of Anaesthesia, 51*(1), 78–83.

Konstantinov, I. E., & Saxena, P. (2010). Independent lung ventilation in the postoperative management of large bronchopleural fistula. *Journal of Thoracic and Cardiovascular Surgery, 139,* e21–e22.

Odish, M. F., Yang, J., Cheng, G., Yi, C., Golts, E., Madani, M., et al. (2021). Treatment of bronchopleural and alveolopleural fistulas in acute respiratory distress syndrome with extracorporeal membrane oxygenation, a case series and literature review. *Critical Care Explorations, 3*(5), e0393.

Shekar, K., Foot, C., Fraser, J., Ziegenfuss, M., Hopkins, P., & Windsor, M. (2010). Bronchopleural fistula: An update for intensivists. *Journal of Critical Care, 25*(1), 47–55.

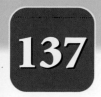

# 137

# High-Frequency Ventilation: Physics, Physiology, and Clinical Applications

KAITLYN BRENNAN, DO, MPH  |  PAUL A. WARNER, MD

## Background

High-frequency ventilation (HFV) delivers small tidal volumes (often less than anatomic dead space) at rates of 60 to 900 or more cycles per minute. Types of HFV include high-frequency positive-pressure ventilation (HFPPV), high-frequency jet ventilation (HFJV), and high-frequency oscillatory ventilation (HFOV).

Table 137.1 compares the common types of HFV. A standard mechanical ventilator can deliver HFPPV with maximal respiratory rates that are generally limited to 60 to 100 per minute. HFJV and HFOV require specialized equipment.

## Physics and Physiology

Both HFPPV and HFJV have active cycles of inspiration and passive cycles of exhalation. These characteristics predispose the lung to overdistension and make accurate measurement of tidal volume ($V_T$) difficult.

HFPPV delivers small tidal volumes at high flow rates and high frequencies. The operator controls the length of the inspiratory cycle in HFJV, and care is required to ensure sufficient time for exhalation. HFOV uses a piston and a diaphragm to create a driving pressure. The driving pressure and $V_T$ are directly related. The frequency controls the distance that the piston moves. The lower the frequency, the greater the volume displaced by the piston. In HFOV, both inhalation and exhalation are active processes. The diaphragm causes a positive deflection in the pressure wave during inhalation and a negative deflection during exhalation, causing a pressure to be applied during both phases. Frequency in HFOV is measured in hertz (Hz) and can range between 3 and 15 Hz (200–900 breaths) per minute.

Gas transport (i.e., oxygen [$O_2$] insufflation and carbon dioxide [$CO_2$] elimination) at very high frequencies depends on mechanisms that differ from those in conventional mechanical ventilation (CMV). These include bulk flow, longitudinal flow, and pendelluft. Cardiogenic mixing and molecular dispersion may provide additional mechanisms of ventilation.

Bulk flow, also described as convective transport, allows for gas exchange in HFV in a manner similar to that in conventional mechanical ventilation. This type of ventilation primarily occurs in the most proximal alveoli in the tracheobronchial tree. Longitudinal flow occurs when convective flow and dispersion are combined. This may increase gas exchange through the development of eddy currents that allow fresh gas flow and alveolar gas to mix, seen in velocity profile distortion and asymmetry. Pendelluft is a phenomenon that occurs when alveoli fill and empty at different times. Pendelluft allows for mutual gas exchange between adjacent alveoli thought to result from time constant inequality. Time constant inequality facilitates gas flow from fast units, with short time constants, to slow units, or those with long time constants. Cardiogenic mixing allows for a small amount of gas exchange, simply from mechanical movement in areas of lung adjacent to the beating heart. The smallest airways use molecular diffusion for gas exchange during HFV.

$CO_2$ elimination occurs at tidal volumes that are much lower than the volume of air contained in the anatomic dead space. However, $CO_2$ elimination increases linearly as ventilation rate increases up to only a certain point (3–6 Hz; 180–360 breaths/min); at higher rates, dead space–to–tidal volume ratio and alveolar minute ventilation are constant.

The goal of HFV is to improve oxygenation; improved ratios of partial pressure of oxygen to fraction of inspired oxygen have been reported with this mode of ventilation. Fluctuations in intracranial pressure are typically lower with HFV than CMV, but the mean intracranial pressure does not decrease.

## Clinical Applications

### HIGH-FREQUENCY JET VENTILATION

HFJV has several routine and emergency clinical applications. The most frequent clinical applications are in otolaryngology procedures. Anesthesia providers frequently use HFJV in laryngeal and tracheal operations because it can be delivered through a cannula much smaller than a traditional tracheal tube. This technique minimizes compromise of the working space available to the otolaryngologist or thoracic surgeon. HFJV also improves operating conditions for the surgeon by decreasing ventilatory excursion.

HFJV is useful in the management of patients with large persistent bronchopleural fistulae. The goal is to limit motion and overdistension of alveoli to promote bronchopleural fistula closure.

Percutaneous transtracheal HFJV is described as a technique to manage emergent difficult airways by inserting a small cannula through the cricothyroid membrane. Connecting the cannula to one of several jet ventilators or to a handheld flush valve connected to an adequate pressure source, such as the $O_2$ flush valve on an anesthesia machine, provides sufficient pressure to

| TABLE 137.1 | General Comparison of the Major Types of High-Frequency Ventilation | | |
|---|---|---|---|
| Feature | HFPPV | HFJV | HFOV |
| Frequency (Hz) | 1–2 | 2–6 | 10–20 |
| Breaths/minute | 60–120 | 120–400 | 600–1200 |
| Tidal volume (mL/kg) | 3–5 | 1–1.5 | ?* |

*Actual value unknown because of entrainment.
*HFJV*, High-frequency jet ventilation; *HFOV*, high-frequency oscillation; *HFPPV*, high-frequency positive-pressure ventilation.

ventilate. Pressing the valve briefly (≤0.3 second) delivers a pulse of $O_2$ at high pressure that dissipates quickly into the airway with slight chest expansion observed. If the valve is held open too long (≥0.5 second), a large volume of $O_2$ fills the airway and airway pressure rises. High airway pressures from overdistention may lead to barotrauma. This technique is associated with a high rate of serious complications and has been largely replaced by alternative approaches to emergent difficult airways.

## HIGH-FREQUENCY OSCILLATORY VENTILATION

Clinical applications of HFOV in the treatment of adults remain controversial. However, HFOV is an established technique that has been used for decades to treat newborn and premature infants with respiratory distress syndrome.

The key physiologic concepts in HFOV include a constant airway pressure and a superimposed oscillating wave. The frequency of the superimposed waveform is similar in neonates and adults. The airway pressure delivered to the alveoli is low; however, the pressure delivered to the conducting airways can be much higher. Under optimal conditions, HFOV could theoretically recruit the entire lung. HFOV with maintenance of a constant airway pressure provides an "open lung" strategy of ventilation intended to improve oxygenation. Studies have shown that oxygenation often improves, but the improvement may come at the expense of hemodynamic stability, including decreases in left and right ventricular cardiac output. More patients ventilated with HFOV require vasopressor support than their CMV counterparts. The pressure needed to support HFOV is usually 4 to 8 cm $H_2O$ higher than the mean airway pressure of patients who are ventilated conventionally. HFOV, in essence, creates continuous positive airway pressure during oscillation. HFOV appears to be associated with increased mortality. The primary cause of death is typically end organ damage rather than direct lung injury or an inability to provide effective oxygenation.

HFOV been implemented more commonly in adult patients, in part caused by the ARDSNet recommendations for lung-protective, low tidal-volume ventilation strategies. Two large randomized controlled trials (RCTs)—the Oscillation for Acute Respiratory Distress Syndrome (ARDS) Treated Early (OSCILLATE) and the OSCillation in ARDS (OSCAR) trials—have attempted to determine whether HFOV improves mortality in ARDS patients. The OSCAR trial demonstrated no mortality benefit or gain with HFOV. The OSCILLATE trial was terminated early because of apparent harm in the HFOV arm. A Cochrane review analyzed these studies and an additional eight RCTs. It found no difference between HFOV and CMV in morbidity, mortality, duration of mechanical ventilation, barotrauma, and hypotension. The authors noted that heterogeneity in these studies resulted in low-quality evidence, suggesting further trials could better define potential benefits of different modes of ventilation.

## Potential Risks and Benefits

Box 137.1 lists potential risks and benefits associated with the use of HFV.

### BOX 137.1 POTENTIAL RISKS AND BENEFITS ASSOCIATED WITH USE OF HIGH-FREQUENCY VENTILATION

| Risks or Drawbacks | Potential Benefits |
| --- | --- |
| Barotrauma | ↓Chest wall and tracheobronchial movement |
| Inability to monitor $V_T$ (HFJV) | ↓Intrathoracic pressures |
| Need for specialized equipment | ↓Intracranial pressures |
| Need for specially trained personnel (HFOV) | Improved oxygenation |
| Decreased right ventricular output | Low tidal volume ventilation |
| Need for neuromuscular blockade (HFOV) | |
| Auto PEEP | |

*HFJV*, High-frequency jet ventilation; *HFOV*, high-frequency oscillation ventilation; *PEEP*, positive end-expiratory pressure; $V_T$, tidal volume.

## SUGGESTED READINGS

Cools, F., Askie, L. M., Offringa, M., Asselin, J. M., Calvert, S. A., Courtney, S. E., et al. (2010). Elective high-frequency oscillatory versus conventional ventilation in preterm infants: A systematic review and meta-analysis of individual patients' data. *Lancet, 375,* 2082–2091.

Fassl, J., Jenny, U., Nikiforov, S., Murray, W. B., & Foster, P. A. (2010). Pressures available for trans-tracheal jet ventilation from anesthesia machines and wall-mounted oxygen flowmeters. *Anesthesia and Analgesia, 110,* 94–100.

Ferguson, N. D., Cook, D. J., Guyatt, G. H., Mehta, S., Hand, L., Austin, P., et al. (2013). High-frequency oscillation in early acute respiratory distress syndrome. *New England Journal of Medicine, 368,* 795.

Kaczka, D. W., Chitilian, H. V., & Vidal Melo, M. F. (2020). Respiratory monitoring. In *Miller's Anesthesia* (Vol. 41, pp. 1298–1339.e11). Elsevier.

Louise, R. (2010). Clinical application of ventilator modes: Ventilatory strategies for lung protection. *Australian Critical Care, 23,* 71–80.

Sud, S., Sud, M., Freidrich, J. O., Wunsch, H., Meade, M. O., Ferguson, N. D., et al. (2016). High-frequency oscillatory ventilation versus conventional ventilation for acute respiratory distress syndrome. *Cochrane Database of Systematic Reviews, 4*(4):CD004085.

Young, D., Lamb, S. E., Shah, S., MacKenzie, I., Tunnicliffe, W., Lall, R., et al. (2013). High-frequency oscillation for acute respiratory distress syndrome. *New England Journal of Medicine, 368*(9), 806–813.

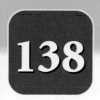

# 138 Thoracotomy Pain Management

SOOJIE YU, MD  |  TARRAH FOLLEY, MD

Pain after thoracic surgery can be some of the most severe and difficult-to-manage postsurgical pain. The consequences of inadequate pain control after thoracic surgery can result in significant patient morbidity (Table 138.1). Thoracotomy patients frequently present in a deconditioned state because of pulmonary dysfunction that contributes to further morbidity. Postoperative lung volumes can be decreased by as much as 50% as a result of chest wall pain that leads to a restrictive pattern of ventilation. Decreased functional residual capacity as a result of altered mechanics of breathing caused by pain may result in atelectasis, decreased clearance of secretions, and pulmonary infections.

## Mechanism of Postthoracotomy Pain

Postthoracotomy chest pain has somatic, neuropathic, and visceral components. Somatic pain, mediated by intercostal nerves, is perceived as chest wall pain that may be triggered by factors such as surgical incisions, stretch of ligaments, placement of intercostal rib retractors, and manipulation of the chest and pleural spaces that leads to an acute inflammatory response. This inflammatory response leads to cytokine release and signals that activate nociceptors, causing centrally mediated pain. Visceral pain is caused by manipulation of the pleural space and airways (bronchi). The pain stimulus is mediated centrally through the vagus and phrenic nerves, often resulting in nonincisional pain and frequently presenting as ipsilateral shoulder pain. Chronic postthoracotomy pain syndrome is a frequent problem, occurring in 25% to 57% of patients, and can include continued chest wall pain, neuropathic pain, sensory loss, or hypersensitivity. Aggressive analgesia in the perioperative setting can decrease the development of chronic pain syndromes.

## Thoracic Epidural Analgesia

Although a variety of techniques have been used to manage postthoracotomy pain, the use of thoracic epidural analgesia (TEA) remains the gold standard. TEA has been shown to blunt the stress response to surgery and provide superior pain relief compared with systemic opioids alone. Placement within the T3–T6 region provides optimal analgesia for thoracic surgery but can be technically challenging due to steep angulation of the spinous processes in this region. The provider must frequently use a paramedian approach to the epidural space at this level. In contrast to the lumbar region, where most success is achieved by placing the needle 1 cm lateral and 1 cm caudal to the palpated spinous process, it is advisable for needle placement to occur directly 1 cm lateral to the spinous process in the thoracic region when using the paramedian approach. This allows the provider to contact the lamina—an important landmark for the paramedian approach—with the needle perpendicular to the skin at all angles and to then walk the needle slightly medial and cephalad.

## Medication Choice

Often a combination of local anesthetic and opioids is used intraoperatively via continuous infusion for optimal pain control. Combining local anesthetic and opioids aims to have a synergistic analgesic effect while minimizing the dose-related adverse effect of using either drug alone. Commonly used local anesthetics include ropivacaine, levobupivacaine, and bupivacaine. Local anesthetics play a dual role in the epidural space. In addition to the local anesthetic effect resulting in blockade of somatic nerves, local anesthetics also facilitate transfer of opioids into the cerebrospinal fluid (CSF). When selecting an epidural opioid, it is important to consider lipid solubility, because variability in diffusion through the spinal membrane alters the plasma and CSF concentrations. Few studies have compared clinical outcomes when infusing a hydrophilic versus a lipophilic opioid for TEA. Commonly used hydrophilic opioids include morphine and hydromorphone, and lipophilic opioids include fentanyl and sufentanil. Administration of systemic opioids while the patient is receiving centrally administered opioids should be done with caution because of the potential for delayed respiratory depression.

## Risks of Thoracic Epidural Analgesia

Risks of TEA can be categorized as procedure related and medication related. The procedure-related risks include unsuccessful catheter placement, dural puncture, bleeding, infection, and nerve injury. Although rare, the risk of neurologic injury is a possibility when placing a thoracic epidural from hemorrhagic or infectious etiologies. It is recommended that the epidural be placed in an awake or lightly sedated patient to minimize the risk of neurologic injury and epidural site monitored daily. Additionally, adhering to American Society of Regional Anesthesia and Pain Medicine consensus statements regarding anticoagulants is recommended for all patients.

Epidural opioids can have systemic side effects. Common side effects include pruritus, nausea, respiratory depression, constipation, urinary retention, and confusion. Because the mechanism of pruritis and nausea is centrally mediated, these symptoms can often be effectively treated with an opioid

| TABLE 138.1 | Consequences of Pain After Thoracic Surgery | |
|---|---|
| **Hypoxemia** | **Respiratory Failure** |
| Increased myocardial oxygen demand | Increased catecholamine response |
| Deep venous thrombosis | Urinary retention |
| Decreased gastrointestinal motility | Poor glycemic control |
| Prolonged hospitalization | Development of chronic pain |

agonist/antagonist, such as nalbuphine, while maintaining adequate pain relief.

Side effects from epidural local anesthetics include hypotension, bradycardia, and the theoretical risk of blockade of accessory muscles of respiration. Reports of dysesthesia, paresthesia, weakness, and local anesthetic toxicity are rare.

## Other Analgesic Techniques

### PARAVERTEBRAL BLOCK

Paravertebral blockade has been demonstrated to be effective at treating pain after thoracic surgery. In fact, some authors have suggested that this technique should replace TEA as the gold standard because of single-side localization, the option to place the catheter at the end of the procedure, and less frequent side effects, most notably sympathetic blockade. It should be noted that epidural absorption of local anesthetic is a possibility after paravertebral blockade. Varying degrees of epidural spread have been shown to occur in up to 70% of percutaneous paravertebral blocks. Most of the local anesthetic spread is unilateral but can be bilateral and could possibly result in total spinal anesthesia. Depending on the surgical approach, a paravertebral catheter placed preoperatively may be near the surgical incision, resulting in decreased acceptance by the surgical team.

### INTERCOSTAL BLOCK

Intercostal blockade is another acceptable technique to treat pain related to thoracic surgery. Intercostal blocks can be performed intraoperatively by the surgeon under direct vision, resulting in significant anesthesia of the dermatomes blocked. Unfortunately, the duration of action of this modality is limited by the duration of local anesthesia. The use of liposomal bupivacaine has shown promise in extending the duration of analgesia provided by this technique. Instead of local anesthetic, cryoablation can be used to freeze the intercostal nerves to provide extended analgesia. Intercostal blockade is an excellent option as a rescue technique after a failed epidural approach or unexpected conversion from a thoracoscopic to open procedure.

### ERECTOR SPINAE PLANE BLOCK

Erector spinae (ESP) single-shot blocks or catheters can be placed for thoracotomies. Advantages of the ESP include that they can be placed under general anesthesia or postoperatively and used for patients receiving anticoagulation. Although evidence suggests they do not anesthetize as many dermatomes as paravertebral blockade, they seem to have clinically similar analgesia.

## PECTORALIS I, PECTORALIS II, AND SERRATUS ANTERIOR PLANE BLOCKS

Other options include the fascial plane blocks, pectoralis I, pectoralis II, and serratus anterior plane blocks. These blocks are useful for anterior chest wall surgery and placement of chest tubes and drains.

### SPINAL OPIOIDS

The use of intrathecal opioids using hydrophilic medications has also been demonstrated to provide significant analgesia after thoracic surgery. Although studies have demonstrated adequate analgesia at rest, patients treated with spinal opioids have significantly more pain with movement (e.g., during deep breathing, coughing) than patients treated with TEA. The risk of delayed respiratory depression is higher for intrathecal opioids compared with epidural placement. Therefore these patients warrant respiratory monitoring for 24 hours after administration.

## Multimodal Analgesia

In addition to regional anesthesia techniques, patients benefit from a multimodal analgesic approach (Table 138.2), particularly when treating nonincisional visceral pain. The use of multiple classes of medications including opioids, nonsteroidal antiinflammatory drugs (NSAIDs), acetaminophen, and α-2 agonists are important aspects of achieving adequate pain control. NSAIDs, such as ketorolac, inhibit cyclooxygenase (COX)1 and COX2 receptors, whereas acetaminophen is more selective for COX2 receptors. Ketorolac should be avoided or used with caution in patients with preexisting renal disease. Ketamine may also be a helpful adjunct, as it works by inhibition of sodium channels at the $N$-methyl-D-aspartic acid receptor. Dexmedetomidine, an α-2 agonist, has been shown to decrease the amount of opioids required and aid with better pain control (see Table 138.2).

| TABLE 138.2 | Pain Medications After Thoracic Surgery | |
|---|---|
| **Drug** | **Mechanism of Action** |
| NSAIDs | Inhibition of COX1/COX2 |
| Acetaminophen | Inhibition of COX2 |
| Ketamine | NMDA receptor antagonist |
| Dexmedetomidine | α-2 agonist |
| Opioids | μ/κ receptor agonist (use caution if received neuraxial opioid) |

*COX*, Cyclooxygenase; *NMDA*, N-methyl-D-aspartic acid; *NSAIDs*, nonsteroidal antiinflammatory drugs.

## SUGGESTED READINGS

Abdelmageed, W. M. (2011). Analgesic properties of a dexmedetomidine infusion after uvulopalatopharyngoplasty in patients with obstructive sleep apnea. *Saudi Journal of Anaesthesia, 5*(2), 150–156.

Bottiger, B., Esper, S., & Stafford-Smith, M. (2013). Pain management strategies for thoracotomy and thoracic pain syndromes. *Seminars in Cardiothoracic and Vascular Anesthesia, 18*, 45–46.

De Cosmo, G., Aceto, P., & Gualtieri, E. (2009). Analgesia in thoracic surgery: Review. *Minerva Anestesiologica, 75*, 393–400.

Gerner, P. (2008). Post-thoracotomy pain management problems. *Anesthesiology Clinics, 26*(2), 355–367.

Gottschalk, A., Cohen, S. P., Yang, S., & Ochroch, E. A. (2006). Preventing and treating pain after thoracic surgery. *Anesthesiology, 104*, 594–600.

Gupta, R., Van de Ven, T., & Pyati, S. (2020). Post-thoracotomy pain: Current strategies for prevention and treatment. *Drugs, 80*(16), 1677–1684. doi:10.1007/s40265-020-01390-0.

Manion, S. C., & Brennan, T. J. (2011). Thoracic epidural analgesia and acute pain management. *Anesthesiology, 115*, 181–188.

Park, S. K., Yoon, S., Kim, B. R., Choe, S. H., Bahk, J. H., & Seo, J. H. (2020). Pre-emptive epidural analgesia for acute and chronic post-thoracotomy pain in adults: A systematic review and meta-analysis. *Regional Anesthesia and Pain Medicine, 45*(12), 1006–1016. doi:10.1136/rapm-2020-101708.

Pyati, S., & Lindsay, D. R. (2012). Acute and chronic post-thoracotomy pain. In *Thoracic anesthesia*. New York, NY: McGraw-Hill. [Ch. 24].

Scherer, R. (2011). Complications related to thoracic epidural analgesia: A prospective study in 1071 surgical patients. *Acta Anaesthesiologica Scandinavica, 37*, 370–374.

# Lung Transplantation

ASHLEY V. FRITZ, DO | ARCHER KILBOURNE MARTIN, MD

## Indications

Lung transplantation is the ultimate treatment for end-stage lung disease (ESLD). Patients with obstructive disease, suppurative disease, restrictive disease, primary pulmonary hypertension, and retransplant are the predominant candidates for lung transplantation. Patients with obstructive and restrictive disease encompass 60% of all lung transplants performed. When tailoring anesthetic management, underlying patient etiology should be considered throughout the perioperative period to optimize patient care and outcomes.

## Preoperative Management and Preparation

Preoperative assessment of the lung transplantation patient should include an in-depth history and a physical exam. Often, patients have a history of prior cardiothoracic surgery secondary to their underlying conditions, including lung volume reduction surgery, pleurodesis, and placement of chest tubes. These patients can present an additional surgical challenge including adhesions, which can increase the risk of bleeding. A complete physical exam should be performed with emphasis on examining the patient's physical status, airway, and vascular access points. A tailored investigation of interval cardiopulmonary deterioration, recent laboratory and echocardiography results, and imaging will assist in guiding perioperative management. The underlying etiology for the patient's ESLD should be considered when formulating a perioperative plan. Specifically, patients with obstructive disease can present with hypotension intraoperatively secondary to hyperinflation. In the setting of single-lung transplant, the compliance differential between the donor and native lung should be considered for postoperative ventilation. Often, patients with suppurative disease require decontamination protocols and therapeutic bronchoscopy. Restrictive lung disease patients are at risk for developing pulmonary hypertension and increased inspiratory pressures leading to hypotension with positive pressure ventilation. The perioperative plan should be tailored to considerations for right ventricular (RV) dysfunction and RV hypertrophy, as it is common in patients with ESLD secondary to primary pulmonary hypertension. Not infrequently, deteriorating physical status can be an indication of worsening pulmonary disease or RV dysfunction. Patients are often mildly hypoxemic despite oxygen supplementation, with some highly decompensated patients requiring high-flow nasal cannula, mechanical ventilation, or extracorporeal membrane oxygenation (ECMO). The type of ECMO used for preoperative bridging depends on patient comorbidities, with venovenous ECMO deployed for isolated pulmonary failure and venoarterial ECMO for ongoing cardiopulmonary failure. These factors, in conjunction with the patient's underlying etiology, should be considered to optimize the perioperative anesthetic management plan.

In preparation for lung transplantation, appropriate medications, equipment, and supplies should be secured with the goal of minimizing anesthesia delays and graft ischemic times. It is vital to determine all necessary antibiotic and immunosuppressant medications and have them easily accessible. Special equipment and supplies are used in lung transplantation. Lung isolation is imperative for the surgical procedure and can be obtained by several methods. Most commonly, a double-lumen endobronchial tube is used, as it offers the advantage of easy manipulation between lung isolation of the left and right lung. A bronchial blocker can be used but can be cumbersome to manipulate intraoperatively. Regardless of the lung isolation technique used, a fiberoptic bronchoscope is needed to quickly confirm tube placement, check bronchial anastomoses, and clear mucus; in some cases it is used for awake fiberoptic intubations in precarious airways. Central venous access should be obtained. The use of a pulmonary arterial catheter to assess pulmonary arterial pressures and mixed venous oxygenation is helpful to guide the administration of inotropes and vasodilators. The use of intraoperative transesophageal echocardiography (TEE) is indispensable and provides for the ability of real-time hemodynamic monitoring and assessment of cardiac function and pharmacologic interventions. In addition, TEE provides the ability to evaluate pulmonary artery and venous anastomoses for obstruction or stricture.

## Intraoperative Anesthetic Management

Induction of anesthesia can present the most precarious challenges for the anesthesiologist, as patients often have tenuous respiratory reserve and compromised RV systolic function. Thus great care should be paid to the anesthetic plan for induction with the goals of securing the airway, maintaining adequate RV preload, and avoiding increases in afterload. Avoiding hypercarbia, hypoxemia, depression of myocardial contractility, and increases in intrathoracic pressure are all pillars of anesthetic induction. To adequately monitor and achieve these goals, often an awake arterial line is placed before induction to allow for continuous monitoring and immediate intervention. Adequate preoxygenation is critical in these patients, as often they present with diminutive respiratory reserve. In addition, patients can often present with difficult airway given an underlying etiology or known airway abnormality. For instance, patients with connective tissue disease are at a risk for difficulty airway given their predilection for a small mouth opening and decreased cervical range of motion. The patient's airway should be secured in a rapid and safe manner, and the use of rapid sequence intubation is reasonable in most patients as not all may present with adequate fasting times. The selection of induction medications should be made deliberately with consideration that profound hemodynamic instability can present with decreases in afterload, increases in RV afterload, and myocardial depression. Propofol should be used judiciously, and often the use of etomidate or other balanced anesthetic technique can provide a safe anesthetic induction. The most fragile patients may benefit from the initiation of preinduction inotrope or even a multidisciplinary preinduction plan for awake ECMO cannulation placement. Ventilation management in lung transplant patients should be tailored to their underlying etiology for ESLD; often permissive hypercapnia, decreased tidal volumes, low respiratory rates, and prolonged expiratory times are used. One-lung ventilation (OLV) can present with separate challenges including increased pulmonary arterial pressures with subsequent decreased RV systolic function and intrapulmonary shunting. Patients with the inability to tolerate OLV or clamping of the pulmonary arteries due to hypoxemia, hypercarbia, or RV dysfunction may require the use of cardiopulmonary bypass or ECMO to safely proceed with surgery. The use of TEE is instrumental to assess for intraoperative hemodynamic stability and can aid in the early decision for the need of extracorporeal life support (ECLS). After reperfusion of the donor lung, attention should be directed to management strategies that minimize primary graft dysfunction (PGD). Lung protective ventilation strategies are of the utmost importance. Increased blood product transfusion, fluid administration, oxygen administration greater than $Fio_2$ 40%, and plateau pressures greater than 30 cm $H_2O$ are all independently associated with an increased risk of PGD. After implantation and separation from any ECLS, it is imperative to assess the new grafts for compliance, gas exchange, and vascular obstruction. Assessing the pulmonary veins and artery for obstruction is crucial; however, there is often some difficulty in the assessment of the left pulmonary artery with TEE.

Surgical approach and considerations should be tailored to the individual patient and planned method of intraoperative support. Single, bilateral, and lobar lung transplant procedures can be considered for the treatment of ESLD. However, current data suggest the use of bilateral-lung transplant provides for increased long-term survival, quality of life, and physiologic outcomes for recipients. To function as a key member of the multidisciplinary lung transplant team, it is vital to understand the key steps involved in lung transplant surgery; this discussion is beyond the scope of this review.

## Postoperative Management

Care in the postoperative period should be provided in the intensive care unit with continuous monitoring of cardiopulmonary and hemodynamic stability. Antibiotic and immunosuppressant regimens should be reviewed and carefully implemented, monitoring for toxicity closely. Vigilance for graft rejection should remain a priority, with continual monitoring for acute chest radiographic changes and worsening gas exchange. Enhanced recovery and postoperative pain control regimen are specific to each transplant center. Despite the dearth of current consensus guidelines or recommendations for enhanced recovery protocols, the translation of thoracic surgery protocols can be used for patient care optimization. Some key points of consideration for enhanced recovery include liberal use of antiemetics, early mobilization and physiotherapy, and adequate pain control. Although traditionally thoracic epidural has been considered the gold standard for postoperative pain control, alternative techniques such as bilateral paravertebral nerve catheters, erector spinae block, and bilateral serratus anterior block have been suggested.

## SUGGESTED READINGS

Abrams, B., Melnyk, V., Allen, W., Subramaniam, K., Scott, C. D., Mitchell, J. D., et al. (2020). TEE for lung transplantation: A case series and discussion of vascular complications. *Journal of Cardiothoracic and Vascular Anesthesia, 34*(3), 733–740.

Fessler, J., Davignon, M., Sage, E., Roux, A., Cerf, C., Feliot, E., et al. (2021). Intraoperative implications of the recipients' disease for double-lung transplantation. *Journal of Cardiothoracic and Vascular Anesthesia, 35*(2), 530–538.

Leard, L., Holm, A., Valapour, M., Glanville, A. R., Attawar, S., Aversa, M., et al. (2021). Consensus document for the selection of lung transplant candidates: An update from the International Society for Heart and Lung Transplantation. *Journal of Heart and Lung Transplantation, 40,* 1349–1379.

Martin, A., Fritz, A., & Wilkey, B. (2020). Anesthetic management of lung transplantation: Impact of presenting disease. *Current Opinion in Anaesthesiology, 33*(1), 43–49.

McLean, S., von Homeyer, P., Cheng, A., Hall, M. L., Mulligan, M. S., Cain, K., et al. (2018). Assessing the benefits of preoperative thoracic epidural placement for lung transplantation. *Journal of Cardiothoracic and Vascular Anesthesia, 32*(6), 2654–2661.

Moreno, G. J., Cypel, M., McRae, K., Machuca, T., Cunningham, V., & Slinger, P. (2019). The evolving role of extracorporeal membrane oxygenation in lung transplantation: Implications for anesthetic management. *Journal of Cardiothoracic and Vascular Anesthesia, 33*(7), 1995–2006.

Pena, J., Bottiger, B. A., & Miltiades, A. N. (2020). Perioperative management of bleeding and transfusion for lung transplantation. *Seminars in Cardiothoracic and Vascular Anesthesia, 24*(1), 74–83.

Yusen, R. D., Edwards, L., Dipchand, A., Goldfarb, S. B., Kucheryavaya, A. Y., Levvey, B. J., et al. (2016). The Registry of the International Society for Heart and Lung Transplantation: Thirty-third Adult Lung and Heart-Lung Transplant Report-2016; Focus Theme: Primary Diagnostic Indications for Transplant. *Journal of Heart and Lung Transplantation, 35*(10), 1170–1184.

# Multispecialty Anesthesia; General Urologic ENT

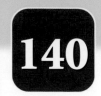

# Thermoregulation and Perioperative Hypothermia

RACHEL CORBITT, MD | BRIDGET P. PULOS, MD

Perioperative changes in body temperature occur frequently, and hypothermia, typically defined as a core body temperature less than 36°C, is a common occurrence. Perioperative hypothermia is caused by environmental exposure and anesthesia-induced impaired thermoregulation and vasodilation. As a general rule, core temperature will decrease 1°C to 1.5°C during the first hour under anesthesia because of redistribution of heat from the core to the periphery. After the initial drop in temperature, subsequent heat loss from the periphery is caused by radiation, convection, conduction, and evaporation. Preventing perioperative hypothermia is an important role of the anesthesia provider.

## Heat Balance and Thermoregulation

Body heat is distributed unevenly, with a typical core-to-peripheral temperature gradient of 2°C to 4°C. As a neurologically mediated physiologic process, thermoregulation involves afferent thermal sensing, central processing, and efferent responses. Thermal receptors are distributed throughout the body (e.g., skin, abdominal and thoracic tissues, spinal cord, hypothalamus), with impulses in response to hypothermia and hyperthermia transmitted to the central nervous system primarily via spinothalamic tracks in the anterior spinal cord on Aδ and C fibers, respectively. Thermoregulatory control depends on instantaneous core temperature rather than core temperature rate of change. Central processing (primarily in the hypothalamus) stimulates voluntary responses (e.g., wearing appropriate attire, adjusting ambient temperature) and involuntary (autonomic) efferent responses.

In awake patients, cold-induced autonomic responses progress from vasoconstriction to nonshivering thermogenesis to shivering thermogenesis. Vasoconstriction and arteriovenous shunting decrease cutaneous blood flow and heat loss via radiation, primarily in the fingers and toes. Although its effects are minimal in adults, nonshivering thermogenesis, which is an increased in basal metabolic rate sympathetically induced by cold stress, can double metabolic heat production in the mitochondria-rich brown fat of neonates and infants. Shivering thermogenesis results from involuntary skeletal muscle activity that increases metabolic rate and heat production for 3 to 4 hours. Muscle fatigue subsequently diminishes the shivering response.

The threshold for warmth-induced autonomic responses, such as active vasodilation and sweating, is similar. Each gram of evaporated sweat dissipates approximately 540 calories of heat to the environment. An adult is able to produce about 1 L of sweat per hour in a dry, convective environment.

Core temperatures between the first cold-induced (i.e., vasoconstriction) and warmth-induced (i.e., vasodilation) responses define the interthreshold range (ITR), or hypothalamic set-point, which normally spans 0.2°C to 0.4°C. Temperature variations within the ITR do not trigger thermoregulatory defense mechanisms.

## Measuring Temperature Intraoperatively

A patient's core temperature should be monitored when general or neuraxial anesthesia is longer than 30 minutes or when clinically significant changes in the patient's core temperature are anticipated or suspected. The gold standard for determination of body temperature is invasive measurement in the pulmonary artery. However, placement of a pulmonary artery catheter is not reasonable for most surgeries. Alternatives include esophageal, nasopharyngeal, and tympanic membrane temperature. Skin, rectal, and bladder temperatures may also be used, but they are considered less reliable and lag behind changes in core temperature.

### GENERAL ANESTHESIA EFFECTS ON THERMOREGULATION

Intravenously administered and inhaled anesthetic agents inhibit thermoregulation in a dose-dependent manner. These agents increase the thresholds for warmth-induced thermoregulatory responses and decrease the thresholds for cold-induced defenses, with a more pronounced effect on the cold-induced thresholds. Accordingly, there is a 20-fold increase (i.e., from 0.2°C to 4.0°C) in the ITR. As a result, anesthetized patients are poikilothermic over this 4°C range, resulting in the vasoconstriction threshold decreasing to around 34.5°C. This loss of tight temperature control renders patients susceptible to heat loss and hypothermia intraoperatively. In contrast, sweating remains largely intact during general anesthesia.

It is important to recognize postoperative shivering increases oxygen ($O_2$) consumption, decreases arterial $O_2$ saturation, and may be associated with increased risk of myocardial ischemia. In addition, postoperative rigors may disrupt delicate surgical incisions, leading to increased pain, and can interfere with accurate hemodynamic monitoring. Meperidine is frequently administered in the recovery area for postoperative shivering.

### REGIONAL ANESTHESIA EFFECTS ON THERMOREGULATION

Thermoregulatory defenses are neurally mediated. Nerve blocks disrupt these neural pathways and interfere with thermoregulation.

Neuraxial anesthesia inhibits central thermoregulatory control by an extent that depends on the level of the block; higher sensory blockade corresponds with a greater decrease in core temperature. Because thermoregulation remains intact above the level of the neuraxial block, increases in the ITR are not as dramatic as those observed during general anesthesia (e.g., from 0.2°C to 0.8°C). Vasodilation from the sympatholytic effects of spinal or epidural anesthesia also leads to redistribution of heat.

## Systemic Side Effects of Perioperative Hypothermia

### CARDIOVASCULAR

Decreased core temperature can slow intracardiac conduction, predisposing patients to developing heart block, QTc prolongation, and lethal cardiac arrhythmias, and can decrease myocardial contractility and cardiac output. Hypothermia can induce catecholamine release, leading to increased pulmonary and systemic vascular resistance and tachycardia, causing increased myocardial stress. Some studies have associated perioperative hypothermia with increased risk of postoperative myocardial ischemia, likely secondary to the adrenergic response, as well as shivering-induced increases in whole-body metabolism. Hypothermia can interfere with platelet aggregation and the coagulation cascade (e.g., decreased thrombin production), causing increased transfusion requirements. Even mild hypothermia (34–36°C) is associated with increased blood loss.

Despite these effects, therapeutic hypothermia has been used to protect organs during various surgeries and after cardiac arrest. According to the 2016 Advanced Life Support Task Force, current recommendations are to maintain a constant temperature between 32°C and 36°C for at least 24 hours after cardiac arrest. This is meant as a protective strategy to slow cellular metabolism and reduce oxygen demand, slow ischemia-induced free radical production, and inhibit apoptosis.

### CENTRAL NERVOUS SYSTEM

Hypothermia decreases brain activity, as measured by electroencephalography, and increases latency in somatosensory evoked potentials. Changes in the amplitude of somatosensory evoked potentials are defined less clearly. The minimal alveolar concentration of volatile agents is decreased at lower temperatures, resulting in decreased inhalational anesthetic requirements. As enzymatic function is temperature dependent, hypothermia can interfere with the metabolism of anesthetic drugs and prolong their action. Mild intraoperative hypothermia has been reported to delay emergence and can prolong postoperative recovery. In regard to neuroprotection, however, hypothermia may protect the brain from ischemic and traumatic injury. In contrast, fever may worsen outcomes after cerebral ischemia or head trauma.

### WOUND INFECTIONS

Hypothermia leading to peripheral vasoconstriction and decreased cutaneous blood flow can impair regional tissue $O_2$ delivery, neutrophil function (e.g., impaired leukocyte mitogenesis, motility, and phagocytosis, resulting in impaired oxidative bacterial killing), and delivery of systemic antibiotics to the wound site. These hypothermia-mediated perturbations increase the risk of wound infection and prolong wound healing from impaired protein metabolism. These complications can increase the duration of hospitalization.

### MISCELLANEOUS

Systemic hypothermia causes a leftward shift of the oxyhemoglobin dissociation curve, decreases $O_2$ consumption and carbon dioxide ($CO_2$) production, slows metabolism of anesthetic drugs, increases the duration of neuromuscular blockade, may delay discharge from the postanesthesia care unit, and predisposes patients to developing citrate toxicity during blood transfusion.

## Mechanisms and Prevention of Perioperative Hypothermia

Perioperative hypothermia occurs via several heat-loss mechanisms: radiation, convection, conduction, and evaporation. Although all of these mechanisms are important to some extent, the initial drop in core temperature—and the most important cause of perioperative hypothermia—is radiation after redistribution of blood and subsequently heat from the core to peripheral tissues (Fig. 140.1). Rapid core-to-peripheral heat transfer produces hypothermia in nearly all patients regardless of the type of anesthesia delivered (e.g., general or regional) and is likely caused by impairment of central thermoregulatory control rather than direct peripheral effects of anesthetics.

Prevention and treatment of hypothermia may be achieved using passive techniques (e.g., applying cotton blankets, sterile drapes, reflective "space" blankets and caps) or active techniques (e.g., using forced-air convective warmers, resistive-heating blankets, conductive circulating water mattresses, intravenous fluid warmers, radiant infrared lamps, and airway heating and humidification). Of these techniques, heat conservation is most effective using forced-air convective surface warming or carbon-fiber resistive heating blankets. Prewarming a patient, such as by using a forced-air device in the preoperative area before induction, can reduce the incidence of inadvertent perioperative hypothermia by decreasing the temperature gradient between the core and the periphery, thus attenuating the initial drop in temperature from redistribution. Simply increasing the ambient room temperature can also help manage intraoperative hypothermia.

Given their larger surface area to volume ratio, children are especially vulnerable to the effects of heat loss during anesthesia. Infants are at particular risk for intraoperative hypothermia caused by minimal insulating subcutaneous fat and a more limited ability to compensate for hypothermic stress. Thus close monitoring of temperature and applying the strategies listed earlier is vital. Areas of the body that cannot be actively warmed should at least be insulated. Neonates and preterm infants may also be transported in a warmed incubator perioperatively.

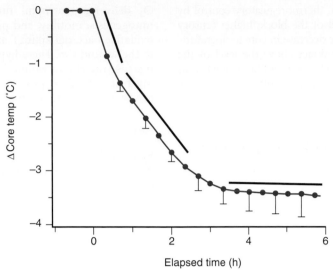

**Fig. 140.1 Heat loss during anesthesia.** Almost all anesthetics are vasodilators; core temperature decreases 1.0°C to 1.5°C during the first hour of anesthesia owing to heat redistribution from the core to the periphery. Subsequent decreases occur less precipitously for the next 2 to 3 hours. This drop results from heat loss exceeding metabolic heat production. During this phase, heat is lost via skin surfaces, with radiant and convective losses contributing far more than evaporative or conductive losses. After 3 to 5 hours of anesthesia, the core temperature plateaus in a thermal steady state, with heat loss equaling heat production.

## SUGGESTED READINGS

Donnino, M. W., Andersen, L. W., Berg, K. M., Reynolds, J. C., Nolan, J. P., & Morley, P. T., et al. (2015). Temperature management after cardiac arrest. *Circulation, 132*, 2448–2456.

Kurz, A. (2008). Thermal care in the perioperative period. *Best Practice and Research. Clinical Anaesthesiology, 22*, 39–62.

Lascarrou, J. B., Merdji, H., Gouge, A. L., Colin, G., Grillet, G., Girardie, P., et al. (2019). Targeted temperature management for cardiac arrest with nonshockable rhythm. *New England Journal of Medicine, 381*(24), 2327–2337.

Rajagopalan, S., Mascha, E., Na, J., & Sessler, D. I. (2008). The effects of mild perioperative hypothermia on blood loss and transfusion requirement. *Anesthesiology, 108*, 71–77.

Ruetzler, K., & Kurz, A. (2018). Consequences of perioperative hypothermia. *Handbook of Clinical Neurology, 157*, 687–697.

Sessler, D. I. (2021). Perioperative temperature monitoring. *Anesthesiology, 134*, 111–118.

Sessler, D. I. (2016). Perioperative thermoregulation and heat balance. *Lancet, 387*, 2655–2664.

Steendijk, P. (2011). Cardiovascular consequences of cooling in critical care. *Critical Care, 15*, 119.

Urits, I., Jones, M. R., Orhurhu, V., Sikorsky, A., Seifert, D., Flores, C., et al. (2019). A comprehensive update of current anesthesia perspectives on therapeutic hypothermia. *Advances in Therapy, 36*(9), 2223–2232.

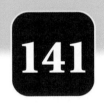

# 141

# The Role of the Anesthesia Provider in Wound Infection

SINDHUJA R. NIMMA, MD | STEVEN B. PORTER, MD

Of the estimated 80 million surgeries performed in the United States each year, surgical site infections (SSI) occur in nearly 2% to 5% of patients and contribute to a significant financial burden on the health care system. According to the Centers for Disease Control and Prevention (CDC), the estimated annual cost of health care–associated infections is $3.5 billion to $10 billion. In addition to causing distress to the patients, SSIs also prolong initial hospitalization, lead to poor wound healing, and increase chances of unplanned readmission. Although some infections are likely unavoidable because of circumstances of injury and preexisting wound contamination, a majority are preventable. According to the CDC, 55% of SSIs are avoidable. Thus there is an inherent responsibility for multidisciplinary teams to reduce the incidence of infection.

Multiple risk factors for SSI have been identified. Although some lie beyond the control of the anesthesia provider, others are directly within our purview, because most prophylactic measures begin in the operative room. Laparoscopic procedures have been demonstrated to have a lower risk of SSI than corresponding open procedures. In the case of emergent colon, esophageal, rectal, or small bowel surgery, the emergency modifier almost doubled the odds of SSI. Longer operative time has also been associated with an increased incidence of SSI. Factors that are more directly affected by anesthesiologists include timing and selection of preoperative antibiotic administration, and maintenance of normothermia, normoglycemia, and sterility while performing various procedures in the perioperative setting.

## Preoperative Optimization

As most SSIs result from translocation of cutaneous flora to the surgical site, interventions to reduce the surface bacterial load have been explored. Showering with 4% chlorhexidine gluconate soap for 2 days before surgery and once on the morning of surgery was shown to effectively reduce bacterial skin flora. There is a dose- and frequency-dependent relationship between exposure to chlorhexidine and reduction in colony-forming units. Despite microbiologic evidence of decontamination, demonstrable reduction in SSIs remains elusive. In addition, nasal colonization with methicillin-resistant *Staphylococcus aureus* (MRSA) may place patients at risk of MRSA SSI. Multiple studies have examined the effectiveness of nasal decontamination with mupirocin, a carboxylic acid derivative. Although a metaanalysis examining the effectiveness of this strategy failed to show a reduction of MRSA SSI in general surgical procedures, a reduction was demonstrated in cardiothoracic, orthopedic, and neurosurgical procedures. Therefore it is important, in conjunction with our surgical colleagues, to reiterate the importance of using surgical soap and decolonization techniques before day of surgery.

## Hand Hygiene

There is strong evidence demonstrating the clinical importance of hand hygiene in health care settings; nevertheless, compliance with hand hygiene is less than 50%. Although it is difficult to generalize these findings to all institutions, the anesthesia provider can directly influence infection outcomes by meticulously adhering to personal hand hygiene and educating others of the importance of hand hygiene and sterility. Anesthesiologists have an active role not only in the operating room but also in various settings throughout the hospital, including pre- and postoperative care unit and intensive care unit. They are dynamically involved in peripheral, central, and arterial line placement, peripheral nerve blocks, neuraxial procedures, airway manipulation, and chronic pain procedures. Therefore contamination in the anesthesia work area can increase health care-associated infections. Providers must be mindful of the potential to contaminate and spread fomites from objects such as the anesthesia work cart, stopcocks, laryngeal masks and laryngoscope blades, and touchscreens and keyboards, as well as on providers' hands.

For invasive procedures, in addition to proper hand hygiene and field sterility, it is also imperative to maintain cleanliness postprocedure with appropriate dressings, as retained blood can serve as an agar medium for bacterial growth. Despite a perceived lack of time, skin factors, and hand hygiene–related work flow interruptions, the anesthesia provider can play a pivotal role not only in their own hand hygiene but in changing the safety culture of other health care workers.

## Hyperglycemia

Hyperglycemia has been extensively studied for its effect on the immune system such as altering the microenvironment of immune cells, the inflammatory response, and oxidative stress (Fig. 141.1). Hyperglycemia also deactivates immunoglobulins by nonenzymatic glycosylation of the C3 component of the complement system. In fact, several preclinical and clinical studies have suggested that hyperglycemia may not only increase the incidence of SSIs, but that a hyperglycemic state seems to also negatively affect the body's ability to respond to antimicrobial therapy. Although tight glycemic control is not recommended and precise optimal glucose levels are unknown, experts agree that serum glucose levels should ideally be maintained at less than 180 mg/dL in the perioperative setting. Although hyperglycemia is commonly encountered in diabetic patients, surgical stress–induced hyperglycemia independently also has a negative effect on perioperative outcomes.

Specifically, in cardiac surgery, a continuous infusion of insulin has shown to improve the phagocytic function of neutrophils compared with the use of intermittent insulin boluses to treat hyperglycemia. In a frequently cited retrospective study of diabetic patients undergoing cardiac procedures, it was also shown that maintenance of blood glucose levels between 150 and 200 mg/dL decreased the incidence of sternal wound infections by 66% versus historical control subjects who were treated with sliding-scale insulin with the goal of maintaining blood glucose levels less than 200 mg/dL.

## Nutritional Status

Perioperative nutrition is of vital importance yet can be an overlooked aspect of surgical care. The metabolic response to surgical stress is complex, and poor nutrition has been demonstrated to correlate with adverse surgical outcomes. It is postulated that adequate nutritional reserve, particularly sufficient protein synthesizing capacity, assists the immune system in combating bacterial microorganism growth. As a multidisciplinary team, it is important to identify at-risk patients who can benefit from preoperative nutritional assessment and supplementation. Traditional teaching emphasized the use of albumin as an important marker of nutritional status with values less than 3 g/dL associated with poor surgical outcomes. A large metaanalysis of orthopedic patients showed those with a low serum albumin had a higher risk of superficial and deep wound infection. This risk factor, however, did not hold up in studies from other surgical disciplines, indicating that additional research is necessary before definitive recommendations can be made.

The serum prealbumin level was later thought to provide a more accurate assessment of nutritional status because of its shorter half-life; however, during surgical stress, albumin and prealbumin are negative-phase proteins and are subject to unreliability. Therefore rather than relying on a highly variable serum marker, the North American Surgical Nutrition Summit recommended a multifactorial, broad-based assessment. This

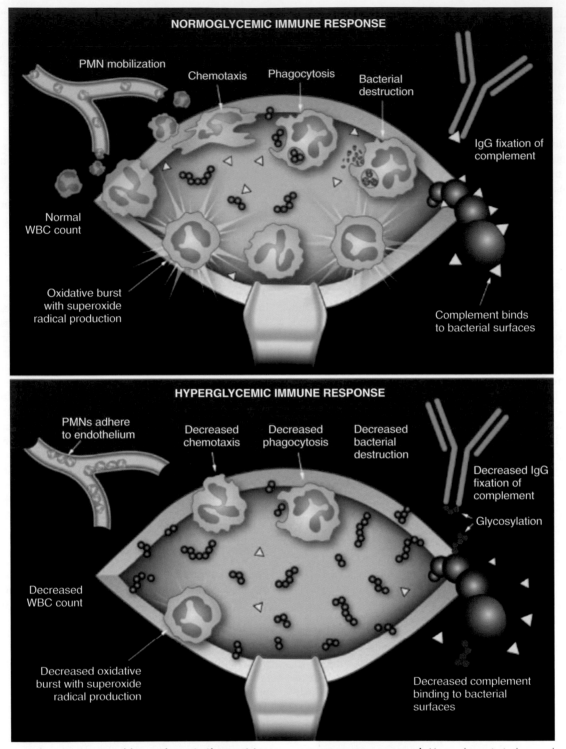

**Fig. 141.1** **Normoglycemic (*top*) and hyperglycemic (*bottom*) immune responses are compared.** Hyperglycemia induces a host of negative effects on the normal immune response in surgical wounds. *IgG*, Immunoglobulin G; *PMN*, polymorphonuclear cell; *WBC*, white blood cell. (Reprinted, with permission, from Mauermann WJ, Nemergut EC. The anesthesiologist's role in the prevention of surgical site infections. *Anesthesiology.* 2006;105:413–421.)

includes gathering details about oral intake, body weight, recent weight loss, and body mass index, as well as biomarkers such as serum C-reactive protein, albumin, prealbumin, and glycated hemoglobin to broaden our assessment of preoperative nutritional status. Additionally, it is also important to emphasize early postoperative initiation of enteral nutrition to enhance recovery and wound healing.

## Intraoperative Factors

### PERIOPERATIVE ANTIBIOTIC ADMINISTRATION

Appropriate perioperative antimicrobial prophylaxis against infection is standard practice. Numerous guidelines have been published regarding the timing, dose, duration, and agents recommended for various surgical procedures. A few general principles should be adhered to when considering antibiotic use. To combat the growing problem of resistance, medications should be selected that have a narrow activity against the most likely organisms at the surgical site, short duration of therapy, and minimal side effects. In procedures where the anticipated flora are primarily skin-derived organisms such as *S. aureus* and *S. epidermidis,* first-generation cephalosporins such as cefazolin are recommended. In contaminated sites or in the cases of implanted prosthetic material, broader-spectrum agents such as ampicillin-sulbactam, piperacillin-tazobactam, or ceftriaxone may be beneficial.

Pharmacologic prophylaxis should be administered within 60 minutes of incision, except in cases where rapid infusion of medication may lead to deleterious side effects such as with vancomycin or fluoroquinolones. These agents may be infused up to 120 minutes before incision. Dosing of antibiotics within 60 minutes before incision has been shown to significantly reduce the incidence of SSIs. Anesthesia providers can reduce SSIs by not only selecting the appropriate antibiotic but also administering it within the time-sensitive window.

## BLOOD TRANSFUSION

Blood product transfusion has increasingly been associated with increases in SSI. Although many studies are subject to inherent limitations in retrospective study design, the body of literature supporting this association is growing. In a retrospective cohort study of patients undergoing Ivor Lewis esophageal resection, transfusion of red blood cells (RBCs) was associated with an odds ratio of 3.1 for wound infection (95% CI, 1.9–5.0). Interestingly, this study also examined administration of other blood components such as frozen plasma (FP) and platelets. In these fractions, the risk of SSI was even higher. With FP, the reported odds ratio of infection, in univariate analysis, was 13.9 (95% CI, 2.8–70.2), and for apheresis platelet units the odds ratio was 12.7 (95% CI, 3.3–48.8). The association of transfusion with wound infections has also been observed in vascular surgical cases. A similar increase in infection risk was reported when patients receiving 3 or more units of RBCs had 3.5 times greater odds of a wound infection (95% CI, 1.8–6.7) compared with patients who did not receive blood. Additional retrospective analyses of gynecologic, orthopedic spine, and general surgical cases all echo similar findings suggesting that transfusion of blood product FP is associated with an increased likelihood of SSI.

The mechanism of increased risk has yet to be determined. However, mounting evidence demonstrates that blood products undergo a transformation during storage referred to as the *storage lesion.* Oxidative damage to RBCs, cell membrane fragments, donor white blood cells, and inflammatory mediators have all been implicated in the immunomodulatory effects of transfusion.

## OXYGEN TENSION

The immune response to bacteria relies on both cellular and humoral components to eradicate potential infection. Neutrophils and macrophages are the primary cells responsible for elimination of bacterial invasion. After phagocytic consumption, bacteria are exposed to reactive oxygen species that disrupt the cellular wall and kill the bacteria. Oxygen is a necessary substrate for several metabolic reactions involving nicotinamide adenine dinucleotide phosphate oxidase and myeloperoxidase that result in the creation of superoxide anions,

hypochlorous acid, chloride anion, and hydrogen peroxide, all of which are cytotoxic to invading bacteria.

Optimization of tissue oxygenation at the cellular level is essential for proper immune function. This relies on adequate RBC mass, hemoglobin saturation, and cardiac output to ensure adequate delivery. Although extremes of oxygen delivery, hyperoxia versus hypoxia, are not recommended, there is no consistent evidence on an ideal oxygen tension to prevent SSIs. A recent systemic review of more than 10,000 patients showed no statistically significant difference in postoperative SSI when comparing patients receiving an inspired fraction of $O_2$ ($Fio_2$) of 80% to those receiving an $Fio_2$ of 30%. During surgical stress, disruption of capillary membranes, tissue edema, and hypothermia-induced vasoconstriction also contribute to abnormal oxygen diffusion and diminished availability of oxygen at the cellular level. The obvious solution would seem to be to optimize tissue oxygenation, which is managed directly by the anesthesia provider. However, the precise $Fio_2$ to maximize tissue oxygenation to reduce SSI remains elusive.

## TEMPERATURE MANAGEMENT

Several studies have demonstrated a correlation between intraoperative hypothermia and increased SSI. The putative mechanism was hypothermia-induced vasoconstriction resulting in reduced perfusion at the site of injury. Diminished blood flow was assumed to cause reduced oxygen tension, perfusion, and immune function, resulting in wound infections. Consequently, national efforts to maintain normothermia using forced air warming devices were adopted. Compliance with these measures was nearly universal. However, the national rate of SSI remained essentially unchanged.

Recent evidence has cast doubt on the role of intraoperative hypothermia as a significant contributor to SSI. A recent case control study examined SSI in general, neurosurgical, orthopedic, spine, and vascular surgical patients. Neither temperature nadir, duration of hypothermia, percent time exposed to hypothermia, nor cumulative hypothermia was found to result in increased SSI. In subgroup analysis, only the neurosurgical population showed reduced SSI with forced-air warming. General surgical patients showed a paradoxical increase in wound infections with forced-air warming. In addition, a large cohort of 1008 colorectal surgical patients similarly failed to demonstrate any correlation between intraoperative hypothermia and increased SSI. Despite mounting doubt of the contribution of hypothermia to wound infection, normothermia remains a goal for other physiologic reasons, including proper coagulation function, metabolic enzyme function, and oxyhemoglobin dissociation.

## Conclusion

As a quality indicator, vigilance must be taken to reduce the risk of SSI. Multiple factors contribute to wound infection, with no clear, universally applicable solution. Avoiding unnecessary blood transfusion, avoiding perioperative hyperglycemia, and timely administration of appropriate antibiotic therapy have been associated with a reduction in infectious complications in surgical patients. It is our responsibility as part of a multidisciplinary team to ensure that we minimize the risk of SSI for our patients by optimizing host immunity. This can be done by ensuring normoglycemia, normothermia, adequate oxygenation, timely administration of antibiotics, and adequate nutritional status, as well as meticulous hand hygiene and sterility.

## SUGGESTED READINGS

Brown, M. J., Curry, T. B., & Hyder, J. A. (2017). Intraoperative hypothermia and surgical site infections in patients with class I/clean wounds: A case-control study. *Journal of the American College of Surgeons, 224*, 160–171.

Forbes, S. S., & McLean, R. F. (2013). Review article: The anesthesiologist's role in the prevention of surgical site infections. *Canadian Journal of Anaesthesia, 60*(2), 176–183.

Hod, E. A., Zhang, N., & Sokol, S. A. (2010). Transfusion of red blood cells after prolonged storage produces harmful effects that are mediated by iron and inflammation. *Blood, 115*, 2365–2371.

Mahdi, H., Goodrich, S., & Lockhart, D. (2014). Predictors of surgical site infection in women undergoing hysterectomy for benign gynecologic disease: A multicenter analysis using the national surgical quality improvement program data. *Journal of Minimally Invasive Gynecology, 21*, 901–909.

Melton, G. B., Vogel, J. D., & Swenson, B. R. (2013). Continuous intraoperative temperature measurement and surgical site infection risk. *Annals of Surgery, 258*(4), 606–611.

Munoz-Price, L. S., Bowdle, A., Johnston, B. L., Bearman, G., Camins, B. C., Dellinger, E. P., et al. (2019). Infection prevention in the operating room anesthesia work area. *Infection Control and Hospital Epidemiology, 40*(1), 1–17. doi:10.1017/ice.2018.303. Epub 2018 Dec 11. Erratum in: Infect Control Hosp Epidemiol. 2019 Apr;40(4):500.

Torgersen, Z., & Balters, M. (2015). Perioperative nutrition. *Surgical Clinics of North America, 95*(2), 255–267.

Wetterslev, J., Meyhoff, C. S., Jørgensen, L. N., Gluud, C., Lindschou, J., & Rasmussen, L. S. (2015). The effects of high perioperative inspiratory oxygen fraction for adult surgical patients. *Cochrane Database of Systematic Reviews, 2015*(6), CD008884. doi:10.1002/14651858.CD008884.pub2.

Yuwen, P., Chen, W., Lv, H., Feng, C., Li, Y., Zhang, T., et al. (2017). Albumin and surgical site infection risk in orthopaedics: A meta-analysis. *BMC Surgery, 17*(1), 7. doi:10.1186/s12893-016-0186-6.

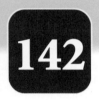

# 142

# Anesthesia in the Patient With Extreme Obesity

YVETTE N. MARTIN MCGREW, MD, PhD

## General

As the prevalence of obesity in the United States and other countries increases, so has the frequency of encountering an obese patient for elective or emergent surgery. Observational studies from UK have shown a greater incidence of obesity in the elective surgical population compared with the general population. Good care for these patients, although perhaps more complex, is obtainable if the implications of obesity and its related disease states are fully recognized.

The World Health Organization and the Centers for Disease Control and Prevention have defined categories of obesity (Table 142.1) based on body mass index (BMI). BMI is calculated as body weight (in kilograms) divided by height (in meters) squared. Additional classifications include *morbid obesity* (defined as BMI >35 and <54.9) and *super* or *extreme morbid obesity* (defined as BMI >55). Categorization of obesity becomes important when considering postoperative morbidity and mortality. Class 3 obesity and higher BMI are associated with increased postoperative morbidity compared with class 1 and class 2 obesity. BMI does not take into consideration adipose distribution; therefore a waist-to-hip ratio of >0.9 for men and >0.85 for women have been proposed as indices for central obesity.

Compared with nonobese patients, obese patients are at increased risk for developing a wide variety of comorbid conditions,

including diabetes, hypertension, cerebrovascular disease, and ischemic heart disease. Obese patients are also predisposed to develop metabolic syndrome (consisting of hypertension, hyperglycemia, and dyslipidemia), obstructive sleep apnea (OSA), apnea hypoventilation syndrome, and cardiomyopathy of obesity. Undoubtedly, the effect of obesity on cardiorespiratory physiology, airway management, pharmacology, and positioning presents multiple concerns for the anesthesia provider. Many of these comorbidities are known to increase perioperative risk for patients.

| TABLE 142.1 | Classification of Obesity | |
|---|---|---|
| **Category** | **BMI (kg/m²)** | **Obesity Class** |
| Underweight | <18.5 | |
| Normal weight | 18.5–24.9 | |
| Overweight | 25.0–29.9 | |
| Obesity | 30.0–34.9 | Class 1 obesity |
| | 35.0–39.9 | Class 2 obesity |
| | >40 | Class 3 obesity |

Data from *Obesity: Preventing and Managing the Global Epidemic.* Geneva, Switzerland, World Health Organization; 1997. Report No. 894.

# Physiology and Pathophysiology of Morbid Obesity

Once considered merely storage of fat from excess caloric intake, adipocytes are now recognized as key effectors in the pathophysiology of obesity. These adipocytes are metabolically active and generate proinflammatory substrates. This activity and effect on disease is more pronounced in truncal fat distribution compared with peripheral fat deposits. One of the functional consequences of these metabolically active adipocytes is the metabolic syndrome.

Two of the primary organ systems affected by obesity are the cardiovascular and respiratory systems. Their dysfunction has significant implication and requires optimization pre- and intraoperatively.

## CARDIOVASCULAR EFFECTS

Obesity is strongly associated with direct effects on hemodynamics and cardiovascular structure and function. Obese patients have increased blood volume, which results in increased cardiac preload and afterload. The subsequent increase in cardiac output is primarily driven by increases in stroke volume, but heart rate may also be mildly increased. Over time, the accompanying structural abnormalities such as left ventricular hypertrophy and left atrial dilation increase the risk for arrhythmias and obesity-induced cardiomyopathy as diastolic and systolic dysfunction progressively ensue.

Systemic hypertension is a common comorbidity in morbidly obese patients and has a strong association with cardiovascular events such as myocardial infarction and stroke. The etiology of the hypertension is from increases in circulating blood volume and cardiac output as mentioned previously. Pulmonary hypertension can also be observed in obese patients. Increased circulating blood volume, increased sympathetic tone, left heart dysfunction, chronic thromboembolism, and arterial hypoxemia from OSA or obesity hypoventilation syndrome are all risk factors for developing pulmonary hypertension in the obese patient.

## AIRWAY AND PULMONARY EFFECTS

The pulmonary function changes caused by obesity are a result of the restrictive effect of mass on the chest wall leading to a tendency to breathe at low lung volumes. The excess chest and abdominal body fat impair chest wall and diaphragmatic excursion and therefore increase work of breathing and reduces pulmonary compliance. Reduction in compliance can also result from increased pulmonary blood volume. Pulmonary compliance decreases exponentially with BMI, waist circumference, and waist-hip ratio. Reductions in compliance can lead to decreased total lung capacity and functional residual capacity (FRC). If the reduction in FRC is severe enough to result in lung volumes below closing capacity, this can lead to small airway closure, ventilation-perfusion mismatch, and arterial hypoxemia. However, most morbidly obese patients maintain $Paco_2$ through hyperventilation.

These physiologic changes are worsened in the supine position and under general anesthesia because of further diaphragm impedance and change in lung volumes. This leads to intolerability for apneic episodes and early desaturation.

Obesity adversely affects the upper airway anatomy. An enlarged face, large tongue, short neck, impaired mouth opening, decreased cervical range of motion, or limited mouth opening suggests the potential for difficult mask ventilation or difficult intubation.

Obesity is the most commonly known risk factor for the development of OSA. OSA consists of a reduction or interruption of airflow, which occurs despite inspiratory effort during stage 4 and rapid eye movement sleep. This eventually causes poor alveolar ventilation and oxyhemoglobin desaturation and in cases of prolonged events, a progressive increase in the arterial partial pressure of carbon dioxide. Eventually, physiologic changes develop that consist of secondary polycythemia, pulmonary hypertension, and right ventricular failure.

# Anesthesia for the Morbidly Obese Patient

As a consequence of the alterations in body habitus and physiology, obese patients present special challenges for the anesthesiologist in airway management, positioning, monitoring, choice of anesthetic technique and anesthetic agents, pain control, and fluid management. As the percentage of obese people in the population continues to increase, studies are ongoing to provide evidence-based approaches for the most optimal care.

## PREOPERATIVE ASSESSMENT

Optimal perioperative care of the obese patient begins in the preoperative period. A thorough health examination focusing on cardiac, pulmonary, airway, and metabolic issues (Table 142.2) should be performed preoperatively.

## INTRAOPERATIVE ANESTHETIC TECHNIQUES

Obesity increases the risk of a difficult airway during induction over the general population. Optimization before induction is necessary to minimize complications. "Ramping" a patient to a "sniffing" position has become a standard technique to facilitate intubation. This entails positioning the patient where the sternal notch and external auditory meatus are in parallel. This position accomplishes the best alignment of the three axes needed for successful intubation: oral, pharyngeal, and laryngeal. Successful intubation with direct laryngoscopy or with video laryngoscopy can be achieved. Currently, there is no evidence to support that videolaryngoscopy is superior to direct laryngoscopy in obese patients without evidence of a difficult airway. If a history of difficult intubation or major concerns regarding difficult ventilation or intubation exists, an awake fiberoptic or awake video laryngoscopy can be performed as an alternative option. If an awake intubation is planned, adequate topical anesthesia and sedation with short-acting drugs, such as remifentanil, should be selected.

A critical step before induction of general anesthesia in the morbidly obese patient is preoxygenation. Techniques to prolong time to desaturation include preoxygenation for 3 to 5 minutes in the reverse Trendelenburg position. In addition, adding 10 cm $H_2O$ of continuous positive airway pressure plus 10 cm $H_2O$ of peak end-expiratory pressure (PEEP) during mask ventilation has been shown to significantly mitigate the initial drop in FRC on induction. Equipment such as multiple-sized oral and nasal airways and supraglottic airway devices

| TABLE 142.2 | Preoperative Assessment of the Morbidly Obese Patient |
|---|---|
| **System** | **Assessment** |
| Cardiovascular | Assess blood pressure control |
| | Examine for symptoms or evidence of right or left ventricular dysfunction |
| | Examine for presence of CAD (noninvasive or invasive evaluation of coronary circulation) |
| | Obtain appropriate guided studies of heart function (ECG, echocardiography) |
| | Ensure appropriate preoperative drug administration for any cardiovascular comorbid conditions |
| Pulmonary | Assess exercise tolerance |
| | Evaluate for symptoms of OSA (e.g., using STOP-Bang or ASA questionnaire) |
| | Determine compliance with CPAP or BiPAP |
| Airway | Perform basic airway examination |
| | Look for evidence of impaired oral or cervical ROM |
| | Determine Mallampati score and neck circumference |
| | Inquire about previous difficult mask airway or intubation |
| Laboratory studies | Obtain electrolyte, blood glucose, and serum hemoglobin concentrations when appropriate |
| Gastrointestinal | Inquire about reflux symptoms |
| Monitoring | Consider the need for adequate intravenous access. A central venous catheter may be needed to obtain reliable venous access |
| | BP cuffs should be of appropriate size. In some cases, the use of direct arterial monitoring may be more reliable or necessary |
| Miscellaneous | Ensure that plans are made for the use of an appropriately sized OR bed that can accommodate the patient's weight and size. |

*ASA,* American Society of Anesthesiologists; *BiPAP,* bilevel positive airway pressure; *BP,* blood pressure; *CAD,* coronary artery disease; *CPAP,* continuous positive airway pressure; *ECG,* electrocardiogram; *OR,* operating room; *OSA,* obstructive sleep apnea; *ROM,* range of motion.

should be available in the event of difficult mask ventilation or difficult intubation.

Intraoperatively, patients with morbid obesity have a high risk for atelectasis formation and are at higher risk for hypoxemia. The severity of the atelectasis extends longer in the postoperative phase in the obese population. Alveolar recruitment maneuvers and use of PEEP improves partial pressure of oxygen/fraction of inspired oxygen ratios and should be used. Head-up (beach-chair) positioning should also be considered. There are no demonstrated advantages of using pressure versus volume-controlled ventilation.

## PHARMACOLOGIC IMPLICATIONS

The physiologic changes produced by obesity such as the apparent volume of distribution, increase in total blood volume and cardiac output, alteration in protein binding, and greater adipose tissue can affect the distribution, binding, and elimination of drugs. Therefore drug doses should be adjusted to provide anesthesia while minimizing side effects.

Lean body mass (ideal body weight +20%) is a good estimate for determining the dose of hydrophilic drugs. The dose of lipid soluble drugs should be based on the patient's total body weight (TBW). Example dosing strategies of commonly used anesthetic agents are in Table 142.3. Induction dose of propofol should be based on lean body weight, which contrasts with the TBW dosing for nonobese patients.

Because of the increased plasma cholinesterase activity, the dose of succinylcholine should be based on the patient's TBW.

| TABLE 142.3 | Dosing Strategies for Commonly Used Intravenous Anesthetics | |
|---|---|---|
| **Drug** | **Base Initial Dose on** | **Infusion** |
| Propofol | LBM | TBW |
| Succinylcholine | TBW | |
| Rocuronium, vecuronium, cisatracurium | LBM | |
| Neostigmine | Not to exceed a total dose of 5 mg | |
| Sugammadex | TBW | |
| Fentanyl | LBM | LBM |
| Remifentanil | LBM | LBM |

*LBM,* Lean body mass, *TBW,* total body weight.

The other neuromuscular blocking agents should be dosed on lean body mass.

Complete reversal and recovery from neuromuscular blockade are critical in the morbidly obese population to minimize risk of postoperative respiratory complications and allow early mobility. The acetylcholinesterase inhibitor neostigmine can be dosed based on TBW, but the total dose is not to exceed 5 mg. Full recovery of neuromuscular blockade after neostigmine has been reported to be prolonged in obese patients.

The modified γ-cyclodextrin sugammadex is a recently approved U.S. Food and Drug Administration reversal agent for neuromuscular blockade. This reversal agent binds to the aminosteroids rocuronium and vecuronium resulting in a rapid and complete recovery from profound neuromuscular blockade. TBW dosing of sugammadex provides safe and effective reversal in obese patients.

All volatile anesthetics can be used in the obese patient. Sevoflurane or desflurane may be preferred over isoflurane because of the more rapid uptake and elimination in morbidly obese patients. Nitrous oxide may be avoided in the setting of pulmonary hypertension.

The effect of obesity on the respiratory system decreases the margin of safety of anesthetic agents and increases the risk of respiratory failure. Given the compromised respiratory system of the morbidly obese, postoperative residual anesthetic drug effect that affects the respiratory system will be poorly tolerated. This is especially pronounced for sedatives and opioids. If these agents are used, appropriate monitoring should be implemented. Non-opioids should be considered in the analgesic plan. Nonsteroidal antiinflammatory drugs, acetaminophen, dexmedetomidine, and ketamine are all viable options for a multimodal analgesia plan in the morbidly obese population.

## EMERGENCE FROM ANESTHESIA

Emergence from general anesthesia is as significant as induction and requires comparable vigilance. Studies have shown increased risk of complications with longer recovery time after anesthesia for the morbidly obese population. Therefore early and full recovery of consciousness and reflexes in the morbidly obese is of utmost importance. Complete reversal of neuromuscular blockade should be achieved. The inhalation agent or intravenous anesthetic infusion should be titrated at the end of the operation to allow prompt emergence and return of airway reflexes and tone. The patient should be returned to the reverse Trendelenburg position to improve airway mechanics. Criteria for extubation of the obese patient are the same as the nonobese. Postextubation, obese patients may benefit from early initiation of continuous positive airway pressure.

## REGIONAL ANESTHESIA

Regional anesthesia offers many potential advantages for the obese patient. Regional anesthesia as an adjunct for pain management can be efficient in reducing opioid-related complications, especially in a population that is vulnerable to respiratory complications. In addition, when selected as the primary anesthetic, obese patients are spared the negative respiratory effects of general anesthesia. However, regional anesthesia can be technically challenging in the obese patient because of the obscured landmarks. Obesity is an independent risk factor for block failure. Ultrasound guidance and experience can markedly enhance success and accuracy.

When dosing local anesthetic for neuraxial block, a reduction in dose may be necessary but is not universally recommended. Studies have shown more extensive cephalad spread with the same dose of local anesthetic in obese versus nonobese patients. This difference is caused in part by reduced cerebrospinal fluid and epidural volumes because of venous engorgement. Equipment for management of a high spinal should be accessible.

## SUGGESTED READINGS

Alpert, M. A., Omran, J., & Bostick, B. P. (2016). Effects of obesity on cardiovascular hemodynamics, cardiac morphology, and ventricular function. *Current Obesity Reports, 5*, 424–434.

Brodsky, J. B., & Mariano, E. R. (2011). Regional anaesthesia in the obese patient: Lost landmarks and evolving ultrasound guidance. *Best Practice and Research. Clinical Anaesthesiology, 25*, 61–72.

Gaddam, S., Gunukula, S. K., & Mador, M. J. (2014). Post-operative outcomes in adult obstructive sleep apnea patients undergoing non-upper airway surgery: A systematic review and meta-analysis. *Sleep & Breathing, 18*, 615–633.

Harbut, P., Gozdzik, W., Stjernfalt, E., Marsk, R., & Hesselvik, J. F. (2014). Continuous positive airway pressure/pressure support pre-oxygenation of morbidly obese patients. *Acta Anaesthesiologica Scandinavica, 58*, 675–680.

Hebbes, C. P., & Thompson, J. P. (2018). Pharmacokinetics of anaesthetic drugs at extremes of body weight. *BJA Education, 18*(12), 364–370.

Moon, T. S., Fox, P. E., Somasundaram, A., Minhajuddin, A., Gonzales, M. X., Pak, T. J., et al. (2019). The influence of morbid obesity on difficult intubation and difficult mask ventilation. *Journal of Anesthesia, 33*(1), 96–102.

Moon, T. S., Van de Putte, P., De Baerdemaeker, L., & Schumann, R. (2021). The obese patient: Facts, fables, and best practices. *Anesthesia and Analgesia, 132*(1), 53–64.

Sharma, S., & Arora, L. (2020). Anesthesia for the morbidly obese patient. *Anesthesiology Clinics, 38*(1), 197–212.

Shaw, M., Waiting, J., Barraclough, L., Ting, K., Jeans, J., Black, B., et al. (2021). Airway events in obese vs. non-obese elective surgical patients: A cross-sectional observational study. *Anaesthesia, 76*(12), 1585–1592.

Subramani, Y., Riad, W., Chung, F., & Wong, J. (2017). Optimal propofol induction dose in morbidly obese patients: A randomized controlled trial comparing the bispectral index and lean body weight scalar. *Canadian Journal of Anaesthesia, 64*, 471–479.

# Weight Loss Procedures

TOBY N. WEINGARTEN, MD | RYAN E. HOFER, MD

Obesity and its associated diseases present a considerable burden on patients and the health care system. Weight loss surgery (WLS) and endoscopic weight loss procedures are proven, effective means of producing substantial and sustained weight loss and favorably affecting obesity-associated diseases such as diabetes, hypertension, dyslipidemia, obstructive sleep apnea (OSA), and other conditions. With widespread adoption of a laparoscopic versus open surgical approach to WLS, these procedures have gained popularity with more than 200,000 surgeries performed in the United States per annum. These patients often have numerous obesity-associated diseases (see Chapter 142, Anesthesia in the Patient With Extreme Obesity) that have implications for the anesthesiologist. Fortunately, these patients typically undergo extensive medical evaluation and optimization before surgery, and rates of perioperative complications is surprisingly low. Currently, WLS is typically performed laparoscopically; however, endoscopic weight loss procedures (endoscopic sleeve gastroplasty, intragastric balloon therapy, and aspiration therapy) are also gaining in popularity.

## Surgical Procedures for Weight Loss

Current WLS involves restrictive or restrictive-malabsorption components. Restrictive procedures create a small stomach but do not alter how food is digested. The two most common restrictive procedures are the laparoscopic adjustable gastric banding procedure and the gastric sleeve resection.

In the banding procedure, a limited dissection of connective tissue is performed at the top of the stomach, and an inflatable band is passed that encircles the upper stomach (Fig. 143.1A). The band can be adjusted via a port attached to the body wall by adding or withdrawing saline. The surgical risk is very low, and in select patients it is performed as an outpatient procedure.

The gastric sleeve resection is typically performed laparoscopically and reduces stomach volume to approximately 100 mL by externally stapling the stomach to exclude the fundus and greater curvature to form a narrow tube along the lesser curvature of the stomach (Fig. 143.1B). Surgical duration is relatively brief and complications are infrequent with minimal blood loss.

The laparoscopic Roux-en-Y gastric bypass is a commonly performed restrictive-malabsorptive WLS procedure. This procedure creates a small gastric pouch (30 mL) that empties into a limb of bowel that excludes a large portion of the small intestine (Fig. 143.1C). As a result, satiety is achieved at relatively low volumes (restriction), and the surface area of small bowel that can absorb calories and nutrients is bypassed (maldigestion), resulting in reliable, sustained weight loss. Blood loss is minimal.

The biliopancreatic diversion/duodenal switch procedure is a more complex restrictive-malabsorptive procedure normally reserved for use in patients with a body mass index (BMI) in excess of 50 kg/m$^2$. With this procedure, a gastric sleeve resection is performed, the stomach is separated from the duodenum, and the small bowel is divided at a point proximal (approximately 100 cm) to the terminal ileum. The stomach is reanastomosed to the distal limb of small bowel, creating an "alimentary channel" where food enters but is not digested. Biliary and pancreatic fluids drain into the duodenum (now separated from the stomach) and contact food where this "biliopancreatic limb" of proximal small bowel is anastomosed to the limb of the alimentary channel (Fig. 143.1D). Digestive enzymes contact food late in the process, and the short segment of small bowel that is available to absorb nutrients and calories is significantly restricted. Compared with the Roux-en-Y gastric bypass, the biliopancreatic diversion/duodenal switch procedure requires considerably longer time, but blood loss and fluid shifts are not significantly different.

Endoscopic bariatric procedures are gaining in popularity by providing successful weight loss with a presumed low rate of negative outcomes. Several approaches have been described: sleeve gastroplasty, intragastric balloon, and aspiration therapy. The endoscopic sleeve gastroplasty is a primary, restrictive endoscopic procedure using a suture system that results in the creation of a tube-shaped gastric lumen with reduced volume. Intragastric balloons can be placed endoscopically as a restrictive procedure to create the sensation of early satiety. Contents of these balloons often include methylene blue so that the patient's urine will appear green if the balloon was to rupture. Aspiration therapy involves the endoscopic placement of a percutaneous gastrostomy tube that allows for the aspiration of gastric contents 20 to 30 minutes after eating.

## ANESTHETIC MANAGEMENT OF PATIENTS UNDERGOING WEIGHT LOSS SURGERY

Patients undergoing WLS require a thorough preoperative evaluation with focus on obesity-related diseases. Patients should be screened and, if indicated, evaluated for OSA. The prevalence of OSA in this patient population is very high, but if recognized and managed appropriately, it does not seem to be associated with increased risk after WLS. Evaluation of the cardiovascular system does not require advanced testing (e.g., echocardiogram, stress electrocardiogram) unless there are clinical signs (e.g., heart murmurs, angina) that warrant evaluation independent of the anticipated operation.

There are several caveats for the induction of anesthesia for WLS. Obesity decreases lung compliance, reduces expiratory reserve volume, and decreases functional residual capacity. These changes promote the development of atelectasis and result in a greater ventilation-perfusion mismatch than normal weight patients. Also oxygen demand and carbon dioxide production are greater in obese patients. These physiologic changes result in accelerated oxyhemoglobin desaturation during periods of apnea. In addition, obesity can result in anatomic changes of the upper airway anatomy, which may complicate airway management.

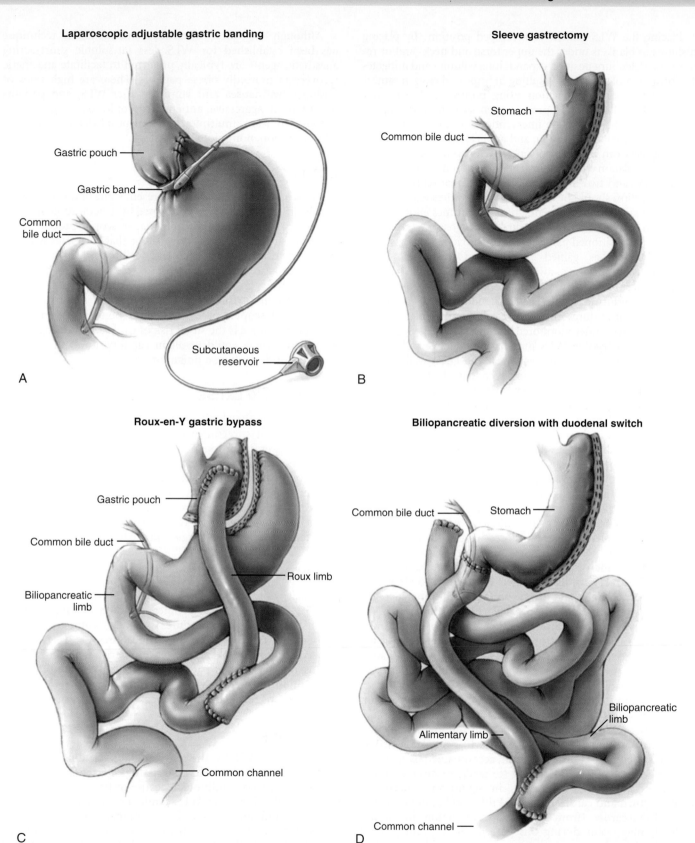

**Laparoscopic adjustable gastric banding**

Gastric pouch

Gastric band

Common
bile duct

Subcutaneous
reservoir

A

**Sleeve gastrectomy**

Stomach

Common bile duct

B

**Roux-en-Y gastric bypass**

Gastric pouch

Common bile duct

Biliopancreatic
limb

Roux limb

Common channel

C

**Biliopancreatic diversion with duodenal switch**

Common bile duct

Stomach

Biliopancreatic
limb

Alimentary limb

Common channel

D

**Fig. 143.1 Common Surgical Procedures for Weight Loss.** Restrictive operations for the treatment of morbid obesity and its coexisting conditions, popular today particularly because of laparoscopic surgical approaches, include adjustable gastric banding **(A)** and vertical (sleeve) gastrectomy **(B)**. Roux-en-Y gastric bypass **(C)**, a procedure that combines restriction and malabsorption, is considered by many to be the gold standard because of its high level of effectiveness and its durability. More extreme malabsorption accompanies biliopancreatic diversion procedures, commonly performed with a duodenal switch **(D)**, in which a short, distal, common-channel length of small intestine severely limits caloric absorption. This procedure also includes a sleeve gastrectomy. (Reprinted, with permission, from DeMaria EJ. Bariatric surgery for morbid obesity. *N Engl J Med.* 2007;356:2176–2183. © 2007 Massachusetts Medical Society. All rights reserved.)

Placing the WLS patient in a ramped position (by placing cushions or blankets under the upper torso and neck) and/or reverse Trendelenburg position expands lung volumes and mitigates the formation of atelectasis resulting in improved oxygen saturations. Preoperative oxygenation using positive end-expiratory pressure (PEEP) can also improve oxygen saturations during induction. Reestablishing these interventions (i.e., torso elevation, reverse Trendelenburg position, and application of PEEP) at the end of surgery can improve postoperative oxygenation.

Mask ventilation can be difficult and may require an oral and/or nasal airway and two-handed mask. Esophageal reflux is common, so suction should be available. WLS requires endotracheal intubation and mechanical ventilation. Oftentimes endotracheal intubation can be achieved with direct laryngoscopy (especially in a carefully positioned patient), but use of video laryngoscopes for intubation has gained popularity. Occasionally, more advanced techniques (e.g., awake fiberoptic intubation) are required to secure the airway. Endoscopic procedures are most commonly performed under general endotracheal anesthesia, though some procedures (intragastric balloon placement) can be safely performed under monitored anesthesia care.

Patients undergoing WLS may have restrictive pulmonary physiology from excess intraperitoneal and chest wall adipose tissue and diaphragmatic elevation secondary to the pneumoperitoneum. These factors reduce pulmonary compliance, which promotes atelectasis and worsens the ventilation-perfusion mismatch. These changes can present challenges to mechanical ventilation (e.g., high pressures required to achieve adequate tidal volumes) and can lead to oxyhemoglobin desaturation. Pulmonary compliance can be improved using an "open-lung ventilation" ventilation strategy. This method combines periodic "alveolar recruitment maneuvers" to recruit collapsed alveoli combined with PEEP to prevent recollapse of open alveoli. Recruitment maneuvers are commonly achieved by either the application of sustained pressure to closed lung fields (typically for 10–15 seconds with an inspiratory pressure of 35–40 cm $H_2O$) or incremental increases in PEEP in a stepwise manner (e.g., from 4 to 20 cm $H_2O$ of PEEP). Open-lung ventilation improves pulmonary mechanics and can be useful in achieving adequate ventilation and oxygenation, especially patients with extremes in BMI. However, postextubation blood gases are not significantly different from baseline or from values from patients ventilated using standard techniques. The clinician should base ventilator-management strategies on individual patient information and the results of laboratory studies and clinical examination.

Insufflation of the peritoneum represents an important period for anesthetic management. Intraperitoneal pressure potentially obstructs venous return from the lower body and also encroaches on intrathoracic space. In most laparoscopic WLS, insufflation of the peritoneum, accompanied by maximal reverse Trendelenburg positioning (to facilitate surgical visualization of the stomach), results in significantly decreased venous return and cardiac preload. Profound hypotension and reflex bradycardia (from the abrupt reduction in cardiac preload) may occur during this period and warrant prompt recognition and treatment; the patient should be rapidly returned to the supine position, the peritoneum desufflated, and vasopressor, vagolytic, or both agents administered, as indicated. These physiologic responses to pneumoperitoneum can be attenuated by fluid loading the patient before insufflation. Once the pneumoperitoneum is established, tachycardia and increased mean arterial pressure are common.

Although no ideal anesthetic maintenance technique has been established for WLS, less fat-soluble short-acting anesthetic agents are typically preferred to facilitate anesthetic recovery in morbidly obese patients. There are high rates of postoperative nausea and vomiting after WLS, and patients benefit from aggressive antiemetic prophylaxis (e.g., use of propofol infusion, multiple classes of prophylactic antiemetic administration, nonopioid analgesics).

## COMPLICATIONS

Laparoscopic WLS procedures represent some of the most technically difficult procedures performed by general surgeons. The surgeon's experience performing laparoscopic procedures is likely the single most important factor that correlates with the frequency of complications. The facility in which WLS is performed also plays a significant role. Because these two aspects of WLS are, by far, the greatest contributors to complication rates, emphasis will be placed on these aspects of WLS. Because endoscopic procedures use carbon dioxide insufflate the stomach, there is the small risk of gas leakage during suture placement, which could result in capnoperitoneum with the potential of developing a pneumothorax.

## SURGEON EXPERTISE

Several studies that have evaluated outcome after WLS have concluded that surgeon experience with laparoscopic gastric bypass is inversely proportional to the incidence of postoperative complications. The most common complications (e.g., anastomotic leaks, internal hernia) occur most frequently when the surgeon has performed fewer than 75 laparoscopic WLS procedures. As surgeon experience exceeds 100 WLS procedures, major complication rates become comparable to those associated with low-risk surgical procedures.

## FACILITY EXPERTISE

Hospitals with high WLS volumes have overall mortality rates of 0.5%. Mortality rate is significantly lower in a high-volume facility (>100 WLS procedures per year) compared with a low-volume facility (<50 WLS procedures per year). These observed differences likely reflect familiarity with the postoperative management of patients undergoing WLS and the early recognition of the signs and symptoms suggestive of surgical complications (e.g., anastomotic leaks, internal hernia).

## Summary

Laparoscopic WLS is the only therapy yielding sustained, significant weight loss and eliminating or attenuating weight-related comorbid conditions. Because of the thorough preoperative evaluations that WLS candidates undergo, anesthesia providers infrequently require additional studies or evaluations to ensure that these patients are safe for surgery. Inducing anesthesia with the patient ramped on blankets and in a modest reverse Trendelenburg position allows for improved oxygenation and ventilation. Open-lung ventilation can be useful when intraoperative ventilation is encountered. Surgeon and facility experience with WLS play significant roles in the morbidity and mortality rates associated with these procedures.

## SUGGESTED READINGS

Buchwald, H., Estok, R., Fahrback, K., Banel, D., Jensen, M. D., Pories, W. J., et al. (2009). Weight and type 2 diabetes after bariatric surgery: Systematic review and meta-analysis. *American Journal of Medicine, 122*, 248–256.

Burns, E. M., Naseem, H., Bottle, A., Lazzarino, A. I., Aylin, P., Darzi, A., et al. (2010). Introduction of laparoscopic bariatric surgery in England: Observational population cohort study. *BMJ, 341*, c4296.

DeMaria, E. J. (2007). Bariatric surgery for morbid obesity. *New England Journal of Medicine, 356*, 2176–2183.

Dixon, B. J., Dixon, J. B., Carden, J. R., Burn, A. J., Schachter, L. M., Playfair, J. M., et al. (2005). Pre-oxygenation is more effective in the 25° head up position than the supine position in severely obese patients. *Anesthesiology, 102*, 1110–1115.

Gander S, Frascarolo P, Suter M, Spahn, D. R., & Magnusson, L. (2005). Positive end-expiratory pressure during induction of general anesthesia increases duration of nonhypoxic apnea in morbidly

obese patients. *Anesthesia and Analgesia, 100*, 580–584.

Nguyen, N. T., Paya, M., Stevens, C. M., Mavandadi, S., Zainabadi, K., & Wilson, S. E. (2004). The relationship between hospital volume and outcome in bariatric surgery at academic medical centers. *Annals of Surgery, 240*, 586–593.

Nguyen, N. T., Silver, M., Robinson, M., Needleman, B., Hartley, G., Cooney, R., et al. (2006). Result of a national audit of bariatric surgery performed at academic centers. *Archives of Surgery, 141*, 445–449.

Puzziferri, N., Austrheim-Smith, I. T., Wolfe, B. M., Wilson, S. E., & Nguyen, N. T. (2006). Three-year follow-up of a prospective randomized trial comparing laparoscopic versus open gastric bypass. *Annals of Surgery, 243*, 181–188.

Sprung, J., Whalley, D. G., Falcone, T., Warner, D. O., Hubmayr, R. D., Hammel, J., et al. (2002). The impact of morbid obesity, pneumoperitoneum, and posture on respiratory system mechanics and

oxygenation during laparoscopy. *Anesthesia and Analgesia, 94*, 1345–1350.

Tabboush, Z. S. (2017). Endoscopic sleeve gastroplasty: A concern of anesthesiologists. *Anesthesia and Analgesia, 125*, 365.

Weingarten, T. N., Flores, A. S., McKenzie, J. A., Nguyen, L. T., Robinson, W. B., Kinney, T. M., et al. (2011). Obstructive sleep apnoea and perioperative complications in bariatric patients. *British Journal of Anaesthesia, 106*, 31–39.

Weingarten, T. N., Hawkins, N. M., Beam, W. B., Brandt, H. A., Koepp, D. J., Kellogg, T. A., et al. (2015). Factors associated with prolonged anesthesia recovery following laparoscopic bariatric surgery: A retrospective analysis. *Obesity Surgery, 25*, 1024–1030.

Whalen, F. X., Gajic, O., & Thompson, G. B. (2006). The effects of alveolar recruitment maneuver and positive end-expiratory pressure on arterial oxygenation during laparoscopic bariatric surgery. *Anesthesia and Analgesia, 102*, 298–305.

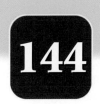

# 144

# Complications of Transurethral Resection of the Prostate

ROBERT L. MCCLAIN, MD

## Introduction

Benign prostatic hypertrophy (BPH) is the most common benign neoplasm in men, with approximately 50% of men over the age of 60 years and 90% by the age of 85 years affected. This equates to about 15 million men who suffer from lower urinary tract symptoms related to BPH in the United States alone. Transurethral resection of the prostate (TURP) remains the standard surgical treatment for BPH when the prostate is less than 80 mL in symptomatic patients. A variety of factors have led to decreasing mortality and morbidity rates associated with this procedure, including increased awareness of BPH, which has led to earlier treatment, and the availability of new drugs and surgical techniques that are associated with lower rates of complications.

In a traditional TURP, resection of the prostate is performed during cystoscopy using a resectoscope with an electrocautery loop. The morbidity rate of 7% to 20% is associated with longer resection times (>90 min), larger gland size (>45 g), acute urinary retention, and age greater than 80 years. One of the most serious complications associated with TURP, the TURP syndrome (Box 144.1), occurs in 2% to 15% of patients treated with this approach. Postoperative bleeding with the need for blood transfusion occurs in about 2% to 4.8% of patients who develop TURP syndrome.

The advent of various laser-assisted surgical enucleation techniques instead of the traditional electrocautery loop has led to a tremendous reduction in the complications associated this procedure. TURP syndrome occurs in as few as 1.1% of patients, such that anesthesia providers are now unlikely to encounter patients with this complication.

## Treatment

### MEDICAL OPTIONS

One of the reasons the incidence of complications of TURP is decreasing is that many men are successfully treated medically. For those whose symptoms progress, the prostate may not be as large as it might have been without medical treatment; therefore the operative procedure has a shorter duration and is associated with fewer complications. The medical treatment of BPH includes oral administration of single or in combination medications to relax the smooth muscles of the prostate or inhibit further growth. Such medications include α-adrenergic antagonists (e.g., tamsulosin), 5α-reductase inhibitors (e.g., finasteride), muscarinic receptor antagonists, and β-3 receptor agonists as monotherapy or in combination depending on the patient's symptoms. If medical treatment is unsuccessful or symptoms progress and the patient is a surgical candidate, a TURP may be performed to treat symptoms.

---

**BOX 144.1   SIGNS AND SYMPTOMS OF TRANSURETHRAL RESECTION OF THE PROSTATE SYNDROME**

| Cardiovascular and Respiratory | Central Nervous System | Metabolic | Other |
| --- | --- | --- | --- |
| Hypotension | Agitation/confusion | Hyponatremia | Hypoosmolality |
| Bradyarrhythmias/tachyarrhythmias | Seizures | Hyperglycinemia | Hemolysis |
| Congestive heart failure | Coma | Hyperammonemia | |
| Pulmonary edema and hypoxemia | Visual disturbances (blindness) | | |
| Myocardial infarction | | | |
| Hypertension | | | |

From Malhotra V, Sudheendra V, O'Hara J, Malhotra A. Anesthesia and the renal and genitourinary systems. In: Miller RD, ed. *Anesthesia*. 9th ed. Vol. 2. Churchill Livingstone; 2020:chap. 59.

---

## SURGICAL OPTIONS

TURP is performed under direct vision. The most common procedure in the past was performed with a modified cystoscope (resectoscope) with a monopolar electrically energized wire loop. Bleeding was controlled with a coagulating current. Continuous irrigation was used to distend the bladder and remove blood and dissected prostatic tissue. Because the prostate contains large venous sinuses, it was inevitable that irrigating solution would be absorbed into the vascular system. The volume absorbed depended on three factors: the hydrostatic pressure, duration of the resection, and number and size of the opened venous sinuses. The hydrostatic pressure is determined by the height of the irrigating fluid above the patient. Prostate venous sinuses have a pressure of approximately 10 mm Hg. The duration of the TURP was dependent on the size of the prostate and experience of the surgeon. Approximately 10 to 30 mL of irrigating solution is absorbed per minute of resection time. The choice of irrigation solution is dependent on several factors as discussed later.

Monopolar TURP is still considered by many as the treatment of choice for intermittently enlarged prostates (50–80 g); however, this gold standard is marred by the previously mentioned significant morbidity and mortality rates.

Recently several alternatives have been introduced that are associated with good results and fewer complications (e.g., bleeding and TURP syndrome). The use of a bipolar electrosurgical device allows the urologist to use alternative irrigation solutions, which are associated with fewer complications. *Plasma TURP* refers to a TURP in which a bipolar electrode, in the shape of a mushroom, generates a "plasma" corona on its surface. The energy simultaneously vaporizes tissue and coagulates all but the largest blood vessels; because of the type of energy used, the procedure can be performed with saline as the irrigation solution, which all but eliminates the possibility of TURP syndrome developing.

Newer technology allows for the use of a laser cautery to vaporize the prostate tissue and create an eschar to minimize bleeding. The laser devices include the green-light laser (a high-power [80W] potassium-titanyl-phosphate laser), holmium laser, and thulium laser devices. For some urologists, laser vaporization techniques have become the treatment option of choice for TURP and are associated with fewer short-term (i.e., perioperative) complications.

## IRRIGATION SOLUTIONS

The choice of which irrigating fluid to use when performing a TURP depends on many factors, including the optical properties of the fluid, its degree of ionization, its potential for inducing hemolysis, and the technology being used to resect the prostate. Distilled water was often used in the past as an irrigation solution because of its excellent optical properties and low cost, but distilled water is not often used in current practice because of its potential for inducing marked dilutional hyponatremia and intravascular red blood cell hemolysis.

Lactated Ringer and normal saline solutions cannot be used if a monopolar electrosurgical probe is used because these solutions are highly ionized and promote current dispersion from the monopolar resectoscope. However, the newer surgical techniques mentioned earlier that use a bipolar probe or a laser device can be performed with normal saline as the irrigating solution, which results in a much lower incidence of TURP syndrome. Normal saline is well tolerated when absorbed intravascularly.

Glycine (1.5%) is a low-cost, nonelectrolytic, and only slightly hypoosmolar fluid that can be used during monopolar therapy. However, if large amounts of glycine are absorbed, transient blindness and encephalopathy can evolve, as can potential complications associated with increased fluid load.

Sorbitol (2.7%) and mannitol (0.54%) have the advantage of being nonelectrolytic, isosmolar, and rapidly cleared from the plasma but are expensive and can lead to complications resulting from increased intravascular fluid load.

## Specific Complications

### TRANSURETHRAL RESECTION OF THE PROSTATE SYNDROME

TURP syndrome, a constellation of symptoms and signs caused by excessive absorption of the irrigating fluid, may occur at any time perioperatively and complicates 0.7% to 1.4% of prostate resections. Early manifestations of TURP syndrome in the conscious patient under neuraxial anesthetic include nausea, headache, dizziness, apprehension, disorientation, and visual disturbances. Progression to agitation often ensues, associated with elevated blood pressure and bradycardia; if no treatment is implemented, seizures, coma, and cardiac arrest may follow and is associated with a mortality rate of approximately 25% (see Box 144.1). Diagnosing TURP syndrome in patients who undergo TURP with general anesthesia may be difficult because the first signs are hypertension and severe refractory bradycardia, followed in short order by seizure and cardiac arrest. These signs develop most often in patients with preexisting compromised myocardial function whose compromise leaves them unable to handle the increased intravascular absorption of the irrigating solution.

The TURP syndrome develops because of circulatory overload and hyponatremia. The former is associated with the amount of irrigating solution that is absorbed, which in turn depends on cardiovascular status, amount and rapidity of absorption of irrigating solution, and amount of surgical blood loss. Dilutional hyponatremia associated with TURP is a hypervolemic hyponatremic condition representing excess total body water with normal total body sodium. If resection time is longer than 90 minutes or the patient has mild symptoms of TURP syndrome, such as nausea, headache, dizziness, or mild confusion, serum sodium should be measured. If hyponatremia is present, the patient should be treated with fluid restriction and a loop diuretic (furosemide 5–20 mg administered intravenously). If serum sodium concentration is less than 120 mEq/L or the patient develops severe signs and symptoms of water intoxication (twitching, visual disturbance, hypotension, dyspnea, seizures), treatment should be instituted immediately with hypertonic (3%) saline at a rate of 100 mL/hour or less, allowing the most rapid correction of plasma sodium concentration. The volume of distribution of sodium equals total body water, so free water excess can be estimated from the following formula:

$$\text{Total body water} = \text{weight}\,(\text{kg}) \times 0.6$$

From this, an estimation of the mEq of sodium ($Na^+$) necessary to normalize the plasma sodium concentration can be obtained:

$$\text{Sodium deficit} = \left(140 - \text{observed plasma Na}^+\right) \\ \times \text{total body water}$$

Hypertonic 3% saline contains 513 mEq of $Na^+$ per liter and should be administered at a rate no faster than 100 mL/hour. Once the symptoms have abated (or the sodium concentration rises above 120 mEq/L), the hypertonic saline should be stopped, and furosemide (40–60 mg) should be intravenously administered to aid free-water excretion by the kidneys. Frequent serum sodium measurements should be obtained. Too rapid correction of hyponatremia can cause seizures, central pontine myelinolysis, and permanent brain damage.

## GLYCINE TOXICITY

Glycine toxicity usually manifests as visual disturbances and transient blindness but may also include other signs and symptoms seen in TURP syndrome. The mechanism of action may be attributed to glycine acting as an inhibitory neurotransmitter because it has a distribution similar to γ-aminobutyric acid in the retina, spinal cord, and brainstem.

## AMMONIA TOXICITY

Ammonia is a major by-product of glycine metabolism. Hyperammonemia usually manifests with nausea and vomiting, followed by encephalopathy.

## BLOOD LOSS

Assessment of blood loss is difficult during a TURP because of dilution of blood with the absorbed irrigation fluid, which maintains intravascular volume, so that the usual hemodynamic responses to blood loss are not seen. The amount of blood loss is directly proportional to the vascularity of the prostate, the length of the operation, and the weight of the prostate gland resected. Continuous postoperative bleeding may indicate a coagulopathy, because patients undergoing TURP have a higher incidence of fibrinolysis. Dilutional thrombocytopenia should also be considered in the differential diagnosis.

## HYPOTHERMIA

Hypothermia, which has not been shown to be influenced by anesthetic technique, could be another cause of confusion in the elderly patient undergoing a TURP.

## BACTEREMIA

Despite preoperative intravenous administration of antibiotics, bacteremia commonly occurs during a TURP and can lead to the development of sepsis. However, bacteremia is usually asymptomatic and is treated with antibiotics to cover gram-positive and gram-negative organisms. Sepsis has been reported to occur in as many as 6% to 7% of patients undergoing a TURP, with septic shock being the first manifestation of the condition.

## PERFORATION OF BLADDER OR URETHRA WITH EXTRAVASATION

Bladder perforation most often occurs during difficult resections by the cutting loop or knife electrode. These perforations can be either extraperitoneal (most common) or intraperitoneal. In the awake patient, extraperitoneal perforation may present as pain in the periumbilical, inguinal, or suprapubic region. Intraperitoneal perforation usually occurs through the bladder wall. Pain may be generalized to the upper abdomen or referred from the diaphragm to the shoulder. Other signs and symptoms include pallor, sweating, nausea, vomiting, shortness of breath, abdominal rigidity, hypotension, and hypertension.

# Prevention of Complications

In general, a TURP is an elective procedure. Therefore optimizing the patient's preoperative state before surgery is always recommended and may minimize anesthetic risks. Surgical risks can be reduced by limiting the duration of the operation, using isosmotic solutions, limiting the depth of dissection, and limiting the pressure of irrigating solution (60 cm $H_2O$ is suggested). Advantages of the use of spinal anesthesia include the earlier detection of complications such as electrolyte disturbances manifested as mental status changes, reduced incidence of deep vein thrombosis, and reduced blood loss. Early detection of bladder perforation can be recognized in patients with a neuraxial block no higher than T9 as they will likely complain of pain. Another advantage of regional anesthesia over general anesthesia for TURP is a decreased requirement of opioids and other analgesic supplementation both during and immediately after surgery. This can theoretically translate to shorter postanesthesia care unit stays.

## SUGGESTED READINGS

Gill, H. S., Chung, B., Deem, S. A., & Pearl, R. G. (2020). Transurethral resection of the prostate (TURP). In R. A. Jaffe, S. I. Sammuels (Eds.), *Anesthesiologist's manual of surgical procedures* (6th ed., pp. 979–984). Philadelphia: Lippincott, Williams & Wilkins.

Hawary, A., Mukhtar, K., Sinclair, A., & Pearce, I. (2009). Transurethral resection of the prostate syndrome: Almost gone but not forgotten. *Journal of Endourology*, 23(12), 2013–2020.

Parsons, J. K., Dahm, P., Köhler, T. S., Lerner, L. B., & Wilt, T. J. (2020). Surgical management of lower urinary tract symptoms attributed to benign prostatic hyperplasia: AUA Guideline Amendment 2020. *Journal of Urology*, 204(4), 799–804.

Rassweiler, J., Teber, D., Kuntz, R., & Hofmann, R. (2006). Complications of transurethral resection of the prostate (TURP): Incidence, management, and prevention. *European Urology*, 50, 969–979.

# Extracorporeal Shock Wave Lithotripsy

JULIAN NARANJO, DO

Urolithiasis is a common condition with a lifetime prevalence of 10.6% among men and 7.1% among women in the United States. Obesity and diabetes are strongly associated with a history of urolithiasis, which most often presents in the third to fourth decade of life. Non-Hispanic Whites are more likely to report kidney stones compared with other races. Nephrolithiasis is less common in children compared with adults, but some have noted increasing incidence of pediatric urolithiasis worldwide, especially in adolescent girls, in a group that historically carries a high probability of recurrence. Urolithiasis presents in all age groups and may even be discovered during prenatal visits with ultrasound. Most urinary stones can pass spontaneously; however, 10% to 30% require urologic intervention. The treatment options for urolithiasis include percutaneous nephrolithotomy (PCNL), retrograde intrarenal surgery (RIRS), and extracorporeal shock wave lithotripsy (ESWL). Should intervention be required, the decision between these treatments is based mainly on stone location and size, but other factors that must be considered include the patient's age, comorbidities and preferences, cost, and available resources. Since the introduction of the first lithotripter in 1980, ESWL (Fig. 145.1) and other minimally invasive stone extraction procedures have become the treatment of choice for most urinary stones requiring intervention in the kidney or upper ureter, having gradually replaced the open and percutaneous surgical approaches. ESWL continues to play an important role in essentially all guidelines worldwide despite reports of higher stone-free rates with other methods. Additionally, ESWL remains the first-line treatment for pediatric urolithiasis. The large role for ESWL in management of urolithiasis in all age groups is likely due to lower reported morbidity and favorable economic aspects. European Association of Urology guidelines state that more than 90% of renal calculi are suitably managed by ESWL.

## Technical Aspects

All lithotripters consist of (1) an energy source that creates a shock wave, (2) a system to focus the energy of the shock wave, (3) a coupling medium that facilitates transfer of the shock wave energy to the patient, and (4) an imaging system to provide localization of the stone and to guide energy delivery to the stone. First-generation lithotripters, such as the Dornier HM-3, are electrohydraulic-type lithotripters that require patients to be immersed in a water bath as the coupling medium and use a spark plug to generate an 18- to 24-kV discharge. Modern lithotripters, such as piezoelectric crystal and electromagnetic shock wave lithotripters, no longer require patient immersion in a water bath because the shock is generated within a water-filled compartment and transferred through a membrane to the patient using a coupling gel (see Fig. 145.1). ESWL is typically performed via ultrasound or fluoroscopic imaging guidance.

Piezoelectric crystal lithotripters generate shock waves via a high-voltage discharge applied across piezoelectric crystals that cause rapid expansion of the crystals and a resultant pressure wave. Electromagnetic shock lithotripters produce pressure waves from a high-voltage current running through an electromagnetic coil. The pressure waves generated from these lithotripsy modalities (electrohydraulic, piezoelectric, electromagnetic) cause rapid expansion and contraction of water bubbles, which then violently collapse and generate a shock wave in a process called *cavitation.*

The origin of the wave is termed the $F_1$ *focal point.* The semiellipsoid reflector focuses the energy wave to converge at the stone (located at the $F_2$ *focal point*) under the guidance of fluoroscopy or ultrasound. The acoustic impedances of the lithotripter, water batch/coupling gel, and the patient's tissues are similar, thus there is little attenuation of the shock wave's energy as it travels from the lithotripter to the stone. The urinary stone presents a change in impedance, resulting in the release of compressive energy and a mechanical stress on the stone. Repeated shocks (1000 or more shocks) lead to disintegration of the stone, and stone fragments are excreted in the urine. Piezoelectric lithotripters have the advantage of having a wider aperture, resulting in lower energy density at the skin and, therefore, less patient discomfort. Some lithotripters can synchronize shock delivery with respiration or the cardiac cycle, although this may limit the maximal rate of shock delivery.

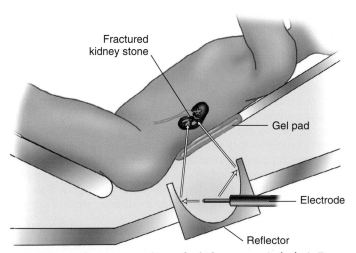

**Fig. 145.1 Lithotripsy, crushing of a kidney stone (calculus).** Extracorporeal shock wave lithotripsy, illustrated here, is used to crush certain types of urinary stones. The reflector focuses a high-energy shock wave on the stone. The stone disintegrates into particles and is passed in the urine. (From Leonard PC. Urinary System. In: *Building a Medical Vocabulary: With Spanish Translations.* 11th ed. Saunders; 2022:fig. 7.27.)

## Patient Selection

ESWL has been used successfully to manage urinary stones in infants, children, and adults. Absolute and relative contraindications to the procedure are listed in Box 145.1. Performing ESWL on patients with untreated urinary infection and urinary obstruction distal to the location of the target stone increases the risk for the development of urosepsis. Pregnancy is considered an absolute contraindication because the effects of shock waves on the fetus have been shown to be harmful in animal studies and have been associated with case reports of spontaneous miscarriages after ESWL, although ESWL has been inadvertently performed on pregnant women without apparent adverse effects on the fetus. The calcified wall of an abdominal aortic aneurysm provides an acoustic interface that can result in liberation of shock wave energy, which can result in release of emboli, aneurysm dissection, or rupture. Various authors have recommended a minimum safe aneurysm diameter (e.g., 5–5.5 cm) and aneurysm-to-stone distance (e.g., at least 5 cm) along with maximum voltage settings and number of shock waves that can be safely delivered. ESWL in patients who are morbidly obese can be technically challenging because of difficulty with positioning, the distance limitations between the F1 and F2 focal points, and large amounts of interposed fat and muscle tissue adjacent to the target site, and therefore tend to have lower success rates. ESWL can be safely performed in patients with pectorally located implanted cardiac devices (i.e., pacemakers and automated implantable cardioverter-defibrillators), provided certain conditions are met (Box 145.2). Performing ESWL in a patient with abdominally located cardiac devices is not recommended.

## Complications

Common side effects reported in the immediate postoperative period include colicky flank pain (40%), gross hematuria (32%), and multiple small stone fragments blocking the ureter, known as *Steinstrasse* (24.2%). Other common side effects include nausea and vomiting, hypertension, skin bruising at the site of shock wave entry, and flank pain lasting several days. Hematuria is almost universally present because of shock wave–induced urothelial, endovascular, or renal parenchymal injury. Preexisting hypertension and preexisting renal disease may

> **BOX 145.1 CONTRAINDICATIONS TO THE USE OF EXTRACORPEAL SHOCK WAVE LITHOTRIPSY**
>
> **ABSOLUTE CONTRAINDICATIONS**
>
> Uncorrected coagulopathy or anticoagulation
> Obstruction distal to the renal calculi
> Pregnancy
> Acute or untreated urinary tract infection
> Urosepsis
>
> **RELATIVE CONTRAINDICATIONS**
>
> Large calcified aortic or renal artery aneurysm
> Morbid obesity
> Implanted cardiac devices
>
> Adapted, with permission, from O'Hara JF, Cywinski JB, Monk TG. The renal system and anesthesia for urologic surgery. In: Barash PG, Cullen BF, Stoelting RK, eds. *Clinical Anesthesia*. 5th ed. Lippincott, Williams & Wilkins; 2006:1030–1031.

> **BOX 145.2 RECOMMENDATIONS FOR MANAGEMENT OF CARDIAC IMPLANTABLE ELECTRONIC DEVICES IN PATIENTS UNDERGOING EXTRACORPEAL SHOCK WAVE LITHOTRIPSY**
>
> Preoperatively determine the type of device and its functional status
> Have a magnet available (and an understanding of the effect of the magnet on the device) or a programming device and a person skilled in its use
> If the patient is pacemaker dependent, ensure that an alternative method of pacing is available
> Position the patient so that the device is not in the shock wave path
> Disable automated implantable cardioverter-defibrillator functions
> Consider reprogramming the device to a nonsensing (asynchronous) mode
>
> Adapted, with permission, from O'Hara JF, Cywinski JB, Monk TG. The renal system and anesthesia for urologic surgery. In: Barash PG, Cullen BF, Stoelting RK, eds. *Clinical Anesthesia*. 5th ed. Lippincott, Williams & Wilkins; 2006:1030–1031.

predispose to endovascular and renal injury after ESWL. Subcapsular hematoma is uncommon, with an incidence of 0.5%. Bleeding complications are more likely to occur in patients with hypertension, diabetes, or coronary artery atherosclerosis; the elderly; and patients with altered coagulation. Substantial bleeding requiring transfusion is rare. Stone fragments are generally excreted in the urine but can, occasionally, accumulate in the ureter, resulting in total obstruction (1%–5%). Air-filled alveoli within the lung present an impedance interface, and therefore shock waves directed toward the lungs result in liberation of shock wave energy, alveolar rupture, and hemoptysis. In children or adults of short stature (<48 in.), polystyrene can be used to protect the lungs from shock waves.

In addition, the amount of energy per shock, which is higher in earlier lithotripters, and the number of shock waves used for treatment have been associated with a greater degree of tissue damage. Cardiac arrhythmias—including atrial and ventricular premature complexes, atrial fibrillation, and supraventricular and ventricular tachycardias—have been reported. Arrhythmias were extremely common in patients who had been treated with the first-generation lithotripters but are now thought to be quite rare. Some lithotripters can be programmed to deliver shock waves using "electrocardiogram gating" to minimize the risk of an R-on-T phenomenon and subsequent ventricular arrhythmia. Pancreatitis and bowel injury resulting in rectal bleeding have been reported. There is conflicting evidence on the long-term effects of ESWL, but some studies suggest that patients who undergo ESWL may develop increased blood pressure and decreased renal function compared with patients undergoing other treatments or observation. Elderly patients appear to be at higher risk for developing these complications.

## Anesthetic Considerations

ESWL is a stimulating procedure that produces pain with cutaneous, somatic, and visceral origins. The continuous shock waves stimulate cutaneous nociceptors, elevated intrapelvic pressure stimulates visceral nociceptors, and the migration of stone fragments causes colic pain. Pain during ESWL that is not well managed may cause patient movement and irregularities in breathing that lead to a defocused shock wave, reduced stone fragmentation and clearance, and possibly a higher rate of kidney hematomas due to a rise in blood pressure. The amount of pain is directly related to the energy density of the shock wave at the skin entry site and the size of the $F_2$ focal zone. Modern lithotripters generally deliver shock waves of lower energy, compared with first-generation machines, and result in less patient discomfort. In addition, piezoelectric lithotripters have a wider aperture and lower energy density at the skin entry point.

A wide variety of anesthetic techniques have been used alone and in combination for ESWL, including general, epidural, and spinal anesthesia; flank infiltration; intercostal and paravertebral nerve blocks; topical application of eutectic mixture of local anesthetic (EMLA) cream; transcutaneous electric nerve stimulation (TENS); and intravenously and orally administered sedative and analgesic agents. Patient-controlled analgesia has also been used successfully. Because of the multifactorial nature of pain associated with urolithiasis and ESWL, combinations of different analgesic modalities have been studied and have noted improved pain control when used together. For example, application of EMLA cream or TENS to address cutaneous somatic pain, in conjunction with intravenous opioid to manage visceral pain and colic, seemed to be more effective than any of these modalities in isolation. First-generation lithotripters generally required general or neuraxial anesthesia, whereas procedures using modern lithotripters in adults may be completed with moderate sedation and, if the patient has comorbid conditions, monitored anesthesia care. There is some data suggesting lithotripsy is slightly more effective under general anesthesia, but further studies are needed to ascertain whether the difference is clinically significant. Notably, a survey of a small group of European physicians at the start of the COVID-19 pandemic uncovered a change in preference in favor of spinal anesthesia to avoid aerosol-generating procedures such as endotracheal intubation. A concern raised at the start of the pandemic was whether the upregulation of Angiotensin Converting Enzyme 2 (ACE2) receptors in the lungs, heart, kidneys, and arteries via use of nonsteroidal antiinflammatory drugs (NSAIDs), such as ibuprofen, to treat colicky pain from urolithiasis would portend more severe COVID-19. To date, there has been no evidence that use of NSAIDs result in worse outcomes from COVID-19, therefore NSAIDs are still widely used for management of renal colic.

ESWL can be performed safely in children, and there is no evidence of long-term kidney morbidity. The approach to the pediatric patient differs substantially from the adult patient with the largest difference being the more frequent use of general and dissociative anesthesia. Although older children may be able to tolerate ESWL under sedation, if additional sedation is required to complete the procedure, the recovery time may exceed that of a carefully planned general anesthetic. High-frequency, low–tidal volume ventilation is commonly used to reduce the range of respiratory movement during ESWL and consequently increase the efficacy of treatment. Incidence of postoperative cognitive dysfunction has been compared between ESWL performed via general and spinal anesthesia with no significant differences noted. Neuraxial techniques should be performed with care to avoid the injection of air, which could provide an acoustic interface, resulting in the release of energy and tissue destruction. When neuraxial blockade is used, a sensory level of T6 is required.

## SUGGESTED READINGS

Auersperg, V., & Trieb, K. (2020). Extracorporeal shock wave therapy: An update. *EFFORT Open Reviews, 5*(10), 584–592.

Constanti, M., Calvert, R. C., Thomas, K., Dickinson, A., & Carlisle, S. (2020). Cost analysis of ureteroscopy (URS) vs extracorporeal shockwave lithotripsy (ESWL) in the management of ureteric stones < 10 mm in adults: A UK perspective. *BJU International, 125*(3), 457–466.

Gadelmoula, M., Elderwy, A. A., Abdelkawi, I. F., Moeen, A. M., Althamthami, G., & Abdel-Moneim, A. M. (2019). Percutaneous nephrolithotomy versus shock wave lithotripsy for high-density moderate-sized renal stones: A prospective randomized study. *Urology Annals, 11*(4), 426–431.

Huang, Y., Chai, S., Wang, D., Li, W., & Zhang, X. (2020). Efficacy of eutectic mixture of local anesthetics on pain control during extracorporeal shock wave lithotripsy: A systematic review and meta-analysis. *Medical Science Monitor, 26*, e921063.

Large, T., & Krambeck, A. (2019). Emerging technologies in lithotripsy. *Urologic Clinics of North America, 46*(2), 215–223.

Shinde, S., Al Balushi, Y., Hossny, M., Jose, S., & Al Busaidy, S. (2018). Factors affecting the outcome of extracorporeal shockwave lithotripsy in urinary stone treatment. *Oman Medical Journal, 33*(3), 209–217.

Shoukry, R. A., & Al-Ansary, A. M. (2019). Transcutaneous Electric Nerve Stimulation (TENS) for pain relief during Extracorporeal Shock-Wave Lithotripsy (ESWL). *Egyptian Journal of Anaesthesia, 35*(1), 71–76.

Tefik, T., Guven, S., Villa, L., Gokce, M. I., Kallidonis, P., Petkova, K., et al. (2020). Urolithiasis practice patterns following the COVID-19 pandemic: Overview from the EULIS collaborative research working group. *European Urology, 78*(1), e21.

Zumstein, V., Betschart, P., Abt, D., Schmid, H. P., Panje, C. M., Putora, & P. M. (2018). Surgical management of urolithiasis–A systematic analysis of available guidelines. *BMC Urology, 18*(1), 1–8.

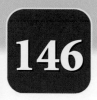

# 146

# Anatomy of the Larynx

LEAL G. SEGURA, MD

## Description

The larynx connects the inferior pharynx with the trachea and serves three functions (Box 146.1): maintain a patent airway, guard against aspiration of liquids or solids into the trachea, and permit vocalization. It is about 5 cm in length, and in adults it lies at the level of C4 to C5. In cross section at the level of the laryngeal prominence (Adam's apple), the larynx is triangular because of the shape of the thyroid cartilage. At the level of the cricoid cartilage, the larynx becomes more round. The larynx provides the area of greatest resistance to passage of air to the lungs.

## Laryngeal Skeleton

The laryngeal skeleton has one bone, the hyoid bone, and nine cartilages (Table 146.1): three sets of paired cartilages (arytenoids, corniculates, cuneiforms) and three unpaired cartilages (thyroid, cricoid, and epiglottic) (Fig. 146.1). The thyroid cartilage, the largest laryngeal cartilage, protects the vocal cords, which attach to its internal surface. The cricoid is the only complete rigid ring in the airway and has a smaller diameter than the trachea; thus it may represent a vulnerable point in the airway for foreign body obstruction or postintubation edema.

## Joints, Ligaments, and Membranes of the Larynx

The joints of the larynx include the cricothyroid joint, which articulates the lateral surfaces of the cricoid cartilage and the inferior horns of the thyroid cartilage, and the cricoarytenoid joint, which provides articulation between the bases of the arytenoid cartilage and the upper surface of the cricoid lamina. The thyrohyoid membrane is an extrinsic ligament that connects the thyroid cartilage to the hyoid bone. The larynx includes three sets of ligaments: the cricothyroid and cricotracheal, which connect the cricoid to the thyroid cartilage and the first tracheal ring, respectively; the vocal ligament, which extends from the thyroid cartilage to the arytenoid cartilage; and the vestibular ligament, which extends from the thyroid cartilage to the arytenoid cartilage above the vocal fold. The cricothyroid ligament is the target site for emergent cricothyrotomy.

## Interior of the Larynx

The glottis is composed of the vocal cords, which mark its anterior edge, and the rima glottidis, which is the opening between the vocal cords. The false vocal folds sit above and

### BOX 146.1 FUNCTIONS OF THE LARYNX

Maintain a patent airway
Guard against aspiration of liquids or solids into the trachea
Permit vocalization

| TABLE 146.1 | Cartilages of the Larynx |
|---|---|
| **Cartilage** | **Description and Location** |
| **PAIRED** | |
| Arytenoid | Shaped like a three-sided pyramid that articulates with the upper border of the cricoid lamina |
| Corniculate | At the apices of the arytenoid cartilage in the posterior part of the aryepiglottic folds |
| Cuneiform | In the aryepiglottic folds, but not always present |
| **UNPAIRED** | |
| Thyroid | Largest cartilage, comprising two laminae that are fused anteriorly to form the laryngeal prominence |
| Cricoid | Ring shaped, with a posterior part (lamina) and an anterior part (arch), and located at the level of C6 in adults; the arytenoids articulate with the lateral parts of the superior border of the lamina |
| Epiglottic | Thin and leaflike, and located behind the root of the tongue and in front of the inlet of the larynx; the mucous membrane covering the epiglottis continues onto the base of the tongue, forming two depressions (epiglottic valleculae) |

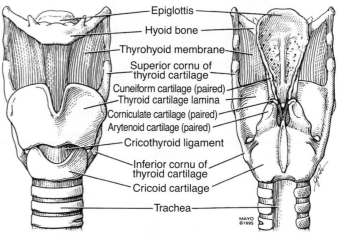

**Fig. 146.1** Anterior and posterior views of the larynx. (Used with permission of Mayo Foundation for Medical Education and Research, all rights reserved.)

lateral to the vocal cords. Both the true and false vocal folds attach to the arytenoids posteriorly.

The laryngeal cavity itself can be divided into three regions. The vestibule, the most superior region, lies above the false cords. The epiglottis marks the superior portion of the larynx. The ventricle is a space formed by the false vocal folds above and the true vocal cords below. The infraglottic cavity is the most inferior region, lying from the true vocal cords to the trachea.

The vocal folds (vocal cords) themselves consist of the vocal ligament; the conus elasticus, which provides support; the vocalis muscle fibers; and an overlying mucous membrane. The false vocal folds are ligaments covered by folds of mucous membrane. They meet during swallowing to prevent aspiration. The rima vestibuli is the space between the false cords.

## Innervation

Innervation to the larynx is supplied by the vagus nerve (X) via two branches: the superior laryngeal nerve (SLN) and the recurrent laryngeal nerve (RLN) (Fig. 146.2). The SLN has two terminal branches: the internal laryngeal nerve, which is purely sensory and innervates from the mucosa of the tongue to the vocal folds (including the superior surface of these folds), and the external laryngeal nerve, which is purely motor and innervates the cricothyroid muscle. The RLN provides branches to all of the other muscles of the larynx and provides sensory innervation below the vocal cords, from the subglottis and trachea. Some anatomic studies suggest that this model of motor innervation may be overly simplified and that the motor contribution of the SLN to other laryngeal muscles may be more variable and complex. The sensory innervation of the laryngeal mucosa is richly developed, and the larynx actually has more sensory receptors than the lungs, despite its markedly smaller surface area.

## Muscles

Laryngeal motion is caused by intrinsic and extrinsic muscles. The extrinsic muscle group connects the larynx to outside

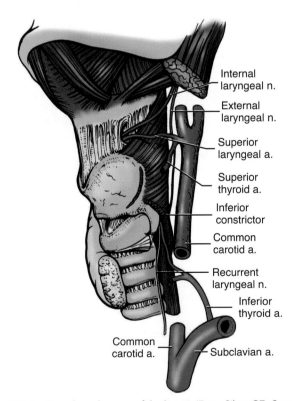

**Fig. 146.2** Vessels and nerves of the larynx. (From Silver CE. *Surgery for Cancer of the Larynx and Related Structures.* 2nd ed. WB Saunders; 1996.)

Internal laryngeal n.
External laryngeal n.
Superior laryngeal a.
Superior thyroid a.
Inferior constrictor
Common carotid a.
Recurrent laryngeal n.
Inferior thyroid a.
Common carotid a.
Subclavian a.

---

> ### BOX 146.2   EXTRINSIC MUSCLES OF THE LARYNX
>
> **DEPRESSORS**
> Omohyoid
> Sternohyoid
> Sternothyroid
>
> **ELEVATORS**
> Stylohyoid
> Digastrics
> Mylohyoid
> Geniohyoid
> Stylopharyngeus

structures and either elevates or depresses the larynx or moves it in the anterior or posterior dimension (Box 146.2). The intrinsic laryngeal muscle group primarily affects vocal cord motion. Each of the intrinsic muscles exerts a unique motion on the arytenoid cartilage, but these muscles work together to move the vocal cords in three dimensions. Contraction of the posterior cricoarytenoid muscle, the only abductor of the glottis, rotates the arytenoid externally and opens the vocal cords. Conversely, the lateral cricoarytenoid muscle, the primary adductor of the larynx, acts to close the vocal cords.

## Blood Supply

The superior laryngeal artery is a branch of the superior thyroid artery off of the external carotid artery. The inferior laryngeal artery is a branch of the inferior thyroid artery off of the thyrocervical trunk off of the subclavian artery.

## Considerations With the Infant Larynx

The infant larynx is higher and more anterior than the adult larynx. The infant cricoid lies at the level of C3 to C4 compared with C4 to C5 in an adult. Historically, airway references have described the infant tongue as relatively larger than an adult tongue; however, this dogma has been challenged by radiologic studies, and other authors have suggested that airway obstruction in anesthetized children may be attributable instead to nasopharyngeal or epiglottic collapse. The distance between the infant tongue, hyoid, and epiglottis is shorter than in an adult, producing an acute angle between the tongue and the laryngeal inlet. Relative to the adult epiglottis, the infant epiglottis is narrow, omega shaped, and retroflexed relative to the trachea. This orientation may make it more difficult to lift the infant epiglottis during direct laryngoscopy. The larynx is cylindrical in both adults and children, but this shape is more pronounced in pediatric patients; classic teaching describes a funnel-shaped larynx ending at the cricoid, the narrowest point of the larynx. This view of the larynx has been challenged by radiologic studies that suggest that the narrowest part of the larynx is at or immediately below the vocal cords. Regardless, the cricoid cartilage is the sole complete rigid ring in the airway that is nondistensible; therefore its small diameter may be the most clinically relevant.

## SUGGESTED READINGS

Moore, K. L. (2010). *Clinically oriented anatomy* (6th ed.). Philadelphia: Lippincott Williams & Wilkins.

Redden, R. J. (2000). Anatomic considerations in anesthesia. In C. A. Hagberg (Ed.), *Handbook of difficult airway management* (pp. 1–13). Philadelphia: Churchill Livingstone.

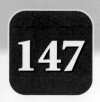

# Anesthesia for Laryngeal Surgery

BARRY A. HARRISON, MBBS, FRACP, FANZCA | RYAN CHADHA, MD

In operations involving the larynx, both the surgeon and the anesthesiologist must share the patient's airway, making an understanding of the operative and anesthesia requirements essential and ongoing communication among team members imperative. Indications for laryngeal operations include congenital conditions and acquired conditions such as trauma, inflammation, and tumors (Box 147.1). Laryngeal signs and symptoms vary from a sore throat and hoarseness to difficulty in breathing, stridor, and potential complete upper airway obstruction. Common laryngeal operations include direct laryngoscopy for diagnosis and treatment of vocal cord lesions, vocal cord surgery, laryngectomy, and trauma to the larynx.

## Airway Anatomy and Physiology

The human larynx has three basic functions: inspiration, tracheobronchial protection, and phonation. A complex system of neuronal innervation to intrinsic and extrinsic laryngeal musculature suspended on cartilaginous structures achieves these functions. The vagus nerve (cranial nerve X), via the superior and recurrent laryngeal nerves, is responsible for the sensory and motor innervation of the larynx. The internal branch of the superior laryngeal nerve provides ipsilateral sensation to the supraglottic (i.e., above the true vocal cords) larynx. The recurrent laryngeal nerve provides ipsilateral sensation below the vocal cords. The posterior half of the vocal cords has the highest density of touch receptors. This is important to remember when regional or topical anesthesia is used, such as before elective fiberoptic intubation.

The recurrent laryngeal nerve provides the motor supply to all intrinsic laryngeal muscles except the cricothyroid muscle. The cricothyroid muscle receives motor innervation from the external branch of the superior laryngeal nerve. A summary of the actions of each muscle is presented in Fig. 147.1. Recurrent laryngeal nerve injury may occur during thyroid and parathyroid surgery. To minimize the possibility of nerve injury, surgeons may monitor recurrent laryngeal nerve function by stimulating this nerve using a special endotracheal tube with

stimulation occurring at the level of the larynx and the recording electrodes positioned at the level of the vocal cords.

## Direct Laryngoscopy

Direct laryngoscopy may assess and/or treat supraglottic, glottic, subglottic, and tracheal conditions. Preoperative cardiac assessment is important because 1.5% to 4% of perioperative deaths in this patient population are attributed to preexisting cardiac disease. Preoperative airway assessment is equally important and may include physical examination, indirect laryngoscopy, and various imaging studies of the larynx. If the ability to secure an airway conventionally is questionable, awake fiberoptic intubation or tracheotomy should be performed under local anesthesia. General anesthesia may be induced for surgical procedures with either spontaneous ventilation (using a nonirritating inhalation anesthetic) or intravenously administered medications if airway difficulty is not anticipated. Topical application of local anesthetic on the vocal cords and adjacent mucosa can decrease the requirements for inhalational anesthesia. Oxygenation is maintained with the use of insufflation in a spontaneously breathing patient with or without the use of an endotracheal tube.

Although dental injury can occur with any technique, patients with difficult airways are at particular risk for incurring these injuries. Otorhinolaryngologic surgeons often use dental guards in patients to reduce the risk of dental injury during direct laryngoscopy. Postsurgical hemoptysis, obstruction, laryngeal edema, and laryngospasm are serious risks associated with direct laryngoscopy.

### WITHOUT A TRACHEAL TUBE

#### Apneic Oxygenation

Patients are hyperventilated with 100% oxygen ($O_2$) and an inhalation anesthetic agent followed by a period of no ventilation during which the surgeon is allowed airway access in 3- to 5-minute epochs or until desaturation occurs. Carbon dioxide ($CO_2$) monitoring is not possible with this technique; accordingly, hypercapnia is a potential problem.

Periods of apneic oxygenation have been extended with the use of a transnasal humidified rapid-insufflation ventilatory exchange (THRIVE) device for laryngeal surgery. This device supports gas flows of warmed, humidified oxygen up to 70 L administered via nasal cannula. This device, initially used in laryngeal surgery in patients with difficult airways, is now being used in everyday practice.

#### Jet Ventilation

Air is entrained by the Venturi effect when a 30- to 50-psi blast from the jet ventilator insufflates $O_2$ into the airway to provide

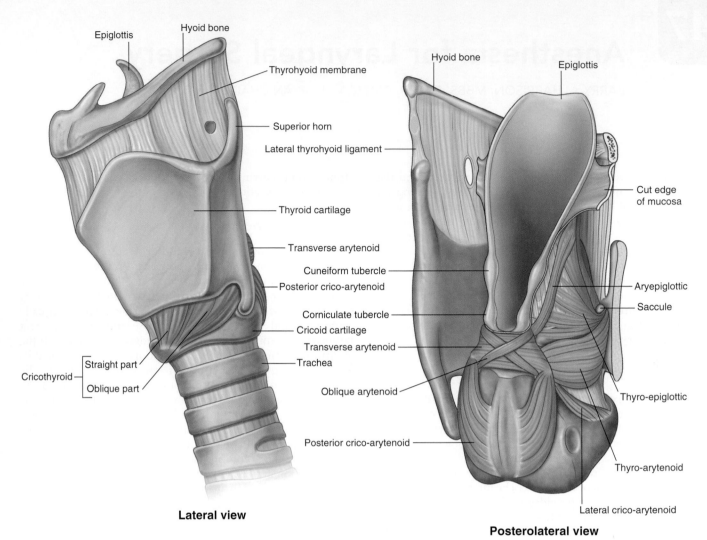

**Lateral view**

- Epiglottis
- Hyoid bone
- Thyrohyoid membrane
- Superior horn
- Lateral thyrohyoid ligament
- Thyroid cartilage
- Transverse arytenoid
- Cuneiform tubercle
- Posterior crico-arytenoid
- Corniculate tubercle
- Cricoid cartilage
- Transverse arytenoid
- Trachea
- Oblique arytenoid
- Cricothyroid — Straight part / Oblique part
- Posterior crico-arytenoid

**Posterolateral view**

- Hyoid bone
- Epiglottis
- Cut edge of mucosa
- Aryepiglottic
- Saccule
- Thyro-epiglottic
- Thyro-arytenoid
- Lateral crico-arytenoid

**Superior view**

- Thyro-arytenoid
- Vocal ligament
- Cricothyroid — Straight part / Oblique part
- Conus elasticus
- Lateral crico-arytenoid
- Transverse arytenoid
- Oblique arytenoid
- Thyroid cartilage
- Vocalis
- Aryepiglottic
- Vocal process of arytenoid
- Superior horn
- Muscular process of arytenoid
- Posterior crico-arytenoid

A

**Fig. 147.1  A,** Muscles of the larynx.

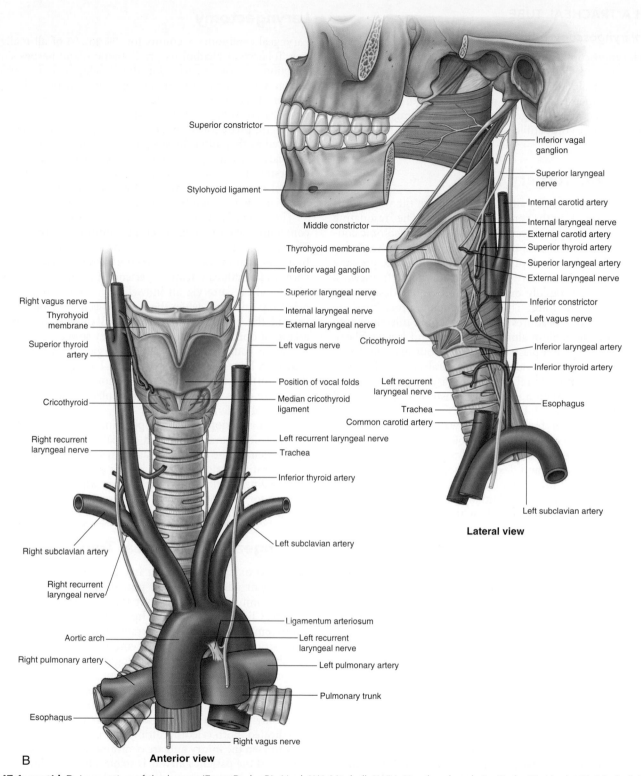

Superior constrictor

Stylohyoid ligament

Middle constrictor

Thyrohyoid membrane

Inferior vagal ganglion

Superior laryngeal nerve

Internal laryngeal nerve

External laryngeal nerve

Left vagus nerve

Position of vocal folds

Median cricothyroid ligament

Left recurrent laryngeal nerve

Trachea

Inferior thyroid artery

Left subclavian artery

Ligamentum arteriosum

Left recurrent laryngeal nerve

Left pulmonary artery

Pulmonary trunk

Right vagus nerve

Inferior vagal ganglion

Superior laryngeal nerve

Internal carotid artery

Internal laryngeal nerve

External carotid artery

Superior thyroid artery

Superior laryngeal artery

External laryngeal nerve

Inferior constrictor

Left vagus nerve

Cricothyroid

Inferior laryngeal artery

Inferior thyroid artery

Esophagus

Left subclavian artery

**Lateral view**

Right vagus nerve

Thyrohyoid membrane

Superior thyroid artery

Cricothyroid

Right recurrent laryngeal nerve

Right subclavian artery

Right recurrent laryngeal nerve

Aortic arch

Right pulmonary artery

Esophagus

**B**   **Anterior view**

**Fig. 147.1, cont'd  B,** Innervation of the larynx. (From Drake RL, Vogl AW, Mitchell AWM. Head and neck. In: Drake RL, Vogl AW, Mitchell AWM, eds. *Gray's Atlas of Anatomy.* 3rd ed. Elsevier; 2021.)

jet ventilation. A properly placed jet allows visualization of chest wall movement. Inhalation anesthesia is not possible during jet ventilation. Intravenously administered anesthesia is better suited for this oxygenation technique.

Jet ventilation systems were initially simple, providing little control of ventilation and limited monitoring while exposing patients to high $O_2$ concentrations. More sophisticated jet ventilators are now commercially available (Monsoon II and III; Acutronic, Hirzel, Switzerland). Some advantages of modern jet ventilators include settings to control frequency (4–1600 breaths per minute) inspired $O_2$ concentration, heating, humidification of gases, airway pressure, and end-tidal $CO_2$ monitoring.

## WITH A TRACHEAL TUBE

### *Microlaryngoscopy Tubes*

Microlaryngoscopy tubes are endotracheal tubes of small diameter and adult length. Available sizes include 4 mm, 5 mm, and 6 mm in diameter and require stylet-guided placement. General anesthesia should be maintained with short-acting medications because emergence can be challenging. A tracheal tube that is laser compatible must be used if laser resection is planned.

## Vocal Cord Surgery

Phonation is produced by air expelled through the vocal cords producing sound with periodic vibration. The resonating chambers of the upper airway modify this sound. Isotonic contraction of the cricothyroid muscle determines voice frequency and changes in the length of the cords and subglottic pressure determine pitch. Vocal cord surgery or laryngeal framework surgery (LFS) are rapidly expanding techniques designed to improve or restore voice. The most frequent procedures are glottic narrowing procedures that often require injections into the vocal cord to achieve glottis narrowing and laryngoplasty, which consists of thyroplasty with or without arytenoid manipulation to treat unilateral vocal cord paralysis, which is usually secondary to injury to the recurrent laryngeal nerve.

Preoperative evaluation includes sophisticated tests of vocal cord function to establish baselines. The anesthesiologist needs to evaluate the larynx for potential airway obstruction and to assess the procedure. Coexisting morbid conditions are common because of the age and etiology of the vocal cord problem. Intravenous antibiotics and dexamethasone are often administered preoperatively. Many of these surgeries require local anesthetic skin infiltration with minimal sedation. The success of the anesthesia requires partnership with the surgeon to ensure sufficient topical anesthesia is obtained in the surgical field. Light sedation may be achieved using incremental doses of midazolam and fentanyl or carefully administered propofol. A propofol infusion may provide deeper sedation during infiltration of local anesthetics. Dexmedetomidine, with its unique sedative properties and lack of respiratory depression, has been described as a successful technique in many reports. Although minimal sedation is the most commonly used technique, general anesthesia using a laryngeal mask airway has also been reported to be successful.

The most serious immediate postoperative complication is airway obstruction. Partial airway obstruction may respond to conservative measures such as racemic epinephrine, intravenous dexamethasone, and inhalation of heliox. However, tracheostomy may be required to treat severe or complete obstruction. Patients with a history of previous LFS surgery who require general anesthesia should not be intubated with an endotracheal tube unless absolutely necessary. Supraglottic airway devices should be considered as an alternative.

## Laryngectomy

Laryngeal carcinoma accounts for 2% to 3% of all malignancies. Tobacco or alcohol use, radiotherapy, and herpes simplex infection are risk factors for the development of laryngeal carcinoma. Patients are predominantly men over the age of 50 years. Laryngeal carcinoma may be supraglottic (30%), glottic (60%), or subglottic (10%) in location.

Careful preoperative patient assessment of these patients is required as they often have significant comorbid disease (e.g., chronic obstructive pulmonary disease, coronary artery disease, congestive heart failure, hypertension, nicotine dependence, alcohol abuse). Measurement of liver function may be indicated in patients with a significant history of alcohol intake.

The airway is often secured using an awake technique with conscious sedation (e.g., fiberoptic intubation, tracheotomy). The type of anesthesia (e.g., sedation vs. general) is determined by airway anatomy, severity of comorbid diseases, patient preference, and health care team experience. Continuous monitoring of arterial pressure via an indwelling arterial cannula is often helpful, particularly when the neck dissection involves the area around the carotid sinus. An arterial catheter also provides access for obtaining blood for laboratory studies (e.g., serial hemoglobin concentrations), during surgical procedures associated with large blood loss (e.g., total laryngectomy with neck dissection). Central venous cannulation is rarely indicated. In these rare cases the catheter can be placed via the subclavian, antecubital, or femoral route.

Potential perioperative complications include air embolism, hypertension, parathyroid and cranial nerve dysfunction, and facial edema. The use of a nasogastric tube is helpful in the postoperative period for both gastric drainage and postoperative feeding. Preliminary experience with transoral robotic surgery for head and neck cancer is encouraging, suggesting that this modality may be more frequent in the future.

## Laryngeal and Tracheal Trauma

Laryngeal or tracheal trauma is rare (1 in 43,000 emergency department admissions) but potentially deadly. The mechanism of injury is usually blunt (85%) or penetrating (15%) trauma. Clinical signs include hoarseness, tenderness, subcutaneous emphysema (an important sign), respiratory distress (e.g., stridor), dysphagia, and hemoptysis. The best outcomes are observed when an otolaryngologist is involved in managing the patient's airway and any treatment is performed in the operating room. If the patient's airway is unstable, the laryngeal mucosa disrupted, or a laryngo-skeletal fracture is present, tracheotomy under local anesthesia followed by neck exploration is indicated. Both cricothyrotomy and endotracheal intubation may worsen the injury and are contraindicated in these circumstances. If the patient's airway is stable, fiberoptic intubation or direct oral intubation under general anesthesia, with either rapid sequence or inhaled induction, may be considered.

## SUGGESTED READINGS

Barakate, M., Maver, E., Wotherspoon, G., & Havas, T. (2010). Anaesthesia for microlaryngeal and laser laryngeal surgery: Impact of subglottic jet ventilation. *Journal of Laryngology and Otology, 124,* 641–645.

Li, L. T., Chitilian, H. V., Alfille, P. H., & Bao, X. (2021). Airway management and anesthesia for airway surgery: A narrative review. *Translational Lung Cancer Research, 10*(12), 4631–4642.

Patel, A., & Nouraci, A. R. (2015). Transnasal humidified rapid-insufflation ventilatory exchange (THRIVE): A physiological method of increasing apnoea time in patients with difficult airways. *Anaesthesia, 70,* 323–329.

Schieren, M., Wappler, F., & Defosse, J. (2022). Anesthesia for tracheal and carinal resection and reconstruction. *Current Opinion in Anaesthesiology, 35*(1), 75–81.

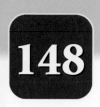

# 148

# Management of the Difficult Airway

MARIANA RESTREPO-HOLGUIN, MD | BRIDGET P. PULOS, MD

The successful management of a difficult airway requires a combination of forethought, proper equipment, and decisiveness. Concentrating on the first two factors makes the third less stressful. The first steps in airway management are to obtain a thorough patient history and perform a physical examination with particular emphasis on the airway. Although difficult to estimate precisely, the reported incidence of an unanticipated difficult intubation remains approximately 10%. Several guidelines exist to assist with difficult airway management, and all anesthesia providers should be familiar with them.

## Defining the Difficult Airway

According to the American Society of Anesthesiologists (ASA) practice guidelines, a difficult airway is defined as a clinical situation in which a trained anesthesia provider experiences anticipated or unanticipated difficulty with facemask ventilation of the upper airway, direct laryngoscopy and tracheal intubation, ventilation with a supraglottic airway, invasive airway management, extubation, or some combination of these (Table 148.1).

The first ASA practice guidelines, including an algorithm for management of the difficult airway, were developed by an ASA panel of experts in the 1990s and have been updated approximately every 10 years since (Fig. 148.1). These guidelines emphasized the importance of learning multiple airway management techniques. This instruction led to anesthesia providers' increased familiarity with multiple airway instruments and a willingness to switch techniques sooner rather than later, when encountering a difficult airway. The 2022 update of the ASA Difficult Airway Algorithm mentions the use of alterative non-invasive devices, such as video laryngoscopy, flexible intubation scopes, alternative rigid laryngoscopic blades, supraglottic devices, and rigid bronchoscopes, as another useful approach. This mirrors the widespread adoption of video laryngoscopy techniques by most anesthesia providers as their favored approach to anticipated difficult airways.

Finally, some indicators of inadequate ventilation include absent or inadequate exhaled carbon dioxide, chest movement and/or breath sounds, auscultatory signs of severe obstruction, cyanosis, gastric air entry or dilatation, decreasing or inadequate oxygen saturation, spirometry with absent or inadequate exhaled gas flow, anatomic lung abnormalities on lung ultrasound, hemodynamic changes secondary to hypoxemia or hypercarbia, and clinical symptoms such as changes in mental status.

## Preoperative Evaluation

A thorough airway evaluation includes both risk assessment and airway examination. The anesthesia provider should preoperatively interview the patient and review the medical record to determine whether the patient has had any previous difficulty while being intubated, has a history of anatomic distortion of the airway, snoring, obstructive sleep apnea, or additional comorbidities that might suggest difficult ventilation. Three classic bedside measurements should be obtained: the size of the tongue, compared with the pharynx and visibility of the uvula; the extension of the atlantooccipital joint; and the size of the anterior mandibular space. A 2019 systematic review found that the best predictor of a difficult airway was an inability to bite the upper lip with the lower incisors (upper lip bite test) and that this increased the probability of a difficult airway to 60%. Importantly, although none of the aforementioned parameters is a definitive predictor of airway difficulty, evaluation of as many bedside measures as possible is recommended to increase the predictive power of the preoperative examination. In addition to obtaining the three classic measurements and upper lip bite test, length of upper incisors, the relationship of maxillary and mandibular incisors during normal jaw closure and during voluntary protrusion of the mandible, shape of the palate, length and thickness of the neck, and cervical spine range of motion should also be evaluated. Nonreassuring findings include relatively long upper incisors, a prominent "overbite" or inability to bring

| TABLE 148.1 | Important Definitions From 2022 ASA Practice Guidelines for Management of the Difficult Airway |
|---|---|
| **Term** | **Definition** |
| Difficult facemask ventilation | Inadequate ventilation, secondary to an inadequate mask seal, excessive gas leakage, or resistance in the flow of gas |
| Difficult laryngoscopy | Impossibility to visualize, after multiple attempts, any portion of the vocal cords |
| Difficult supraglottic airway ventilation | Inadequate ventilation due to a difficult supraglottic airway placement, placement requiring multiple attempts, inadequate seal, excessive gas leak, or resistance to the flow of gas |
| Difficult or failed intubation | When tracheal intubation requires multiple attempts or fails after multiple attempts |
| Difficult or failed invasive airway | A reduction or prevention in the likelihood of successfully placing an airway into the trachea through the anterior aspect of the neck by anatomic features or abnormalities |
| Difficult or failed extubation | The loss of airway patency and adequate ventilation after removal of a tracheal or supraglottic airway from a patient with a known or suspected difficult airway |

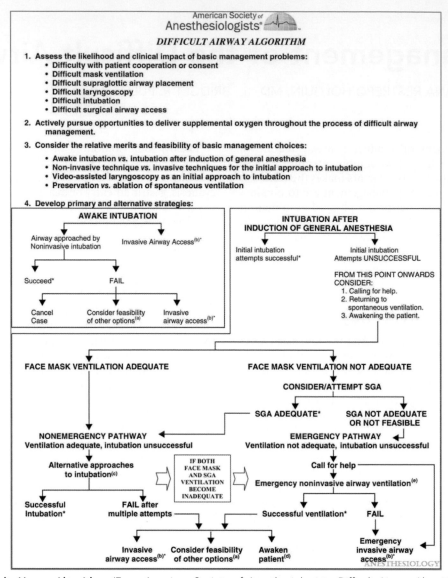

**Fig. 148.1   ASA Difficult Airway Algorithm.** (From American Society of Anesthesiologists. Difficult Airway Algorithm. *Anesthesiology.* 2013; 118(2):251–270. Reprinted with permission of the American Society of Anesthesiologists, Park Ridge, IL.)

mandibular incisors in front of maxillary incisors, a highly arched or very narrow palate, and a short and thick neck. Some additional measurements that can be found on ultrasound evaluation are skin-to-hyoid distance, tongue volume, and distance from the skin to the epiglottis.

## TONGUE VERSUS PHARYNGEAL SIZE

Preinduction visualization of the faucial pillars, soft palate, and base of the uvula, with the patient in a sitting position, is used to classify patients according to how well pharyngeal structures can be seen (Table 148.2 and Fig. 148.2). Mallampati classes III and IV are predictive of a difficult airway.

## ATLANTOOCCIPITAL EXTENSION

Mobility of the atlantooccipital joint enables alignment of the oral, pharyngeal, and laryngeal axes, facilitating mask ventilation and tracheal intubation. Extension of the atlantooccipital joint can be quantified by observing the angle of the occlusal surface

| TABLE 148.2 | Mallampati Classification of the Upper Airway | |
|---|---|
| **Class** | **Visible Structures** |
| I | Palate, faucial pillars, entire uvula |
| II | Palate, faucial pillars, base of uvula |
| III | Palate, some of the faucial pillars |
| IV | Palate |

of the upper teeth with respect to horizontal when the patient is upright and extending the neck; 35 degrees of extension is a normal value.

## ANTERIOR MANDIBULAR SPACE

The anterior mandibular space refers to the thyromental distance: the distance from the thyroid notch to the mental prominence, when the neck is fully extended. A convenient way to assess this finding is a thyromental distance of less than three fingerbreadths

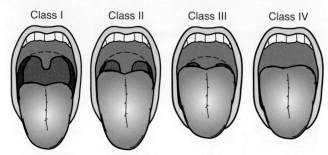

**Fig. 148.2 Mallampati classification of the upper airway.** See Table 148.2 for explanation of each class. (Modified from Mallampati SR, Gatt SP, Gugino LD, et al. A clinical sign to predict difficult tracheal intubation: a prospective study. *Can Anaesth Soc J.* 1985;32: 429–434.)

predicts a more difficult intubation. This is often referred to as an "anterior" airway.

## Preparation for Management of the Difficult Airway

In preparation for airway management, ensure monitoring is in place as established by the ASA Standards for Basic Anesthesia Monitoring, airway management equipment is readily accessible in the room with further difficult airway management equipment available, and additional anesthesia providers are present if possible. This may include alerting otorhinolaryngology or general surgery to the potential need for a surgical airway. All health care providers involved should be aware of the potential difficult airway and chosen plan. Position the patient appropriately and administer supplemental oxygen.

## Management of the Difficult Airway

The implementation of the ASA Difficult Airway Algorithm will differ depending on patient factors such as comorbidities and surgical requirements, the availability of equipment, and perhaps most critically, the skill of the anesthesia provider.

A morbidly obese patient (i.e., body mass index >40 kg/m²) may be more difficult to mask ventilate, but morbid obesity does not, per se, lead to difficulty in intubating the trachea unless the patient has other factors such as increased periglottic tissue, limited neck mobility, or is not properly positioned. In addition, obese patients rapidly develop hypoxemia during apnea. These factors can be ameliorated by placing the patient in a "ramped up" position (see Chapter 142, Anesthesia in the Patient With Extreme Obesity).

Depending on whether an anticipated versus unanticipated difficult airway occurs, different pathways in the algorithm will be used. Identification of a difficult airway after the induction of general anesthesia and administration of neuromuscular blocking drugs leads to the arm of the algorithm that is most stressful for the anesthesia provider. If ventilation is adequate in an unanticipated difficult tracheal intubation, a nonemergent approach can be taken. The goal is to establish a secure airway. This is done by using an alternate device such as a video laryngoscope, flexible intubation scope, or laryngeal mask airway as a temporizing measure. Limit attempts to three by the primary airway manager plus one by a secondary airway manager, and ventilate the patient between attempts. If ventilation becomes inadequate or is not able to be established, an emergency approach is taken to establish ventilation. Attempt to ventilate the patient with a facemask and obtain a supraglottic airway or tracheal tube while limiting attempts as previously described. If ventilation remains inadequate, consider an emergency invasive airway such as cricothyrotomy or surgical tracheostomy, rigid bronchoscopy, and finally, if appropriate, extracorporeal membrane oxygenation.

Only rarely is a surgical airway the first choice for securing an airway. The most common reasons include trauma to the face or cervical spine or a neoplastic disease involving the airway or neck.

The anesthesia provider must always be prepared to manage the airway with transoral supraglottic techniques (e.g., laryngeal mask airway, Combitube) and with techniques involving emergency invasive airway access (surgical or percutaneous cricothyrotomy plus transtracheal jet ventilation) while moving toward achieving a more definitive airway. Patient safety depends on planning ahead and progressing rapidly down the appropriate arms of the algorithm. Studying the algorithm and being aware of the potential pathways before encountering airway difficulties is likely to result in the best outcome.

## Specific Patient Populations

There are some modified difficult airway algorithms that address specific differences in select patients.

### TRAUMA PATIENTS

The Difficult Airway Algorithm is modified for use in trauma patients (Fig. 148.3). Some unique challenges include altered airway anatomy, the need for cervical spine protection, positioning difficulty, and potential hemodynamic instability. It is important to remember that in a trauma patient, it will likely not be possible to wake up the patient or cancel the procedure, and therefore a surgical airway may be the best first approach to the difficult airway in certain situations.

Frequent reevaluation of the traumatized airway should be performed, and presence of inspiratory stridor should suggest impending loss of airway. Traumatized airways can be evaluated via direct laryngoscopy, video laryngoscopy, fiberoptic bronchoscopy, or ultrasonic imaging. Imaging also provides information about the airway and structures and can be done if intubation is nonemergent or once the airway is secured. Nasal airways should be avoided in the setting of possible basilar skull or nasal fracture. In the presence of facial fractures, facemask ventilation may lead to displacement of the bone fragments and increase airway obstruction. Also, cricoid pressure, rigid laryngoscopy, stylets, and endotracheal intubation should be used with caution given the possibility of worsening the injury due to the avulsion of mucous membranes and pseudolumen creation.

In patients with extensive airway disruption, a surgical airway distal to the injury will be the best initial approach. Practitioners should use the technique they feel most comfortable with and move toward emergent cricothyrotomy or surgical tracheostomy if there is an inability to intubate. If possible, patients with airway trauma should be managed in collaboration with surgical colleagues.

### OBSTETRIC PATIENTS

In 2015, the Obstetric Anesthetists' Association and the Difficult Airway Society published guidelines for management of the difficult airway in the obstetric population. They emphasize

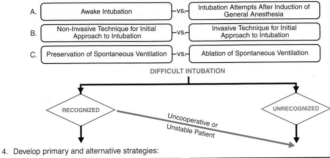

ASA AMERICAN SOCIETY OF ANESTHESIOLOGISTS

**2003 DIFFICULT AIRWAY ALGORITHM (MODIFIED FOR TRAUMA)**

1. Assess the likelihood and clinical impact of basic management problems.
   A. Difficult Ventilation
   B. Difficult Intubation
   C. Difficulty with Patient Cooperation or Consent
   D. Difficult Tracheostomy
2. Actively pursue opportunities to deliver supplemental oxygen throughout the process of difficult airway management.
3. Consider the relative merits and feasibility of basic management choices:

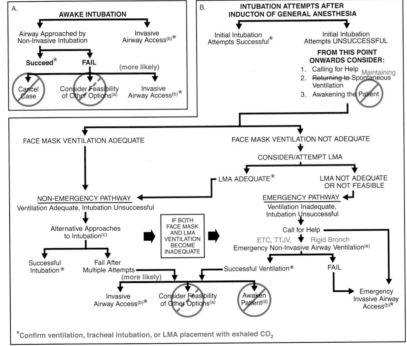

\*Confirm ventilation, tracheal intubation, or LMA placement with exhaled $CO_2$

a. Other options include (but are not limited to): surgery utilizing face mask or LMA anesthesia, local anesthesia infiltration or regional nerve blockade. Pursuit of these options usually implies that mask ventilation will not be problematic. Therefore, these options may be of limited value if this step in the algorithm has been reached via the Emergency Pathway. Judgment required, Rarely appropriate for trauma patients.

b. Invasive airway access includes surgical or percutaneous tracheostomy or cricothyrotomy.

c. Alternative non-invasive approaches to difficult intubation include (but are not limited to): use of different laryngoscope blades, LMA as an intubation

conduit (with or without fiberoptic guidance), fiberoptic intubation (FOB), intubation stylet or tube changer (airway exchange catheter, (AEC) light wand, retrograde intubation, and blind oral or nasal intubation.

d. Consider re-preparation of the patient for awake intubation or canceling surgery. Rarely applicable in the trauma patient.

e. Options for emergency non-invasive airway ventilation include (but are not limited to): rigid bronchoscope (Rigid Bronch), esophageal-tracheal combitube ventilation (ETC), or transtracheal jet ventilation (TTJV).

f. Extubation strategies include: evaluation of the airway with FOB and extubation over an airway exchange catheter (AEC).

**Fig. 148.3**  The 2003 American Society of Anesthesiologists Difficult Airway Algorithm Modified for Trauma. *LMA,* Laryngeal mask airway. (From Wilson WC. Trauma: airway management. *Am Soc Anesthesiol Newslett.* 2005;69(11):10. Reprinted with permission of the American Society of Anesthesiologists, Park Ridge, IL.)

prevention of the rapid desaturation that is often seen in pregnant woman, consideration for the early release of cricoid pressure if difficulty with intubation is encountered, and recommendation for cesarean section if the "can't intubate, can't oxygenate" situation arises.

## PEDIATRIC PATIENTS

In the pediatric population, special considerations include congenital anomalies affecting the airway, acute obstructions such

as a foreign body, infections such as retropharyngeal abscess or croup, and the unanticipated difficult airway. The 2022 ASA Practice Guideline for Management of the Difficult Airway included an algorithm for pediatric airway management.

## EXTUBATION OF THE DIFFICULT AIRWAY

It is critical to also have a plan when facing a potentially difficult extubation. As with intubation, extubation will depend on patient factors, availability of equipment, and provider skills.

The first step is to assess the patient's readiness for extubation and perform the extubation in an appropriate location (i.e., in the operating room). Consider the use of a supraglottic airway as a transition and guide for reintubation if needed, and the risks and benefits of an elective surgical tracheostomy and awake extubation.

## SUGGESTED READINGS

Apfelbaum, J. L., Hagberg, C. A., Connis, R. T., Abdelmalak, B. B., Agarkar, M., Dutton, R. P., et al. (2022). 2022 American Society of Anesthesiologists Practice Guidelines for Management of the Difficult Airway. *Anesthesiology, 136*(1), 31–81.

Detsky, M. E., Jivraj, N., Adhikari, N. K., Friedrich, J. O., Pinto, R., Simel, D. L., et al. (2019). Will this patient be difficult to intubate? The rational clinical examination systematic review. *JAMA, 321*(5), 493–503.

Frerk, C., Mitchell, V., McNarry, A., Mendonca, C., Bhagrath, R., Patel, A., et al. (2015). Difficult Airway Society 2015 guidelines for management of unanticipated difficult intubation in adults. *British Journal of Anaesthesia, 115*, 827–848.

Hagberg, C. A., & Kaslow, O. (2014). Difficult airway management algorithm in trauma updated by COTEP. *ASA Newsletter, 78*(9), 56–60.

Mallampati, S. R., Gatt, S. P., Gugino, L. D., Desai, S. P., Waraksa, B., Freiberger, D., et al. (1985). A clinical sign to predict difficult tracheal intubation: A prospective study. *Canadian Anaesthetists' Society Journal, 32*, 429–434.

Mushambi, M., Kinsella, S., Popat, M., Swales, H., Ramaswamy, K. K., Winton, A. L., et al. (2015). Obstetric Anaesthetists' Association and Difficult Airway Society guideline for the management of difficult and failed tracheal intubation in obstetrics. *Anaesthesia, 70*, 1286–1306.

Ruetzler, K., Guzzella, S., Tscholl, D., Restin, T., Cribari, M., Turan, A., et al. (2017). Blind intubation through self-pressurized, disposable supraglottic airway laryngeal intubation masks: An international, multicenter, prospective cohort study. *Anesthesiology, 127*, 307–316.

Shiga, T., Wajima, Z., Inoue, T., & Sakamoto, A. (2005). Predicting difficult intubation in apparently normal patients: A meta-analysis of bedside screening test performance. *Anesthesiology, 103*, 429–437.

Wilson, W. C. (2005). Trauma: Airway management. *ASA Newsletter, 69*(11), 10.

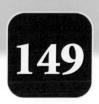

# 149

# Enhanced Recovery Pathways (ERPS)

TONIA M. YOUNG-FADOK, MD, MS, FACS, FASCRS

## History and Development

The concept of improving postoperative recovery was developed in the 1990s by colorectal surgeon and pathophysiologist Henrik Kehlet, who recognized that the body's perception of injury directly controlled surgical stress response. In 2005, he showed that evidence-based interventions aimed at attenuating the neurohormonal response to surgery produced significant and reproducible decreases in morbidity, mortality, and length of stay (LOS) in patients undergoing colorectal operations. All members of the team needed to be involved: anesthesia providers, nurses, and therapists, not only the surgeon. The Enhanced Recovery After Surgery (ERAS) Society was founded in 2001 with the dual aims of providing evidence-based guidelines (Table 149.1 and Box 149.1) and promoting real-time feedback regarding outcomes, to recognize and address areas of concern. This differed from early publications on "fast-track" surgery, a term that is now discredited. Manuscripts were sparse on details, fewer than seven elements of the guidelines were incorporated, and readmission rates were predictably high.

## Preoperative Considerations

### PREHOSPITAL PREPARATION

Enhanced recovery protocols should begin preoperatively. Preparation has four major components: preoperative optimization, preoperative nutrition screening, prehabilitation, and patient counseling.

### Preoperative Optimization

Optimization of the patient's physical status should be planned once the decision for surgical intervention is made. The most common modifiable comorbidities include obesity, tobacco intake, excessive alcohol intake, anemia, and hyperglycemia.

The majority of obese patients are capable, with encouragement and motivation, to lose 10 to 20 lb in a 2- to 4-week period before surgery. ERAS guidelines for bariatric surgery recommend calorie-restricted diets for 2 to 4 weeks preoperatively to reduce visceral obesity, and this can be helpful in other abdominal procedures. Improved outcomes in some specialties (e.g., hernia repair, breast reconstruction) are associated with a body mass index (BMI) less than 30.

Tobacco intake is associated with pulmonary complications, postoperative comorbidities, and intensive care unit admission. Although 20% to 30% risk reduction is noted after 4 to 6 weeks of abstinence, reduced carboxyhemoglobin levels can be noted as early as 1 day after quitting. Smokers should receive counseling regarding cessation as early as possible and stop preoperatively for at least 4 weeks to reduce respiratory and wound complications.

Chronic, excessive alcohol intake (>2 units daily for women, >3 for men) has metabolic, nutritional, hematologic, and

| TABLE 149.1 | Guidelines for Pre-, Intra-, and Postoperative Care in Colorectal Surgery: Enhanced Recovery After Surgery Society Recommendations | | |
|---|---|---|---|
| **Item** | **Recommendations** | **Evidence Level** | **Recommended Grade** |
| **PREADMISSION ITEMS** | | | |
| Preoperative information education and counseling | Patients should routinely receive dedicated preoperative counseling | Moderate | Strong |
| Preoperative optimization | Medical risk assessment | Low | Strong |
| | Smoking and alcohol consumption (alcohol abusers) should be stopped 4 weeks before surgery | Smoking: High | Strong |
| | | Alcohol: Low | Strong |
| | Anemia should be actively identified, investigated, and corrected preoperatively | High | Strong |
| Prehabilitation | Effect on functional capacity | Moderate | Weak |
| | Effect on postoperative outcomes | Low | Weak |
| Preoperative nutritional care | Preoperative screening | Low | Strong |
| | Preoperative nutrition | Moderate | Strong |
| Anemia correction | Screening and treatment | High | Strong |
| | Restricted transfusion practice | High | Strong |
| **PREOPERATIVE ITEMS** | | | |
| Prevention of PONV | Multimodal PONV prophylaxis | High | Strong |
| | Rescue with different drug class | High | Strong |
| Preanesthetic medication | Avoid routine sedative medication | Moderate | Strong |
| Thromboembolism prophylaxis (not in current guidelines) | Patients at risk of VTE should receive prophylaxis with either LMWH or heparin, commenced preoperatively, combined with mechanical methods | High (Preoperative administration: moderate) | Strong |
| | Patients should be advised to consider stopping HRT or consider alternative preparations before surgery | Low | Weak |
| | Patients should discontinue oral contraception before surgery and switch to another form | High | Strong |
| Antimicrobial prophylaxis and skin preparation | IV antibiotics (cephalosporin and metronidazole) within 60 minutes before skin incision | High | Strong |
| | Performed (if necessary) with clippers | None | None |
| | Chlorhexidine-alcohol–based skin preparation | High | Strong |
| Bowel preparation | MBP alone has no clinical advantage | High | Strong |
| | Combined MBP and oral antibiotics | Low | Weak |
| Preoperative fasting and carbohydrate drink | Adherence to fasting guidelines | High | Strong |
| | CHO drink improves insulin resistance | Moderate | Strong |
| | CHO drink in diabetics | Low | Weak |
| **INTRAOPERATIVE ITEMS** | | | |
| Standard anesthetic protocol | Short-acting anesthetic agents | Low | Strong |
| | A ventilation strategy using tidal volumes of 5–7 mL/kg with a PEEP of 4–6 cm $H_2O$ should be used to reduce postoperative pulmonary complications (old guidelines) | Moderate | Strong |
| | Cerebral monitoring | High | Strong |
| | Reduce intraabdominal pressure with neuromuscular block | Low | Weak |
| | Monitor level and reversal of neuromuscular block | High | Strong |
| Minimally invasive surgery | Recommended when possible | High | Strong |
| Pelvic and peritoneal drains | No effect and clinical outcome and should not be used routinely | High | Strong |
| Nasogastric intubation | Routine nasogastric intubation should be avoided. Orogastric tubes during surgery: should be removed before reversal of anesthesia | High | Strong |
| Preventing intraoperative hypothermia | Prewarming | Moderate | Strong |
| | Maintenance of normothermia | High | |
| | Monitoring of temperature | High | |

| TABLE 149.1 | Guidelines for Pre-, Intra-, and Postoperative Care in Colorectal Surgery: Enhanced Recovery After Surgery Society Recommendations—cont'd | | |
|---|---|---|---|
| **Item** | **Recommendations** | **Evidence Level** | **Recommended Grade** |
| Perioperative fluid management | Perioperative near-zero fluid balance<br>Goal-directed fluid therapy | High<br>High | Strong<br>Strong in high-risk patients and large fluid losses<br>Weak in low-risk patients and low-risk surgery |
| **POSTOPERATIVE ITEMS** | | | |
| Postoperative analgesia | Avoid opioids, apply multimodal analgesia, in combination with blocks when indicated | Moderate | Strong |
| | Thoracic epidural analgesia | High: in laparotomy<br>Moderate: not used in laparoscopy | High<br>High (not used) |
| | Spinal analgesia, option for laparoscopic surgery | Moderate | Strong |
| | Lidocaine infusion reduces opioid use | High | Strong |
| | Abdominal wall blocks reduce opioid use | Moderate | Strong |
| Postoperative thromboprophylaxis | Stockings/SCDs in hospital<br>LMWH<br>LMWH, longer duration (28 days for high-risk patients) | High<br>High<br>Low | Strong<br>Weak<br>Strong |
| Postoperative fluid and electrolyte therapy | "Net zero" fluid balance<br>Balanced salt solutions, not 0.9%<br>Maintenance: hypotonic crystalloids | High<br>Low<br>Low | Strong<br>Strong<br>Strong |
| Urinary drainage | Low risk: remove POD 1<br>Moderate/high risk for retention: up to 3 days | High | Strong |
| Prevention of ileus | Multimodal prevention<br>μ-opioid receptor antagonists<br>Bisacodyl, magnesium oxide, coffee | High<br>Moderate<br>Low | Strong<br>Weak<br>Weak |
| Glycemic control | Stress reducing ERAS elements<br>Insulin treatment in ICU<br>Insulin treatment on ward | Moderate<br>Moderate<br>Low | Strong<br>Strong<br>Weak |
| Nutritional care | Early resumption of diet<br>Immunonutrition | Moderate<br>Low | Strong<br>Strong |
| Early mobilization | Early mobilization, discourage bed rest | Moderate | Strong |
| Audit | Collect key outcome and process data; regular feedback | High | Strong |

*CHO,* Carbohydrate; *ERAS,* enhanced recovery after surgery; *HRT,* hormone replacement therapy; *ICU,* intensive care unit; *IV,* intravenous; *LMWH,* low-molecular-weight heparin; *MBP,* mechanical bowel preparation; *PEEP,* positive end-expiratory pressure; *POD,* postoperative day; *PONV,* postoperative nausea and vomiting; *SCD,* sequential compression device; *VTE,* venous thromboembolism.
Adapted from Gustafsson UO, Scott MJ, Hubner M, et al. Guidelines for perioperative care in elective colorectal surgery: Enhanced Recovery After Surgery (ERAS®) Society recommendations: 2018. *World J Surg.* 2019;43:659–695.

neurologic consequences. Although evidence regarding its effect on perioperative morbidity are moderate, ERAS guidelines strongly recommend 4 weeks of preoperative reduction or abstinence.

Preoperative anemia should be identified. The World Health Organization definition of anemia is a hemoglobin concentration of less than 13 g/dL for men and less than 12 g/dL for women, although recent studies suggest a value of less than 13 g/dL should be considered anemic for all adults. Anemia is common in surgical patients (31% in men and 27% in women), with multiple causes, such as acute or chronic blood loss, vitamin $B_{12}$ or folate deficiency, and anemia of chronic disease. Anemia is a risk factor for postoperative complications and mortality and should be corrected when possible. Perioperative blood transfusion can decrease cancer survival in patients with colorectal cancer and is a risk factor for poor outcomes in liver resection for metastatic colorectal cancer. As perioperative transfusion and erythropoietin-stimulating medications are all associated with risks, anemia should be addressed preoperatively as an outpatient. Oral iron supplements are frequently poorly tolerated, and many patients will not respond, due to either chronic illness or ongoing blood loss. Current versions of intravenous iron are unlikely to cause adverse reactions and are more effective than oral iron in addressing anemia from both iron deficiency and chronic disease.

Poorly controlled diabetes is associated with increased surgical site infections, thromboembolic events, cardiovascular complications, renal insufficiency, and prolonged LOS. Elevated hemoglobin $A_{1c}$ (HbA$_{1c}$) is associated with complications, and current recommendations are to achieve a level less than 8%. The urgency of operative intervention determines whether this can be achieved preoperatively. All patients with diabetes and patients with an elevated random blood glucose should have a HbA$_{1c}$ preoperatively. A value greater than 8% may require referral to a diabetes specialist. Intraoperatively, blood glucose levels should be less than 180 mg/dL while avoiding hypoglycemia. Postoperatively, the goal is 80 to

150 mg/dL. In the absence of known gastroparesis or suggestive symptoms, standard fasting guidelines can be applied. Whether or not a preoperative carbohydrate loading drink is beneficial or detrimental is to be determined.

### Preoperative Nutrition Screening

Malnutrition and sarcopenia are common in operative patients. Malnutrition occurs through two main mechanisms: the effect of disease on gastrointestinal (GI) function (e.g., obstruction or inflammation of the GI tract) and by tissue catabolism (e.g., from cancer cachexia). Current practice is to screen all hospitalized patients for malnutrition on admission, but patients should be screened preoperatively to allow intervention if indicated. There are multiple screening tools available. The Malnutrition Universal Screening Tool (MUST) produces a score based on the severity of a low BMI, the percentage of unplanned weight loss over 3 to 6 months, and whether the patient has been acutely ill or will not be able to take oral intake for more than 5 days. A modification of this score is the Peri-Operative Nutritional Score, which treats the variables of the MUST score as binary variables and adds serum albumin less than 3 g/dL as a parameter. Patients with a BMI less than 20, weight loss greater than 10%, and 50% reduction in oral intake or low albumin should be referred for nutritional assessment and intervention. Serum markers alone are not a reliable screening tool.

Sarcopenia is a generalized loss of skeletal muscle mass, strength, and function. It is associated with poor outcomes after major surgery. Sarcopenia is not detected by nutritional screening questionnaires but requires functional testing, such as measurement of gait speed and hand grip strength. Patients with impaired muscle function on these two measures can then undergo further assessment. Computed tomographic imaging is under evaluation as a screening tool for sarcopenia.

### Prehabilitation

Compromised physical status is a risk factor for postoperative complications. Depending on the urgency of an operation, there may be time to address modifiable risk factors. Prehabilitation describes preoperative interventions to increase functional capacity, typically focusing on physical and nutritional approaches. Early studies of intense exercise showed poor compliance, modest improvements in functional capacity, and unclear postoperative

benefit. Subsequent trials using structured prehabilitation protocols, incorporating exercise, protein supplementation, and a focus on compliance have shown improvements in preoperative physiologic reserve and returning to baseline function postoperatively. Other studies have shown an association between an increase in preoperative aerobic capacity after a 4-week prehabilitation program, and a reduction in postoperative complications. The current ERAS guidelines for colorectal surgery do not consider prehabilitation a mandatory item, as these programs are resource intensive and the cadre of patients that they benefit is not clearly defined.

### Patient Counseling

Patient counseling begins at the earliest patient interactions. To increase retention, information can be dispensed in verbal, written, or video formats depending on the patient's learning style. Aside from the standard risk/benefit discussion, the patient should be informed of goals of recovery, and key elements of enhanced recovery protocols, such as the preoperative carbohydrate drink, early feeding, early mobilization, and multimodal pain management.

## PREOPERATIVE MANAGEMENT

### Preoperative Nutrition and Fasting

The American Society of Anesthesiologists guidelines have recommended the 8/6/2-hour rule (fatty foods/light meal/clear liquids) since 1999, but the ingrained dictum of nothing to eat or drink after midnight has been remarkably resistant to change. Patients, however, are often pleasantly surprised to find that they can have clear liquids up until 2 hours before surgery time. A solution of complex carbohydrate and maltodextrin (800 mL on the evening before surgery and 400 mL 2 hours preoperatively) improves preoperative well-being, reduces postoperative insulin resistance with lower insulin requirements, and decreases protein breakdown. A Cochrane review showed a shorter time to passage of flatus and a modest decrease in LOS.

### Bowel Preparation

Mechanical bowel preparation (MBP), in the form of an oral solution, was once performed routinely for most abdominal surgery but is now quite contentious, with different practices in Europe compared with the United States. Early ERAS guidelines recommended avoiding MBP for colonic surgery but acknowledged it might be advantageous in rectal surgery. In a metaanalysis of 36 studies of MBP versus no MBP, the former was not associated with any significant difference in anastomotic leak rate, surgical site infection, mortality, reoperative rate, or LOS. In the absence of any demonstrable advantage of MBP, the guidelines reflected that it could be discontinued, which would avoid side effects of dehydration and electrolyte abnormalities. The use of enemas for rectal surgery was still retained to facilitate a low anastomosis. This recommendation was widely adopted in Europe but less so in the United States.

Avoiding MBP has since been questioned because of large database studies from the United States. Metaanalysis observational data from the American College of Surgeons National Surgical Quality Improvement Program (ACS NSQIP) included 40,446 patients and compared no preparation, MBP alone, oral antibiotic alone, and MBP with oral antibiotics. Oral antibiotic alone was protective of surgical site infection, anastomotic leak, ileus, and major morbidity. Interestingly, combined oral antibiotics and MBP conveyed no benefit over oral antibiotics alone. This differed from a metaanalysis of 23 randomized controlled trials (RCTs) and 8 cohort studies of 63,432 patients, which demonstrated that systemic antibiotic alone produced a reduction in surgical site infections versus oral antibiotics alone. The addition of oral antibiotics to MBP in conjunction with systemic antibiotics significantly reduced the instance of surgical site infection.

The most recent guidelines indicate that MBP with systemic antibiotics has no clinical advantage and should not be routinely used. It was also noted that there is some evidence from RCTs to support a combination of MBP and oral antibiotics, and in the United States this would be in addition to intravenous antibiotics, which are a standard part of surgical site infection prevention.

### Postoperative Nausea and Vomiting Prophylaxis

Prevention of postoperative nausea and vomiting (PONV) is a fundamental aspect of a smooth recovery. It can affect up to 50% of patients and is multifactorial, with patient-related, anesthesia-related, and surgery-related factors. Patient factors are female gender and past history of PONV or motion sickness. The risk associated with volatile anesthetic gases and nitrous oxide can be ameliorated with total intravenous anesthesia (TIVA) and minimizing opioids. The type and duration of the operation and GI pathology are also factors.

Optimal PONV prophylaxis should start preoperatively. A preoperative carbohydrate loading drink may help minimize symptoms. A scoring system for predicting PONV should guide how many prophylactic medications to use, with a simple guide that the number of medications should be the same or one greater than the number of risk factors. A multimodal approach employing selections from the different classes of antiemetic drugs, both first line (e.g., dopamine antagonists, serotonin antagonists, corticosteroids) and second line (e.g., antihistamines, motility agents such as metoclopramide), is encouraged. Additional medications such as gabapentin and pregabalin do reduce PONV, but side effects limit their use. A neurokinin-1 antagonist is used in high-risk patients, although extensive use has been constrained by expense concerns; in high-risk patients, the expense is justified as it is outweighed by the cost of a prolonged LOS. If nausea or vomiting occur despite prophylaxis, salvage therapy should include different classes of drugs from those already used.

## Intraoperative Interventions

### MINIMIZING SURGICAL STRESS

The aim behind the ERAS intraoperative protocol is to minimize stress. Some of the measures to achieve this are under the purview of the surgical team, and others are managed by the anesthesia team.

The surgical team may use preemptive local anesthetic by infiltration, nerve block, or plane block before making the incision or shortly afterward. Minimally invasive procedures, whether endoscopic, laparoscopic, or robotic, all minimize the length of the incision, with a decrease in inflammatory markers, surgical pain, and metabolic catabolism in addition to improved pulmonary hygiene, reduced paralytic ileus, shorter recovery, and decreased LOS. Minimizing the use of drains intraoperatively is encouraged where possible. In laparoscopic and robotic cases, using the lowest pneumoperitoneal pressure that allows adequate working space reduces postoperative pain. Studies of warmed and humidified carbon dioxide for the pneumoperitoneum have shown mixed results, but it is widely used.

### ANESTHETIC PROTOCOL

Maintaining normothermia ($\geq$36°C) is important. Even mild hypothermia increases blood loss and blood transfusion rates

in addition to vasoconstriction, increased afterload, myocardial ischemia, arrhythmias, reduced splanchnic blood flow, and reduced drug biotransformation. Postoperatively, it is associated with increased infection rates. Prevention begins in the preoperative area with the use of forced-air warming blankets. The forced-air warming blanket must be disconnected for transport to the operating room, but it should be reconnected and active warming resumed as soon as possible to minimize the drop in core temperature that can occur with induction. Reliable and accurate temperature-monitoring techniques should be used.

Avoiding benzodiazepines and using short-acting general anesthetic agents allow rapid awakening. The use of intraoperative opioids should be minimized, and if used, short-acting opioids are preferred. Using propofol for TIVA and avoiding prolonged use of nitrous oxide also reduces the risk of PONV.

Cerebral function monitoring using bispectral index reduces risk of awareness in high-risk patients and avoids overdose of anesthetic agents in the elderly, reducing the risk of postoperative delirium and cognitive dysfunction, which is increasingly being recognized as a significant problem in elderly patients.

Many operations require the use of muscle relaxants, and neuromuscular monitoring is the standard of care. In laparoscopic and robotic cases, providing deep muscle relaxation may allow use of a lower pressure for the pneumoperitoneum, but optimizing this approach requires excellent communication between the anesthesia and surgical teams. Decreasing the intraabdominal pressure below 10 to 12 mm Hg may reduce the adverse physiologic effects of pneumoperitoneum. Reversal of neuromuscular blockade to a train-of-four ratio of 90% is important to avoid residual paralysis and postoperative pulmonary complications.

Intravenous fluid therapy should maintain intravascular volume, cardiac output, and tissue perfusion while avoiding fluid and salt overload. Intraoperative fluid management trials have become increasingly confusing, with terms such as *liberal fluid use* and *restrictive fluid use* without clear and consistent definitions. Current guidelines indicate a preference for the term *goal-directed fluid therapy* (GDFT). At the beginning of the case, with minimally invasive devices monitoring cardiac output, patients are optimized on the individual Frank-Starling curve using goal-directed boluses of intravenous solution, usually colloid, and then using GDFT to determine the maintainance rate of crystalloid during the procedure. A metaanalysis of 23 studies with almost 2100 patients in either traditional or ERAS programs showed that, overall, GDFT was associated with a significant reduction in morbidity, LOS, and time to bowel function. When analyzed by setting, patients managed within an enhanced recovery pathway showed only reduction in intensive care LOS and time to bowel function compared with significant reductions in overall morbidity and total hospital LOS if managed in a traditional care setting. Hence, GDFT can likely be used selectively for high-risk patients and high-risk procedures.

The current recommendation is to avoid perioperative weight gain of more than 2.5 kg with the goal of perioperative near-zero fluid balance. GDFT is recommended for high-risk patients and for operations with large intravascular fluid loss. Vasopressors are used for hypertension if fluid boluses do not improve stroke volume by 10% or more.

### PAIN MANAGEMENT

Pain management is a primary principle of enhanced recovery. Excellent pain control requires a preemptive and multimodal, opioid-sparing strategy to combat postoperative pain. A common preoperative protocol included preemptive acetaminophen, with or without concomitant cyclooxygenase-2 inhibitors or other nonsteroidal antiinflammatory drugs (NSAIDs), in combination with γ-aminobutyric acid analogs for neuropathic pain. More recently, however, gabapentin has been removed because of the risk of sedation and falls, especially in the elderly. Aside from traditional intraoperative opioids (which should be short-acting and minimized), adjunctive medications such as steroids and α-2 adrenoceptor agonists have shown potential. Additional intraoperative techniques include local anesthetic infusions, and boluses or infusions of ketamine and/or magnesium (both N-methyl-D-aspartate receptor antagonists) have demonstrated decreased postoperative pain and ileus. β-Blockers such as esmolol are another area of research.

Regional anesthetics including subarachnoid, epidural, and local anesthesia inhibit or reduce transmission of the initial surgical noxious stimuli. This can limit cortisol, catecholamines, and inflammatory markers and avoid the catabolic state, insulin resistance, and fluid retention. ERAS pathways encourage regional anesthesia when possible. Early guidelines recommended thoracic epidural for abdominal procedures to reduce postoperative ileus and decrease opioid use. This was removed from recent guidelines after evidence that thoracic epidural appears to prolong LOS in patients undergoing laparoscopic colorectal procedures.

The desire to limit opioids has prompted surgeons in addition to anesthesiologists to perform regional blocks. Surgeons use transversus abdominis plane (TAP), transversalis fascia, subcostal, and rectus blocks, with the TAP block best performed under ultrasound guidance, as the "two-click" laparoscopic TAP block is deposited in the correct plane less than 25% of the time. Anesthesiologists are adding paravertebral and other blocks to their repertoire.

## Postoperative Management

The primary goal of the postoperative period is to facilitate expedited recovery. This is best achieved with communication of the anticipated timeline of recovery, with as many facets as possible of the protocol being encapsulated within order sets, to maximize compliance. Good outcomes require excellent teamwork involving nursing staff, allied health staff, trainees such as residents and fellows, and, of course, the patient.

## MULTIMODAL ANALGESIA

Opioid sparing is associated with early mobilization, return of bowel function, fewer complications, and reduced LOS. Using multiple pain-reducing medications minimizes opioids and avoids their side effects. Scheduled acetaminophen and NSAIDs are commonly used. Some institutions have protocols that allow for lidocaine or ketamine infusions postoperatively. The intraoperative use of long-acting local anesthetics for blocks also assists with pain management for up to 72 hours postoperatively. Although epidurals are less frequently used postoperatively, intraoperative spinal anesthesia with a combination of local anesthetic and long-acting opioid reduces morphine requirements postoperatively for approximately 24 hours allowing early mobilization.

## EARLY FEEDING

Patients can drink liquids once awake and without nausea. An oral diet can often be started on postoperative day 0 or the morning of day 1, and intravenous fluids can be discontinued.

## AUDIT

The monitoring of outcomes is another central principle of enhanced recovery, as audit is vital to improve outcomes. In the United States, the American College of Surgeons runs the ACS NSQIP, which involves several hundred hospitals collecting sample outcome data across all surgical specialties. This has resulted in a large database that is a resource for outcomes research. It does have limitations in that not all hospitals can afford to participate, a sample is taken of surgical patients rather than including all of them, and the data are reported at intervals and are not available in real time.

The ERAS Society had previously developed an online data and analytic system that allows data on all chosen subjects to be entered, and the data are available online. The database reports outcomes data, collects information that tracks the adequacy of surgical processes, and calculates compliance with the protocol. All this information is available in real time for timely feedback to all members of the team.

## SUGGESTED READINGS

Baimas-George, M., Cochran, A., Watson, M., Murphy, K. J., Iannitti, D., Martinie, J. B., et al. (2020). Vertical Compliance: A novel method of reporting patient specific ERAS compliance for real-time risk assessment. *International Journal of Medical Informatics*, 141, 104194.

Ban, K. A., Gibbons, M. M., Ko, C. Y., Wick, E. C., Cannesson, M., Scott, M. J., et al. (2019). Evidence review conducted for the agency for healthcare research and quality safety program for improving surgical care and recovery: Focus on anesthesiology for colorectal surgery. *Anesthesia & Analgesia*, 128(5), 879–889.

Dort, J. C., Farwell, D. G., Findlay, M., Huber, G. F., Kerr, P., Shea-Budgell, M. A., et al. (2017). Optimal perioperative care in major head and neck cancer surgery with free flap reconstruction: A consensus review and recommendations from the enhanced recovery after surgery society. *JAMA Otolaryngology Head & Neck Surgery*, 143(3), 292–303.

Elsarrag, M., Soldozy, S., Patel, P., Norat, P., Sokolowski, J. D., Park, M. S., et al. (2019). Enhanced recovery after spine surgery: A systematic review. *Neurosurgical Focus*, 46(4), E3.

ERAS® Society Guidelines. Retrieved from https://erassociety.org/guidelines/. Accessed March, 2022.

Gustafsson, U. O., Scott, M. J., Hubner, M., Nygren, J., Demartines, N., Francis, N., et al. (2019). Guidelines for perioperative care in elective colorectal surgery: Enhanced Recovery After Surgery (ERAS®) Society recommendations: 2018. *World Journal of Surgery*, 43, 659–695.

New York School of Regional Anesthesia (NYSORA). *Thoracic and Abdominal Wall Blocks*. Retrieved fom https://www.nysora.com/techniques/truncal-and-cutaneous-blocks/. Accessed March, 2022.

Peden, C. J., Aggarwal, G., Aitken, R. J., Anderson, I. D., Bang Foss, N., Cooper, Z., et al. (2021). Guidelines for perioperative care for emergency laparotomy Enhanced Recovery After Surgery (ERAS) Society recommendations: Part 1—preoperative: Diagnosis, rapid assessment and optimization. *World Journal of Surgery*, 45, 1272–1290.

Tinguely, P., Morare, N., Ramirez-Del Val, A., Berenguer, M., Niemann, C. U., Pollok, J. M., et al. (2021). Enhanced recovery after surgery programs improve short-term outcomes after liver transplantation-A systematic review and meta-analysis. *Clinical Transplantation*, 35(11), e14453.

# Anesthesia for Unique Situations

# 150

# Anesthesia During a Pandemic

NARJEET KHURMI, MD

## Introduction

In December 2019, a pneumonia-like illness of unknown origin befell residents of Wuhan in Hubei Province, China. Within several days, Chinese scientists identified the virus as a member of the Coronaviridae, viruses that can infect humans and other animals. The name of the virus evolved from 2019-nCoV to severe acute respiratory syndrome–related coronavirus 2 (SARS-CoV-2) to coronavirus disease 2019 (COVID-19). According to the World Health Organization (WHO), the first confirmed case in the United States was identified on January 20, 2020. Based on prior experience with severe acute respiratory syndrome (SARS) in 2002 and Middle East respiratory syndrome (MERS) in 2012, considerable concern for the safety of health care workers is warranted. During the SARS outbreak, WHO data showed that 21% of infected people (globally) were health care workers. Furthermore, Canadian data from the SARS outbreak revealed 43% of SARS cases were health care providers. Because of continued mutations of the COVID-19 virus and persistent community prevalence, hospitals are obligated to remain vigilant and maintain appropriate plans and protocols to care for these patients while protecting the safety of health care providers.

Pandemic preparedness to maintain safe surgical and anesthesia practices requires centralized coordination. Health care facilities must address capacity concerns during a pandemic with efforts to match capacity to community prevalence of the disease. Deliberate coordination with local and state authorities is needed to ensure that hospitals can safely treat all patients requiring hospitalization without resorting to crisis standards of care. Regular assessment to ensure sufficient intensive care unit (ICU) and non-ICU beds, personal protective equipment (PPE), testing reagents and supplies, anesthetic drugs, medical and surgical supplies, ventilators, and trained staff to treat patients seeking surgical care is critical to ensuring maximal patient and staff safety. During a pandemic, optimal and timely forecasting is necessary to pursue an elective surgical practice that requires postoperative inpatient beds. Daily assessment by hospital and surgical/perioperative leadership is essential to pursue elective surgical care when hospital capacity becomes concerning.

## Supply Chain

Supply chain disruptions can rapidly lead to low levels of essential components of a surgical and anesthesia practice. One should ensure suppliers are able to meet the demands of the health care facility before committing to busier surgical schedules. Collaborating with other health care organizations, the U.S. Food and Drug Administration (FDA), and local, state, and federal governments to mitigate shortages of essential drugs, PPE, and medical/surgical equipment may be needed. Facilities

should take advantage of times of lower pandemic activity and make deliberate efforts to stockpile essential equipment such as PPE, medications, and testing materials. Minimizing medication waste helps avoid using nonpreferred agents that practitioners are less familiar with, that are less effective, and that may have more side effects. When a supply chain disruption is identified that results in critical shortages of PPE, one can consider options for health care providers to obtain and wear their personal, facility-approved PPE during times of PPE shortages.

## COVID-19 Testing

Pandemic-related testing is a crucial component of maintaining a safe anesthesia practice. One should determine with laboratory leadership an optimal timeline for presurgical testing that substantially reduces the risk of inadvertent infection to caregivers by asymptomatic patients. Knowledge of test accuracy, specificity, and sensitivity along with expected turnaround time for test results play a role in establishing the timeline for presurgical testing. If a nonreassuring test result or no test result is available, a protocol to proceed with nonelective surgery should be established, which includes implementation of evidence-based infection prevention and use of all appropriate pandemic-related PPE.

## Personal Protective Equipment

To keep patients and staff safe during a pandemic, it is essential to obtain adequate levels of PPE for the practice.

### N95 RESPIRATORS

An N95 respirator is a facemask that can effectively filter airborne microbial particles down to 0.3 microns, including bacteria and viruses (95% of time). For the N95 masks to be optimally effective, achieving an adequate seal to the face is essential. Manufacturers, U.S. regulatory agencies, and health care facilities require that health care workers undergo an annual fit test. Importantly, people with facial hair may be unable to achieve a proper fit. Therefore the N95 may not provide full protection in individuals with beards, goatees, or mustaches.

All FDA-cleared N95 respirators are labeled as "single-use, disposable devices." Policies for extended use and reuse of PPE should comply with Centers for Disease Control and Prevention (CDC) and FDA recommendations. The N95 mask can be reused by the same employee if covered with a surgical mask or full-length face shield. The surgical mask should be discarded at room exit or PPE doffing. A full-length polycarbonate face shield may be reused if appropriately cleaned and disinfected with hospital-grade disinfectant. N95 masks can be reused over multiple shifts if intact, free of damage and visible soil, and still able to pass a fit check. One should store the N95 mask in a clean and protected area (e.g., a paper bag labeled with the employee's name or a plastic container with a few holes in the lid to allow for air circulation).

If the N95 mask is reused over multiple shifts while maintaining its integrity, a new paper bag should be used for storage. When redonning, use clean gloves before removing the facemask from the bag, while applying to the face, and during the fit check. Discard gloves after donning N95 and reapply clean gloves. Other PPE that can be reused include glasses/goggles for eye protection, controlled air purifying respirators (CAPRs) and powered air purifying respirators (PAPRs). Gowns and gloves should be single-use only. Protocols for resterilization and decontamination should follow CDC and FDA emergency use authorizations. These respirators can be resterilized and reused. This is feasible by several methods, such as repeated thermal disinfection, ultraviolet illumination, irradiation, or hydrogen peroxide vapor exposure.

## CONTROLLED AIR PURIFYING RESPIRATORS AND POWERED AIR PURIFYING RESPIRATORS

A CAPR is a helmet with face shield respirator that can filter large and small particulates (0.04–0.06 μm) with higher efficiency (99.97%). The high-efficiency particulate air (HEPA) filter in the device has a National Institute of Occupational Safety and Health (NIOSH)–defined filter efficiency of N100, which indicates filtration of 99.97% of airborne particles 0.3 μm and larger. The CAPR is composed of four elements: (1) a helmet with power cord, (2) a battery, (3) a belt, and (4) a charger. There are no belt-mounted hoses or blower units, as seen with PAPRs. The filter cartridge is housed within the helmet, which can be sized for optimal fit. A switch on the helmet regulates airflow. The full-face shield is first attached to the helmet at three connection points. The face shield is then pulled toward the face and the elastic membrane is wrapped around the face to create a tight seal.

A PAPR is an alternate helmet with face shield respirator with filtration efficiencies similar to the CAPR. The essential components include a full-face piece, a battery-operated blower, and a HEPA filter. The blower pushes contaminated air through the HEPA filter before supplying clean air into the contained helmet and face piece. PAPRs are approved for use in the operating room or other venues where a sterile field is maintained. CAPRs are not approved for this environment and should be used in ICU, endoscopy, and other areas where maintaining a sterile environment is not required. Reuse of PAPR and CAPR face shields is encouraged by wiping them down using hospital-grade cleaning wipes. Any streaking that results can be wiped off using soap and water.

## TRAINING OF STAFF

Staff should receive proper training with donning and doffing of PPE. This can be achieved by web-based educational videos, written recommendations from CDC, and live and recorded simulation and educational sessions created by members of the perioperative staff. Many health care workers self-contaminate during the doffing process. Frequent hand hygiene, especially before and after donning and doffing, is expected. Efforts to conserve PPE should be routine.

## Managing the Surgical Schedule

Surgical case scheduling and prioritization are best coordinated by a committee made up of surgical, anesthesia, and nursing leadership. Hospital capacity concerns should be discussed daily when deciding to proceed with elective surgery that will result in a postoperative admission. Prioritizing cases using a tiered system is useful to gain some semblance of order in a chaotic situation. Patients in the higher priority levels include those needing cardiac, cancer, and trauma surgery and any other cases where a delay of 15 to 30 days would result in worsening of patient's condition or lead to worse surgical outcomes.

Surgical preparation can be divided into four phases: preoperative, intraoperative, postoperative, and discharge. In the preoperative setting an anesthesiology-led preoperative assessment team should be established. Use of telemedicine is advocated when preoperative patient access to the hospital is limited. If there is a delay in surgery from time of initial evaluation, have a mechanism in place for appropriate and timely reevaluation, either face-to-face or via telemedicine. During this phase, it is important to assess for appropriate postoperative disposition and if the facility has capacity when a postoperative admission is anticipated.

Relevant pandemic-related preoperative testing should be obtained per established institutional protocols. If a patient has a pandemic-related illness, it is crucial to have a huddle with the operating room (OR) team and surgeon before bringing the patient to the OR. The intraoperative phase should see limited personnel in the operating room. All anesthesia personnel should use appropriate PPE given the proximity to the patient and increased risk of exposure and infection. The anesthesia team should lean on standardized protocols to optimize length of stay, improve efficiencies, and reduce complications.

Postoperative care starts with complying with appropriate isolation needs for patient in the postanesthesia care unit (PACU). One should mimic the patient's preoperative isolation needs in the PACU. Continue with standardized protocols to optimize length of stay, improve efficiencies, and reduce complications. Ensure staff and equipment are in adequate supply for post-PACU disposition (ICU and non-ICU). A postoperative environmental sanitation and decontamination protocol should be in place that is endorsed by the hospital infection prevention and control (IPAC) group. Discharge planning involves ensuring that the appropriate postacute care facility is available. Discharge to home is ideal, if possible, as it is likely safer than a skilled nursing facility or nursing home because there is less exposure to pandemic organisms and viruses. Telemedicine may be used for follow-up and continued patient education.

## The Next Pandemic

Drawing on prior and current local, national, and international experience during epidemics and pandemics including SARS, MERS, and COVID-19, one can better estimate the needs of the perioperative and surgical workplace to safely treat patients during the next pandemic. By consulting with hospital leadership and IPAC, one can determine the availability and appropriate use of scarce PPE to maintain the highest level of protection for all staff. Routine preprocedural and surgical pandemic testing is critical in the effort to preserve scarce PPE. A deliberate and tiered approach to performing elective and nonelective surgery may be necessary if hospital capacity concerns arise. Staff should be educated and trained on appropriate PPE donning and doffing techniques. Perioperative care of patients should involve established protocols to optimize length of stay, improve efficiencies, and reduce complications. Data collection and management is also a needed effort when navigating a pandemic. Facility data that is of high value includes preoperative testing, bed availability, PPE utilization rates, staff exposures, contact tracing, and patient and staff isolation/quarantine policies. Quality metrics, such as mortality, complications, readmission rates, errors, and near misses, are vital in evaluating established processes and the need for revisions to workflows and patient care.

## SUGGESTED READINGS

American Society of Anesthesiologists (ASA). (March 24, 2020). *Joint Statement Recommending a Surgical Review Committee for COVID-19-Related Surgical Triage Decision Making*. Retrieved from https://www.asahq.org/about-asa/newsroom/news-releases/2020/03/joint-statement-recommending-a-surgical-review-committee-for-covid-19-related-surgical-triage-decision-making. Accessed October 31, 2022.

Celina, M. C., Martinez, E., Omana, M. A., Sanchez, A., Wiemann, D., Tezak, M., et al. (2020). Extended use of face masks during the COVID-19 pandemic: Thermal conditioning and spray-on surface disinfection. *Polymer Degradation and Stability, 179*, 109251.

Hegde, S. (2020). Which type of personal protective equipment (PPE) and which method of donning or doffing PPE carries the least risk of infection for healthcare workers? *Evidence-Based Dentistry, 21*(2), 74–76.

Holshue, M. L., DeBolt, C., Lindquist, S., Lofy, K. H., Wiesman, J., Bruce, H., et al. (2020). First case of 2019 novel coronavirus in the United States. *New England Journal of Medicine, 382*(10), 929–936.

Howard, B. E. (2020). High-risk aerosol-generating procedures in COVID-19: Respiratory protective equipment considerations. *Otolaryngology and Head and Neck Surgery, 163*(1), 98–103.

Howard, R. A., Lathrop, G. W., & Powell, N. (2020). Sterile field contamination from powered air-purifying respirators (PAPRs) versus contamination from surgical masks. *American Journal of Infection Control, 48*(2), 153–156.

Huang, C., Wang, Y., Li, X., Ren, L., Zhao, J., Hu, Y., et al. (2020). Clinical features of patients infected with 2019 novel coronavirus in Wuhan, China. *Lancet, 395*(10223), 497–506.

Offeddu, V., Yung, C. F., Low, M. S. F., & Tam, C. C. (2017). Effectiveness of masks and respirators against respiratory infections in healthcare workers: A systematic review and meta-analysis. *Clinical Infectious Diseases, 65*(11), 1934–1942.

Peng, P. W. H., Ho, P. L., & Hota, S. S. (2020). Outbreak of a new coronavirus: what anaesthetists should know. *British Journal of Anaesthesia, 124*(5), 497–501.

Qian, Y., Willeke, K., Grinshpun, S. A., Donnelly, J., & Coffey, C. C. (1998). Performance of N95 respirators: Filtration efficiency for airborne microbial and inert particles. *American Industrial Hygiene Association Journal, 59*(2), 128–132.

# 151

# Monitored Anesthesia Care

SARAH K. ARMOUR, MD   |   TRYGVE K. ARMOUR, MD

The continuum of sedation as defined by the American Society of Anesthesiologists (ASA) ranges from minimal, to moderate, to deep sedation and finally to general anesthesia (Table 151.1). Categories are based upon the patient's responsiveness to various stimuli, ability to maintain a patent airway with adequate ventilation, and degree of hemodynamic stability. With the shift toward more minimally invasive and endovascular approaches, the number of procedures performed under sedation as opposed to general anesthesia is increasing, and therefore understanding of this continuum is important. The most critical differentiation is made between moderate and deep sedation, with the latter requiring additional training to manage patients safely.

Patients undergoing sedation may be managed in one of two ways. In the single-provider model, a proceduralist may supervise both the sedation and procedure being performed. The sedation may be performed by a nurse or by the proceduralist themselves; however, neither of them requires special anesthesia training to do so. Most institutions mandate that such a model be used only in situations where at most moderate sedation will be required. Thus the proceduralist or sedation nurse must be able to identify and rescue patients who unintentionally transition to deeper planes of anesthesia. The quantity and variety of sedating medications are also typically restricted by institutional policy.

Monitored anesthesia care (MAC) is an alternative to the single-provider model that does not place a restriction on the level of sedation. Instead, MAC refers to a collection of services that may be delivered by a separate skilled anesthesia provider during procedures where any level of sedation is required. The services include diagnosis and management of respiratory and/or cardiovascular compromise that can occur with moderate (or even minimal) levels of sedation and, most importantly, the option of converting to a general anesthetic if necessary. Careful periprocedural evaluation, monitoring, and management are also included in MAC.

| TABLE 151.1 Continuum of Depth of Sedation | | | | |
|---|---|---|---|---|
| | **Minimal Sedation** | **Moderate Sedation** | **Deep Sedation** | **General Anesthesia** |
| Responsiveness | Normal verbal stimulation sufficient | Verbal or nonpainful tactile stimulation needed | Repeated verbal or painful tactile stimulation needed | Unarousable |
| Airway | No intervention required | At most mild impairment; no intervention required | May be impaired; intervention often required | Intervention required |
| Spontaneous ventilation | No intervention required | At most mild impairment; no intervention required | May be impaired; intervention often required | Intervention required |
| Hemodynamics | Unaffected | Within 20% of baseline | May be >20% from baseline; intervention may be required | May be >20% from baseline; intervention may be required |

Adapted from Quality Management and Departmental Administration Committee, American Society of Anesthesiologists. Approved October 1999, amended October 2014.

| TABLE 151.2 Common Intravenous Agents Used in Monitored Anesthesia Care | | |
|---|---|---|
| **Agent** | **Common Intravenous Dose for Moderate Sedation** | **Common Side Effects** |
| Fentanyl | 0.5–1.5 mcg/kg per bolus dose | Respiratory depression, nausea/vomiting, constipation, and pruritis |
| Midazolam | 1–5 mg/kg | Respiratory depression (synergistic with fentanyl), amnesia |
| Propofol | 25–100 mcg/kg/min | Respiratory depression, hypotension, pain with injection |
| Ketamine | 0.1–0.5 mcg/kg/min | Hallucinations, increased oropharyngeal secretions |
| Dexmedetomidine | 1 mcg/kg loading dose 0.2–1.5 mcg/kg/hr | Bradycardia, hypotension |
| Remifentanil | 0.05–0.2 mcg/kg/min | Hyperalgesia |
| Remimazolam | 5-mg load over 1 min, then 2.5 mg every 2 min Reduce load to 2.5–5 mg, then 1.25- to 2.5-mg doses for ASA III/IV | |

Not every patient is an appropriate candidate for the single-provider model, and not every patient is appropriate for MAC. Patients with a known or suspected difficult airway, those who cannot be reliably expected to cooperate or tolerate minimal doses of sedating or local anesthetic medications (e.g., those with medication allergies, chronic opioid or benzodiazepine use, or complex cardiovascular or pulmonary disease), may not be candidates for the single-provider model. Depending on the complexity of these issues, MAC may not be adequate. It is therefore critical that each patient be carefully evaluated before any procedure where sedation will be performed. The depth of sedation required to achieve both optimal procedural conditions and patient comfort and satisfaction must also be considered.

MAC begins with a careful and complete preanesthetic evaluation. This includes a review of the patient's medical, surgical, and anesthesia history; current medications; allergies; last oral intake; recent laboratory values; consent for blood transfusion; and a focused physical examination (including at a minimum heart, lungs, and airway). Although typically covered by the surgical consent, a separate consent for general or regional anesthesia may be obtained and relevant risks and benefits of the anesthetic plan should be discussed. Adequate preoperative intravenous access is required.

All equipment needed to convert to a general anesthetic must be present, including airway equipment and an anesthesia workstation. Standard ASA monitors must be used, including capnography. After the procedure, the anesthesia provider must also manage the recovery of the patient and is responsible for deciding when the patient is ready for discharge from the postanesthesia care unit (PACU) or procedural suite. The specific agents used for MAC are typically the same as those used for induction of general anesthesia (Table 151.2). The ideal sedative is easy to use, quickly produces optimal sedation with minimal pain on injection, causes minimal cardiovascular or respiratory depression, and has a short recovery time. Several studies have sought to identify the best agent or combination of agents, but no universally clear patterns have emerged. Propofol, midazolam, and fentanyl are most commonly used, although ketamine, diphenhydramine, dexmedetomidine, and remifentanil are gaining acceptance and utility in particular patient scenarios. Remimazolam is a novel ultra-short-acting benzodiazepine that is emerging as a potential ideal sedative.

Both ketamine and dexmedetomidine have the advantage over propofol and midazolam of producing less respiratory depression. Ketamine, as well, offers greater hemodynamic stability than propofol, although it carries a greater risk of postoperative nausea and vomiting (PONV). Routine use of remifentanil for MAC is limited by the potential development of hyperalgesia. Midazolam and fentanyl in combination have a synergistic effect on respiratory depression and should be used with caution. Dexmedetomidine commonly produces hypotension and bradycardia at doses required for moderate sedation. Remimazolam has many promising characteristics, including minimal hypotension and respiratory depression, rapid onset and recovery, and minimal pain; however, it is so short-acting that it must be frequently redosed or given as an infusion. Several adjunct agents such as nonsteroidal antiinflammatory agents and acetaminophen may also be used as part of MAC.

Compared with general anesthesia, MAC is associated with higher patient satisfaction scores, shorter times to emergence and orientation, decreased PACU times, and decreased time to dismissal from the hospital (for those patients having outpatient procedures). The incidence of PONV is also reduced. A review of the ASA closed claim database showed that MAC performed outside the operating room was more often associated with insufficient oxygenation and ventilation than general anesthesia, and that these cases were more likely to result in patient death. With an ever-increasing focus on the value of health care services, it is also important to consider that MAC carries a significantly higher cost than the sedation model. Improved outcomes to justify the incremental expense, however, have not been universally proven. The single-provider model may be appropriate in many circumstances. The decision as to what model and level of sedation is appropriate for any procedure must depend on careful assessment of both patient and procedural factors.

## SUGGESTED READINGS

American Society of Anesthesiologists Economic Committee. Distinguishing Monitored Anesthesia Care ("MAC") From Moderate Sedation/Analgesia (Conscious Sedation). Approved by the ASA House of Delegates on October 27, 2004, last amended on October 21, 2009, and reaffirmed on October 16, 2013.

American Society of Anesthesiologists Quality Management and Departmental Administration Committee. Continuum of Depth of Sedation:

Definition of General Anesthesia and Levels of Sedation/Analgesia. Approved Oct 1999, amended Oct 2014.

Bayman, E. O., Dexter, F., Laur, J. J., & Wachtel, R. E. (2011). National incidence of use of monitored anesthesia care. *Anesthesia and Analgesia, 113*(1), 165–169.

Checketts, M. R., Alladi, R., Ferguson, K., Gemmell, L., Handy, J. M., Klein, A. A., et al. (2016). Recommendations for standards of monitoring during anaesthesia

and recovery 2015: Association of Anaesthetists of Great Britain and Ireland. *Anaesthesia, 71*(1), 85–93.

Ghisi, D., Fanelli, A., Tosi, M., Nuzzi, M., & Fanelli, G. (2005). Monitored anesthesia care. *Minerva Anestesiologica, 71*, 533–538.

Saunders, R., Struys, M. M. R. F., Pollock, R. F., Mestek, M., & Lightdale, J. R. (2017). Patient safety during procedural sedation using capnography monitoring: A systematic review and meta-analysis. *BMJ Open, 7*(6), e013402.

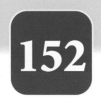

# 152

# Anesthesia for Patients Undergoing Magnetic Resonance Imaging

TASHA L. WELCH, MD

## Magnetic Resonance Imaging Basics

Magnetic resonance images result from the absorption and emission of electromagnetic radiation by atomic nuclei, such as hydrogen atoms, when in the presence of a strong magnetic field. Hydrogen atoms consisting of a single proton are ubiquitous within the human body. The protons become aligned within the magnetic field. A radiofrequency pulse results in a change of the energy state of the protons. Termination of the radiofrequency pulse allows the protons to drift back to their original low-energy state. The transformation back to the low-energy state causes an emission of radiofrequency signals, which are detected within the magnetic resonance imaging (MRI) scanner receiver coil. Digital processing then produces the image.

The magnetic field in MRI is produced by an electric current flowing through a coiled wire that is cooled to a low temperature to provide a low resistance. The magnetic field strength is expressed in gauss and tesla. One tesla (T) is equivalent to 10,000 gauss (G). As a reference, the magnetic field strength of the earth is 0.3 to 0.7 G ($3 \times 10^{-5}$ T to $7 \times 10^{-5}$ T). The magnetic field strength within a clinical MRI scanner is immense and can range from 0.5 T to 9.4 T, with typical clinical scanners having a magnetic field strength of 1.5 to 3.0 T.

## Magnetic Resonance Imaging Safety

*The basic tenet of MRI safety is that the magnet is always on and a magnetic field is always present.* Access to the MRI suite is

| TABLE 152.1 | Safety Zones in the Magnetic Resonance Imaging Environment | | | |
|---|---|---|---|---|
| | **MRI SAFETY ZONES** | | | |
| | **Zone I** | **Zone II** | **Zone III** | **Zone IV** |
| Definition | Areas freely accessible to the public | Interface between unregulated area of Zone I and strictly controlled Zones III and IV | Area near the magnet room<br>Magnetic fields sufficiently strong to present harm to patients and personnel | Room containing the MR scanner<br>Highest exposure to magnetic field |
| Restrictions | None | Unscreened patients to undergo MRI | Access strictly restricted<br>Screened patients to undergo MRI<br>Approved MR personnel | Access strictly restricted<br>Screened patients undergoing MRI under direct supervision by MR personnel |
| Additional Information | Outside the MRI environment | Ferromagnetic items remain in this area<br>Potential anesthetizing location<br>Resuscitation and anesthetic equipment may be left here | Access to Zone IV<br>Potential anesthetizing location<br>Approved resuscitation and anesthetic equipment may be left here | Ferromagnetic objects are strictly excluded |

*MR,* Magnetic resonance; *MRI,* magnetic resonance imaging.

regulated by the U.S. Food and Drug Administration. The American College of Radiology has defined a series of four safety zones (Zones I–IV) with increasing magnetic field exposure, potential safety concerns, and access restrictions (Table 152.1). Fig. 152.1 is a schematic illustrating the safety zone of an MRI facility.

One of the main safety concerns is that nearby ferromagnetic objects can be attracted to the magnetic field. These objects can act as projectiles and cause injury to patients in the bore of the MRI scanner and staff working in the MRI setting. Ferromagnetic objects can cause irreversible damage to the MRI scanner itself. Anesthetic equipment (e.g., intravenous [IV] infusion pumps, IV poles, anesthesia machines) often contains ferromagnetic components and is not exempt from becoming a projectile. In the event of an injury (e.g., a patient is pinned by the projectile) or emergency, the magnet can be shut down. A magnet shutdown (i.e., a "quench") can be completed by the MRI technician. If the MRI must be quenched, the patient and all personnel should leave the scan room because of the risk for hypothermia and hypoxia.

Gadolinium-based contrast may be needed for enhancement of MRI scans. Gadolinium-based agents are not considered nephrotoxic in typical doses. As with any contrast material, a potential for allergic reactions exists. The frequency of adverse reactions is estimated to be 0.07%–2.4% with severe life-threatening reactions very rare (0.001%–0.01%). Patients with prior reactions to gadolinium are at higher risk of having a subsequent reaction. If a patient with a known allergy necessitates contrast administration, premedication with steroids and antihistamines should be considered.

## Monitors and Equipment Compatibility

During anesthetics performed in the MRI setting, all monitors must be MRI compatible and used according to manufacturer's guidelines. In addition to requiring MRI-compatible monitors, the noise in the MRI setting necessitates visual and usual audio alarms. Anesthesia providers must also have visual access to all vital sign monitors and the ability to view the patient directly through a window, with a video camera, or both.

Special care must be taken when arranging the wires and cables of the monitors. Direct contact of wires or cables with the patient's skin can produce electric currents due to electromagnetic induction, which can cause patient burns. Precordial electrocardiogram (ECG), typically used as conventional ECG, will not function properly unless precordial leads are placed close together on the chest to minimize distortion of the signal by the magnetic field. Because of this placement, precordial ECG leads may less reliably monitor ST segments for detection of myocardial ischemia. Standard pulse oximeters are not compatible with the MRI environment. Therefore only an MRI-compatible fiberoptic pulse oximeter should be used. Patients who are critically ill may necessitate the use of an arterial line. Note the strain gauge transducer is MRI compatible, but clamps and other devices used to secure the transducer to a pole may not be compatible. Radiofrequency pulses from the MRI may cause artifact in the arterial waveform and an erroneous pressure reading.

## Anesthetic Management

A preanesthetic evaluation must be completed by the anesthesiologist. The MRI technician must ensure that the patient has no contraindication to entering the MRI environment. The patient should not be premedicated or anesthetized before this assessment. Several anesthetic techniques have been successfully used in the MRI environment, including sedation, monitored anesthesia care, and general anesthesia. Given the remote location of the patient and the potential for motion artifact associated with sedation, general anesthesia is often selected.

Induction of anesthesia often occurs in a separate location from the MRI scanner. A separate anesthetizing location (Zone II) allows for non-MRI-compatible equipment (e.g., fiberoptic bronchoscope, videolaryngoscope) to be used during induction. After induction, the patient is transferred into Zone IV and into the scanner. In this zone, only MRI-compatible equipment is allowed and should be used. After the anesthetic, a postanesthesia recovery unit must be available to recover patients from the MRI suite.

## Unique Considerations

MRI is often the imaging modality of choice to evaluate back pain. It is not uncommon for patients with severe pain that

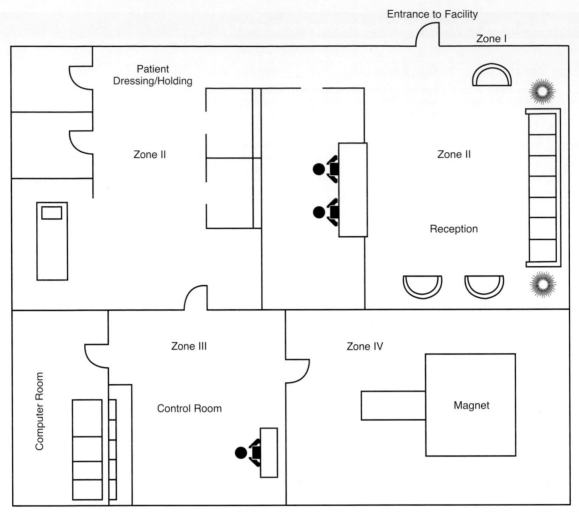

**Fig. 152.1** Schematic demonstrating the four safety zones in facilities with magnetic resonance imaging scanners. (Figure modified with permission from Allen Elster, MD FACR, MRIquestions.com.)

limits ability to tolerate the supine position for the time required for scanning. However, anesthesia may mask the warning signs and symptoms of developing neurologic deficits. There are case reports of the development of new-onset permanent neurologic deficits after anesthesia performed for MRI. Patients with preexisting spine disease, who are unable to tolerate supine positioning, should receive counseling regarding the risks to undergoing the MRI under anesthesia, are recommended to undergo MRI without anesthesia, or should consider alternative imaging options that do not require the patient to assume the supine position for lengthy periods of time.

The presence of implantable devices, such as cardiac pacemakers, internal cardiac defibrillators (ICD), vagal nerve stimulators, spinal cord stimulators, and programmable ventriculoperitoneal (VP) shunts, also may complicate the performance of an MRI scan. These devices may contain ferromagnetic and conductive components with potential to cause injury to the patient, interference with the imaging, device malfunction, and potential damage to the implantable device if exposed to the strong magnetic field of the MRI. Any patient presenting with an implanted device should be screened by the radiologists and MRI technologists to confirm the safety of MRI.

Further, the magnetic field may interfere with programming of a pacemaker and ICD. A tachyarrhythmia detection

mode must be disabled. Pacemakers should be reprogrammed to an asynchronous pacing mode in those who are pacemaker dependent and an inhibited mode in those who are not pacemaker dependent. A cardiac electrophysiology technician should be present during imaging, and an MRI physicist should adjust imaging parameters to minimize risk for interference.

Vagal nerve stimulators and deep brain stimulators should be turned off before imaging; stimulation can be resumed after the patient is removed from the scan room. The overflow pressure setting on programmable VP shunts can be altered by the magnetic field. The device must be interrogated before and after imaging to confirm no change in the overflow pressure setting. Otherwise, a standard x-ray image of the head before and after MRI can also be used to confirm no changes in the overflow setting. Nonprogrammable VP shunts are generally safe in the MRI scanner.

Emergencies in the MRI scanner can be daunting and devastating. If an emergency does occur, the patient should be promptly removed from the magnet room. Additional physicians, nurses, and other health care workers who arrive to aid in the resuscitation should not enter the scanner room under any circumstance. Resuscitation equipment that is ferromagnetic may be used in a Zone II location, and moving the patient into Zone I or II will allow for more care providers to be present to assist in the care of the patient.

## SUGGESTED READINGS

*ACR Manual on MR Safety.* Version 1.0, 2020. ACR Committee on MR Safety. Accessible on the American College of Radiology (ACR). Retrieved from https://www.acr.org/Clinical-Resources/Radiology-Safety/MR-Safety. Accessed June 12, 2021.

American Society of Anesthesiologists. (2015). Practice advisory on anesthetic care for magnetic resonance imaging. *Anesthesiology, 122,* 495–520.

Veenith, T., & Coles, J. P. (2011). Anaesthesia for magnetic resonance imaging and positron emission tomography. *Current Opinion in Anaesthesiology, 24,* 451–458.

Weglinski, M. R., Berge, K. H., & Davis, D. H. (2002). New-onset neurologic deficits after general anesthesia for MRI. *Mayo Clinic Proceedings, 77,* 101–103.

# 153

# Anesthesia for Robotic Surgery

ALEXANDRA L. ANDERSON, MD │ MATTHEW N. VOGT, MD │ WILLIAM BRIAN BEAM, MD

## Introduction

Robotic-assisted surgery has increased in frequency and breadth of application across surgical specialties over the last 20 years. Robotic technique has the advantages of laparoscopic minimally invasive surgery with the added benefits of improved visibility, increased maneuverability of instruments, decreased surgical tremor, and improved surgical ergonomics. Increased visualization and instrument manipulation make the robotic system well suited to operations on difficult to reach structures, such as those housed in the pelvis (Box 153.1). Urologic and gynecologic surgical specialties were early adopters of robotic technique, but use of this technology is expected to continue to expand with current use in colorectal, general, thoracic, cardiac, orthopedic, and otolaryngologic surgical procedures. For the purposes of this chapter, emphasis will be placed on urologic and gynecologic robotic-assisted surgery.

Current robotic systems (Fig. 153.1) include a surgeon console with the high-resolution stereo viewer and main controls, the patient cart with instrument and camera arms, and a vision cart with image processing and ancillary surgical instruments. Additional screens provide real-time visualization of the surgical field to the room. As with laparoscopic surgery, small incisions are made and trochars inserted. To improve visualization and access within the surgical field, insufflation is performed using $CO_2$. Through the trochars, or ports, laparoscopic instruments attached to the robot are inserted. The surgeon views the surgical field and manipulates instruments from the console.

Robotic surgery creates unique challenges for the anesthesia team. In additional to the usual complications associated with invasive surgery and general anesthesia, robotic surgery adds potential complications related to insufflation and patient positioning. A variety of physiologic disturbances should be anticipated. With the robotic unit docked, there is limited access to the patient and limited ability to assess invasive access sites, monitors, and patient position.

## Technique

After induction of general anesthesia, the patient is positioned, prepped, and draped in usual sterile fashion according to the surgical procedure. The initial laparoscopic trochar or Veress needle is placed, and insufflation is performed. Additional access ports are placed according to surgical need.

Gravity is often used to optimize exposure of the surgical field; patient position is determined by the surgery being performed. The anesthesia team should be aware of the possibility for extreme positions, such as steep Trendelenburg for pelvic surgery or lateral tilt of the bed during colon surgery. Special attention must be paid to securing the patient to the surgical table; this typically involves a non-slip pad beneath and straps across the patient's body (e.g., chest straps). A face shield is placed to protect the face and airway from robotic arms. Once table position is finalized, robotic arms are attached to the ports and both the robot and the patient cart are locked into position or docked. Once the robot is docked, the operating table must not be moved independently, as arm positions are fixed and serious harm could occur. Contemporary systems may allow for the robotic unit and the surgical table to move together in a safe synchronous mode.

---

**BOX 153.1  BENEFITS OF ROBOTIC SURGERY FOR PATIENTS AND PROVIDERS**

↓ Tissue trauma and incision size
↓ Postoperative pain
↓ Wound infections
Improved recovery and ↓ hospital length of stay
Improved visualization of the surgical field
↑ Maneuverability of surgical instruments
Improved ergonomics for surgeon
↓ Blood loss for certain procedures

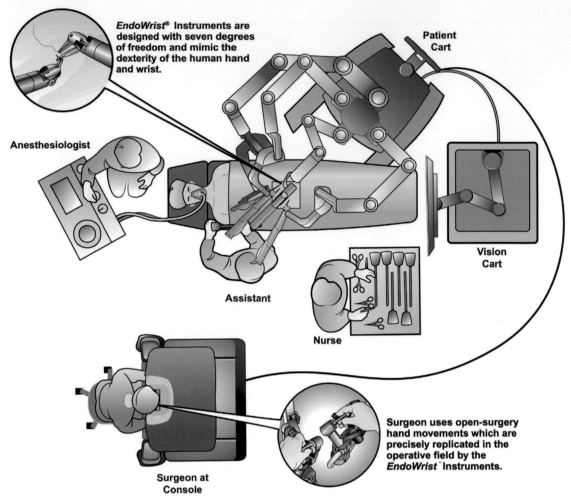

**Fig. 153.1   Operating room schematic of a robotic surgery system.** (Reprinted from Ellis D, Albrecht M. Anesthesia for robotic surgery. In: Gropper MA, Cohen NH, Eriksson LI, Fleisher LA, Leslie K, Wiener-Kronish JP (eds.). *Miller's Anesthesia.* 9th ed. Elsevier, 2020:2236–2250. With permission from Elsevier/Courtesy Intuitive Surgical, Sunnyvale, CA.)

## Physiology

Physiologic changes with robotic-assisted surgery are primarily related to changes resulting from abdominal insufflation and extremes of patient positioning; these are summarized in Box 153.2.

For abdominal and pelvic surgeries, pneumoperitoneum is induced by insufflating the abdominal cavity to pressures of 12 to 15 mm Hg with $CO_2$ via needle or trochar access. Both intraperitoneal insufflation and $CO_2$ have physiologic consequences. Insufflation rapidly expands the abdominal cavity. Acute peritoneal stretch can cause a vagal response resulting in profound bradycardia and even asystole. Extra vigilance is required during initial trochar placement and insufflation as there is also potential for vascular injury, gas embolism, or acute hypercarbia with $CO_2$ absorption. Subcutaneous emphysema can develop leading to prolonged $CO_2$ absorption postoperatively, as well as distortions of anatomy. Increased intraabdominal pressure can result in an initial increase in venous return followed by venous pooling and increased systemic vascular resistance (SVR) due to pressure on the aorta and abdominal arterial vasculature. In the supine position, decreased venous return may cause a decrease in cardiac output and hypotension.

---

**BOX 153.2   EXPECTED PHYSIOLOGIC CHANGES RELATED TO PNEUMOPERITONEUM AND THE TRENDELENBURG POSITION FOR PATIENTS UNDERGOING ROBOTIC SURGERY**

Initial ↑ venous return / ↑ CVP
No change or small ↓ in CO (in normal heart)
↑ SVR
↓ Chest wall and lung compliance
↑ IOP
↑ ICP
↓ Renal perfusion pressure
↑ Intragastric pressure
↑ Vagal tone related to peritoneal stretch

*CO*, Cardiac output; *ICP*, intracranial pressure; *IOP*, intraocular pressures; *SVR*, systemic vascular resistance.

---

Hypercarbia and acidosis may also affect cardiac function and irritability. Increased abdominal pressure transmits across the diaphragm to cause decreased respiratory compliance, increased airway pressures, decreased functional residual capacity of the lungs, and atelectasis. Hypercarbia from $CO_2$ absorption and atelectasis cause pulmonary vasoconstriction. Pneumoperitoneum leads to decreased renal perfusion and increased gastric pressure. Hypercarbia leads to cerebral vasodilation and a potential increase in intracranial pressure.

Patient positioning for robotic surgery has unique implications for patient safety and physiology. Steep Trendelenburg position with more than 30 degrees of head-down tilt is often employed to expose pelvic anatomy by shifting abdominal contents cephalad. Steep Trendelenburg causes increased venous return. Generally, in healthy patients no significant net change in stroke volume or cardiac output are noted. Hypertension is often observed with increased venous return combined with increased SVR caused by pneumoperitoneum. Upward shift of the diaphragm along with the external compression of chest wall by safety belts leads to decreased lung and chest wall compliance, furthering atelectasis and increased airway pressures. The head-down position also increases intracranial pressure (ICP) and intraocular pressure (IOP). Prolonged Trendelenburg can lead to dependent edema of the facial structures and airway (Box 153.2).

## Anesthetic Considerations

The anesthetic assessment and plan must reconcile patient comorbidities and their inherent risks with the physiology and positioning of robotic surgery. General anesthesia is required with deep neuromuscular blockade to optimize pneumoperitoneum and surgical conditions. Gastric decompression with an orogastric tube is warranted given the increase in gastric pressure with abdominal insufflation. Intravenous access must be reliable with confirmation of patency after final positioning. Invasive blood pressure monitoring may be prudent depending on patient comorbidities, access to extremities, and length of surgery as blood pressure cuffs may cause pressure injuries during prolonged cases or be subject to positioning artifact and inaccurate readings. Furthermore, monitoring arterial $CO_2$ and $O_2$ may assist with ensuring adequate ventilation and oxygenation with the anticipated challenges of $CO_2$ absorption and the effect of pneumoperitoneum and positioning on respiratory mechanics.

### HEMODYNAMICS

Patient position and the contribution of insufflation have major effects on hemodynamics. Hemodynamic instability during trochar placement or insufflation should be quickly evaluated to rule out vascular injury or air embolism. Bradycardia with insufflation should be recognized and treated promptly. In severe cases, bradycardia can progress to asystole. Treatment includes discussion with the surgical team to release pneumoperitoneum, administration of vagolytics, and slower staged reinsufflation. Bradycardia with the vagal stimulation of peritoneal stretch and manipulation of pelvic organs can also be anticipated and treated. Patients may become hypertensive due to increased SVR from increased intraabdominal pressure and increased venous return in the Trendelenburg position. Conversely, hypotension may occur with pneumoperitoneum and decreased venous return in supine or reverse Trendelenburg position.

Cardiovascular comorbidities must be considered when evaluating patients for robotic-assisted procedures. Patients with right ventricular dysfunction or pulmonary hypertension are at risk for decompensation, as increased preload and hypercapnia can further increase pulmonary vascular resistance. Patients

with diastolic dysfunction, coronary artery disease, or valvular pathology may also be affected by the physiologic demands of pneumoperitoneum, hypercarbia, and positioning. In patients with cardiac disease, trial insufflation and positioning may be performed, and the possibility of converting to an open technique should be discussed. Invasive monitors may be indicated.

### OXYGENATION AND VENTILATION

Ventilation strategy should follow "lung-protective" parameters when possible. Although peak and plateau pressures for robotic surgery in the Trendelenburg position can exceed traditional lung-protective parameters, increased pleural pressure must be acknowledged as a major contributor to elevated airway pressures. The combination of patient factors (e.g., excess chest wall/abdominal weight related to obesity), abdominal insufflation, tight chest straps, and steep Trendelenburg position lead to elevated pleural pressures and decreased lung compliance. Increased pleural pressure decreases functional residual capacity and can cause atelectasis. With atelectasis and hypercarbia-induced pulmonary vasoconstriction, ventilation/perfusion mismatch increases and hypoxemia may develop. The flow dynamics associated with pressure control ventilation allow for an overall lower peak airway pressure compared to a volume control mode of ventilation. To improve oxygenation and lung mechanics, open lung strategy with increased positive end-expiratory pressure (PEEP) and frequent lung recruitment should be considered in hemodynamically stable patients. Review of parameters that assess alveolar strain, such as driving pressure (DP = Pplat − PEEP) and transpulmonary pressure (TP = Pplat – Ppleural) along with pressure volume loops, may be helpful in defining optimal individualized PEEP. Measurement of transpleural pressure using an esophageal balloon has been explored but is not currently considered standard of care. An increased minute ventilation may be required to maintain normocapnia in the setting of $CO_2$ absorption from insufflation. With obstructive lung disease, compensation with increased respiratory rate may be limited due to prolonged expiratory phase and risk of developing intrinsic PEEP. Anticipating challenges to ventilation and oxygenation may prompt placement of an arterial line as arterial blood gases can guide ventilation strategy.

Position-dependent factors also affect ventilation and airway management. With abdominal insufflation and/or Trendelenburg position, upward shift of the diaphragm may lead to endobronchial positioning of the endotracheal tube. Tube position should be confirmed after insufflation and again after positioning. Dependent swelling of the face and airway should be monitored, and checking for a cuff leak before extubation should be considered when significant swelling is noted. Extreme subcutaneous emphysema, facial or airway swelling, and persistent hypercarbia may preclude extubation at the end of a procedure. These patients should receive ongoing mechanical ventilation until they meet appropriate extubation criteria.

### VOLUME STATUS/FLUID MANAGEMENT

Fluid administration should aim for euvolemia and take into consideration lower insensate losses, impaired venous return, and decreased cardiac output associated with pneumoperitoneum. Urine output may be difficult to monitor, as it is often in the surgical field with urologic procedures. Urine output may also be decreased from impaired renal perfusion or pooling of urine in the dome of the bladder with extreme Trendelenburg position. During a long procedure with high intraperitoneal pressure in Trendelenburg position, blood pressure may not be a reliable indicator of actual volume status, as a volume deficit may be masked by increased SVR and augmentation of preload in head-down position. Attention to the surgical field with monitoring blood loss and lab values can assist in identifying suspected hypovolemia or bleeding. Again, invasive blood pressure monitoring with an arterial line may be of use.

## POSITIONING

Patient positioning is central to robotic surgery and can be extreme in the degree of head-down Trendelenburg position. Thus risk for patient migration and positioning injury is increased. Methods to secure patients, such as firm chest straps or shoulder bolsters, can also cause restricted ventilation, pressure point damage, and nerve traction injuries. Tests are often performed to ensure the patient is adequately secured on the operating table before the start of the operation. Endotracheal tube position should be confirmed once the patient is in the final position as steep Trendelenburg and cephalad shift of thoracic structures may lead to endotracheal tube migration and mainstem intubation. Patient position is further complicated by restricted access to the patient with the position of the robotic arms and screens, the face shield, possible tucked arms, and lack of access to lower extremities that may be in boots or fins. After placement of the face shield, the anesthesia team should assure the face is free of any contact or pressure points. This shield significantly limits access to the patient's face and airway. The patient's head and face should be regularly evaluated and pressure points relieved, as alopecia is a known complication of prolonged robotic surgery. Facial swelling may also progressively cause pressure points where gastric tubes or endotracheal tubes are secured. Lines and monitors must be double-checked and padded. Intravenous access and invasive monitors should be tailored to the surgery and patient medical comorbidities, considering restricted access to assess or place lines going forward. Accurate blood pressure cuff readings may be impaired by tucked arms or kinking of the tubing, and prolonged surgical time may increase the risk of compression injury from repeat blood pressure cuff measurements. Lack of access to the patient, especially with tucked arms, may increase risk of pressure injuries and difficulty in detecting infiltration of intravenous lines. Joint or extremity contractures may make safe positioning difficult. Patients with increased ICP, closed-angle glaucoma, or high baseline IOP are likely at increased risk for adverse outcomes from robotic surgery in the Trendelenburg position and may not be appropriate candidates for this approach. Although rare, there are case reports of postoperative vision loss after robotic surgery in prolonged Trendelenburg; usually this is attributed to ischemic optic neuropathy. Bleeding from the ears (usually bilateral) has also been reported; this is hypothesized to be associated congestion of the subcutaneous vasculature of the ear. Epistaxis can also occur with increased congestion of the nasal passages, and caution should be used with placement of nasogastric tubes, nasal temperature probes, or nasal trumpets.

## POSTOPERATIVE MANAGEMENT

Patients should receive multimodal analgesia along with local anesthetic infiltration of surgical incisions where relevant, particularly those with risk factors for postoperative respiratory depression. The need for deep neuromuscular blockade for these procedures makes monitoring and reversal of neuromuscular blocking drugs critical to avoid residual postoperative residual neuromuscular blockade. Patients may be at risk for postoperative nausea and vomiting and should receive multimodal prophylactic agents. In recovery, residual intraperitoneal $CO_2$ may lead to referred shoulder pain with diaphragmatic irritation, and patients should be assessed for peripheral nerve injury or corneal abrasion. Head-up position should assist with draining facial edema, and patients should be monitored regarding subcutaneous emphysema.

## Other Adverse Effects/Risks

The adverse effects and risks unique to robotic-assisted surgery are listed in Box 153.3. As detailed in previous sections, positioning injuries resulting from pressure, traction, and lack of access to the patient undergoing robotic surgery are of concern. In extreme cases, risk of patient migration with steep table position is possible. In tables not synchronized with the robotic unit, changes in table position can be catastrophic. A trial period of insufflation and final position should be performed to ensure patients will be able to tolerate the physiologic demands of pneumoperitoneum and positioning. Should a patient decompensate or become unstable during robotic surgery, converting to an open technique should be considered.

Other disadvantages of robotic surgery include potentially increased operative times compared with open approaches, increased cost, increased training involved for the technology, and the space required for storing these systems. Many of these disadvantages are mitigated over time with increased surgical experience and efficiency and must be weighed against the potential advantages of decreased patient recovery times, increased patient satisfaction, improved patient outcomes, and decreased length of stay.

## Summary

Robotic-assisted surgery has a wide range of increasing applications across surgical specialties and can yield many advantages for patient outcomes in terms of recovery, pain control, and length of hospital stay. The anesthesia provider must be cognizant of the unique physiologic effects caused by insufflation and position required for robotic-assisted surgery to effectively identify patients at risk, mitigate harmful effects, and optimize perioperative care and outcomes.

---

**BOX 153.3 SPECIAL CONSIDERATIONS AND RISKS ASSOCIATED WITH ROBOTIC SURGERY**

Facial and airway edema (in Trendelenburg position)
Respiratory acidosis/hypercarbia related to insufflation and decreased lung compliance
Hypoxemia related to atelectasis
Trochar injury
Subcutaneous emphysema
Venous $CO_2$ embolism
Restricted access to airway, invasive access, monitors, and cardiopulmonary resuscitation
Need for special attention to securing/positioning patient
Risk for nerve/soft tissue injury related to securement devices/position
Risk of endobronchial intubation with Trendelenburg position
Otorrhagia related to congestion of subcutaneous ear vasculature
Alopecia related to pressure injury
Learning curve and required training for surgeons

## SUGGESTED READINGS

Aceto, P., Beretta, L., Cariello, C., Claroni, C., Esposito, C., Forastiere, E. M., et al. (2019). Società Italiana di Anestesia Analgesia Rianimazione e Terapia Intensiva (SIAARTI), Società Italiana di Ginecologia e Ostetricia (SIGO), and Società Italiana di Urologia (SIU). Joint consensus on anesthesia in urologic and gynecologic robotic surgery: Specific issues in management from a task force of the SIAARTI, SIGO, and SIU. *Minerva Anestesiologica, 85*(8), 871–885.

Ashrafian, H., Clancy, O., Grover, V., & Darzi, A. (2017). The evolution of robotic surgery: Surgical and anaesthetic aspects. *British Journal of Anaesthesia, 119*(S1), i72–i84.

Assessment of Ventilation during general AnesThesia for Robotic surgery (AVATaR) Study Investigators, for the PROtective VEntilation (PROVE) Network: Queiroz, V.N.F., da Costa, L.G.V., Takaoka, F., et al. (2021). Ventilation and outcomes following

robotic-assisted abdominal surgery: An international, multicentre observational study. *British Journal of Anaesthesia, 126*(2), 533–543.

Brandão, J. C., Lessa, M. A., Motta-Ribeiro, G., Hashimoto, S., Paula, L. F., Torsani, V., et al. (2019). Global and regional respiratory mechanics during robotic-assisted laparoscopic surgery: A randomized study. *Anesthesia and Analgesia, 129*(6), 1564–1573.

Ellis, D., & Albrecht, M. (2020). Anesthesia for robotic surgery. In M. A. Gropper (Ed.), *Miller's Anesthesia* (9th ed., pp. 2236–2250). Philadelphia, PA: Elsevier.

Fantola, G., Brunaud, L., Nguyen-Thi, P. L., Germain, A., Ayav, A., & Bresler, L. (2017). Risk factors for postoperative complications in robotic general surgery. *Updates in Surgery, 69*(1), 45–54.

Lestar, M., Gunnarsson, L., Lagerstrand, L., Wiklund, P., & Odeberg-Wernerman, S. (2011).

Hemodynamic perturbations during robot-assisted laparoscopic radical prostatectomy in 45° Trendelenburg position. *Anesthesia and Analgesia, 113*(5), 1069–1075.

Tharp, W. G., Murphy, S., Breidenstein, M. W., Love, C., Booms, A., Rafferty, M. N., et al. (2020). Body habitus and dynamic surgical conditions independently impair pulmonary mechanics during robotic-assisted laparoscopic surgery. *Anesthesiology, 133*(4), 750–763.

Yoon, H. K., Kim, B. R., Yoon, S., Jeong, Y. H., Ku, J. H., & Kim, W. H. (2021). The effect of ventilation with individualized positive end-expiratory pressure on postoperative atelectasis in patients undergoing robot-assisted radical prostatectomy: A randomized controlled trial. *Journal of Clinical Medicine, 10*(4), 850.

# 154

# Anesthesia for Electroconvulsive Therapy

ERICA D. WITTWER, MD, PhD

Convulsive therapy for psychiatric disorders has been used since 1934. Electroconvulsive therapy (ECT), modified over the years to incorporate monitoring, intravenous (IV) administration of anesthetic drugs, neuromuscular blockade, and the use of supplemental oxygen ($O_2$), is both safe and effective for the treatment of endogenous depression in patients whose symptoms have failed to respond to an adequate course of antidepressant drugs; who may be jeopardized by adverse events associated with the use of pharmacologic agents; who have psychosis, bipolar disorder, or catatonia; or who are suicidal.

## Mechanism of Action

Seizures induced by ECT are generalized seizures. Configurations of electrode placement include bilateral, right unilateral, and bifrontal. The initial session may require a dose titration to determine the appropriate electrical stimulus to evoke a seizure, which requires an appropriate duration of anesthesia and neuromuscular blockade. A 2- to 3-second latent phase is followed by a tonic phase lasting 10 to 12 seconds, then a clonic phase of 30 to 50 seconds. Both the duration of individual seizures and cumulative seizure time correlate with clinical improvement of depression. The number of treatments is determined by the patient's clinical response.

## Physiology

The physiologic mechanisms responsible for the therapeutic benefit of ECT are unknown; however, a variety of theories have been posited (Box 154.1). The cardiovascular response to ECT is secondary to autonomic nervous system discharge. Parasympathetic discharge, secondary to vagus nerve stimulation, is immediate and may cause asystole, bradycardia, premature

---

**BOX 154.1   THEORIES OF THE PHYSIOLOGIC MECHANISM RESPONSIBLE FOR THE THERAPEUTIC EFFECTS OF ELECTROCONVULSIVE THERAPY**

**CHANGES IN THE FOLLOWING**

Ion transport
Permeability of the blood-brain barrier
Regional cerebral blood flow
Concentrations of
  Biogenic amines
  Electrolytes
  Neurotransmitters

**RELEASE OF HORMONES AND CYTOKINES**

Corticotropin
Hypothalamic peptides
Prolactin

ventricular contractions, hypotension, and a ventricular escape rhythm. The parasympathetic effect can be blunted by a small dose of glycopyrrolate in patients who have a profound response. Sympathetic tone increases with seizure generation, possibly manifesting as increased heart rate, premature ventricular contractions, bigeminy, trigeminy, sinus tachycardia, and severe hypertension. A marked increase in myocardial $O_2$ consumption frequently occurs. The increase in sympathetic tone often resolves quickly, but if the patient requires intervention, esmolol or labetalol may be used for tachycardia or hypertension, respectively. An initial constriction of cerebral vessels is followed by increased cerebral blood flow (1.5–7 times baseline) from increased cerebral $O_2$ consumption and elevated blood pressure. Preoxygenation is used to prevent cerebral hypoxia. The neuroendocrine response to ECT is manifest by increased levels of corticotropin, cortisol, and catecholamines. The effects on glucose levels vary; thus patients with diabetes mellitus should have their glucose levels monitored before and after ECT. Miscellaneous effects of ECT of importance to the anesthesia provider include increased intragastric pressure and increased intraocular pressure.

## Morbidity and Mortality Rates

The mortality risk from ECT is estimated at less than 1 in 75,000 treatments. Other complications include transient arrhythmias (10%–40%), gastric aspiration (2.5%), and musculoskeletal disorder (0.4%), including fractures. In addition, adverse events after ECT may include pulmonary edema, headache, memory disturbance, and agitation. Very rarely takotsubo cardiomyopathy, febrile reactions, or neurologic dysfunction may occur.

## Anesthetic Management

### CONTRAINDICATIONS

A variety of contraindications to ECT, both absolute and relative, are of particular note to anesthesia providers (Box 154.2).

### PREOPERATIVE ASSESSMENT

Preoperative assessment should document cardiopulmonary, neurologic, and endocrine status; risk of gastrointestinal reflux; and history of earlier drug therapy. Monoamine oxidase inhibitors (MAOIs), tricyclic antidepressants, selective serotonin reuptake inhibitors, and antipsychotics can be continued during ECT therapy. If the decision is made to stop MAOIs, they should be discontinued 2 weeks before ECT. Patients receiving lithium may experience delayed awakening, memory loss, and postictal confusion; thus it is recommended to hold for 12 hours before ECT. Benzodiazepines should also be held for 12 hours prior because of the negative effect on seizures.

---

> **BOX 154.2   RELATIVE AND ABSOLUTE CONTRAINDICATIONS TO THE USE OF ELECTROCONVULSIVE THERAPY**
>
> **ABSOLUTE CONTRAINDICATIONS**
> - Intracranial mass
> - Recent myocardial infarction
> - Recent stroke
>
> **RELATIVE CONTRAINDICATIONS**
> - Angina pectoris
> - Chronic obstructive pulmonary disease
> - Congestive heart failure
> - Glaucoma
> - High-risk pregnancy
> - Retinal detachment
> - Severe osteoporosis
> - Thrombophlebitis

---

Management of a patient with a cardiac implantable electronic device is influenced by device type, if the device is a pacemaker versus an implantable cardioverter-defibrillator (ICD). If the patient has a pacemaker but is not dependent on the device, a magnet should be available in event of device failure. However, if the patient is dependent on the pacemaker, consideration should be made to program the device into an asynchronous mode and a backup mode of pacing should be immediately available. If the device is an ICD, there is a risk that the device misinterprets muscle movements as an abnormal cardiac rhythm, and a discharge is possible. Therefore the device should be deactivated and an external defibrillator should be immediately available with placement of external defibrillator pads strongly considered. For a patient with an ICD and who is pacemaker dependent, the electrophysiology (EP) service should be consulted. EP should also be consulted in any cases with pacing concerns.

### ANESTHESIA TECHNIQUE

Depending on the patient's comorbidities, pharmacologic intervention to reduce the risks of aspiration of gastric contents may be indicated. At a minimum, the American Society of Anesthesiologists' standards for fasting and monitoring should be followed. Patients should be adequately preoxygenated before induction of anesthesia. Anesthesia may be induced via inhalational agent (sevoflurane) or IV agents. A small dose of IV anesthetic is often given to produce hypnosis with a goal of rapid awakening after the procedure. A variety of agents can be used, including methohexital, ketamine, propofol, ketofol (combination of ketamine and propofol), remifentanil, and etomidate. Table 154.1 highlights IV medications commonly

---

| TABLE 154.1 | Medications Commonly Used in Electroconvulsive Therapy | | | | |
|---|---|---|---|---|---|
| **Premedication** | **Dose (IV)** | **Benefits** | **Side Effects** | **Suggested Use** | |
| Glycopyrrolate | 0.1–0.2 mg | Attenuates bradycardia | Tachycardia Dry mouth | Significant bradycardia or asystole with ECT | |
| **INDUCTION MEDICATIONS** | | | | | |
| Methohexital | 1 mg/kg | Short duration of action Low anticonvulsant properties | Myoclonus Nausea | First-line choice | |

| TABLE 154.1 | Medications Commonly Used in Electroconvulsive Therapy—cont'd | | | |
|---|---|---|---|---|
| **Premedication** | **Dose (IV)** | **Benefits** | **Side Effects** | **Suggested Use** |
| Ketamine | 1 mg/kg | Potential for augmenting ECT effects | Increased salivation | Use in research for enhancing ECT |
| Propofol | 1 mg/kg | Decreased nausea/vomiting | Increased anticonvulsant properties | Nausea/vomiting post-ECT |
| Etomidate | 0.3 mg/kg | No effect on seizure threshold | Nausea | Hemodynamic instability |
| **COMBINATION AGENTS** | | | | |
| Ketamine/ propofol | 0.5 mg/kg and 0.5 mg/kg | Positive effects of each medication | Reduced negative effects | Nausea/vomiting post-ECT or hemodynamic instability |
| Remifentanil | | Less anticonvulsant properties | Risk of awareness, not for use as sole agent | Difficult to elicit seizure |
| **PARALYTIC** | | | | |
| Succinylcholine | 1 mg/kg | Rapid onset/offset | Potential for muscle soreness or hyperkalemia | Safe for majority of patients |
| Rocuronium | 0.6 mg/kg | Rapid onset/reversible | Prolonged apnea | Safe for majority of patients |
| **ADJUNCTS** | | | | |
| Ketorolac | 15–30 mg | Antiinflammatory | Potential for renal dysfunction in susceptible patients | Headache prophylaxis |
| Ondansetron | 4 mg | Antiemetic | Constipation | Nausea/vomiting prophylaxis |
| Lorazepam | 1–4 mg | Anxiolysis | Sedation | Post-ECT agitation |
| Midazolam | 1–2 mg | Anxiolysis | Sedation | Post-ECT agitation |
| **ANTIHYPERTENSIVE AGENTS** | | | | |
| Labetalol | 5–10 mg | Rapid onset | Hypotension | Postseizure hypertension |
| Hydralazine | 2.5–5 mg | Longer time to onset | Hypotension | Postseizure hypertension |
| **β-BLOCKERS** | | | | |
| Esmolol | 10–30 mg | Rapid onset/short acting | Hypotension/bradycardia | Post-ECT tachycardia |

*ECT,* Electroconvulsive therapy; *IV,* intravenous.

used for ECT. Muscle relaxation is often achieved with succinylcholine (~0.5–1 mg/kg) to prevent musculoskeletal injuries while allowing rapid return of respirations. With sugammadex available to reverse nondepolarizing neuromuscular blockade, the use of this medication class will likely increase. Patients with a contraindication to succinylcholine will require an alternative agent such as rocuronium with sugammadex reversal. Patients may experience headaches or muscle aches after treatment, and ketorolac may be used in appropriate patients for prophylaxis. Ondansetron is commonly used as an antiemetic in patients who experience nausea and/or vomiting after treatment. Occasionally, patients may have seizures that last longer than the desired interval, and additional anesthetic agent may be given to help stop the seizure. Postictal agitation may be treated by a benzodiazepine, antipsychotic medication, or propofol in patients who are unsafe to themselves or others.

Methohexital (~1 mg/kg) is often the anesthetizing agent of choice secondary to the short duration of action combined with the property of fewer anticonvulsant effects. Combining ketamine with ECT for enhanced treatment is an active area for research. In fact, ketamine selection may have added advantages for use in patients with major depression or bipolar depression refractory to other therapies secondary to the drug's inherent pharmacodynamic antidepressant properties. Of note, ketamine may result in increased salivation and pretreatment with glycopyrrolate may be beneficial. Propofol can be especially useful for patients with postprocedure nausea and vomiting, although propofol has more seizure-suppressing properties. Ketofol, a combination of ketamine and propofol, can be used to take advantage of the positive effects of each medication while minimizing the negative effects. Remifentanil may be of particular benefit for patients in whom it is difficult to induce an acceptable seizure as it has little effect on the seizure threshold. Because of risk for awareness, it is not ideal as a sole agent, but it can allow a lower dose of another anesthetic agent to be given. Etomidate has little effect on the seizure threshold and is a hemodynamically stable induction agent, although it may result in increased nausea. After the emergence of COVID-19 concerns regarding providing mask ventilation arose in many areas of anesthesia practice. ECT is considered a necessary procedure as it is used in patients with severe mental illness. Thus efforts to minimize the need for bag-mask ventilation are advised such as reducing both the anesthetic and paralytic dosage to allow for return of respiratory function as quickly as possible. This requires careful titration and accurate record of doses during former treatments. Postseizure hemodynamic changes, including hypertension and tachycardia, often resolve quickly. However, if persistent or in patients with significant cardiovascular comorbidities, treatment with either beta-blockage or a calcium-channel blocker may be indicated.

## SUGGESTED READINGS

Chawla, N. (2020). Anesthesia for electroconvulsive therapy. *Anesthesiology Clinics, 38,* 183–195.

Hermida, A. P., Glass, O. M., Shafi, H., & McDonald, W. M. (2018). Electroconvulsive therapy in depression: Current practice and future direction. *Psychiatric Clinics of North America, 41,* 341–353.

Peroski, M. S., Chu, M. M., Doddi, S. R., & Regenold, W. T. (2019). The safety of electroconvulsive therapy in patients with implanted deep brain stimulators: A review of the literature and case report. *Journal of ECT, 35,* 84–90.

Rose, S., Dotters-Katz, S. K., & Kuller, J. A. (2020). Electroconvulsive therapy in pregnancy: Safety, best practices, and barriers to care. *Obstetrical & Gynecological Survey, 75,* 199–203.

Soehle, M., Bochem, J., Kayser, S., Weyerhäuser, J., & Valero, R. (2021). Challenges and pitfalls in anesthesia for electroconvulsive therapy. *Best Practice and Research. Clinical Anaesthesiology, 35,* 181–189.

Thiruvenkatarajan, V., Dharmalingam, A., Armstrong-Brown, A., Weiss, A., Waite, S., & Van Wijk, R. (2020). Uninterrupted anesthesia support and technique adaptations for patients presenting for electroconvulsive therapy during the COVID-19 era. *Journal of ECT, 36,* 156–157.

# 155

# Myasthenia Gravis and Lambert-Eaton Myasthenic Syndrome

RYAN E. HOFER, MD

## Myasthenia Gravis

### BACKGROUND

Myasthenia gravis is a chronic autoimmune disorder of the neuromuscular junction characterized by skeletal muscle weakness and easy fatigability that typically worsens throughout the day. Voluntary muscles are rapidly exhausted with repetitive use, and often only partial recovery is obtained with rest. Prevalence is roughly 1 in 7500 with a bimodal pattern of age involvement. Women in their third to fourth decade of life are most commonly affected. Men are often older than 60 years when symptoms start, and more men than women are affected in this advanced age group. Acetylcholine receptor antibodies are present in more than 80% of patients with myasthenia gravis. The origin of these antibodies is not entirely clear, but the thymus gland seems to be involved because two-thirds of patients with myasthenia gravis have thymic hyperplasia and 10% to 15% have thymomas, the incidence of which increases with age.

### PATHOPHYSIOLOGY

Autoantibodies to the alpha-subunit of the muscle-type nicotinic acetylcholine receptor, or functionally related molecules, lead to transmission failure and, ultimately, the muscle weakness of myasthenia gravis. Up to 80% of receptors can be lost through inactivation or destruction by these antibodies leaving an inadequate number of functional receptors at the neuromuscular junction. Neuronal-type nicotinic acetylcholine receptors are not affected. Therefore this disease only affects skeletal muscle and there is no autonomic or central nervous system involvement. Those muscles innervated by cranial muscles are the most susceptible. This is demonstrated by the most common initial complaints being the bulbar symptoms of ptosis, diplopia, and dysphagia.

### DIAGNOSIS

Diagnosis of myasthenia gravis involves a combination of specific signs and symptoms along with a positive test for certain antibodies. The natural course of the disease involves waxing and waning periods of exacerbation and remission. Exercise and repetitive muscle use quickly promote weakness. Truncal and extremity weakness is often asymmetric, more proximal than distal, and without muscle atrophy. The vast majority of patients with myasthenia gravis will have antibodies for acetylcholine receptors, muscle-specific kinase, or lipoprotein receptor related protein 4. When antibodies are not detectable, a thorough neurologic examination can confirm the diagnosis. An edrophonium (Tensilon) test involves the administration of a short-acting anticholinesterase. An increase in strength, though temporary, supports the diagnosis of myasthenia gravis. Electromyography will classically show a decrease in muscle action potential after repetitive nerve stimulation. In patients being considered for myasthenia gravis, the differential diagnosis includes congenital myasthenic syndrome, Lambert-Eaton myasthenic syndrome (LEMS), hyperthyroidism, Graves disease, botulism, neuromyotonia, progressive external ophthalmoplegia, and intracranial mass compression of cranial nerves.

### TREATMENT

Several treatment options exist with the goal of symptom improvement and even elimination. They include anticholinesterase

| TABLE 155.1 | Differentiating Myasthenic Crisis and Cholinergic Crisis | |
|---|---|---|
| Differentiating Factor | Myasthenic Crisis | Cholinergic Crisis |
| Use of anticholin-ergics | Steady/decreased dose | Overdose |
| Pupil size | Mydriasis/normal | Miosis |
| Heart rate | Normal/tachycardia | Bradycardia |
| Edrophonium (Tensilon) test | Improves symptoms | Worsens symptoms |
| Parasympathomi-metic effects | Uncommon | Salivation, lacrimation, urination, defection, gastrointestinal cramps, emesis |

medications, thymectomy, immunosuppressive therapy, and plasmapheresis/immunoglobulin. Anticholinesterase drugs are considered to be first-line therapy. They derive their efficacy by inhibiting the cholinesterase enzymes responsible for the break-down of acetylcholine. This results in an increase in the amount of acetylcholine available in the neuromuscular junction lead-ing to more successful muscle contraction. Pyridostigmine is most commonly used for this purpose. Dosing is derived from a balance of improving muscle strength and limiting the side effect profile, which most often involves the gastrointestinal tract. Typical dosing rarely exceeds 120 mg every 6 hours. Higher doses can actually have a paradoxical effect on muscle strength known as the cholinergic crisis. Though this can be difficult to differentiate from a myasthenic crisis, it is important to do so because the treatments differ and appropriate actions for one will worsen the other. Cholinergic crisis will be worsened with an edrophonium test and will involve miosis, bradycardia, and other parasympathomimetic symptoms not commonly seen in a myasthenic crisis (Table 155.1).

Thymectomy is indicated in myasthenia gravis patients with generalized symptoms and thymoma. The goal is symptom remission or reduction in the required dose of immunosup-pressive medications through a reduction in circulating antibodies. Though often successful, the full benefit may not be realized for months.

Immunosuppressive therapy is often added to a patient regimen when anticholinesterases fail to adequately control symptoms. First-line therapy often involves a combination of corticosteroids and azathioprine. Secondary medications include cyclosporine, mycophenolate, and tacrolimus. These immunosuppressives can lead to side effects limiting their use, for example, osteoporosis, weight gain, hyperglycemia, hyper-tension, cancer risk, and renal failure. Patients using these medications are at an increased risk of perioperative infection.

Plasmapheresis involves the removal of antibodies from circulation leading to a short-term improvement for those pre-paring for surgery or for those in a myasthenic crisis. Immuno-globulin is used for the same indications and has effects that are also temporary.

## ANESTHETIC IMPLICATIONS

The preoperative evaluation of patients with myasthenia gravis should include the severity and duration of symptoms along with their treatment regimen. Pulmonary function testing may be helpful to determine the need for postoperative ventilator support. Myasthenia gravis patients should be forewarned regarding their increased risk of requiring postoperative venti-lator support and developing postoperative respiratory compli-cations. Several factors have been linked to this increased risk: (1) disease duration longer than 6 years; (2) other pulmonary disease; (3) daily total pyridostigmine dose greater than 750 mg; (4) vital capacity less than 2.9 L; and (5) negative inspiratory pressure not less than $-20$ cm $H_2O$. Patients with myasthenia gravis, compared with those without, are most likely to have other coexisting autoimmune diseases including thyroiditis, systemic lupus erythematosus, rheumatoid arthritis, and perni-cious anemia. Fifteen percent of neonates born to mothers with myasthenia gravis demonstrate skeletal muscle weakness at times lasting up to 1 month. Factors known to exacerbate symptoms include infection, electrolyte abnormalities, preg-nancy, emotional stress, surgery, and certain antibiotics: amino-glycosides, fluoroquinolones, and macrolides. These patients should be continued on home anticholinesterase drugs during the perioperative period.

Patients with myasthenia gravis often have significant sensi-tivity to nondepolarizing muscle relaxants caused by the de-creased number of functional acetylcholine receptors. Dosing these medications should be 0.1 to 0.2 times the effective dose $(ED)_{95}$ dose. Because of this sensitivity, pretreatment with these medications should be avoided as well to prevent the profound weakness that can follow. The decreased number of functional receptors also results in an increased resistance to depolarizing muscle relaxants. The $ED_{95}$ dose for succinylcholine has been measured at 2.6 times higher than normal. Anticholinesterase drugs will also inhibit pseudocholinesterase potentially leading to a prolonged block when succinylcholine is administered. Tracheal intubation, however, can often be achieved without the use of any muscle relaxants, for example, using an intubat-ing bolus dose of remifentanil. It should be taken into consid-eration that these patients can be at high risk for aspiration if pharyngeal and laryngeal muscles are involved with their disease process. The asymmetric involvement and uneven distribution of muscle weakness can lead to inaccuracies with nerve stimulators.

Sugammadex, a γ-cyclodextrin, has improved the manage-ment of neuromuscular blockade in patients with myasthenia gravis. It promotes reversal of blockade via two mechanisms. First, sugammadex will encapsulate aminosteroid neuromuscular blockers leading to their inactivation. Second, this will foster a concentration gradient at the neuromuscular junction resulting in the dissociation of rocuronium from receptors. Unlike pyr-idostigmine use, there is no effect on the neuromuscular junction or the metabolism of pseudocholinesterase. Numerous case reports have demonstrated quick and complete reversal of rocuronium neuromuscular blockade. However, randomized controlled trials are needed to evaluate the effects of sugammadex versus acetylcholinesterase inhibitors in this patient population.

Inhalational agents have also been successfully used to pro-vide an adequate degree of muscle relaxation thus decreasing or eliminating the need for muscle relaxants. Medications with a respiratory depressant effect, such as narcotics and benzodiaz-epines, should be used judiciously in these patients at a high risk of respiratory compromise.

Neuraxial blocks can be safely used as long as muscle function and ventilation can be adequately monitored in the

| TABLE 155.2 | Myasthenia Gravis and Lambert-Eaton Myasthenic Syndrome Comparison | |
| --- | --- | --- |
| **Characteristic** | **Myasthenia Gravis** | **Myasthenic Syndrome** |
| Signs and symptoms | Extraocular, bulbar, and facial muscles most commonly affected<br>Exercise increases weakness<br>Normal reflexes | Proximal > distal muscles<br>Legs > arms<br>Repetitive movement improves strength<br>Reflexes decreased |
| Sex | Females > males | Males > females |
| Coexisting conditions | Thymoma | Small cell lung cancer |
| Muscle relaxants response | Sensitive to nondepolarizing muscle relaxants<br>Resistant to depolarizing muscle relaxants<br>Good response to anticholinesterases | Sensitive to both depolarizing and nondepolarizing muscle relaxants<br>Poor response to anticholinesterases |

perioperative period. Peripheral blocks can also be safely used. However, risks with certain blocks need to be considered. For example, interscalene blockade results in phrenic nerve paresis, which may be relatively contraindicated in patients with symptomatic dyspnea or poor respiratory reserve. Aminoester local anesthetics may have prolonged duration of action as these drugs are metabolized by pseudocholinesterase, which would be inhibited by anticholinesterase drugs.

Extubation should not occur until solid evidence exists of adequate return of respiratory function. Consideration should also be given to the potential to develop weakness in the initial postoperative hours after first appearing to have sufficient strength.

## Lambert-Eaton Myasthenic Syndrome

### BACKGROUND

LEMS is an acquired autoimmune channelopathy that resembles myasthenia gravis. Some patients also develop autonomic dysfunction. Myasthenic syndrome is often associated with paraneoplastic disease, most commonly with small-cell lung cancer. Antibodies are created that bind to presynaptic calcium channels. This results in a deficiency of calcium entry when depolarization occurs and thus an inadequate release of acetylcholine. Similar to myasthenia gravis, patients will demonstrate muscle weakness and fatigability. However, unlike myasthenia

gravis, lower limb muscles are most commonly affected and less common is bulbar involvement in LEMS. Weakness is often worse in the morning and improves throughout the day as exercise and repetitive movements will lead to increasing accumulations of presynaptic calcium. Anticholinesterase drugs, though a mainstay in myasthenia gravis, do not provide a beneficial effect to patients with LEMS. 3,4-Diaminopyridine, however, has been shown to increase acetylcholine release and improve strength. Plasmapheresis and immunoglobulin therapy will provide an improvement in symptoms, albeit temporary (6–8 weeks). A comparison of myasthenia gravis with LEMS can be seen in Table 155.2.

### ANESTHETIC IMPLICATIONS

Patients should be counseled on the increased risk for requiring postoperative ventilator support and developing perioperative respiratory complications. Myasthenic syndrome patients have been shown to be sensitive to both depolarizing and nondepolarizing muscle relaxants. Autonomic dysfunction is often mild but can lead to hemodynamic instability. Patients with bulbar symptoms are at an increased risk for aspiration. Myasthenic syndrome should be considered in patients undergoing procedures related to lung carcinoma. Neuromuscular blockade can have a poor response to anticholinesterase drugs resulting in incomplete reversal.

## SUGGESTED READINGS

Carron, M., De Cassai, A., & Linassi, F. (2019). Sugammadex in the management of myasthenic patients undergoing surgery: Beyond expectations. *Annals of Translational Medicine, 7*(Suppl. 8), S307.

Gilhus, N. E. (2016). Myasthenia gravis. *New England Journal of Medicine, 375*(26), 2570–2581.

Hines, R. L., & Marschall, K. E. (2018). *Stoelting's Anesthesia and Co-Existing Disease* (7th ed.). Philadelphia: WB Saunders.

Miller, R. D., Cohen, N. H., Eriksson, L. I., Fleisher, L. A., Weiner-Kronish, J. P., & Young, W. L. (2015). *Miller's Anesthesia* (8th ed.). Philadelphia: WB Saunders.

Mouri, H., Jo, T., Matsui, H., Fushimi, K., & Yasunaga, H. (2020). Effect of sugammadex on postoperative myasthenic crisis in myasthenia gravis patients: Propensity score analysis of a Japanese Nationwide Database. *Anesthesia and Analgesia, 130*(2), 367–373.

Vymazal, T., Krecmerova, M., Bicek, V., & Lischke, R. (2015). Feasibility of full and rapid neuromuscular blockade recovery with sugammadex in myasthenia gravis patients undergoing surgery—A series of 117 cases. *Therapeutics and Clinical Risk Management, 11*, 1593–1596.

Weingarten, T. N., Araka, C. N., Mogensen, M. E., Sorenson, J. P., Marienau, M. E., Watson, J. C., et al. (2014). Lambert-Eaton myasthenic syndrome during anesthesia: A report of 37 patients. *Journal of Clinical Anesthesia, 26*(8), 648–653.

# 156

# Anesthesia for Endoscopic Procedures

RICHARD K. PATCH III, MD  |  MATTHEW N. VOGT, MD

## Introduction

Non–operating room anesthesia (NORA) is becoming a larger part of many anesthesia practices as the demand for coverage outside the traditional operating room (OR) increases. Gastrointestinal (GI) endoscopy is one area where the demand for anesthesia services is rapidly evolving. In the National Anesthesia Clinical Outcomes Registry, 81% of NORA cases occurred in the GI endoscopic suite. Endoscopic and technical advancements have allowed endoscopists to perform interventional procedures for multiple conditions that require deep sedation or general anesthesia. Additionally, the complexity and at times critical nature of patients has created an area of need for advanced and specialized anesthesia skills.

## Operational Considerations

As is the case with many NORA cases, the procedure suite is designed around the proceduralist and endoscopic procedure. It does not account for specific anesthetic needs. Endoscopic suites may be remotely located; thus additional supplies and assistance are not accessible in a timely manner. Additionally, equipment found in a traditional OR environment may not be present in the endoscopic suite. Examples include gas scavenging systems, a backup oxygen supply, difficult airway equipment, or emergency supplies such as a malignant hyperthermia kit. The patient's body habitus must also be considered, as some procedure suites may not have tables that can accommodate the patient. The anesthesia team must ensure all the potential issues are addressed either before the beginning of the case or, ideally, before the creation of an anesthesia-endoscopic service. The American Society of Anesthesiologists (ASA) has a statement on minimum standards regarding NORA (Tables 156.1 and 156.2).

Staffing for endoscopic procedures can be difficult, particularly in comprehensive and rapidly expanding practices. Including all NORA cases within the daily OR electronic case list creates the ability to allocate appropriate resources. Block scheduling can also assist with ensuring anesthesiologist coverage for cases that run late. The anesthesiologist also needs to have an active role in the periprocedural triage and postprocedure recovery areas. In many cases the patient is referred to the endoscopist only for the procedure. Unexpected admissions, prolonged recovery, and management of periprocedural complications likely fall within the anesthesia team's scope of practice, and an anesthesiologist's oversight is vital.

Non–anesthesiologist-administered propofol (NAAP) under the direction of the endoscopist and administered by a registered nurse may create contention and "boundary" issues between anesthesia and endoscopy practices. The American Gastroenterological Association (AGA) and American Society for Gastrointestinal Endoscopy (ASGE) position statement on NAAP for GI

| TABLE 156.1 | Adapted American Society of Anesthesiologists Statement on Non–Operating Room Anesthesia Locations |
|---|---|
| A reliable source of oxygen with a backup supply in each location |
| Adequate and reliable source of suction |
| Adequate and reliable scavenging system for locations with inhalation anesthetics |
| A self-inflating resuscitator bag, adequate anesthesia medications, and ASA standard monitoring |
| Sufficient electrical outlets and power supplies including an emergency power supply |
| Adequate illumination of the patient, anesthesia machine, and monitoring equipment |
| Sufficient space to allow expeditious access to the patient, anesthesia machine, and monitoring equipment |
| Emergency cart with defibrillator, emergency medications, and CPR equipment |
| Adequate support staff for the anesthesiologist |
| Observation of applicable building and safety codes |
| Appropriate postanesthetic management and access to a PACU if required |

*ASA*, American Society of Anesthesiologists; *CPR*, cardiopulmonary resuscitation; *PACU*, postanesthesia care unit.

endoscopy asserts that the safety profile is equivalent to that of standard sedation with respect to the risks of hypoxemia, hypotension, and bradycardia. Additionally, the statement discusses monitoring, but capnography is only suggested during NAAP, as the evidence is not definitive. This is in stark contrast to ASA standards. Moreover, as illustrated in the patient safety section, absence of capnography resulted in poor outcomes. Finally, the AGA/ASGE statement mentions that personnel using NAAP need to be trained in emergency airway management. However, airway management is not a component of gastroenterology and endoscopy training. NAAP has the potential for significant medical-legal ramifications for providers and hospital systems and anesthesiologists should be aware of its impact.

## Monitoring

Regardless of the location of the endoscopic suite, standard ASA monitoring for the assessment of oxygenation, ventilation, and circulation is required. Continuous pulse oximetry, capnography, electrocardiogram, temperature, and noninvasive blood pressure are included as in the OR. However, depending on the complexity of the case and patient's history, additional monitoring may be required. For example, a patient undergoing

| TABLE 156.2 | Gastrointestinal Endoscopic Procedures Requiring Anesthesia Management | |
|---|---|---|
| **Routine** | **Advanced** | |
| Esophagogastroduodenoscopy | Esophageal or colonic stent placement | |
| Colonoscopy | Endoscopic retrograde cholangiopancreatography | |
| Sigmoidoscopy | Endoscopic ultrasound | |
| | Double balloon enteroscopy | |
| | Stricture dilation | |
| | Tracheal-esophageal stricture closure | |
| | Percutaneous gastrostomy tube placement | |
| | Variceal banding | |
| | Pancreatic pseudocyst drainage | |
| | Mucosal ablation and/or resection | |
| | Fine needle biopsy | |
| | Natural orifice transluminal endoscopic surgery | |
| | Peroral endoscopic myotomy | |

an urgent endoscopic retrograde cholangiopancreatography (ERCP) for severe acute gallstone pancreatitis may require invasive hemodynamic monitoring if distributive shock is also present. Bispectral index monitoring may be used in patients requiring a general anesthetic for their endoscopic procedure who cannot receive a volatile anesthetic.

## Patient Safety

Although common, GI endoscopy is not without risk. Adverse events such as cardiopulmonary arrest, bleeding, perforation, postprocedural pain, and post-ERCP pancreatitis have all been reported. These events occur with anesthesia- and non-anesthesia-directed care. The ASA closed claim analysis provides some data regarding the safety and adverse events associated with anesthesia for endoscopic procedures. Of 20 NORA cases associated with oversedation, 13 occurred in the GI endoscopic setting. Twelve of the 13 cases did not have capnographic monitoring, and in all 20 cases the oversedation resulted in significant morbidity and mortality to the patient. In each of the cases, propofol was either used alone or in combination with other sedating medications. Aspiration is also a very important concern. As the complexity of upper endoscopic procedures increases, so does the depth of anesthesia required to perform the procedure and the potential loss of protective airway reflexes. In one large database of over 60,000 patients, a statistically significant association between the type of anesthetic and incidence of aspiration was found to be highest with monitored anesthesia care (MAC). Moreover, a systematic review of aspiration cases during GI endoscopy revealed that the severity of illness and use of propofol were significant factors. Finally, a prospective cohort study in Australia of anesthetist-managed sedation revealed that hypotension was the most

common side effect and that ASA status III and IV, as well as emergency procedure, were predictors of death.

## Anesthetic Management

A significant and important distinction may exist between patients presenting for surgery in the traditional OR setting and those presenting for endoscopy: the absence of a preanesthesia evaluation. Patients are referred to the endoscopist for the procedure, and most of the time the endoscopist is neither the patient's primary care provider nor the referring provider. Patient evaluation is important before any delivered anesthetic. However, in this patient population the anesthesiologist's role is crucial. Patients with significant comorbidities requiring complex procedures may not have had an adequate perioperative evaluation, and that evaluation may need to occur before the procedure. Moreover, the nothing-by-mouth status must be established, as occasionally this is not adequately explained to patients before their endoscopy.

Multiple anesthetic techniques are used for endoscopic procedures. A detailed description of the pharmacology of specific agents is provided in other sections of this textbook. Propofol alone or in combination with other agents is the most common anesthetic agent. Ketamine, midazolam, and dexmedetomidine are also options. Some centers use topical anesthesia sprays such as benzocaine to facilitate upper endoscopic esophageal intubation. Glycopyrrolate can be employed to reduce secretion burden. Multimodal analgesia with opioids, ketorolac, and acetaminophen is as important in the endoscopic setting as it is in the traditional OR. Patients in this setting may have chronic abdominal pain, such as those with chronic pancreatitis, and take long-acting opioids at home. Postoperative nausea prophylaxis is also important given the manipulation and required insufflation of the GI tract for the endoscopic procedure. At times, general endotracheal anesthesia (GETA) is required depending on patient characteristics and the planned procedure.

Postanesthesia care is similar in the endoscopy suite as in the OR environment with management of hemodynamics, oxygenation, pain control, and nausea. However, as previously mentioned, some important differences exist. Patients undergoing procedures for either severe acute gallstone pancreatitis or infected pancreatic pseudocysts may be in septic shock or develop sepsis after the procedure. Appropriate sepsis management will depend on the anesthesiologist, and if admission to the hospital or an intensive care unit is required, coordination may fall to the anesthesia team. Similarly, if admission is required for pain control in a patient with chronic pain secondary to a GI etiology, the anesthesia team may also be responsible for admission.

## Procedures

A comprehensive description of each procedure and supporting evidence is out of the scope of this review. However, a brief description of each procedure is provided to give the practicing anesthesia provider information to better care for these patients.

### ESOPHAGOGASTRODUODENOSCOPY

Esophagogastroduodenoscopy (EGD) is used for diagnostic, therapeutic, and advanced procedures. Routine evaluations include abdominal pain, reflux, and unexplained nausea, although acute indications such as upper GI bleeding are also common. Forceps can be used to assist in biopsies for diagnosis. Esophageal varices can be banded and stents deployed for palliation in the case of malignant gastric obstructions. Strictures are can be dilated and percutaneous gastrostomy (PEG) tubes placed with an EGD. Dilation with either a bougie or balloon is very stimulating and requires a deep level of sedation and many times, a general anesthetic. The management of these patients depends on the clinical context and patient comorbidities. Patients with an acute upper GI bleed and retained blood likely require intubation for airway protection. A general anesthetic may also be indicated for PEG tube placement or esophageal stent deployment. Additionally, EGD can be used for submucosal dissection for which a general anesthesia may be required.

## DOUBLE BALLOON ENTEROSCOPY

Double balloon enteroscopy employs extended-length endoscopes with a sliding tube overlaying the endoscope with balloons attached at the distal end. The balloons are intermittently inflated, allowing for insertion of the endoscope into the small intestine. It is used to evaluate patients with obscure GI bleeding and surgically altered anatomy. Although the procedure can be successfully performed under MAC, more often it requires a general anesthetic because of the length and stimulation of the procedure.

## ENDOSCOPIC ULTRASOUND

Endoscopic ultrasound (EUS) uses an endoscope with a high-frequency transducer at the tip. It can evaluate lesions in the upper digestive tract, surrounding structures near the GI tract, and allow for fine-needle aspiration (FNA) of the upper GI tract wall, mediastinal structures, and pancreas. Depending on the indication and planned procedure, EUS can be performed under MAC with propofol or general anesthesia.

## ENDOSCOPIC RETROGRADE CHOLANGIOPANCREATOGRAPHY

ERCP combines endoscopic and fluoroscopic techniques to visualize the pancreatic and biliary systems. The scope is modified with side-viewing optics, and an accessory channel allows catheter advancement. The most common indications for ERCP are choledocholithiasis, palliation of malignant biliary obstruction, bile leaks, and management of benign biliary strictures. The patient is typically positioned in a modified prone position or occasionally supine. The procedure is longer and more intense than a routine EGD. It can be performed under MAC with propofol; however, GETA with airway protection should be considered.

## NATURAL ORIFICE TRANSLUMINAL ENDOSCOPIC SURGERY

Natural orifice transluminal endoscopic surgery (NOTES) is a form of minimally invasive surgery and endoscopy. Endoscopic cystgastrostomy is currently the most common NOTES seen in the endoscopy setting. It is performed in an ERCP suite and is a combination of EUS and fluoroscopy. Additionally, it is now first-line treatment for symptomatic pancreatic pseudocyst and infected pancreatic walled-off necrosis. Endoscopic cystgastrostomy can be technically intense, and optimal patients need to be well sedated. Many times, the sedation requirements necessitate endotracheal intubation with a general anesthetic. Depending on the clinical context and patient comorbidities, MAC with propofol could be sufficient.

## PERORAL ENDOSCOPIC MYOTOMY

Peroral endoscopic myotomy (POEM) is intended to replicate a Heller myotomy for patients with achalasia. The procedure is most performed in the traditional operative setting. However, advanced centers with experienced endoscopists and comprehensive resources are performing the procedure in an endoscopy suite. General anesthesia with endotracheal intubation is most appropriate for these patients.

## COLONOSCOPY/SIGMOIDOSCOPY

As with EGD, there are routine and advanced aspects to endoscopic evaluation of the lower GI tract. The most common indications are colon cancer screening, anemia, and lower GI bleeding. Procedures such as EUS with or without FNA, mucosal resection, stent deployment, stricture dilation, and NOTES can be performed with a lower GI tract endoscope. The most common indication for colonoscopies is colon cancer screening. MAC with propofol is sufficient for most of the procedures. Again, general anesthesia with endotracheal intubation is likely necessary for NOTES to achieve optimal conditions.

## SUGGESTED READINGS

Allen, M. L. (2017). Safety of deep sedation in the endoscopy suite. *Current Opinion in Anesthesiology*, 30(4), 501–506.

Bohman, J. K., Jacob, A. K., Nelsen, K. A., Diedrich, D. A., Smischney, N., Olatoye, O., et al. (2018). Incidence of gastric-to-pulmonary aspiration in patients undergoing elective upper gastrointestinal endoscopy. *Clinical Gastroenterology and Hepatology*, 16(7), 1163–1164.

Early, D. S., Lightdale, J. R., Vargo, J. J., Acosta, R. D., Chandrasekhara, V., Chathadi, K. V., et al.

(2018). Guidelines for sedation and anesthesia in GI endoscopy. *Gastrointestinal Endoscopy*, 87, 327–337.

Leslie, K., Allen, M. L., Hessian, E. C., Peyton, P. J., Kasza, J., Courtney, A., et al. (2017). Safety of sedation for gastrointestinal endoscopy in a group of university-affiliated hospitals: A prospective cohort study. *BJA: British Journal of Anaesthesia*, 118(1), 90–99.

Sharp, C. D., Tayler, E., & Ginsberg, G. G. (2017). Anesthesia for routine and advanced upper

gastrointestinal endoscopic procedures. *Anesthesiology Clinics*, 35(4), 669–677.

Tetzlaff, J. E., Vargo, J. J., & Maurer, W. (2014). Non-operating room anesthesia for the gastrointestinal endoscopy suite. *Anesthesiology Clinics*, 32(2), 387–394.

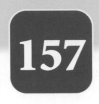

# Anesthesia Outside of the Operating Room

MISTY A. RADOSEVICH, MD

## Introduction

A steadily increasing demand for sedation and anesthesia outside of the operating room (OR) has developed over the past 20 years. With this increased demand, anesthesia providers are treating older and sicker patients who increasingly require complex procedures that are performed outside of the OR. In fact, a greater percentage of American Society of Anesthesiologists (ASA) Physical Class III through V patients receive care in the non–operating room anesthesia (NORA) setting than in the operating room (37.6% vs. 33.0%, respectively). Challenges of NORA include remote and unfamiliar anesthetizing locations, limited equipment and supplies, variable training levels of providers (not always anesthesia providers), unique procedural considerations, and patient complexity. Institution-wide guidelines should be in place to ensure the consistent delivery of safe anesthesia and sedation by appropriately trained individuals with sufficient support (equipment, monitoring, and personnel), regardless of location.

## Monitoring, Equipment, and Patient Evaluation

Patients who are to undergo procedures requiring sedation or anesthesia should be evaluated with the same scrutiny as if undergoing a general anesthetic. Guidelines for the provision of NORA in terms of the minimal requirements for staffing, equipment, and environment were described in a statement published by the ASA and are outlined in Table 157.1. Basic monitoring as outlined by the ASA, including pulse oximetry, ventilation monitoring (including end-tidal carbon dioxide monitoring unless not possible), blood pressure measurement (at least every 5 minutes), and electrocardiogram monitoring, must be provided. Adequate monitoring cannot be overemphasized, because most deaths in NORA settings have been attributed to lack of adequate monitoring (see "Complications" section).

## Spectrum of Sedation and Anesthesia

Sedation and anesthesia can be thought of as a spectrum with progressively increasing effects on the cardiopulmonary system. Light sedation corresponds to a calm, nonanxious state in which the patient remains able to verbally respond to providers. With moderate sedation, a patient is sedate but able to purposefully respond to a provider's voice or touch. Deep sedation requires painful or repeated stimuli to elicit a response from a patient. Oxygenation, ventilation, and hemodynamics may need to be supported at this level of sedation. Under general anesthesia, the patient no longer responds to painful stimuli. Deep sedation and general anesthesia should only be administered by those trained to intervene and support the airway and hemodynamics.

## Providers

Light and moderate sedation for many procedures with minimal to no invasiveness (e.g., imaging studies, simple interventional

---

**TABLE 157.1  Minimal Standards for the Provision of Anesthesia Outside the Operating Room**

**EQUIPMENT**
Source of oxygen (central source preferred) with a backup supply (E-cylinder or equivalent)
Suction apparatus
Waste gas scavenging system (if inhaled anesthetics are used in that location)
Anesthesia machine (if inhalation anesthesia provided in that location)
Self-inflating bag valve mask for positive pressure mask ventilation
Monitoring equipment consistent with the ASA Standards for Basic Anesthesia Monitoring
Sufficient number and type (isolated if appropriate) of electrical outlets for all necessary equipment
Adequate lighting to visualize the patient, monitors, and anesthesia machine, including an additional battery-powered source of light such as a flashlight
Sufficient space to accommodate the patient, equipment, monitors, and personnel that also enables easy access to the patient

**EMERGENCIES**
Immediate access to an emergency cart that has cardiopulmonary resuscitation equipment including a defibrillator and emergency medications including medications to treat malignant hyperthermia (e.g., dantrolene)

**PERSONNEL**
Adequate staff to support the anesthesia provider
Reliable means of two-way communication
Adequate numbers of personnel and equipment to safely transport patients to the postanesthesia care unit

*ASA*, American Society of Anesthesiologists.
(Adapted from the ASA Statement on Nonoperating Room Anesthetizing Locations, 2013.)

radiology procedures), and a large percentage of gastrointestinal (GI) endoscopy, is provided by nonanesthesia personnel under the direction of the proceduralist. These providers must be trained sufficiently to intervene and support the patient at a level of sedation deeper than intended; that is, if moderate or deep sedation is being provided, the provider should be trained to support a patient under deep sedation or general anesthesia, respectively. The appropriate basic monitoring and equipment previously mentioned must be in place. Anesthesiologists must be involved in the oversight and establishment of institutional standards regarding the appropriate provision of sedation and anesthesia, both in terms of providers and resources. NORA cases directed by anesthesiologists have been shown to have fewer deaths related to failure to rescue.

## Complications

The ASA closed claims database has provided insight into the complications associated with NORA. More than other non-OR locations, GI endoscopy procedures were associated with closed claim filings. Risks associated with GI procedures

include crowding of the airway with the endoscope, aspiration, bleeding, oversedation, inappropriate use of a nonanesthesia provider, and lack of vigilance. Additional NORA complications include cardiovascular, equipment-related, and medication-related events. The next most common locations for NORA claims were the cardiology catheterization and electrophysiology laboratory followed by radiology. Inadequate oxygenation and ventilation was found responsible for many claims, which may reflect a higher proportion of cases under monitored anesthesia care or sedation with no definitive airway device. According to Woodward and colleagues, claims related to death were reported more frequently for NORA than anesthesia care in the OR, and most of these deaths were caused by respiratory events judged potentially preventable by adequate monitoring.

## Nonoperating Room Locations

Common locations in which sedation and anesthesia are often required and the specific considerations related to procedures in those locations are listed in Table 157.2.

| TABLE 157.2 | Special Considerations for Non-Operating Room Anesthesia by Location |
|---|---|
| **Nonoperating Room Location** | **Special Considerations** |
| Cardiac catheterization laboratory | Wide spectrum of patient acuity (scheduled angiograms vs. cardiogenic shock and respiratory failure in the setting of an acute STEMI). The expanding role of non–OR-based cardiac procedures (e.g., TAVR) emphasizes the importance of anesthesiologist involvement in this setting. Complications in this location can be catastrophic and require high-level intervention (e.g., VAD or ECMO initiation, emergent transfer to the OR, emergent pericardiocentesis). Appropriate resources (e.g., invasive monitoring equipment) and protocols should be in place anticipating such events. |
| Neuroradiology | Frequent requirement for GETA (limit patient movement, secure airway in event of a complication). May require rapid wake-up. Complex management may be necessary (e.g., intracranial hypertension management maneuvers, neuromonitoring). |
| MRI | Unique environment: specialized equipment (no ferromagnetic objects), screening, monitoring are vital. Despite these limitations, must comply with the ASA's Standards for Basic Anesthesia Monitoring. Patient is remote from providers for lengths of time. High noise level. Staff should undergo annual MRI safety education. |
| CT imaging and interventional procedures | Patients requiring anesthesia assistance in the CT area are usually presenting for CT-guided procedures. Often these patients are complex and often "too ill" for a more invasive procedure to manage a disease process. May require nonstandard positioning (e.g., prone) to perform the procedure. Contrast is often used and preparations for responding to an allergic reaction should be readily available. The spectrum of interventions in this area is broad (invasive line placement, liver biopsy, sclerotherapy, coil embolizations), and the complications associated with each should be well understood. |
| Gastroenterology (endoscopy) | Upper endoscopy presents the challenge of sharing access to the patient's airway with the proceduralist. Complications such as aspiration of gastric contents, loss of airway, and bleeding may occur. |
| Radiation therapy/proton beam | Immobility is key to the precise delivery of radiation to the targeted tissue while minimizing damage to nearby normal tissues. Frequently, this therapy is planned as a series of daily treatments. Providers must be remote from the patient during treatments to avoid exposure to radiation. Appropriate means of monitoring the patient remotely must be in place. Neuraxial anesthesia with sedation may be considered for brachytherapy treatments in some abdominal and pelvic malignancies. |

*ASA,* American Society of Anesthesiologists; *CT,* computed tomography; *ECMO,* extracorporeal membrane oxygenation; *GETA,* general endotracheal anesthesia; *MRI,* magnetic resonance imaging; *OR,* operating room; *STEMI,* ST-elevation myocardial infarction; *TAVR,* transcatheter aortic valve replacement; *VAD,* ventricular assist device.

## SUGGESTED READINGS

Abenstein, J. P., & Warner, M. A. (1996). Anesthesia providers, patient outcomes, and costs. *Anesthesia and Analgesia, 82,* 1273–1283.

Robbertz, R., Posner, K. L., & Domino, K. B. (2006). Closed claims review of anesthesia for procedures outside the operating room. *Current Opinion in Anaesthesiology, 19,* 436–442.

*Standards for Basic Anesthetic Monitoring.* (2020). The American Society for Anesthesiologists.

www.asahq.org/standards-and-guidelines/standards-for-basic-anesthetic-monitoring.

*Statement on Nonoperating Room Anesthetizing Locations.* (2018). The American Society for Anesthesiologists. www.asahq.org/standards-and-guidelines/statement-on-nonoperating-room-anesthetizing-locations.

Wong, T., Georgiadis, P. L., Urman, R. D., & Tsai, M. H. (2020). Non-operating room anesthesia:

Patient selection and special considerations. *Local and Regional Anesthesia, 13,* 1–9.

Woodward, Z. G., Urman, R. D., & Domino, K. B. (2017). Safety of non-operating room anesthesia: A closed claims update. *Anesthesiology Clinics, 35,* 569–581.

Youn, A. M., Ko, Y. K., & Kim, Y. H. (2015). Anesthesia and sedation outside of the operating room. *Korean Journal of Anesthesiology, 68,* 323–331.

# 158

# Anesthesia for Interventional Neuroradiology

ARNOLEY S. ABCEJO, MD | JEFFREY J. PASTERNAK, MS, MD

Interventional neuroradiology encompasses a range of diagnostic and therapeutic techniques used to assess or treat disorders involving the brain, brainstem, spinal cord, and cerebral vasculature. As technology advances, the practice of interventional neuroradiology expands while the number of patients requiring these procedures continues to increase. This chapter will aim to summarize and review the anesthetic concerns and management goals for patients having neurologic interventional radiologic (NIR) procedures.

## Neurologic Interventional Radiologic Imaging Exposure and Considerations

Most NIR procedures involve the use of fluoroscopy, although some use computerized tomography and magnetic resonance imaging. Fluoroscopy is an x-ray–based technique that allows for real-time imaging due to differential scattering of x-rays by different tissues and contrast. Fluoroscopy exposes the patient and providers to x-rays with radiation dose directly proportional to the duration of imaging. Thus health care providers should exercise measures to minimize exposure to both the patient and themselves. This should include standing as far from the radiation source as possible and using lead aprons, lead shields, and eye protection. Given the high sensitivity of eye lenses to radiation exposure, lead shields offer an advantage over standard aprons at potentially minimizing long-term risk for cataracts in health care providers.

## Contrast Drugs

Radiopaque contrast drugs are iodinated organic compounds that scatter x-rays and are used to delineate vascular structures and define anatomy. When administered intravascularly, these drugs will cause blood to appear hypodense on conventional fluoroscopic images. Although their use is often critical to the success of NIR procedures, they are associated with some adverse effects that are of interest to anesthesia providers.

- *Acute contrast reactions:* These occur within 1 hour of contrast administration and present as an anaphylactic or anaphylactoid reaction characterized by mild to severe urticaria, bronchospasm, and hypotension.
- *Delayed contrast reactions:* These adverse reactions occur after 1 hour and up until 1 week after contrast drug exposure. They usually manifest as mild and nonspecific signs and symptoms including nausea, vomiting, diarrhea, and pruritis. Severe delayed contrast reactions, such as Stevens-Johnsons syndrome, can occur.
- *Contrast-induced nephropathy:* This is defined as an increase in baseline serum creatinine concentration of greater than 25% within 3 days of receiving contrast. Preexisting renal dysfunction is the strongest risk factor

| TABLE 158.1 | Risk Factors for Contrast-Induced Nephropathy |
| --- | --- |

Preexisting renal dysfunction
Hypovolemia, dehydration
Increased age
Diabetes mellitus
Hypertension
Conditions of poor renal perfusion:
   Congestive heart failure
   Myocardial infarction
   Hemodynamic instability
   Concurrent use of nephrotoxic drugs
   ACE inhibitors
Use of high-osmolality contrast drugs
Use of high volumes of contrast drugs

*ACE,* Angiotensin converting enzyme.

(Table 158.1). Although its etiology is likely multifactorial, contrast-induced nephropathy likely results from direct nephrotoxicity and contrast-induced renal vasoconstriction. Prevention includes minimizing contrast dose, use of *N*-acetylcysteine, and periprocedural hydration. Prophylactic intravenous bicarbonate is controversial, and forced diuresis should be avoided.

## Ischemic Stroke

In suitable candidates, endovascular therapy has become the standard of care for management and treatment of acute ischemic stroke. Expeditious time to treatment is critical to improving neurologic morbidity.

Anesthetic management for endovascular ischemic stroke management focuses on optimizing cerebral physiologic and hemodynamic conditions to improve cerebral perfusion and prevent secondary neurologic complications. Table 158.2 describes the recommended management for patients undergoing stroke revascularization from the Society for Neuroscience in Anesthesiology and Critical Care. Avoidance of hypotension and hypertension in patients undergoing general anesthesia is critical. Anesthetic-induced hypotension can worsen cerebral perfusion, whereas hypertension, such as during emergence from anesthesia, can potentiate the risk for hemorrhagic transformation after restoration of flow. This latter complication is associated with high morbidity and mortality. Every 10 minutes of cumulative time that mean arterial pressure is either less than 70 mm Hg or greater than 90 mm Hg intraprocedurally can significantly and adversely alter neurologic outcome. Other risk factors for hemorrhagic conversion are greater stroke severity, edema after administration of tissue plasminogen activator (tPA), hyperglycemia, coagulopathy, and prolonged time to revascularization. If hemorrhagic conversion is suspected,

| TABLE 158.2 | Perioperative Management for Anesthesia for Acute Ischemic Stroke Revascularization Adapted From the 2016 Society for Neuroscience in Anesthesiology and Critical Care (SNACC) Recommendations |
|---|---|

**Society for Neuroscience in Anesthesiology and Critical Care Perioperative Recommendations for Acute Ischemic Stroke Revascularization**

**ANESTHESIA TECHNIQUE**

- Preoperative exam: focused preanesthetic examination to prevent delay of treatment
- Monitors: American Society of Anesthesiologists standard monitors
- The choice of anesthesia technique should be individualized, however:
  - Consider general anesthesia
    - In uncooperative patients
    - In patients with posterior circulation strokes
    - In patients with decreased level of consciousness
    - In patients with active nausea or emesis
    - In patients at risk for hypoxia, hypercarbia, or airway obstruction
  - If local anesthesia with sedation is provided
    - The patient must be cooperative and able to protect their airway
    - General anesthesia can be rapidly administered emergently, if needed

**MANAGEMENT OF OXYGENATION AND VENTILATION**

- Titrate fraction of inspired oxygen to maintain an oxygen saturation of hemoglobin >92% and arterial oxygen partial pressure of >60 mm Hg
- Ventilation should be adjusted to maintain normocapnia if under general anesthesia (arterial partial pressure of carbon dioxide of 35–40 mm Hg)
- Avoid respiratory depression secondary to oversedation

**PERIPROCEDURAL HEMODYNAMIC MANAGEMENT**

- Hemodynamic and cardiac rhythm monitoring should be used as soon as stroke has been diagnosed
- Continuous invasive intraarterial pressure measurement may be performed as long as arterial cannulation does not delay therapy
- Systolic blood pressure should be maintained between 140 and 180 mm Hg
- Do not allow systolic blood pressure <140 mm Hg during induction of anesthesia
- After successful recanalization or thrombectomy, blood targets may be adjusted

**OTHER PERIPROCEDURAL MANAGEMENT GOALS**

- Hyperthermia and hypothermia should be aggressively treated
  - Target temperatures between 35°C and 37°C
  - Antipyretics should be provided if patient febrile
- Hyperglycemia and hypoglycemia should be aggressively treated
  - A serum glucose should be obtained before the procedure if not already obtained
  - Maintain serum glucose between 70 and 140 mg/dL
  - Treat hypoglycemia <50 mg/dL

Data from Talke PO, Sharma D, Heyer FJ, et al. Society for Neuroscience in Anesthesiology and Critical Care expert consensus statement: anesthetic management of endovascular treatment for acute ischemic stroke: endorsed by the Society of NeuroInterventional Surgery and the Neurocritical Care Society. *J Neurosurg Anesthesiol.* 2014;26(2):95-108.

maintaining adequate cerebral perfusion and treating intracranial hypertension are paramount.

General anesthesia and conscious sedation can both be used to facilitate revascularization for ischemic stroke. General anesthesia offers the advantage of a motionless patient but may be associated with hypotension. Conscious sedation allows for intraprocedural, real-time neurologic assessment but may be suitable for all patients, especially those with severe stroke. At the current time, there is no strong data to support the use of one technique over another.

## Carotid Artery Stenting

Transient ischemic attacks and stroke can occur in patients with significant carotid atherosclerosis. In addition to carotid endarterectomy, carotid artery stenting can also be used to treat carotid atherosclerosis. Many patients undergoing carotid artery stenting have significant comorbidities and should be medically optimized for this elective procedure, if possible.

Monitored anesthetic care with or without intravenous sedation is often used to facilitate carotid angioplasty with stenting. Though general anesthesia can also be used in patients in whom it is medically indicated, a neurologic exam is often desired throughout the entire periprocedural setting. Local anesthesia for arterial puncture is often sufficient for procedural analgesia. Nonetheless, there are several critical, high-risk portions of the procedure that should be anticipated and well understood.

- *Balloon angioplasty:* Balloon inflation can exert pressure against the carotid sinus. Vagally mediated bradycardia can ensue, and an anticholinergic medication (atropine, glycopyrrolate) may be needed prophylactically to attenuate this reflex. Transcutaneous pacing may be required if the patient's comorbidities cannot tolerate relative tachycardia associated with anticholinergic agents.
- *Recurrent or new distal stroke:* Embolization of plaque material can occur at several key points during carotid stenting: (1) catheter advancement through the stenotic area, (2) deployment of the distal protection device, (3) balloon angioplasty, (4) stent deployment, and (5) retraction of the distal protection device. The distal protection device is an embolic trap that prevents particulate matter from traveling distally. However, manipulation of the trap itself can initiate embolism. Gross neurologic examination is essential during these critical times.
- *Reperfusion syndrome:* Cerebral autoregulation may be impaired within the vessels distal to the atherosclerotic lesion. After carotid revascularization, increases in systemic

blood pressure may not be attenuated in brain regions perfused by the ipsilateral carotid artery. Thus absolute or relative systemic hypertension can cause cerebral hyperemia. This reperfusion syndrome is characterized by cerebral edema, altered mental status, and new neurologic deficit. Treatment involves blood pressure reduction.

## Cerebral Aneurysms

Cerebral aneurysm rupture is often associated with significant morbidity and mortality. Thus treatment of unruptured and ruptured aneurysm is often performed to reduce risk of rupture and rerupture, respectively. Treatments include NIR-based techniques such as coil embolization, pipeline placement (Fig. 158.1), or surgical aneurysm clipping. The decision to perform an NIR-based technique or surgical clipping depends on many factors including aneurysm location, aneurysm anatomy, and patient comorbidities.

General anesthesia is preferred over monitored anesthesia care to facilitate NIR treatment of a cerebral aneurysm, as general anesthesia can ensure a motionless patient. Patient movement during NIR aneurysm treatment increases risk for aneurysm rupture or coil embolization distal to the aneurysm. General anesthesia is also warranted in patients with poor-grade subarachnoid hemorrhage to facilitate airway protection and possible hyperventilation to treat acute intracranial hypertension.

Anesthetic and physiologic goals for patients undergoing NIR-based cerebral aneurysm treatment include:

- Controlling intracranial hypertension (i.e., maintenance of cerebral perfusion), especially in those with subarachnoid hemorrhage
- Maintaining a motionless patient
- Avoiding sudden increases in blood pressure before aneurysm treatment, especially during laryngoscopy
- Ensuring metabolic hemostasis, such as avoiding extremes in core temperature and serum glucose concentration

## Brain Arteriovenous Malformations

Arteriovenous malformations (AVMs) consist of pathologic anastomosis between arteries and veins without intervening capillaries, forming a nidus of low-resistance, high-flow vessels amenable to mass effect, edema formation, and rupture. NIR-based embolization of AVMs can rarely lead to complete obliteration of the AVM. Instead, NIR techniques are often employed to decrease AVM size before stereotactic radiosurgery (i.e., gamma knife) or before surgical resection.

General anesthesia or sedation can be administered for NIR-based AVM embolization. The choice of anesthetic is largely dependent on the patient, patient comorbidities, and risk of AVM rupture. Invasive blood pressure monitoring is not absolutely necessary. However, large-bore intravenous access should be strongly considered.

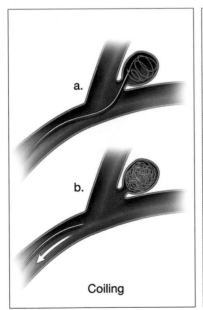 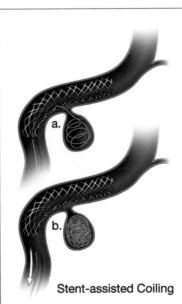 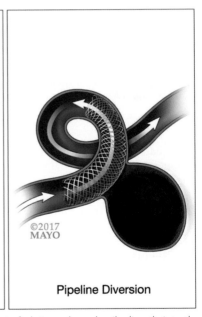

| Coiling | Stent-assisted Coiling | Pipeline Diversion |

**Fig. 158.1 Endovascular treatment options for intracerebral aneurysms.** *(Left)* Placement of platinum-based coils directly into the aneurysmal sac obstructs blood flow and minimizes risk for rupture. *(Middle)* In stent-assisted coiling, a fenestrated stent can act as a conduit for coil placement into the aneurysmal sac while preventing coil reentry back into the feeding artery. *(Right)* A pipeline stent isolates the blood contained in the aneurysmal sac from the systemic circulation promoting thrombosis of the aneurysmal sac.

## SUGGESTED READINGS

Berkhemer, O. A., Fransen, P. S., Beumer, D., van den Berg, L. A., Lingsma, H. F., Yoo, A. J., et al. (2015). A randomized trial of intraarterial treatment for acute ischemic stroke. *New England Journal of Medicine, 371*, 11–20.

Brott, T. G., Hobson, R. W., II, Howard, G., Roubin, G. S., Clark, W. M., Brooks, W., et al. (2010). Stenting versus endarterectomy for treatment of carotid-artery stenosis. *New England Journal of Medicine, 363*, 11–23.

Campbell, D., Diprose, W. K., Deng, C., & Barber, P. A. (2021). General anesthesia versus conscious sedation in endovascular thrombectomy for stroke: A meta-analysis of 4 randomized controlled trials. *Journal of Neurosurgical Anesthesiology, 33*, 21–27.

Hindman, B. J. (2019). Anesthetic management of emergency endovascular thrombectomy for acute ischemic stroke, part 1: Patient characteristics, determinants of effectiveness, and effect of blood pressure on outcome. *Anesthesia and Analgesia, 128*(4), 695–705.

Hoefnagel, A. L., Rajan, S., Martin, A., Mahendra, V., Knutson, A. K., Uejima, J. L., et al. (2019). Cognitive aids for the diagnosis and treatment of neuroanesthetic emergencies: Consensus guidelines on behalf of the Society for Neuroscience in Anesthesiology

and Critical Care (SNACC) Education Committee. *Journal of Neurosurgical Anesthesiology, 31*(1), 7–17.

Powers, W. J., Rabinstein, A. A., Ackerson, T., Adeoye, O. M., Bambakidis, N. C., Becker, K., et al. (2019). Guidelines for early management of patients with acute ischemic stroke: 2019 update to the 2018 guidelines for the early management of acute ischemic stroke: A guideline for healthcare professionals from the American Heart Association/ American Stroke Association. *Stroke, 50*(12), e344–e418.

Rasmussen, M., Schonenberger, S., Henden, P. L., Valentin, J. B., Espelund, U. S., Sørensen, L. H., et al. (2020). Blood pressure thresholds and neurologic outcomes after endovascular therapy for acute ischemic stroke: An analysis of individual patient data from 3 randomized clinical trials. *JAMA Neurology, 77*(5), 622–631.

Sharma, D. (2020). Perioperative management of aneurysmal subarachnoid hemorrhage. *Anesthesiol, 133*(6), 1283–1305.

# 159

# Anesthesia for Patients With Diabetes Mellitus

MICAH T. LONG, MD  |  ALEXANDRA L. ANDERSON, MD  |  ERIC R. SIMON, MD

## Introduction

Diabetes mellitus (DM) is a severe disease with significant societal impact. The incidence of DM type 2 (DM2) has reached epidemic proportions, with a nearly 50% increase in prevalence over the past 20 years. Currently an estimated 14.6% of U.S. adults (>30 million Americans) have been diagnosed with diabetes, including nearly 5% of adults aged 45 years and younger and 20% of adults aged 45 to 65 years. Importantly, 1 out of every 4 patients with DM2 are undiagnosed. A retrospective review of approximately 40,000 patients who underwent noncardiac surgery found that 10% of patients had undiagnosed diabetes. These patients may not be optimized for surgery and may be at greater risk for perioperative morbidity and even mortality.

Both DM type 1 (DM1) and DM2 result in impaired cellular glucose uptake causing cellular starvation and stress in the face of hyperglycemia, the common end point for all diabetes subtypes. Hyperglycemia is injurious, causing oxidative stress, inflammation, hypovolemia, and more. Autoimmune or idiopathic destruction of insulin secreting islet β cells in the pancreas causes DM1 and results in an absolute insulin deficiency. These patients require a constant supply of exogenous insulin, or cellular starvation will result. In extreme states of insulin deficiency, patients can develop diabetic ketoacidosis (DKA), a state of intense cellular starvation and stress with life-threatening hyperglycemia, hypovolemia, and ketoacidosis.

DM2 is the result of progressive insulin resistance with progression to relative deficiency in insulin release. In extremis, patients enter a hyperglycemic hyperosmolar state (HHS), a critical state of relative insulin deficiency and massive hyperglycemia with severe hypovolemia. Individuals with higher than normal glucose levels not high enough to meet diabetes

criteria are said to have prediabetes, characterized by impaired fasting glucose and/or impaired glucose tolerance. DM2 is typically caused by obesity, poor diet, and inactivity. Other factors may contribute, including hereditary characteristics, genetic defects of β-cell function, glucose-transport or insulin action abnormalities, exocrine pancreas dysfunction, polyglandular endocrinopathies, pregnancy, medications, infections, or chronic inflammation. Other, less common subtypes of diabetes exist. A summary of the American Diabetes Association definitions for DM, prediabetes, and stress hyperglycemia in hospitalized patients is presented in Table 159.1.

## Complications of Diabetes

Chronic hyperglycemia causes multiple organ system dysfunction due to nonenzymatic glycosylation (glycation), oxidative stress, inflammation, and other factors. Traditionally, chronic injury in diabetes is broadly categorized as macrovascular (e.g., coronary, cerebral, and peripheral artery disease) and microvascular (e.g., nephropathy, retinopathy, neuropathy). Specific perioperative considerations for these complications are reviewed in Table 159.2.

Cardiovascular disease is the leading cause of morbidity and mortality in patients with DM. Perioperatively, diabetes (on insulin therapy) is a major contributor to risk in the Revised Cardiac Risk Index (RCRI), with increased risk for major adverse cardiac events (reviewed in Chapter 75, Preoperative Evaluation of the Patient With Cardiac Disease for Noncardiac Operations). Oxidative stress, inflammation, acute hyperglycemia, and glycation contribute. Glycation is a phenomenon that is time and glucose concentration dependent, in which glucose progressively attaches to cells and proteins. This causes progressive vessel narrowing and vascular compromise. Further, resultant

| TABLE 159.1 | Definitions for Diabetes Mellitus, Prediabetes, and Stress Hyperglycemia |
| --- | --- |
| **Diagnosis*** | **Criteria** |
| **DIABETES MELLITUS** | |
| Fasting PG | ≥126 mg/dL |
| Random PG | ≥200 mg/dL + symptoms of hyperglycemia† |
| 2-hour PG during 75-g OGTT | ≥200 mg/dL |
| HbA$_{1c}$ | ≥6.5% |
| **PREDIABETES** | |
| Fasting PG | 100–125 mg/dL (impaired fasting glucose) |
| 2-hour PG during 75-g OGTT | 140–199 mg/dL (impaired glucose tolerance) |
| HbA$_{1c}$ | 5.7%–6.4% |
| **STRESS HYPERGLYCEMIA‡** | |
| Fasting PG | ≥126 mg/dL |
| Random PG | ≥200 mg/dL |

*Testing should be performed with the patient in an unstressed state, and a second test should confirm the diagnosis unless a clear diagnosis is present (e.g., a hyperglycemic crisis).
†Classic symptoms of hyperglycemia include polyuria, polydipsia, and fatigue, and can include presentation with hyperglycemic crisis.
‡The PG is obtained in a patient without evidence of previous diabetes mellitus while the patient is in a stressed state and reverts to a normal value after recovery.
*HbA$_{1c}$*, Hemoglobin A$_{1c}$; *OGTT*, oral glucose tolerance test; *PG*, plasma glucose.

advanced glycation end products are metabolically active and contribute to ongoing injury, such as the characteristic highly atherogenic, very-low-density lipoprotein dyslipidemia of DM. Further, glycation contributes to stiffened joints and soft tissue, which may impair wound healing and make direct laryngoscopy more difficult.

Microvascular injury includes diabetic neuropathy, a complex process that results in small-fiber glycation-related nerve damage. Peripheral neuropathy classically presents as sensory deficits in a "stocking and glove" distribution pattern and can increase risk for positioning injury and chronic wound development. Central autonomic neuropathy, on the other hand, can lead to delayed gastric emptying, thus increasing the risk of aspiration, and contribute to silent myocardial infarctions. Importantly, autonomic disease and dysfunction can cause depressed or absent responses to stimulation and physiologic aberrancies, such as hypotension or hypercarbia.

Diabetic nephropathy results from chronic microvascular injury to the kidneys, which increases the risk of chronic kidney disease (CKD) and perioperative acute kidney injury (AKI) independent of baseline creatinine. This is partly related to impaired autoregulation of glomerular blood flow and hyperglycemia-induced afferent glomerular vasoconstriction. The earliest sign of diabetic nephropathy is microalbuminuria and an elevated urinary protein-to-creatinine ratio, with eventual elevation of serum creatinine.

Acutely poor glycemic control may result in life-threatening complications, such as DKA in DM1 and HHS in DM2, or more insidious complications, such as immune dysfunction, surgical or other site infection, poor wound healing, and overall oxidative stress and inflammation. Immune dysfunction is multifactorial with deficits in nearly all immune pathways. This is amplified by chronic wounds that are prone to resistant microbes and poor healing from tissue glycation. Acute or acute-on-chronic stress-induced hyperglycemia may be an even more important contributor to negative perioperative outcomes than the diagnosis of diabetes itself.

## Preoperative Assessment

The preoperative evaluation of patients with diabetes should begin with a comprehensive risk assessment prior to surgery. First, the type of diabetes should be clearly delineated. Patients

| TABLE 159.2 | Perioperative Considerations for the Complications of Diabetes Mellitus | |
| --- | --- | --- |
| **Complication** | **Perioperative Risk** | **Considerations** |
| **MACROVASCULAR INJURY** | | |
| Cerebrovascular, coronary, and peripheral arterial disease | Increased risk of CAD, PAD, and CVA. Increased risk of perioperative MACE.* | Careful risk assessment and consent. Consider advanced monitoring (e.g., arterial line). Maintain BP within 20% of baseline. |
| **MICROVASCULAR INJURY** | | |
| Nephropathy | Increased risk of CKD and perioperative AKI. | Avoid hypotension and nephrotoxins; maintain euvolemia. |
| Neuropathy | Autonomic neuropathy can result in delayed gastric emptying and decreased physiologic responses to hypotension, hypercarbia, stress, or stimulation. Peripheral neuropathy increases risk for positioning-related injury. | Consider rapid sequence induction. Use appropriate drugs for hemodynamic support. Cautious operative positioning. |
| Diffuse glycation of joints and soft tissue | Stiff joint syndrome can increase risk of difficult direct laryngoscopy. Healing and wound strength is at risk. | Employ a cautious airway management plan. |
| Hyperglycemia and other dysglycemia | Hyperglycemia (absolute and stress) increases perioperative morbidity and mortality. Fasted patients may develop perioperative hypoglycemia. Certain home medications have unique perioperative risks. Immune dysfunction can increase risk of surgical site and postoperative infections. Patients with DM1 require constant exogenous insulin. | Consider first-case (morning) scheduling. Review preoperative medications and hold/administer medications accordingly. Employ a glucose monitoring and treatment plan with a hospital-wide algorithm. |

*MACE includes myocardial infarction, arrhythmia, CVA, and death.
*AKI*, Acute kidney injury; *BP*, blood pressure; *CAD*, coronary artery disease; *CKD*, chronic kidney disease; *CVA*, cerebrovascular accident; *DM1*, diabetes mellitus type 1; *MACE*, major adverse cardiac event; *PAD*, peripheral arterial disease.

with DM1 have an absolute insulin deficiency and require constant exogenous insulin to prevent cellular starvation. Next, screening for micro- and macrovascular disease processes should be performed. The cardiovascular assessment warrants focused attention: signs and symptoms of coronary artery disease, congestive heart failure, and cerebrovascular disease should be reviewed. Note that myocardial ischemia can present silently or with atypical symptoms, particularly in those with dysautonomia. Similarly, cerebrovascular disease may present as subtle cognitive decline. Signs and symptoms of autonomic neuropathy including orthostasis, resting tachycardia, chronic diarrhea, and early satiety should be elicited. A baseline blood pressure should be noted to guide intraoperative blood pressure goals.

Airway assessment should consider stiff joints and soft tissue, noting that direct laryngoscopy is more difficult in patients with DM compared with those without, even with equal airway examinations and body mass index (BMI). The "prayer sign," or the inability to bring together palms and fingers, can signify advanced tissue glycosylation that may be indicative of limited joint mobility in the neck. Dysautonomia including delayed gastric emptying contributes to the aspiration risk assessment, and gastric emptying studies may be indicated. Finally, creatinine, trend in creatine, and the urine protein-to-creatinine ratio can offer insight into renal health and the risk of perioperative kidney injury. As discussed earlier, the risk for patients undergoing moderate- to high-risk procedures should be stratified using the RCRI or other risk assessment tools discussed in Chapter 75, Preoperative Evaluation of the Patient with Cardiac Disease for Noncardiac Operations.

Recent glycemic control can be assessed with measuring glycated hemoglobin or hemoglobin $A_{1C}$ ($HbA_{1c}$), which estimates the average serum glucose over the prior 3 months. For those with known diabetes, an $HbA_{1c}$ measurement should be obtained within 3 to 6 months of surgery. Measuring $HbA_{1c}$ may also help identify patients at risk for undiagnosed diabetes; standardized recommendations for screening for diabetes are displayed in Table 159.3. After screening, for those with a new diagnosis of DM ($HbA_{1c} > 6\%$), poorly controlled DM ($HbA_{1c} > 8\%$), or an $HbA_{1c}$ less than 8% but at high risk of complications of dysglycemia (DM1, insulin pump or U500 insulin use, CKD stage IV, or cirrhosis), preoperative consultation likely benefits from a dedicated endocrinology or diabetes team (see Palermo & Garg, 2019).

Data are mixed regarding the absolute risk contribution from an elevated $HbA_{1c}$ (poor control of glucose over the prior

3 months) in terms of surgical outcomes, though most studies support worse outcomes with progressive elevations in $HbA_{1c}$. No clear "optimal" $HbA_{1c}$ target has been determined, though a goal of less than 8% is frequently used for preoperative optimization. There is only limited evidence to support delaying elective surgery to lower a patient's $HbA_{1c}$; the optimal $HbA_{1c}$ target, risks of aggressive acute glycemic control, and duration of adequate control required to reverse chronic injury or decrease perioperative risk remain unclear. The likelihood and time needed for improved glycemic control also needs to be balanced with specific perioperative and procedural risks and considerations for each patient.

A patient's current therapies for diabetes should be reviewed and medication instructions given. In general, oral antihyperglycemics are held the day of surgery. The incidence, symptoms, and severity of hypoglycemic events should be reviewed as should the patient's typical eating habits. Grazers, as opposed to those who eat in defined meal windows, may be more prone to hypoglycemia when fasting. The degree of hypoglycemia causing symptoms may be different in those with chronically elevated glucose; these should be noted. The scheduled and corrective doses of insulin should be listed; higher correction ratios suggest increased insulin resistance. Long-acting insulin is generally maintained at 50% to 70% of the home regimen based on the risk of hypoglycemia and average glucose control for those patients on insulin. In general, other oral antihyperglycemics are held the day of surgery. Table 159.4 reviews preoperative medication instructions, including for insulin, for patients with diabetes.

Glucose monitoring and therapeutic technology is expanding rapidly. Patients may present with personal devices including insulin pumps, continuous glucose monitors, or artificial pancreas devices. Standardized assessments and protocols for these should be considered at the hospital-wide level with close engagement of endocrinology teams.

## Hyperglycemia

Hyperglycemia is associated with an increased risk of perioperative complications and mortality in both cardiac and noncardiac surgery. This risk relates to both absolute hyperglycemia and to acute-on-chronic hyperglycemia—the elevation in glucose above the patient's baseline. Accordingly, a perioperative glucose management algorithm should be employed to address perioperative glycemic monitoring, treatment of hyperglycemia, and discharge planning. Management of perioperative hyperglycemia

---

| TABLE 159.3 | Preoperative Screening Recommendations |
| --- | --- |

Screen for diabetes in all patients with multiple risk factors, and all patients aged ≥45 years regardless of risk factors. Screen patients aged 35–70 years with BMI ≥25 kg/m² (≥23 kg/m² in Asian Americans) with at least one risk factor:
  a. Known prediabetes with $HbA_{1c}$ ≥ 5.7%, impaired glucose tolerance test, or impaired fasting glucose
  b. Chart review with any random blood glucose ≥ 200 mg/dL
  c. Cardiovascular disease history
  d. Conditions associated with insulin resistance: hypertension, dyslipidemia, or polycystic ovarian syndrome
  e. Symptoms of insulin resistance (e.g., acanthosis nigricans)
  f. Maternal history of gestational diabetes
  g. Family history of DM2 in first- or second-degree relative
  h. High-risk race or ethnicity (African American, Latino, Native American, Asian American, or Pacific Islander)

*BMI,* Body mass index (normal 18.5–24.9 kg/m²); *DM2,* diabetes mellitus type 2; *$HbA_{1c}$,* glycated hemoglobin.
Data from American Diabetes Association. 2. Classification and diagnosis of diabetes: standards of medical care in diabetes – 2018. *Diab Care.* 2018;41(suppl 1):S13-S27; U.S. Preventive Services Task Force. Screening for prediabetes and type 2 diabetes: USPSTF recommendation statement. *JAMA.* 2021;326(8):736-743.

| TABLE 159.4 | Preoperative Medication Recommendations |

This assumes normal diet the day before surgery and nothing by mouth after midnight the day of surgery, allowing clears up to 2 hours preoperatively.

| Medication Class | Examples | Day Before Surgery | Morning of Surgery |
|---|---|---|---|
| Biguanides | Metformin | Continue.* *Rare risk of metformin-associated lactic acidosis.* | Hold* |
| Sulfonylureas | Glimepiride Glipizide Glyburide | Continue | Hold |
| Meglitinides | Repaglinide | Continue | Hold |
| Thiazolidinediones | Pioglitazone Rosiglitazone | Continue | Continue |
| Alpha glucosidase inhibitors | Acarbose | Continue | Hold |
| Sodium-glucose cotransporter-2 inhibitors | Canagliflozin Dapagliflozin Empagliflozin Ertugliflozin | Hold for 3 days (4 days for ertugliflozin). *Rare risk of perioperative euglycemic ketoacidosis.* | Hold |
| Dipeptidyl peptidase-4 inhibitors | Alogliptin Linagliptin Saxagliptin Sitagliptin | Continue | Continue |
| Glucagon-like peptide 1 receptor agonists | Dulaglutide Exenatide Liraglutide Semaglutide | Continue | Hold if dosed daily. Continue if dosed weekly, unless prone to hypoglycemia when fasting. |
| Insulin Class | Examples | Day Before Surgery | Morning of Surgery† |
| Long-acting (basal) insulin | Glargine Degludec Detemir | *Daily morning dosing:* Continue normal dose *Daily evening dosing:* 75%–80% of normal dose *Twice daily dosed:* Continue normal AM dose; 75%–80% of normal PM dose | *Daily morning dosing:* 80% of normal dose *Twice daily dosed:* 80% of normal AM dose |
| Intermediate-acting (basal) insulin | NPH | 80% of normal AM dose 80% of normal PM dose | 50% of normal AM dose (hold if PG < 120 mg/dL) |
| Combination intermediate- and short-acting | NPH/Regular 70/30 | 80% of normal AM dose 80% of normal PM dose | 50% of normal AM dose (hold if PG < 120 mg/dL) |
| Short-acting (correction) | Regular | Continue normal doses | Hold |
| Rapid-acting (correction) insulin analogs | Aspart Glulisine Lispro | Continue normal doses | Hold |
| Insulin pump | Variable | Continue minimum outpatient basal rate. Consider reduction of 25%–50% or transition to insulin infusion at this rate. | Continue prior rate. Hold prandial doses. |

*Hold metformin the day of and the day before surgery if the procedure includes intravenous dye administration, particularly if the patient's glomerular filtration rate is <45 mL/min. In patients without renal dysfunction undergoing minor surgery with low risk of acute kidney injury, metformin may be continued the day of surgery.
†For patients at risk of hypoglycemia, with a history of hypoglycemia or with hypoglycemia unawareness, insulin doses should be further reduced.
*NPH*, Neutral protamine hagedorn; *PG*, plasma glucose.

is discussed in Chapter 211, Perioperative Management of Blood Glucose. Patients with poorly controlled diabetes, challenges to medication follow-through, extreme or difficult-to-control hyperglycemia, or significant complications of diabetes warrant close engagement of an expert in diabetes or a diabetes management team.

## Management of Anesthesia

The anesthesiologist must determine the types of physiologic monitoring to be used during anesthesia. Diabetic patients with dysautonomia may be more susceptible to the vasodilating and

myocardial-depressant effects of anesthetic agents and may benefit from invasive physiologic monitoring, such as an arterial line. Blood pressure should generally be kept within 20% of the patient's baseline. An arterial line can also serve as access to monitor serum glucose should operating conditions, patient position, or physiology make point-of-care fingerstick capillary measurements suboptimal. Regional anesthesia may improve overall hemodynamics, but consideration must be given to the risk of nerve injury in patients with diabetic neuropathy. Airway management should anticipate difficult direct laryngoscopy. For patients with gastroparesis, metoclopramide, nonparticulate antacids, $H_2$-receptor blockers, and/or proton pump inhibitors may be indicated, and a rapid sequence intubation should be considered. Preoperative gastric ultrasound is a growing area of interest. Strict attention should be given to patient positioning because of the increased risk of nerve and position-related injury.

Glucose monitoring is challenging in the operating room, and a myriad of operative and perioperative factors affect point-of-care testing negatively. Specific algorithms and strategies for glucose monitoring and management should be followed and are addressed in Chapter 211, Perioperative Management of Blood Glucose.

Patients should be monitored closely in the postoperative window for dysglycemia, autonomic instability, airway compromise, stroke, and myocardial ischemia. In the outpatient setting, a conservative consideration for discharge should be deployed. For patients with an elevated preoperative HbA$_{1c}$, severe hyperglycemia, or difficult-to-control hyperglycemia, the primary physician and endocrinologist, or an inpatient diabetes team, should be closely engaged.

## Summary

Diabetes is a serious disease of abnormal glucose metabolism that affects every organ system. It is the most common endocrinopathy, and its prevalence is at epidemic proportions. Clinicians must be intimately familiar with the disease and its perioperative implications. Glycosylation affects all tissues and can cause difficult direct laryngoscopy, increased risk of positioning-related injury, impaired wound healing, increased risk for surgical site infections, and complications of associated end-organ disease. Macrovascular disease increases the risk of stroke, myocardial ischemia, and other major adverse cardiac events. Microvascular disease increases the risk of perioperative AKI, whereas autonomic neuropathy can yield aspiration risk and hemodynamic instability. With appropriate diagnosis, identification of risks, preoperative optimization, cautious anesthetic planning, and appropriate monitoring, there is great opportunity to improve postoperative outcomes in patients with diabetes.

## SUGGESTED READINGS

Duggan, E. W., Carlson, K., & Umpierrez, G. E. (2017). Perioperative hyperglycemia management: An update. *Anesthesiology, 126*(3), 547–560.

Duggan, E., & Chen, Y. (2019). Glycemic management in the operating room: Screening, monitoring, oral hypoglycemics, and insulin therapy. *Current Diabetes Reports, 19*(11), 134.

Duggan, E. W., Klopman, M. A., Berry, A. J., & Umpierrez, G. (2016). The Emory University perioperative algorithm for the management of hyperglycemia and diabetes in non-cardiac surgery patients. *Current Diabetes Reports, 16*, 34.

Hashim, K., & Thomas, M. (2014). Sensitivity of palm print sign in prediction of difficult laryngoscopy in diabetes: A comparison with other airway indices. *Indian Journal of Anaesthesia, 58*(3), 298–302.

Long, M. T., & Coursin, D. B. (2020). The perils of perioperative dysglycemia. *International Anesthesiology Clinics, 58*(1), 21–26.

Palermo, N. E., & Garg, R. (2019). Perioperative management of diabetes mellitus: Novel approaches. *Current Diabetes Reports, 19*, 14.

Preiser, J. C., Provenzano, B., Mongkolpun, W., Halenarova, K., & Cnop, M. (2020). Perioperative management of oral glucose-lowering drugs in the patient with type 2 diabetes. *Anesthesiology, 133*(2), 430–438.

Simha, V., & Shah, P. (2019). Perioperative glucose control in patients with diabetes undergoing elective surgery. *JAMA, 321*(4), 399–400.

Sreedharan, R., & Abdelmalak, B. (2018). Diabetes mellitus: Preoperative concerns and evaluation. *Anesthesiology Clinics, 36*, 581–597.

Wang, L., Li, X., Wang, Z., Bancks, M. P., Carnethon, M. R., Greenland, P., et al. (2021). Trends of prevalence of diabetes and control of risk factors in diabetes among US adults, 1999-2018. *JAMA, 326*(8), 704–716.

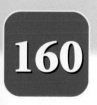

# 160 Anesthesia for Thyroid Surgery

ROBERT L. McCLAIN, MD

Although operations on the thyroid gland are often viewed as routine procedures, they can present a unique combination of problems for the anesthesia provider. For example, difficulties in securing the airway in the presence of a large mass or surgical trauma to the recurrent laryngeal nerve (RLN), especially if bilateral, may cause dysphonia and stridor after extubation.

The presence of coexisting thyroid hyper- or hypofunction, particularly if severe, affects morbidity and mortality. Anesthesia, by itself, may precipitate "thyroid storm" in patients with hyperfunction of the thyroid. Also, hypofunction of unknown severity may present multisystem clinical challenges during both the intraoperative and postoperative periods. Close cooperation between the anesthesia provider, surgeon, and perhaps an endocrinologist is imperative in achieving optimal outcomes in patients undergoing thyroid operations.

## General Considerations

### PREOPERATIVE ASSESSMENT

Thyroid operations have been successfully completed under local, regional, and monitored care anesthesia. However, most thyroid surgery is performed under general anesthesia. For an endotracheal intubation, a regular polyvinyl chloride (PVC) endotracheal tube (ETT) will usually suffice. However, a wire-reinforced ETT may be considered if airway patency compromise is anticipated; even ETT adapted for RLN monitoring may be requested for surgery (see the next section).

Airway management issues in patients with goiters should be anticipated. Patients should be asked about positional dyspnea and hypotension when supine because these symptoms may suggest clinically relevant airway or superior vena cava mechanical compression. High suspicion for possible difficult intubation exists in many cases, and consideration should be given to requesting preoperative ultrasonography or computerized tomography (CT) of the neck in patients with thyroid disease. Preoperative evaluation may be required to guide the anesthesia provider's initial airway management decisions to perform an awake intubation or facilitate perioperative discussions with surgeons regarding elective tracheostomy in severe cases. Although a chest x-ray may provide evidence of tracheal deviation or airway collapse, a CT scan may be more informative regarding retrosternal extension of thyroid disease, tracheal ring compression, and/or airway tortuosity.

### PRESERVING AND ASSESSING FUNCTION OF THE RECURRENT LARYNGEAL NERVE

The overall incidence of RLN damage during thyroid operations is 2% to 5%. Visual identification and preservation of the RLN by surgery remains the gold standard for protection; however, dynamic real-time nerve integrity monitoring (NIM) of RLN function during airway management has emerged as the preferred method to reduce the incidence of damage. Commonly requested with NIM, the anesthesia provider substitutes the usual PVC ETT with an endotracheal tube impregnated with electrodes near the balloon cuff. When this ETT is correctly inserted (which may require indirect laryngoscopy tools), the electrodes of the ETT are aligned with the vocal cords. The surgeon will often verify the integrity of contact by using a small stimulating current. NIM provides both an audible and visual display of action potential generation whenever the RLN is stimulated during surgery. Although false positives do occur, studies have shown NIM alerts the surgeon to potential RLN damage more than 70% of the time, reducing the incidence of unilateral RLN injury to 0.77% and bilateral RLN injury to 0.3%.

### POSTOPERATIVE COMPLICATIONS

At the end of surgery, direct visual or indirect laryngoscopy may be necessary to evaluate vocal cord movement; laryngoscopy may be necessary to identify glottic edema linked to postoperative stridor. Unilateral RLN paralysis, resulting in a midline ipsilateral cord collapse of the affected side on inspiration, is more common and is rarely clinically apparent. In contrast, bilateral RLN paralysis, in which both cords deviate to midline, is associated with aphonia, stridor, and often requires reintubation.

Excessive postoperative bleeding resulting in hematoma formation occurs in 1% to 2% of cases and is the most common cause of airway obstruction within the first 24 hours after surgery. Returning the patient to the operating room may be necessary, and consultation with the surgeon should occur upon any suspicion of this complication.

Last, thyroid surgery can be complicated by iatrogenic injury to the parathyroid glands either from disruption of vascular supply leading to ischemia to the glands or inadvertent excision of the glands themselves. The resultant hypoparathyroidism can lead to acute hypocalcemia postoperatively. Symptomatic postoperative hypocalcemia may be encountered in 3% to 5% of thyroid surgeries and usually presents between 24 and 48 hours after surgery. Symptoms of acute hypocalcemia include QT prolongation, muscle spasms, laryngospasm, airway obstruction, seizures, and even cardiac arrest if not identified early.

## The Patient With Known Thyroid Disease

Patients presenting for elective surgery, commonly for thyrotoxicosis, goiter, and/or thyroid cancer, should ideally be assessed preoperatively for clinical symptomatology or for subclinical signs. Evidence of excess circulating thyroid hormone may present in patients as tremor, palpitation anxiety, and even angina pectoris. Ideally before elective surgery, a patient with hyperthyroidism should consider serology testing and perhaps endocrinology consultation. If a euthyroid state is not present, further optimization with antithyroid medication may be advised. Commonly prescribed antithyroid medications include thioamide drugs such as methimazole, which inhibits thyroxine ($T_4$) synthesis, and propylthiouracil, which both inhibits synthesis of $T_4$ and also reduces the peripheral conversion of $T_4$ to triiodothyronine ($T_3$). Iodine to reduce vascularity, antiadrenergics, and steroids may be prescribed. Patients should be euthyroid before surgery to minimize complications. Generally, 6 weeks of therapy may be necessary to appropriately reduce free $T_4$ or $T_3$ levels and to normalized hemodynamic values before surgery. In patients with Graves disease, the presence of exophthalmos may require additional eye care measures (e.g., lubrication) to avoid corneal-conjunctival desiccation and damage.

Preoperatively discovering mild hypothyroidism is not uncommon, but rarely does mild or even moderate hypothyroid disease result in significant perioperative adverse events. Patients with severe hypothyroidism, or myxedema, are prone to hypothermia and have potential for postoperative refractory circulatory collapse. Other potential problems linked to hypothyroidism include an increased risk of aspiration, increased sensitivity to opioids and inhaled anesthetic agents, and hypoglycemia. It may be prudent to postpone elective surgery until the patient is optimized by an endocrinologist. Myxedematous patients are at added risk of developing adrenal insufficiency and therefore should be given prophylactic steroids intraoperatively. It should be noted that $T_4$ and $T_3$ have approximate half-lives of 7 and 1.5 days, respectively. Therefore even if both are administered preoperatively for the treatment of severe cases of myxedema, the immediate clinical benefits may not be appreciated for several days. The cardiac effects of $T_3$ and $T_4$ may have a faster onset relative to their other thyroid hormone actions and may be detrimental, possibly manifesting as increased risk for arrhythmias and even acute coronary syndrome. The risk of preoperative treatment with $T_4$ in myxedema needs to be weighed on a case-by-case basis and may require coordination with endocrinology.

## The Patient With Occult Thyroid Disease

Atrial fibrillation may be the initial presentation for up to 20% of patients with occult hyperthyroidism. Hypertension, tachycardia, tremor, sweating, diarrhea, and extreme animation or even agitation should elevate one's level of suspicion. Myxedema may be seen in elderly, sedentary patients with bradycardia, constipation, and/or altered mental status. For the patient with myxedema requiring emergency surgery, the degree of elevation of the thyroid-stimulating hormone level and the clinical status should be further investigated before treating with $T_4$. However, the concept of using a bolus of $T_4$ preoperatively (as discussed earlier) may be acceptable. Further evaluation for thyroid gland derangements should be considered in any patient displaying postoperative agitation, restlessness, tachycardia, or delayed emergence from anesthesia. Cognizance of perioperative thyroid dysfunction, even if remote on a differential diagnosis list, is often the key to diagnosis and prompt management.

## Thyroid Storm

Thyroid storm is a potentially life-threatening clinical diagnosis in which manifestations of hyperthyroidism are exacerbated by the sudden release of $T_3$ and $T_4$. A chemical euthyroid state lessens the risk of thyroid storm but does not negate it. It can be induced by surgery, trauma, pregnancy, or any severe illness. Thyroid storm in the operating room may be confused with malignant hyperthermia (MH), neuroleptic malignant syndrome, or the signs manifested by a pheochromocytoma. However, in contrast to MH and other mimickers, thyroid storm is more likely to develop *postoperatively* (on occasion taking up to 24 hours). The signs and symptoms of thyroid storm include hypokalemia, metabolic acidosis, high fever, tachycardia, and confusion, and even congestive heart failure has been reported. However, unlike MH, thyroid storm is typically *not* associated with rigidity, elevated creatine kinase, or lactic acidosis. Once the diagnosis is made, the goal is to treat the underlying cause and to provide simultaneous supportive therapy. The patient's body should be cooled with ice packs and cold intravenous fluids. Propranolol has been the β-blocking agent of choice both for heart rate control and for the inhibition of peripheral conversion of $T_4$ to $T_3$. Titrating esmolol intravenously up to 300 mcg/kg/min has also been shown to be efficacious. Vasopressors for hypotension and inotropes for heart failure may be used judiciously. Magnesium has been shown to be helpful in controlling catecholamine-induced arrhythmias provoked by $T_4$. Hydrocortisone may be administered for coexisting adrenal hypofunction. Carbimazole (not available in the United States), methimazole, and propylthiouracil have all been used successfully to inhibit thyroid hormone secretion and peripheral conversion of $T_4$ to $T_3$. Patients with thyroid storm carry a significant mortality risk. They should be monitored in an intensive care unit postoperatively until their condition stabilizes.

Finally, advancements in surgical technique have led to the emergence of robotic-assisted thyroid surgery. This has added another level of complexity and often physical equipment barriers to the patient, which means further restricting access the airway shared. In summary, exemplary anesthesia care during thyroid surgery requires vigilance during all parts of the perioperative process and awareness of possible complications faced when caring for a patient with thyroid disease.

## SUGGESTED READINGS

Bajwa, S. J., & Sehgal, V. (2013). Anesthesia and thyroid surgery: The never ending challenges. *Indian Journal of Endocrinology and Metabolism, 17*, 228–234.

Chen, A. Y., Bernet, V. J., Carty, S. E., Davies, T. F., Ganly, I., & Inabnet III, W. B., et al. (2014). American Thyroid Association Statement on optimal surgical management of goiter. *Thyroid, 24*, 181–189.

MacDonald, D. B., Skinner, S., Shils, J., & Yingling, C. (2013). Intraoperative motor evoked potential monitoring: A position statement by the American Society of Neurophysiological Monitoring. *Clin Neurophysiology, 124*(12), 2291–2316.

Patel, A. (2020). Anesthesia for otolaryngologic and head-neck surgery. In R. D. Miller (Ed.), *Anesthesia* (9th ed., Vol. 2, pp. 2210–2235). Philadelphia: Churchill Livingstone.

Shindo, M. L., Caruana, S. M., Kandil, E., McCaffrey, J. C., Orloff, L. A., Porterfield, J. R., et al. (2014). Management of locally invasive well-differentiated thyroid cancer: An American Head and Neck Society consensus statement. *Otolaryngology – Head and Neck Surgery, 36*, 1379–1390.

Steurer, M., Passler, C., Denk, D. M., Schneider, B., Niederle, B., & Bigenzahn, W. (2012). Advantages of recurrent laryngeal nerve identification in thyroidectomy and parathyroidectomy and the importance of preoperative and postoperative laryngoscopic examination in more than 1000 nerves at risk. *Laryngoscope, 112*, 124–133.

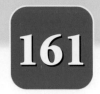

# 161

# Anesthesia for Patients With Carcinoid Syndrome

MICHELLE A. OCHS KINNEY, MD | JOHN A. DILGER, MD

## Small Bowel Neuroendocrine Tumors

The incidence of small bowel neuroendocrine tumors (SBNETs) is 1.05 per 100,000 population in the United States, and these tumors can cause debilitating signs and symptoms. SBNETs arise from enterochromaffin tissues and release various vasoactive substances (e.g., histamine, serotonin, kallikreins). Because these substances are cleared from the circulation by the liver, tumors that are isolated to the gastrointestinal tract usually do not result in the systemic manifestations of the carcinoid syndrome. The carcinoid syndrome occurs when these substances are secreted into the systemic venous system from an SBNET that has metastasized to the liver (thus bypassing the portal circulation) or a neuroendocrine tumor that has originated in the ovaries, lungs, or thyroid. Clinical signs and symptoms of carcinoid syndrome include bronchoconstriction, episodic cutaneous flushing, abdominal pain, diarrhea, hemodynamic instability, hepatomegaly, hyperglycemia, dysrhythmias, and decreased plasma albumin concentrations. Physiologic stress can stimulate tumors to release these substances and result in a carcinoid crisis. Cardiac valvular manifestations result from chronic exposure to high levels of serotonin. Cardiac valvular lesions are usually isolated to the right heart and include thickening and shortening of the leaflets resulting in decreased mobility with both regurgitation and stenosis of the tricuspid and pulmonary valves.

## Anesthetic Management

### PREOPERATIVE ANESTHETIC MANAGEMENT

Octreotide acetate is a long-acting analog of the naturally occurring peptide somatostatin. It inhibits release by tumor cells of serotonin, gastrin, vasoactive intestinal peptide, secretin, motilin, and pancreatic polypeptide. Octreotide can be administered intravenously or subcutaneously, depending on the desired time of onset and duration. Intravenous (IV) administration results in peak serum concentrations within approximately 3 minutes. Subcutaneous injections of octreotide result in peak concentrations 30 to 60 minutes after injection, with a plasma half-life of 113 minutes. The biologic duration of effect may last 12 hours.

Administering octreotide before and/or during surgical procedures in an attempt to prevent a carcinoid crisis is generally safe and does not appear to increase complication rates. The usual preoperative dose of octreotide is 500 mcg IV or subcutaneously 1 to 2 hours before surgery. Acute octreotide administration may be lifesaving in an acute carcinoid crisis and is generally given in 50- to 300-mcg IV doses. Octreotide doses of 500 to 1000 mcg have been reported in cardiac valvular surgery. However, IV bolus doses of octreotide and doses of 100 mcg or greater may result in bradycardia and atrioventricular conduction abnormality, presumably by acting directly on the cardiac conduction system. Dilution of octreotide, slow infusion, and continuous electrocardiogram monitoring may be advisable to minimize potential cardiac side effects of octreotide. Given the plasma half-life of 113 minutes, IV infusions of octreotide have been successfully used for operative cases lasting more than 2 hours. Administering a 500-mcg IV bolus of octreotide preoperatively followed by a continuous IV infusion of 500 mcg/hour, with additional bolus doses as clinically indicated, has been associated with a very low incidence of carcinoid crisis (3.4%).

Octreotide is also administered as a once monthly intramuscular long-acting release (LAR) preparation. Patients on octreotide LAR who need surgery may have high sustained levels of octreotide. Nonetheless, these patients may still require subcutaneous or IV octreotide in the perioperative period.

Preoperative sedation may be administered to avoid sympathetic stimulation, which could result in a carcinoid crisis. The presence of hypovolemia, electrolyte abnormalities, and right-sided cardiac valvular lesions should be ascertained. Left-sided cardiac valves are usually spared from carcinoid-related abnormalities, which reflect the ability of the pulmonary parenchyma to inactivate vasoactive substances. Left-sided cardiac valve involvement can occur, though, in the presence of pulmonary tumors, right-to-left intracardiac shunts, or in the presence of overwhelming disease.

Intraarterial hepatic embolization or chemoembolization is sometimes used before partial hepatectomy to reduce tumor burden and/or symptoms. Octreotide administration may be used preoperatively, intraoperatively, and postoperatively to reduce the risk of a carcinoid crisis.

### INTRAOPERATIVE ANESTHETIC MANAGEMENT

Gentle surgical skin preparation to avoid tumor compression is advised (Table 161.1). Consider avoiding histamine-releasing drugs, although these drugs have been used without complications. Very low doses of β-adrenergic agonists (e.g., 5 mcg of IV epinephrine) have been shown to stimulate the release of vasoactive substances; however, phenylephrine and amrinone can be safely used. However, Weingarten and colleagues' cardiac surgery study, the administration of catecholamine drugs in conjunction with octreotide was tolerated, suggesting that vasoactive medications can be given safely to patients with carcinoid syndrome in the presence of octreotide therapy. However, if the etiology of hypotension is secondary to carcinoid activity, the treatment should consist of IV octreotide and fluid.

| TABLE 161.1 | Anesthetic Management in Patients With Carcinoid Syndrome |
|---|---|
| **AVOIDANCE OF:** | |
| Opioids: | Meperidine and morphine |
| Histamine-releasing neuromuscular relaxants: | Atracurium, mivacurium, d-tubocurarine |
| Administration of exogenous catecholamines (controversial, use only in conjunction witsh octreotide): | Epinephrine, norepinephrine, dopamine, isoproterenol |
| Release of endogenous catecholamines: | Anxiety, hypotension, pain, hypothermia, minimize laryngotracheal reflexes on intubation |
| Mechanical tumor stimulation: | Vigorous abdominal scrubbing; succinylcholine (controversial) |

Adapted from Botero, M., Fuchs, R., Paulus, D. A., & Lind, D. S. (2002). Carcinoid heart disease: a case report and literature review. *Journal of Clinical Anesthesia, 14*(1), 57–63.

β-Adrenergic agonists should only be used when the cause of hypotension is not from carcinoid activity.

Octreotide should be readily available for immediate treatment of carcinoid symptoms intraoperatively. Administer octreotide whenever carcinoid symptoms (e.g., bronchospasm, unexpected hypotension, facial flushing) occur, along with volume infusion and phenylephrine as needed. The usual intraoperative IV bolus dose for carcinoid symptoms is 50 to 500 mcg and may need to be repeated. The presence of carcinoid heart disease and previous exposure to octreotide may require higher doses of octreotide to treat carcinoid symptoms. The total intraoperative dose of octreotide administered in noncardiac surgery may reach 4000 mcg, although this is uncommon. In Weingarten's cardiac valvular surgery series, the median intraoperative octreotide dose was 1500 mcg (mean 3666 ± 6461 mcg, range 50–54,000 mcg).

Intraoperative hypotension and other complications can occur despite octreotide LAR, single-dose prophylactic octreotide, or continuous octreotide infusion. Hepatic metastases, hepatic resection, placement of an epidural catheter, blood loss, and transfusion have been correlated with increased intraoperative complications. Anesthesiologists should be prepared to treat intraoperative hypotension with additional octreotide, vasopressors, and IV fluids as needed. In addition, hepatic resection can involve intermittent compression of vascular structures, and transient surgically induced hypotension can occur. Good communication between the anesthesiologist and surgeon is essential and can help guide the appropriate management of hypotension.

## POSTOPERATIVE MANAGEMENT

The humoral effects of metastatic SBNET lesions are usually not eliminated by surgery. Thus octreotide should be continued if the patient was using it preoperatively.

## SUGGESTED READINGS

Botero, M., Fuchs, R., & Paulus, D. A. (2002). Carcinoid heart disease: A case report and literature review. *Journal of Clinical Anesthesia, 14*, 57–63.

Dasari, A., Shen, C., Halperin, D., Zhao, B., Zhou, S., Xu, Y., et al. (2017). Trends in the incidence, prevalence, and survival outcomes in patients with neuroendocrine tumors in the United States. *JAMA Oncology, 3*, 1335–1342.

Dilger, J. A., Rho, E. H., Que, F. G., & Sprung, J. (2004). Octreotide-induced bradycardia and heart block during surgical resection of a carcinoid tumor. *Anesthesia and Analgesia, 98*, 318–320.

Howe, J. R., Cardona, K., Fraker, D. L., Kebebew, E., Untch, B. R., Wang, Y. Z., et al. (2017). The surgical management of small bowel neuroendocrine tumors: Consensus guidelines of the North American Neuroendocrine Tumor Society. *Pancreas, 46*, 715–731.

Kinney, M. A. O., Nagorney, D. M., Clark, D. F., O'Brien, T. D., Turner, J. D., Marienau, M. E., … Martin, D.P. (2018). Partial hepatic resections for metastatic neuroendocrine tumors: Perioperative outcomes. *Journal of Clinical Anesthesia, 51*, 93–96.

Kinney, M. A. O., Warner, M. E., Nagorney, D. M., Rubin, J., Schroeder, D. R., & Maxson, P. M., et al. (2001). Perianaesthetic risks and outcomes of abdominal surgery for metastatic carcinoid tumours. *British Journal of Anaesthesia, 87*, 447–452.

Massimino, K., Harrskog, O., Pommier, S., & Pommier, R. (2013). Octreotide LAR and bolus octreotide are insufficient for preventing intraoperative complications in carcinoid patients. *Journal of Surgical Oncology, 107*, 842–846.

Seymour, N., & Sawh, S. C. (2013). Mega-dose intravenous octreotide for the treatment of carcinoid crisis: A systematic review. *Canadian Journal of Anaesthesia, 60*, 492–499.

Weingarten, T. N., Abel, M. D., Connolly, H. M., Schroeder, D. R., & Schaff, H. V. (2007). Intraoperative management of patients with carcinoid heart disease having valvular surgery: A review of one hundred consecutive cases. *Anesthesia and Analgesia, 105*, 1192–1199.

Woltering, E. A., Wright, A. E., Stevens, M. A., Wang, Y. Z., Boudreaux, J. P., Mamikunian, G., et al. (2016). Development of effective prophylaxis against intraoperative carcinoid crisis. *Journal of Clinical Anesthesia, 32*, 189–193.

# Anesthesia for Patients With Hepatocellular Disease

BENJAMIN T. KOR, MD | TODD M. KOR, MD

The liver is vital for several physiologic and synthetic processes, and dysfunction may lead to a variety of clinically significant complications. Knowledge of the varied physiologic functions of the liver (Table 162.1) allows the anesthesia provider to anticipate potential problems when patients with hepatocellular disease present for surgery.

Patients with hepatocellular disease may have an altered perioperative coagulation status and physiologic derangements such as hypoglycemia, encephalopathy, renal or pulmonary impairment, altered drug metabolism, pancytopenia, and reduced plasma oncotic pressure, as well as hemodynamic challenges like low systemic vascular resistance (SVR) and elevated pulmonary vascular resistance. In early-stage or mild liver dysfunction, the pharmacokinetics and pharmacodynamics of anesthetic drugs may be altered by chemically induced microsomal enzyme induction, which may result in an acceleration of the metabolism of drugs and alter the amount of anesthetic drug necessary to achieve a specific anesthetic depth. Alternatively, in more advanced liver disease, there is significant hepatic dysfunction with hypoalbuminemia and decreased levels of alpha-1-acid glycoprotein. Thus there is increased sensitivity and prolongation of the effects of many anesthetic medications (e.g., opioids, benzodiazepines, muscle relaxants) due to decreased clearance by the liver and/or increased free fraction of drugs that are protein bound.

## Chronic Hepatic Disease

Anesthetic management of patients with chronic liver disease is dictated by the severity of hepatic and extrahepatic conditions. Patients with mild chronic hepatic disease typically tolerate surgery well. Systemic physiologic and pharmacokinetic derangements increase with increasing severity of hepatic disease. Calculation of the Model for End-Stage Liver Disease (MELD) score may provide insight to severity of disease and increased

| TABLE 162.1 | Critical Processes Performed by the Liver |
|---|---|

Drug metabolism
Bilirubin metabolism
Protein synthesis
  Albumin
  Coagulation factors
Protein metabolism
Glucose homeostasis
Fatty acid and cholesterol metabolism
Bile formation and elimination
Blood reservoir and filter of toxins
Iron store for hemoglobin formation
Immune functions
Vitamin and amino acid storage

risk. A low threshold should exist for consideration of placement of invasive arterial catheters for hemodynamic monitoring in patients with meaningful hepatic disease. Additional intravenous (IV) access may also be indicated in anticipation of potential coagulopathy, increased blood loss, and increased risk of requiring a transfusion or vasopressor support. Perioperative glycemic control may be impaired in part due to reduced gluconeogenesis and patients may require glucose containing solutions to treat hypoglycemia, or insulin for hyperglycemia. Patients with chronic hepatic disease are more likely than the general population to have cholestasis and cholelithiasis, either of which increases their susceptibility to developing cholecystitis, cholangitis, pancreatitis. These patients also may have gastroesophageal reflux and intestinal hypomotility. Increased intraabdominal pressure from ascites may also increase aspiration risk.

Portal hypertension and impaired coagulation from thrombocytopenia, factor deficiencies, disseminated intravascular coagulation, and fibrinolysis place these patients at risk for increased intraoperative bleeding. Renal disease may coexist with chronic liver disease. Hepatorenal syndrome may occur as a manifestation of end-stage liver disease but typically would not be present with mild or chronic hepatic disease. Encephalopathy and peripheral neuropathy from nutritional deficiencies may arise.

## Acute Hepatic Failure

The patient with acute hepatic failure or end-stage hepatic disease presents many challenges, and surgery should be performed in patients with acute or end-stage hepatic failure only in an emergency or for liver transplantation. Severe liver dysfunction may affect many other organ systems. Central nervous system manifestations of acute hepatic failure include encephalopathy, in part due to elevated ammonia levels due to dysfunction of the patient's urea cycle, and altered levels of consciousness potentially from cerebral edema. Cardiac output is typically increased from reduced SVR and increased arteriovenous shunting. Concurrent significant cardiac dysfunction is not uncommon in these patients as well. Cardiac dysfunction may further be worsened by the presence of portopulmonary hypertension, which can potentially contribute to right-sided failure. Pulmonary complications include hepatopulmonary syndrome, intrapulmonary shunting, pleural effusions, dyspnea, and decreased respiratory reserve. Patients may develop renal dysfunction including decreased filtration, retention of extracellular fluids, and hepatorenal syndrome, which may require dialysis support. Hypoglycemia may result from impaired gluconeogenesis, depleted glycogen stores, and reduced insulin degradation. Intraabdominal ascites is a common feature of hypoalbuminemia and portal hypertension. Immune function is impaired. Cholesterol and steroid metabolism may be altered.

Significant coagulopathy is a frequent finding. Of the proteins synthesized by the liver, factor VII, has one of the shortest half-lives. Accordingly, the prothrombin time (PT) and international normalized ratio (INR) provide valuable information as to acute changes in hepatic function. Coagulation status should be frequently monitored with laboratory testing including thromboelastography and serologic laboratory analysis of PT/INR used to aid in the correction of coagulopathy. It is important to remember these patients are also susceptible to excessive clotting as well, due to protein C and S being synthesized in the liver and thus may have decreased concentrations. A blood management strategy should be used, as patients with coagulopathies often require multiple blood products (e.g., fresh frozen plasma, cryoprecipitate, specific factor therapy, red blood cells, and platelets). Use of antifibrinolytic medications may be considered if evidence of fibrinolysis exists. Severe coagulopathy may require massive transfusion requirements if significant bleeding occurs.

Because these patients have decreased rates of drug metabolism and higher free drug fractions from decreased serum proteins, anesthetic requirements are significantly reduced, and the effects of IV anesthetics and opiate agents may be prolonged.

## Anesthesia Considerations

Preoperative evaluation of all patients should include an investigation of subjective and objective physical or historical signs of liver disease. Routine liver function testing is not recommended in the general surgical population without evidence or signs of liver dysfunction. The preoperative history and physical examination of patients with known or suspected hepatocellular disease should focus on identifying extrahepatic manifestations of chronic liver failure. The laboratory evaluation of patients with known or suspected liver disease may comprise arterial blood gas analysis, complete blood count, coagulation studies, and a chemistry panel that includes albumin and glucose concentrations. Calculation of a Model for End-stage Liver Disease (MELD) score may be helpful for predicting perioperative risk for patients undergoing either transplant or nontransplant surgery. Increasing MELD scores reflect a corresponding increase in severity of liver disease and surgical and procedural morbidity.

If the patient has limited hepatic dysfunction and no coagulopathy, a regional anesthetic technique may be considered, but exaggerated hypotension may complicate this technique. Hypotension in these patients may result in impaired hepatic perfusion with uncertain benefit from the use of IV vasopressors.

Changes to the synthetic function of the liver may affect pharmacokinetics and pharmacodynamics of many commonly used anesthetic drugs. Benzodiazepines and opiates may have enhanced effect and prolonged duration and should be used with caution. Prolonged propofol administration may result in delayed emergence, whereas standard induction doses typically clear in a similar pattern to healthy patients. Fentanyl or remifentanil may be preferred opiates in this patient population to reduce prolonged and unexpected effects from opiate administration. The effect from succinylcholine may be prolonged due to changes in plasma cholinesterase concentration. Cisatracurium may be preferred over rocuronium or vecuronium because of its Hofmann elimination rather than dependence on hepatic metabolism.

For patients with mild hepatic dysfunction, standard monitoring alone may be sufficient. However, for patients with more advanced liver dysfunction or for surgery on the liver, large-bore or central IV access should be obtained preoperatively; hemodynamic values should be invasively monitored, as appropriate; and anesthetic drugs should be carefully titrated to effect. The placement of an intraarterial catheter should be considered to facilitate careful perioperative monitoring of blood pressure and blood withdrawal for laboratory analysis of arterial blood gases, electrolytes, hemoglobin, glucose concentrations, and coagulation parameters. Monitoring central venous pressure and, occasionally, pulmonary artery pressure aids in perioperative fluid management. Placement of a transesophageal ultrasound transducer to allow for real-time monitoring of cardiac function may be beneficial in complex surgical cases, though it should be placed with caution given these patients may have esophageal varices at risk for bleeding. If surgery is likely to be associated with large-volume blood loss, a rapid-infusion pump should be readily available. A peripheral nerve stimulator should be used to avoid administering excess amounts of neuromuscular blocking agents, so these may be adequately reversed at the conclusion of surgery.

Rapid sequence induction may be considered to mitigate the risk of aspiration due to anatomic, physiologic, and systemic alterations. Doses of induction agents (etomidate, propofol) will often be reduced because of the likelihood of patients having an increased sensitivity to the neurologic and cardiovascular effects of these drugs. Though plasma cholinesterase levels may be decreased, plasma levels are usually still sufficent and succinylcholine typically does not significantly prolong apnea and, therefore, may be used in most cases. Maintenance of adequate systemic blood pressure and cardiac output is critical to prevent additional hepatocyte ischemic injury and alterations to systemic blood flow distribution in patients with systemic shunts. Maintenance of euvolemia or mild hypovolemia may improve hepatic congestion and reduce the risk of blood loss during abdominal surgery. Postoperative analgesic requirements are often reduced in patients with hepatocellular disease because of impaired hepatic metabolism of opiates and must be used carefully to prevent postoperative respiratory complications.

## SUGGESTED READINGS

Adelmann, D., Kronish, K., & Ramsay, M. A. (2017). Anesthesia for liver transplantation. *Anesthesiol Clin, 35,* 491–508.

Crager, S. (2019). Critically ill patients with end-stage liver disease. *Emergency Medicine Clinics of North America, 37*(3), 511–527.

Keegan, M. T., & Kramer, D. J. (2016). Perioperative care of the liver transplant patient. *Critical Care Clinics, 32,* 453–473.

Scarlatescu, E., Marchenko, S., & Tomescu, D. (2022). Cirrhotic cardiomyopathy: A veiled threat. *Cardiology in Review, 30*(2), 80–89. doi:10.1097/CRD.0000000000000377.

Sharma, S., Stine, J. G., Verbeek, T., & Bezinover, D. (2022). Management of patients with non-alcoholic steatohepatitis undergoing liver transplantation: Consideration for the anesthesiologist. *Journal of Cardiothoracic and Vascular Anesthesia, 36*(8 Pt A), 2616–2627.

Simmons, F., Pustavoitau, A., & Merritt, W. T. (2021). Diseases of the liver and biliary tract. In R. L. Hines, & S. B. Jones (Eds.), *Stoelting's Anesthesia and Co-Existing Disease* (8th ed., pp. 333–346). Philadelphia: Elsevier Saunders.

Starczewska, M. H., Mon, W., & Shirley, P. (2017). Anesthesia in patients with liver disease. *Current Opinion in Anaesthesiology, 30,* 392–398.

# Anesthesia for the Patient Undergoing Liver Transplantation

ALEXANDRA L. ANDERSON, MD | JAMES Y. FINDLAY, MB, ChB

Liver transplantation (LT) is an established therapy for end-stage liver disease (ESLD) and acute liver failure, with more than 8000 liver transplants performed yearly in the United States. The overall 3-year survival rate is greater than 80%. Demand continues to significantly exceed availability of quality donor organs despite advances with living donors, split-liver grafts, and revised organ allocation. Approximately 13,000 candidates are on the waiting list for LT at any given time. Ongoing efforts for optimization of donor organ availability include increased use of deceased after circulatory death organs and machine perfusion techniques for donor graft salvage. Orthotopic LT presents challenges to the anesthesiologist with the multisystem organ dysfunction of ESLD and the hemodynamic and physiologic effects of the surgery.

## Preoperative Evaluation

Functional and structural ESLD result in systemically altered metabolism and blood flow that affect each organ system.

Table 163.1 lists some of the relevant multisystem organ dysfunction and physiologic consequences of liver failure. As a result, all patients being considered for LT undergo extensive multidisciplinary evaluation.

All liver transplant candidates undergo cardiopulmonary screening. A resting transthoracic echocardiogram (TTE) assesses cardiac function and allows estimation of systolic pulmonary artery pressures (sPAPs). Evaluation for cirrhotic cardiomyopathy (CM) should be pursued in patients with systolic and diastolic dysfunction, low cardiac output, electrophysiologic changes, and high filling pressures. Patients with advanced cirrhotic CM will have a decreased contractile response to stress. Cirrhotic CM is progressive but may be reversed with LT. Identification of CM preoperatively is important for optimization and management, as patients with CM are at increased risk of perioperative heart failure, arrhythmia, graft failure, and death. Patients with high estimated sPAP on TTE (sPAP >50 mm Hg and/or right ventricle size or functional abnormalities) should undergo further investigation to evaluate

| TABLE 163.1 | Pathophysiologic Changes Associated With Liver Failure | |
|---|---|---|
| **Organ System** | **Change** | **Consequence(s)** |
| Cardiovascular | Low SVR, adrenergic activation, high CO<br>Cirrhotic cardiomyopathy: systolic and diastolic dysfunction, blunted response to vasoactive agents, impaired contractile response to stress<br>Electrophysiologic changes, prolonged QT | Hyperdynamic state with high or preserved EF<br>Hypotension, atrial fibrillation, cardiac failure, dysrhythmias |
| Pulmonary | Ascites, hepatic hydrothorax<br>Hepatopulmonary syndrome: pulmonary vasodilation, intrapulmonary shunting<br>POPH: inflammation, vasoconstriction, remodeling of pulmonary vasculature | Restrictive ventilation defect, atelectasis<br>Hypoxemia, platypnea, orthodeoxia<br>RV dysfunction; in patients with RV dysfunction or severe POPH, LT should be deferred |
| Central nervous system | Accumulation of neurotoxins and portosystemic shunting, ammonia metabolism to glutamine, cerebral edema<br>Impaired metabolism | Hepatic encephalopathy that can deteriorate<br>Increased sensitivity to sedation |
| Renal | Hepatorenal syndrome: increased renal vasoconstriction secondary to intravascular volume depletion with reduced SVR<br>Acidosis, uremia, impaired water and sodium excretion, hyponatremia, hypokalemia | Renal impairment: type I with rapid progression or type II with gradual onset<br>May require renal replacement therapy<br>Potential for ODS if hyponatremia corrected too quickly |
| Gastrointestinal | Portal hypertension | Ascites, bacterial translocation, gastric varices, esophageal varices, GI bleeding |
| Metabolic | Impaired synthetic and metabolic function | Malnutrition, sarcopenia, low serum osmolality, decreased protein binding<br>Impaired metabolism, volume of distribution, and elimination of medications |
| Coagulation | Decreased synthesis of procoagulant factors and decreased synthesis of anticoagulant factors<br>Anemia | Rebalanced hemostasis sensitive to intrinsic and extrinsic factors that may increase bleeding or clotting risk |

*CO,* Cardiac output; *EF,* ejection fraction; *GI,* gastrointestinal; *LT,* liver transplant; *ODS,* osmotic demyelination syndrome; *POPH,* portopulmonary hypertension; *RV,* right ventricle; *SVR,* systemic vascular resistance.

for portopulmonary hypertension, which is a potential contraindication to transplant. Venous administration of agitated saline can be performed; delayed appearance of contrast microbubbles in the left heart may indicate intrapulmonary shunting and hepatopulmonary syndrome. Baseline pulse oximetry also identifies patients for further pulmonary investigation.

With an aging candidate population and increased prevalence of nonalcoholic fatty liver disease, coronary artery disease is a significant concern. Noninvasive testing is frequently performed in those with cardiac risk factors, often using dobutamine stress echocardiography, with cardiac catheterization and intervention as indicated. Severe coronary artery disease or valve pathology not amenable to correction may preclude candidacy. Intervention may be too high risk in patients with decompensated ESLD.

Renal dysfunction often accompanies ESLD from hepatorenal syndrome, acute tubular necrosis, or a combination of both. In patients requiring intermittent hemodialysis or continuous renal replacement therapy, consideration should be given to performing continuous dialysis or ultrafiltration preoperatively or in the operating room (OR) to manage volume or metabolic derangements. Washing red blood cells to reduce potassium may be helpful but has limitations in that it is time and labor intensive and unable to keep up with massive transfusion requirements.

Baseline metabolic derangements such as acidosis, hyponatremia, hypocalcemia, hypomagnesemia, hypoglycemia, and hyperkalemia should be identified and managed accordingly. Patients with ESLD are in a state of rebalanced hemostasis with decreased function of both procoagulant and anticoagulant pathways, along with dysfibrinogenemia. Various factors can tip the state of hemostasis toward bleeding or clotting, as outlined in Table 163.2. The anesthesiologist must monitor and tailor transfusion therapy to the dynamic coagulation status perioperatively, in addition to being prepared for large-volume balanced transfusion. Cell salvage techniques can be frequently be used.

The severity of ESLD is assessed by calculating the Model for End-Stage Liver Disease (MELD) score, which incorporates serum bilirubin, serum creatinine, and the international normalized ratio (INR) for prothrombin time to predict survival. Serum sodium was added to the score in 2016 reflecting the influence of renal dysfunction on severity of decompensation (MELD- Na). Whether the patient requires renal replacement therapy is also entered into the equation.

$$MELD = 3.78[\text{Ln bilirubin (mg/dL)}] + 11.2[\text{Ln INR}]$$
$$+ 9.57[\text{Ln creatinine (mg/dL)}] + 6.43$$
$$MELD\text{-}Na = MELD \text{ score} - Na - 0.025 \times MELD$$
$$\times (140 - Na) + 140$$

A higher MELD score is associated with more severe liver failure and higher wait-list mortality. High MELD is also predictive of a greater rate of intraoperative blood product transfusion and vasopressor requirement. Allocation of livers is prioritized for higher MELD scores, with MELD exception points granted for disease states in which progression and mortality is not reflected by MELD lab values.

## Intraoperative Management

### ANESTHESIA

Induction of anesthesia may be achieved using any of the commonly used agents. Rapid sequence induction and intubation is indicated in the presence of ascites or other risk factors for aspiration, including a presumed full stomach in patients who were called in without time for fasting. Maintenance is achieved with a balanced technique using an inhaled agent and opioid, often fentanyl. Cisatracurium may be preferred for maintenance of neuromuscular blockade because it is not dependent on hepatic metabolism or renal function for elimination, but other neuromuscular blocking agents can be used with appropriate monitoring and reversal.

Invasive monitoring is the norm; direct arterial pressure is best monitored by a brachial or femoral catheter (rather than radial) because these give more accurate and consistent measurements, particularly at reperfusion. Two arterial lines are frequently placed to allow for continuous monitoring with frequent lab draws. Advanced cardiac monitoring is routine. Transesophageal echocardiography (TEE) is frequently employed. TEE allows visual real-time monitoring of cardiac function and volume status. It is also useful to quickly identify intracardiac clot, intracardiac air, or other causes of hypotension such as dynamic left ventricular outflow tract obstruction. See Table 163.3 for some suggested TEE views and uses during LT. Recent evidence supports the safety of TEE despite esophageal varices provided it is placed with caution and if varices have not bled recently. All other absolute and relative contraindications to

| TABLE 163.2 | Rebalanced Hemostasis: Factors That Contribute to Bleeding or Hemostasis in End-Stage Liver Disease | |
|---|---|---|
| | **Antithrombotic (Bleeding Risk)** | **Prothrombotic (Clotting Risk)** |
| Primary hemostasis | Thrombocytopenia<br>Platelet dysfunction | Increased Vwf<br>Decreased ADAMTS 13 |
| Coagulation | Decreased factors II, V, VII, IX, X, and XI<br>Decreased fibrinogen/dysfibrinogenemia | Increased factor VIII<br>Decreased protein C, protein S, antithrombin |
| Fibrinolysis | Increased fibrinolysis<br>Increased tissue plasminogen activator | Decreased plasminogen<br>Increased plasminogen activator inhibitor |
| Other | Alcohol use disorder<br>Portal hypertension<br>Active infection<br>Anticoagulation therapy (DOACS, warfarin)<br>Acute renal failure | PSC, PBC, NASH, HCC<br>Baseline coagulation disorder<br>Inflammation<br>Chronic renal failure |

*ADAMTS 13*, vWF cleaving protease; *DOACS*, direct oral anticoagulants; *HCC*, hepatocellular carcinoma; *NASH*, nonalcohol steatosing hepatitis; *PBC*, primary biliary cirrhosis; *PSC*, primary sclerosing cholangitis; *vWF*, von Willebrand factor.

| TABLE 163.3 | Liver Transplant Transthoracic Echocardiogram: Suggested Views | | |
|---|---|---|---|
| **View** | | **Probe** | **Assessment/Diagnosis** |
| ME 4C 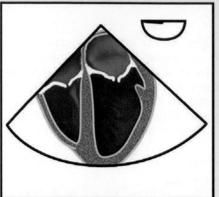 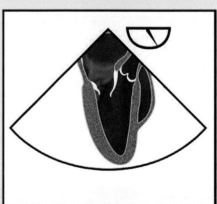 | | Insert 30–35 cm<br>Angle 0–20 degrees | Global RV and LV function<br>Volume status<br>Tamponade |
| ME LV LAX 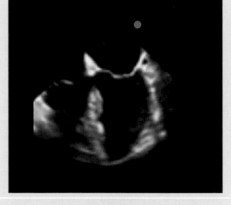 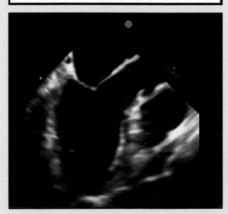 | | Insert 30–35 cm<br>Angle 120–160 degrees | SAM<br>LVOTO |

| TABLE 163.3 | Liver Transplant Transthoracic Echocardiogram: Suggested Views—cont'd | | |
|---|---|---|---|
| **View** | | **Probe** | **Assessment/Diagnosis** |
| ME RV inflow/outflow 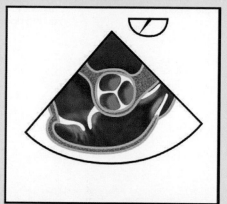 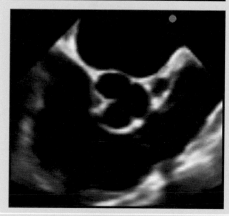 | | Insert 20–30 cm Angle 60–75 degrees | RA, RV, PA catheter placement, tricuspid valve, pulmonic valve, right-sided thrombus |
| ME Bicaval 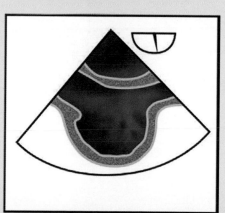 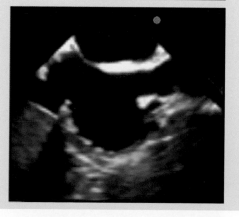 | | Insert 20–30 cm Angle 90–110 degrees | LA, RA, interatrial septum, SVC and IVC, wire placement for central line |

*Continued*

| TABLE 163.3 Liver Transplant Transthoracic Echocardiogram: Suggested Views—cont'd | | |
|---|---|---|
| **View** | **Probe** | **Assessment/Diagnosis** |
| TG Mid SAX 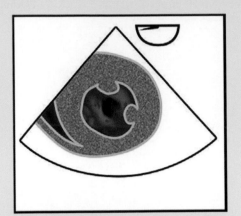 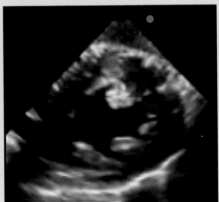 | Insert to stomach, anteflex Angle 0 degrees | LV function and volume status. May be inaccessible during dissection/retraction |

| TABLE 163.3 | Liver Transplant Transthoracic Echocardiogram: Suggested Views—cont'd | | |
|---|---|---|---|
| **View** | | **Probe** | **Assessment/Diagnosis** |
| Hepatic Vein View/TG IVC LAX | | Insert to stomach, rotate right Angle 0–40 degrees | IVC, hepatic vein, anastomosis, hepatic venous congestion, IVC cannula |

*4C*, 4 Chamber; *IVC*, inferior vena cava; *LA*, left atrium; *LAX*, long axis; *LV*, left ventricle; *LVOTO*, left ventricular outflow tract obstruction; *ME*, Midesophageal; *PA*, pulmonary artery; *RA*, right atrium; *RV*, right ventricle; *SAM*, systolic anterior motion; *SAX*, short axis; *SVC*, superior vena cava; *TG*, transgastric.

Modified from Puchalski, M. D., Lui, G. K., Miller-Hance, W. C., Brook, M. M., Young, L. T., Bhat, A., et al. (2019). Guidelines for Performing a Comprehensive Transesophageal Echocardiographic: Examination in Children and All Patients with Congenital Heart Disease: Recommendations from the American Society of Echocardiography. *Journal of the American Society of Echocardiography, 32*(2), 173–215.

TEE apply. Alternatively, or in addition, a pulmonary artery (PA) catheter may be placed to monitor cardiac filling pressures, PA pressures, and cardiac output. A "stat lab" near the OR is useful for rapid and frequent analysis of blood gases, electrolytes, glucose, and coagulation status throughout the procedure. Many centers use viscoelastic testing (thromboelastography or rotational thromboelastometry) to provide a rapid assessment of coagulation and to inform blood component transfusion.

Adequate large-bore venous access is essential given the potential for massive hemorrhage and must be obtained in the upper body as the procedure involves partial or total clamping of the inferior vena cava (IVC). A dedicated peripheral or centrally placed 8 French (or larger) catheter connected to a rapid infusion pump is used. If venovenous bypass (VVB) is planned, a second dedicated large-bore catheter is centrally placed as the VVB return line. Red blood cell salvage is typically used. The blood bank should have massive transfusion capability.

The large surgical incision, prolonged operating time, and implantation of a cold graft make hypothermia a potential problem. The use of fluid warmers and forced-air convective warming blankets can help mitigate perioperative hypothermia.

## TRANSPLANTATION PROCEDURE

Initial dissection and hepatectomy can result in significant blood loss from friable variceal vessels in the abdominal wall, abdomen, and around the liver. Portal hypertension, previous LT, or previous abdominal surgeries can increase blood loss during hepatectomy. Drainage of abdominal ascites can also lead to significant volume shifts in the dissection phase. Fluid restrictive strategies can reduce bleeding during this stage. Hepatectomy involves mobilization followed by clamping and division of the hepatic vasculature (hepatic artery, portal vein, and IVC/hepatic veins). Movement of the liver can transiently occlude the IVC and decrease venous return during this phase. Maintaining cardiac filling pressures and output with caval occlusion and the loss of venous return can be challenging. Techniques to address this include partial IVC clamping ("piggyback" technique) or the use of venovenous bypass. For the latter, cannulas are placed in the portal and femoral veins; blood is drained by gravity to a centrifugal pump and is returned to the upper body via a large-bore venous cannula (Fig. 163.1). Alternatively, volume can be administered before

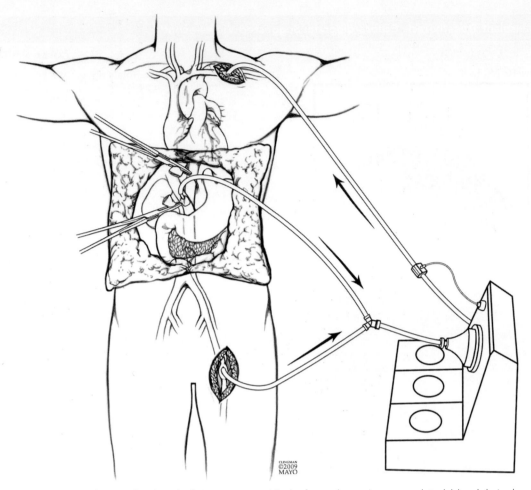

**Fig. 163.1    Venovenous bypass.** The portal vein and inferior vena cava (via the femoral artery) are cannulated; blood drains by gravity to the pump and is then returned to a central vein in the upper body. (© Mayo Foundation for Medical Education and Research. All rights reserved.)

going anhepatic with total caval occlusion, and restricted when clamps are on. Portosystemic shunting may give some venous return. In patients at risk for thrombosis, intravenous heparin may be administered before IVC clamping.

Before portal vein anastomosis or in patients with portal vein thrombosis, blood loss may occur with bleeding the portal vein to get rid of clot and debris below the clamp, or with thrombectomy.

Once vascular anastomoses to the graft are complete, recirculation occurs. Liver inflow is restored by opening the portal vein (with or without the hepatic artery), blood is flushed through the nearly complete anastomosis, and then the IVC clamp is released. Blood flushing may be performed on the neograft before completing the portal or IVC anastomosis depending on surgical technique, resulting in acute blood loss. Opening the IVC results in the abrupt delivery of cold, potassium-containing acidic blood to the heart, and potentially microthrombi or entrained air. Hypotension is common, PA pressures elevate, and cardiac arrhythmia or even arrest may occur. Intravenously administered calcium chloride antagonizes potassium-induced changes, and low-dose epinephrine is frequently used for immediate hemodynamic support. Sodium bicarbonate or tromethamine solution (THAM) can be administered as a buffer with severe acidosis or

as part of managing hyperkalemia. Magnesium may be administered to decrease arrhythmogenicity. Significant ongoing hypotension after recirculation, termed *postreperfusion syndrome*, is most often caused by the aforementioned systemic vasodilation and increased pulmonary vascular resistance; however, myocardial depression is sometimes seen. Vasopressor and/or inotropic support should be used as indicated; resolution typically occurs within 30 minutes. TEE and pulmonary arterial catheter monitoring can provide guidance regarding diagnosis and management of recirculation-related hemodynamic instability. Insulin is useful for acute hyperglycemia with the neograft, along with managing potassium levels. The final stage of transplantation involves hepatic artery anastomosis (if not already performed) and a biliary drainage procedure. Ongoing correction of coagulopathy and metabolic abnormalities occur in this period and should improve as the donor graft begins to function.

## COAGULATION AND TRANSFUSION MANAGEMENT

Although average transfusion requirements have decreased in recent years, catastrophic bleeding still occurs, both surgical and coagulopathic. ESLD is characterized by thrombocytopenia and elevated conventional coagulation tests; however, viscoelastic testing typically reveals a normal coagulation profile. This is caused by the decreased factor synthesis affecting both pro- and anticoagulant factors. The system is unstable; intraoperatively, it typically tips toward coagulopathy, but intravascular and/or intracardiac thrombosis can occur and is well reported. Correction of coagulopathy is dynamic and should not be based purely on conventional coagulation testing but on a combination of viscoelastic testing (when available) and the clinical setting. Management, when indicated, is typically with blood component therapy (fresh frozen plasma, cryoprecipitate, platelets); however, the use of factor therapy (fibrinogen, prothrombin complex concentrate) is increasing.

On recirculation, tissue plasminogen activator activity rises, which can result in marked fibrinolysis. Heparinoids are also released. Although prophylactic use of antifibrinolytic agents is not typical, they may be considered if clinically significant fibrinolysis occurs; again, viscoelastic testing aids identification. A thromboelastogram immediately after recirculation will often reflect the acute fibrinolysis and heparinoid activity. Aggressive correction should be avoided, as this often resolves within 30 minutes, and overcorrection could increase the risk for thromboembolic events. When large volumes of blood and blood products are transfused, ionized hypocalcemia secondary to citrate chelation may occur; this should be anticipated and treated appropriately. Balanced transfusion and avoiding dilutional coagulopathy are prudent. Communication with the surgical team regarding any ongoing surgical bleeding is key.

The quantity of blood and blood products transfused are both independent predictors of poor outcome post-LT, so overtransfusion should be avoided. Appropriate transfusion practices may be aided with clinical pathways, routine monitoring, and targeted component transfusion.

## Postoperative Management

Straightforward cases can often be fast-tracked, with early extubation if appropriate drug and dosing choices are pursued intraoperatively. Immediate postoperative management should be in an area where adequate patient monitoring is available to detect early complications, particularly bleeding. Patients requiring ongoing vasopressor support, ongoing correction of coagulopathy, ongoing correction of metabolic disturbances, and possible renal replacement therapy are best managed in an intensive care unit setting.

## Acute Liver Failure

Patients with acute liver failure can present a significant challenge. Multiple organ failure syndrome can be present, complicating preoperative and intraoperative management. The absence of chronic portal hypertension and the associated portosystemic shunting can make these patients more acutely sensitive to the loss of cardiac venous return with hepatectomy and IVC clamping. A particular concern is the development of cerebral edema and increased intracranial pressure. This is managed as for cerebral edema of other causes. Intraoperatively, the anesthesiologist should be prepared to deal with exacerbations.

## SUGGESTED READINGS

Adelmann, D., Kronish, K., & Ramsay, M. A. (2017). Anesthesia for liver transplantation. *Anesthesiology Clinics, 35,* 491–508.

Forkin, K. T., Colquhoun, D. A., Nemergut, E. C., & Huffmyer, J. L. (2018). The coagulation profile of end-stage liver disease and considerations for intraoperative management. *Anesthesia and Analgesia, 126,* 46–61.

Koulava, A., Sannani, A., Levine, A., Gupta, C. A., Khanal, S., Frishman, W., et al. (2018). Diagnosis, treatment, and management of orthotopic liver transplant candidates with portopulmonary hypertension. *Cardiology in Review, 26*(4), 169–176, doi:10.1097/CRD.0000000000000195.

Liu, H. Jayakumar, S., Traboulsi, M., & Lee, S. S. (2017). Cirrhotic cardiomyopathy: Implications for liver transplantation. *Liver Transplantation, 23,* 826–835.

Manning, M. W., Kumar, P. A., Maheshwari, K., & Arora, H. (2020). Post-reperfusion syndrome in liver transplantation- An overview. *Journal of Cardiothoracic and Vascular Anesthesia, 34,* 501–511.

United Network for Organ Sharing. Retrieved from https://www.unos.org/.

Vanneman, M. W., Dalia, A. A., Crowley, J. C., Luchette, K. R., Chitilian, H. V., & Shelton, K. T. (2020). A focused transesophageal echocardiography protocol for intraoperative management during orthotopic liver transplantation. *Journal of Cardiothoracic and Vascular Anesthesia, 34*(7), 1824–1832.

Wray, C. (2018). Liver transplantation in patients with cardiac disease. *Seminars in Cardiothoracic and Vascular Anesthesia, 22*(2), 111–121.

# 164

# Autonomic Dysreflexia

MICHAEL E. JOHNSON, MD, PhD

Autonomic dysreflexia (AD, also referred to as autonomic hyperreflexia) is a potentially life-threatening emergency. It occurs in at least two-thirds of patients with spinal cord injury (SCI) at T6 or above and is characterized by an acute increase in blood pressure (BP) of 20 mm Hg or above in response to a strong sensory stimulus below the level of the SCI.

## Pathophysiology of Autonomic Dysreflexia

AD results from unopposed sympathetic efferent activation from the spinal cord below the level of the SCI, with reflex activation of central parasympathetic outflow. AD can occur in nontraumatic (e.g., neoplasm) and traumatic SCI. The pathways involved are summarized in Fig. 164.1.

A noxious stimulus below the level of SCI causes discharge of sympathetic preganglionic neurons as an independent reflex at the level of the cord. Ordinarily, this would elicit compensatory bulbospinal sympathetic inhibition via descending spinal pathways, but these are now blocked by the SCI, resulting in unopposed vasoconstriction below the injury. Sensory stimuli can ascend via spinothalamic and posterior columns to activate sympathetic neurons up to the level of the cord injury. Injury at T6 or higher allows involvement of the splanchnic vascular beds with an exaggerated hypertensive response. Cord injury below T10 does not cause AD, whereas injury at the T6–T10 levels may have a mild BP elevation without full-blown AD. AD can occur with incomplete SCI but is more severe with a complete injury.

Baroreceptors in the aortic arch and carotid sinus respond to the hypertension by activating brainstem vasomotor reflexes, resulting in increased parasympathetic activation via the intact cranial nerve X effector pathway, which is unaffected by SCI. Alone, this would cause bradycardia, but tachycardia is also possible, presumably depending on the balance between vasopressors that diffuse into the bloodstream after sympathetic neuron activation below the SCI, and vagal outflow. Recent studies find that tachycardia is as frequent as bradycardia in AD. Parasympathetic activation also causes vasodilation above the level of the SCI.

Although AD has been reported in the acute phase of SCI, it generally becomes evident 1 to 6 months after the initial injury. This is attributed to injury-induced changes in structure and electrophysiology of both primary afferents and spinal neurons. There is also increased sensitivity of the peripheral vasculature to α-adrenergic stimulation, which heightens the exaggerated sympathetic response to noxious stimuli. Animal studies find that treatment with minocycline, and early blockade of tumor necrosis factor α (TNFα) after SCI, decrease development of AD.

## Clinical Features

AD is potentially life-threatening. Blood pressures as high as 250 to 300 mm Hg systolic/200 to 220 mm Hg diastolic have been reported and are the etiology of the major associated acute morbidities (e.g., myocardial ischemia, arrhythmia, congestive failure, cerebral ischemia or hemorrhage, and encephalopathy). Frequent episodes of AD also have a chronic negative effect on cardiac function.

Initial BP elevation may be mild. An acute increase in systolic BP of 20 mm Hg in the context of an at-risk patient and a stimulus below the level of SCI suggests the onset of AD with high probability. It may be disguised by the low resting vasomotor tone and BP in patients with high SCI. A pressure of 120/80 mm Hg in a patient whose normal pressure is 90/60 mm Hg should raise concern that AD has begun and BP may shortly rise to much higher levels.

A dangerous example of AD is "boosting," where Paralympics competitors deliberately induce AD with its catecholamine excess to increase performance, with up to a 10% decrease in wheelchair racing times. Multiple examples of serious heart and brain injury have been reported.

Other signs and symptoms can vary between patients, and even between episodes of AD in the same patient, and may be masked by sedation or anesthesia. In an awake patient, AD often presents with the triad of severe headache, profuse sweating, and cutaneous flushing above the level of the injury. The skin below may be pale and cool with piloerection. Nasal congestion, anxiety and malaise, nausea, and visual disturbances may also occur. These are generally consistent with marked sympathetic activation below the SCI with increased central reflex parasympathetic outflow. However, the hyperhidrosis of AD is most common on the face and neck, above the level of cord injury, rather than below, where sympathetic outflow is maximal. The mechanism is not well understood, although it could involve a direct effect of catecholamines spilling over into the bloodstream, a central effect of excess catecholamines passing the blood-brain barrier, or a direct effect of intense parasympathetic stimulation on the forehead and upper lip, the only area in humans where there is parasympathetic and sympathetic innervation of sweat glands. A recently reported effect of AD is that it impairs the antibacterial immune response. TNFα is involved, although a detailed mechanism is not established.

Usually the diagnosis of AD in the setting of surgery below the SCI in a susceptible patient is straightforward, but other potential causes of acute hypertension should also be considered, particularly if a strong sensory stimulus cannot be identified as the cause of the AD. In a laboring parturient, preeclampsia can also cause severe hypertension, but in AD the BP elevation is usually much more marked during uterine contraction, with decline during relaxation. It should also be kept in mind that urinary catheter constriction and bowel impaction are frequent causes of AD in nonanesthetized patients and can occur in any susceptible patient during any surgical procedure, including those above the level of the SCI.

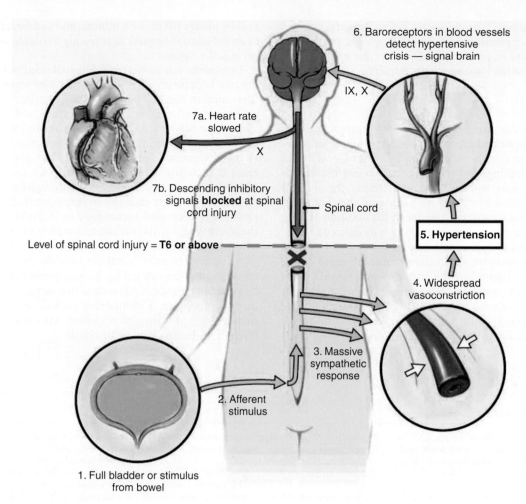

**Fig. 164.1** **Diagram illustrating how autonomic dysreflexia occurs in a person with spinal cord injury.** The afferent stimulus, in this case a distended bladder, triggers a peripheral sympathetic response, which results in vasoconstriction and hypertension. Descending inhibitory signals, which would normally counteract the rise in blood pressure, are blocked at the level of the spinal cord injury. The roman numerals (IX, X) refer to cranial nerves. (Reprinted with permission from Blackmer, J. (2003). Rehabilitation medicine: 1. Autonomic dysreflexia. *Canadian Medical Association Journal, 169,* 931–935.)

## Prevention

AD is a potential concern for any procedure where innervation of the affected site is below the level of the SCI. Anything that would elicit pain or other strong sensory stimulus in a patient without SCI can cause AD in an at-risk patient. A past history of AD is helpful in alerting the anesthesiologist to the risk of AD and its magnitude in a specific patient, but any patient with SCI at T6 or above should be considered at risk, even in the absence of previous episodes of AD. Pelvic visceral pain is a particularly potent stimulus of AD, so that bladder, bowel, gynecologic, and obstetric procedures are the most common causes of AD under anesthesia. These include not only surgery but also other stimulating procedures (e.g., labor and vaginal delivery, urodynamic studies, ejaculation, and wound care). The magnitude of AD increases with the magnitude of the sensory stimulus and with increasing distance between the level of the cord lesion and the level of the dorsal root entry zone of the stimulus.

Prevention of AD is the ideal, and for surgery it usually requires a dense regional block or a deep volatile anesthetic. This may require education of the patient and surgeon to accept the need for an anesthetic for a procedure that may not elicit any conscious sensation of pain in the patient. The most studied

agent is sevoflurane, which prevents AD in at-risk patients undergoing transurethral litholapaxy with EC50 3.1% in 50% nitrous oxide ($N_2O$). This decreases to 2.6% and 2.2% with remifentanil 1 and 3 ng/mL target-controlled infusion. Although propofol intravenous (IV) anesthesia is recommended by some reviews, it has not been fully studied beyond case reports. There is one report of AD occurring during 140 to 240 mcg/kg/min propofol with 66% $N_2O$. Preoperative oral prazosin and terazosin and intrathecal baclofen may be effective in preventing AD, as well as intradetrusor injection of botulinum toxin for urologic procedures.

Although both epidural and spinal anesthetics have been used successfully to prevent AD, epidural anesthesia may not block the larger sacral nerve roots as effectively as spinal anesthesia. It is difficult to assess the level of neuraxial block with a high cord injury, so a spinal anesthetic confirmed by cerebrospinal fluid return during placement may offer more assurance of an adequate block than an epidural technique. Patients with SCI may present a technical challenge in accessing the subarachnoid space, and have low resting BP, but in practice these have not proven problematic in most patients.

Topical local anesthetic alone before superficial rectal and urinary procedures has not been uniformly effective in preventing

AD, although intravesicular lidocaine before urinary catheter change has. Neither parenteral nor epidural opioids, nor $N_2O$, is consistently effective in preventing AD, except for epidural meperidine, which also has local anesthetic properties.

## Treatment

When AD does occur, it is a potentially life-threatening emergency and must be treated rapidly. In awake patients, nonpharmacologic measures such as elevating the head and torso, loosening tight clothing, and relieving inadvertent bladder or bowel distention may suffice. Under anesthesia the surgical stimulus may be paused to allow deepening of anesthesia and other treatment, but it must continue with the addition of drug treatment for AD if the surgery is to achieve its desired result.

Multiple pharmacologic agents have been used to treat AD. The ideal antihypertensive medication would be rapid acting but short-lived, so that when the stimulus inciting AD is removed, there is not prolonged hypotension in a patient with decreased vasomotor tone because of SCI and anesthesia. IV clevidipine is a promising option with extensive studies, although not specifically in AD. Bolus clevidipine (0.125–0.5 mg) rapidly lowers BP, $t_{1/2}$ of 1 minute, and can be repeated or given as an infusion if needed. It is readily available as a shelf-stable, premixed suspension.

Immediate-release oral or sublingual nifedipine has fallen into disfavor because of severe adverse reactions when given for acute BP control in non-AD patients. Nitroglycerin, nitroprusside, and other nitrates have been used effectively, although the use of sildenafil or other PDE5 inhibitors in the previous 24 hours needs to be ruled out first. Sildenafil alone is not effective in treating AD. IV phentolamine is acutely effective, but phenoxybenzamine's effect is inconsistent. IV prostaglandin E1 and hydralazine are effective for acute treatment of AD, although hydralazine appears more likely to cause excessive hypotension. Labetalol and metoprolol have been used successfully in individual cases, although the severe bradycardia that can accompany AD may make the use of any β-blocker problematic.

AD can present or continue into the postoperative period and should be monitored for in susceptible patients. After resolution of an episode of AD related to a surgical or other stimulus during anesthesia, a monitoring period of 2 hours is recommended. If the cause of apparent AD cannot be identified, longer monitoring may be justified.

## SUGGESTED READINGS

Delhaas, E. M., Frankema, S. P. G., & Huygen, F. J. P. M. (2021). Intrathecal baclofen as emergency treatment alleviates severe intractable autonomic dysreflexia in cervical spinal cord injury. *Journal of Spinal Cord Medicine, 44,* 617–620.

Krassioukov, A., Linsenmeyer, T. A., Beck, L. A., Elliott, S., Gorman, P., Kirshblum, S., et al. (2021). Evaluation and management of autonomic dysreflexia and other autonomic dysfunctions: Preventing the highs and lows: Management of blood pressure, sweating, and temperature dysfunction. *Topics in Spinal Cord Injury Rehabilitation, 27,* 225–290.

Lakra, C., Swayne, O., Christofi, G., & Desai, M. (2021). Autonomic dysreflexia in spinal cord injury. *Practical Neurology, 21,* 532–538.

Mazzeo, F. (2015). "Boosting" in Paralympic athletes with spinal cord injury: Doping without drugs. *Functional Neurology, 30,* 91–98.

Mironets, E., Fischer, R., Bracchi-Ricard, V., Saltos, T. M., Truglio, T. S., O'Reilly, M. L., et al. (2020). Attenuating neurogenic sympathetic hyperreflexia robustly improves antibacterial immunity after chronic spinal cord injury. *Journal of Neuroscience, 40,* 478–492.

Shouman, K., & Benarroch, E. E. (2019). Segmental spinal sympathetic machinery: Implications for autonomic dysreflexia. *Neurology, 93,* 339–345.

Solinsky, R., Kirshblum, S. C., & Burns, S. P. (2018). Exploring detailed characteristics of autonomic dysreflexia. *Journal of Spinal Cord Medicine, 41,* 549–555.

Walter, M., Kran, S. L., Ramirez, A. L., Rapoport, D., Nigro, M. K., Stothers, L., et al. (2020). Intradetrusor onabotulinumtoxina injections ameliorate autonomic dysreflexia while improving lower urinary tract function and urinary incontinence-related quality of life in individuals with cervical and upper thoracic spinal cord injury. *Journal of Neurotrauma, 37,* 2023–2027.

Yoo, K. Y., Jeong, C. W., Kim, S. J., Jeong, S. T., Kim, W. M., Lee, H. K., et al. (2011). Remifentanil decreases sevoflurane requirements to block autonomic hyperreflexia during transurethral litholapaxy in patients with high complete spinal cord injury. *Anesthesia and Analgesia, 112,* 191–197.

# Obstetric Anesthesia

# Maternal Physiologic Changes in Pregnancy

KRISTEN VANDERHOEF, MD

Alterations in maternal physiology are caused by hormonal and mechanical changes. They begin approximately 5 weeks after fetal implantation and may not return to normal until 8 weeks after delivery (Table 165.1).

## Respiratory System

Pregnancy-induced changes of increased vascularity coupled with an increase in the parturient's body mass index often result in edema and narrowing of the maternal upper airway, necessitating the use of a smaller endotracheal tube and the heightened risk for upper airway trauma. Further, expected decreases in functional residual capacity (20%) and increased maternal oxygen consumption place the mother at risk for hypoxemia during induction and intubation where apnea is a norm resulting in reduced times to desaturation. Adequate preoxygenation is of crucial importance.

Progesterone stimulates the maternal central chemoreceptors to increase maternal minute ventilation (50%). This results in maternal hypocapnia; however, maternal pH remains within the high normal, nonpregnant range due to renal excretion of bicarbonate (maternal serum bicarbonate is decreased). This slight respiratory alkalosis shifts the oxyhemoglobin dissociation curve to the left, but the 30% rise in 2,3-diphosphoglyceric acid shifts the curve back to the right. A rightward shift of the oxyhemoglobin dissociation curve (P50 = 30.4 mm Hg, non-maternal P50 = 26.7) ensures fetal oxygenation.

## Cardiovascular System

Maternal cardiac output increases (40%) to meet higher metabolic demands of mother and fetus. This increase is initially caused by stroke volume increases and later increases in heart rate. In the presence of comorbid maternal cardiac disease, these cardiovascular changes may pathologically stress the mother and fetus. Progesterone decreases pulmonary and systemic vascular resistance; however, central venous and pulmonary artery pressure remains unchanged. This is influenced by the increase in plasma volume (50%). Red blood cell mass does not increase to the same degree, contributing to a dilutional anemia. Both these increases were physiologically designed to allow for blood and fluid losses associated with the delivery process.

As the size of the gravid uterus increases, maternal hypotension results from compression on the inferior vena cava and aorta. This is treated prophylactically by placing the mother in a 15-degree left lateral tilt. A study using magnetic resonance imaging demonstrated that even at a 45-degree angle, there was not complete resolution of this aortocaval compression. Surprisingly, the study did not report any hemodynamic changes, but interpretation is warranted because of the small sample

size, an absence from changes from regional or general anesthesia, and the parturients were not in active labor.

The gravid uterus pushes the heart cephalad and rotates it leftward. Electrocardiographic changes (e.g., left-axis deviation and T-wave inversion in lead III) occur because of cardiac enlargement in pregnancy.

## Gastrointestinal System

Symptomatic gastroesophageal reflux is reported in nearly every parturient. Lower esophageal sphincter tone is diminished by increased progesterone levels. Gastric pH is decreased because of increased gastrin production by the placenta. The gravid uterus shifts the gastroesophageal junction cephalad and posterior increasing gastric pressure. These changes place the parturient at risk for gastric aspiration during labor and delivery. The incidence of maternal aspiration for parturients undergoing emergency cesarean section is approximately 2%. Fasting guidelines, antacid prophylaxis, and cricoid pressure are all suggested techniques to minimize the potential for gastric aspiration. Previously, all pregnant women were considered to have a "full stomach" from 20 weeks' gestation until 6 weeks after delivery due to the aforementioned changes and delayed gastric emptying. Newer studies using gastric point of care ultrasound (PoCUS) challenge this belief. PoCUS evidence suggests delayed gastric emptying does not begin until after the onset of labor.

## Renal Function

Elevated intraabdominal pressure and changes in bladder size and shape lead to mechanical obstruction and ureteral reflux, which increases the incidence of ascending urinary tract infection. Increased renal blood flow increases glomerular filtration by 50%, causing a 40% reduction in blood urea nitrogen and creatinine levels. A slight increase in creatinine of 1 mg/dL indicates impaired renal function. The increased glomerular filtration rate and decreased proximal tubular reabsorption results in proteinuria (up to 300 mg/24 h). Glycosuria without hyperglycemia develops and is caused by a decrease in renal tubular reabsorption of glucose and an increased secretion of glucose.

## Hepatic Function

Minor changes in hepatic transaminase concentrations may occur. Dilution of plasma proteins causes a decrease in the albumin:globulin ratio. Accordingly, an increase in the free fraction of albumin-bound medications should be expected. Plasma cholinesterase levels are decreased (by dilution), but this does not result in a clinically significant prolongation of succinylcholine-induced neuromuscular blockade.

| TABLE 165.1 | Maternal Physiologic Changes During Pregnancy |
|---|---|

| Parameter | Change During Pregnancy | Normal Pregnancy Value* |
|---|---|---|
| **CARDIAC** | | |
| Rate | ↑ | 75–95 beats/min |
| SV | ↑ | |
| CO | ↑ | 3–8 L/min |
| MAP | ↓ | 80 mm Hg |
| SVR | ↓ | 1200–1500 dyn • $s^{-1}$ • $cm^{-5}$ |
| **RESPIRATORY** | | |
| Rate | None | |
| $V_T$ | ↑ | ↑40%–45% |
| $\dot{V}$ | ↑ | 10.5 L/min |
| ERV | ↓ | 550 mL |
| FRC | ↓ | 1350 mL |
| Blood gas concentrations pH, arterial | None | 7.4–7.45 |
| $P_{CO_2}$ | ↓ | 25–33 mm Hg |
| $P_{O_2}$ | ↑ | 92–107 mm Hg |
| $HCO_3^-$ | ↓ | 16–22 mEq/L |
| **HEMATOLOGIC** | | |
| Blood volume | ↑ | 4500 mL or 100 mL/kg |
| Plasma volume | ↑ | +45% |
| Erythrocyte volume | ↑ | +10%–15% |
| Hemoglobin | ↓ | 11.5–15 g/dL |
| Hematocrit | ↓ | 32%–36% |
| WBC count | ↑ | 6000–20,000/μL |
| Procoagulant factors[†] | ↑ | |
| Anticoagulant activity[‡] | ↓ | |
| PAI 1 and 2 | ↑ | |
| Iron | ↓ | 30–193 mcg/mL |
| TIBC | ↑ | 80.1 μmol/L |

| Parameter | Change During Pregnancy | Normal Pregnancy Value* |
|---|---|---|
| **ELECTROLYTES/RENAL** | | |
| Renal blood flow | ↑ | 700 mL/min |
| GFR | ↑ | 140 mL/min |
| Serum Cr | ↓ | 0.53–0.9 mg/dL |
| Serum BUN | ↓ | 8–10 mg/dL |
| $HCO_3^-$ | None | 15–20 mEq/L |
| $Na^{2+}$ | ↓ | 130–148 mEq/L |
| $K^+$ | None or ↓[§] | 3.3–5.0 mEq/L |
| $Cl^-$ | ↓ | 97–109 mEq/L |
| **METABOLIC** | | |
| Basal body temperature | ↑ | |
| $O_2$ consumption | ↑ | |
| Insulin resistance | ↑ | |
| **GASTROINTESTINAL** | | |
| Lower esophageal sphincter tone | ↓ | |
| Gastric emptying time | None except during labor | |
| Gastric acid secretion | ↑ | |
| **HEPATOBILIARY SYSTEM** | | |
| Gallbladder emptying time | ↑ | |
| Liver size | None | |
| ALP | ↑ | Up to 2–4 times normal value |
| Bilirubin/AST/ALT | None | |
| LDH | ↑ | 650–700 U/L |
| Prothrombin time | None | |
| Albumin | ↓ | 2.3–4.2 g/dL |
| **LIPIDS** | | |
| Cholesterol | ↑ | 141–210/219–349 mg/dL[‖] |
| Triglycerides | ↑ | |

*Values are approximate and vary throughout pregnancy.
[†]Factors XII:c, VII:c, VII, and V; von Willebrand factors; and fibrinogen.
[‡]Activated protein C and protein S.
[§]Although there are total body accumulations of $Na^+$ and $K^+$, because of the retention of fluid and increase in plasma volumes, concentrations decrease.
[‖]First trimester/third trimester.
*ALP*, Alkaline phosphatase; *ALT*, alanine transaminase; *AST*, aspartate aminotransferase; *BUN*, blood urea nitrogen; *CO*, cardiac output; *Cr*, creatinine; *ERV*, expiratory reserve volume; *FRC*, functional residual capacity; *GFR*, glomerular filtration rate; *LDH*, lactate dehydrogenase; *MAP*, mean arterial pressure; *PAI*, plasminogen activator inhibitor; *SV*, stroke volume; *SVR*, systemic vascular resistance; *TIBC*, total iron-binding capacity; *V̇*, minute ventilation; *VT*, tidal volume; *WBC*, white blood cell.

## Hematologic System

Pregnancy causes an activation of platelets, with an increased platelet turnover and shorter half-life. Levels of factors VII, VIII, X, and XII and fibrinogen are increased; in addition, the fibrinolytic system is depressed by a relative reduction of antithrombin III. This results in a hypercoagulable state. Although these changes may minimize blood loss during delivery, they increase the risk of developing thromboembolism sixfold during pregnancy.

## Neurologic System

Local anesthetic requirements for neuraxial blockade are decreased during pregnancy secondary to reduced volume in the epidural space (epidural vein engorgement), decreased volume of cerebrospinal fluid, increased cerebrospinal fluid pH, and enhanced neural sensitivity to local anesthetic agents. Enhanced neural sensitivity is caused by increased plasma endorphins and up to 10- to 20-fold increases in the levels of progesterone, a depressant of central nervous system function. These factors also contribute to a decrease (40%) in the minimum alveolar concentration of inhalation anesthetics in pregnancy.

## Uterine Physiology

Uterine blood flow and placental perfusion are affected by systemic vascular resistance, aortocaval compression, and uterine contraction. Placental blood supply is determined by spiral intervillous arteries, which are maximally dilated (Fig. 165.1). They are supplied by arcuate and radial arteries, ovarian arteries, and uterine arteries. Myometrial tension decreases the caliber of spiral arteries, reducing placental perfusion. Spiral arteries are maximally dilated and sensitive to the effects of α-adrenergic receptor agonists (e.g., phenylephrine). In the treatment of maternal hypotension, both ephedrine and phenylephrine are options. Vasoconstriction can cause dramatic changes in placental blood supply. The surface area and integrity of the placenta are affected by maternal and placental disorders.

Prolonged uterine contraction (hypertonia) can cause fetal asphyxia. Treatment options include fluids, bed rest, oxygen supplementation, and tocolytic agents (e.g., terbutaline). After delivery, uterine contraction is potentiated with massage, oxytocin, methylergonovine maleate, and carboprost tromethamine. Cardiac output rises immediately after delivery with approximately 500 to 750 mL of blood added to the maternal circulation with uterine contractions (placental autotransfusion).

## Fetal Oxygenation

Fetal oxygenation is dependent on placental blood supply, surface area integrity, and fetal cardiac output. Fetal cardiac output is rate dependent. Mechanical compression of the umbilical cord decreases the delivery of oxygen ($O_2$) to the fetus. Maternal–fetal $O_2$ transfer is facilitated by a leftward shifting of the fetal oxyhemoglobin curve. Fetal blood gas concentrations are dependent on placental perfusion and maternal ventilation. Respiratory acidosis occurs with maternal hypoventilation.

## Conclusion

Most of the changes that have occurred in the maternal physiology return to normal within 3 to 4 weeks after parturition but can take up to 8 weeks to return to normal. The changes in maternal physiology have beneficial effects with definite anesthetic implications.

## Acknowledgment

The editor wishes to sincerely thank Barry A. Harrison, MBBS, FRACP, FANACA, for his work in the previous edition of this chapter.

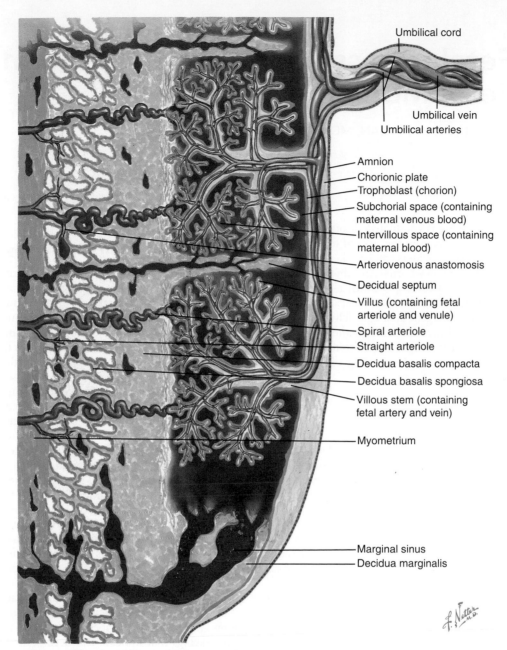

Umbilical cord

Umbilical vein
Umbilical arteries

Amnion
Chorionic plate
Trophoblast (chorion)
Subchorial space (containing maternal venous blood)
Intervillous space (containing maternal blood)
Arteriovenous anastomosis
Decidual septum
Villus (containing fetal arteriole and venule)
Spiral arteriole
Straight arteriole
Decidua basalis compacta
Decidua basalis spongiosa
Villous stem (containing fetal artery and vein)
Myometrium

Marginal sinus
Decidua marginalis

**Fig. 165.1** **Circulation in the placenta.** (Netter illustration from http://www.netterimages.com. © Elsevier Inc. All rights reserved.)

## SUGGESTED READINGS

Chestnut, D. H. (Ed.). (2020). *Chestnut's obstetric anesthesia: Principles and practice* (6th ed., pp. 13–37). Philadelphia: Elsevier.

Higuchi, H., Takagi, S., Zhang, K., Furui, I., & Ozaki, M. (2015). Effect of lateral tilt angle on the volume of the abdominal aorta and inferior vena cava in pregnant and non-pregnant women determined by magnetic resonance imaging. *Anesthesiology, 122*, 286–293.

Howle, R., Sultan, P., Shah, R., Sceales, P., Van de Putte, P., & Bampoe, S. (2020). Gastric point-of-care ultrasound (PoCUS) during pregnancy and the postpartum period: A systematic review. *International Journal of Obstetric Anesthesia, 44*, 24–32.

# 166

# Fetal Assessment and Intrapartum Fetal Monitoring

ROCHELLE J. POMPEIAN, MD

## Overview

Assessment of fetal well-being is conducted throughout pregnancy, labor, and delivery to decrease the risks of fetal morbidity and mortality. Anesthesia providers can be asked to assist in the resuscitation of unhealthy newborns. Anesthetic interventions during labor and delivery can significantly alter maternal and, thus, fetal physiology. Changes in fetal status can result in the need to proceed with emergent cesarean delivery. Understanding the degree of fetal distress informs an anesthesia team how rapidly they must achieve surgical conditions. Therefore anesthesia providers require an understanding of commonly used fetal assessment measures.

## Antepartum Fetal Assessment

During pregnancy, fetal assessment modalities can diagnose congenital anomalies, assess fetal well-being, and provide an idea of gestation age and fetal maturity. Chromosomal abnormalities can be detected during first trimester through maternal serum analysis and ultrasound assessment of nuchal translucency and can be confirmed through chorionic villus sampling. First-trimester aneuploidy tests include commercial cell-free DNA testing of maternal serum and the analysis of trophoblastic cells in cervicovaginal discharge. During second and third trimesters, amniocentesis can detect chromosomal abnormalities and assess fetal lung maturity by measuring the ratio of the phospholipids lecithin to sphingomyelin. A lecithin:sphingomyelin ratio of 2.0 or greater correlates with a low risk of the neonate developing respiratory distress syndrome.

Ultrasonography is an extremely important tool in obstetrics. Early ultrasound scans assist in confirming gestational age and can detect structural abnormalities. As pregnancy progresses, a nonstress test (no contractions stimulated) is used to assess fetal heart rate (FHR) and fetal movements, and a stress test (contractions present or induced) is used to assess the FHR response to the stress of contractions. Vibroacoustic stimulation can be used to shorten the time it takes to achieve a reactive nonstress test. A biophysical profile is a more extensive examination and includes both a nonstress test and a fetal ultrasound. The latter specifically assesses five components: FHR, fetal breathing, fetal movement, fetal tone, and amniotic fluid volume. Each component is scored from 0 to 2, and certain interventions are recommended for specific scores. For example, a score of 8 to 10 is generally considered reassuring, and therefore no intervention is recommended, but a score of 0 to 2 is highly suspicious for asphyxia, and evaluation for immediate delivery is recommended. During labor, ultrasound is used to detect fetal position, placental position, causes of vaginal bleeding, quantity of amniotic fluid, and the presence of significant risk factors for bleeding, including the ability to evaluate likelihood of placental accreta, increta, or percreta.

## Intrapartum Fetal Monitoring

The most common form of fetal monitoring during labor is continuous FHR monitoring (Fig. 166.1). Although intermittent FHR monitoring is reasonable for low-risk pregnancies, most labor and delivery units use continuous monitoring from early labor through delivery. The FHR tracing and concurrently obtained uterine contraction tracings from the tocodynamometer are displayed together so that the relationship of the FHR tracing to uterine contractions can be observed. FHR can be monitored externally (noninvasively through a Doppler) or internally (invasively through a fetal scalp electrode). Internal monitoring is generally indicated if the external monitor tracings are of poor quality or if nonreassuring FHR patterns are evident. Likewise, uterine contractions can either be monitored internally or externally. An external tocodynamometer involves a pressure transducer applied to the abdomen at the level of the fundus to detect changes in tension across the abdominal wall. It indicates the timing and duration of contractions. To measure the strength of contractions, an intrauterine pressure catheter placed into the amniotic space is necessary. This is helpful if the progression of labor is slow and the adequacy of the forces of contraction needs to be evaluated. Internal monitoring of contractions may also be useful when pharmacologic uterine stimulation is used to augment or induce labor.

Patterns of the FHR tracing are evaluated to assess fetal well-being. Table 166.1 describes the individual characteristics of FHR tracings that indicate fetal well-being or fetal distress. In general, assessment of the baseline heart rate, variability, and presence or absence of decelerations or accelerations allows a provider to describe an FHR tracing as category I (indicative of a normal acid-base status), category II (abnormal tracings with an uncertain prognosis), or category III (indicative of an increased likelihood of hypoxia or acidemia). Table 166.2 summarizes these National Institute of Child Health and Human Development categories of FHR tracings.

The normal baseline FHR of a term fetus ranges from 110 to 160 beats per minute (bpm). Normal FHR indicates normal intrinsic cardiac conduction, autonomic innervation, and normal fetal catecholamine levels. The variability of the FHR tracing is the amplitude range of the heart rate's change from baseline. Variability is a highly sensitive indicator of fetal well-being; it indicates that the sympathetic and parasympathetic nervous systems of the fetus are intact and thereby indicates adequate oxygenation of the central nervous system.

Decelerations describe the pattern of FHR slowing in relationship to uterine contractions and are illustrated in Fig. 166.1.

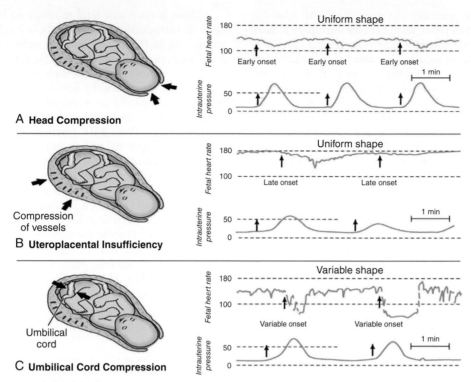

**Fig. 166.1** Periodic changes in fetal heart rate related to uterine contraction. **A,** Early decelerations. **B,** Late decelerations. **C,** Variable decelerations. (Modified and reproduced from Danforth DN, Scott JR. *Obstetrics and Gynecology.* 5th ed. Lippincott; 1986.)

| TABLE 166.1 | Assessment of Intrapartum Fetal Heart Rate Tracings | | |
|---|---|---|---|
| **Characteristic** | **Normal** | **Abnormal** | **Diagnostic Considerations and Significance** |
| Baseline Heart Rate | 110–160 bpm | <110 bpm "fetal bradycardia" | Maternal hypotension, hypoxemia, hypothermia, hypoglycemia, maternal β-blocker therapy, or congenital heart block |
| | | >160 bpm "fetal tachycardia" | Maternal medications or fever, chorioamnionitis, thyrotoxicosis, fetal anemia, fetal tachyarrhythmias, or elevation of fetal catecholamines |
| Variability | 5–25 bpm | 0 "absent" ≤5 bpm "minimal" | Absent or minimal baseline variability can be indicative of acidemia or hypoxia but can also be caused from prematurity, sleep cycle, anesthesia, arrhythmia, neurologic injury, or congenital anomalies |
| | | 5–25 bpm "moderate" | Moderate baseline variability predicts the absence of fetal acidemia or hypoxia |
| | | >25 bpm "marked" | The significance of marked variability is unknown |
| Decelerations | Early | Early decelerations are normal | Head compression |
| | Variable | Variable decelerations are abnormal | Cord compression |
| | Late | Late decelerations are abnormal | Uteroplacental insufficiency |

*Bpm,* Beats per minute.

| TABLE 166.2 | National Institute of Child Health and Human Development Categories of Fetal Heart Rate Tracings | |
|---|---|---|
| **Category** | **FHR Pattern** | **Significance** |
| Category I | Baseline 110–160 bpm Moderate variability Absence of late or variable decelerations | Minimal likelihood of acidemia or ongoing fetal hypoxic injury |
| Category II | All patterns not categorized as Category I or III | Uncertain |
| Category III | Absent variability with recurrent late or variable decelerations Absent variability with bradycardia Sinusoidal pattern | Increased likelihood of hypoxia or acidosis |

*Bpm,* Beats per minute; *FHR,* fetal heart rate.

Early decelerations are generally not associated with fetal distress and may result from reflex vagal activity secondary to head compression as the fetus descends down the vaginal canal during labor. The FHR tracing usually decreases fewer than 20 bpm, and the onset and recovery mirror the uterine contraction. Variable decelerations are of more concern and may result from compression of the umbilical cord, with resulting increased vagal tone. The patterns of variable decelerations may differ regarding onset, depth, duration, and shape. Late decelerations suggest uteroplacental insufficiency. Their onset is typically 10 to 30 seconds after the onset of uterine contractions, and recovery to a normal FHR is equally delayed after the end of a contraction. With a normal baseline, the presence of variable or late decelerations results in a category II FHR tracing. Once variability is lost, this tracing then progresses to a category III tracing. This loss of FHR variability after repeated variable or late decelerations indicates a fetus that has been stressed by the ongoing labor and may now be developing acidosis. This may precipitate an obstetrician's decision to proceed with surgical vaginal or cesarean delivery.

Although electronic fetal monitoring has been used widely since its introduction in the 1960s, it has been associated with an increase in the rate of cesarean deliveries without improvement in perinatal mortality rate or fetal neurologic injury. A likely hypothesis is that although a normal FHR tracing predicts a fetus with a healthy acid-base status, an abnormal FHR tracing is not specific for a compromised fetus. In other words, there are many false positives resulting in cesarean delivery of healthy fetuses. Three FHR tracings are of particular concern: (1) late decelerations and absent variability, (2) a prolonged bradycardic event, and (3) a sinusoidal pattern. A prolonged bradycardic event may be indicative of a catastrophic event (e.g., uterine rupture or placental abruption) and impending fetal demise and may even necessitate rapid cesarean delivery under a general anesthetic if regional anesthesia would require additional time. Despite the shortcomings of continuous FHR tracing, other modalities of intrapartum fetal assessment have been evaluated from fetal pulse oximetry to fetal electrocardiograph, but to date, FHR monitoring remains the standard of intrapartum obstetric care for most obstetric practices.

## SUGGESTED READINGS

American Congress of Obstetricians and Gynecologists. (November 2010, Reaffirmed 2017). Management of intrapartum fetal herat rate tracings. Practice Bulletin No. 106.

Clark, S. L., Hamilton, E. F., Garite, T. J., Timmins, A., Warrick, P. A., & Smith, S. (2017). The limits of electronic fetal heart rate monitoring in the prevention of neonatal metabolic acidemia.

*American Journal of Obstetrics and Gynecology,* 216, 163.e1.

Graham, G. M., Park, J. S., & Norwitz, E. R. (2020). Antepartum fetal assessment and therapy. In D. H. Chestnut, C. A. Wong, L. C. Tsen, W. D. Ngan Kee, Y. Beilin, J. M. Mhyre, & B. T. Bateman (Eds.), *Chestnut's obstetric anesthesia: Principles and practice* (6th ed., pp. 97–131). Philadelphia: Elsevier Saunders.

Livingston, E. G. (2020). Intrapartum fetal assessment and therapy. In D. H. Chestnut, C. A. Wong, L. C. Tsen, W. D. Ngan Kee, Y. Beilin, J. M. Mhyre, & B. T. Bateman (Eds.), *Chestnut's obstetric anesthesia: Principles and practice* (6th ed., pp. 155–170). Philadelphia: Elsevier Saunders.

# 167

# Analgesia for Labor

HOLLY B. ENDE, MD, MS  |  K.A. KELLY MCQUEEN, MD, MPH, FASA

## Labor Pain

The first stage of labor begins with the onset of regular, painful contractions and ends at complete cervical dilation. This stage can be further divided into a latent phase (cervix ≤3 cm dilated) and an active phase (cervix 4–10 cm dilated). Pain in the first stage of labor is visceral (vague, diffuse, and poorly localized) and is caused by uterine contractions and dilation of the cervix and lower uterine segment. Visceral afferent nerves travel along the sympathetic nerves and transmit pain signals via the dorsal horn at T10–L1 (Fig. 167.1). Effective relief of first-stage labor pain is achieved by blocking peripheral afferent nerves (by paracervical, paravertebral, lumbar sympathetic, or epidural blocks) or by spinal cord transmission (intrathecal injection).

The second stage of labor begins when the cervix is completely dilated and ends with delivery of the infant. Pain in the second stage of labor is somatic in nature as stretching and tearing of the pelvic ligaments and muscles occur. The pain signals from this stage are transmitted by the same afferents as the first stage, in addition to afferents that are conducted along

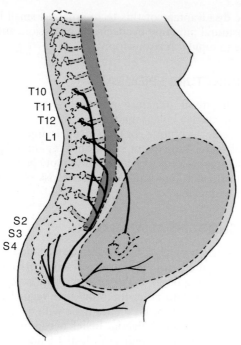

**Fig. 167.1** Parturition pain pathways. Afferent pain impulses from the cervix and uterus are carried by nerves that accompany sympathetic fibers and enter the neuraxis at the T10, T11, T12, and L1 spinal levels. Pain pathways from the perineum travel to S2, S3, and S4 via the pudendal nerve. (Modified from Bonica JJ, Chadwick HS. Labour pain. In: Wall PD, Melzack R, eds. *Textbook of Pain.* 2nd ed. Churchill Livingstone; 1989:482.)

the pudendal nerves at S2–S4. Pain impulses during distention of the vagina and perineum just before delivery are conducted along the genitofemoral (L1, L2), ilioinguinal (L1), and posterior cutaneous nerves of the thighs (S2, S3), although these have a small role in labor pain.

## Preanesthesia Evaluation and Monitoring

Before providing any labor anesthetic intervention, the anesthesia provider should obtain a maternal and perinatal history, complete a chart review, and perform an anesthesia-specific physical examination, including airway evaluation, heart and lung examination, and palpation of the spine. Maternal vital signs (blood pressure, heart rate, oxygen saturation) and fetal heart rate should be monitored during neuraxial placement. Preprocedure intravenous hydration may be considered if a regional technique is used that causes sympathectomy and subsequent hypotension; however, fluid should be administered cautiously to those parturients with preeclampsia or significant cardiac dysfunction.

## Analgesia Options for Parturients During Labor

### EPIDURAL ANALGESIA

Epidural analgesia provides excellent relief of labor pain while preserving maternal motor function and fetal circulation. A continuous epidural technique is most often employed for

labor, with an epidural catheter placed between the L2 and L5 vertebral interspaces. Many medications can be administered epidurally to effectively obliterate or attenuate labor pain (Table 167.1). Used alone, lipid-soluble opioids (e.g., fentanyl) provide good pain relief in early labor and allow maternal ambulation ("walking epidural"). Local anesthetics, used alone or in combination with a lipid-soluble opioid, provide excellent pain relief throughout labor, but the risk of associated motor weakness precludes ambulation. Although both bupivacaine and ropivacaine are commonly used in obstetric anesthesia practice, ropivacaine offers a superior safety profile because of the decreased risk of cardiovascular collapse with inadvertent intravascular injection. Both bupivacaine and ropivacaine are used in dilute solutions, often in combination with fentanyl. Commonly, the analgesic mixture is initially administered as a bolus through the epidural catheter to achieve maternal comfort, followed by continuous infusion or programmed intermittent epidural bolus (PIEB) to maintain the desired dermatomal level of analgesia. The continuous infusion or PIEB may be delivered via a standard epidural pump with or without the addition of patient-controlled epidural analgesia (PCEA), which allows for patient-controlled boluses (time interval, volume, and lock-out interval are set by the anesthesia provider). The addition of PCEA is associated with improved patient satisfaction and decreased need for provider-administered boluses. Adverse effects and complications associated with epidural and other neuraxial techniques are presented in Box 167.1. Contraindications to neuraxial analgesia are listed in Box 167.2.

## COMBINED SPINAL-EPIDURAL ANALGESIA

The combined spinal-epidural (CSE) technique is another option for labor analgesia. A needle-through-needle technique is

| TABLE 167.1 | **Medications Used for Epidural and Spinal Labor Analgesia** | | |
|---|---|---|---|
| | **Epidural Bolus*** | **Epidural Infusion** | **Spinal** |
| **LOCAL ANESTHETICS** | | | |
| Bupivacaine | 0.125%–0.25% 5–10 mL | 0.04%–0.125% 5–15 mL/h | 1.25–2.5 mg |
| Ropivacaine | 0.1%–0.2% 5–10 mL | 0.1%–0.2% 6–8 mL/h | 2.0–3.5 mg |
| Lidocaine | 0.75%–1.0% 5–10 mL | NA | NA |
| **OPIOIDS** | | | |
| Fentanyl | 50–100 mcg | 2–5 mcg/mL | 15–25 mcg |
| Hydromorphone | 0.4–1 mg | 5–10 mg/mL | 50–200 mcg |
| Morphine sulfate | 2–5 mg | 20–40 mcg/mL | 100–200 mcg |
| Sufentanil | 5–10 mcg | 0.5–2 mcg/mL | 1.5–5 mcg |
| **ADJUNCTS** | | | |
| Epinephrine | 50–200 mcg | NA | 50–200 mcg |
| Clonidine | 50–100 mcg | NA | 15–50 mcg |

*Initial epidural bolus may require greater volume.
*NA,* Not applicable.
Ranges provided represent typical dosing, although individual dosing regimens may vary.

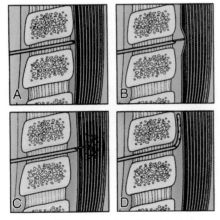

**Fig. 167.2** The combined spinal-epidural technique. An epidural needle is inserted in the epidural space **(A)**, and a spinal needle is inserted through it **(B)**. Because of the presence of air in the epidural space, the pencil-point spinal needle may considerably deform the dura before puncturing it. After the anesthetic agent is injected through the spinal needle **(C)**, the spinal needle is withdrawn, and an epidural catheter is inserted **(D)**. Finally, the epidural needle is withdrawn. (Modified from Eisenach JC. Combined spinal-epidural analgesia in obstetrics. Anesthesiology. 1999; 91:299–302.)

most commonly used (Fig. 167.2), during which the anesthesia provider intrathecally administers opioids, with or without a local anesthetic, and then inserts an epidural catheter. The intrathecal injection results in significantly more rapid sacral coverage compared with a standard epidural (2–5 minutes vs. 10–15 minutes). The CSE technique may also lower the incidence of epidural catheter failure. The epidural catheter can be bolused if additional analgesia is required after the intrathecal dose, with subsequent initiation of continuous infusion or

PIEB. The disadvantage of this technique is a small increased risk of postdural puncture headache, hypotension, and uterine tetany due to rapid sympathectomy.

## DURAL PUNCTURE EPIDURAL

Recently, the dural puncture epidural technique has been described in which a hole is made in the dura using the needle-through-needle technique, but no drug is injected into the intrathecal space. Subsequent injection of epidural local anesthetics and opioids leads to slightly more rapid pain relief compared with standard epidural, with lower risk of hypotension compared with CSE.

## SINGLE-SHOT SPINAL ANALGESIA

Rapid progression of labor in a multiparous patient may make the time required for epidural catheter placement and incremental dosing of an analgesic agent impractical. In a patient who desires pain relief for imminent vaginal delivery, a single intrathecal dose of local anesthetic with or without opioid can provide rapid analgesia. Relief occurs within several uterine contractions and predictably lasts 1.5 hours. The disadvantages of a single-shot spinal include increased risk of postdural puncture headache and the potential that labor outlasts the duration of medication action.

## CONTINUOUS SPINAL ANALGESIA

Complications associated with spinal microcatheters used for continuous spinal analgesia and anesthesia in the 1990s necessitated their removal from the market and decreased the use of continuous spinal techniques in the United States. However, when an inadvertent dural puncture occurs (incidence approximately 1% in teaching institutions), a choice must be made as to how to proceed. Options include (1) removal of the Tuohy needle and replacement of the catheter one lumbar level above or below the space at which the puncture occurred; or (2) placement of the epidural catheter through the dural rent and institution of a continuous intrathecal catheter with dosing at approximately one-tenth the epidural infusion rate. Although both a local anesthetic agent and an opioid are acceptable for continuous spinal infusion, side effects associated with opioids (pruritus) are more common when the agent is delivered into the subarachnoid space compared with the epidural space.

## OTHER REGIONAL BLOCKADE

Several options exist for blockade of specific nerve plexuses during labor. These include paravertebral, lumbar sympathetic, paracervical, and pudendal blocks. Risk-versus-benefit profiles and provider inexperience discourage their mainstream use when other options are available; however, in some circumstances these techniques may prove useful. Paracervical blocks offer good transient relief of pain in the first stage of labor, and pudendal blocks are effective for pain in the second stage.

## NITROUS OXIDE

Nitrous oxide is the most commonly used inhalational agent for labor analgesia worldwide. In the United States it is typically delivered as 50% nitrous oxide in oxygen using a blender device and a mask for delivery. Equipment must be available to ensure a hypoxic mixture is not delivered to the patient, and a scavenging mechanism should be in place to limit environmental pollution and staff exposure. The mechanism of action is believed to be enhancement of the release of opioid peptides from the midbrain and modulation of descending spinal pain pathways. Parturients should be encouraged to start inhalation in anticipation of the next uterine contraction, which can be difficult as uterine contractions are not always regular. Nitrous oxide is a less effective labor analgesic agent compared with epidural analgesia; however, it does provide high levels of patient satisfaction for some parturients. Side effects include nausea, vomiting, drowsiness, dizziness, and a small risk of hypoxemia.

## Systemically Administered Medication

Opioids are the most effective and widely used of the systemically administered medications for labor analgesia; however, use is limited by dose-dependent maternal respiratory depression and other side effects (Box 167.3). Opioids are also readily transported across the placenta, leading to decreased variability in the fetal heart rate and neonatal depression after birth. Therefore systemic opioids are cautiously used in labor to reduce pain when neuraxial analgesia is refused or contraindicated.

Options for systemic opioid therapy include patient-controlled analgesia (PCA) (Table 167.2) or nurse administration at 2- to 4-hour intervals. Although fentanyl PCA was historically used for labor analgesia, newer agents including remifentanil and ketamine have increased in popularity. Remifentanil acts at the μ-opioid receptor with peak onset time of 20 to 30 seconds. Because of rapid metabolism by tissue esterases, the elimination half-life of remifentanil is approximately 9.5 minutes. Although remifentanil does cross to the placenta, the fetus also rapidly metabolizes the drug, and thus there is little fetal effect. This makes it ideal for labor analgesia in the form of a PCA bolus during each contraction.

### BOX 167.3  SIDE EFFECTS OF SYSTEMICALLY ADMINISTERED OPIOIDS

Sedation
Respiratory depression
Hypotension
Pruritus
Nausea and vomiting
Decreased gastric motility
Potential decreased uterine activity in early stages of labor
Decreased variability in fetal heart rate

### TABLE 167.2  Medications Used for Intravenous Patient-Controlled Labor Analgesia

| Medication | Dose | Lock-Out Interval (Min) |
|---|---|---|
| Nalbuphine | 1–3 mg | 5–10 |
| Fentanyl | 10–25 mcg | 5–10 |
| Meperidine | 5–15 mg | 10–20 |
| Alfentanil | 200 mcg | 5–10 |
| Remifentanil | 0.2–0.5 mcg/kg | 2–3 |
| Ketamine | Bolus: 0.1–0.2 mg/kg | 5–10 |

Ketamine is also a newer agent to be used for labor analgesia. With its $N$-methyl-D-aspartate antagonism and mu opioid receptor agonism at high doses, ketamine can produce labor analgesia without the respiratory depressive side effects of opioid medications. It has an onset time of 30 seconds and duration of action around 5 to 10 minutes. Caution should be used in preeclamptic and hypertensive patients, as ketamine's sympathomimetic properties can cause an increase in heart rate, systolic blood pressure, and cardiac output.

## SUGGESTED READINGS

Bucklin, B. A., & Santos, A. C. (2020). Local anesthetics and opioids. In D. H. Chestnut, C. A. Wong, L. C. Tsen, W. D. Ngan Kee, Y. Beilin, J. M. Mhyre, & B. T. Bateman (Eds.), *Chestnut's obstetric anesthesia: Principles and practice* (6th ed., pp. 271–311). Philadelphia: Mosby Elsevier.

Chau, A., Bibbo, C., Huang, C. C., Elterman, K. G., Robinson, J. N., & Tsen, L. C. (2017). Dural puncture epidural technique improves labor analgesia quality with fewer side effects compared with epidural and combined spinal epidural techniques: A randomized clinical trial. *Anesthesia and Analgesia, 124*(2), 560–569.

George, R. B., Allen, T. K., & Habib, A. S. (2013). Intermittent epidural bolus compared with continuous epidural infusions for labor analgesia: A systematic review and meta-analysis. *Anesthesia and Analgesia, 116*(1), 133–144.

Nathan, N., & Wong, C. A. (2020). Spinal, epidural, and caudal anesthesia: Anatomy, physiology, and technique. In D. H. Chestnut, C. A. Wong, L. C. Tsen, W. D. Ngan Kee, Y. Beilin, J. M. Mhyre, B. T. Bateman (Eds.), *Chestnut's obstetric anesthesia: Principles and practice* (6th ed., pp. 238–270). Philadelphia: Mosby Elsevier.

# 168

# Opioid Dependence in the Parturient

HOLLY B. ENDE, MD, MS  |  K.A. KELLY MCQUEEN, MD, MPH, FASA

## Pharmacology

The term *opioid* refers to the class of drugs with structures similar to morphine, including heroin, oxycodone, hydrocodone, methadone, and buprenorphine, among others. Opioids bind to μ-, δ-, and κ-opioid receptors throughout the body and have multiple systemic effects in almost every system (Box 168.1). Their euphoric and analgesic properties primarily result from μ-receptor binding. All opioids cross the placenta in variable amounts depending on factors such as their lipophilicity and protein binding, and opioid transfer to the fetus can lead to changes in fetal heart rate and neonatal depression if delivery occurs.

## Maternal and Fetal Outcomes

Opioid abuse during pregnancy has many potential deleterious effects on both mother and fetus. Compared with pregnancies not affected by opioid abuse or dependence, those pregnancies complicated by opioid abuse are associated with significantly higher mortality and morbidity (Box 168.2). In addition, opioid-addicted parturients are more likely to seek late prenatal care and to exhibit poor compliance with medical treatments.

Fetuses of mothers afflicted with opioid addiction will commonly display signs of neonatal abstinence syndrome (NAS) because of opioid withdrawal. NAS is characterized by autonomic dysfunction, feeding difficulties, hypertonicity, tremors, irritability, and failure to thrive.

## Pregnancy Management for the Opioid-Addicted Parturient

Current standard of care for opioid addiction in pregnancy includes continuation or initiation of opioid-assisted therapy

### BOX 168.1  SYSTEMIC EFFECTS OF OPIOIDS

**NEUROLOGIC**
Decreased sympathetic activity
Increased parasympathetic activity
Miosis
Drowsiness/obtundation

**CARDIOVASCULAR**
Bradycardia
Hypotension
Bradyarrhythmia or tachyarrhythmia

**RESPIRATORY**
Respiratory depression
Decreased ventilatory response to hypercarbia

**GASTROINTESTINAL**
Nausea/vomiting
Gastroesophageal reflux
Constipation

### BOX 168.2  MORBIDITY ASSOCIATED WITH MATERNAL OPIOID ABUSE

Prolonged hospital stay
Premature rupture of membranes
Placental abruption
Fetal growth restriction
Preterm labor
Oligohydramnios
Cesarean delivery
Maternal cardiac arrest

with methadone or buprenorphine (Table 168.1). Because of physiologic changes of pregnancy including increased intravascular volume and renal clearance, doses of opioid replacement therapy may need to be increased during the second and third trimesters. These medications have been shown to improve both maternal and fetal outcomes and should be continued during hospitalization for delivery. While receiving these medications, saturation of μ-opioid receptors may decrease the efficacy of other opioids administered in the peripartum period and make pain control more difficult.

## Labor Analgesia

Although both methadone and buprenorphine function as opioid-receptor agonists, they each have low intrinsic activity at the μ-opioid receptor and thus may not provide adequate analgesia for labor and delivery. Neuraxial anesthesia is safe and effective in this patient population and should be offered as an option for pain control. The efficacy of neuraxially administered local anesthetics will be unaffected by concomitantly administered methadone or buprenorphine; however, opioids by any route will have diminished effects secondary to opioid receptor occupation by these drugs. It is estimated that 25% to nearly 100% of receptors may be occupied, depending on the patient's dose. Higher than normal doses of opioids may be required to displace these low-activity opioid agonists from μ-opioid receptors. Consideration should be given to adjuvant therapy with nonopioid medications to improve overall pain control. In the case of labor analgesia, epidural clonidine may be used in conjunction with local anesthetics, although special attention must be paid to preventing maternal hypotension.

## Anesthetic Management for Cesarean Delivery

Neuraxial anesthesia is the preferred technique for cesarean delivery in the opioid-addicted population, assuming no other contraindications. Doses of local anesthetic do not require adjustment; however, usual doses of opioids may be less efficacious in these patients. For this reason, other adjuvant medications such as intrathecal clonidine may be considered. If

| TABLE 168.1 | Pharmacology of Opioid-Replacement Therapies | | | |
|---|---|---|---|---|
| | Mechanism of Action | Usual Starting Dose | Advantages | Disadvantages |
| Methadone | Racemic mixture of two enantiomers: R-methadone μ-agonist S-methadone NMDA antagonist | 25–10 mg PO | Preferable for polysubstance users More long-term data on fetal neurodevelopmental outcomes | Higher risk of overdose and drug interactions Requires daily visit to licensed treatment program |
| Buprenorphine | Partial μ-agonist κ-antagonist | 2–4 mg sublingual | Lower risk of overdose and drug interactions Daily visits to licensed treatment program unnecessary Less severe NAS | Less experience/evidence of long-term fetal effects Higher patient dropout Higher chance of withdrawal with initiation |

*NAS,* Neonatal abstinence syndrome; *NMDA,* N-methyl-D-aspartate; *PO,* orally.

intraoperative intravenous supplementation is required for pain control, nonopioid medications such as ketamine may confer greater benefit than intravenous opioids. Postoperative pain management is frequently challenging, and increased doses of systemic opioids should be used in conjunction with multimodal analgesia (Box 168.3) to achieve adequate pain control. Mixed opioid agonists/antagonists (e.g., nalbuphine) should be avoided in parturients with a history of opioid abuse, as they may precipitate withdrawal.

> **BOX 168.3  MULTIMODAL ANALGESIC OPTIONS FOR PATIENTS RECEIVING OPIOID-REPLACEMENT THERAPY AFTER CESAREAN DELIVERY**
>
> Neuraxial opioids
> Intravenous patient-controlled opioid analgesia
> Nonsteroidal antiinflammatory medications
> Acetaminophen
> Gabapentin
> Intravenous ketamine
> Transversus abdominis plane blocks
> Quadratus lumborum blocks
> Epidural analgesia

## SUGGESTED READINGS

Leffert, L. R. (2020). Substance Use Disorders. In D. H. Chestnut, C. A. Wong, L. C. Tsen, W. D. Ngan Kee, Y. Beilin, J. M. Mhyre, B.T. Bateman (Eds.), *Chestnut's Obstetrical Anesthesia: Principles and Practice* (6th ed., pp. 1248–1273). Philadelphia: Mosby Elsevier.

Mozurkewich, E. L., & Rayburn, W. F. (2014). Buprenorphine and Methadone for Opioid Addiction During Pregnancy. *Obstetrics and Gynecology clinics of North.* America, 41(2), 241–253.

Opioid Use and Opioid Use Disorder in Pregnancy. Committee Opinion No. 711. American College of Obstetricians and Gynecologists. (2017). *Obstetrics and Gynecology, 130,* e81–e94.

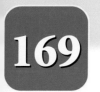

# 169

# Preterm Labor: Tocolytics and Anesthetic Management

HOLLY B. ENDE, MD, MS  |  K.A. KELLY MCQUEEN, MD, MPH, FASA

## Epidemiology

Preterm birth, or delivery before 37 weeks' gestation, accounts for approximately 12% of live births in the United States and is associated with fetal morbidity and mortality (Fig. 169.1). Preterm labor (PTL) is defined by regular uterine contractions in the setting of cervical dilation or effacement and precedes approximately half of these preterm births. PTL is linked to various maternal and fetal risk factors (Box 169.1). Although 30% of PTL episodes spontaneously resolve and 50% of patients hospitalized for PTL remain pregnant until term, PTL occasionally necessitates inpatient monitoring and pharmacologic interventions.

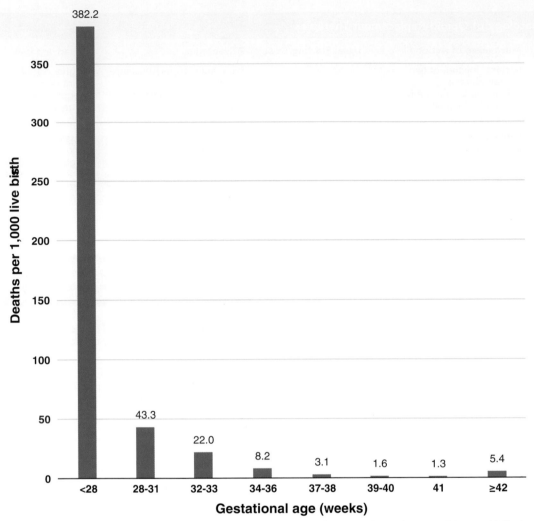

**Fig. 169.1** Infant mortality rates by gestational age at birth. (Ely DM, Driscoll AK. Infant mortality in the United States, 2018: data from the period linked birth/infant death file. Natl Vital Stat Rep. 2020;69(7):1–1.)

---

**BOX 169.1 FACTORS ASSOCIATED WITH DEVELOPMENT OF PRETERM LABOR**

**DEMOGRAPHICS**

Nonwhite race
Advanced maternal age
Low education level
Body mass index <18.5 or >30 kg/m²

**MEDICAL HISTORY**

History of preterm labor
Prior preterm birth
Interpregnancy interval <6 months
Prior uterine curettage or cervical surgery
Abnormal uterine anatomy
Abdominal surgery during pregnancy
Acute or chronic systemic disease

**BEHAVIORAL FACTORS**

Physical or psychological stress
Tobacco use

Alcohol use
Substance abuse

**OBSTETRIC FACTORS**

Shortened cervical length
Vaginal bleeding
Infection (systemic, genital tract, periodontal)
Multiple gestations
Assisted reproduction
Preterm premature rupture of membranes
Abnormal placentation
Polyhydramnios

**FETAL FACTORS**

Genetic abnormalities
Fetal death

Modified from Cobo T, Kacerovsky M, Jacobsson B. Risk factors for spontaneous preterm delivery. *Int J Gynaecol Obstet.* 2020;150(1):17–23; and Bolden JR, Grobman WA. Preterm labor and delivery.
In: Chestnut DH, Wong CA, Tsen LC, et al., eds. *Chestnut's Obstetric Anesthesia: Principles and Practice.* 6th ed. Mosby Elsevier; 2020:798–821.

| TABLE 169.1 | Tocolytic Pharmacologic Agents | |
|---|---|---|
| **Drug** | **Dose and Route** | **Side Effects** |
| Calcium channel blockers<br>  Nifedipine | *Loading:* 25–50 mg PO<br>*Maintenance:* 10–20 mg PO every 4–6 hours | Hypotension, bradycardia, flushing |
| β₂-agonists<br>  Terbutaline | SC: 0.25 mg (can be given every 20 minutes–3 hours)<br>IV infusion: 2.5–10 μg/min | Tachycardia, dysrhythmias, pulmonary edema, anxiety, hyperglycemia |
| Cyclooxygenase inhibitors<br>  Indomethacin<br>  Ketorolac | *Loading:* 50–100 mg PO/PR<br>*Maintenance:* 25–50 mg PO/PR every 4 hours<br>30 mg IM every 6 hours | Maternal: Tachycardia, hypotension, nausea<br>Fetal: Premature closure of the ductus arteriosus, intracranial hemorrhage, necrotizing enterocolitis, oligohydramnios |

*IV*, Intravenous; *IM*, intramuscular; *PO*, orally; *PR*, per rectum; *SC*, subcutaneous.

Tocolytic therapy is the mainstay of treatment. Anesthesia providers must be familiar with the pharmacokinetics and pharmacodynamics of tocolytic agents and the care of the parturient during preterm labor and delivery.

## Tocolytic Agents

Tocolytic medications inhibit contraction of uterine smooth muscle by a variety of mechanisms (Table 169.1). Although long-term maintenance therapy with tocolytics is not effective at decreasing the incidence of preterm birth or improving neonatal outcomes, short-term courses of tocolytics are recommended for up to 48 hours. This provides adequate time for corticosteroid and magnesium administration (see later), as well as transfer to a tertiary care facility with a neonatal intensive care unit equipped to handle preterm neonates. The decision to administer tocolysis should weigh risks and benefits to both mother and fetus, considering specific contraindications.

One of the most common classes of medications used in the treatment of PTL are calcium channel blockers (CCBs), which act by blocking cell membrane channels that are selective for calcium, thereby preventing the coupled release of calcium from the intracellular sarcoplasmic reticulum. This subsequently results in relaxation of uterine smooth muscle. CCBs possess equal efficacy to other tocolytic agents with fewer maternal and fetal side effects.

β₂-Adrenergic receptor agonists (terbutaline and ritodrine) activate adenyl cyclase within myometrial cells, which increases cyclic adenosine monophosphate and ultimately decreases intracellular calcium, resulting in uterine relaxation. β2-Agonists were historically a first-line treatment for PTL; however, they have fallen out of favor because of frequent and significant side effects.

Cyclooxygenase (COX) inhibitors, such as indomethacin, have also been shown to effectively relax uterine smooth muscle by preventing the synthesis of prostaglandins that play an important role in uterine smooth muscle contraction. Fetal concerns in the setting of prolonged use (i.e., premature closure of the ductus arteriosus and renal dysfunction leading to oligohydramnios) limit the use of these drugs; however, if exposure is short (<48 hours), these fetal complications are less likely.

## Magnesium Sulfate for Neuroprotection

Although intravenous magnesium sulfate (MgSO₄) may also inhibit myometrial contraction, its use as a tocolytic is not recommended because of lack of evidence demonstrating prolongation of pregnancy and improved neonatal outcomes. Rather, MgSO₄ is administered in the setting of PTL to reduce the incidence of cerebral palsy in preterm infants ("fetal neuroprotection"). For this indication, the loading dose of MgSO₄ is 4 to 6 g intravenous over 30 minutes, followed by a continuous infusion of 2 g/h.

## Corticosteroids for Fetal Lung Maturity

An antenatal course of corticosteroids is recommended in the setting of PTL if delivery is anticipated within 7 days. Large clinical trials have shown positive fetal effects of maternal corticosteroid administration including decreased incidence of neonatal respiratory distress syndrome, intraventricular hemorrhage, necrotizing enterocolitis, and neonatal death; however, fetal hypoglycemia is more common in these infants. The most commonly administered corticosteroid regimens are two doses of intramuscular betamethasone 12 mg given 24 hours apart or four doses of intramuscular dexamethasone 6 mg given 12 hours apart. The course of steroids is considered "complete" once 24 hours have elapsed from the final dose. This is when maximum fetal benefit is thought to be conferred.

## Anesthesia Management of Parturients With Preterm Labor

Anesthesiologists commonly care for parturients who have received tocolytic medications to slow or stop impending preterm delivery. These patients may request neuraxial analgesia after progression of labor or may present for cesarean delivery after a failed trial of tocolysis in the setting of prior cesarean delivery, nonreassuring fetal status, or severe hemorrhage. The side effects of therapies aimed to stop PTL must be considered when developing the anesthetic plan.

For example, some CCBs, such as nifedipine, can augment the effects of nondepolarizing neuromuscular blockers, leading to prolongation of muscle relaxation. CCBs also cause hypotension, vasodilation, myocardial depression, and myocardial conduction defects, which can be accentuated in the setting of hypotension related to general or neuraxial anesthesia.

Side effects of β-adrenergic receptor agonists occur primarily because of β1 stimulation and include tachycardia, arrhythmias, myocardial ischemia, and pulmonary edema. β2 effects can result in hypotension, hyperglycemia, and hypokalemia.

Each of these complications has significant implications for anesthetic management during labor and delivery.

The maternal side effects of indomethacin are minimal, most commonly nausea and heartburn. Although there is a transient effect on platelet function, administration of indomethacin is not a contraindication to neuraxial analgesia.

Finally, the use of $MgSO_4$ can have significant side effects that may alter maternal physiology. These side effects are similar to β-adrenergic tocolytic therapy and include hypotension, maternal obtundation, pulmonary edema, and muscle weakness. $MgSO_4$ causes muscle relaxation by affecting the uptake and binding of cellular calcium, decreasing the release of acetylcholine, and altering the sensitivity of the neuromuscular junctions to acetylcholine. These effects alter the neuromuscular junction in skeletal muscle, producing prolonged muscle relaxation in the parturient who receives depolarizing or nondepolarizing neuromuscular blockade.

## SUGGESTED READINGS

American College of Obstetricians and Gynecologists. (2016). Practice Bulletin No. 171: Management of preterm labor. *Obstetrics and Gynecology,* *128*(4), e155–e164.

Bolden. J. R., & Grobman, W. A. (2020). Preterm labor and delivery. In D. H. Chestnut, C. A. Wong, L. C. Tsen, W. D. Ngan Kee, Y. Beilin, J. M. Mhyre, & B. T. Bateman (Eds.). *Chestnut's obstetric anesthesia: Principles and practice* (6th ed., pp. 798–821). Philadelphia: Mosby Elsevier.

Cobo, T., Kacerovsky, M., & Jacobsson, B. (2020). Risk factors for spontaneous preterm delivery. *International Journal of Gynaecology and Obstetrics, 150*(1), 17–23.

# 170

# Hypertensive Disorders of Pregnancy

HOLLY B. ENDE, MD, MS | K.A. KELLY MCQUEEN, MD, MPH, FASA

## Definitions

A spectrum of hypertensive disorders, including gestational hypertension, preeclampsia, chronic hypertension, and chronic hypertension with superimposed preeclampsia, affects 2%–8% of pregnant women (Box 170.1). Collectively, these disorders significantly contribute to maternal and fetal morbidity and mortality. Preeclampsia, a syndrome occurring after the 20th week of pregnancy, is diagnosed by new-onset hypertension in addition to proteinuria or systemic findings. Preeclampsia is characterized as severe if end organ damage occurs and can progress to eclampsia if central nervous system involvement results in new-onset seizures. HELLP (hemolysis, elevated liver enzymes, and low platelet count) syndrome is a severe variant of preeclampsia. Disorders of hypertension related to pregnancy usually abate within 48 hours after delivery of the placenta; however, they can also newly present in the postpartum period.

## Etiology and Pathophysiology

Preeclampsia, with or without severe features, is a multisystem disorder defined by maternal cardiovascular, respiratory, central nervous system, renal, and placental dysfunction (Box 170.2).

### BOX 170.1 CLASSIFICATION OF HYPERTENSIVE DISORDERS OF PREGNANCY

| | |
|---|---|
| Chronic hypertension | Hypertension that predates pregnancy or is diagnosed before 20 weeks' gestation |
| Chronic hypertension with superimposed preeclampsia | Chronic hypertension with development of preeclampsia (see below) after 20 weeks' gestation |
| Gestational hypertension | Hypertension after 20 weeks' gestation in the absence of proteinuria or systemic findings |
| Preeclampsia (with or without severe features) | Hypertension after 20 weeks' gestation in addition to proteinuria or systemic findings |

Although associated with some well-defined risk factors (Box 170.3), the etiology of preeclampsia is not completely understood. The pathogenic mechanism for preeclampsia appears to be a combination of immunologic (fetal and maternal), genetic, and endothelial factors and involves abnormalities of the clotting cascade. The final common pathway most likely involves the vascular endothelium—affected by several cytokines and hormones, with a decrease in the production of nitric oxide and vasodilating

| | |
|---|---|
| Blood pressure | • Greater than or equal to 140 mm Hg systolic or greater than or equal to 90 mm Hg diastolic on two occasions at least 4 hours apart after 20 weeks of gestation in a woman with a previously normal blood pressure<br>• Greater than or equal to 160 mm Hg systolic or greater than or equal to 110 mm Hg diastolic; hypertension can be confirmed within a short interval (minutes) to facilitate timely antihypertensive therapy |
| and<br>Proteinuria | • Greater than or equal to 300 mg per 24-hour urine collection (or this amount extrapolated from a timed collection)<br>or<br>• Protein/creatinine ratio greater than or equal to 0.3*<br>• Dipstick reading of 1+ (used only if other quantitative methods not available) |

Or in the absence of proteinuria, new-onset hypertension with the new onset of any of the following:

| | |
|---|---|
| Thrombocytopenia | Platelet count less than 100,000/mcL |
| Renal insufficiency | Serum creatinine concentrations greater than 1.1 mg/dL or a doubling of the serum creatinine concentration in the absence of other renal disease |
| Impaired liver function | Elevated blood concentrations of liver transaminases to twice normal concentration |
| Pulmonary edema | |
| Cerebral or visual symptoms | |

*Each measured as mg/dL.
American College of Obstetricians and Gynecologists. Hypertension in pregnancy: executive summary, *Obstet Gynecol.* 2013;122(5): 1122–1131.

**PARTNER-RELATED RISK FACTORS**

Partner who previously fathered a preeclamptic pregnancy with another woman
Mother has limited preconceptional exposure to paternal sperm
Mother's first pregnancy with this partner

**MATERNAL HISTORY AND DEMOGRAPHIC RISK FACTORS**

Nulliparity
Family history of preeclampsia
History of placental abruption, fetal growth restriction, or fetal death
History of preeclampsia in previous pregnancy
Maternal age >35 years
Non-Hispanic Black

**MATERNAL COMORBIDITY RISK FACTORS**

Behavioral
Chronic hypertension
Diabetes mellitus
Obesity
Smoking
Thrombovascular disease

**PREGNANCY-ASSOCIATED RISK FACTORS**

Hydatidiform mole
Multiple gestation

eicosanoids. The result is a decrease in uterine blood flow and vasoconstriction of the spiral arteries of the myometrium. In addition to the vasoconstriction, damage caused by endothelial cell dysfunction contributes to platelet activation and a further imbalance of two eicosanoids: prostacyclin and thromboxane.

## Treatment

The definitive treatment for preeclampsia is delivery of the fetus and placenta. However, when the fetus is preterm, symptomatic treatment can be used as part of expectant management with close obstetric monitoring. Treatment usually includes administration of antihypertensive agents (e.g., β-adrenergic receptor blocking agents, $\alpha_1$-adrenergic receptor blocking agents, centrally acting $\alpha_2$-adrenergic agonists, methyldopa) or vasodilators (e.g., hydralazine, nitroglycerin). Use of sodium nitroprusside for this indication is generally discouraged because the fetus is susceptible to cyanide toxicity resulting from continuous infusion; however, it may be used for short periods if hypertension cannot otherwise be controlled. Once the patient is hospitalized, magnesium sulfate ($MgSO_4$) can be used to lower the seizure threshold in those with severe features and may also lower blood pressure. Table 170.1 summarizes the effects of increasing plasma $MgSO_4$ levels.

## Anesthetic Management

Once the fetus has reached term or if preeclampsia with severe features cannot be successfully managed with symptomatic treatment, delivery is usually planned, and if eclampsia or HELLP (hemolysis, elevated liver enzymes, and low platelet count) syndrome develops, delivery may be urgent. The goals of the anesthesia provider include management of hypertension, intravascular volume replacement, and control of central nervous system irritability while providing analgesia for labor or anesthesia for cesarean delivery.

Vaginal delivery may be an option, depending on the severity of the hypertension and whether the fetus is distressed. If no contraindications to epidural placement are present, lumbar epidural analgesia provides excellent pain relief, decreases levels of circulating catecholamines, and may reduce blood pressure during labor. For the patient with preeclampsia, early placement of an epidural is indicated because of the increased likelihood that the patient will need to undergo a cesarean delivery, potentially emergently.

**TABLE 170.1  Effects of Increasing Plasma Magnesium Levels**

| Observed Condition | Magnesium Level (mEq/L) |
|---|---|
| Normal plasma level | 1.5–2 |
| Therapeutic range | 4–6 |
| Electrocardiographic changes (prolonged PQ interval, widened QRS complex) | 5–10 |
| Loss of deep tendon reflexes | 10 |
| Sinoatrial and atrioventricular block | 15 |
| Respiratory arrest | 15 |
| Cardiac arrest | 25 |

Before catheter placement, it must be ascertained that the parturient does not have thrombocytopenia (typically $<70,000/mm^3$ is used as a cutoff) or another coagulopathy. Volume preloading should be carefully titrated if the patient has severe preeclampsia because, although these patients are uniformly volume contracted, they are also predisposed to developing additional capillary leakage, which can cause or exacerbate pulmonary edema. Anesthetic agents should be slowly and carefully infused in these patients to avoid a precipitous drop in maternal blood pressure and subsequent decelerations of the fetal heart rate.

Cesarean delivery may be indicated by maternal history, deterioration of the mother's condition, or fetal intolerance to labor, as indicated by a nonreassuring fetal heart tracing. If an epidural catheter is in place, it may be used to provide surgical anesthesia for urgent or emergent cesarean delivery. Spinal anesthesia has also been shown to be a safe technique for cesarean delivery for severely preeclamptic patients. The more precipitous drop in systemic vascular resistance that occurs with spinal anesthesia mandates careful administration of loading fluids, appropriate monitoring of blood pressure, and careful titration of ephedrine or phenylephrine, as parturients with preeclampsia may be hypersensitive to the effects of catecholamines.

General anesthesia is less desirable for anesthetic management of preeclamptic patients because of associated risks of glottic edema that may compromise airway management and acute blood pressure elevations during laryngoscopy. Nonetheless, general anesthesia may occasionally be required when coagulation abnormalities prevent neuraxial use or when terminal fetal bradycardia necessitates emergent delivery in the presence of a reassuring airway. The brief but severe elevations in systemic and pulmonary pressures seen during laryngoscopy and tracheal intubation in preeclamptic parturients can lead to a significant risk of cerebral hemorrhage and pulmonary edema. A rapid-sequence induction technique and intubation are used, with propofol 1 to 2 mg/kg plus succinylcholine 1 to 1.5 mg/kg. Pretreatment with intravenous hydralazine, lidocaine, sodium nitroprusside, nitroglycerin, or esmolol has been used with success to attenuate the hypertensive response to laryngoscopy.

Because of the possibility of glottic edema, the use of a smaller-sized endotracheal tube is recommended. Anesthesia is then maintained with either intravenous or inhalational agents. If uterine atony occurs after delivery, ergot preparations including methylergonovine are considered relatively contraindicated because of potential hypertensive side effects. Coagulopathies are managed with transfusions of platelets, fresh frozen plasma, and cryoprecipitate, as needed. After the operation is completed, the patient may be extubated once she is fully awake.

The amount of intravenously administered fluid should be guided by urine output ($>1$ mL/kg/h) and central venous pressure (4–6 cm $H_2O$) if such monitoring is indicated. Indications for radial artery catheters include poorly controlled blood pressure, need for rapid-acting vasodilator infusions, or frequent arterial blood gas collection in patients with respiratory compromise secondary to pulmonary edema. Loop diuretics are recommended to treat pulmonary edema, and mannitol may be given to treat manifestations of cerebral edema. If $MgSO_4$ has been administered because of the presence of severe features, potential side effects must be considered, including potentiation of neuromuscular blockade and opioid sedative effects. If $MgSO_4$ levels become significantly supratherapeutic, respiratory depression and cardiac arrest can occur. Calcium chloride is first-line treatment to counteract the adverse effects of $MgSO_4$.

Careful postpartum monitoring should occur for parturients with preeclampsia. The risk of developing pulmonary edema is highest in the postpartum period. For the patient with HELLP syndrome, a platelet count should be obtained before removal of the epidural catheter, and the catheter should not be removed until the platelet count is greater than approximately $70,000/mm^3$. Return of normal neuromuscular function should be carefully monitored, and symptoms of an epidural hematoma should be immediately evaluated with imaging studies and a neurosurgical consultation.

## SUGGESTED READINGS

ACOG Committee Opinion No. 623: Emergent therapy for acute-onset, severe hypertension during pregnancy and the postpartum period. (2015). *Obstetrics and Gynecology, 125*, 521–525.

ACOG Practice Bulletin No. 222: Gestational hypertension and preeclampsia. (2020). *Obstetrics and Gynecology, 135*(6), 1492–1495.

American Society of Anesthesiologist. Guidelines for regional anesthesia in obstetrics. Approved by the ASA HOD on Oct. 12, 1988, and last amended on Oct. 17, 2018. Retrieved from https://www.asahq.org/standards-and-guidelines/guidelines-for-neuraxial-anesthesia-in-obstetrics.

Dyer, R. A., Swanevelder, J. L., & Bateman, B. T. (2020). Hypertensive disorders. In D. H. Chestnut, C. A. Wong, L. C. Tsen, W. D. Ngan Kee, Y. Beilin, J. M. Mhyre, & B. T. Bateman (Eds.). *Chestnut's obstetric anesthesia: Principles and practice* (6th ed., pp. 840–878). Philadelphia: Mosby Elsevier.

Ives, C. W., Sinkey, R., Rajapreyar, I., Tita, A. T., & Oparil, S. (2020). Preeclampsia-pathophysiology and clinical presentations: JACC state-of-the-art review. *Journal of the American College of Cardiology, 76*(14), 1690–1702.

Practice Guidelines for Obstetric Anesthesia. (2016). An updated report by the American Society of Anesthesiologists Task Force on Obstetric Anesthesia. *Anesthesiology, 124*(2), 270–300.

# 171

# Anesthesia for Cesarean Delivery

HOLLY B. ENDE, MD, MS  |  K.A. KELLY MCQUEEN, MD, MPH, FASA

## Preoperative Evaluation and Preparation

Performing a maternal evaluation, including a focused history and physical examination, and obtaining informed consent are essential steps before administration of anesthesia for CD. In addition, the anesthesia provider should also ascertain information regarding fetal gestation and pregnancy-related complications. Laboratory studies are obtained as maternal comorbid conditions and surgical variables dictate, and a type and screen should be considered in women with risk factors for hemorrhage. Aspiration prophylaxis should be administered preoperatively, and adequate venous access should be obtained before proceeding with surgery (Box 171.1). The prophylactic use of antibiotics has been shown to decrease the incidence of postsurgical infections after CD, and therefore antibiotics should be administered before abdominal incision.

## Regional Anesthesia

Neuraxial anesthesia is the preferred anesthetic modality for CD. Compared with general anesthesia, neuraxial techniques avoid potentially difficult airway management and prevent the possibility of gastric aspiration and fetal depression. Multiple neuraxial techniques exist, including spinal, epidural, and combined spinal-epidural (Table 171.1). When intrapartum CD is required, indwelling labor epidural catheters can be used to convert to surgical anesthesia. For intrapartum CD without a previously placed epidural catheter or for CD without prior labor, spinal anesthesia is commonly preferred because of rapid onset, as well as reliable and dense sensory block. Combined spinal-epidural techniques can be considered when the duration of the surgical procedure is anticipated to outlast the duration of a single-shot spinal. Local anesthetics (Table 171.2), with or without the addition of opioids or other adjuvants (Table 171.3), may be used for either subarachnoid or epidural injection. Hypotension is a common and anticipated side effect of neuraxial anesthesia. Maternal hypotensive episodes are ideally treated with intravenous hydration, left uterine displacement to prevent aortocaval compression, and vasopressors.

---

### BOX 171.1  PREPARING THE PARTURIENT FOR CESAREAN DELIVERY

Perform a focused maternal history and physician exam
Obtain informed consent
Send a blood sample for type and screen or crossmatch, as indicated
For elective procedures, ensure appropriate fasting status
Obtain large-bore (18-gauge or 16-gauge) intravenous access
Administer aspiration prophylaxis (nonparticulate antacid, H2-receptor blocking agent, and/or metoclopramide as indicated)
Administer prophylactic antibiotics
Ensure availability of uterotonics

---

| TABLE 171.1 | Advantages and Disadvantages of Neuraxial Techniques for Cesarean Delivery | |
|---|---|---|
| **Technique** | **Advantages** | **Disadvantages** |
| Spinal | • Rapid onset<br>• Dense sensory block<br>• Low medication doses<br>• Technically simple | • No ability to extend duration of block |
| Epidural | • Conversion of labor epidural avoids additional procedure<br>• Ability to titrate anesthetic level<br>• No dural puncture | • Slower onset<br>• Larger medication doses required (greater risk of maternal toxicity and fetal exposure) |
| Combined spinal-epidural | • Rapid onset<br>• Dense sensory blockade<br>• Low medication doses<br>• Ability to titrate anesthetic level | • Delayed verification of functioning epidural catheter |

Adapted from Tsen LC, Bateman BT. Anesthesia for cesarean delivery. In Chestnut DH, Wong CA, Tsen LC, et al., eds. *Chestnut's Obstetric Anesthesia: Principles and Practice*. 6th ed. Mosby Elsevier; 2020: 568–626.

Prophylactic phenylephrine infusions have been shown to improve maternal hemodynamics compared with intermittent boluses.

## Emergent or Urgent Cesarean Delivery

The need for an emergency CD is a constant threat during labor, and an operating room should be immediately available with all necessary equipment for provision of anesthesia. Although general anesthesia is usually the most expedient option for use in a true emergency without a preexisting epidural catheter, spinal anesthesia may be a viable option provided that (1) the fetal heart rate returns to normal after obstetric management of nonreassuring fetal status (e.g., optimize maternal position, provide supplemental $O_2$, improve maternal circulation, discontinue oxytocin, administer a tocolytic agent for uterine hypertonus) and (2) an experienced anesthesia provider can place a subarachnoid block in a timely fashion, with ongoing monitoring of the fetal heart rate. Communication between the anesthesia and obstetric teams is essential in these scenarios.

If general anesthesia is required, the abdomen should first be prepped and draped, and subsequent rapid-sequence induction should proceed with cricoid pressure, intravenously administered propofol and succinylcholine, and placement of endotracheal tube by the most experienced provider. Video laryngoscopy should be considered for the first intubation attempt. The surgical team is then notified when they can safely proceed as soon as proper endotracheal tube placement is

| TABLE 171.2 | Neuraxial Local Anesthetics Used for Cesarean Delivery | | | |
|---|---|---|---|---|
| **Local Anesthetic** | **Intrathecal Dose** | **Epidural Dose** | **Comments** | |
| Bupivacaine | 10–15 mg | 75–150 mg | 0.75% hyperbaric bupivacaine is the most commonly used spinal anesthetic for cesarean delivery in the United States | |
| Ropivacaine | 15–25 mg | 75–150 mg | Improved safety profile compared with bupivacaine after inadvertent intravascular injection | |
| Lidocaine | 60–100 mg | 300–500 mg | Intrathecal administration can lead to transient neurologic symptoms | |
| Chloroprocaine | 45–60 mg | 450–750 mg | Commonly used to convert epidural analgesia to cesarean anesthesia in emergencies (rapid onset); rarely used intrathecally for cesarean delivery because of short duration; may reduce efficacy of neuraxial opioids | |

| TABLE 171.3 | Neuraxial Opioids and Adjuvant Medications Used for Cesarean Delivery | |
|---|---|---|
| **Medication** | **Intrathecal Dose** | **Epidural Dose** |
| Fentanyl | 10–25 mcg | 50–100 mcg |
| Morphine | 100–200 mcg | 2–5 mg |
| Hydromorphone | 50–150 mcg | 0.5–1 mg |
| Sufentanil | 2.5–5 mcg | 10–30 mcg |
| Clonidine | 15–530 mcg | 50–100 mcg |
| Epinephrine | 100–200 mcg | 5–10 mg |

### BOX 171.2 · MEASURES TO IMPROVE UTERINE TONE AFTER DELIVERY

Minimize volatile anesthetic concentration by supplementing with additional anesthetics
- Intravenous midazolam
- Intravenous opioid
- Intravenous propofol infusion
- Inhaled nitrous oxide

Immediately initiate oxytocin (Pitocin) infusion after delivery

Consider additional uterotonics (methylergonovine, 15-methylprostaglandin F2α, misoprostol) as indicated

confirmed. Maintenance with low-concentration volatile anesthetic (e.g., isoflurane or sevoflurane) and 50% $O_2/N_2O$ mixture can be safely used; however, consideration should be given to transitioning to total intravenous anesthetic for improved uterine tone after delivery. Nondepolarizing neuromuscular blocking agents may be given as needed. Frequently, opioid administration is delayed until umbilical cord clamping, when there is no longer concern for neonatal respiratory depression; however, earlier administration can occur when clinically indicated. In addition, midazolam may be administered after cord clamping to prevent patient awareness under anesthesia, the incidence of which is increased during emergent CD. Steps should be taken to improve uterine tone (Box 171.2), including oxytocin infusion for active management of the third stage of labor. If uterine hypotonia persists, additional uterotonics (see Chapter 174, Peripartum Hemorrhage, Table 174.2) may be given. Both oxytocin and methylergonovine produce hemodynamic sequelae. If endotracheal intubation is required, the patient should be fully awake before extubation to minimize the risk of aspiration.

## SUGGESTED READINGS

American Society of Anesthesiologists Task Force on Obstetric Anesthesia. (2016). Practice guidelines for obstetric anesthesia: An updated report by the American Society of Anesthesiologists Task Force on Obstetric Anesthesia. *Anesthesiology*, 124, 270–300.

Dahl, J. B., Jeppesen, I. S., Jorgensen, H., Wetterslev, J., & Moiniche, S. (1999). Intraoperative and postoperative analgesic efficacy and adverse effects of intrathecal opioids in patients undergoing Cesarean section with spinal anesthesia: A qualitative and quantitative systematic review of randomized controlled trials. *Anesthesiology*, 91(6), 1919–1927.

Ngan Kee, W. D. (2017). The use of vasopressors during spinal anaesthesia for caesarean section. *Current Opinion in Anaesthesiology*, 30(3), 319–325.

Tsen, L. C., & Bateman, B. T. (2020). Anesthesia for cesarean delivery. In D. H. Chestnut, C. A. Wong, L. C. Tsen, W. D. Ngan Kee, Y. Beilin, J. M. Mhyre, et al., (Eds.), *Chestnut's obstetric anesthesia: Principles and practice* (6th ed., pp. 568–626). Philadelphia: Mosby Elsevier.

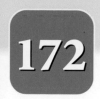

# 172 Nonobstetric Surgery in Pregnancy

EMILY E. SHARPE, MD

Approximately 2% of parturients will have surgery during their pregnancy. Pregnant patients may require surgery for many indications, including appendicitis, cholecystitis, traumatic injuries, adnexal masses, fetal surgery, malignancies, and cervical incompetence; however, major procedures such as cardiopulmonary bypass, craniotomy, and organ transplantation may also be necessary. Providing anesthesia during pregnancy requires an understanding of the complex maternal physiologic changes associated with pregnancy and attention to the maintenance of fetal well-being. The type of anesthesia should take into consideration maternal indications and the site and nature of surgery. There is no association between any specific anesthetic technique and improved fetal outcome. When appropriate, however, local or regional anesthesia is preferred. Anesthetic considerations for the pregnant patient are summarized in Box 172.1.

## Physiology of Pregnancy

Maternal physiologic changes during pregnancy affect every organ system and are discussed in Chapter 165, Maternal Physiologic Changes in Pregnancy. Those most significant to anesthetic management are described below.

### CARDIOVASCULAR

Cardiac output increases up to 50% because of an increase in both heart rate and stroke volume while systemic vascular resistance is decreased. A dilutional anemia occurs because of plasma volume expansion relative to erythrocyte volume.

---

**BOX 172.1 ANESTHETIC CONSIDERATIONS IN THE PREGNANT PATIENT**

Postpone elective surgery until after pregnancy
Consult with a maternal fetal medicine specialist or obstetrician
Aspiration prophylaxis after 18 to 20 weeks' gestational age
Left uterine displacement to relieve aortocaval compression after 20 weeks' gestational age
Consider intraoperative fetal monitoring
Maintain normal pregnant physiology
General anesthesia
- Maximal preoxygenation
- Rapid sequence induction
- Minimum alveolar concentration of inhalational agents is decreased 25% to 40% by second trimester
- Avoid hyperventilation as hypocarbia can result in uterine vasoconstriction and decrease placental blood flow
- Extubate when fully awake
Regional anesthesia
- Provide an appropriate dose: local anesthetic requirements one-third less
Provide effective postoperative analgesia
Monitor fetal heart rate and uterine tone postoperatively

---

Perfusion to the uterus is not autoregulated, and therefore a decrease in maternal blood pressure will impair uteroplacental blood flow. Aortocaval compression from the enlarging uterus can result in hypotension.

### RESPIRATORY

By midpregnancy, alveolar ventilation increases by 30%, resulting in chronic respiratory alkalosis (pH ~7.44) with a $Paco_2$ of 28 to 32 mm Hg. Functional residual capacity decreases and total body oxygen consumption increases; therefore desaturation occurs more quickly during periods of apnea. Capillary engorgement and edema of airway structures may lead to increased potential for bleeding and greater chance for difficulty with both mask ventilation and intubation.

### GASTROINTESTINAL

The stomach is displaced cephalad and lower esophageal sphincter tone is decreased, increasing risk for aspiration. Gastric emptying and pH are unlikely changed during pregnancy.

### CENTRAL NERVOUS SYSTEM

Anesthetic requirements are reduced in pregnancy. The minimum alveolar concentration for volatile anesthetics is decreased 25% to 40%. Also, pregnant women require approximately one-third less local anesthetic for neuraxial anesthesia.

## Teratogenicity of Anesthetic Agents

Current anesthetic drugs, when used in standard concentrations, have not been shown to be teratogenic in humans. An association between diazepam use in the first trimester and cleft palate was reported in the 1970s. However, later studies were unable to confirm the association between benzodiazepines and oral cleft anomalies. Nitrous oxide affects deoxyribonucleic acid synthesis and has shown to be teratogenic in rats, but it has been used in human pregnancy without any evidence of teratogenicity. Recent animal studies on intravenous and inhalational anesthetics have demonstrated neuronal cell loss and behavior and memory impairment. However, the clinical relevance of the effects of exposure to anesthesia of the developing brain in humans is less clear. A recent study in Australia found exposure to general anesthesia during pregnancy was associated with childhood externalizing behavior problems. This was only one study, and further studies are needed.

## Preoperative Preparation

The American College of Obstetricians and Gynecologists (ACOG) recommends that pregnant women should not be denied a medically indicated surgery or procedure; however, it is recommended to delay elective surgery until after delivery. When surgery cannot be postponed, ideal timing for surgery is the second trimester because organogenesis occurs in the first trimester and risk for preterm delivery is higher in the third trimester. In premature fetuses at a viable gestational age, corticosteroid administration should be considered before the procedure.

Aspiration prophylaxis may include an $H_2$-receptor antagonist, metoclopramide, and a clear nonparticulate antacid to be administered after 18 to 20 weeks' gestational age. The guidelines for preoperative fasting developed by the American Society of Anesthesiologists should be followed when possible. After 20 weeks' gestational age, patients should be positioned with left uterine displacement to avoid aortocaval compression.

## Fetal Monitoring

The well-being of the fetus should be evaluated in the perioperative period. In a previable pregnancy, ACOG recommends measurement of the fetal heart rate by Doppler before and after the surgical procedure. If the fetus is viable, then the minimum recommendations include assessment of fetal well-being with electronic fetal heart rate monitoring and simultaneous contraction monitoring before and after the procedure. The decision for type of fetal monitoring, including continuous intraoperative fetal monitoring, should be made in consultation with an obstetrician based on an individualized assessment of the gestational age, type of surgery, and facilities available.

The intraoperative management of fetal distress is summarized in Table 172.1. Fetal oxygenation is preserved by maintaining normal maternal arterial oxygen tension, partial pressure of carbon dioxide, and uteroplacental blood flow. Although short periods of hypoxia may be tolerated, severe maternal hypoxia may lead to fetal acidosis and demise. Hypercapnia can cause acidosis in the fetus, and hypocapnia from hyperventilation decreases uterine blood flow by direct vasoconstriction. Maternal hypotension should be avoided. Uterine blood flow is not auto-regulated and systemic hypotension will result in a decrease in uteroplacental blood flow and fetal ischemia.

## Anesthetic Technique

Pregnant women beyond the first trimester should be treated as though they have a full stomach. Monitoring should include blood pressure, pulse oximetry, electrocardiogram, capnography, and temperature. If general anesthesia is planned, the placement of an endotracheal tube and performance of a rapid-sequence intravenous induction are recommended. Preoxygenation before induction is important because pregnant patients have increased oxygen consumption and decreased functional residual capacity, which may lower oxygen reserve such that a short period of apnea may lead to a precipitous drop in the partial pressure of oxygen. Pregnant women are also at increased risk of a difficult intubation, so careful airway examination and planning should occur with consideration of the use of a video laryngoscope or other difficult airway adjuncts readily available.

Laparoscopy during pregnancy may be used as a surgical technique. Studies have shown fetal outcomes to be similar when laparotomy and laparoscopy are compared. If a laparoscopic approach is planned, maintain low pneumoperitoneum pressures (10–15 mm Hg) and monitor maternal end-tidal carbon dioxide to avoid fetal hypercarbia and acidosis.

Before removing the endotracheal tube, it is important the pregnant patient is fully awake with intact airway reflexes to minimize the risk of aspiration. Pain management during surgery and after should be managed using multimodal analgesia. Nonsteroidal antiinflammatory drugs are usually avoided for concern of premature closure of the fetal ductus arteriosus. Early mobilization is important to reduce the risk of venous thromboembolism, and the appropriate perioperative prophylaxis should be administered. Fetal heart rate and uterine tone monitoring should be assessed postoperatively.

| TABLE 172.1 | **Intraoperative Management of Fetal Distress** |
|---|---|
| **Evaluate** | **Treatment** |
| Maternal position | Ensure left uterine displacement. |
| Oxygenation | Increase $Fio_2$. |
| Blood pressure | Treat hypotension. Phenylephrine and ephedrine okay. |
| Maternal $Paco_2$ | Change ventilation for goal $ETCO_2$ 28–32 mm Hg. Ensure appropriate acid-base status. |
| Surgical factors | Release surgical retraction, surgical manipulation, or pneumoperitoneum |

$ETCO_2$, End-tidal carbon dioxide; $Fio_2$, fraction of inspired oxygen; $Paco_2$, partial pressure of carbon dioxide.

## SUGGESTED READINGS

American College of Obstetricians and Gynecologists Committee Opinion No. 775. Nonobstetric surgery during pregnancy. (2019). *Obstetrics and Gynecology, 133*(4), e285–e286.

Bauchat, J. R., & Van de Velde, M. (2020). Nonobstetric surgery during pregnancy. In D. H. Chestnut (Ed.), *Chestnut's obstetric anesthesia principles and practice* (6th ed., pp. 368–391). Philadelphia: Elsevier.

Heesen, M., & Klimek, M. (2016). Nonobstetric anesthesia during pregnancy. *Current Opinion in Anaesthesiology, 29*(3), 297–303.

Ing, C., Landau, R., DeStephano, D., Miles, C. H., von Ungern-Sternberg, B. S., Li, G., et al. (2021). Prenatal exposure to general anesthesia and childhood behavioral deficit. *Anesthesia and Analgesia, 133*(3), 595–605.

Reitman, E., & Flood, P. (2011). Anaesthetic considerations for non-obstetric surgery during pregnancy. *British Journal of Anaesthesia, 107*, 172–178.

# 173

## Anesthesia for Fetal Surgery

HANS P. SVIGGUM, MD

Performing surgery on a fetus while still in utero has rapidly evolved into a realistic option for patients whose fetuses are affected by several conditions. The aim of intrauterine fetal surgery is to improve neonatal outcomes in comparison with postdelivery surgery (Box 173.1). Advances in the understanding of fetal pathophysiology and disease progression, coupled with improvements in diagnostic and therapeutic technologies, have created the ability for prenatal surgical interventions to lessen disease progression, prevent organ damage, and even reduce fetal demise. Fetal intervention has shown promising results for several conditions, including obstructive uropathy, congenital diaphragmatic hernia (CDH), congenital pulmonary airway malformations, myelomeningocele, sacrococcygeal teratoma, twin-to-twin transfusion syndrome, and some congenital heart defects (e.g., aortic stenosis with evolving hypoplastic left heart syndrome).

Fetal surgery is most often performed in the middle/late second trimester or early third trimester. Performing intrauterine surgery before mid-gestation is usually not possible because of the small size of the fetus, immaturity of fetal tissue, and imprecise characterization of the lesion. Intrauterine surgery is usually not performed after the early part of the third trimester because there is less overall benefit of intervention to the fetus and an increased risk of triggering preterm labor. Ex utero intrapartum treatment (EXIT) procedures are a unique subset of fetal surgeries that are performed concurrently with cesarean delivery.

Although there are no clear standardized guidelines for the exclusion of candidates for fetal surgery, there are important considerations for fetal surgery to be a reasonable option (Box 173.2). Any coexisting disease that places the mother at greater surgical or anesthetic risk may be reason to forgo the procedure. Thus women with pregnancy-induced disease states (e.g., preeclampsia) or other significant comorbidities are usually not considered candidates for fetal interventions. Fortunately,

serious maternal complications from intrauterine fetal surgery are relatively uncommon. Anesthesiologists must participate in multidisciplinary presurgical assessment efforts to determine whether maternal risk is acceptably low for the potential fetal benefit. In fact, the American Society of Anesthesiologists Committees on Obstetric and Pediatric Anesthesiology recently collaborated with members of the North American Fetal Therapy Network on a consensus statement describing the integral role of the anesthesiologist in this multidisciplinary team.

In contrast to low maternal risk, the fetal risks of intrauterine surgery are relatively high. Preterm delivery is the most significant complication, and when it occurs, it often mitigates the benefits of the fetal procedure. Other complications include physical injury, chorioamniotic membrane separation, amniotic fluid leaks, preterm rupture of membranes, and preterm contractions.

General considerations for the maternal anesthetic management during fetal surgery are similar to those for other cases of nonobstetric surgery during pregnancy (see Chapter 172, Nonobstetric Surgery in Pregnancy). However, providing anesthesia for fetal surgery presents a unique challenge because more than one patient needs to be considered. Although the purpose of the surgery is to promote fetal health, it is imperative to protect the mother from potential harm. A thorough understanding of the anatomic and physiologic changes that occur during pregnancy, and their potential effect on anesthetic management, is necessary for anesthesiologists to provide safe maternal care.

General, neuraxial, and local anesthesia with sedation are all options depending on the type of procedure and patient characteristics. The three main categories of fetal surgery procedures have similarities and differences regarding characteristics and management (Table 173.1). Although care should be individualized, there are a few principles that apply to nearly all patients undergoing fetal surgery (aspiration prophylaxis; left lateral decubitus positioning, if possible; restrictive use of

| TABLE 173.1 Comparing Management of Different Types of Fetal Surgery | | | |
|---|---|---|---|
| | **Open Surgery** | **Minimally Invasive** | **EXIT** |
| Gestational age | Late second/early third trimester | Late second/early third trimester | Time of delivery |
| Maternal anesthesia | General, epidural for postoperative analgesia | Local or neuraxial anesthesia* ± IV sedation | General ± epidural for postoperative analgesia |
| Desired uterine tone | Complete relaxation | Minimal relaxation | Complete relaxation |
| Fetal anesthesia | Transplacental inhalation agents, direct (IM or umbilical cord) opioids and muscle relaxants | Direct (IM or umbilical cord) opioids and muscle relaxants or transplacental opioids† | Transplacental inhalation agents, direct (IM or umbilical cord) opioids and muscle relaxants |
| Preterm labor risk | Increased | Minimal | Not applicable |
| Invasive blood pressure monitoring | Yes | No | Yes |
| Amnio-infusion | Yes | No | Yes |
| Future labor allowed | No | Yes | Yes |

*Local anesthesia is used mostly for surgery *on* the placenta or membranes. Neuraxial anesthesia is used for more complex fetoscopic procedures.
†Remifentanil is most reliable.
*EXIT*, Ex utero intrapartum therapy; *IM*, intramuscular; *IV*, intravenous.
Sviggum HP, Kodali BS. Maternal anesthesia for fetal surgery. *Clin Perinatol.* 2013;40:421; used with permission.

intravenous [IV] fluids; maintenance of end-tidal carbon dioxide in normal range for pregnancy [30–34 mm Hg]; aggressive blood pressure [BP] treatment; plan for postoperative pain control; necessary teams/equipment available should delivery become imminent). Prevention of preterm labor is essential. Tocolytic agents are used before, during, and after surgery. Although well tolerated by most patients, these agents can contribute to maternal complications, including development of pulmonary edema.

Fetal surgeries can be classified into three different categories: open fetal surgery, minimally invasive fetal surgery, and EXIT procedures. The type of anesthesia used is dictated primarily by the category of fetal surgery.

## Anesthesia for Open Fetal Surgery

Open fetal surgery involves a laparotomy incision and hysterotomy, and general anesthesia is nearly always used. Important perioperative considerations for open fetal surgery are detailed in Table 173.2. Significant maternal blood loss is possible during open fetal surgery because of the high blood flow to the uterus, reduced uterine tone, and difficulty in achieving intraoperative hemostasis. Fetal blood loss is also possible, and because of the low total blood volume in the preterm fetus, the anesthesiologist should always be prepared for both maternal and fetal resuscitation.

Preoperatively, a low-thoracic or high-lumbar epidural may be placed without administration of a loading dose of local anesthetic because its main role is for postoperative analgesia. Care should be taken to limit intravenous fluid administration before surgery to prevent subsequent pulmonary edema. Tocolytic agents (e.g., rectal indomethacin) are often administered as well. Sedative medications are used judiciously before induction to allow use of higher doses of volatile agents intraoperatively for uterine relaxation if needed. After preoxygenation, a rapid sequence induction and intubation with an endotracheal tube is performed. Fetal heart rate (FHR) monitoring, umbilical blood flow assessment, and/or direct fetal echocardiography are used before, after, and sometimes during the induction period.

After intubation, additional large-bore IV access and direct arterial monitoring are obtained, and the surgical team begins using ultrasound to assess fetal lie and placental location. It is usually the task of the anesthesia team to prepare fetal medications for analgesia (e.g., fentanyl 0.01–0.02 mg/kg), immobility (e.g., vecuronium 0.2 mg/kg), and resuscitation (epinephrine 0.01 mg/kg, atropine 0.02 mg/kg, and crystalloid 10 mL/kg) in weight-based doses in individual sterile syringes.

It is imperative to prepare for intraoperative hemorrhage. Cross-matched blood should be obtained for the mother and kept in a cooler in the operating room. One unit of O-negative, cytomegalovirus-negative, irradiated, leukocyte-depleted, potassium- and glucose-reduced, maternally cross-matched blood should also be available for fetal transfusion if necessary. Intraoperative fluids are often restricted to 2 L or less to reduce risk for postoperative pulmonary edema. The use of tocolytic medications (magnesium, nitroglycerin) is associated with maternal pulmonary edema, but benefits in reducing the incidence and impact of preterm contractions outweigh the risks.

Traditionally, high doses of volatile anesthetics (2–3 minimum alveolar concentration [MAC]) have been used for open fetal surgery. Not only does this provide complete fetal anesthesia, but it also allows for profound uterine relaxation, optimizing surgical conditions. After skin incision, the volatile anesthetic agent is slowly increased while closely monitoring maternal vital signs, with the goal of reaching the desired volatile concentration before uterine incision. Sevoflurane is the most commonly used halogenated agent. A phenylephrine infusion may be used to maintain BP at baseline. Bolus administration of ephedrine and glycopyrrolate can be used as dictated by maternal heart rate to increase maternal cardiac output. Neuromuscular blocking agents are not needed with deep volatile anesthesia.

Although providing optimal operating conditions, high-dose volatile anesthesia has been shown to contribute to detrimental side effects in some instances. Specifically, high concentrations

## TABLE 173.2 Perioperative Considerations for Open Fetal Surgery

### PREOPERATIVE CONSIDERATIONS

- Complete maternal history and physical examination
- Fetal work-up to exclude other anomalies and imaging studies to determine fetal lesion, placental location, and estimated fetal weight
- Maternal counseling by multidisciplinary team and preoperative team meeting
- Lumbar epidural catheter placed and tested
- Prophylactic premedication for aspiration and tocolysis
- Blood products available for potential maternal and fetal transfusion
- Sequential compression devices on lower extremities for thrombosis prophylaxis

### INDUCTION AND INTRAOPERATIVE CONSIDERATIONS

- Left uterine displacement and standard monitors
- Preoxygenation for 3 minutes before induction
- Rapid-sequence induction and intubation
- Maintain maternal $FiO_2$ >50% and $ETCO_2$ 28–30 mm Hg
- Ultrasonography to determine fetal and placental positioning
- Urinary catheter placed; additional large-bore IV access placed ± arterial line
- Prophylactic antibiotics administered
- Fetal resuscitation drugs and fluid transferred to scrub nurse in unit doses
- After skin incision, high concentration of volatile anesthetic administered
- Blood pressure maintained (± 10% baseline with IV phenylephrine, ephedrine, and/or glycopyrrolate)
- Consider IV nitroglycerin if uterine relaxation not adequate
- IM administration of fetal opioid and neuromuscular blocking agent by surgeons
- Fluid restriction to <2 L to reduce risk for maternal pulmonary edema
- IV loading dose of magnesium sulfate once uterine closure begins
- Discontinue volatile agent once magnesium sulfate load is complete
- Administer propofol, opioids, nitrous oxide as needed
- Activate epidural catheter for postoperative analgesia
- Monitor neuromuscular blockade carefully because of magnesium sulfate administration
- Extubate trachea when patient is fully awake

### EARLY POSTOPERATIVE CONSIDERATIONS

- Continue tocolytic therapy
- Patient-controlled epidural analgesia
- Monitor uterine activity and fetal heart rate
- Ongoing fetal evaluation

$ETCO_2$, End-tidal carbon dioxide; $FiO_2$, fraction of inspired oxygen; *IM*, intramuscular; *IV*, intravenous.

From Rollins MD, Rosen MA. Anesthesia for fetal surgery and other intrauterine procedures. In: Chestnut DH, ed. *Chestnut's Obstetric Anesthesia: Principles and Practice*. Elsevier Saunders; 2014:136, used with permission.

of volatile agents can depress fetal myocardium and have been shown to lead to progressive fetal acidosis in animal models. They can also cause significant reductions in maternal cardiac output with a subsequent decrease in uterine blood flow. Although this has not been shown to have definitive clinical detriment, some practitioners have proposed moving away from high-dose volatile anesthesia techniques.

At this time, maternally administered volatile anesthetics remain the primary anesthetic agent for most open fetal surgeries. However, recently a more balanced anesthesia technique has shown promise in providing adequate surgical conditions for many intrauterine procedures as an alternative to high-dose volatile anesthesia. Reducing volatile agent concentrations to 0.5 to 1.0 MAC in combination with combined or isolated infusions of remifentanil, propofol, and/or dexmedetomidine provides acceptable maternal and fetal anesthesia and often adequate uterine relaxation. Although only approximately half of open fetal surgery cases use supplemental IV anesthesia, future practice may see higher use as this technique has been shown to reduce the dose of the volatile agent needed, resulting in less fetal cardiac dysfunction and maternal hemodynamic instability. IV anesthetics and opioids can decrease FHR variability but do not lead to significant fetal morbidity if maternal cardiac output remains normal. In cases where further uterine relaxation is needed, additional medications that can relax the uterine muscle, such as nitroglycerine, atosiban, or a volatile agent, can be

titrated to effect. Although open fetal surgery could technically be performed under primary neuraxial anesthesia, this is not routinely practiced because of difficulties with maintaining maternal comfort with positioning, optimizing uterine tone, maintaining effective spontaneous ventilation, and the potential need for blood transfusion. Further studies are needed to determine the optimal anesthetic technique for ensuring maternal and fetal cardiovascular stability, optimal uteroplacental perfusion, and adequate fetal anesthesia.

After optimizing maternal anesthesia and hemodynamics and verifying fetal position, medications are often delivered to the fetus intramuscularly before fetal incision. This can either be done under ultrasound guidance before hysterotomy or under direct vision after hysterotomy. Although the fetus may already be partially or completely anesthetized from maternal transfer of anesthetic agents, fentanyl (0.01–0.02 mg/kg) is often administered for further fetal analgesia/anesthesia, vecuronium (0.2 mg/kg) to ensure fetal immobility, and sometimes atropine (0.02 mg/kg) to prevent medication- or stimulation-induced bradycardia.

Of utmost importance during the procedure is timely and effective assessment of fetal well-being. Although there is no standard for fetal assessment, many centers use continuous assessment of the fetus during the procedure. Several different modalities can be used, including electronic FHR monitoring, pulse oximetry, echocardiography to assess ventricular contractility, Doppler assessment of umbilical cord blood flow, blood gas and acid-base tests, or any combination of these. Newer devices with little clinical experience to date may allow for measurements of fetal cerebral oxygenation, fetal electroencephalogram, and fetal BP.

After the initial uterine incision is made, a special stapling device is used to extend the incision while simultaneously sealing the membranes to the endometrium to limit blood loss. The exposed fetus and uterus are continually bathed in warmed fluids and the intrauterine temperature is monitored closely to prevent fetal hypothermia.

An infusion of magnesium sulfate is often started concomitantly with uterine closure. A bolus dose of 4 to 6 g is followed by an infusion of 1 to 2 g/h for 24 to 72 hours. As the magnesium is started, the volatile agent (if used in high doses) is titrated down. If muscle relaxant is used, close monitoring of neuromuscular relaxation is needed because magnesium potentiates neuromuscular blockade. After ensuring hemodynamic stability, epidural analgesia can be initiated, usually by a small bolus of dilute bupivacaine followed by an infusion (e.g., 0.1% bupivacaine + 5 mcg/mL of hydromorphone at 10 mL/h).

The most common complication after open fetal surgery is preterm labor. Profound analgesia and tocolysis are essential to prevent uterine activity. The epidural catheter is maintained postoperatively for 1 to 4 days. IV opioids can provide supplemental analgesia if needed, understanding that their use may decrease fetal heart variability. Uterine activity is continuously monitored along with FHR. Other postoperative concerns include infection, maternal pulmonary edema, fetal heart failure, and fetal demise. Most patients will stay in hospital for at least 4 to 5 days after surgery and remain close to the fetal surgery center for 1 to 2 weeks. Barring complications, patients can be discharged if the fetal monitoring is reassuring, amniotic fluid levels are adequate, there is no evidence of preterm labor, and the patient has support from a nearby perinatology practice. These patients are at increased risk for uterine rupture and/or emergent cesarean delivery. A cesarean delivery via classical uterine incision is required for patients undergoing fetal surgery. This is usually done at 37 weeks at the institution where the fetal surgery was performed, if possible.

## Anesthesia for Minimally Invasive Fetal Surgery

Minimally invasive fetal interventions are the most commonly performed fetal surgeries. All fetal therapy centers in the United States perform ultrasound-guided fetal interventions, and almost all perform fetoscopic interventions. The most common minimally invasive procedures performed are amniocentesis, cyst aspiration, percutaneous umbilical blood sampling, radiofrequency ablation, selective fetoscopic laser photocoagulation for twin-twin transfusion syndrome, shunt placement (e.g., bladder, thorax), and tracheal balloon placement for CDH. For most minimally invasive procedures, local anesthetic infiltration of the abdominal wall is sufficient to provide primary anesthesia for the procedure, with maternal IV sedation providing additional analgesia and anxiolysis. Maternal sedation and anxiolysis can be achieved with an opioid and/or midazolam combined with an infusion of propofol titrated to patient comfort. Local anesthesia plus sedation has been shown to reduce vasopressor use, operating room time, and intraoperative fluid administration compared with neuraxial anesthesia. In select procedures where local anesthetic infiltration plus maternal sedation will not provide enough patient comfort (e.g., large needles, multiple access points, long duration of case, minilaparotomy), neuraxial anesthesia can be used effectively. Epidural anesthesia is typically preferred over spinal anesthesia in case the procedure lasts longer than anticipated.

Many minimally invasive procedures rely on precise location and placement of the needle and/or catheter, making any fetal movement potentially catastrophic. Although placental transfer of maternal sedative drugs (e.g., opioids, benzodiazepines, propofol) can reduce fetal movement, complete fetal immobility cannot be guaranteed. For these cases without general anesthesia, direct intramuscular or umbilical vein administration of a nondepolarizing muscle relaxant (e.g., vecuronium) produces reliable fetal relaxation within a few minutes. A remifentanil infusion (starting at 0.1 mcg/kg/min with titration up to 0.2 mcg/kg/min as tolerated) or small boluses of fentanyl can be used to improve operating conditions and provide additional fetal analgesia/anesthesia when desired. Just as in open fetal surgery, the surgical and anesthetic teams should be prepared to treat intraoperative fetal compromise, including a plan for emergent cesarean delivery if indicated.

## Anesthesia for Ex Utero Intrapartum Treatment Procedures

EXIT procedures are performed far less commonly than open fetal procedures or minimally invasive fetal procedures. However, the EXIT procedure has proven useful for several disorders, primarily for neonates with lesions that compress their airway and make tracheal intubation difficult. Common cases performed as EXIT procedures include intubation/tracheostomy with subsequent removal of a neck mass (e.g., teratoma), thoracotomy for pulmonary airway malformations, and assistance in the transition to extracorporeal membrane oxygenation. Because the fetus maintains gas exchange through the placenta, profound and sustained uterine relaxation is needed to prevent premature placental separation from the uterine wall. Thus nearly all EXIT procedures are performed under general anesthesia. Use of an arterial catheter is recommended, as the mother may experience abrupt hemodynamic changes. Fetal pulse oximetry and fetal echocardiography are often used in conjunction for fetal monitoring during EXIT surgery and may be superior to FHR monitoring because they may be an earlier sign of fetal compromise. Fetal analgesia and anesthesia can be achieved directly or indirectly. Inhalational and IV anesthetics are transferred to the fetus via the placenta. In addition, direct IV or intramuscular medication administration to the fetus can also be performed using similar doses as for open fetal surgery.

In summary, fetal surgery is growing in both scope and numbers of procedures. The anesthetic management for fetal surgery begins with the fundamentals for safely caring for a pregnant patient. However, because fetal surgery involves two patients, the anesthesiologist must be attentive to the needs and responses to surgery of both the mother and fetus. Depending on the procedure, maternal anesthesia can involve IV sedation, local anesthesia infiltration, neuraxial anesthesia, general anesthesia, or a combination of these techniques. The surgical and anesthetic teams should always be prepared to treat intraoperative fetal compromise, and if the fetus is deemed viable in preoperative care conferences, preparations should be in place for immediate cesarean delivery if in utero resuscitation proves futile. Preoperative multidisciplinary planning, including preparation for maternal and fetal emergencies, is important for safe and effective care for both mother and fetus.

## SUGGESTED READINGS

Adzick, N. S., Thom, E. A., Spong, C. Y., Brock, J. W., Burrows, P. K., Johnson, M. P., et al. (2011). A randomized trial of prenatal versus postnatal repair of myelomeningocele. *New England Journal of Medicine, 364*(11), 993–1004.

Arens, C., Koch, C., Veit, M., Greenberg, R. S., Lichtenstern, C., Weigand, M. A., et al. (2017). Anesthetic management for percutaneous minimally invasive fetoscopic surgery of spina bifida aperta: A retrospective, descriptive report of clinical experience. *Anesthesia and Analgesia, 125*(1), 219–222.

Chatterjee, D., Arendt, K. W., Moldenhauer, J. S., Olutoye, O. A., Parikh, J. M., Tran, K. M., et al. (2021). Anesthesia for maternal-fetal interventions: A consensus statement from the American Society of Anesthesiologists Committees on Obstetric and Pediatric Anesthesiology and the North American Fetal Therapy Network. *Anesthesia and Analgesia, 132*(4), 1164–1173.

Ferschl, M., Ball, R., Lee, H., & Rollins, M. D. (2013). Anesthesia for in utero repair of myelomeningocele. *Anesthesiology, 118*(5), 1211–1223.

Hoagland, M. A., & Chatterjee, D. (2017). Anesthesia for fetal surgery. *Paediatric Anaesthesia, 27*(4), 346–357.

Ngamprasertwong, P., Michelfelder, E. C., Arbabi, S., Choi, Y. S., Statile, C., Ding, L., et al. (2013). Anesthetic techniques for fetal surgery: Effects of maternal anesthesia on intraoperative fetal outcomes in a sheep model. *Anesthesiology, 118*(4), 796–808.

Sviggum, H. P., & Kodali, B. S. (2013). Maternal anesthesia for fetal surgery. *Clinics in Perinatology, 40*(3), 413–427.

Tran, K. M., Smiley, R., & Schwartz, A. J. (2013). Anesthesia for fetal surgery: Miles to go before we sleep. *Anesthesiology, 118*(4), 772–774.

Wood, C. L., Zuk, J., Rollins, M. D., Silveira, L. J., Feiner, J. R., Zaretsky, M., & Chatterjee, D. (2021). Anesthesia for maternal-fetal interventions: A survey of fetal therapy centers in the North American Fetal Therapy Network. *Fetal Diagnosis and Therapy, 48*(5), 361–371.

# 174

# Peripartum Hemorrhage

HOLLY B. ENDE, MD, MS | K.A. KELLY MCQUEEN, MD, MPH, FASA

## Antepartum Hemorrhage

### PLACENTA PREVIA

#### Background

Placenta previa is defined as implantation of the placenta overlying the internal cervical os and is a common cause of antepartum hemorrhage (Box 174.1). It occurs in 1 in 200 pregnancies, and risk factors include prior previa, prior cesarean delivery (CD) or uterine surgery, increasing maternal age, increasing parity, smoking, and multiple gestation. The chance of recurrence in a subsequent pregnancy is approximately 5%.

#### Anesthetic Management

Patients with placenta previa most commonly present in the antepartum period with vaginal bleeding or for scheduled CD (vaginal delivery is contraindicated in the setting of placenta previa) between 36 and 37 weeks' gestation. All patients presenting with vaginal bleeding in the setting of known placenta previa should be evaluated by an anesthesia provider as soon as possible after admission. A complete evaluation should include assessment of volume status and detailed history of prior CD or uterine surgery, which may prompt further investigation if there is concern for placenta accreta spectrum disorder (Table 174.1). Treatment for acute bleeding should include large-bore peripheral intravenous (IV) access, fluid resuscitation, and pretransfusion testing in anticipation of possible transfusion. Once stabilized and if delivery is not immediately indicated, many women with placenta previa remain hospitalized for expectant management after second or third bleeding episodes. During this time, adequate IV access should be maintained, and type-and-screen should remain up to date in the event of recurrent bleeding or emergency delivery. Neuraxial anesthesia is typically preferred for eventual CD, except for patients with hypovolemic shock.

### PLACENTAL ABRUPTION

#### Background

Placental abruption results from separation of a normally implanted placenta from the myometrium after 20 weeks' gestation and before birth. It occurs in 1 in 75 to 1 in 226 deliveries. Risk factors include hypertensive disorders, high

---

> **BOX 174.1 ETIOLOGIES OF ANTEPARTUM AND POSTPARTUM HEMORRHAGE**
>
> **ANTEPARTUM HEMORRHAGE**
> Placenta previa
> Placental abruption
> Uterine rupture
>
> **POSTPARTUM HEMORRHAGE**
> Uterine atony
> Retained placenta
> Genital tract trauma
> Placenta accreta spectrum disorders

| TABLE 174.1 | Association Between Placenta Accreta and Number of Prior Cesarean Births in Patients With Known Placenta Previa | |
| --- | --- | --- |
| **Cesarean Delivery** | **Percent of Patients With Placenta Accreta** | |
| First | 3% | |
| Second | 11% | |
| Third | 40% | |
| Fourth | 61% | |
| Fifth | 67% | |
| Sixth or more | 67% | |

Adapted from Silver RM, Landon MB, Rouse DJ, et al. Maternal morbidity associated with multiple repeat cesarean deliveries. *Obstet Gynecol.* 2006;107(6):1226–1232.

parity, uterine abnormalities, trauma, intravenous drug use, and history of previous abruption. Bleeding may be apparent (external) or concealed (internal) and varies in severity from mild (<100 mL) to severe (>500 mL).

### Anesthetic Management

The type and timing of delivery will depend on the severity of hemorrhage. With limited blood loss, vaginal delivery is often possible, and neuraxial analgesia is not contraindicated. If the mother or fetus is in distress, then emergent CD is required. Neuraxial anesthesia is preferred; however, general anesthesia may be required if emergency delivery is warranted in the absence of a preexisting epidural catheter. In the setting of intrauterine fetal demise secondary to placental abruption, maternal coagulation must be evaluated before regional anesthesia is administered because disseminated intravascular coagulation may occur within 8 hours of fetal death.

### UTERINE RUPTURE

#### Background

Uterine rupture is a rare but serious cause of hemorrhage occurring in 0.1% to 0.3% of pregnancies. Risk factors include previous uterine surgery, history of prior uterine rupture, abnormal fetal presentation, operative vaginal delivery, and use of uterotonic agents. Maternal mortality rate approaches 5%, and fetal mortality rate is as high as 50%.

#### Anesthetic Management

The most common clinical scenario for uterine rupture includes active uterine contractions in the setting of a uterine scar (e.g., during a trial of labor after cesarean delivery). Vaginal bleeding from uterine rupture is typically associated with extreme abdominal pain (out of proportion to prior pain levels and not associated with uterine contractions), nonreassuring fetal heart rate tracing, loss of fetal station, and maternal hypotension. Emergency cesarean delivery is indicated. If a preexisting epidural catheter is in place for neuraxial analgesia, rapid administration of chloroprocaine or lidocaine can be used to convert to epidural anesthesia for CD. Otherwise, general anesthesia with rapid-sequence induction should be used in the absence of concern for difficult airway. Significant intraoperative bleeding may occur, so early consideration should be given

to obtaining additional IV access (peripheral or central) and blood products.

## Postpartum Hemorrhage

Postpartum hemorrhage (PPH) is defined as a blood loss of ≥1000 mL accompanied by signs or symptoms of hypovolemia after vaginal delivery or CD. Regardless of etiology, standard treatment for PPH includes obtaining additional large-bore IV access, fluid resuscitation with crystalloid or colloid solutions, vasopressor administration for symptomatic treatment of hypotension, laboratory investigations (hemoglobin, hematocrit, coagulation studies, and fibrinogen), and preparation of blood products for possible transfusion. Transfusion ratios should mimic other scenarios requiring massive transfusion; however, early consideration should be given to cryoprecipitate administration given the rapid drop in fibrinogen characteristic of PPH. Blood warmers should be used to prevent hypothermia. The use of invasive hemodynamic monitoring (arterial catheterization, central venous pressure monitoring) should be considered on a case-by-case basis, as should the use of a rapid-infusion device. While implementing these general resuscitative measures, providers should identify the likely etiology of PPH so that etiology-specific therapies can be added (see below).

### UTERINE ATONY

Uterine atony is the most common cause of postpartum hemorrhage and accounts for up to 70% of cases. There are numerous recognized risk factors (Box 174.2). Etiology-specific treatments include uterine massage and uterotonic medications (Table 174.2). These agents stimulate the smooth muscle of the uterus, thereby augmenting uterine contraction and

---

**BOX 174.2 RISK FACTORS FOR UTERINE ATONY**

**HISTORY AND DEMOGRAPHIC RISK FACTORS**
Advanced maternal age
Nulliparity
Prior postpartum hemorrhage

**MATERNAL COMORBIDITIES**
Hypertension
Diabetes

**PREGNANCY-RELATED RISK FACTORS**
Multiple gestation
Placenta previa
Placental abruption

**LABOR-RELATED RISK FACTORS**
Chorioamnionitis
Uterine rupture
Predelivery oxytocin exposure
Induction of labor
Prolonged labor

**DELIVERY-RELATED RISK FACTORS**
Genital tract trauma
Instrumented vaginal delivery
Cesarean delivery

Adapted with permission from Ende HB, Lozada MJ, Chestnut DH, et al. Risk factors for atonic postpartum hemorrhage: a systematic review and meta-analysis. *Obstet Gynecol.* 2021;137(2):305–323.

| TABLE 174.2 | Uterotonic Medications for Treatment of Uterine Atony | |
|---|---|---|
| **Medication** | **Dose** | **Predominant Side Effects** |
| Oxytocin | 0.3–0.9 IU/min IV infusion | Hypotension, tachycardia, hyponatremia |
| Methylergonovine maleate* | 0.2 mg IM | Hypertension, nausea, vomiting |
| 15-Methylprostaglandin $F_{2\alpha}$† | 0.25 mg IM | Bronchospasm, nausea, vomiting, diarrhea, fever |
| Misoprostol | 600–1000 µg PR, sublingual, or buccal | Shivering, nausea, vomiting, diarrhea, fever |

*Relatively contraindicated in patients with hypertension or preeclampsia.
†Relatively contraindicated in patients with reactive airway disease
*IM,* Intramuscular; *IU,* international units; *IV,* intravenous; *PR,* per rectum.

improving uterine tone. Persistent uterine atony accompanied by severe PPH may necessitate massive blood transfusions and, in extreme cases, hysterectomy.

## RETAINED PLACENTA

The placenta and membranes are retained in about 1% of vaginal deliveries. Treatment usually includes manual exploration of the uterus, which may require transfer to the operating room. If pharmacologically induced uterine relaxation is required to facilitate manual evacuation or dilation and curettage, intravenous nitroglycerin or volatile anesthetic (if general anesthesia is used) may be used. Depending on the procedure required to remove remaining tissues, regional anesthesia, sedation with ketamine or opioids, or induction of general anesthesia may be necessary.

## GENITAL TRACT TRAUMA

Genital tract trauma includes lacerations of the vagina, perineum, cervix, or body of the uterus and can occur spontaneously or iatrogenically (e.g., episiotomy) during delivery. Most lacerations are repaired primarily in the labor room immediately after delivery; however, occasionally, more extensive lesions will require transfer to the operating room for repair and control of ongoing bleeding.

## PLACENTA ACCRETA SPECTRUM

Placenta accreta spectrum (PAS) is a term used to describe a range of invasive placentation disorders including placenta accreta, placenta increta, and placenta percreta. The incidence of PAS has been steadily increasing, potentially because of the increasing rates of CD. Placenta accreta, the most common form, is present when the placenta is adherent to the myometrium without invasion into the uterine muscle. Placenta increta involves myometrial adherence with invasion into the muscle, and placenta percreta involves invasion into the uterine serosa and beyond—often involving other pelvic structures. Multidisciplinary approach should be considered in preparation for delivery of a patient with known placenta accreta (Box 174.3).

---

**BOX 174.3  CESAREAN DELIVERY CONSIDERATIONS FOR ANTENATALLY DIAGNOSED PLACENTA ACCRETA SPECTRUM**

Prenatal counseling regarding risk of:
- Hemorrhage
- Blood transfusions
- Need for hysterectomy
- Intensive care admission

Consider transfer to Center of Excellence for placenta accreta
Scheduled daytime delivery with availability of all necessary subspecialties
- Obstetrics/maternal fetal medicine
- Additional surgical specialties: urogynecology, urology, gynecologic oncology, general surgery, vascular surgery
- Anesthesiology
- Neonatology
- Interventional radiology
- Blood bank specialists
- Perfusionists
- Nursing staff

Preoperative preparation
- History
- Physical exam

- Informed consent
- Intravascular access (central or multiple large-bore peripheral)
- Confirmed availability of adequate red blood cells, fresh frozen plasma, cryoprecipitate, and platelets
- Consider preoperative balloon catheterization or arterial embolization of uterine vessels to decrease intraoperative blood loss

Intraoperative management
- Consider general anesthesia given risk for massive blood loss
- Consider cell saver intraoperatively
- Uterine conservation versus hysterectomy on case-by-case basis

Postoperative care
- Intensive care unit bed should be available
- Continued intubation and ventilatory support may be necessary
- Vasopressor support and invasive hemodynamic monitoring as clinically indicated
- Analgesic management—consider regional blockade if no long-acting neuraxial opioid administered

---

## SUGGESTED READINGS

Banayan, J. M., Hofer, J. E., & Scavone, B. M. (2020). Antepartum and postpartum hemorrhage. In D. H. Chestnut, C. A. Wong, L. C. Tsen, W. D. Ngan Kee, Y. Beilin, J. M. Mhyre, et al., (Eds.), *Chestnut's obstetric anesthesia: principles and practice* (6th ed., pp. 901–936). Philadelphia: Mosby Elsevier.

Committee on Practice Bulletins-Obstetrics. (2017). Practice Bulletin No. 183: Postpartum Hemorrhage. *Obstetrics and Gynecology, 130*(4), e168–e186.

# 175

# Anesthesia for Tubal Ligation

ROCHELLE J. POMPEIAN, MD

Tubal ligation is a commonly preferred method of permanent contraception. The procedure may be performed either in the immediate postpartum period or as an interval procedure unrelated to a recent delivery. Although tubal ligations may be safely performed at any time, there are several considerations that may factor into the timing. Postpartum tubal ligation (PPTL) is typically convenient for the patient and may reduce costs by eliminating the need for a second hospital visit. Operating conditions may be more optimal in the postpartum period, as the uterine fundus remains near the level of the umbilicus, creating better exposure of the fallopian tubes. Some data suggests that patients undergoing PPTL, especially young patients under the age of 25, are more likely to regret their decision, so it is important to ensure patient certainty before performing the procedure.

## Interval Tubal Ligations

Laparoscopy is the most common surgical approach for interval tubal ligations. Anesthetic considerations include those related to pneumoperitoneum, Trendelenburg positioning, and related cardiovascular and pulmonary complications.

Pneumoperitoneum is typically achieved by inserting a needle at the lower margin of the umbilicus, which is a relatively thin and avascular portion of the abdominal wall. Bradydysrhythmias may occur upon abdominal insufflation or with manipulation of the fallopian tubes. Treatment includes pausing the procedure, deflating the abdomen, and often administering an anticholinergic agent such as atropine. An incorrectly placed needle can lead to insufflation of the abdominal wall, retroperitoneum, mesentery, omentum, or bowel, which may lead to a perforated viscus, venous air embolism, and cardiopulmonary collapse. Because of the latter, carbon dioxide is the gas of choice to perform pneumoperitoneum because it is highly soluble, is rapidly absorbed postoperatively, is nonflammable, and provides a margin of safety if injected intravascularly.

Trendelenburg positioning is associated with decreased functional residual capacity, decreased pulmonary compliance, and elevated peak inspiratory pressures, which can lead to atelectasis, inadequate ventilation, hypercapnia, and hypoxia. Main-stem intubation may result from cephalad shift of the mediastinum and carina, requiring repositioning of the endotracheal tube. Trendelenburg positioning is also associated with brachial plexus injury if shoulder rests are used because of clavicular compression of nerve roots. Consequently, current guidelines recommend that shoulder rests not be used. Cardiovascular changes result from increased intraabdominal pressure, patient position, anesthesia, and hypercarbia. Decreased cardiac output, increased peripheral and pulmonary vascular resistance, increased arterial pressure, and arrhythmias may result.

## ANESTHETIC TECHNIQUES

### General Anesthesia

For procedures done under general anesthesia, an inhaled or intravenous anesthetic, or a combination thereof, is used to maintain anesthesia. This is supplemented with short-acting opioids and neuromuscular blocking agents. Common postoperative complications of general anesthesia are abdominal and shoulder pain and postoperative nausea and vomiting (PONV). Increasing the volume of infused preoperative and intraoperative fluids reduces the incidence of PONV and improves hemodynamic response to pneumoperitoneum and postoperative recovery. Metoclopramide (10–20 mg, administered intravenously 15–30 minutes before induction) may decrease nausea, vomiting, and recovery time. Droperidol (0.625–2.15 mg) administered after induction is an effective antiemetic that may shorten time in the postanesthesia care unit. Ondansetron (4–8 mg, administered intravenously) also significantly reduces the incidence of PONV. Dexamethasone (4–8 mg, administered intravenously) after induction has been shown to reduce PONV, especially when coadministered with another antiemetic.

### Neuraxial Anesthesia

Regional anesthesia, though less common, may be used for interval tubal sterilization. Postdural puncture headaches are more likely to occur in this patient group; a smaller-gauge (25 or 27 gauge), pencil-point needle may be used to reduce the risk. Because a steep head-down position may be required, isobaric bupivacaine (vs. hyperbaric) should be used. The ability to maintain spontaneous ventilation may be difficult for the patient, especially in the case of obesity in the steep head-down position. However, the incidence of PONV is lower in patients who receive neuraxial anesthesia, compared with general anesthesia.

### Local Anesthesia

Although local anesthesia is not commonly used for laparoscopy in the United States, it is used elsewhere in the world for either interval or PPTL. The use of local anesthesia for tubal ligation produces fewer hemodynamic changes (less likelihood of hypertension, hypotension, or tachycardia), less PONV, quicker recovery, and earlier diagnosis of complications. It is also associated with shorter surgical time and is significantly less expensive. Success of local anesthesia is contingent upon gentle and precise surgical technique. Sedation improves management of patient anxiety and pain from organ and tissue manipulation.

## Postpartum Tubal Ligation

PPTLs are commonly preferred over interval tubal ligations because of convenience and cost effectiveness. Occasionally, there may be scheduling concerns that delay or prohibit a desired PPTL from being performed during a delivery hospitalization such that only 50% of patients desiring a PPTL successfully undergo the procedure. Unfortunately, nearly 50% of those with unfulfilled PPTL requests are pregnant within 1 year, which is twice that of patients who do not request PPTL. Thus the American College of Obstetricians and Gynecologists considers PPTLs "urgent," not elective, procedures. The American Society of Anesthesiologists provides published guidelines concerning PPTLs in section VI of their Practice Guidelines for Obstetric Anesthesia (Box 175.1). Ideally, the obstetric anesthesiologist can facilitate these procedures in the postpartum period, ensuring effective contraception for those who desire it.

## ANESTHETIC TECHNIQUES

### General Anesthesia

Postpartum patients are at increased risk for aspiration because of progesterone-related decreased lower esophageal sphincter tone and delayed gastric emptying. Because the placenta is the primary producer of progesterone, progesterone levels begin to decline at 2 hours postpartum and typically return to normal within 24 hours. Delayed gastric emptying is most pronounced in the setting of parenteral opioid use. The increased risk of aspiration warrants consideration for the prophylactic use of an $H_2$-receptor antagonist, a nonparticulate antacid, and/or metoclopramide with rapid-sequence induction and application of cricoid pressure. As with pregnant patients, intubation in the

---

BOX 175.1  **SUMMARY OF POSTPARTUM TUBAL ANESTHESIA GUIDELINES FROM AMERICAN SOCIETY OF ANESTHESIOLOGISTS PRACTICE GUIDELINES FOR OBSTETRIC ANESTHESIA**

STATEMENTS

- There is insufficient literature to evaluate the benefits of neuraxial, compared with general, anesthesia.
- There is insufficient literature to evaluate the effect of timing of procedure on maternal outcome.

NEURAXIAL, COMPARED WITH GENERAL, ANESTHESIA REDUCES COMPLICATIONS

- The consultants agree that performing postpartum tubal ligation within 8 hours of delivery does not increase maternal complications.

RECOMMENDATIONS

1. For postpartum tubal ligation, the patient should have no oral intake of solid foods within 6 to 8 hours of the surgery, depending on the type of food ingested (e.g., fat content).
2. Aspiration prophylaxis should be considered.
3. Both the timing of the procedure and the decision to use a specific anesthetic technique (i.e., neuraxial vs. general) should be individualized, based on anesthetic risk factors, obstetric risk factors (e.g., blood loss at delivery), and patient preferences.
4. Neuraxial techniques are preferred to general anesthesia for most postpartum tubal ligations. The anesthesia provider should be aware that gastric emptying will be delayed in patients who have received opioids during labor, and that an epidural catheter placed for labor may be more likely to fail with longer postdelivery time intervals.
5. If a postpartum tubal ligation is to be performed before the patient is discharged from the hospital, the procedure should not be attempted at a time when it might compromise other aspects of patient care on the labor and delivery unit.

---

postpartum patient may prove more challenging because of obesity and increased laryngeal edema secondary to Valsalva maneuvers during the second stage of labor.

Halogenated inhaled anesthetic agents cause dose-related uterine relaxation and therefore increase the risk of hemorrhage, especially in multiparous parturients. Although pregnancy results in reduced minimum alveolar concentration (MAC) of an inhaled anesthetic agent, MAC requirements return to normal 12 to 36 hours after delivery. Propofol anesthesia (induction and maintenance) provides a lower incidence of PONV and rapid awakening, with low concentrations in breast milk at 4 and 8 hours postoperatively.

Plasma cholinesterase activity is significantly lower in postpartum patients compared with their nonpregnant counterparts. Therefore blockade with succinylcholine, rocuronium, mivacurium, or vecuronium may be slightly prolonged in the postpartum period. Neuromuscular blockade is unchanged with atracurium and is shortened with cisatracurium. Metoclopramide inhibits plasma cholinesterase and prolongs succinylcholine neuromuscular blockade by 100% to 200%.

### Neuraxial Anesthesia

Neuraxial anesthesia provides excellent operating conditions and is the most common anesthetic technique used for PPTL in the United States. Airway risk (obstruction, hypoventilation, and aspiration) is significantly reduced, compared with general anesthesia. A T4 block provides optimal operating conditions and pain relief. Of note, a T10 block may be inadequate, especially if it is difficult to mobilize the uterus during surgery. Sedation that prolongs postoperative amnesia should be avoided to improve early maternal-neonate interaction and bonding.

Although it is possible to use labor epidural catheters to provide surgical anesthesia for a PPTL, failure to reactivate the catheter is possible. Some anesthesia providers leave labor epidurals indwelling for up to 24 hours to use in a forthcoming PPTL procedure, with variable reactivation success rates ranging from 66% to 92%. Risk factors for epidural failure include poor epidural function during labor and long duration of time between epidural placement and reactivation attempt. Starting at 18 hours postpartum, there is a progressive decrease in dermatomal spread of epidural anesthesia, compared with the spread in patients given epidurals for cesarean section. At 36 hours postpartum, there is no significant difference in spread between patients who have recently delivered and nonpregnant patients.

Spinal anesthesia has a very positive risk-benefit profile. The risk of local anesthetic toxicity is low compared with epidural anesthesia. Rapidity of onset (and offset) and density of block are favorable. The risk of a postdural puncture headache when using small-gauge or pencil-point-design spinal needles is low. Local anesthetic requirements (which are lessened by 30% in pregnant patients) return to nonpregnant levels within 12 to 36 hours after delivery and appear to be associated with rapid decline in progesterone levels. There is a faster onset, higher level, and longer duration of spinal anesthesia in term patients than in young gynecologic patients. There is also a progressive decline in duration of block during the first 3 days postpartum. Cardiovascular effects of spinal anesthesia are markedly decreased in postpartum patients (no aortocaval compression and maternal autotransfusion at delivery), compared with pregnant patients. The need for treatment of hypotension after spinal anesthesia is lower (<10%) compared with patients undergoing cesarean section (>80%).

Historically, hyperbaric 5% lidocaine was frequently used for PPTLs because of its short duration, though this has largely fallen out of favor because of the risk of transient neurologic symptoms (TNS). Preservative-free mepivacaine (intrathecal formulation) or hyperbaric bupivacaine is now used. TNS is more likely with spinal mepivacaine than bupivacaine, but it provides for a short duration for this relatively short procedure. Alternatively, preservative-free meperidine may be used at a dose of 1 mg/kg based on the patient's prepregnancy weight (usual range 50–80 mg); the onset time is 3 to 5 minutes, with a duration of 30 to 60 minutes.

### Local Anesthesia

Although uncommon in the United States, as with interval tubal ligations, local anesthesia alone can be used to provide anesthesia for a PPTL. See earlier discussions on Anesthetic Techniques in Interval Tubal Ligation for a discussion of the use of local anesthesia in tubal ligation.

## SUGGESTED READINGS

American College of Obstetricians and Gynecologists' Committee on Health Care for Underserved Women. (2021). Access to postpartum sterilization: ACOG Committee Opinion, Number 827. *Obstetrics and Gynecology, 137*(6), e169–e176.

American Society of Anesthesiologists, & Task Force on Obstetric Anesthesia. (2007). Practice guidelines for obstetric anesthesia: An updated report by the American Society of Anesthesiologists Task Force on Obstetric Anesthesia. *Anesthesiology, 106,* 843–863.

Drasner, K. (2005). Epidural chloroprocaine-standard of care for postpartum bilateral tubal ligation. *Anesthesia and Analgesia, 101*(4), 1241.

Gupta, L., Sinha, S., Pande, M., & Vajifdar, H. (2011). Ambulatory laparoscopic tubal ligation: A comparison of general anaesthesia with local anaesthesia and sedation. *Journal of Anaesthesiology Clinical Pharmacology, 27*(1), 97–100.

Hawkins, J. L. (2014). Postpartum tubal ligation. In D. H. Chestnut, L. S. Polley, L. C. Tsen, & C. A. Wong (Eds.), *Obstetric anesthesia* (5th ed., pp. 530–542). Philadelphia: Saunders Elsevier.

Lawrie, T. A., Nardin, J. M., Kulier, R., & Boulvain, M. (2011). Techniques for the interruption of tubal patency for female sterilisation. *Cochrane Database of Systematic Reviews,* (2), CD003034.

McKenzie, C., Akdagli, S., Abir, G., & Carvalho, B. (2017). Postpartum tubal ligation: A retrospective review of anesthetic management at a single institution and a practice survey of academic institutions. *Journal of Clinical Anesthesia, 43,* 39–46.

Panni, M. K., George, R. B., Allen, T. K., Olufolabi, A. J., Schultz, J. R., Okumura, M., et al. (2010). Minimum effective dose of spinal ropivacaine with and without fentanyl for postpartum tubal ligation. *International Journal of Obstetric Anesthesia, 19*(4), 390–394.

Suelto, M. D., Vincent, R. D., Jr., Larmon, J. E., Norman, P. F., & Werhan, C. F. (2000). Spinal anesthesia for postpartum tubal ligation after pregnancy complicated by preeclampsia or gestational hypertension. *Regional Anesthesia and Pain Medicine, 25*(2), 170–173.

# 176

# Maternal Diabetes: Neonatal Effects

EMILY E. SHARPE, MD

As the obesity epidemic continues in the United States, the incidence of diabetes mellitus is also increasing, with a prevalence of 9% of the general adult population in the United States. Approximately 7% of pregnancies in the United States and 17% of pregnancies globally are complicated by diabetes. Approximately 86% of pregnant women with diabetes have gestational diabetes mellitus (GDM). Diabetes can lead to both maternal and fetal complications. Diabetes diagnosed before pregnancy is classified as either type 1 or type 2. Type 1 results from deficiency of insulin secretion, and type 2 is caused by a combination of resistance to insulin action and inadequate insulin secretion. GDM is defined as glucose intolerance that is newly diagnosed in pregnancy. The mechanism is caused by both inadequate insulin supply and insulin resistance that occurs secondary to physiologic changes in pregnancy.

Risk factors for GDM include greater maternal age, obesity, and family history of type 2 diabetes mellitus. All pregnant women should undergo screening for GDM. Box 176.1 describes a typical approach to screening for GDM. GDM typically resolves after delivery, but patients with GDM are at increased risk of developing type 2 diabetes mellitus later in life. After delivery, women with GDM should undergo screening for diabetes at 4 to 12 weeks postpartum.

Traditionally, maternal diabetes mellitus has been linked to increased maternal and fetal risks (Box 176.2), particularly associations with fetal macrosomia, fetal anomalies, shoulder dystocia, neonatal hypoglycemia, and a higher incidence of operative delivery. There is evidence that identifying and treating GDM can decrease the incidence of macrosomia, reduce serious newborn complications, and reduce hypertensive

## BOX 176.1  CRITERIA FOR SCREENING AND DIAGNOSIS OF GESTATIONAL DIABETES MELLITUS

### SCREEN AT 24 TO 28 WEEKS' GESTATION

**Initial Screen:**

   50-g oral glucose solution
   1-hour venous glucose determination
   If glucose exceed institutional screening threshold (vary from
      130–140 mg/dL), then diagnostic test

**Diagnostic Oral Glucose Tolerance Test:**

   Overnight fast
   100-g oral glucose solution
   Glucose at fasting, 1 hour, 2 hours, and 3 hours
   Diagnosis requires two or more glucose thresholds be met or
      exceeded

## BOX 176.2  NEONATAL AND MATERNAL MORBIDITY ASSOCIATED WITH MATERNAL DIABETES MELLITUS

### FETAL

   Fetal macrosomia (>4–4.5 kg)
      Shoulder dystocia
      Birth trauma
   Fetal pulmonary hypoplasia
   Increased risk of congenital anomalies*
   Increased risk of intrauterine or neonatal death
   Increased risk of autism
   Neonatal hypoglycemia
   Nonreassuring fetal status
   Polyhydramnios
   Reduction in uteroplacental perfusion[†]

### MATERNAL

   Operative delivery (cesarean or assisted vaginal)
   Intrauterine infections
   Maternal diabetic ketoacidosis[‡]
   Maternal hypoglycemia[‡]
   Hypertensive diseases of pregnancy (i.e., preeclampsia, gesta-
      tional hypertension)
   Future development of cardiovascular disease and type 2 diabetes

*Especially cardiovascular and central nervous system anomalies.
[†]Compared with parturients without diabetes, 35% to 40% lower.
[‡]In parturients with type 1 diabetes.

disorders. GDM management typically begins with dietary modifications, exercise, and glucose monitoring. If target glucose levels cannot be achieved with lifestyle modifications alone, pharmacologic treatment should be initiated. Insulin and oral antidiabetic medications are both commonly used to achieve better glycemic control in pregnancy.

Antepartum fetal testing is recommended in parturients with pregestational diabetes and may be beneficial in women with GDM with poor glycemic control. There is not a consensus on antenatal testing in patients with well-controlled GDM. Women with GDM, good glycemic control, and normal antenatal testing are commonly managed expectantly until term. Expert opinion supports earlier delivery in women with poorly controlled GDM and pregestational diabetes. Optimal timing of delivery should balance trade-offs between the risks of prematurity and the risks of worsening maternal and fetal health, typically between 37 0/7 weeks' and 38 6/7 weeks' gestation. Timing of delivery for women with GDM well controlled with medications should occur between 39 0/7 and 39 6/7 weeks' gestation.

Intrapartum management of maternal glucose usually differs between GDM and pregestational diabetics. Patients with GDM often do not require insulin during labor; however, women with type 1 or type 2 diabetes mellitus may require insulin. During active labor, glucose control can be difficult and intravenous insulin may be required. After delivery, the most common complication neonates of mothers with diabetes may face is hypoglycemia, occurring in 15% to 25% of cases. The proposed cause relates to increased secretion of insulin by the fetus in response to maternal hyperglycemia, which can lead to hypoglycemia after interruption of the umbilical supply of nutrients. Neonatal hypoglycemia should be monitored, and local protocols should be established. Infants born to women with pregestational diabetes are at increased risk of fetal anomalies compared with those born to women with GDM. The former group is associated with a 6% to 18% incidence of major anomalies (most commonly cardiovascular and central nervous system), whereas the latter group is associated with a lower 3% to 8% incidence—still higher than in nondiabetic parturients. Clinical data, although inconclusive, point to a benefit of strict glycemic control in diabetic parturients—in terms of preventing neonatal adverse outcomes and anomalies.

## SUGGESTED READINGS

Caughey, A. B., & Turrentine, M. (2018). Practice Bulletin No. 190: Gestational Diabetes Mellitus. *Obstetrics and Gynecology*, 131(2), e49–e64.

Caughey, A. B., & Valent, A. M. (2016). When to deliver women with diabetes in pregnancy? *American Journal of Perinatology*, 33(13), 1250–1254.

Horvath, K., Koch, K., Jeitler, K., Matyas, E., Bender, R., Bastian, H., et al. (2010). Effects of treatment in women with gestational diabetes mellitus: Systematic review and meta-analysis. *BMJ (Clinical Research)*, 340, c1395.

Pillay, J., Donovan, L., Guitard, S., Zakher, B., Gates, M., Gates, A., et al. (2021). Screening for gestational diabetes: Updated evidence report and systematic review for the US Preventive Services Task Force. *JAMA*, 326(6), 539–562.

Wissler, R. N. (2020). Endocrine disorders. In D. H. Chestnut (Ed.), *Chestnut's obstetric anesthesia principles and practice* (6th ed., pp. 1056–1065). Philadelphia: Elsevier.

# SECTION X

# Pediatric Anesthesia

# 177

# Impact of Anesthesia on Neural Development

MICHAEL VEGA, MD

## Relevance

Increased concern about possible deleterious effects of anesthesia on the neurocognitive development of children is a current topic of interest in the mainstream media. These concerns include long-term effects on language development, increased incidence of attention-deficit/hyperactivity disorder, learning disabilities, and memory issues. The media sometimes raises the possibility of negative outcomes associated with exposure to anesthesia without clearly evaluating the data, which often leaves the public with more questions than answers.

In addition to attention from the news media, the U.S. Food and Drug Administration (FDA) made a statement in December 2016 "warning that repeated or lengthy use of general anesthetic and sedation drugs during surgeries or procedures in children younger than 3 years or in pregnant women during their third trimester may affect the development of children's brains." Practicing physicians face increasing questions about the safety of general anesthesia in children and are challenged by the expanding literature addressing this topic. Awareness of the most up-to-date data guides physicians on how to best counsel parents and inform their own practice.

## U.S. Food and Drug Administration Statement

In the recently published FDA Drug Safety Communication, the FDA specifically highlights that children younger than 3 years old and procedures lasting more than 3 hours carry the highest risk of possible negative side effects from general anesthesia. The communication also advises parents and caregivers to ask about adverse effects of anesthesia on brain development and the timing of procedures to avoid "jeopardizing" their child's health.

## Data: Nonclinical Studies

Animal studies have demonstrated that early exposure to general anesthesia drugs can have deleterious neurotoxic effects on the rapidly developing brain. These effects specifically include nerve cell loss in the brains of animals in utero and in young animals exposed to general anesthesia. Long-term effects included alterations in behavior and learning. Neuronal apoptosis and changes in synaptogenesis correlated with persistent deficits in learning and memory. Most notably, these changes reflected a deficit in recollection in the surrounding days after anesthetic administration. These studies were conducted in a variety of species and across a range of ages. Inference from these studies suggests the most vulnerable time in humans ranges from the third trimester of pregnancy up to 3 years old. However, not all anesthetic drugs resulted in cell loss, and some effects appeared to be dependent on cumulative dose or length of exposure. Short exposure times were less likely to result in long-term deficits. The clinical significance of these studies and their application to humans is currently unclear.

## Data: Clinical Studies

Current studies published on the effects of anesthesia on children are approximately evenly divided between finding and not finding an association (Table 177.1). The common themes of these studies are limitations in study design and generalizability. It is challenging to clearly ascribe neurodevelopmental delays entirely to anesthesia exposure when there are other important variables in play such as the surgery itself, the underlying pathology requiring multiple surgeries, uncontrolled confounding variables, and epidemiologic factors. Other issues with these studies include the variance in age groups, anesthesia exposure (dose and length of exposure), and outcome definitions. Many of the studies also lack sufficient power to draw meaningful conclusions.

Two recent studies have added greater credence that a brief, single exposure to general anesthesia in healthy children is not likely to cause clinically significant cognitive deficits. The General Anaesthesia Compared to Spinal Anaesthesia trial is an international, multicenter, randomized controlled trial that compared neurocognitive outcomes after randomization with either awake-regional anesthesia or with sevoflurane-based general anesthesia in children younger than 60 weeks born at more than 26 weeks' gestation undergoing inguinal hernia repair. The primary outcome is measured using the Wechsler Preschool and Primary Scale of Intelligence Third Edition Full Scale Intelligence Quotient at age 5 years. The secondary outcome is measured using the Bayley Scales of Infant and Toddler Development III at age 2 years. The 2-year follow-up results were published in early 2016 and showed no difference between the two study groups on the Bayley Scales of Infant and Toddler Development III assessment. Initial interpretation is that sevoflurane anesthesia of less than 1 hour does not appear to increase the risk of adverse neurodevelopmental outcome at age 2 years compared with awake-regional anesthesia. Most recently, the trial completed its 5-year follow-up on the same cohort of children. Using the same scales and questionnaires, the investigators concluded that after 5 years, these patients still did not show any signs of delay in their neurodevelopment that was inappropriate with their age.

The second study, the Pediatric Anesthesia Neurodevelopment Assessment (PANDA) study, is a sibling-matched, observational cohort study that evaluated whether a single exposure to anesthesia in healthy children younger than 3 years old is associated with an increased risk of impaired global cognitive function as the primary outcome, and abnormal neurocognitive functions and behavior as secondary outcomes at ages 8 to 15 years. The PANDA study found that average IQ scores were not significantly different between the exposed and unexposed

| TABLE 177.1 | Current Studies Published on the Effects of Anesthesia on Children |
|---|---|

### NO ASSOCIATION

| Author | Study Type | Outcome | PMID/Journals |
|---|---|---|---|
| Andropoulos, 2018 | Review | Effect of anesthesia on the developing brain: infant and fetus | 28586779/*Fetal Diagn Ther* |
| Bartels, 2009 | Twin study | No difference between exposed and unexposed twin; anesthetic parameters and causality unclear | 19456216/*Twin Res Hum Genet* |
| Bong, 2013 | Retrospective | The odds of a formal diagnosis of LD by age 12 years in healthy children exposed to general anesthesia for minor surgery during infancy were 4.5 times greater than their peers who had never been exposed to anesthesia; however, study precision inadequate to detect relevant difference | 24132012/*Anesth Analg* |
| Creagh, 2015 | Sibling cohort | No association between early exposure and autism spectrum disorder | 26742193/*Bol Asoc Med P R* |
| Elsinga, 2013 | Retrospective | Associated deficits but confounding variables and underpowered | 23084574/*Early Hum Dev* |
| Fan, 2013 | Self-controlled | No association between volatile anesthetic exposure and cognitive function, small sample size, ages 4–7 years old | 23386252/*J Anesth* |
| Filan, 2012 | Retrospective | No association when confounding variables adjusted | 22048043/*J Pediatr* |
| Guerra, 2011 | Prospective | No association with dose/duration of sedation/analgesia and neurodevelopmental outcome | 21507125/*Paediatr Anaesth* |
| Hansen, 2011 | Retrospective | No association with single exposure after known confounders adjusted | 21368654/*Anesthesiology* |
| Hansen, 2013 | Retrospective | No association with single exposure in children under 3 months old on adolescent educational performance tests after known confounders adjusted | 23863116/*Paediatr Anaesth* |
| Kalkman, 2009 | Retrospective | Study underpowered, behavioral differences identified but not statistically significant | 19293699/*Anesthesiology* |
| Ko, 2014 | Retrospective | No association for ADHD diagnosis with single or multiple exposures | 24612161/*Paediatr Anaesth* |
| McCann, 2019 | Prospective | Less than 1 h of general anesthesia in early infancy does not alter neurodevelopmental outcome at age 5 years compared with awake-regional anaesthesia in a predominantly male study population. | 30782342/*Lancet* |
| Sun, 2016 | Sibling match cohort | No association for healthy children with single exposure | 27272582/*JAMA* |
| Yang, 2012 | Prospective | No association for children 5–10 years old with single exposure, study underpowered | 22244524/*Am J Ophthalmol* |

### ASSOCIATION

| Author | Study Type | Outcome | PMID/Journals |
|---|---|---|---|
| Block, 2012 | Retrospective | Findings consistent with possible adverse effects of anesthesia and surgery during infancy on subsequent academic achievement; duration of anesthesia and surgery correlated negatively with scores, not all confounders accounted for | 22801049/*Anesthesiology* |
| DiMaggio, 2009 | Retrospective | Children status post-hernia repair >2 times as likely to be diagnosed with developmental or behavioral disorder | 19955889/*J Neurosurg Anesthesiol* |
| DiMaggio, 2011 | Retrospective | Exposed group risk of diagnosis of developmental or behavioral disorders 60% higher than matched siblings who were unexposed, more tightly matched pairwise analysis needed to determine causality | 21415431/*Anesth Analg* |
| Flick, 2011 | Retrospective | Multiple exposures to anesthesia increases risk of LD, but no intervention required for LD | 21969289/*Pediatrics* |
| Ing, 2012 | Retrospective | Adjusted for demographic characteristics, exposure to anesthesia was associated with increased risk of disability in language. Children exposed when under 3 years of age had higher relative risk of language and abstract reasoning deficits at age 10 years than unexposed children | 22908104/*Pediatrics* |
| Ing, 2014 | Retrospective | Exposure associated with language and abstract reasoning deficits; assessment tool used may influence whether association is identified | 24694922/*Anesthesiology* |

*Continued*

| TABLE 177.1 | Current Studies Published on the Effects of Anesthesia on Children—cont'd | | |
|---|---|---|---|
| | **ASSOCIATION** | | |
| **Author** | **Study Type** | **Outcome** | **PMID/Journals** |
| Morriss, 2014 | Retrospective | Major surgery in very low-birth-weight infants independently associated >50% increased risk of death or neurodevelopmental impairment at 18–22 months' corrected age. Exposure implicates anesthesia but does not prove it | 24934607/*JAMA Pediatr* |
| Naumann, 2012 | Retrospective | Average neurodevelopmental scores were lower among children experiencing longer surgeries and higher exposures to inhaled anesthesia | 22502768/*Paediatr Anaesth* |
| Sprung, 2012 | Retrospective | Single exposure no increased risk, multiple exposures associated with increased risk for ADHD when adjusted for comorbidities | 22305025/*Mayo Clin Proc* |
| Stratmann, 2014 | Retrospective | Exposure to anesthetics associated with difficulty in recollection, but not in IQ | 24910347/*Neuropsychopharmacology* |
| Walker, 2010 | Prospective | Lower than expected developmental scores for infants after surgery for infantile hypertrophic pyloric stenosis than for healthy control infants | 21129547/*J Pediatr Surg* |
| Walker, 2012 | Prospective | Major surgery in infants found to be significantly associated with developmental delay at 1 year of age compared with control infants | 22578999/*J Pediatr* |
| Wilder, 2009 | Retrospective | Multiple exposures associated with increased risk of LD, no association with single exposure, anesthesia exposure was significant risk factor | 19293700/*Anesthesiology* |

*ADHD,* Attention-deficit/hyperactivity disorder; *GAS,* General Anaesthesia Compared to Spinal Anaesthesia trial; *LD,* learning disability.

siblings. The secondary outcome did not show significant differences in the average scores.

Although these studies help assure the physician that single, brief exposures likely do not result in clinically significant neurocognitive deficits, more research is needed to investigate the effects of prolonged or multiple exposures to anesthesia, the effects of anesthesia in a less healthy pediatric population, and to be sufficiently powered to evaluate meaningful differences at specific ages of exposure, length of exposure, or possible gender differences.

## What to Tell Parents and Caregivers

SmartTots is a partnership between the FDA and the International Anesthesia Research Society whose mission is to coordinate and fund research programs to deliver safe surgery for children who undergo general anesthesia or sedation.

SmartTots advises that, when answering questions from parents and caregivers regarding the risks of general anesthesia in children, the physician should elucidate the differences between research findings in animals and children and the uncertainty of any effect in children. Main recommendations include:

- No specific medications or technique can be chosen that are safer than any other
- Discuss necessity of procedure
- Carefully evaluate the timing of planned procedure
- Weigh risks/benefits
- Single versus multiple exposures

## SUGGESTED READINGS

Battaglin, F., Schirripa, M., Buggin, F., Pietrantonio, F., Morano, F., Boscolo, G., et al. (2018). The PANDA study: a randomized phase II study of first-line FOLFOX plus panitumumab versus 5FU plus panitumumab in RAS and BRAF wild-type elderly metastatic colorectal cancer patients. *BMC Cancer, 18*(1), 98.

Creagh, O., Torres, H., Rivera, K., Morales-Franqui, M., Altieri-Acevedo, G., & Warner, D. (2015). Previous Exposure to Anesthesia and Autism Spectrum Disorder (ASD): A Puerto Rican Population-Based Sibling Cohort Study. *Boletin de la Asociacion Medica de Puerto Rico, 107*(3), 29–37.

FDA Drug Safety Communication. *FDA review results in new warnings about using general anesthetics and sedation drugs in young children and pregnant women.* Retrieved from https://www.fda.gov/Drugs/DrugSafety/ucm532356.htm.

McCann, M. E., de Graaff, J. C., Dorris, L., Disma, N., Withington, D., Bell, G., et al. (2019). Neurodevelopmental outcome at 5 years of age after general anaesthesia or awake-regional anaesthesia in infancy (GAS): an international, multicentre, randomised, controlled equivalence trial. *Lancet (London, England), 393*(10172), 664–677.

SmartTots. *FAQ: Frequently asked questions.* Retrieved from http://smarttots.org/resources/faq/. Accessed November 7, 2022.

Wilder, R. T., Flick, R. P., Sprung, J., Katusic, S. K., Barbaresi, W. J., Mickelson, C., et al. (2009). Early exposure to anesthesia and learning disabilities in a population-based birth cohort. *Anesthesiology, 110*(4), 796–804.

# 178

# Anesthetic Risks Associated With Prematurity

LINDSAY ROYCE HUNTER GUEVARA, MD

The World Health Organization currently defines prematurity as a gestational age (GA) of less than 37 weeks regardless of birth weight. Premature infants can be further classified as late preterm (GA between 34 and 36 6/7 weeks), moderate preterm (GA between 32 and 33 6/7 weeks), very preterm (GA between 28 and 31 6/7 weeks), and extremely preterm (GA <28 weeks). Additionally, infants can be categorized by birth weight, including low birth weight (<2500 g), very low birth weight (<1500 g), and extremely low birth weight (<1000 g). Lower birth weights and increased prematurity are associated with increased morbidity and mortality. Preterm birth is often caused by a combination of fetal, placental, and uterine factors (Table 178.1).

Premature infants presenting for anesthesia and surgery require special attention because they often have multiorgan dysfunction, including severe cardiopulmonary, gastrointestinal, neurologic, endocrinologic, or hematologic derangements (Table 178.2). Premature infants have higher-than-expected perioperative complication rates after even minor procedures. Anesthetic morbidity rate increases directly with the degree of prematurity.

## Respiratory Distress Syndrome

Respiratory distress syndrome (RDS) is common in preterm infants and is caused by a decrease in quantity and quality of surfactant in underdeveloped lungs. The more premature the infant is, the more likely they are to have RDS. Surfactant lines alveoli and reduces surface tension within the alveoli, which decreases the risk of atelectasis. Without surfactant, alveoli can collapse, resulting in respiratory acidosis, hypoxemia, intrapulmonary and extrapulmonary shunting, and need for mechanical ventilation, which further stimulates inflammation. Diagnosis of RDS is based on clinical features, including progressive respiratory failure after birth and chest radiographic data, which show low lung volumes with reticulogranular, ground-glass appearance and air bronchograms. Current treatment goals of RDS focus on use of exogenous surfactant and early nasal continuous positive airway pressure (CPAP). Infants who fail noninvasive therapy progress to endotracheal intubation and mechanical ventilation. Very or extremely preterm neonates, those with moderate or severe RDS, or those with other significant comorbidities are more likely to require endotracheal intubation and administration of exogenous surfactant. Several systematic reviews, many including the Surfactant Positive Airway Pressure and Pulse Oximetry Randomized Trial (SUPPORT study), have shown that CPAP over intubation with or without exogenous surfactant administration is associated with lower mortality, less respiratory morbidity, and reduced risk of bronchopulmonary dysplasia. Of note, a pneumothorax should also be considered in any neonate whose oxygenation deteriorates suddenly.

| TABLE 178.1 | Factors That Increase the Risk of Preterm Birth |
|---|---|
| **FETAL** | |
| Fetal distress | |
| Multiple gestation | |
| **PLACENTAL** | |
| Abruptio placentae | |
| Placenta previa | |
| **UTERINE** | |
| Incompetent cervix | |
| **MATERNAL** | |
| Preeclampsia | |
| Heart disease | |
| Drug abuse (cocaine, nicotine) | |
| African American | |
| Lower socioeconomic status | |
| Younger or older age | |
| **OTHER** | |
| Premature rupture of membranes | |
| Polyhydramnios | |

## Bronchopulmonary Dysplasia

Bronchopulmonary dysplasia (BPD), as defined by the U.S. National Institute of Child Health and Development, occurs when an infant requires oxygen supplementation beyond 28 days of life or 36 weeks postmenstrual age (GA plus chronologic age). BPD can further be classified by severity grades, including I (mild), II (moderate), and III (severe), depending on need for noninvasive and invasive positive pressure ventilation and oxygen supplementation (flow and fraction of inspired oxygen [$Fio_2$]). BPD is a chronic disorder, usually occurring in infants with a history of RDS. Although studies evaluating incidence of BPD have demonstrated conflicting results, it appears that the incidence of BPD has not decreased in recent times despite improved neonatal care.

The cause of BPD is thought to be multifactorial with both antenatal and postnatal factors that result in injury to the premature lung. Risk factors associated with BPD include prematurity, intrauterine growth restriction, maternal smoking, increased inspired concentration of oxygen, the use of mechanical ventilation, and history of postnatal infection. Additional risk factors that have inconsistent evidence include patent ductus arteriosus (PDA), antenatal infection, and genetic factors.

BPD is characterized by increased airway resistance, decreased pulmonary compliance, ventilation/perfusion mismatch, decreased

| TABLE 178.2 | Organ System Pathology in Premature Neonates |
|---|---|

**NEUROLOGIC**
Intraventricular hemorrhage*

Delayed development

Seizures

Hydrocephalus

Cerebral palsy

**CARDIOVASCULAR**
Congenital malformation

Persistent patent ductus arteriosus

**RESPIRATORY**
Apnea

Respiratory distress syndrome*

Bronchopulmonary dysplasia*

Pneumothorax

Pneumonia

**GASTROINTESTINAL**
Necrotizing enterocolitis*

Hyperbilirubinemia

Disordered swallowing/sucking

Gastroesophageal reflux

Bowel obstruction

**HEPATIC**
Hepatic failure

Hyperalimentation hepatitis

**HEMATOLOGIC**
Anemia

Vitamin K deficiency

**ENDOCRINOLOGIC**
Hypoglycemia

Hypocalcemia

**RENAL**
Chronic renal failure

Renal tubular acidosis

Electrolyte abnormalities

   Hyponatremia

   Hypernatremia

   Hyperkalemia

**VISUAL**
Retinopathy of prematurity

**OTHER**
Malnutrition

Sepsis*

*Major causes of morbidity.

partial pressure of oxygen, tachypnea, increased oxygen consumption, and an increased number of pulmonary infections. Pulmonary artery hypertension is a complication associated with moderate and severe BPD.

## Apnea

All premature infants have some degree of periodic breathing because of their immature respiratory control systems. Apnea of prematurity is defined as cessation of breathing that lasts for 20 seconds or longer or a shorter respiratory pause associated with oxygen desaturation and/or bradycardia. The risk of apnea after anesthesia may be increased in infants with anemia, history of apneic spells, neurologic diseases (seizures, intracranial hemorrhage), or those with significant comorbidities. The American Academy of Pediatrics recommends hospital admission and monitoring for former preterm patients until they are 50 to 60 weeks postmenstrual age for at least 12 hours after a preterm infant has undergone anesthesia. Caffeine therapy is used in the treatment of apnea of prematurity to reduce episodes of apnea.

## Patent Ductus Arteriosus

The ductus arteriosus, a vascular connection between the aorta and pulmonary artery, is present during fetal circulation and bypasses the high resistance of the pulmonary vascular beds. At birth, as the infant transitions from fetal circulation, pulmonary vascular resistance (PVR) decreases, systemic vascular resistance (SVR) increases, and the partial pressure of oxygen in arterial blood increases, which helps close the ductus arteriosus. Preterm infants are at risk of having a persistent PDA, which typically causes a left-to-right shunt, left ventricular hypertrophy, and increased pulmonary blood flow. If left untreated, a PDA can lead to congestive heart failure. The amount of flow through the PDA depends on the size of the PDA, and the direction of blood flow depends on the SVR and PVR. Although PDA shunting is usually left to right, if the neonate has significantly elevated PVR (i.e., persistent pulmonary hypertension of the newborn and some congenital heart diseases), the flow through the PDA can be reversed, and the shunt becomes right to left. Treatment of PDA includes supportive management with moderate fluid restriction; pharmacologic therapy with cyclooxygenase inhibitors, such as indomethacin, to block prostaglandin E2 (a potent PDA vasodilator); cardiac catheterization-based closure; or surgical ligation through a left posterolateral thoracotomy.

Neonates that require PDA ligation may be very ill, and PDA ligation is commonly performed in the neonatal intensive care unit. Special anesthetic considerations for surgical PDA ligation include preductal and postductal pulse oximetry. These monitors can be helpful to ensure correct vessel ligation, because the aorta and PDA are near each other and are often comparable in size. Monitoring blood pressure in both preductal and postductal limbs is also helpful for determining pressure gradients and ensuring appropriate perfusion. Once the PDA is ligated, the diastolic pressure should increase immediately, which is another indicator that the correct vessel was ligated. Recurrent laryngeal nerve paralysis is a possible complication.

## Necrotizing Enterocolitis

Primarily a disease of preterm and very and extremely low-birth-weight infants, the cause of necrotizing enterocolitis

(NEC) is thought to be multifactorial. Additional risk factors include the use antibiotics and medications that decrease gastric acidity and nonhuman milk feeding. It is characterized by ischemic necrosis and inflammation of intestinal mucosa with enteric organisms that cause gas to form in the muscularis and portal venous system. There are three stages of NEC; the first stage is based on clinical signs of abdominal distention, feeding intolerance, and hematochezia or melena with additional signs of temperature instability and apnea/bradycardia. In the first stage of NEC, radiographs of the abdomen may be normal or may show mild intestinal dilation or ileus. The treatment is supportive and includes cessation of enteral feedings and decompression of the gastrointestinal tract in addition to initiation of parental nutrition and antibiotics. The second stage of NEC has the same clinical presentation (described earlier) *with the addition of radiologic findings* including pneumatosis intestinalis (air within the wall of the intestine) or portal venous gas. Similarly, treatment is supportive. In the third stage of NEC, the infant develops intestinal perforation or necrotic bowel with cardiopulmonary, hematologic, or metabolic decompensation and requires surgical intervention. These infants may develop diffuse intravascular coagulopathy and/or septic shock requiring treatment with fluid resuscitation and vasopressor therapy. Peritoneal drainage may be performed as a temporizing measure to stabilize the infant before operation; sometimes peritoneal drainage may be adequate enough to avoid surgery. Surgical management includes laparotomy to remove diseased bowel.

Potent inhaled anesthesia gases may cause hemodynamic instability in these sick infants, and the use of high-dose opioid techniques with muscle relaxant may be preferred. The use of nitrous oxide should be avoided, and normal blood pressure in the perioperative period should be maintained. Rapid fluid administration in preterm neonates may cause intracranial hemorrhage or reopening of the ductus arteriosus. Close monitoring of metabolic, hematologic, circulatory, and respiratory function is required during the operation.

## Intracranial Hemorrhage

Intraventricular hemorrhage (IVH), also known as *periventricular*, *germinal matrix*, or *subependymal hemorrhage*, is the most common type of intracranial hemorrhage in preterm infants. The small, underdeveloped capillary beds of the germinal matrix are the typical location of intracranial bleeds in preterm infants. Newborn prematurity is the single most important risk factor for the development of intracranial hemorrhage. IVH presents in the first days of life and rarely occurs after the infant is 10 days old. There are four grades of IVH that correlate with neurodevelopmental outcomes, with grade IV being the most severe. Posthemorrhagic hydrocephalus can develop, requiring drainage via ventriculoperitoneal shunt.

A variety of mechanisms are involved in intracranial hemorrhage. Impaired autoregulation of cerebral blood flow (CBF) occurs in preterm neonates, and CBF may become pressure dependent with hypotension resulting in hypoperfusion. Hypertension can cause elevation of CBF resulting in hemorrhage. Hyperosmolarity is also a contributing factor. Therefore the use of hyperosmolar fluids should be avoided (e.g., dilute sodium bicarbonate and infuse slowly). It is prudent to prevent hypoxemia and hypercapnia, maintain blood pressure in the normal range, and provide adequate analgesia to avoid changes in CBF in infants with IVH undergoing an anesthetic.

## Infection

Infection (e.g., pneumonia, sepsis, and meningitis) in premature infants who are known to have reduced cellular and tissue immunity is a constant threat to life. Of note, sepsis in these infants can develop in the absence of a positive blood culture, elevated white blood cell count, or fever. The first clinical indication of infection may be apnea, bradycardia, or acidosis. Strict compliance with handwashing and maintenance of universal precautions is mandatory when providing care.

## Retinopathy of Prematurity

Premature infants are at increased risk for developing retinopathy of prematurity (ROP), characterized by abnormal retinal vascularization that can lead to visual impairment. The risk of ROP increases with prematurity and low birth weight, with the highest risk in infants weighing less than 1000 g. The cause of ROP is multifactorial with many risk factors implicated, including assisted ventilation, surfactant therapy, severe illness, and high blood transfusion volume, in addition to low GA and birth weight. There is evidence suggesting abnormal tissue oxygen levels (when comparing fetal oxygen levels with those a preterm infant is exposed to) can cause alterations of angiogenesis resulting in hypoxic and ischemic changes of the retina. Minimizing inspired oxygen exposure is prudent until 44 weeks postmenstrual age because this time is when retinal vascularization is completed. The goal for oxygen saturation readings should be 90% to 95% when oxygen supplementation is used, with the $Fio_2$ minimized as able. There is little convincing evidence that brief exposures to $Fio_2$ of 100% is a risk factor for the development of ROP in susceptible infants. Although many retinal changes regress spontaneously, severe cases of ROP can lead to retinal detachment and blindness.

## Temperature Instability

Impaired temperature regulation in premature infants results from a variety of factors, including increased surface area–to–mass ratio, limited insulating adipose tissue, decreased number of brown fat cells that can generate heat, and thin skin from lack of keratinization causing loss of heat and water. The epidermis is not mature until after 32 weeks gestation. Premature infants lose heat through four mechanisms, with radiation and convection being the biggest factors followed by evaporation and conduction. Hypothermia is associated with hypoglycemia, acidosis, respiratory distress, increased oxygen consumption, decreased cardiac output, increased peripheral vascular resistance, and sepsis. Outcomes are improved if premature (and sick) infants are cared for in a normothermic environment. Using forced warming air devices and radiant warmers, covering the infant in a plastic body covering, providing a head covering for the infant, and warming the operating theater are suggested ways to decrease the risk of hypothermia. Careful monitoring is required because infants may develop iatrogenic hyperthermia.

## Pharmacologic Concerns

Neurotoxicity resulting in long-term behavioral and cognitive effects from sedation and general anesthesia in infants and young children is a popular area of research. In 2016, the U.S. Food and Drug Administration (FDA) issued a drug safety communication regarding repeated and/or prolonged anesthetics in children less than 3 years of age and fetal exposure during the third trimester over the concern for potential neurotoxicity. All potent inhaled anesthetics and many intravenous medications, including propofol, ketamine, etomidate, methohexital, lorazepam, midazolam, and phenobarbital, were included in this FDA announcement. Animal studies have shown apoptosis of neurons after exposure to a variety of commonly used medications for sedation and general anesthesia. This research has evolved to primarily retrospective and observational studies in pediatric patients, with some research showing associations of behavioral and/or cognitive effects as the result of surgery and anesthesia, particularly in infants and children exposed to multiple anesthetics.

Independent of these concerns over anesthesia exposures on the developing brain, other important issues affect pharmacokinetics and pharmacodynamics within preterm infants. Hepatic metabolism and renal clearance are decreased in premature infants. Reduced elimination may cause prolongation of some anesthesia medications. Total body water weight is higher in preterm infants resulting in a larger volume of distribution per unit weight for most drugs. Premature infants have decreased protein binding, including albumin (acidic medications) and alpha-1 glycoprotein (basic medications), resulting in increased potency and lower dose requirements of certain medications (e.g., local anesthetics).

## Acknowledgment

The author and editors wish to sincerely thank Kelly Dolittle, MD, for her work on the previous edition of this chapter.

## SUGGESTED READINGS

Andropoulos, D. B. (2018). Effect of anesthesia on the developing brain: infant and fetus. *Fetal Diagnosis and Therapy, 43*(1), 1–11.

Carlo, W. A., & Polin, R. A. (2013). Respiratory support in preterm infants at birth. *Pediatrics, 133*, 171–174.

Davis, P. J., & Cladis, F. P. (2021). Smith's anesthesia for infants and children. In *Neonatology for anesthesiologists* (10th ed.). Philadelphia: Elsevier.

Kuan, C. C., & Shaw, S. J. (2020). Anesthesia for major surgery in the neonate. *Anesthesiology Clinics, 38*(1), 1–18.

Lerman, J., Coté, C. J., & Steward, D. J. (2016). Manual of pediatric anesthesia with an index of pediatric syndromes. In *Anatomy and physiology* (7th ed., pp. 10–42). Philadelphia: Churchill Liviçngstone.

McCann, M. E., & Soriano, S. G. (2019). Does general anesthesia affect neurodevelopment in infants and children? *BMJ, 367*, l6459.

Polaner, D. M., & Houch, C. S. (2015). Critical elements for the pediatric perioperative anesthesia environment section on anesthesiology and pain medicine. *Pediatrics, 136*, 1200–1205.

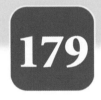

# 179

# Meconium Aspiration and Meconium Aspiration Syndrome

MOLLY M.H. HERR, MD

Meconium aspiration syndrome (MAS) is defined as respiratory distress developing shortly after birth in an infant born through meconium-stained amniotic fluid (MSAF) whose symptoms cannot otherwise be explained. MAS can vary substantially from mild respiratory distress to life-threatening respiratory failure. It is a leading cause of morbidity and mortality in term infants. MSAF requires coordination of the obstetric and neonatal teams to reduce the incidence of MAS and to provide emergent therapy in those infants who develop MAS.

MSAF is a common obstetric situation, occurring in 10% to 22% of laboring women and up to 23% to 52% after 42 weeks' gestation. MAS occurs in roughly 2% to 10% of infants exposed to MSAF, with an incidence of about 0.1% to 0.4% of live births. Infants born through MSAF are 100 times more likely than infants born through clean amniotic fluid to develop respiratory distress in the neonatal period. When MSAF is accompanied by nonreassuring fetal heart rate tracing, neonatal distress and morbidity are even more likely. There are many fetal and maternal conditions associated with an increased incidence of meconium aspiration (Box 179.1). The risk of MAS and MSAF is greatest in postmature (>41 weeks) and small for gestational age (SGA) infants. Fortunately, the incidence of MAS has been decreasing over the last several decades, largely caused by changes in obstetric care, primarily with the reduction of postmature births.

MAS has been characterized according to its severity, with infants having mild MAS requiring less than 40% oxygen for less than 48 hours; moderate MAS infants needing greater than

40% oxygen or supplemental oxygen for more than 48 hours without a pulmonary air leak; and severe MAS infants requiring mechanical ventilation for more than 48 hours and/or developing pulmonary hypertension.

## Pathophysiology of Meconium Passage in Utero

Meconium is a thick, green-black material first seen in the fetus during the third month of gestation. It results from the accumulation of desquamated cells from the intestine and skin, lanugo hair, fatty material from the vernix caseosa, amniotic fluid, and intestinal secretions. It gets its green-black color from bile pigments. Fetal passage of meconium is infrequent in early pregnancy and occurs rarely before 34 weeks' gestation. Meconium passage may be caused by increased peristalsis and relaxation of the rectal sphincter with umbilical cord compression or fetal hypoxia. In many circumstances, however, passage of meconium is a manifestation of a mature gastrointestinal tract. The incidence of meconium staining increases with fetal maturity, affecting only 2% of infants born at less than 37 weeks' gestation but as much as 44% to 52% of infants born over 42 weeks' gestation.

## Consequences of Meconium Passage or Aspiration

Meconium aspiration can occur before, during, or after birth. Under normal conditions, fetal breathing results in the movement of amniotic fluid into the trachea. With times of prolonged fetal stress or hypoxia, fetal breathing and "gasping" is increased, leading to the increased aspiration of amniotic fluid. Fetal hypoxic stress also stimulates colonic activity resulting in the passage of meconium. Thus this increased fetal gasping can lead to meconium aspiration in utero. Mounting evidence suggests that chronic in utero insults may be responsible for the most severe cases of MAS as opposed to an acute peripartum event. However, in some cases, if meconium remains in the pharynx or trachea after delivery, it may also be aspirated with the first breaths.

Meconium, although sterile, provides an excellent bacterial growth medium in amniotic fluid, especially for *Escherichia*

*coli*, increasing the risk of perinatal bacterial infection and neonatal pneumonia. It also irritates fetal skin, which, in turn, increases the incidence of erythema toxicum. However, of greatest consequence to the fetus are the effects on the respiratory and cardiac systems. Aspirated meconium can cause partial or complete airway obstruction. Distal atelectasis may occur because of particulate obstruction. Partial mechanical obstruction of the airway from meconium aspiration includes ball-valve effects, causing air trapping, overdistention of the lung, and alveolar rupture causing pneumothorax. Complete tracheal obstruction may result in death.

Chemical irritation and inflammation of the lung often occurs relatively quickly because of the composition of meconium. This direct injury results in an inflammatory and exudative pneumonitis. Meconium can also inactivate surfactant and cause a decrease in surfactant synthesis, worsening lung function. Hypoxemia can result from decreased alveolar ventilation related to lung injury, and ventilation-perfusion mismatching with perfusion of poorly ventilated lung alveoli. Persistent pulmonary hypertension of the newborn frequently accompanies MAS, caused by abnormally elevated pulmonary vascular resistance after birth, resulting in a right-to-left shunt and resultant hypoxemia. See Fig. 179.1 for pulmonary effects associated with MAS.

## Treatment

Prevention is a key component of treatment and remains a primary aspect of care. Because meconium aspiration can occur before the time of delivery, perhaps the most critical preventive strategy is good prenatal care, including the detection and prevention of fetal hypoxemia and the avoidance of postdate deliveries. During labor, it has become the standard of care in the United States for continuous or periodic intrapartum fetal heart rate monitoring, especially those pregnancies at higher risk for fetal hypoxemia including postterm pregnancy, intrauterine growth restriction, and preeclampsia. In addition, because the risk of MAS is greatest in infants born after 41 weeks,

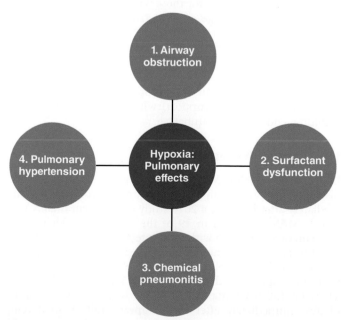

**Fig. 179.1** The potential pulmonary effects associated with meconium aspiration syndrome.

induction of labor in those women rather than expectant management has shown to reduce the incidence of MAS.

## TREATMENT BEFORE DELIVERY

In the past, amnioinfusion, the transvaginal instillation of warm sterile saline into the amniotic cavity, was used in hopes of diluting the thick clumps of meconium in those women with MSAF and reducing the risk of MAS. However, studies have shown that amnioinfusion is neither beneficial nor recommended for the prevention of MAS. It is hypothesized that many fetuses have already aspirated meconium before the meconium passage has been noted during labor, or, in some cases, aspiration may predate labor. Of note, amnioinfusion may be recommended for other reasons, such as repetitive variable decelerations, regardless of the presence of meconium or in low-resource settings where fetal monitoring is not available.

## TREATMENT DURING DELIVERY

In 2015, the American Heart Association (AHA) and the American Academy of Pediatrics (AAP) updated the guidelines for infant resuscitation, and in 2016 the Neonatal Resuscitation Program with these new recommendations, including the management of delivery of a newborn with MSAF, became available. They state that infants born with MSAF, regardless of whether they are vigorous or not, should no longer routinely receive intrapartum suctioning (delivery of the head but before the delivery of the shoulders), as this practice did not decrease the risk of developing MAS. Before these guidelines, the 2005 guidelines recommended routine intubation and suctioning of meconium or other aspirated material from beneath the glottis in nonvigorous newborns. However, current recommendations for the infant with MSAF with poor muscle tone and respiratory effort state the initial steps of resuscitation should be under the radiant warmer and efforts to support ventilation and oxygenation, including bag-mask ventilation, should be initiated without delay. Resuscitation should follow the same principles for infants with MSAF as for those with clear fluid.

The American College of Obstetricians and Gynecologists Committee on Obstetric Practice's Committee Opinion on Delivery of a Newborn with Meconium-Stained Amniotic Fluid, written in 2017 and reaffirmed in 2021, agrees with the AHA and AAP that MSAF is a condition that requires the notification and availability of an appropriately credentialed team (neonatal advanced life support) with full resuscitation skills, including endotracheal intubation.

## Diagnosis After Delivery

Infants who develop MAS usually show signs of respiratory distress (tachypnea, grunting, retractions, and/or cyanosis) immediately after birth. In a 2010 study of 394 term infants with MSAF, MAS developed in 19 of the 394 infants. Eighteen of those infants were born with 5-minute Apgar scores less than or equal to 8, and only one infant with a 5-minute Apgar greater than or equal to 9 developed MAS. All 19 infants with MAS had signs of respiratory distress within 15 minutes after birth. Therefore full-term infants with MASF without any respiratory distress immediately after birth appear unlikely to develop MAS. However, it is common to monitor infants born with MASF for 6 to 24 hours after delivery for signs of respiratory

---

> ### BOX 179.2   MECONIUM ASPIRATION SYNDROME DIAGNOSTIC CRITERIA
>
> 1. Respiratory distress in a newborn born through meconium-stained amniotic fluid
> 2. Oxygen requirement to maintain a $SpO_2$ greater than 92%
> 3. The need for oxygen within in the first 2 hours of life and for more than 12 hours
> 4. The absence of malformations of the airway, lungs, or heart
>
> Reprinted with permission from Elsevier (Vain NE, Szyld EG, Prudent LM, et al. Oropharyngeal and nasopharyngeal suctioning of meconium-stained neonates before delivery of their shoulders: multicentre, randomised controlled trial. *Lancet.* 2004;364(9434):597–602.)

---

distress. (See Box 179.2 for diagnostic criteria of MAS.) Other physical clues of MAS include signs of postmaturity (cracked or peeling skin, weight loss), SGA, and yellow staining of the fingernails and skin. Classical chest x-ray (CXR) findings in MAS are overexpansion of the lungs with diffuse patchy infiltrates; however, if meconium is aspirated primarily in utero, more uniform infiltrates are seen on CXR.

## Management

The management of MAS is supportive. All infants with signs of respiratory distress should be admitted to the neonatal intensive care unit (NICU). Goals include keeping an infant warm in a nonstimulating environment to avoid agitation, which can cause more right-to-left shunting, leading to increased hypoxia and acidosis. Maintenance of adequate blood pressure and perfusion, with correction of acidosis and hypoglycemia, are required. Respiratory management consists of maintaining adequate oxygenation and ventilation. The goals include limiting oxygen ($O_2$) consumption and optimizing partial pressure of $O_2$ in arterial blood ($Pao_2$) with minimal airway pressures and preventing air trapping.

Supplemental $O_2$ is useful in mild to moderate disease to maintain a goal $O_2$ saturation in arterial blood greater than 90%. Continuous positive airway pressure may be used when the fraction of inspired $O_2$ needs is greater than 0.4 to 0.5; however, care must be used in infants with hyperinflation because it may worsen air trapping. Mechanical ventilation is required in more severe cases with the goals of achieving optimal gas exchange with minimal respiratory trauma, often allowing partial pressure of carbon dioxide in arterial blood levels to be in the 45 to 55 mm Hg range. When conventional mechanical ventilation fails, rescue therapies include high-frequency oscillation and surfactant therapy. Inhaled nitric oxide may be used to prevent persistent pulmonary hypertension of the newborn, which may occur in neonates who have MAS. In the developed world, extracorporeal membrane oxygenation (ECMO) is the standard of care for infants with MAS who fail maximum ventilation therapy including high frequency ventilation and inhaled nitric oxide. Roughly 35% of infants requiring ECMO have MAS.

Cardiac complications, which are the result of chronic in utero hypoxia, include persistent fetal circulation and persistent pulmonary hypertension of the newborn. Minimizing right-to-left pulmonary shunting by keeping systemic pressures greater than pulmonary pressures will decrease the incidence of patent ductus arteriosus. Persistent pulmonary hypertension of the newborn is associated with the greatest risk of death in neonates with MAS.

## Outcomes

Current outcomes after the 2016 revised Neonatal Resuscitation Program, stating nonvigorous infants born through MSAF should be treated the same as those infants born through clear fluid—that is, without immediate tracheal suctioning but with immediate positive pressure ventilation and resuscitation as needed—are starting to be analyzed. In one study, the California Perinatal Quality Care Collaborative (CPQCC) database has been analyzed pre- and postguideline changes. All NICUs belonging to the CPQCC (93% of California's NICUs) were included, and data was compared between 2013 to 2015 versus 2017. In their analysis, the diagnosis of MAS included all of the following: (1) presence of MSAF at birth, (2) respiratory distress within the first hour of birth, (3) central cyanosis on room air or supplemental oxygen requirement to maintain $Pao_2$ greater than 50 mm Hg, (4) abnormal CXR compatible with a diagnosis of MAS, and (5) absence of culture-proven early-onset bacterial sepsis or pneumonia.

With analysis of roughly 365,000 infant births per year at Californian centers having participating NICUs, it was found that the incidence of MAS decreased significantly from the base years 2013 to 2015 (average of 1.02 cases/1000 births) compared to 2017 (0.78 cases/1000 births) with the application of new resuscitation guidelines that did not include immediate tracheal suctioning. Among the infants who developed MAS, the severity was not different with the new guidelines between 2013 to 2015 and 2017 regarding invasive ventilation (80.1% vs. 80.8%), inhaled nitric oxide (28.8% vs. 28.4%) or ECMO (0.81% vs. 0.35%). There was a significant increase in noninvasive ventilation for MAS during the study period (24.5% vs. 36.5%). The incidence of morbidity including moderate to severe hypoxic-ischemic encephalopathy (10% vs. 9.7%) and pneumothorax (10% vs. 11%) and mortality (6.1% vs. 5.3%) remained unchanged.

It is hypothesized that prompt resuscitation and positive pressure ventilation of the lungs without delaying for tracheal intubation and suctioning could potentially limit hypoxic-ischemic damage to the heart and brain, necessitating fewer NICU admissions because of MAS.

## SUGGESTED READINGS

ACOG Committee on Obstetric Practice. (2017). ACOG Committee Opinion No. 689, Delivery of a newborn with meconium-stained amniotic fluid. *Obstetrics and Gynecology, 129*(3), e33–e34. Reaffirmed, 2021.

Argyridis, S., & Arulkumaran, S. (2016). Meconium stained amniotic fluid. *Obstetrics Gynaecology and Reproductive Medicine, 26*(8), 227–230.

Aziz, K., Lee, H. C., Escobedo, M. B., Hoover, A. V., Kamath-Rayne, B. D., Kapadia, V. S., et al. (2020).

Part 5: Neonatal Resuscitation: 2020 American Heart Association Guidelines for Cardiopulmonary Resuscitation and Emergency Cardiovascular Care. *Circulation, 142*(16_suppl_2), S524–S550.

Kalra, V. K., Lee, H. C., Sie, L., Ratnasiri, A. W., Underwood, M. A., & Lakshminrusimha, S. (2020). Change in neonatal resuscitation guidelines and trends in incidence of meconium aspiration syndrome in California. *Journal of Perinatology, 40*(1), 46–55.

Olicker, A. L., Raffay, T. M., & Ryan, R. M. (2021). Neonatal respiratory distress secondary to meconium aspiration syndrome. *Children (Basel, Switzerland), 8*(3), 246. doi:10.3390/children 8030246.

Vain, N. E., & Batton, D. G. (2017). Meconium "aspiration" (or respiratory distress associated with meconium-stained amniotic fluid?). *Seminars in Fetal & Neonatal Medicine, 22*(4), 214–219.

# 180

# Risks of General Anesthesia and Sedation Drugs in Pediatric Patients

DEVON AGANGA, MD   |   MICHAEL E. NEMERGUT, MD, PhD   |
RANDALL PAUL FLICK, MD, MPH

## Introduction

Anesthetic drugs are potent modulators of the central nervous system (CNS) and reversibly render patients insensate to surgical procedures. Most anesthetic drugs are either γ-aminobutyric acid (GABA) receptor agonists or N-methyl-D-aspartate (NMDA) glutamate receptor antagonists, or a combination of the two. Both GABA agonists and NMDA antagonists have been implicated in causing anesthetic-induced developmental neurotoxicity (AIDN). AIDN refers to the apoptosis and resultant reduction in neural density observed in experimental animal studies and by disturbances in memory, attention, and learning observed in preclinical and clinical studies looking at the effect of commonly used anesthetic drugs on the developing brain. Retrospective human studies have reported an association between exposure of young children to general anesthesia and an

| TABLE 180.1 | List of General Anesthetic and Sedation Drugs Affected by FDA Label Change | |
|---|---|---|
| **Generic Name** | **Brand Name** | |
| Desflurane | Suprane | |
| Halothane | Only generic available | |
| Isoflurane | Forane | |
| Sevoflurane | Ultane, Sojourn | |
| Etomidate | Amidate | |
| Ketamine | Ketalar | |
| Lorazepam injection | Ativan | |
| Methohexital | Brevital | |
| Midazolam injection, syrup | Only generic available | |
| Pentobarbital | Nembutal | |
| Propofol | Diprivan | |

increased risk of developing learning deficits; however, recent human studies suggest that a single, relatively short exposure to general anesthesia with inhaled and/or intravenous anesthetic drugs in infants and young children is unlikely to have negative effects on their behavior or learning. Further research is needed to fully characterize what effect, if any, exposure to sedatives/anesthetics has on children's brain development. To inform the public about the potential risk, the FDA now requires warning labels to be added to general anesthetic and sedation drugs (Table 180.1). This chapter will discuss the evidence of the effects of anesthetic agents on neuronal structure and neurocognitive function in laboratory animals and evaluate its relevance to the practice of pediatric anesthesia.

## Development Neuroscience

Neonatal brains are estimated to contain approximately 100 billion neurons and weigh between 300 and 400 g. Increased myelination, synapse formation, neuron maturation, and proliferation of glial cells increase the weight of the brain to 1100 g at 3 years of age and up to 1400 g by adulthood. In utero, the CNS goes through extensive neurogenesis, which is almost completed by the end of the second trimester. CNS development is marked by massive growth in the last trimester of gestation and through the first 3 years of postnatal life. In the first year of life, there is extensive dendritic branching, myelination, and glia proliferation. During this time there is also ongoing synaptogenesis, a process requiring key synchronized events to occur. The formation of synapses then leads to neuronal maturation, differentiation, and creation of neuronal circuits via processes tightly controlled by glial cells. Synaptogenesis, which has been characterized as among the most critical periods of brain development, consists of five phases. Phase 3, which marks the peak of synapse formation, corresponds to the neonatal period. Phase 4, which has synapse formation occurring at nearly the same speed as during phase 3, occurs during infancy to adolescence. It is important to note that the brain's sensitivity to environmental stimuli is at a maximum during the neonatal and infancy periods when synaptogenesis is at its peak.

The neurotransmitter glutamate promotes all key aspects of neuronal development, and the balance between GABA-mediated and glutamate-mediated neurotransmission is important for the timely formation of synapses and neuronal circuits. Neurons that do not make consequential connections are marked as redundant and undergo programmed cell death, or *apoptosis*. Apoptosis of neurons is a normal, tightly controlled, and essential phase in CNS development; gene mutations that render laboratory animals unable to undergo this process are lethal. Disruption in the GABA and glutamate-mediated signaling balance during this phase of brain development may promote excessive activation of neuro-apoptosis and death of large populations of developing neurons. General anesthetics have been reported to cause widespread neuroapoptotic degeneration of developing neurons in a variety of mammals in animal studies, including nonhuman primates. Of note, the peak of vulnerability to AIDN in each species was found to coincide with its peak of synaptogenesis, with much less vulnerability observed in later stages.

## Description of Anesthetic-Induced Developmental Neurotoxicity

Accelerated apoptosis is the hallmark of AIDN (Table 180.2). Although neuroapoptosis is a vital pathway in regulating neural development, it has also been reported to be in response to cellular stresses such as hypoxia, radiation, heat, exogenous glucocorticoids, starvation, infection, and pain. Apoptosis is commonly mediated through a cascade of cysteine-dependent aspartyl proteases called *caspases*. These caspases are activated by two pathways: the mitochondrial-dependent apoptotic cascade (the *intrinsic pathway*) and the death receptor–dependent apoptotic cascade (the *extrinsic pathway*). The intrinsic pathway, in response to stress, causes the release of proapoptotic proteins such as cytochrome c into the cytoplasm, which activates the caspase cascade resulting in apoptosis. Exposure to general anesthetic agents impairs mitochondrial function, which has been reported to induce the intrinsic apoptotic pathway. Interestingly, melatonin, a sleep hormone, has been reported to offer some protection in laboratory animals by inhibition of cytochrome c leakage and caspase activation, although evidence of clinical efficacy is absent. Apoptosis can also proceed via the extrinsic pathway involving the formation of a death-inducing signaling complex (DISC),

| TABLE 180.2 | Key Features of Anesthetic-Induced Developmental Neurotoxicity | |
|---|---|---|
| **Feature** | **Description** | |
| Pathologic apoptosis | The hallmark of AIDN Can be induced by intrinsic or extrinsic pathways | |
| Impeded neurogenesis | Effect of anesthetics on neurogenesis is age dependent | |
| Altered dendritic development | Anesthetics affect dendritic morphogenesis in age-dependent manner | |
| Aberrant glial development | Isoflurane can interfere with release of trophic factors by astrocytes affecting synaptogenesis | |

Taken from McCann ME, Soriano II SG. Anesthetic neurotoxicity. In: Pardo MC Jr, Miller RD, eds. *Basics of Anesthesia*. 7th ed. Elsevier; 2018:176–188.

which results in activation of the caspase cascade and neuronal cell death. Exposure to general anesthetics can also promote DISC formation; however, studies show that there is anesthesia-induced activation of the intrinsic pathway first.

Anesthetics affect neurogenesis in animals in an age-dependent manner. Isoflurane causes loss of neural stem cells and reduced neurogenesis in neonatal but not adult rats. Propofol is reported to decrease hippocampal cell proliferation in young rats but not in adults. Exposure to isoflurane impairs growth and delayed maturation of astrocytes in young animals. Anesthetics have also been found to affect dendritic morphogenesis in a similar age-dependent manner. Dendritic spines are small protrusions of neurons that receive input from a single synapse of an axon and are invaluable components of synaptogenesis. Mice pups exposed to isoflurane were found to have decreases in synapse and dendritic spine density; likewise, rat pups exposed to propofol at postnatal days 5 and 10 also showed significantly decreased dendritic spine density, whereas older rat pups showed a significant increase in spine density with the same propofol exposure. The implications of this observation are unclear. Isoflurane can interfere with release of trophic factors by astrocytes, which are essential in guiding migration and synaptogenesis during neuronal development. Isoflurane is also thought to interfere with the release of brain-derived neurotrophic factor by astrocytes, which leads to deprivation of neurons of trophic support for axonal growth. Decrements in neurocognitive function occur after fetal and neonatal exposure to anesthetic agents in animal studies. Exposed rodents were found to have decreased performance compared with rodents that were not exposed to general anesthesia in standard behavioral measuring tests.

## Anesthetic and Sedative Drugs

Anesthetic drugs elicit their effects by enhancing the activity of major inhibitory neurotransmitters such as GABA and/or antagonizing the NMDA receptors of the major excitatory neurotransmitter glutamate. During brain development, GABA facilitates cell proliferation, neuroblast migration, and dendritic maturation and acts as an excitatory neurotransmitter during infancy rather than an inhibitory neurotransmitter. When the GABA receptor is engaged, the immature Na/K/2Cl transporter protein NKCC1 produces a chloride influx leading to neuron depolarization. As a result of this depolarization, GABA remains excitatory until the GABA neurons switch to the normal inhibitory mode. This occurs when the mature chloride transporter, KCC2, is expressed, which results in active transport of chloride out of the neural cell. This switch to the normal inhibitory mode is completed at about 1 year of age in human infants. Alternatively, the NMDA receptor is activated when bound by glutamate, glycine, or D-serine and is important for synaptic plasticity and needed for learning and memory. Ketamine, an NMDA receptor antagonist, has been associated with AIDN in animals and has been shown to cause an upregulation of subunits of the NMDA receptor. Opioids generally do not increase neuroapoptosis, but under experimental conditions, repeated morphine administration over 7 days is associated with increased apoptosis in the sensory cortex and amygdala of neonatal rats. However, a single dose of morphine administered on postnatal day 7 did not cause this increase in neuroapoptosis in developing rats.

The duration and the dosage of medications are key factors in any toxicity study and appear to be important factors in

AIDN. Almost all animal studies involved an anesthetic exposure of at least 4 hours, with some trials exposing animals to up to 24 hours of continuous anesthesia. Exposures of less than 1 hour, regardless of the animal model studied, did not result in an increase in neuroapoptosis.

It is also important to note that studies have also reported several drugs to confer some neuroprotective properties to alleviate AIDN. These drugs include dexmedetomidine, melatonin, erythropoietin, estrogen, lithium, pilocarpine, xenon, L-carnitine, and estradiol. At clinical doses, dexmedetomidine has been found to mitigate isoflurane-induced neuroapoptosis and behavioral impairment.

## Clinical Evidence for Anesthesia-Induced Developmental Neurotoxicity

Although many animal studies have been conducted studying AIDN, extrapolation of this data to the human neonate and the practice of pediatric and obstetric anesthesia is very problematic. There is wide variability in the developmental timelines of mammalian brains, from a few weeks in a rat brain to the many years required for human brain maturation. Also of important consideration is the dose and duration of anesthetics used in these experimental animal models as these doses may not directly correlate with anesthetic exposure times used in clinical practice. For example, adjusted for the life span of a rat, 6 hours of anesthesia would correspond to 1 month of continuous anesthesia using a human lifespan. Finally, the implication that exposure to general anesthesia may be harmful to young children has been limited to retrospective epidemiologic studies, which can be confounded by the effects of surgery, as well as the patient's underlying medical and surgical conditions. Table 180.3 lists a sampling of recent clinical studies that have looked at AIDN in clinical practice.

Two recent studies that looked at AIDN in children were the Pediatric Anesthesia NeuroDevelopment Assessment (PANDA) and the General Anesthesia Compared with Spinal Anesthesia (GAS) trial. The PANDA study is a sibling-matched observational cohort study that examined whether a single exposure to general anesthesia in healthy children younger than 3 years is associated with an increased risk of impaired global cognitive function. The GAS study is an international, multicenter, randomized controlled trial comparing neurocognitive outcomes of children after they were assigned to receive either sevoflurane-based general anesthesia versus awake-neuraxial anesthesia for inguinal herniorrhaphy. In both studies, the authors reported no significant difference between the two study groups. In the Mayo Anesthesia Safety in Kids (MASK) matched cohort study, children who had no anesthetic exposure, a single exposure, and multiple exposures to general anesthesia before 3 years of age were tested for general intelligence and neuropsychologic parameters. There was no difference in intelligence scores between the groups. However, children with multiple anesthetic exposures were more likely to have modest decreases in fine motor coordination, behavioral problems, and processing speed.

## Conclusion

Evidence for AIDN has been reported in multiple preclinical studies from many animal species including nonhuman primates. Evidence from human studies is more limited and largely retrospective. Many retrospective studies have reported learning

| TABLE 180.3 | Sample of Clinical Studies Looking at Anesthetic-Induced Developmental Neurotoxicity in Clinical Practice | |
|---|---|---|
| **NO ASSOCIATION** | | |
| Kalkman 2009 | Retrospective, Netherlands | No ability to confirm an effect<br>Study underpowered |
| Bartels 2009 | Twin study, Netherlands | No difference between exposed and unexposed twin |
| Hansen 2011 | Retrospective, Denmark | No evidence of any effects of a single exposure |
| Guerra 2011 | Prospective, Canada | No association between dose/duration of sedation/analgesia and neurodevelopmental outcome |
| Ko 2014 | Retrospective, Taiwan | No increased risk of ADHD diagnosis for single or multiple exposure |
| Sun 2016 | Sibling match cohort, United States (PANDA) | No risk for healthy children with single exposure |
| Davidson 2016 | Randomized controlled trial, multinational (GAS) | General anesthesia vs. neuraxial anesthesia<br>Median general anesthesia time was 54 minutes<br>No significant difference between two groups at age 2 years in cognitive testing |
| **ASSOCIATED NEGATIVE OUTCOME** | | |
| Wilder 2009 | Retrospective, United States | Significant increased risk of learning disability with multiple but not single exposure |
| DiMaggio 2009 | Retrospective, United States | Children who had hernia repair more than two times more likely to be diagnosed with a developmental or behavioral disorder |
| DiMaggio 2011 | Retrospective, United States | Anesthesia-exposed group risk of diagnosis 60% higher; no causal connection can be made<br>Higher risk with multiple exposures |
| Flick 2011 | Retrospective, United States | Multiple exposures to general anesthesia increases risk for a learning disorder, but no associating with single exposure |
| Sprung 2012 | Retrospective, United States | No increased risk with single exposure, but increased risk for attention-deficit/hyperactivity disorder with repeated exposure |
| Ing 2014 | Retrospective, Australia | Deficits in language and abstract reasoning associated with anesthesia exposure |

deficits in children exposed to multiple anesthetics at an early age, although such a finding has not been universal. One recent prospective trial compared neuraxial to general anesthesia in infants undergoing a single surgery (inguinal herniorrhaphy) and was unable to find differences in cognitive testing at 2 years of age. Of note, many cognitive domains cannot be evaluated at such an age and the primary outcome of the study involved cognitive testing at 5 years of age, which are years into the future. Thus although evidence in laboratory animals is robust and concerning, evidence in humans is limited and unclear and therefore future research is required for clarification. Additional research is also needed to explore possible subtle behavioral effects, vulnerable ages of exposure, potential gender differences, and potential variability among specific anesthetic drugs and protocols.

## SUGGESTED READINGS

Bartels, M., Althoff, R. R., & Boomsma, D. I. (2009). Anesthesia and cognitive performance in children: no evidence for a causal relationship. *Twin Research and Human Genetics, 12*(3), 246–253. doi:10.1375/twin.12.3.246.

Davidson, A. J., Disma, N., de Graaff, J. C., Withington, D. E., Dorris, L., Bell, G., et al. (2016). Neurodevelopmental outcome at 2 years of age after general anaesthesia and awake-regional anaesthesia in infancy (GAS): An international multicentre, randomised controlled trial. *Lancet (London, England), 387*(10015), 239–250.

DiMaggio, C., Sun, L. S., Kakavouli, A., Byrne, M. W., & Li, G. (2009). A retrospective cohort study of the Association of Anesthesia and Hernia Repair Surgery with behavioral and developmental disorders in young children. *Journal of Neurosurgical Anesthesiology, 21*(4), 286–291. doi:10.1097/ANA.0b013e3181a71f11.

DiMaggio, C., Sun, L. S., & Li, G. (2011). Early childhood exposure to anesthesia and risk of developmental and behavioral disorders in a sibling birth cohort. *Anesthesia and Analgesia, 113*(5), 1143–1151. doi:10.1213/ANE.0b013e3182147f42.

Eckenhoff, R., & Jevtovic-Todorovic, V. (2020). Perioperative and anesthesia neurotoxicity. In R. Miller, N. Cohen, L. Eriksson, L. Fleisher, J. Wiener-Kronish, & W. Young (Eds.), *Miller's anesthesia* (9th ed., pp. 2420–2459). Philadelphia, PA: Elsevier.

Fda, Cder. FDA Drug Safety Communication. *FDA review results in new warnings about using general anesthetics and sedation drugs in young children and pregnant women.* Retrieved from https://www.fda.gov/downloads/Drugs/DrugSafety/UCM533197.pdf.

Flick, R. P., Katusic, S. K., Colligan, R. C., Wilder, R. T., Voigt, R. G., Olson, M. D., et al. (2011). Cognitive and behavioral outcomes after early exposure to anesthesia and surgery. *Pediatrics, 128*(5), e1053–e1061. doi:10.1542/peds.2011-0351.

Guerra, G. G., Robertson, C. M., Alton, G. Y., Joffe, A. R., Cave, D. A., Dinu, I. A., et al. (2011). Neurodevelopmental outcome following exposure to sedative and analgesic drugs for complex cardiac surgery in infancy. *Paediatric Anaesthesia, 21*(9), 932–941. doi:10.1111/j.1460-9592.2011.03581.x.

Hansen, T. G., Pedersen, J. K., Henneberg, S. W., Pedersen, D. A., Murray, J. C., Morton, N. S., et al. (2011). Academic performance in adolescence after inguinal hernia repair in infancy: A nationwide cohort study. *Anesthesiology, 114*(5), 1076–1085. doi:10.1097/ALN.0b013e31820e77a0.

Ing, C. H., DiMaggio, C. J., Whitehouse, A. J., Hegarty, M. K., Sun, M., von Ungern-Sternberg, S. B., et al. (2014). Neurodevelopmental outcomes after initial childhood anesthetic exposure between ages 3 and 10 years. *Journal of Neurosurgical Anesthesiology, 26*(4), 377–386. doi:10.1097/ANA.0000000000000121.

Kalkman, C. J., Peelen, L., Moons, K. G., Veenhuizen, M., Bruens, M., Sinnema, G., et al. (2009). Behavior and development in children and age at the time of first anesthetic exposure. *Anesthesiology, 110*(4), 805–812. doi:10.1097/ALN.0b013e31819c7124.

Ko, W. R., Liaw, Y. P., Huang, J. Y., Zhao, D. H., Chang, H. C., Ko, P. C., et al. (2014). Exposure to general anesthesia in early life and the risk of attention deficit/hyperactivity disorder development: A nationwide, retrospective matched-cohort study. *Paediatric Anaesthesia, 24*(7), 741–748. doi:10.1111/pan.12371.

Montana, M. C., & Evers, A. S. (2017). Anesthetic neurotoxicity: New findings and future directions. *Journal of Pediatrics, 181,* 279–285.

Sprung, J., Flick, R. P., Katusic, S. K., Colligan, R. C., Barbaresi, W. J., Bojanić, K., et al. (2012). Attention-deficit/hyperactivity disorder after early exposure

to procedures requiring general anesthesia. *Mayo Clinic Proceedings, 87*(2), 120–129. doi:10.1016/j.mayocp.2011.11.008.

Sun, L. S., Li, G., Miller, T. L., Salorio, C., Byrne, M. W., Bellinger, D. C., et al. (2016). Association between a single general anesthesia exposure before age 36 months and neurocognitive outcomes in later childhood. *JAMA, 315*(21), 2312–2320.

Warner, D. O., Zaccariello, M. J., Katusic, S. K., Schroeder, D. R., Hanson, A. C., Schulte, P. J., et al. (2018). Neuropsychological and behavioral outcomes after

exposure of young children to procedures requiring general anesthesia: The Mayo Anesthesia Safety in Kids (MASK) Study. *Anesthesiology, 129*(1), 89–105.

Wilder, R. T., Flick, R. P., Sprung, J., Katusic, S. K., Barbaresi, W. J., Mickelson, C., et al. (2009). Early exposure to anesthesia and learning disabilities in a population-based birth cohort. *Anesthesiology, 110*(4), 796–804. doi:10.1097/01.anes.0000344728.34332.5d.

# 181

# Neonatal Cardiovascular Physiology

ROXANN BARNES PIKE, MD

To properly care for patients in the neonatal period, it is necessary to understand normal fetal circulation, the physiology of the neonatal heart and circulation, and the transition between the two, during and after the birth process.

## Fetal Circulation

In the fetal circulation the right (RV) and left ventricles (LV) are in parallel, whereas in the postnatal circulation the ventricles are in series. Because the fetal lungs are not inflated, the placenta is responsible for gas exchange, and therefore there must be mixing and redirection of blood flow. The fetal parallel circulation is created by several shunts and preferential blood flow patterns that deliver relatively well-oxygenated blood from the placenta to those fetal organs that have increased metabolic demand, such as the brain and heart. The most important structures that provide mixing and preferential blood flow in the fetal circulation are the ductus venosus (DV), the foramen ovale (FO), and the ductus arteriosus (DA).

From the placenta, blood with a partial pressure of oxygen ($Po_2$) of 30 to 35 mm Hg flows to the fetus via the umbilical vein (UV) (Fig. 181.1), which, in the liver of the fetus, separates into two branches, with one branch joining the portal vein and the other becoming the DV, which joins the inferior vena cava (IVC). Approximately 50% to 60% of the oxygenated UV blood flowing will bypass the hepatic circulation and flow directly through the DV into the IVC, mixing with deoxygenated IVC blood flowing along its posterior wall, toward the FO. The FO is a hole in the atrial septum formed by the overlapping of the septum primum inferiorly/leftward and the septum secundum superiorly/rightward. As this oxygenated blood enters the right atrium, more than half the blood is directed across the FO into the left atrium by the eustachian valve, being ejected out of the

LV into the proximal aorta, which immediately supplies the coronaries and coronary arteries primarily.

The deoxygenated blood returning from the superior vena cava, and from the myocardium via the coronary sinus (mixed with the remainder of the IVC blood), tends to stream directly at the tricuspid valve into the RV, where it is ejected out the pulmonary artery (PA). Because the lungs are not inflated and pulmonary vascular resistance (PVR) is high in the lungs, blood is preferentially shunted through the DA. Most of this deoxygenated blood returns to the proximal descending aorta via the DA, and only a small percentage of the cardiac output passes through the high-resistance pulmonary circulation. Blood in the descending aorta either flows through the umbilical arteries to be reoxygenated in the placenta or continues to supply the lower body and limbs. This fetal streaming is advantageous for the fetus because the oxygen is directed to where it is metabolically needed the most, namely the heart and brain. The fetal circulation therefore runs in parallel, with the LV providing 35% and the RV providing 65% of cardiac output.

These three major shunts are under autonomic, neural, and hormonal control. The DV, for example, is not a passive shunt: the vessel is trumpet-shaped, with a sphincter at its distal end that regulates flow by β-adrenergic dilation or α-adrenergic constriction. Hypoxemia, presumably caused by release of endothelial nitric oxide, results in significant vasodilation. Prostaglandins ostensibly have an important role, as they do in the DA, in maintaining patency and in closure after birth.

The DA is a wide muscular vessel that connects the PA to the descending aorta. Most of the blood ejected from the RV into the PA crosses the DA and flows to the lower torso, lower extremities, and the umbilical arteries. At this point, 5% to 10% of the right ventricular output flows beyond the DA into the pulmonary circulation because, before inflation of the lungs at

**Fetal circulation**

**Neonatal circulation**

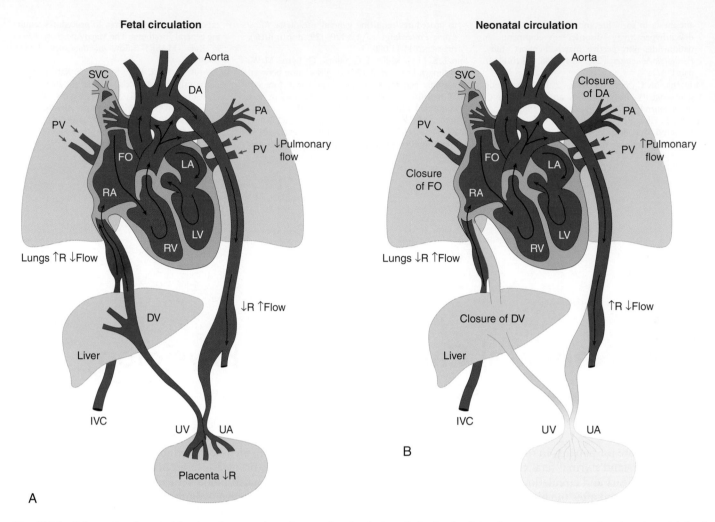

**Fig. 181.1** Schematic of normal fetal and neonatal cardiovascular circulation. **A,** During fetal development, oxygenated and nutrient-rich fetal blood from the placenta passes to the fetus via the umbilical vein. Approximately half of this blood bypasses the liver via the ductus venosus *(DV)* and enters the inferior vena cava *(IVC)*. The remainder enters the portal vein to supply the liver with nutrients and oxygen. Blood entering the right atrium *(RA)* from the IVC bypasses the right ventricle *(RV)*, as the lungs are not yet functioning, and then enters the left atrium *(LA)* via the foramen ovale *(FO)*. Blood from the superior vena cava *(SVC)* enters the RA, passes to the RV, and moves into the pulmonary artery *(PA)* trunk. Most of this blood enters the aorta via the ductus arteriosus *(DA)*, a right-to-left shunt. The partially oxygenated blood in the aorta returns to the placenta via the paired umbilical arteries *(UAs)* that arise from the internal iliac arteries. **B,** Under normal physiologic conditions, when pulmonary respiration begins at birth, pulmonary blood pressure falls, causing blood from the main PA trunk to enter the left PA and right PA, become oxygenated at the lungs, and then return to the LA via the pulmonary veins *(PVs)*. The FO and DA close, eliminating the fetal right-to-left shunts. The pulmonary and systemic circulations in the heart are now separate. As the infant is separated from the placenta, the UAs occlude (except for the proximal portions), along with the umbilical vein and DV. Blood to be metabolized now passes through the liver. (Permission granted from Tan CMJ, Lewandowski AJ. The transitional heart: from early embryonic and fetal development to neonatal life. *Fetal Diagn Ther.* 2020;47(5):373–386.)

the time of birth, the PVR is quite high secondary to collapsed alveoli compressing the interstitium of the lung. Despite the small amount of supplied blood, it is sufficient to meet the metabolic needs for development and growth of the lungs.

Fetal cardiac output increases from 210 mL/min at 20 weeks' gestation to 1900 mL/min at term. Two-thirds of the total aortic flow goes to the placenta because the systemic vascular resistance (SVR) within the placental blood vessels is relatively low, compared with the resistance in the blood vessels within the fetal organs and tissues. Placental blood flow is relatively stable, unaffected by autonomic or neural inputs, and correlates best with maternal arterial blood pressure.

The fetal ventricles are stiff and poorly compliant, with the RV less so than the LV, in part from the constraint of the pericardium, collapsed lungs, and constrained chest wall. They are therefore limited in their ability to increase stroke volume, so

that an increase in cardiac output is achieved by an increase in heart rate. Thus, if heart rate decrease is significant, cardiac output drops significantly. During fetal life, there is very little difference between fetal right and left ventricular pressures, unlike in the postnatal state.

## Transition to Neonatal Circulation

For seamless transition from the placenta to the lung as the primary source of gas (oxygen and carbon dioxide) exchange, two abrupt changes occur: (1) a dramatic increase in SVR caused by removal of the placenta (which has a low SVR); and (2) inflation of the lungs, causing an equally dramatic lowering in PVR mediated by increased production of endogenous nitric oxide via up-regulation of nitric oxide synthase. Because the direction of flow across the DA is determined by SVR and PVR, these changes lead to a shift from fetal right-to-left flow to the newborn left-to-right flow. Normally, smaller vessels in the lungs continue to dilate for 24 to 48 hours after birth. Through a combination of change in directional flow, an increase in Po$_2$ with lung inflation, and a drop in prostaglandin E (which is synthesized in the placenta) along with chemicals such as bradykinin, the unique contractile elements in the DA start to constrict. However, the pulmonary vasculature of the neonate is very sensitive to hypoxia, acidosis, and hypercarbia, which may trigger pulmonary vasoconstriction and dilation, respectively, rather than closure of the DA. If the precipitating factors are left untreated, life-threatening conditions such as persistent hypertension of the newborn (PPHN) and persistent fetal circulation (PFC) may develop.

The closure of the FO is based on pressure differences between the right and left atria. The RV compliance gradually increases, and the resultant difference in compliances between the RV and LV allow the "flap" of FO to gradually close, decreasing mixing. After birth, SVR rises, PVR declines. The output of the RV goes through the lungs, increasing pulmonary venous return to the left atrium. The significantly increased left atrial pressure forces the flap of the FO to press against the septum, functionally closing the opening between the right and left atria, and this combined with changes in oxygenation, SVR, and PVR that occur at birth functionally close the fetal shunts, and the ventricles begin working in series. The flow in the DV starts to diminish once the UV flow disappears after placental separation and occurs functionally between 3 and 7 days after birth and is obliterated by 1 to 3 weeks. Unlike the DA, there is no identifiable trigger for its closure.

Flow through the DA changes from a right-to-left shunt to a left-to-right shunt until functional closure occurs, usually within 24 to 48 hours. Anatomic closure normally occurs within 4 to 8 weeks of life; however, the DA will remain patent in the presence of hypoxemia, PPHN, sepsis, and other pathologic conditions.

## Neonatal Cardiovascular Physiology

Fetal myocytes are morphologically different from those of pediatric and adult myocytes in that they are smaller and more immature with less cellular and structural organization and have fewer contractile proteins and are less compliant. This means neonatal cells have less cellular mitochondria and DNA, fewer myofibrils, and display greater myofibril disorganization, and they also have less actin and myosin, making the fetal heart much stiffer. The implication of this is that it is less able to respond to volume loading on the Frank-Starling curve. Growth of the fetal heart occurs by hyperplasia (cell proliferation) of the myocytes, accounting for the increased size of the heart temporarily after birth. The RV is larger than the LV at birth because of the nature of the fetal circulation, but within a few months after birth the LV increases in size by a factor of 3 secondary to its increased afterload.

Immediately after birth, the neonate's stroke volume nearly doubles because of an increased preload (removal of the placenta) and because of increased thoracic compliance (decreased mechanical encroachment on the mediastinum).

Diastolic function of the heart depends on myocardial relaxation and compliance. Initially, the neonatal heart is much less compliant than the adult heart because of immaturity of the sarcoplasmic reticulum and its inability to sequester calcium during diastole. The decreased compliance limits the ventricular response to preload; excessive preload places the ventricle on the downslope to the right of the Starling curve. Although diastolic function improves with age, neonatal cardiac output is as dependent on heart rate as it was in utero. The typical neonatal heart rate is usually above 140 beats/min to achieve a cardiac output (150–200 mL · kg$^{-1}$ · min$^{-1}$); this is twice the adult value based on weight because of the need to meet high neonatal oxygen requirements. Heart rate is typically 160 to 180 beats/min the first 30 minutes after birth, but then settles around 100 to 160 beats/min after that.

Because of the decreased compliance of the ventricles and immaturity of the autonomic nervous system, cardiac output in neonates is more affected by changes in SVR than it is in infants, and much more so than in the adult heart. Beat-to-beat variability improves over time as the autonomic nervous system matures.

Mean arterial pressure is more dependent on vascular tone than myocardial function. Baroreflexes are impaired after birth, manifested by hypotension with relatively small decreases in preload. Because of the immature autonomic nervous system, direct agonists, compared with indirect agonists, are more effective for increasing heart rate and blood pressure in neonates.

Neonatal PVR remains relatively high after birth because the pulmonary arterioles have a thicker layer of muscle relative to their diameter, compared with infants or adults, which results in greater sensitivity to hypoxemia and hypercarbia, sometimes causing PFC. When diagnosing PFC, the clinician must exclude parenchymal lung disease or congenital heart disease as causes of the patient's symptoms and signs. There are many causes of PFC, but once PFC is diagnosed, the administration of nitric oxide or a vasodilating prostaglandin decreases PVR; attenuates, if not abolishes, the PFC; and eliminates the right-to-left shunt.

Finally, after birth there is a switch to cardiomyocyte hypertrophy. The neonatal myocardium has an underdeveloped sarcoplasmic reticulum and is significantly more dependent on extracellular calcium sources. A decrease in contractility and hypotension can ensue when ionized calcium levels are low, so careful attention must be paid to calcium levels in the neonatal period.

## Acknowledgment

The author wishes to acknowledge William C. Oliver Jr., MD, for his valuable contributions to previous versions of this chapter.

## SUGGESTED READINGS

Abdulla, R., Blew, G. A., & Holterman, M. J. (2004). Cardiovascular embryology. *Pediatric Cardiology*, *25*(3), 191–200.

Benson, D. W. (2000). Advances in cardiovascular genetics and embryology: Role of transcription factors in congenital heart disease. *Current Opinion in Pediatrics*, *12*(5), 497–500.

Hines, M. H. (2013). Neonatal cardiovascular physiology. *Seminars in Pediatric Surgery*, *22*(4), 174–178.

Kiserud, T. (2005). Physiology of the fetal circulation. *Seminars in Fetal & Neonatal Medicine*, *10*(6), 493–503.

Lake, C. L., & Booker, P. D. (Eds.). (2005). *Pediatric Cardiac Anesthesia* (4th ed., pp. 1–22). Philadelphia: Lippincott, Williams & Wilkins.

Rudolph, A. M. (2000). Myocardial growth before and after birth: Clinical implications. *Acta Paediatrica (Oslo, Norway: 1992)*, *89*(2), 129–133.

Soufan, A. T., van den Berg, G., Moerland, P. D., Massink, M. M., van den Hoff, M. J., Moorman, A. F., et al. (2007). Three-dimensional measurement and visualization of morphogenesis applied to cardiac embryology. *Journal of Microscopy*, *225*(Pt 3), 269–274.

Tan, C. M. J., & Lewandowski, A. J. (2020). The transitional heart: From early embryonic and fetal development to neonatal life. *Fetal Diagnosis and Therapy*, *47*(5), 373–386.

# Differences Between the Infant and Adult Airway

LEAL G. SEGURA, MD | DANIEL THUM, MD

Subtle yet significant differences exist between the infant and adult airway in both structure and function (Fig. 182.1). Comprehensive understanding of these differences is vital for effective airway management of pediatric patients.

## Anatomy

### HEAD SIZE

The infant's head is proportionately larger than that of an adult because of a prominent occiput. The prominent occiput may contribute to neck flexion and subsequent airway obstruction when an infant is supine. When such obstruction occurs, a small, folded towel under the shoulders and neck may slightly elevate the thorax and reduce excessive flexion. Elevation of the head to produce an anatomic sniffing position is usually unnecessary in most infants and children because of the prominent occiput. The head should be stabilized during laryngoscopy to prevent excessive side-to-side motion produced by the typical infant head shape.

### LARYNGEAL POSITION

The infant's larynx is significantly more cephalad and anterior than the adult larynx. Imaging studies confirm an elevated laryngeal position at C3–C4 in the infant, compared with the adult level of C4–C5. The anterior and cephalad position of the larynx create an acute angle between the plane of the tongue and the larynx, with a decreased distance between the tongue,

hyoid bone, and epiglottis. If these differences are not appreciated, this short distance and anterior position may lead to difficult glottic visualization during direct laryngoscopy. Further, placement of a shoulder roll may bring the already anterior and high larynx even more anterocephalad, preventing a glottic view on laryngoscopy.

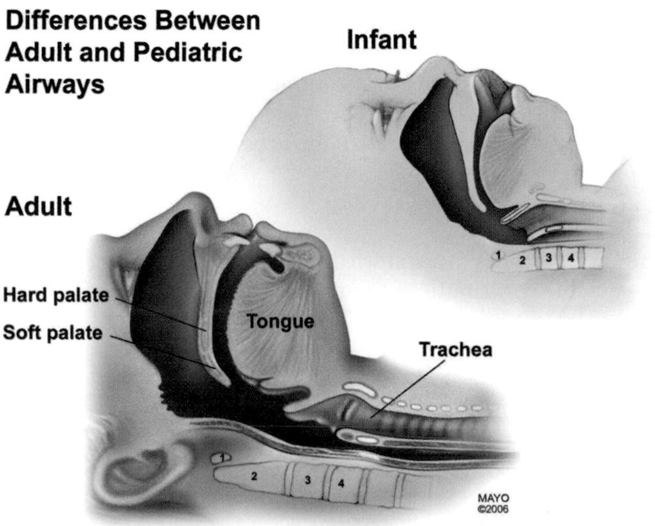

Functionally, this anatomic arrangement allows the tongue to oppose the palate more easily, providing a functional separation between breathing and swallowing, and allowing the infant to suck, swallow, and breathe without aspiration. The larynx ultimately descends throughout childhood, eventually reaching an adult position between ages 5 and 8 years. By this time, the spatial relationships between the tongue, hyoid bone, epiglottis, and other oral structures become similar to those in an adult.

### TONGUE

The infant's tongue has historically been described as proportionately larger than the adult tongue and thus has been identified as a common cause of airway obstruction. However, recent radiologic studies challenge this assertion and suggest that the infant tongue may contribute less to upper airway obstruction than nasopharyngeal or epiglottic collapse. Oral airways often relieve upper airway obstruction during mask ventilation in infants and children, regardless of cause.

### EPIGLOTTIS

The infant's epiglottis is proportionally longer and narrower compared with the adult epiglottis. It is often described as omega-shaped, whereas the adult epiglottis is typically flatter and more flexible. Because the infant hyoid bone overlaps the superior aspect of the thyroid cartilage, the base of the infant tongue depresses the epiglottis and causes it to protrude into the pharyngeal cavity in a more retroflexed position than the parallel position found in adult airways. With age, the hyoid bone and the thyroid cartilage separate, and the epiglottis becomes more flexible.

### VOCAL FOLDS

The vocal folds are composed of the vocal ligament anteriorly and the cartilaginous vocal process of the arytenoid posteriorly. The anterior insertion of the vocal fold is attached in a more caudal position in an infant, causing an angled position relative to the perpendicular position of adult vocal cords. This angled position, lower anteriorly than posteriorly, can make passage of endotracheal tubes (ETTs) difficult if the tip of an ETT gets caught at the more caudal anterior commissure. This difficulty can often be overcome with gentle rotation of the tracheal tube's tip away from the commissure.

**Differences Between Adult and Pediatric Airways**

Infant

Adult

Hard palate

Soft palate

Tongue

Trachea

**Fig. 182.1** Differences between the pediatric and adult airway. (By permission of Mayo Foundation for Medical Research and Education. All rights reserved.)

## SUBGLOTTIS

Classic teaching, based on anatomic and cadaveric studies, states that the infant airway is funnel-shaped relative to the cylindrical adult airway, with the narrowest point at the level of the cricoid cartilage instead of the vocal folds, the narrowest point in the adult airway. Indeed, the cricoid ring is the only complete cartilage ring in the airway and is nonexpandable, whereas the trachea has a membranous muscle posteriorly that allows for increased compliance. However, this dogma describing a funnel-shaped infant larynx tapering to its narrowest point at the cricoid has been challenged by recent radiologic studies. These studies, performed in spontaneously breathing children with natural airways, suggest that the narrowest part of the airway is not the cricoid cartilage but the glottic opening or the immediate subglottis. In addition, some anatomic studies describe an ellipsoid cricoid outlet; others, a circular or near-circular shape.

Although these seemingly contradictory studies can be confusing for the pediatric anesthesia provider, the most functionally relevant point may be that the cricoid cartilage is the only complete ring in the larynx; therefore it is nondistensible (unlike the pliable vocal folds) and therefore often the site of postextubation complications such as trauma, edema, croup, and subglottic stenosis, particularly when an inappropriately large ETT has been placed or an ETT cuff has been overinflated.

## Intubation

Anatomic differences may make mask ventilation and intubation more difficult for inexperienced providers. Although the overall incidence of difficult tracheal intubation in children is low, many childhood syndromes and sequences are associated with additional anatomic characteristics that may make intubation difficult (i.e., Pierre-Robin sequence, Treacher-Collins syndrome). Infants younger than 1 year are also more likely to have a difficult airway, and neonates less than 60 weeks corrected gestational age are at particular risk. One multicenter European study demonstrated a risk of difficult tracheal intubation in this neonatal age group of almost 6%, and the majority were unexpected. Recent analyses of the Pediatric Difficult Intubation Registry suggest children less than 10 kg are at high risk and early transition to video laryngoscopy may improve results.

## Tracheal Tube

### SIZE AND TYPE

Choosing the correct size and type of ETT in infants and children is critical and dependent on the size of the child and the procedure taking place. Poiseuille's law dictates that airway resistance is inversely proportional to the radius of the lumen to the fourth power for laminar flow. This law translates to significant consequences in the infant airway; 1 mm of airway edema from a large ETT or overly inflated cuff will increase airway resistance by more than 40%. An ETT that is too small may lead to problematic circuit leaks, impaired ventilation, or increased aspiration risk. Age-based formulas are most

| TABLE 182.1 | Sizes of Tracheal Tubes |
| --- | --- |
| **Age** | **Size** |
| Premature (<2.5 kg) | 2.5 |
| Term neonate | 3.0 |
| 2–8 months | 3.5 |
| 8–12 months | 4.0 |
| 18–24 months | 4.5 |
| Older than 24 months | (Age in years/4) + 4 |

frequently used for ETT size selection (see Table 182.1) but are imperfect.

A "leak test" measures the presence of an air leak around the ETT and is critically important in preventing postintubation edema. An air leak should be present at less than 20 to 25 cm $H_2O$ peak inflation pressure, approximately equivalent to the capillary pressure of the tracheal mucosa. If no leak is present, providers should consider replacing the tube with the next half-size smaller, although a provider may tolerate leaks at higher pressures for short-term intubation rather than risk reintubation. Manufacturers are required to standardize the inner diameter of ETTs, but the outer diameter may vary, further reinforcing the important of a leak test.

If an ETT is too small or if a cuff needs more air, a leak will be present at very low inflation pressures (<10 cm $H_2O$); this may interfere with the ability to generate positive pressure to ventilate a child. In this case a larger tube may be indicated if an uncuffed tube was used or more air may be needed in the cuff.

Historically, uncuffed ETTs were preferred by many pediatric providers to avoid excessive pressure on the subglottis, but modern cuffed ETTs are available with short balloons, which are more distal on the tube, allowing a tracheal position below the subglottis and avoiding the nondistensible cricoid ring. These ETTs have ultrathin cuffs that allow a tracheal seal at low pressures.

## LENGTH

The position of the ETT in the trachea is critically important in infants because even small movements can cause either mainstem bronchus intubation or accidental extubation. Term newborns have an insertion distance of approximately 9 to 10 cm; a 1-year-old child, 11 cm; and a 2-year-old child, 12 cm. Preterm infants have an insertion distance that varies dramatically depending on their size. One approximate formula to estimate tube insertion distance is three times the size of the ETT. Many other formulas exist for estimating insertion distance, but it remains important to clinically assess and confirm the position in each individual child with bilateral auscultation and observation of equal anterior chest wall movement. Even small but persistent changes in oxygen saturation in an infant should prompt a reassessment of the position of the ETT.

## SUGGESTED READINGS

Disma, N., Virag, K., Riva, T., Kaufmann, J., Engelhardt, T., Habre, W., et al. (2021). Difficult tracheal intubation in neonates and infants. NEonate and Children audiT of Anaesthesia pRactice IN Europe (NECTARINE): A prospective European multicentre observational study. *British Journal of Anaesthesia, 126*(6), 1173–1181.

Fiadjoe, P., Litman, R., Serber, J. F., Stricker, C., & Cote, C. (2019). The pediatric airway. In C. Cote,

J. Lerman, & B. Anderson (Eds.), *A practice of anesthesia for infants and children* (6th ed., pp. 297–339). Philadelphia: Elsevier.

Holzki, J., Brown, K. A., Carroll, R. G., & Coté, C. J. (2018). The anatomy of the pediatric airway: Has our knowledge changed in 120 years? A review of historic and recent investigations of the anatomy of the pediatric larynx. *Paediatric Anaesthesia, 28*(1), 13–22.

Peyton, J., Park, R., Staffa, S. J., Sabato, S., Templeton, T. W., Stein, M. L., et al. (2021). A comparison of videolaryngoscopy using standard blades or non-standard blades in children in the Paediatric Difficult Intubation Registry. *British Journal of Anaesthesia, 126*(1), 331–339.

# 183

# Fluid Management in Infants

ASHLEY V. WONG GROSSMAN, MD | RANDALL PAUL FLICK, MD, MPH

## Fluid Management in Infants

Neonates and infants are particularly prone to developing fluid and electrolyte derangements, particularly in the setting of critical illness or surgery. Total body water in neonates and infants contributes to a substantially larger proportion of body mass than in the older child or adult (80% vs. 60%). Body surface area compared with body mass is also increased in neonates and infants and contributes to greater insensible fluid losses, especially when a major body cavity is opened. Finally, limited ability to communicate thirst makes the infant dependent on thoughtful fluid and electrolyte management by a vigilant anesthesia provider throughout the perioperative period.

## Maintenance Fluids

Reliance on the method of Holliday and Segar continues, despite concern regarding its relevance to the perioperative care of young children. In their seminal 1957 paper, the authors provided a simplified method for estimating maintenance fluids and electrolytes based on energy requirements: 1- to 10-kg infants need about 100 cal $\cdot$ kg$^{-1}$ $\cdot$ 24 h$^{-1}$; each kilogram over 10 kg and up to 20 kg requires an additional 50 cal $\cdot$ kg$^{-1}$ $\cdot$ 24 h$^{-1}$; after 20 kg, each additional kilogram requires 20 cal $\cdot$ kg$^{-1}$ $\cdot$ 24 h$^{-1}$. Approximately 1 mL of water is needed for each calorie expended. This method can be simplified (Table 183.1). These recommendations were intended to guide maintenance fluid therapy for hospitalized children and not for intraoperative management.

| TABLE 183.1 | Maintenance Fluid Therapy for Hospitalized Neonates and Infants* | |
|---|---|---|
| **Weight (kg)** | **Fluid Needed (mL $\cdot$ kg$^{-1}$ $\cdot$ h$^{-1}$)** | |
| <10 | 4 | |
| 10–20 | 2 | |
| >20 | 1 | |

*Based on the method of Holliday and Segar.
*Note:* These recommendations are not intended to be used intraoperatively.

## Fluid Replacement

The fluid deficit in a fasting patient can be calculated by multiplying the number of hours that the patient is fasting by the maintenance fluid requirement described previously. Although a scientific basis for the following recommendation is lacking, common practice is to not only provide maintenance requirements but also replace half of the fluid deficit in the first hour, one-fourth of the deficit in the second hour, and the final one-fourth of the deficit in the third hour. Importantly, perioperative pediatric nothing-by-mouth guidelines have liberalized in recent years making routine fluid deficit replacement in the otherwise healthy child presenting for elective surgery less common. In addition, limited data exist to support the practice of replacing third-space losses as has been described in most standard texts of pediatric anesthesia (Table 183.2). Many factors

| TABLE 183.2 | Guidelines for Third-Space Fluid Replacement | |
|---|---|---|
| Probability of Fluid Translocation | Example Procedure | Additional Fluid Replacement ($mL \cdot kg^{-1} \cdot h^{-1}$) |
| Little or no | Tympanostomy tube placement | 0 |
| Mild | Inguinal hernia | 2 |
| Moderate | Thoracotomy | 4 |
| Severe | Bowel obstruction | 6 |

| TABLE 183.3 | Mechanisms of Complications of Massive Transfusion |
|---|---|
| Complication | Mechanism |
| Acidosis | Poor oxygen delivery, lactate accumulation |
| Alkalosis | Citrate metabolism to bicarbonate by the liver |
| Hypocalcemia | Citrate binding of calcium |
| Hyperglycemia | Dextrose preservative in packed red blood cells |
| Hypothermia | Transfusion of cold blood products |
| Hyperkalemia | Multifactorial |

may influence fluid requirements in neonates and infants making the use of simplified formulas problematic and potentially dangerous. In the neonate, insensible water loss is increased by fever, crying, sweating, hyperventilation, phototherapy, and radiant warmers. Adequacy of fluid therapy is best monitored by clinical signs (heart rate, blood pressure, urine output, capillary refill) rather than by blind adherence to a poorly validated formula. A few simple rules follow that will hopefully help avoid problems encountered in fluid management:

- Intravenously administered hypotonic fluids in general should not be used in the operating room. Hyponatremia in the perioperative setting is a concern and has been associated with mortality; however, replacement of sodium should rarely be undertaken in the operating room. Alterations in serum sodium are more often a reflection of abnormalities in total body water than in sodium, and, importantly, rapid replacement of sodium can result in devastating neurologic injury.
- Literature supporting the use of colloids (albumin) for fluid resuscitation in children is minimal and may be harmful in certain pediatric populations (e.g., children with traumatic brain injuries).
- Metabolic acidosis is most often a reflection of poor tissue perfusion and should first prompt the anesthesia provider to evaluate the patient's volume status.
- Potassium replacement is rarely indicated in young children and carries significant risk. If undertaken, replacement should be accomplished slowly with frequent monitoring of serum potassium concentration at a maximum of $3 \text{ mEq} \cdot kg^{-1} \cdot 24 \text{ h}^{-1}$ at a rate not to exceed $0.5 \text{ mEq} \cdot kg^{-1} \cdot h^{-1}$. Adequate renal function should be identified before the initiation of potassium replacement, typically by the presence of adequate urine output ($0.5$–$1.0 \text{ mL} \cdot kg^{-1} \cdot h^{-1}$).
- Hypocalcemia is a frequent complication of massive transfusion secondary to citrate concentration in banked blood products (Table 183.3). Tissue loss from extravasation of calcium chloride given through a peripheral intravenous (IV) line is an unfortunate occurrence that can be avoided by ensuring adequate functioning IV access, central venous access, or using calcium gluconate. The typical dose of IV calcium chloride is 10 mg/kg and calcium gluconate is 30 mg/kg.

## Blood Replacement

During the transition of fetal hemoglobin to adult hemoglobin that occurs in the first 3 months of life, infants experience a physiologic anemia; the mean hemoglobin decreases from approximately 16.8 g/dL at term to a nadir of 10.5 to 11.5 g/dL at 8 to 12 weeks of age. In premature infants, this decrease may be even more profound and may occur earlier around 6 weeks of age. Infants undergoing surgical interventions during their physiologic nadir do not require transfusion therapy unless there are clinical indications. There are only two accepted indications for the transfusion of red blood cells (RBCs): (1) to increase oxygen ($O_2$)-carrying capacity ($O_2$ delivery = cardiac output × hemoglobin × $O_2$ saturation) or to avoid an impending inadequate $O_2$-carrying state and (2) to suppress production, or dilute the amount, of endogenous hemoglobin in selected patients with thalassemia or sickle cell disease.

The American Society of Anesthesiologists Task Force on Blood Component Therapy updated transfusion practice guidelines in 2015 that are likely applicable to pediatric patients without cardiopulmonary disease. The points regarding RBC transfusions are summarized subsequently:

- Transfusion is rarely indicated when hemoglobin concentration is above 10 g/L and is almost always indicated when the hemoglobin concentration is less than 6 g/L, especially if the anemia is acute.
- The determination of whether intermediate hemoglobin concentrations (6–10 g/L) justify transfusion should be based on the patient's risk for developing complications related to inadequate oxygenation.
- The use of a single hemoglobin trigger for all patients is not recommended.

Several calculations have been presented for the evaluation of transfusion thresholds. One such formula proposes that the maximum allowable blood loss should equal the estimated blood volume multiplied by the hematocrit minus the target hematocrit divided by the hematocrit. In clinical practice, these calculations have limited utility as they are dependent on estimates of blood loss that have been repeatedly shown to be inaccurate. In children, transfusion is best guided by close monitoring of hemodynamic parameters and frequent determination of hemoglobin concentration. Estimated blood volume for various ages is shown in Table 183.4.

## Red Blood Cell Products

The transfusion of fresh whole blood (≤5 days old) would appear to be the obvious choice for resuscitation of a bleeding child because it replaces all the components being lost. If fresh whole blood is not obtainable but its use is required, stored RBCs can be reconstituted with fresh frozen plasma. It may be

| TABLE 183.4 | Estimated Blood Volume in Infants and Children | |
| --- | --- | --- |
| Age Group | | Estimated Blood Volume (mL/kg) |
| Premature infants | | 90–100 |
| Term newborns | | 80–90 |
| Infants younger than 1 year | | 75–80 |
| Older children | | 60–75 |

appropriate to ask the blood bank to split units to limit donor exposure and waste. For neonates, it is recommended that RBCs be cytomegalovirus negative and leukocyte reduced via filtration or irradiation to prevent infection and graft-versus-host disease.

## Glucose Management

Controversy exists over the need for the perioperative administration of supplemental glucose in infants and children. Historically, all children under anesthesia were thought to be at risk of hypoglycemia and received glucose-containing fluid; however, more recently, hyperglycemia is also a recognized risk and care is now taken to avoid both prolonged hyperglycemia and hypoglycemia. Infants receiving glucose solutions preoperatively should continue to receive this dextrose rate in the operating room to prevent hypoglycemia; this is especially applicable to any child receiving preoperative parenteral nutrition when this nutrition is discontinued in the intraoperative setting. Children with liver insufficiency, metabolic disease, or extended fasting are also at increased risk of perioperative hypoglycemia and should receive appropriate supplementation. When in doubt, the serum glucose concentration should be measured at regular intervals. Current literature does not support tight intraoperative glucose control in children because of the risk of hypoglycemia and subsequent neurologic injury.

## SUGGESTED READINGS

American Society of Anesthesiologists Task Force on Perioperative Blood Management. (2015). Practice guidelines for perioperative blood management. *Anesthesiology, 122*(2), 241–275.

Holliday, M. A., & Segar, W. E. (1957). Maintenance need for water in parenteral fluid therapy. *Pediatrics, 19*, 823.

Myburgh, J., Cooper, D. J., Finfer, S., Bellomo, R., Norton, R., Bishop, N., et al. (2007). Saline or albumin for fluid resuscitation in patients with traumatic brain injury. *New England Journal of Medicine, 357*(9), 874–884.

Nemergut, M. E., Haile, D. T., Mauermann, W. J., & Flick, R. P. (2017). Blood conservation in infants and children. In E. Motoyoma & P. Davis (Eds.), *Smith's anesthesia for infants and children* (9th ed., pp. 399–422). Philadelphia: Mosby.

Neville, K. A., Sandeman, D. J., Rubinstein, A., Henry, G. M., McGlynn, M., & Walker, J. L. (2010). Prevention of hyponatremia during maintenance intravenous fluid administration: A prospective randomized study of fluid type versus fluid rate. *Journal of Pediatrics, 156*(2), 313–319.

Roseff, S. D., Luban, N. L., & Manno, C. S. (2002). Guidelines for assessing appropriateness of pediatric transfusion. *Transfusion, 42*(11), 1398–1413.

Smith, H. M., Farrow, S. J., Ackerman, J. D., Stubbs, J. R., & Sprung, J. (2008). Cardiac arrests associated with hyperkalemia during red blood cell transfusion: a case series. *Anesthesia and Analgesia, 106*(4), 1062–1069.

# 184

# Neuromuscular Blocking Agents in Infants

JASON M. WOODBURY, MD

Neonates are generally more sensitive to the effects of neuromuscular blocking agents (NMBAs), which may be attributable to a variety of factors. Neuromuscular transmission is incompletely developed at birth and is immature in neonates and infants until around 2 months of age. Neonates deplete acetylcholine reserves more quickly than older infants and children. In addition, animal models suggest that neonatal motor end plates release a much smaller amount of acetylcholine in response to motor nerve stimulation. It has also been shown that NMBAs occupy only one of the two α-subunits on the postjunctional acetylcholine receptor in neonates as opposed to both α-subunits in older children and adults, resulting in more efficient blockade in neonates.

The onset time for NMBAs is faster in neonates compared with older children and adults. The more rapid onset time is a function of the relatively greater cardiac output seen in neonates. Children with low cardiac output or decreased muscle perfusion will experience prolonged onset times. Total body water and extracellular fluid are comparatively higher in preterm infants and neonates. The larger volume of distribution for NMBAs necessitates a higher initial dose due to more rapid redistribution. Subsequent doses, however, often need to be decreased in comparison with adults, as neonates and infants are at risk for prolonged blockade due to increased sensitivity and reduced elimination.

## Specific Agents and Unique Characteristics in Neonates and Infants

### DEPOLARIZING NEUROMUSCULAR BLOCKING AGENT: SUCCINYLCHOLINE

Succinylcholine is currently the only depolarizing NMBA in clinical use. Infants are more resistant to the effects of succinylcholine, requiring up to two times the initial dose compared with adults and older children. In addition, infants have a shorter onset time, faster clearance, and more rapid distribution because of larger extracellular fluid volume. An intravenous (IV) dose of 3 to 4 mg/kg is typically required to achieve complete blockade within 30 to 40 seconds. Fasciculations may be observed in older children and adolescents but are rarely seen in infants. Succinylcholine is metabolized rapidly by the enzyme butyrylcholinesterase. The fact that this enzyme activity is reduced in neonates does not appear to have any clinical effect on duration of action.

In emergency situations where IV access is not immediately available, succinylcholine can be administered via the intramuscular (IM) route or intralingually through a sublingual or submental approach. An IM dose of 5 mg/kg will typically result in profound relaxation in 210 to 290 seconds. Intralingual dosing is the same as the IV route and has a more rapid onset compared with IM, with complete relaxation occurring in 75 to 130 seconds. Regardless of route, vocal cords will begin to relax in as quickly as 30 to 40 seconds.

Succinylcholine structurally resembles two acetylcholine molecules joined by an ester linkage, which may result in vagotonic effects on administration, particularly in infants. Significant bradycardia or asystole may develop after a single IV dose. Administration of atropine 10 to 20 mcg/kg provides adequate prophylaxis against bradyarrhythmias in all age groups including infants.

Serum potassium concentration can be expected to rise 0.5 to 1 mEq/L after administration of succinylcholine in normal children. In children with prolonged immobilization, neuromuscular diseases, crush injuries, motor neuron lesions, or burns (more than 8% body surface area), a single dose of succinylcholine may result in life-threatening hyperkalemia due to proliferation of extrajunctional acetylcholine receptors. However, infants born with myelomeningocele or cerebral palsy with spastic quadriparesis will respond with a normal rise in potassium.

Succinylcholine is a known triggering agent for malignant hyperthermia (MH). Triggering episodes are extremely rare in neonates and infants, even those with MH susceptibility. There have been, however, several case reports of MH or MH-like reactions in infants as young as 6 months.

The U.S. Food and Drug Administration issued a black box warning for succinylcholine in 1994 prompted by case reports of cardiac arrest due to massive hyperkalemia in male children with undiagnosed muscular dystrophies. Current recommendations are to avoid the use of succinylcholine in infants and children except for emergency intubation and situations where the airway must be rapidly secured, such as a difficult airway, laryngospasm, or full stomach.

## NONDEPOLARIZING NEUROMUSCULAR BLOCKING AGENTS

### Vecuronium

Vecuronium is a monoquaternary aminosteroid that produces intermediate-duration neuromuscular blockade in adults. It primarily undergoes hepatic metabolism and has multiple active metabolites. There is no vagolytic effect or associated histamine release. Infants are much more sensitive to the effects of vecuronium compared with older children and adults, experiencing faster onset, prolonged duration of action, and prolonged recovery time. Vecuronium is therefore considered a long-acting NMBA in neonates and infants.

### Rocuronium

Rocuronium is an aminosteroid similar to vecuronium but with one-tenth the potency, resulting in more rapid onset. Recovery time is almost twice as long in infants compared with older children. Rocuronium mainly undergoes hepatic metabolism like vecuronium, though there are no active metabolites. There are no vagolytic effects or histamine release in infants. However, rocuronium is known to block $M_2$ and $M_3$ muscarinic receptors, which may result in clinically variable bronchoconstriction.

### Pancuronium

Pancuronium is a long-acting bis-quaternary aminosteroid. Infants typically require comparatively smaller doses than older children or adults. Metabolism is dependent on hepatic and renal mechanisms, and a prolonged duration of action is observed with dysfunction of either organ system. Pancuronium is not associated with histamine release but will increase circulating levels of catecholamines due to inhibition of presynaptic uptake. Increases in heart rate and blood pressure are commonly observed, leading to concerns that pancuronium may contribute to the risk of intracerebral hemorrhage in premature infants and neonates.

### Atracurium

Atracurium is a benzylisoquinolinium that decomposes via ester hydrolysis and Hofmann degradation into inactive metabolites. Both processes are pH and temperature dependent; therefore duration of action is prolonged in infants who are hypothermic or acidotic. Neonates younger than 48 hours require lower doses for complete relaxation and have a longer recovery time. Doses of 0.3 to 0.6 mg/kg will provide effective intubating conditions in almost all infants. Higher doses or rapid IV administration may result in clinically significant histamine release.

### Cisatracurium

Cisatracurium is an isolated stereoisomer of atracurium and shares many of its properties including metabolism and Hofmann degradation. Cisatracurium is 1.5 times more potent than atracurium, resulting in a slightly slower onset time. Unlike atracurium, high doses and rapid administration of cisatracurium will not result in histamine release or cardiovascular changes.

### Mivacurium

Mivacurium is a short-acting benzylisoquinolinium that is rapidly metabolized by butyrylcholinesterase. The onset time to complete relaxation in infants is very similar to succinylcholine; however, there is a higher comparative incidence of coughing and diaphragmatic movement with mivacurium resulting in less ideal intubating conditions. Recovery is faster in infants than in children, but the duration of action is still prolonged compared with succinylcholine. Like atracurium, high doses of mivacurium may result in histamine release and associated cardiovascular effects. Mivacurium had not been available in the United States since 2006. It was reintroduced in 2016 but is not widely used. Mivacurium is, however, more commonly used in many other countries.

## Reversal of Neuromuscular Blockade

Even mild depression of respiratory muscle function in infants may result in hypoxia and hypercarbia. Infants, particularly those with higher ASA scores or those undergoing short procedures, are at much higher risk of postoperative respiratory complications with the use of NMBAs. It is therefore vitally important that full neuromuscular function is restored before extubation. Neonates and infants are at particular risk for residual neuromuscular blockade for several reasons including immaturity of the neuromuscular junction and slower metabolism and elimination of agents. However, because of the decreased percentage of type I muscle fibers in the neonatal diaphragm, respiratory function will be relatively more preserved and will recover more rapidly than the peripheral musculature. Recovery of train-of-four (TOF) at a monitored peripheral site will safely indicate recovery of the diaphragm in an infant.

Neostigmine is a cholinesterase inhibitor that has been the classical agent of choice for NMBA reversal in adults and children of all ages for many decades. The dose requirement for neostigmine in infants and children is 30% to 40% less than for adults. With partial spontaneous recovery of TOF, full recovery of muscle strength has been achieved with doses of neostigmine as low as 20 to 30 mcg/kg. Administration of neostigmine in an infant should always be preceded by an antimuscarinic agent (atropine 10–20 mcg/kg or glycopyrrolate 5–10 mcg/kg) to

> ### BOX 184.1 FACTORS PROLONGING NEUROMUSCULAR BLOCKADE IN INFANTS
>
> Abnormal variant or deficient pseudocholinesterase
> Antibiotics
>    Aminoglycosides
>    Tetracyclines
>    Lincomycins
>    Polymyxins
> Chemotherapy agents
> Dantrolene
> Hepatic or renal dysfunction
> Hypermagnesemia
> Hypokalemia
> Hypothermia
> Lithium
> Local anesthetic agents
> Phase II block with succinylcholine
> Residual inhalation agent
> Respiratory or metabolic acidosis

attenuate the risk of bradycardia. Edrophonium is no longer recommended as a reversal agent in pediatrics as neostigmine has been shown to be more efficacious and less variable in its effect. Failure of reversal or recurarization postoperatively may indicate the presence of other factors that can prolong neuromuscular blockade (Box 184.1).

Sugammadex is a relatively new reversal agent that was approved for adult use in the United States in 2015. Sugammadex is a modified γ-cyclodextrin that selectively binds aminosteroid NMBAs (rocuronium and vecuronium), providing rapid and complete reversal in a dose-dependent manner. As there is no activity at the muscarinic receptor, sugammadex avoids the well-known and potentially problematic side effects of cholinesterase inhibitors.

Though sugammadex is currently approved only for adults, off-label use in children has become more frequent. Data have emerged over the last several years supporting its safety and efficacy in all age groups. Multiple studies comparing sugammadex and neostigmine have demonstrated no difference in the incidence of anaphylaxis, bronchospasm, and hypotension in infants and children. The risk of bradycardia appears to be substantially mitigated with sugammadex in pediatric populations. Sugammadex has been shown to result in faster and more complete reversal with reduced incidence of residual neuromuscular blockade in all pediatric groups, particularly neonates and infants.

## SUGGESTED READINGS

Anderson, B. J., Lerman, J., & Coté, C. J. (2019). Pharmacokinetics and pharmacology of drugs used in children. In C. J. Coté, J. Lerman, & B. J. Anderson (Eds.), *A practice of anesthesia for infants and children* (6th ed., pp. 100–176). Philadelphia: Elsevier Saunders.

Gaver, R. S., Brenn, B. R., Gartley, A., & Donahue, B. S. (2019). Retrospective analysis of the safety and efficacy of sugammadex versus neostigmine for the reversal of neuromuscular blockade in children. *Anesthesia and Analgesia, 129*(4), 1124–1129.

Nnamani, N. P., & Moss, D. R. (2015). Babies in distress: Malignant hyperthermia in infancy explored. *Clinical Pediatrics, 54*(6), 557–562.

Ozmete, O., Bali, C., Cok, O. Y., Turk, H. E., Ozyilkan, N. B., Civi, S., et al. (2016). Sugammadex given for rocuronium-induced neuromuscular blockade in infants: A retrospective study. *Journal of Clinical Anesthesia, 35*, 497–501.

Scheffenbichler, F. T., Rudolph, M. I., Friedrich, S., Althoff, F. C., Xu, X., Spicer, A. C., et al. (2020). Effects of high neuromuscular blocking agent

dose on post-operative respiratory complications in infants and children. *Acta Anaesthesiologica Scandinavica, 64*(2), 156–167.

Woelfel, S. (2017). Neuromuscular blocking agents. In P. J. Davis & F. P. Cladis (Eds.), *Smith's anesthesia for infants and children* (9th ed., pp. 239–257). St. Louis: Elsevier Mosby.

# Congenital Diaphragmatic Hernia

MOLLY M.H. HERR, MD

Congenital diaphragmatic hernia (CDH) most commonly presents as respiratory distress and cyanosis in a baby shortly after birth. Because the diaphragmatic malformation originates early in fetal development, the presence of abdominal contents in the thorax inhibits lung development, resulting in the primary problems in CDH—hypoplasia of the lung parenchyma and pulmonary vasculature—which can lead to persistent pulmonary hypertension of the newborn (PPHN).

## Incidence and Classification

CDH occurs in about 1 in every 2500 to 3000 live births. Classification is based on location of the defect, with the most common and significant being the posterolateral aspect of the diaphragm, through the foramen of Bochdalek (about 75%–80% of CDH). Of Bochdalek hernias, roughly 85% are left-sided, 13% right, and 2% are bilateral. Other types are anterior or Morgagni hernias (roughly 15%–25%), and 2% are central paraesophageal hernias, which are generally small, without compromised pulmonary function, and do not usually present in the neonatal period. Sometimes a weakness of the diaphragm can cause diaphragmatic eventration to occur, resulting in the development of a hernia sac in the thorax. This usually occurs on the right side and is often asymptomatic, but severe cases may present identically to CDH (Fig. 185.1).

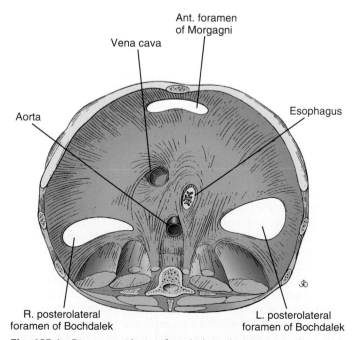

**Fig. 185.1** Diagram, with view from below, showing sites of congenital diaphragmatic hernia. (From Davis PJ, Cladis FP, eds. *Smith's Anesthesia for Infants and Children.* 9th ed., Elsevier; 2017.)

## Etiology, Embryology, and Pathophysiology

CDH is a complex developmental defect that appears to be multifactorial, and in most cases the etiology is unknown. Rare familial cases of CDH have been reported, although many genetic defects among sporadic cases have been identified. Environmental exposures to an herbicide called *nitrofen* have been implicated in rodent studies, where pregnant rodents exposed to nitrofen result in most offspring developing CDH. In addition, nutritional deficiencies have also been proposed for possible etiologies. There appears to be a disturbance in the vitamin A pathway in CDH infants with low retinol and retinol-binding protein levels from cord blood samples.

Although CDH is usually an isolated lesion, approximately 40% are associated with anomalies, including congenital heart disease (ventricular septal defects, atrial septal defects, tetralogy of Fallot) as a more frequent comorbidity. Syndromes associated with CDH include Beckwith-Wiedemann; CHARGE (coloboma, heart defects, atresia choanae, growth retardation, genital abnormalities, and ear abnormalities); Cornelia de Lange; Marfan; and trisomies 13, 18, 21, and 45X aneuploidies. CDH can also be associated with various gastrointestinal (intestinal atresia and malrotation), genitourinary (hypospadias), and neurologic (spina bifida, hydrocephalus) abnormalities.

In the fetus, the pleuroperitoneal cavity begins as a single compartment. The development of the diaphragm begins around the fourth week of gestation and is usually complete by 10 to 12 weeks' gestation. It is unclear if failure of the normal fusion of the pleuroperitoneal folds of the diaphragm causes CDH; there is new speculation that the developing lung buds are disturbed, resulting in lung hypoplasia, which then leads to the defective diaphragm and herniation of abdominal contents into the thorax. Regardless of the cause, the presence of abdominal viscera in the thorax leads to abnormal lung development and hypoplasia. The shifted mediastinum compresses the contralateral lung and contributes to its abnormal development. The diaphragmatic defect leads to abnormal fetal breathing movements resulting in the loss of stretch induced lung maturation. Lung hypoplasia also manifests in fewer alveoli and decreased branching of the bronchioles with thickened membranes for gas exchange. In addition, the vasculature of the lungs is affected, with fewer vessels per unit of lung, and vascular remodeling with medial hyperplasia leads to thickened vessels distally with abnormal vascular smooth muscle response. This fixed, nonresponsive vasculature can lead to PPHN.

Severe left-sided CDH is also often associated with left ventricular (LV) hypoplasia, which contributes to significantly increased mortality. It is thought that abdominal contents within the left chest cause a rotation of the heart, decreasing blood flow across the foramen ovale, leading to underfilling of the left ventricle resulting in decreased LV growth. Additionally, it appears that increased blood flow on the right side of the heart leads to right ventricular hypertrophy and diastolic dysfunction.

## Prenatal Diagnosis and Management

Prenatal diagnosis by ultrasound detects 50% to 70% of CDH cases at a mean of 24 weeks' gestation. Three-dimensional ultrasound, fetal echocardiography, and fetal magnetic resonance imaging (MRI) are used to assess the severity of CDH, along with other fetal anomalies including congenital heart or neural tube defects. Fetal MRI is especially useful in assessing the position of the liver and estimating lung volumes, which affects prognosis. Lung-to-head ratio (LHR) is a method of assessing severity of pulmonary hypoplasia. LHR measures the area of the contralateral lung at the level of the atria divided by the circumference of the head but varies greatly upon gestational age. Observed to expected LHR standardizes LHR for gestational age by expressing the LHR as a percentage compared with normal fetuses. These measurements are important indicators for prognosis of the CDH infant (Table 185.1).

## Prenatal Management: Fetal Endoscopic Tracheal Occlusion

Because the fundamental pathophysiology of CDH is pulmonary hypoplasia, various fetal surgical techniques have been investigated to improve the growth of hypoplastic lungs in utero. Currently, fetal endoscopic tracheal occlusion (FETO) remains the only clinically relevant in utero intervention. Fetal lungs secrete approximately 100 mL/kg/day of fluid that normally exits the trachea and mouth to enter the amniotic fluid. FETO is accomplished by endoscopically placing a balloon through the mouth of the fetus, through the vocal cords, and inflating it in the trachea. By preventing lung fluid from exiting the lung, tracheal occlusion aims to manipulate lung development by stretching the lung to accelerate growth. It also increases the intrathoracic pressure, which tends to move the viscera out of the thorax.

FETO is generally performed on fetuses with severe isolated CDH who are likely to have poor outcomes if repaired after birth. A study by Ruano and colleagues in 2012 randomized

fetuses with severe isolated CDH with LHR less than 1 or liver herniation to either FETO or no FETO. FETO was performed under maternal epidural between 26 and 30 weeks' gestation with fetal intramuscular paralytics, pain medication, and atropine using ultrasound guidance to place a tracheal balloon. All FETO cases were delivered by the ex utero intrapartum therapy (EXIT) procedure with removal of the tracheal balloon while the fetus was still on placental circulation, and all non-FETO infants were delivered via cesarean section. Postnatal therapy was the same for both groups. The study found that 10 of 19 (52.6%) infants assigned to FETO survived to 6 months, whereas only 1 of 19 (5.3%) infants survived to 6 months. The frequency of severe pulmonary arterial hypertension was significantly lower in the FETO group, 50% versus 86% in the non-FETO group.

Recently, FETO surgery involves placement of the tracheal balloon at 26 to 30 weeks' gestation with the mother under monitored anesthetic care with local infiltration and then ultrasound surveillance every 1 to 2 weeks to assess balloon integrity and to measure fetal lung response. At approximately 34 weeks, the balloon is deflated and removed via a second in utero procedure. Studies have shown that release of tracheal occlusion at least 24 hours before delivery appears to improve neonatal outcomes further by allowing recovery of type II pneumocytes, which are responsible for the secretion of surfactant. By removing the balloon electively earlier in gestation, an emergent EXIT procedure can be avoided.

Delivery should be planned at a tertiary medical center with extracorporeal membrane oxygenation (ECMO) capabilities when possible. Close monitoring of the fetus with regular ultrasound is paramount. It appears that delivery near or at term (38–40 weeks) allows infants with isolated CDH the highest survival, but some studies show CDH infants with associated anomalies and low lung volumes have a slightly better survival if a cesarean section is performed at 37 weeks.

## Postnatal Diagnosis and Management

The CDH infant presents with the classic triad of cyanosis, respiratory distress, and apparent dextrocardia. Physical findings include a scaphoid abdomen, barrel-shaped chest, shifted cardiac sounds, diminished breath sounds on the affected side, and bowel sounds in the chest. Radiographs are usually confirmatory showing a bowel gas pattern in the chest with a mediastinal shift.

Management consists of immediate tracheal intubation without bag and mask ventilation to avoid distending the intrathoracic stomach, which can worsen pulmonary function. Mechanical ventilation with low peak pressures (<25 cm $H_2O$) is essential to avoid lung damage. An orogastric tube is placed to decompress the gut, and central or peripheral venous and arterial lines are placed. Preductal oxygen ($O_2$) saturations of 80% to 95% and postductal saturation >70% are targeted while blood pressure is maintained at levels acceptable for gestational age using fluid boluses and inotropes. Upon transfer to the neonatal intensive care unit, ventilation management consists of minimizing lung barotrauma with permissive hypercapnia and gentle ventilation. In general, management consists of respiratory rates of 40 to 60 breaths/min, peak inspiratory pressure <25 cm $H_2O$, positive end-expiratory pressure (PEEP) of 3 to 5 cm $H_2O$, and allowing partial pressure of carbon dioxide in arterial blood ($Paco_2$) to be in the 50 to 70 mm Hg range. Inhaled nitric oxide, a selective pulmonary vasodilator, is used

| TABLE 185.1 | Prenatal Predictors of Outcome in Congenital Diaphragmatic Hernia |
|---|---|
| LHR >1.35 | 100% survival |
| LHR 1.25–0.6 | 61% survival |
| LHR <0.6 | 0% survival |
| O/E LHR >35% | 65%–88% survival |
| O/E LHR <25% (severe CDH) | 10% survival liver up; 25% survival liver down |
| O/E LHR <15% | 0% survival liver up |
| Liver up | 35%–60% survival; 80% risk of needing ECMO |
| Liver down | 74%–93% survival; 25% risk of needing ECMO |

*ECMO,* Extracorporeal membrane oxygenation; *LHR,* lung-to-head ratio; *O/E,* observed to expected.

selectively with patients with marked preductal desaturation secondary to right-to-left shunting and for stabilization before ECMO. The routine use of inhaled nitric oxide in CDH patients has been shown in a Cochrane review to lead to increased ECMO utilization and no survival benefit. High-frequency ventilation is used for CDH neonates who have hypoxia and hypercarbia ($Paco_2$ >70 mm Hg) refractory to conventional ventilation.

## The Use of Extracorporeal Membrane Oxygenation

Roughly 33% to 50% of CDH infants who do not respond to pharmacologic and ventilatory therapy proceed to ECMO to provide time for pulmonary growth and remodeling. Selection criteria for ECMO include hypoxia with the inability to keep preductal $O_2$ saturation greater than 80%, hemodynamic instability caused by left ventricular systolic dysfunction with poor urine output, persistent acidosis, and severe pulmonary hypertension unresponsive to pharmacologic intervention. However, the use of ECMO is associated with significant risks, and contraindications exist (Box 185.1). ECMO is discontinued if irreversible brain damage or lethal organ failure occurs or when lung function improves.

## Surgery and Timing

Surgery consists of open or thoracoscopic primary closure of the diaphragmatic defect, a prosthetic patch in larger hernias, a staged closure with a Silastic silo if the abdomen cannot be closed, or, in very large hernias, split abdominal wall muscle flaps are used. Patch repair includes the risks of increased infection and CDH recurrence; however, it is often necessary in large hernias. The timing of surgery for CDH repair has shifted from emergent surgical intervention to delayed surgical repair after the patient has been stabilized medically. Survival rates using this preoperative management and selective use of ECMO has improved survival rates to 79% to 92%. Infants with mild symptoms and no evidence of pulmonary hypertension are usually repaired at 2 to 3 days of life. Patients with mild reversible pulmonary hypertension are repaired when medically stable at 5 to 10 days of life. In patients with severe pulmonary hypertension, with no response to medical management or with the use of ECMO, support is often withdrawn. Patients who respond favorably on ECMO can be repaired after weaning from ECMO, in the ideal situation. If they are unable to be weaned, hernia repair can be performed while on ECMO. This leads to increased bleeding because of the heparinization required; however, antifibrinolytics have been used and shown to improve success. Several studies have shown earlier repair on ECMO within 2 to 3 days of cannulation appears to have better success than late repair on ECMO, which has the highest bleeding and complication rate.

---

**BOX 185.1  CONTRAINDICATIONS TO THE USE OF EXTRACORPOREAL MEMBRANE OXYGENATION**

Gestational age <35 weeks
Weight <2000 g
Preexisting intracranial hemorrhage
Congenital or neurologic anomalies incompatible with good outcome

---

## Anesthetic Management

Most infants with CDH are urgently intubated in the delivery room and then medically stabilized before surgery. However, if the infant is not intubated before coming to the operating room, the endotracheal tube can be placed while the infant is awake, or a rapid sequence intravenous induction can be planned. The neonate is preoxygenated, cricoid pressure is applied, and precautions are taken to prevent aspiration of stomach contents. Positive-pressure ventilation with bag and mask before intubation should be avoided because it may cause further distention of the gut. The use of standard monitors, along with arterial and central venous pressure catheters, is recommended. Because heat loss is rapid, the operating room should be warmed, and a forced air device should be used.

Selection of anesthetic agent and technique depends on the infant's condition. The usual technique is $O_2$/high-dose opioid/neuromuscular blocking agent. The use of nitrous oxide is contraindicated. Some infants may be receiving inhaled nitric oxide during the repair. Sudden deterioration in heart rate, blood pressure, blood $O_2$ saturation ($SpO_2$), or lung compliance suggests a contralateral pneumothorax, which should be promptly treated by inserting a chest tube. Some practitioners advocate the prophylactic insertion of a contralateral chest tube. A peak inspiratory pressure less than 25 cm $H_2O$, PEEP of 3 to 5 cm $H_2O$, and adequate oxygenation without hyperoxia ($SpO_2$ 90%–95%) are recommended. Permissive hypercapnia is used while maintaining the pH above 7.25. Profound hypercapnia often develops during thoracoscopic repair; therefore hand ventilation, increased respiratory rate, and increased tidal volumes are sometimes required.

## Postoperative Care

After surgery, the infant should be transferred to an intensive care unit and remain intubated, mechanically ventilated, and occasionally paralyzed in a warmed incubator unit. Attempts to expand the ipsilateral lung may lead to excessive airway pressure and pneumothorax. Infants with relatively normal lungs usually do well, but those with varying degrees of pulmonary hypoplasia may have difficulty maintaining adequate oxygenation because of persistent fetal circulation. In some cases, ECMO may be required. Bilateral chest tubes are also frequently needed, and gastric suctioning should be continued. Pain management is important and may include epidural or caudal analgesia or opioid infusions.

## Outcome

As many as 87% of infants with CDH face long-term sequelae including respiratory, nutritional, developmental, and musculoskeletal issues. Overall, infants who required ECMO have had patch or flap repairs (indicative of larger defects) and have higher risks of these impairments than those without ECMO or who have had primary repairs. Respiratory issues include bronchopulmonary dysplasia, pulmonary hypertension, obstructive pulmonary disease, asthma, and increased respiratory infections, especially in early childhood. Fortunately, most school age and adolescent CDH survivors recover lung function achieving near-normal lung volume and mechanics without significant obstructive lung disease, pulmonary hypertension, or exercise intolerance. Nutritional issues occur in over half of CDH survivors, including gastroesophageal reflux disease, oral aversion, and failure to thrive, predominantly in those with larger hernias with patch repairs. Neurodevelopmental issues can include mild to profound motor and cognitive delays, with more than half of CDH survivors having some type of delay, and are typically worse in those with larger defects. Sensorineural hearing loss is also very common in CDH patients, ranging from 5% up to 60% in some studies. Orthopedic problems, including pectus excavatum and scoliosis, often become more apparent in adolescence. Pectus deformities occur in 9% of primary repairs and up to 50% in patch or flap repairs, and scoliosis occurs in 7% of primary repairs and 15% in patch or flap repairs. Recurrent hernias occur in 2% to 20% of CDH patients and are more likely in patch repairs, larger hernias, or in thoracoscopically repaired CDH.

## Mortality Rate

With the advances in medical and surgical management over the years, the overall survival rate of those born with CDH is about 70% to 90%. Those CDH infants not requiring ECMO have up to 90% survival, whereas ECMO CDH infants have survival rates around 50% to 75% depending on the study. Other indicators of poorer prognosis include prematurity; associated congenital defects, especially cardiac, persistent, and severe pulmonary hypertension; right-sided hernias; and liver in the thorax (indicating a larger defect). FETO procedures done at high-volume tertiary institutions appear to improve survival among those CDH infants with severe defects who are unlikely to do well with postnatal management alone.

## SUGGESTED READINGS

Bojanić, K., Woodbury, J. M., Cavalcante, A. N., Grizelj, R., Asay, G. F., Colby, C. E., et al. (2017). Congenital diaphragmatic hernia: Outcomes of neonates treated at Mayo Clinic with and without extracorporeal membrane oxygenation. *Paediatric Anaesthesia, 27*(3), 314–321.

Chandrasekharan, P. K., Rawat, M., Madappa, R., Rothstein, D. H., & Lakshminrusimha, S. (2017). Congenital Diaphragmatic hernia–a review. *Maternal Health Neonatology and Perinatology, 3*, 6.

Chatterjee, D., Ing, R. J., & Gien, J. (2020). Update on congenital diaphragmatic hernia. *Anesthesia and Analgesia, 131*(3), 808–821.

Danzer, E., & Hedrick, H. L. (2014). Controversies in the management of severe congenital diaphragmatic hernia. *Seminars in Fetal & Neonatal Medicine, 19*(6), 376–384.

Davis, P. J., & Cladis, F. P. (2017). *Smith's Anesthesia for Infants and Children* (9th ed.). St. Louis, MO: Elsevier.

Gupta, V. S., Harting, M. T., Lally, P. A., Miller, C. C., Hirschl, R. B., Davis, C. F., et al. (2023). Mortality in congenital diaphragmatic hernia: A multicenter registry study of over 5000 patients over 25 years. *Annals of Surgery, 277*(3), 520–527. doi:10.1097/SLA.0000000000005113.

Hoagland, M. A., & Chatterjee, D. (2017). Anesthesia for fetal surgery. *Paediatric Anaesthesia, 27*(4), 346–357.

Ruano, R., Yoshisaki, C. T., da Silva, M. M., Ceccon, M. E., Grasi, M. S., Tannuri, U., et al. (2012). A randomized controlled trial of fetal endoscopic tracheal occlusion versus postnatal management of severe isolated congenital diaphragmatic hernia. *Ultrasound in Obstetrics & Gynecology, 39*(1), 20–27.

# 186

# Congenital Pediatric Airway Problems

ELIZABETH R. VOGEL, MD, PhD

## Congenital Pediatric Airway Problems

Congenital airway abnormalities frequently complicate pediatric airways and may result in difficulty with airway management. Both bony and soft tissue components of the airway may be involved and should be carefully evaluated preoperatively. Alterations in bony anatomy may involve mandibular and maxillary hypoplasia, as well as restrictions in temporomandibular joint mobility. The cervical spine should be evaluated for atlantoaxial instability, or limited mobility because of cervical fusion or arthritic anomaly. Soft tissue abnormalities may include macrosomia, mass effect because of tumor or arteriovenous

malformations, and stiff, immobile tissues because of conditions such as myositis ossificans, dermatomyositis, or mucopolysaccharidosis. In this chapter, potential challenges associated with specific syndromes involving congenital airway abnormalities and strategies for management are discussed.

## Congenital Abnormalities of the Airway

### CLEFT LIP AND PALATE

Considered together, cleft lip and palate represent the most common craniofacial abnormality and are associated with more than 300 syndromes. The incidence of cleft lip with or without cleft palate is approximately 1 in 750 births, while that of cleft palate alone is approximately 1 in 2500 births.

Anesthetic management depends on the degree of malformation and the presence of associated syndromes and can be relatively straightforward in uncomplicated cases. Isolated cleft lip typically does not result in complications for airway management. Large palate defects, however, may result in airway obstruction or difficult mask ventilation if the defect is extensive enough to allow the tongue to prolapse into the nasopharynx. Placement of an oral airway will typically prevent this. Palate defects may also cause difficulty with intubation if the defect is large enough for the laryngoscope blade to slip easily into the cleft. In an intubated patient, the endotracheal tube may also migrate into the cleft, potentially resulting in extubation. Of note, bilateral clefts may result in an anterior angle of the premaxilla that may alter the line of site during laryngoscopy, complicating intubation. Additionally, postoperative airway problems are common after palatoplasty as surgical edema in children with small oral cavities can result in airway obstruction, requiring reintubation.

## PIERRE ROBIN SEQUENCE

Pierre Robin sequence (PRS) is characterized by micrognathia and glossoptosis (posterior displacement of the tongue). A subset of patients may present with syndromic diagnoses such as Stickler syndrome (poor vision and hypermobile joints) or velocardiofacial syndrome (cleft palate, congenital cardiac anomalies, short stature). Infants with PRS can present with significant airway problems almost immediately after birth due to airway obstruction caused by the combination of glossoptosis and micrognathia. Both intubation and mask ventilation may be difficult in PRS. Airway obstruction may be relieved by prone positioning, pulling the tongue forward with gauze, or using a nasopharyngeal airway. If necessary, a suture may be placed to maintain a forward tongue position. A difficult intubation should be anticipated, and awake fiberoptic intubation should be considered. If intubation after induction of anesthesia is planned, a fiberoptic scope or video laryngoscope is the first choice for airway securement, as the failure rate of direct laryngoscopy is high. Laryngeal mask airways (LMAs) have been used with increased frequency in this population and may be particularly useful to both assist with ventilation and relief of airway obstruction during induction and to provide a pathway for fiberoptic intubation. Because of the potential difficulties in airway management, early consideration should be given to tracheostomy, particularly if severe obstruction is present at baseline. In general, airway management becomes easier as these patients age and the mandible grows or when they undergo surgical interventions such as mandibular distraction.

## TREACHER COLLINS SYNDROME

This syndrome is the most common of the mandibulofacial synostoses. Clinical features include maxillary, zygomatic, and mandibular hypoplasia; microstomia (small mouth); high-arched palate; choanal atresia; hearing loss; and congenital heart disease. Cleft palates are also common in this population. Because of the mandibulofacial hypoplasia, mask ventilation and intubation may be very difficult, and many of these patients will require techniques other than direct laryngoscopy to secure the airway. A combination of LMA placement and fiberoptic intubation may

help alleviate obstruction to ventilation and provide a conduit for successful fiberoptic intubation. Of note, a subset of these patients also present with mandibular immobility resulting in limited mouth opening. In these patients, awake or sedated nasal fiberoptic intubation should be strongly considered because their mouth opening may not accommodate an LMA and likely will not allow for placement of a laryngoscopy blade. In a subset of patients, significant airway obstruction may necessitate tracheostomy for definitive airway management.

## CRANIOFACIAL DYSOSTOSES

Craniofacial dysostoses encompass many syndromes including Apert, Pfeiffer, and Crouzon syndromes. Apert and Pfeiffer syndromes are characterized by acrocephalosyndactyly, a combination of cranial and limb anomalies. Overall, syndromes associated with craniofacial dysostoses are characterized by craniosynostosis (premature fusion of one or more cranial sutures), varying midface hypoplasia, and proptosis. A high-arched palate and malocclusion commonly occur. These patients may also have limited neck mobility because of vertebral abnormalities, with cervical fusion being common in Apert and Crouzon syndromes. Tracheal ring abnormalities may result in decreased airway caliber. These patients are typically mouth breathers because of small nasal passages with choanal stenosis. Midface hypoplasia results in upper airway obstruction and sleep apnea symptoms in about half of patients and can make mask ventilation difficult. Typically, an oral or nasal airway is sufficient to alleviate the obstruction and allow adequate mask ventilation. Intubation is typically not a challenge apart from patients with significant cervical immobility. LMA placement can be helpful both to relieve obstruction and improve ventilation and to provide a conduit for fiberoptic intubation in particularly challenging airways. Because of the potentially smaller size of the nasal and tracheal passage, downsizing of the nasal or oral endotracheal tubes should be considered.

## GOLDENHAR SYNDROME

Patients with Goldenhar syndrome are characterized by hemifacial microsomia associated with mandibular hypoplasia, congenital heart disease, macrostomia, and eye, ear, and vertebral abnormalities on the affected side. Neck flexion and extension may be limited because of fused vertebrae or hemivertebrae. Mask ventilation may be challenging because of difficulty maintaining a seal in the setting of facial asymmetry. The difficulty of tracheal intubation is highly variable in these patients and ranges from minimal to extreme difficulty depending on the severity of presentation. Some patients may present with bilateral symptoms, which can be mistaken for PRS.

## BECKWITH- WIEDEMANN SYNDROME

This syndrome is characterized by exophthalmos, macroglossia, and gigantism. A large, protuberant tongue is the primary source of airway compromise for these patients. This compromise may be so severe that partial glossectomy is required to maintain airway patency. At baseline, placement of a nasopharyngeal airway or prone positioning may help alleviate upper airway obstruction. Mask ventilation is often difficult because of obstruction secondary to macroglossia. Pulling the tongue forward or using a nasopharyngeal airway may assist in mask ventilation. If an LMA can be maneuvered past the tongue, it can provide both relief of obstruction and a potential conduit for fiberoptic intubation. Nasotracheal intubation is typically indicated when these patients undergo partial glossectomies, particularly as postoperative tongue swelling, and the resultant oropharyngeal airway obstruction, may require persistent intubation for several days after surgery.

## KLIPPEL-FEIL SYNDROME

Patients with this syndrome demonstrate severe limitation in neck flexion and extension because of fusion of cervical vertebrae, as well as atlantooccipital abnormalities. Although mask ventilation is typically easy, intubation may be very difficult because of limitations in neck positioning. Careful manipulation of the neck is necessary as cervical stenosis is also often present and neurologic injury is possible with forceful extension or flexion. Use of a fiberoptic or video laryngoscope is strongly recommended to compensate for limitations in neck mobility and to minimize neck manipulation to help prevent injury.

## TRISOMY 21/DOWN SYNDROME

Patients with Down syndrome have several airway considerations. Features of this syndrome include a narrowed nasopharynx, possible cleft lip/palate, macrosomia, tracheomalacia, and a small larynx and cricoid ring. Acquired subglottic stenosis is common. Atlantoaxial instability is also common in this patient population and preoperative x-rays should be considered before anesthesia if there is concern for this. Considering the smaller caliber larynx and risk for acquired subglottic stenosis, downsizing the endotracheal tube is recommended.

## MUCOPOLYSACCHARIDOSES

In the mucopolysaccharidoses, enzyme production deficiencies lead to mucopolysaccharide accumulation in tissues throughout the body. Accumulation in airway tissues results in blockage of nasal passages, enlarged tongue, and swelling of the soft tissues of the oropharynx. Thick secretions are often present. A difficult airway should be expected and, as the child ages, the airway may become even more difficult to manage because of progression of the disease.

Multiple syndromes fall under mucopolysaccharidosis, each with specific features. Hurler syndrome is associated with significant intellectual developmental disorder, gargoyle facies, deafness, stiff joints, dwarfism, pectus excavatum, kyphoscoliosis, abnormal tracheobronchial cartilage, hepatosplenomegaly, severe cardiac valvular disease, and early coronary artery disease. Hunter syndrome is an X-linked recessive syndrome characterized by coarse facial features, macrocephaly, a protruding tongue, stiff joints, stunted growth, skeletal abnormalities, and developmental delay. Children with Morquio syndrome often appear healthy at birth; however, as the child ages, manifestations may include coarse facial features, prognathism, odontoid hypoplasia, atlantoaxial instability resulting from thoracic or lumbar kyphosis, aortic valve incompetence, hepatomegaly, inguinal hernias, mixed hearing loss, ocular complications, and limb abnormalities.

# Anesthetic Management of the Difficult Pediatric Airway

Regardless of the congenital anomaly associated with a difficult pediatric airway, problems should be anticipated and managed expectantly. Preoperative evaluation should include careful assessment of potential barriers to successful mask ventilation, including assessment of history of snoring or sleep apnea. Evaluation for limited cervical mobility or instability should also be performed. Documentation of prior airway instrumentation should be reviewed. However, it should be noted that pediatric airway concerns are typically dynamic. The rapid growth and anatomic changes that take place during infancy and early childhood mean that prior airway interventions may not be indicative of future conditions. Some conditions may improve over time as the child grows, whereas others may progressively worsen. A careful history and physical exam should be performed before every anesthetic to evaluate for any changes.

The upper airway may be more easily compromised in infants and children compared with adults because of the unique anatomy and physiology of the pediatric airway. The tongue of an infant or child is relatively larger within the mouth, the larynx more cephalad, the glottic opening and airways narrower, the arytenoid cartilages more prominent, and the occiput larger. Pediatric respiratory physiology may further complicate airway management. Oxygen consumption and carbon dioxide production rates are higher because of higher weight-adjusted basal metabolic rates in infants and young children. In addition, the functional residual capacity of infants, per kilogram, is less than that of adults. This combination of increased oxygen consumption and decreased reserve means that pediatric patients are less able to tolerate apnea during airway management and will desaturate much more quickly than adult patients. In this regard, apneic oxygenation via high-flow nasal cannula may be helpful during airway manipulation.

Pediatric patients typically cannot cooperate or tolerate airway management with minimal sedation. An anesthetic is usually required before airway manipulation, which means common techniques to secure the airway awake, as are often performed in adult patients, are not feasible. As in adult patients, pediatric patients can be divided into those who will be difficult to intubate but can be ventilated by mask and those who are difficult or impossible to ventilate by mask. If a child can be ventilated by mask, then numerous options can be safely used until the trachea is successfully intubated. In mask-able patients, administration of muscle relaxant may improve conditions for potentially difficult intubations and should be strongly considered. In patients where mask ventilation is anticipated to be difficult, spontaneous ventilation should be prioritized and a deep plane of anesthesia established before attempting intubation in an unparalyzed patient. In this latter population, strong consideration should be given to establishing deep sedation with agents such as midazolam and dexmedetomidine, which maintain spontaneous breathing and establish a plane of sedation that may facilitate fiberoptic intubation before initiating general anesthesia.

Asleep or sedated fiberoptic intubation remains a mainstay for securing the difficult pediatric difficult airway. Increasingly, LMAs are being used as a track for fiberoptic intubation, with the advantage that oxygenation and ventilation may be continued through the LMA during the fiberoptic intubation, avoiding periods of apnea. In addition, LMAs may provide better ventilation and oxygenation in patients who are difficult to mask ventilate because of upper airway obstruction. Indirect video laryngoscopes are increasingly used as well, with pediatric specific blades and adaptors now readily available. Both traditionally shaped straight and curved blades are available in addition to hyperangulated curved blades.

Suggestions for management include the following:
- Evaluate the patient's history and physical exam. Determine whether you anticipate difficult intubation, difficult mask ventilation, or both.
- Several intubation approaches should be considered (e.g., awake, fiberoptic, video laryngoscope), but alternative methods must be immediately available, including facilities for cricothyrotomy or tracheostomy.
- Strongly consider premedication to facilitate intravenous access before induction.
- Consider whether to secure the airway under general anesthesia or deep sedation.
- Induction with sevoflurane via spontaneous ventilation is preferred if awake or sedated intubation is not possible.
- Spontaneous ventilation should be maintained until the ability to mask ventilate is confirmed. If able to mask ventilate,

muscle relaxant may improve intubation conditions and should be strongly considered.
- An LMA may be warranted to assist ventilation if mask ventilation is difficult.
- Laryngoscopy should be performed under deep anesthesia with spontaneous ventilation if muscle relaxant is not used.
- A variety of laryngoscopy blades, tracheal tubes, and stylets should be readily available.
- Fiberoptic equipment or an indirect video laryngoscope is the first choice for many congenital airway anomalies. If not used on the first attempt, it should be readily available if direct laryngoscopy fails.
- Consider combining techniques such as using an LMA as a conduit for fiberoptic intubation or using a video laryngoscope to guide fiberoptic intubation.
- Because children are prone to developing laryngospasm at the time of extubation, all equipment for ventilation and reintubation should be available before extubation is attempted. Careful consideration should be given as to when and where extubation should occur, especially if surgery-induced swelling or edema of the airway is present.

## SUGGESTED READINGS

Burjek, N. E., Nishisaki, A., Fiadjoe, J. E., Adams, H. D., Peeples, K. N., Raman, V. T., et al. (2017). Videolaryngoscopy versus Fiber-optic Intubation through a Supraglottic Airway in Children with a Difficult Airway: An Analysis from the Multicenter Pediatric Difficult Intubation Registry. *Anesthesiology, 127*(3), 432–440.

Cladis, F., Kumar, A., Grunwaldt, L., Otteson, T., Ford, M., & Losee, J. E. (2014). Pierre Robin Sequence: A perioperative review. *Anesthesia and Analgesia, 119*(2), 400–412.

Garcia-Marcinkiewicz, A. G., & Stricker, P. A. (2020). Craniofacial surgery and specific airway problems. *Paediatric Anaesthesia, 30*(3), 296–303.

Hardcastle, T. (2009). Anaesthesia for repair of cleft lip and palate. *Journal of Perioperative Practice, 19*(1), 20–23.

Krishna, S. G., Bryant, J. F., & Tobias, J. D. (2018). Management of the difficult airway in the pediatric patient. *Journal of Pediatric Intensive Care, 7*(3), 115–125.

Miller, K. A., & Nagler, J. (2019). Advances in emergent airway management in pediatrics. *Emergency Medicine Clinics of North America, 37*(3), 473–491.

Oliveira, C. R. D. (2020). Pediatric syndromes with noncraniofacial anomalies impacting the airways. *Paediatric Anaesthesia, 30*(3), 304–310.

Vijayasekaran, S., Lioy, J., & Maschhoff, K. (2016). Airway disorders of the fetus and neonate: An overview. *Seminars in Fetal & Neonatal Medicine, 21*(4), 220–229.

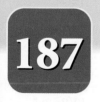

# 187

# Congenital Heart Disease: Congestive Heart Failure

ROXANN BARNES PIKE, MD

Anesthetic management of a patient with congenital heart disease (CHD) and heart failure (HF) requires a thorough understanding of anatomy and physiology. Anesthesia is more frequently used in the setting of cardiac surgery for patients with CHD and HF; however, as life expectancy increases in this patient population, anesthesia is increasingly necessary for the performance of noncardiac procedures as well. Patients with CHD and HF frequently need diagnostic and therapeutic interventional and invasive procedures.

Certain congenital heart lesions typically result in poor ventricular function and hemodynamics with progression to HF. Unfortunately, the cause of HF is not always readily apparent in neonates and infants. In addition to HF, patients with CHD may have secondary effects, such as pulmonary hypertension. Two consensus statements regarding HF in pediatric and adult patients with CHD have recently been published (Hinton, 2017; Stout, 2016) and are both comprehensive reviews of the topic. A review of anesthesia for patients with CHD undergoing non-cardiac surgery is also a useful resource.

CHD is classified according to the presence or absence of cyanosis. Cyanotic lesions are caused by shunting of blood from the pulmonary circulation to the systemic circulation, which results in poor pulmonary blood flow and progressive arterial desaturation. In contrast, acyanotic lesions are characterized by pulmonary overcirculation because of shunting from the systemic to pulmonary circulation that eventually causes HF. Excessive blood flow to the lung reduces lung compliance and increases the work of breathing by increasing left atrial pressure resulting in pulmonary venous congestion and pulmonary edema, which decreases the compliance of the lung itself. The increased size of pulmonary vessels also causes greater obstruction to airflow in both large and small airways.

A typical example of acyanotic CHD with HF is the preterm infant with a patent ductus arteriosus (PDA). A large left-to-right (L-to-R) shunt causes systemic circulatory steal and subsequent diastolic hypotension and pulmonary overcirculation. Pharmacologic, percutaneous, or surgical closure of the PDA is required to resolve the HF. The orifice of the shunt in a PDA may be described as *restrictive* or *nonrestrictive*. If the orifice is restrictive, the primary determinant of shunt fraction is the radius of the orifice and the resultant pressure gradient. If the orifice is nonrestrictive, the shunt direction and magnitude depend on the relative resistances of the pulmonary and systemic vascular circulations, which can be manipulated as part of the care of individuals until closure of the PDA.

In addition to HF resulting from shunts, HF can also occur from obstructive cardiac defects and may progress to circulatory collapse without immediate intervention. Obstructive defects are characterized as subvalvular, primary valvular, or supravalvular obstructions causing reduced ventricular function, hypotension, and eventually ventricular hypertrophy. Furthermore, myocardial ischemia is especially common in obstructive lesions of both ventricles. Patients with obstructive defects are at increased risk for developing arrhythmias in part because of the tenuous myocardial oxygen ($O_2$) supply-to-demand ratio. Isolated obstructive lesions can occur in the right ventricle and are exacerbated by increased pulmonary vascular resistance (PVR), resulting in right-sided HF.

## Anesthetic Management

Identification of surgical and anesthetic risk is critical to improve outcomes in the CHD patient population. Risk factors include single ventricle physiology, Williams syndrome, pulmonary hypertension, cardiomyopathies (hypertrophic, restrictive, and dilated), and the presence of ventricular assist devices. These risk factors in a patient with CHD should raise concern, because these patients are at increased risk for experiencing serious perioperative morbidity and death. In some patients, the stress of surgery may be enough to cause acute cardiac decompensation. There is no single anesthetic technique that has been identified as "ideal" for these patients. Anesthetic management for each patient must be individualized and must include knowledge of the individual physiologic aspects of the cardiac

| TABLE 187.1 | Manipulations That Alter Pulmonary Vascular Resistance | |
|---|---|
| **↑ PVR** | **↓ PVR** |
| Hypoxia | Oxygen |
| Hypercarbia | Hypocarbia |
| Acidosis | Alkalosis |
| Hyperinflation | Normal FRC |
| Atelectasis | Low hematocrit |
| Sympathetic stimulation | Blocking sympathetic stimulation |
| High hematocrit | Nitric oxide |
| Surgical constriction | |

*FRC,* Functional residual capacity; *PVR,* pulmonary vascular resistance.

anatomy and a plan to minimize myocardial depression and maintain baseline hemodynamic parameters.

Central to the anesthetic management of patients with HF secondary to L-to-R shunting is to *avoid* increasing the shunt and thereby increasing pulmonary overcirculation (Table 187.1). Hemodynamic goals include maintaining or decreasing systemic vascular resistance (SVR) and avoiding decreases in PVR. One of the foremost responsibilities of the anesthesia team is to consider factors that may adversely affect shunt flow. However, the team must be cautious about the degree to which the L-to-R shunt is manipulated to reduce pulmonary overcirculation. Efforts to aggressively reduce SVR or increase PVR to reduce pulmonary overcirculation and, hence, improve HF will lessen the L-to-R shunt; however, the ensuing hypotension or pulmonary hypertension, respectively, may reduce coronary perfusion and stress a poorly functioning right ventricle, leading to hemodynamic deterioration. In contrast, cyanotic CHD with a right-to-left (R-to-L) shunt can be improved dramatically with aggressive measures to increase SVR or decrease PVR, often in association with immediate hemodynamic improvement.

Altering ventilation and oxygenation are important ways to influence either L-to-R or R-to-L shunts. The pulmonary vasculature is very sensitive to changes in partial pressure of carbon dioxide in arterial blood ($Paco_2$). Values of $Paco_2$ between 28 and 32 mm Hg are associated with pulmonary vasodilation that will worsen HF in patients with L-to-R shunts. A $Paco_2$ above 55 mm Hg raises PVR and lessens pulmonary overcirculation in these patients. However, the patient will tolerate hypercarbia only until the associated respiratory acidosis results in worsening myocardial function and compromised hemodynamics, overcoming any benefit from reduced L-to-R shunt. The effect of $O_2$ as a potent pulmonary vasodilator often goes underappreciated in patients with shunts. The patient's inspired $O_2$ concentration should be lowered incrementally after induction of anesthesia to avoid hyperoxia, which decreases PVR and could worsen pulmonary overcirculation.

Patients with HF secondary to L-to-R shunts or obstructive lesions will benefit from anesthetic medications that do not change or only minimally decrease myocardial contractility. Administering appropriate doses of synthetic opioids (e.g., fentanyl), ketamine, or both (which have minimal to no negative inotropic effects) provides excellent hemodynamic stability for these patients. Ketamine is widely used for neonates and infants with HF because it maintains cardiac output and perfusion pressures by enhanced sympathetic stimulation secondary to its sympathomimetic effects. Contractility and SVR are thereby maintained or increased, whereas PVR and heart rate are minimally affected. Propofol can cause severe hypotension and low cardiac output as a result of decreased preload, SVR, and diminished contractility (effects of which can be more pronounced in children with HF), and so has been used infrequently in this patient population. Even with careful dose adjustments, the use of propofol poses the risk of hemodynamic instability. Etomidate can also be used as an induction agent in patients with CHD because it causes minimal myocardial depression in CHD patients, but a single dose can potentially cause adrenal suppression, which can be problematic in these patients.

Preservation of baseline heart rate is essential in the neonate or infant because neonates and infants, unlike adults, are unable to augment cardiac output via increases in stroke volume. Ketamine preserves the heart rate and prevents the bradycardia often associated with the administration of fentanyl alone. There are benefits to the use of synthetic opioids in patients with CHD and HF; fentanyl has been shown to decrease the stress response in children undergoing cardiac surgery, and it also has the ability to attenuate increases in PVR. Although patients with CHD and HF may have hypertrophied pulmonary vasculature, the vasculature can be very reactive. Any insult that increases PVR may cause severe systemic hypotension by decreasing left ventricular preload and hypoxemia by decreasing perfusion of the lungs.

Dexmedetomidine can also be used safely as a sedative and analgesic agent in children with CHD in HF, because the hemodynamic profile is considered safe. Dexmedetomidine can, however, cause dose-related hypotension and bradycardia in rare instances and especially in those patients receiving digoxin, so should be used with caution.

If the intravenous route is not an option for induction of anesthesia, inhalation techniques may be used.

Halogenated inhalation agents have been used for induction for years in pediatric patients with CHD and HF. An echocardiographic assessment of patients with CHD receiving volatile anesthetics has shown that cardiac output and contractility are maintained while using sevoflurane and isoflurane, but isoflurane did cause tachycardia and a decrease in SVR. Even low doses of volatile anesthetics can cause myocardial depression and cardiac decompensation when administered to CHD patients in HF. Hypotension can then occur, as a result of a combination of reduced myocardial contractility, decreased SVR, lower heart rate, and inhibition of compensatory reflex mechanisms.

Unlike desflurane, sevoflurane has been evaluated repeatedly in neonates and infants with either cyanotic or acyanotic CHD and has been found to be acceptable in terms of cardiopulmonary side effects when used appropriately for induction and maintenance of anesthesia. Sevoflurane is the agent of choice for inhalation induction because it results in more rapid inductions, reasonably well-maintained hemodynamics, fewer arrhythmias, better contractility, and more rapid emergence and possesses the nonirritating airway effects. Furthermore, the use of sevoflurane has been shown to be associated with less breath holding, coughing, and laryngospasm, compared with other inhalational agents.

Anesthesia can be induced by sevoflurane in patients with obstructive lesions, but at the concentration often used for an inhalation induction, the negative inotropic effect and risk of hypotension may present a risk of hemodynamic collapse, a phenomenon not seen when ketamine is used to induce anesthesia. However, compared with the hypotension associated with the use of other inhalation agents, hypotension from sevoflurane can be quickly corrected by decreasing the concentration of inhaled drug as soon as intravenous access is obtained.

Finally, there is a proliferation of mechanical ventricular assist devices now available in pediatric sizes, which are being used much more frequently in the CHD population with HF. Anesthesia providers will find the article by Newington and colleagues (2021) a useful guide to manage the anesthetic for pediatric ventricular assist device implantation.

## Acknowledgment

The author wishes to recognize William C. Oliver Jr., MD, professor of anesthesiology and perioperative medicine, for contributions to previous versions of this chapter.

## SUGGESTED READINGS

Brown, M. L., DiNardo, J. A., & Nasr, V. G. (2020). Anesthesia in pediatric patients with congenital heart disease undergoing noncardiac surgery: Defining the risk. *Journal of Cardiothoracic and Vascular Anesthesia, 34*(2), 470–478.

Hinton, R. B., & Ware, S. M. (2017). Heart failure in pediatric patients with congenital heart disease. *Circulation Research, 120*(6), 978–994.

Jooste, E., & Machovec, K. Anesthesia for adults with congenital heart disease undergoing noncardiac surgery. In UpToDate, J. B. Mark, L. S. Sun, & M. Greutmann (Eds.), *UpToDate*. Waltham, MA. Accessed November 24, 2021.

Newington, D. F. T., De Rita, F., McCheyne, A., & Barker, C. L. (2021). Pediatric ventricular assist device implantation: An anesthesia perspective. *Seminars in Cardiothoracic and Vascular Anesthesia, 25*(3), 229–238.

Riveros, R., & Riveros-Perez, E. (2015). Perioperative considerations for children with right ventricular dysfunction and failing fontan. *Seminars in Cardiothoracic and Vascular Anesthesia, 19*(3), 187–202.

Stout, K. K., Broberg, C. S., Book, W. M., Cecchin, F., Chen, J. M., Dimopoulos, K., et al. (2016). Chronic heart failure in congenital heart disease: A scientific statement from the American Heart Association. *Circulation, 133*(8), 770–801.

Sungur Ulke, Z., Kartal, U., Orhan Sungur, M., Camci, E., & Tugrul, M. (2008). Comparison of sevoflurane and ketamine for anesthetic induction in children with congenital heart disease. *Paediatric Anaesthesia, 18*(8), 715–721.

Walker, A., Stokes, M., & Moriarty, A. (2009). Anesthesia for major general surgery in neonates with complex cardiac defects. *Paediatric Anaesthesia, 19*(2), 119–125.

# Other Neonatal Emergencies: Tracheoesophageal Fistula and Omphalocele

ROBERT J. FRIEDHOFF, MD

## Tracheoesophageal Fistula

Tracheoesophageal fistula (TEF) occurs as the result of failure of the tracheal bud to develop normally from the primitive foregut. TEF occurs in several forms (Fig. 188.1); type C—esophageal atresia (more correctly agenesis because the proximal part of the primitive foregut develops primarily into a trachea rather than an esophagus) with a distal TEF—is the most common form (accounts for 90% of all TEFs). Maternal polyhydramnios may indicate the presence of the lesion before birth. Diagnosis is suspected at birth when the neonate has excessive drooling, cyanotic episodes, or coughing relieved by suctioning or the clinician is unable to pass a soft catheter into the infant's stomach. TEF can be confirmed by radiography by showing a curled catheter in the upper esophageal pouch with an air bubble in the stomach. Contrast medium is unnecessary and contraindicated because the neonate may aspirate the medium. Associated conditions include prematurity (20%–25%), congenital heart disease (20%–25%), and other midline defects.

### PREOPERATIVE MANAGEMENT

Preoperative assessment is directed at detecting associated congenital lesions and assessing the patient's pulmonary status. The infant should be fed in the semiupright position, and continuous suction should be applied to the upper esophageal pouch to prevent aspiration. Respiratory support with humidified oxygen should be provided. Routine newborn preoperative laboratory studies (i.e., hemoglobin, electrolytes, glucose, and calcium concentration with or without arterial blood gases) and echocardiography to detect cardiac anomalies, including a right aortic arch (5% of neonates with TEF), should be performed. Pulmonary complications of TEF will not resolve until the fistula is ligated. A preliminary gastrostomy is often performed under local anesthesia.

### INTRAOPERATIVE MANAGEMENT

Induction techniques for repair of a TEF include the use of inhalation agents with a rapid sequence or awake intubation. The use of nitrous oxide ($N_2O$), which will add to gastric distention, should be avoided. Care must be taken to avoid intubating the fistula. A tracheal tube with the Murphy eye facing anteriorly should be inserted into the right main bronchus while listening for unilateral breath sounds; the tracheal tube is then pulled back until bilateral breath sounds are heard. Some clinicians prefer to cut the distal end of the tracheal tube, eliminating the Murphy eye. Use of a cuffed tracheal tube to both ventilate and occlude the fistula has been reported. Placement of a Fogarty catheter to identify and occlude the fistula using a pediatric bronchoscope can be attempted. Spontaneous ventilation, to avoid gastric distention until the fistula has been ligated, should be performed, and then controlled ventilation can be used.

Thoracoscopic repair of the fistula will avoid a thoracotomy and its sequelae. Use of a Fogarty catheter placed in the right main bronchus with the aid of a bronchoscope will facilitate one-lung

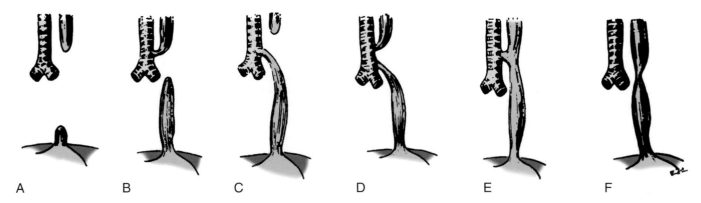

**Fig. 188.1** Types of congenital abnormalities of the esophagus. **A,** Esophageal atresia, no esophageal communication with the trachea. **B,** Esophageal atresia, the upper segment communicating with the trachea. **C,** Esophageal atresia, the lower segment communicating with the back of the trachea. More than 90% of all esophageal malformations fall into this group. **D,** Esophageal atresia, both segments communicating with trachea. **E,** Esophagus has no disruption of its continuity but has a tracheoesophageal fistula. **F,** Esophageal stenosis. (Modified from Gross RE. *The Surgery of Infancy and Childhood.* WB Saunders; 1953.)

ventilation. An alternative technique is to manipulate the tracheal tube to the left main bronchus with a bronchoscope. Surgical insufflation of carbon dioxide (5–6 mm Hg) into the right hemithorax will cause right lung collapse and possible hypercapnia and hypoxemia. Time to extubation and discharge from the neonatal intensive care unit are decreased with thoracoscopic repair. Patients less than 2000 g can undergo successful repair via the thoracoscopic technique but have an increased incidence of gastroesophageal reflux needing a Nissen fundoplication later in life.

A precordial stethoscope should be placed under the dependent lung. Routine intraoperative monitors and an arterial catheter are typically used. Regional anesthesia can be added as an adjuvant.

## POSTOPERATIVE CARE

Respiratory status in the intensive care unit can be optimized with the use of tracheal intubation and mechanical ventilation. Damage to the esophageal anastomosis can be avoided by marking a suction catheter so that it is not inadvertently extended past the anastomosis during nasopharyngeal suctioning.

## POSTOPERATIVE COMPLICATIONS

Tracheal compression secondary to tracheomalacia may occur. Infants with TEF typically have abnormal swallowing; 68% have gastroesophageal reflux, leading to possible aspiration. Esophageal stricture is common. A tracheal diverticulum may persist, causing problems with subsequent intubations.

# Omphalocele

Anesthetic management for omphalocele and gastroschisis are essentially the same, but knowledge of the associated anomalies will influence anesthetic decisions. Omphalocele and gastroschisis are congenital defects of the anterior abdominal wall, permitting external herniation of abdominal viscera. Gastroschisis is not midline (usually occurs on the right), has a normally situated umbilical cord (not covered with a hernia sac), and is rarely associated with other congenital anomalies but is associated with an increased incidence of prematurity.

Omphalocele has a 75% incidence of other congenital defects, including cardiac anomalies (ventricular septal defects most common), trisomy 21, and Beckwith-Wiedemann syndrome (omphalocele, organomegaly, macroglossia, and hypoglycemia). Epigastric omphaloceles are associated with cardiac and lung anomalies. Hypogastric omphaloceles are associated with exstrophy of the bladder and other genitourinary anomalies.

## PREOPERATIVE CARE

The exposed viscera must be covered with a sterile plastic bag or film to limit evaporative heat loss from exposed bowel. Deficits of fluid and electrolytes (often excessive) need to be replaced before operative repair. Hypoglycemia should be corrected slowly with a glucose infusion (6–8 mg/kg/min). Severe rebound hypoglycemia may occur after bolus doses of glucose. The stomach should be decompressed using a nasogastric tube.

## INTRAOPERATIVE MANAGEMENT

General tracheal anesthesia, using a combination of an inhaled anesthetic agent ($N_2O$ should be avoided) and a parenteral opioid, along with controlled ventilation is required. Preoxygenation followed by awake or rapid sequence intubation is preferred.

Routine monitors, along with an arterial catheter and central venous line for measurement of intravascular pressures, are recommended. Elevated intraabdominal pressures, high ventilatory pressures, and inferior vena cava compression, which can result in circulatory stasis in the lower limbs, should be avoided.

## POSTOPERATIVE MANAGEMENT

Problems seen intraoperatively with ventilation, elevated intraabdominal pressure causing compression of the inferior vena cava and impaired visceral blood flow, prolonged ileus, and decreased hepatic clearance of drugs can continue postoperatively. Urine output should be monitored closely.

## SUGGESTED READINGS

Alabbad, S. I., Shaw, K., Puligandla, P. S., Carranza, R., Bernard, C., & Laberge, J. M. (2009). The pitfalls of endotracheal intubation beyond the fistula in babies with type C esophageal atresia. *Seminars in Pediatric Surgery*, 18(2), 116–118.

Broemling, N., & Campbell, F. (2011). Anesthetic management of congenital tracheoesophageal fistula. *Paediatric Anaesthesia*, 21(11), 1092–1099.

Deanovic, D., Gerber, A. C., Dodge-Khatami, A., Dillier, C. M., Meuli, M., & Weiss, M. (2007). Tracheoscopy assisted repair of tracheo-esophageal fistula (TARTEF): a 10-year experience. *Paediatric Anaesthesia*, 17(6), 557–562.

Gayle, J. A., Gómez, S. L., Baluch, A., Fox, C., Lock, S., & Kaye, A. D. (2008). Anesthetic considerations for the neonate with tracheoesophageal fistula. *Middle East Journal of Anaesthesiology*, 19(6), 1241–1254.

Ho, A. M., Wong, J. C., Chui, P. T., & Karmakar, M. K. (2007). Case report: Use of two balloon-tipped catheters during thoracoscopic repair of a type C tracheoesophageal fistula in a neonate. *Canadian Journal of Anaesthesia*, 54(3), 223–226.

Knottenbelt, G., Costi, D., Stephens, P., Beringer, R., & Davidson, A. (2012). An audit of anesthetic management and complications of tracheo-esophageal fistula and esophageal atresia repair. *Paediatric Anaesthesia*, 22(3), 268–274.

Kinottenbelt, G., Skinner, A., & Seefelder, C. (2010). Tracheo-oesophageal fistula (TOF) and oesophageal atresia (OA). *Best Practice & Research Clinical Anaesthesiology*, 24(3), 387–401.

Son, J., Jang, Y., Kim, W., Lee, S., Jeong, J. S., Lee, S. K., et al. (2021). Thoracoscopic repair of esophageal atresia with distal tracheoesophageal fistula: is it a safe procedure in infants weighing less than 2000 g? *Surgical Endoscopy*, 35(4), 1597–1601.

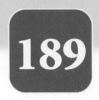

# Neonatal Resuscitation

STEPHANIE C. MAVIS, MD  |  JENNIFER L. FANG, MD, MS

An anesthesiologist may become involved in a neonatal resuscitation unexpectedly and may be the most qualified team leader given their experience with critical care, airway management, and medications. Therefore it is prudent to have a basic understanding of neonatal resuscitation. This chapter will provide a brief summary of (1) the transition from fetal to neonatal circulation; (2) preparing for a neonatal resuscitation; (3) Neonatal Resuscitation Program (NRP) basics including airway management, ventilation, chest compressions, and medications; and (4) other unique considerations. The intent of this chapter is to provide an overview of neonatal resuscitation and is not all-inclusive. We strongly recommend referring to the suggested readings at the end of this chapter for more in-depth learning. Anesthesiologists who have a high likelihood of being involved in neonatal resuscitation (e.g., pediatric or obstetric anesthesiologists) should take the NRP Provider Course through the American Academy of Pediatrics (AAP) and American Heart Association (AHA) to become trained in newborn resuscitation as may be required by individual hospital policies.

## Transition From Fetal to Neonatal Circulation

Most newborns undergo a relatively smooth physiologic transition at birth and do not require active intervention to establish adequate cardiorespiratory function. However, approximately 10% of all births will require some form of resuscitation beyond basic care. Neonatal resuscitation differs from adult and pediatric resuscitation in several ways. Most notably, neonatal resuscitation involves the unique physiology involved in the transition from fetal to extrauterine life. An understanding of this transition and how to effectively assist the process guides the practice of newborn resuscitation.

The elements necessary for successful transition involve effective respiration, circulation, and thermoregulation. In utero, the fetus lives in a fluid-filled environment and is dependent on the placenta for gas exchange. Upon delivery, the neonate must initiate continuous breathing and establish the lungs as the site of gas exchange by facilitating clearance of lung fluid and establishing functional residual capacity (FRC). The establishment of FRC is thought to occur with the first few breaths in spontaneously breathing neonates. Lung expansion stimulates surfactant release; ventilation, through decreases in $Pco_2$ and increases in $Pao_2$ and pH, leads to decreased pulmonary vascular resistance (PVR) and increased pulmonary blood flow. Clamping of the cord after birth removes the low-resistance placenta from the systemic circuit, increasing systemic blood pressure (SBP). The increase in SBP, decrease in PVR, and rise in $Pao_2$ promote closure of the ductus arteriosus and foramen ovale, thus facilitating the transition from fetal to neonatal circulation. Without strict attention to thermoregulation, neonates (especially low-birth-weight and premature infants) are susceptible to hypothermia. Cold stress is associated with significant delays in transitional physiology, including metabolic acidosis, increased oxygen consumption, and hypoglycemia. Although the initial steps in a normal transition occur within the first few minutes of birth, the entire process may not be completed for hours or even several days.

## Preparing for a Neonatal Resuscitation

Although certain antepartum and intrapartum risk factors will identify most newborns that require resuscitation after birth, some newborns without any apparent risk factors will require resuscitation. Therefore the AHA/AAP *Textbook of Neonatal Resuscitation* and the Guidelines for Perinatal Care have advised, "At least one person skilled in initiating neonatal resuscitation should be present at every delivery. An additional person capable of performing a complete resuscitation should be immediately available." An area in or near the delivery room should be designated as the resuscitation area. Adequate equipment and resources should be available and checked before delivery. At minimum, this should include:

- A warming device
- Suction catheters connected to a suction system
- Stethoscope, pulse oximeter, cardiac monitor, and electrocardiogram leads
- Ability to provide positive-pressure ventilation (PPV) (device for delivering PPV, term and preterm masks, compressed air and oxygen sources, and oxygen blender)
- Airway supplies (e.g., laryngoscopes, endotracheal tubes [ETTs], carbon dioxide detector, laryngeal masks [LMAs])
- Emergency medications

Use of a standardized equipment checklist to ensure that all necessary supplies and equipment are present and functioning may facilitate preparedness.

## Neonatal Resuscitation Program Basics

NRP interventions are based on the evaluation of respiratory effort and heart rate, so both must be continually assessed throughout the resuscitation. The process involves evaluation of the neonate's condition, a decision based on that evaluation, implementation of an action, and reevaluation of the patient's response to that action. *Adequate ventilation is the most important and effective action during neonatal resuscitation.* In addition, an increase in heart rate is the most important indicator of effective ventilation and response to resuscitative interventions. Fig. 189.1 is the NRP 8th edition Flow Diagram and should serve as a visual reference for the interventions described in the following paragraphs.

In addition to effective ventilation, adequate preparation and teamwork are emphasized as key behavioral skills within NRP. A report from The Joint Committee found that poor teamwork and communication are the most frequently cited root causes for potentially preventable infant death in the

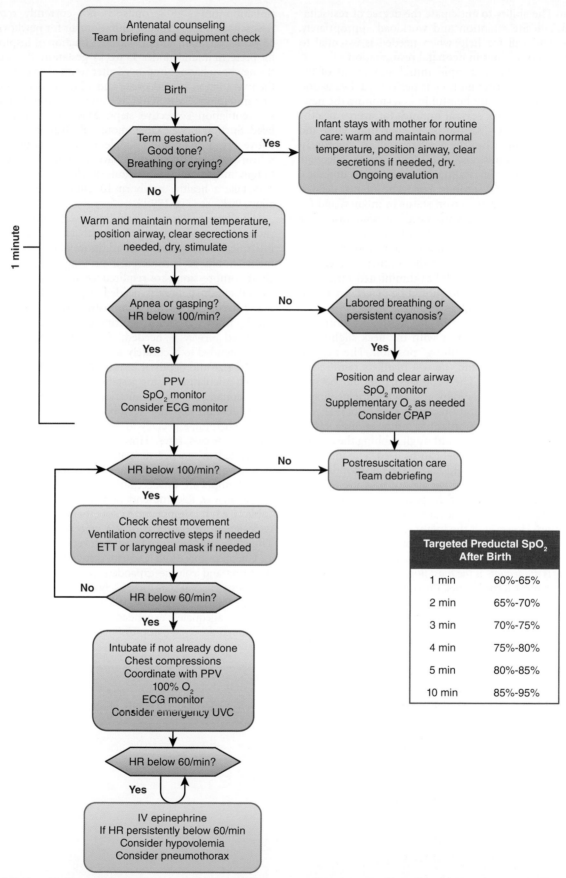

**Fig. 189.1** NRP Flow Diagram. *CPAP,* Continuous positive airway pressure; *ECG,* electrocardiographic; *ETT,* endotracheal tube; *HR,* heart rate; *IV,* intravenous; *O₂,* oxygen; *PPV,* positive-pressure ventilation; *SpO₂,* oxygen saturation; *UVC,* umbilical venous catheter. (Reprinted with permission from American Academy of Pediatrics and American Heart Association. Weiner GM and Zaichkin J, eds. *Textbook of Neonatal Resuscitation.* 8th ed. American Academy of Pediatrics; 2021.)

delivery room. The ability to anticipate the degree of resuscitation required, allocate attention and workload appropriately, communicate, and call for help when needed is essential to achieving optimal outcomes in neonatal resuscitation.

When an infant is born, a rapid initial assessment of the newborn's respiratory effort and tone is performed. Evaluation of color at birth is usually not helpful in determining the newborn's status, as it may take several minutes for even a healthy term infant to achieve $O_2$ saturation greater than 90% and "become pink." Typically, a healthy newborn will cry vigorously, maintain effective respirations, and demonstrate adequate muscle tone. In this case it is appropriate to delay umbilical cord clamping for 30 to 60 seconds. For term infants, delayed cord clamping (DCC) improves iron status in infancy, and for premature infants, DCC reduces the need for both vasoactive support and transfusions and lowers the risk of intraventricular hemorrhage. The term neonate with good tone and spontaneous breathing or crying can stay with the mother, whereas the neonate who is not breathing well, has diminished tone, does not appear vigorous, or is preterm should be placed on a radiant warmer for a more thorough assessment.

The neonate should be placed in the supine position with the head in the neutral position or with the neck slightly extended so the head is in the "sniffing" position. The neonate should be thoroughly dried and the wet blankets removed to avoid evaporative heat loss. The oropharynx should be suctioned if needed (mouth followed by nose) while the neonate is stimulated and assessed (respirations, heart rate, color). The act of drying and suctioning the infant is often enough tactile stimulation to initiate respiration, although rubbing the infant's back or flicking the soles of the feet can be used. The initial assessment and interventions should take 30 to 60 seconds. Subsequently, facial continuous positive airway pressure (CPAP) may be considered in neonates with spontaneous respirations who demonstrate labored respirations, grunting, and/or low oxygen saturation. However, if the infant remains apneic or has a heart rate below 100 bpm, then PPV should be initiated.

*Providing effective assisted ventilation when the infant's spontaneous breathing is inadequate is the most important step in newborn resuscitation.* For most term infants, initial inflation pressures of 25 to 30 cm $H_2O$ are adequate, although pressures as high as 30 to 40 cm $H_2O$ may be required. Breaths should be administered at a rate of 40 to 60 breaths/min. An initial sustained inflation (inflation time >5 seconds) is not currently recommended. Resuscitation should begin with room air for newborns at or over 35 weeks' gestation and 21% to 30% fraction of inspired $O_2$ ($Fio_2$) for preterm infants under 35 weeks' gestation. If the condition of the newborn has not improved after ventilation has been initiated, then ventilation is inadequate and adjustments should be made. The mnemonic "MR SOPA" is commonly used to remember the six ventilation corrective steps: **M**ask adjustment, **R**eposition head, **S**uction airway, **O**pen mouth, **P**ressure increase, and **A**lternative airway. In addition, supplemental $O_2$ should be considered if heart rate and oxygenation have not improved. It is important to remember that $O_2$ saturations slowly increase over time, and it may take a healthy newborn 10 minutes to reach saturations above 90% (see Fig. 189.1).

An alternative airway, including insertion of an ETT or LMA, should be considered when PPV with a face mask does not result in clinical improvement. In addition, alternative airway placement should be considered if prolonged PPV is necessary, if chest compressions are required, or if reliable airway access in special circumstances is needed (e.g., for suspected diaphragmatic hernia, surfactant administration, or obstruction of airway by thick secretions requiring direct tracheal suction). If an advanced airway is needed, electronic cardiac monitoring is recommended to accurately assess the newborn's heart rate.

ETT size and depth of insertion are based on birthweight, although calculations using gestational age also exist (Table 189.1). The neonatal airway lies anteriorly, and cricoid pressure during the intubation step may be of benefit. Use of video laryngoscopy may be helpful, especially for trainees, where use improves first-attempt success rates. However, video laryngoscopy use may be limited in smaller neonates due to device size. Intubation should be completed within approximately 30 seconds. If intubation attempts are unsuccessful, a LMA can provide a successful rescue airway. Recommendations for LMA size are included in Table 189.1. It is important to note that the smallest (size-1) LMA is designed for use in neonates who weigh more than 2000 g. Therefore LMAs cannot be used in very small neonates.

Chest compressions and emergency medications such as epinephrine and volume expanders are rarely needed during newborn resuscitation. The most likely cause of cardiovascular collapse in a newborn is asphyxia/inadequate gas exchange. Thus if the lungs are adequately expanded and ventilated, it is rare for a neonate to require chest compressions. Chest compressions should not

| TABLE 189.1 | Endotracheal Tube and Laryngeal Mask Recommendations | | | | |
|---|---|---|---|---|---|
| Gestational Age (Weeks) | Infant's Weight (g) | ETT Size | ETT Insertion Depth at Lip (cm) | Laryngeal Mask Size* |
| 23–24 | 500–600 | 2.5 | 5.5 | |
| 25–26 | 700–800 | | 6.0 | |
| 27–29 | 900–1000 | | 6.5 | |
| 30–32 | 1100–1400 | 3.0 | 7.0 | |
| 33–34 | 1500–1800 | | 7.5 | |
| 35–37 | 1900–2400 | | 8.0 | 1 |
| 38–40 | 2500–3100 | 3.5 | 8.5 | |
| 41–43 | 3100–4200 | | 9.0 | |

*Currently, the smallest laryngeal mask is intended for use in infants who weigh >2000 g, although many reports support its use in infants who weigh between 1500 and 2000 g, and some reports document success in infants who weigh <1500 g.
*ETT*, Endotracheal tube.

be initiated until chest movement with ventilation attempts has been achieved. Neonates who do not respond to adequate ventilation likely suffer from hypoxia, acidosis, and impaired coronary artery perfusion. Chest compressions can improve coronary artery blood flow and restore heart function. If the heart rate remains below 60 bpm after at least 30 seconds of PPV that moves the chest (ideally through an ETT or LMA), then chest compressions should be initiated and Fio₂ should be increased to 100%. Compressions should be delivered at a depth of approximately one-third of the anterior-posterior diameter of the chest via the two-hand encircling technique at a rate of 90 compressions per minute. This results in three compressions and one ventilation every 2-second cycle (One-and-Two-and-Three-and-Breathe …). The heart rate is reassessed after 60 seconds of coordinated compressions and ventilation. Chest compressions are discontinued when the heart rate is above 60 bpm. Additional interventions such as medication administration are indicated if the heart rate remains below 60 bpm.

Epinephrine is the first-line agent to be used if heart rate remains below 60 bpm, and it can be given intravenously (IV) (preferred), intraosseously (IO), or endotracheally (less effective). Note, only the 1:10,000 preparation (0.1 mg/mL) of epinephrine should be used for neonatal resuscitation and can be repeated every 3 to 5 minutes. The recommended starting dose of 1:10,000 epinephrine is 0.2 mL/kg (0.02 mg/kg) IV/IO and 1 mL/kg (0.1 mg/kg) via ETT. If epinephrine is given via IV/IO, it should be followed by 3 mL normal saline flush. For epinephrine given via the ETT, the medication should be given directly into the tube followed by several positive pressure breaths. Volume expanders such as normal saline and packed red blood cells are given if there are signs of shock or a history of acute blood loss (e.g., delivery after acute placental abruption). Volume expanders should be administered at an initial dose of 10 mL/kg over 5 to 10 minutes. Nonresponse to these efforts should prompt evaluation of all efforts (e.g., chest movement with each breath, coordination of compressions and respirations, 100% oxygen) and for an acute pneumothorax.

If the newborn has an undetectable heart rate after complete and adequate resuscitation efforts, discontinuation of resuscitation may be appropriate. NRP recommends to "consider cessation of resuscitative efforts around 20 minutes after birth" if absence of a heart rate is confirmed after all appropriate steps have been performed. This decision must be individualized on patient and contextual factors. Other situations, such as prolonged bradycardia without improvement, may also serve as indications for discontinuation of resuscitation. Emergency consultation with a colleague or individual with additional expertise may be helpful in these situations.

## Additional Considerations: Meconium

Meconium staining of amniotic fluid represents a special circumstance, and management of such infants has undergone multiple changes over the past several decades. Routine intubation for tracheal suction is no longer recommended. If an infant born through meconium-stained fluid has good respiratory effort and muscle tone, the infant can stay with the mother to receive the initial steps of newborn care. Gentle suction with a bulb syringe may be all that is needed. If an infant has depressed respirations or poor muscle tone, the initial steps of newborn resuscitation should ensue starting with clearing secretions from the mouth and nose by suction. If the infant has poor respiratory effort or the heart rate remains below 100 bpm, then PPV should be initiated and resuscitation should continue per the NRP Flow Diagram (see Fig. 189.1). *Routine* endotracheal suctioning in nonvigorous neonates born through meconium-stained amniotic fluid is not recommended. Endotracheal suction *may be* needed if PPV does not move the chest and airway obstruction is suspected.

## Additional Considerations: Prematurity

Premature infants are significantly more likely to require resuscitation than term infants, as there are additional physiologic challenges after birth (e.g., respiratory distress syndrome [RDS]). Attention to thermoregulation is especially important in preterm infants. A polyethylene wrap and a thermal mattress should be available for any infant under 32 weeks' gestation. CPAP should be considered in a spontaneously breathing preterm infant to facilitate alveolar recruitment, stabilize the airways, minimize the need for intubation, and reduce the risk of lung injury. Intubation and surfactant administration are often required in extremely premature infants (those born at less than 28 weeks' gestation) to treat RDS. Hypoglycemia is common in premature infants, so glucose levels must be monitored.

## Unique Neonatal Assessments: Apgar Scores and Umbilical Cord Gases

The Apgar score is a rapid assessment tool based on physiologic responses to birth at specific time intervals. It can be used objectively to define the condition of a neonate, but the score itself is not used to determine the need for interventions. At intervals of 1 minute and 5 minutes after birth, an experienced and qualified examiner evaluates five physiologic parameters (heart rate, respiratory effort, tone, color, and reflex irritability) (Table 189.2). Newborns who fail to achieve an Apgar score of 7 by 5 minutes

| TABLE 189.2 | Apgar Scoring System | | |
|---|---|---|---|
| | **POINTS ASSIGNED** | | |
| **Score Component** | **0** | **1** | **2** |
| Heart rate (bpm) | 0 | <100 | >100 |
| Respiration | Apnea | Shallow, irregular, or gasping respirations | Vigorous and crying |
| Muscle tone | Absent | Weak, passive tone | Active movement |
| Reflex irritability | Absent | Grimace | Cry, cough, withdraw from stimulus |
| Color | Pale, central cyanosis | Blue extremities, centrally pink (acrocyanosis) | Pink |

of age should have the Apgar score repeated every 5 minutes until the score is at least 7 or the neonate is 20 minutes of age.

Umbilical cord blood gas measurements are often obtained when a newborn requires advanced resuscitation and can serve to assess the fetal condition at the time of delivery. Umbilical artery measurements represent the fetal condition and fetal acid-base status immediately before birth. Umbilical vein measurements represent the maternal condition and uteroplacental gas exchange. The umbilical artery measurement is used by clinicians to evaluate for hypoxic ischemic encephalopathy and the need for therapeutic hypothermia. In general, a newborn with an umbilical cord pH of 7.0 or less or a base deficit of 16 mmol/L or greater should have a neurologic examination performed to determine eligibility for therapeutic hypothermia. Newborns with an umbilical cord pH between 7.01 and 7.15 or base deficit between 10 mmol/L and 15.9 mmol/L may also need a neurologic evaluation depending on perinatal events and neonatal resuscitation requirements.

## Conclusions

In summary, establishing effective ventilation is the most important intervention during neonatal resuscitation. Because inadequate gas exchange is the most common cause of cardiovascular collapse of a newborn, corrective steps to improve ventilation (MR SOPA) should be optimized before proceeding to chest compressions and emergency medications. The NRP Flow Diagram requires reevaluation of the newborn's status at 30- to 60-second intervals and is guided by respiratory effort and heart rate. The authors of this chapter recommend referring to the most current *Textbook of Neonatal Resuscitation* published by AHA/AAP for a more thorough understanding of the neonatal resuscitation. These guidelines are updated and published every 5 years. Anesthesiologists who could be called to a neonatal resuscitation should be trained in NRP.

## SUGGESTED READINGS

American Academy of Pediatrics and American Heart Association, Weiner, G. M., & Zaichkin, J. (Eds.). (2021). *Textbook of neonatal resuscitation* (8th ed.). Itasca: American Academy of Pediatrics.

Aucott, S. W., & Murphy, J. D. (2020). Neonatal assessment and resuscitation. In D. H. Chestnut, C. A. Wong, L. C. Tsen, & Ngan W. D. (Eds.), *Chestnut's obstetric anesthesia* (6th ed., pp. 171–198). Philadelphia: Elsevier.

Aziz, K., Lee, C. H. C., Escobedo, M. B., Hoover, A. V., Kamath-Rayne, B. D., Kapadia, V. S., et al. (2021).

Part 5: Neonatal Resuscitation 2020 American Heart Association Guidelines for Cardiopulmonary Resuscitation and Emergency Cardiovascular Care. *Pediatrics, 147*(Suppl. 1), e2020038505E.

Kirpalani, H., Ratcliffe, S. J., Keszler, M., Davis, P. G., Foglia, E. E., Te Pas, A., et al. (2019). Effect of sustained inflations vs intermittent positive pressure ventilation on bronchopulmonary dysplasia or death among extremely preterm infants: The SAIL Randomized Clinical Trial. *JAMA, 321*(12), 1165–1175.

Lingappan, K., Arnold, J. L., Fernandes, C. J., & Pammi, M. (2018). Videolaryngoscopy versus direct laryngoscopy for tracheal intubation in neonates. *Cochrane Database of Systematic Reviews, 6*(6), CD009975.

Owen, L., & Davis, P. (2020). Role of positive pressure ventilation in neonatal resuscitation. In R. J. Martin & A. A. Fanaroff (Eds.), *Fanaroff and Martin's neonatal-perinatal medicine* (11th ed.). Philadelphia: Elsevier.

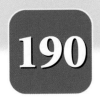

# 190

# Pyloric Stenosis

ROBERT J. FRIEDHOFF, MD

Pyloric stenosis is one of the most common gastrointestinal abnormalities occurring during the first 4 months of life. The incidence is 1 in 500 live births in the White population and 1 in 2000 in the Black population. Pyloric stenosis is four times more common in males than females. It is especially common in firstborn males of parents who had pyloric stenosis.

Pyloric stenosis usually presents at 3 to 5 weeks of age in the preterm or term infant. The etiology is unknown.

Proposed mechanisms include an imbalance in the autonomic nervous system, humoral imbalances, infection, or edema with muscular hypertrophy. Pyloric stenosis was first described in 1888 by Hirschsprung, although he could offer no effective treatment. Ramstedt described the optimal surgical therapy in 1912. Since then, improvements in fluid therapy and anesthetic technique have decreased the morbidity from 25% to 0.1% to 0.01%.

# Presentation

Pyloric stenosis is caused by thickening of the circular muscular fibers in the lesser curvature of the stomach and pylorus that result in obstruction of the pyloric lumen. There is both hypertrophy and an increased number of muscle fibers and deficiency of nerve terminals. The typical presentation is characterized by persistent, bile-free vomiting. The infant is dehydrated and lethargic. The skin is cool to the touch, capillary refill is usually greater than 15 seconds, and the eyes are sunken. The infant may present at less than or equal to its birth weight. Vomiting can be projectile (2–3 feet), occurring after every feeding, thus resulting in loss of hydrogen and chloride ions and sodium and potassium ions from the stomach. The vomitus does not contain any of the alkaline secretions of the small intestine because the obstruction is proximal (at the gastric outlet). Bicarbonate will remain in the plasma (instead of being secreted by the pancreas).

Initially, the kidneys secrete bicarbonate and potassium from the distal tubules and collecting ducts, producing alkaline urine to maintain a normal systemic pH. This results in hypokalemic, hypochloremic metabolic alkalosis. Eventually acidic urine is produced because of the preferential conservation of sodium from the increased aldosterone secretion secondary to volume depletion. Maximal chloride ion conservation in the kidney results in a urinary chloride less than 20 mEq/L.

On physical examination, an olive-sized, palpable mass may be palpated in the midepigastrium. This, along with history, is diagnostic in 99% of the cases. Noninvasive diagnostic tests include ultrasound, which can confirm the diagnosis. The "string-sign" on barium swallow shows elongation and narrowing of the pyloric canal. Elevated levels of unconjugated bilirubin are seen in 20% of the patients.

Pyloric stenosis is a medical emergency, not a surgical emergency. Assessment of the degree of dehydration is made by noting the infant's weight loss and measuring bicarbonate and chloride levels. Treatment is instituted with intravenous (IV) normal saline or lactated Ringer solution. Addition of 40 mmol/L of potassium can be added after urine output is established. The solution is administered at a rate of 3 L/m$^3$/day. Therapy is aimed at repletion of intravascular volume and correction of electrolyte and acid-base abnormalities. Urine chloride concentration greater than 20 mEq/L implies the volume status has been corrected. The plasma chloride concentration should then be greater than 105 mEq/L.

# Management of Anesthesia

Anesthetic considerations for pyloric stenosis include the usual neonatal anesthetic concerns; fluid, electrolyte, and glucose balance; and those for a patient with a full stomach and consideration postoperative apnea. Patients with pyloric stenosis are at increased risk of pulmonary aspiration of gastric contents. After administration of IV atropine (20 mcg/kg), the stomach should be emptied as completely as possible by passing a large-bore (14F multiorifice) orogastric tube two to three times immediately before the induction of anesthesia. After the application of the routine monitors, the induction of anesthesia is variable. It can be accomplished through a modified rapid sequence IV induction with or without cricoid pressure. Induction via an awake oral endotracheal intubation or inhalation induction has been described.

After the induction of general anesthesia, a nasogastric tube should be inserted and left in place during the operative procedure. This will allow testing of the integrity of the pyloric wall after pyloromyotomy by the surgeon. Anesthesia is maintained with volatile agents without nitrous oxide. Skeletal muscle relaxation is usually not needed after induction. Narcotic analgesia is necessary, but in this age group increased respiratory sensitivity to narcotics must be appreciated. Thoracic epidural anesthesia has recently been described with higher oxygen saturations and less oxygen desaturation events and shorter operating room occupancy times. Caudal anesthesia is effective for intraoperative analgesia and muscle relaxation, and a rectus sheath block is an option for postoperative pain management.

Postoperatively, the infant may be lethargic. Respiratory depression and apnea may occur and are related to an alkaline cerebrospinal fluid pH and hypoventilation. For these reasons, the infant should be fully awake and able to sustain a regular respiratory pattern before extubation. Hypoglycemia may occur 2 or 3 hours after surgical correction. This can be caused by cessation of IV glucose infusions and the depletion of glycogen stores from the liver. Small, frequent feeding is usually begun 4 to 6 hours postoperatively. An uneventful recovery should result in discharge from the hospital in 12 to 36 hours.

---

**PEARLS FOR INTRAOPERATIVE MANAGEMENT**

Begin with operating room preparation for a neonate.
Administer atropine 0.1 mg intravenously (IV), followed by fentanyl 0.5 mcg/kg IV before orogastric suctioning of the stomach.
This should be repeated in both lateral decubitus positions until the aspiration is negative.
Follow with a modified rapid sequence intravenous induction.
The stomach must be aspirated whether an orogastric tube is in place or not.

---

## SUGGESTED READINGS

Hines, R. J., & Jones, S. B. Pediatric diseases. (2022). In R. L. Hines, & S. B. Jones (Eds.), *Anesthesia and co-existing disease* (8th ed.). Philadelphia: Elsevier.

Kamata, M., Cartabuke, R. S., & Tobias, J. D. (2015). Perioperative care of infants with pyloric stenosis. *Paediatric Anaesthesia, 25*(12), 1193–1206.

Opfermann, P., Wiener, C., Schmid, W., Zadrazil, M., Metzelder, M., Kimberger, O., et al. (2021). Epidural versus general anesthesia for open pyloromyotomy in infants: A retrospective observational study. *Paediatric Anaesthesia, 31*(4), 452–460.

Park, R. S., Rattana-Arpa, S., Peyton, J. M., Huang, J., Kordun, A., Cravero, J. P., et al. (2021). Risk of hypoxemia by induction technique among infants and neonates undergoing pyloromyotomy. *Anesthesia and Analgesia, 132*(2), 367–373.

Scrimgeour, G. E., Leather, N. W., Perry, R. S., Pappachan, J. V., & Baldock, A. J. (2015). Gas induction for pyloromyotomy. *Paediatric Anaesthesia, 25*(7), 677–680.

Whitaker, E. E., Williams, R. K., Lauro, H. V., Chaudary, R., & Davis, P. J. (2022). Anesthesia for general abdominal, urologic surgery. In P. J. Davis & F. P. Cladis (Eds.), *Smith's anesthesia for infants and children* (10th ed.). Philadelphia: Elsevier.

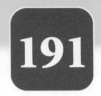

# Pediatric Breathing Circuits

DAWIT T. HAILE, MD

Anesthetic breathing circuits function to deliver oxygen ($O_2$) and anesthetic gases to patients and to eliminate carbon dioxide ($CO_2$) from patients. They are classified according to (1) the presence or absence of unidirectional valves, (2) the presence and the position of a reservoir bag, (3) how $CO_2$ is eliminated, and (4) the ability of the circuit to permit or prevent rebreathing.

## Mapleson Circuits

The first anesthesia breathing systems delivered a nitrous oxide–oxygen ($N_2O$)-$O_2$ mixture for dental anesthesia via a reservoir bag directly connected to an expiratory valve and a facemask. Sir Ivan Magill improved this circuit by distancing the reservoir bag from the expiratory valve and facemask with a reservoir tube to improve surgical access for facial operations. The Magill attachment, also referred to as Mapleson A, was popular for more than 50 years.

By the 1950s, several types of semiclosed circuits were used to deliver anesthetic gases. Semiclosed circuits under optimal conditions prevent rebreathing of alveolar gases. In 1954, the physicist William W. Mapleson analyzed five of these circuits and proposed optimal conditions that would prevent rebreathing. The efficiency of a nonrebreather is determined by the amount of fresh-gas flow and by the positions of the inflow of fresh gas, the expiratory valve, and the reservoir bag. Mapleson labeled these circuits A, B, C, D, and E (Fig. 191.1); subsequently, these circuits have been referred to as the Mapleson circuits, and Mapleson's theoretical analyses have been verified empirically by others.

The five Mapleson circuits lack unidirectional valves and a $CO_2$ absorber. They have the advantage of reduced airflow resistance, which is ideal for use in pediatric patients. The Mapleson circuit removes $CO_2$ by venting exhausted gas to the atmosphere, in contrast with circle systems, in which $CO_2$ is removed by a $CO_2$ absorber. Because Mapleson circuits lack a unidirectional valve, the fresh gas and alveolar gases mix, and significant rebreathing occurs if the fresh-gas flow is not adequate. The Mapleson A and D circuits have been analyzed most extensively, the B and the C circuits are rarely used, and the E circuit is basically a T-piece system. The D circuit is the most commonly used Mapleson circuit, and the A circuit is infrequently used but has a historical and a functional significance.

### MAPLESON A CIRCUIT

The Mapleson A circuit, as described earlier, contains a reservoir tubing (corrugated tubing) separating, at one end, the fresh-gas flow passing through a reservoir bag and, at the opposite end, an adjustable pressure-limiting valve (APL valve) near the facemask. The system is the most efficient and, with spontaneous ventilation, requires less fresh-gas flow than with

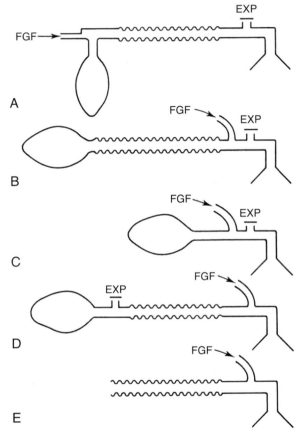

**Fig. 191.1** Mapleson breathing circuits **A** through **E**. Note that **E** is a T-piece system. *EXP*, Expiratory valve; *FGF*, fresh-gas flow. (Redrawn from Ward CS. *Anaesthetic Equipment: Physical Principles and Maintenance.* 2nd ed. Bailliere Tindall WB Saunders; 1985:122–126.)

controlled ventilation. To explain these differences, the breathing cycle can be artificially divided into three phases: the inspiratory, the expiratory, and the expiratory-pause phase.

Immediately before the inspiratory phase of spontaneous ventilation occurs, continuous fresh gas flows into the reservoir bag and the circuit (Fig. 191.2). As the patient inhales, the reservoir bag begins to empty. The lower the fresh-gas flow, or the higher the tidal volume, the emptier the reservoir bag becomes. During the expiratory phase, the reservoir bag completely fills with fresh gas, and when the fresh-gas flow exceeds 70% of minute ventilation, enough pressure develops to vent alveolar and fresh gas through the APL valve. At the last stage of the expiratory phase, a pause occurs before the initiation of the next cycle. During the expiratory pause, fresh-gas flow further drives alveolar gas through the APL valve and virtually eliminates rebreathing.

How can a fresh-gas flow that is only 70% of minute ventilation prevent rebreathing? The answer is "dead-space gas." The

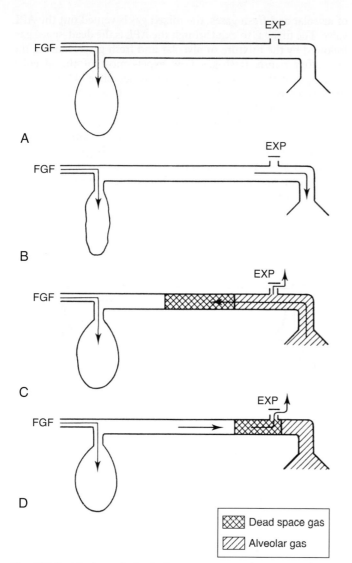

**Fig. 191.2** Mapleson A circuit: Spontaneous ventilation. **A,** Before the inspiratory phase, continuous fresh gas flows into the reservoir bag and the circuit. **B,** The reservoir bag empties during inspiration. **C,** During expiratory phase, the reservoir bag fills with fresh gas, and when it exceeds 70% of minute ventilation, alveolar gas is pushed through the adjustable pressure-limiting *(APL)* valve. **D,** During the last phase of expiration, fresh gas further pushes alveolar gas through the APL and virtually eliminates rebreathing. *EXP,* Expiratory valve; *FGF,* fresh-gas flow. (Redrawn from Ward CS. *Anaesthetic Equipment: Physical Principles and Maintenance.* 2nd ed. Bailliere Tindall WB Saunders; 1985:122–126.)

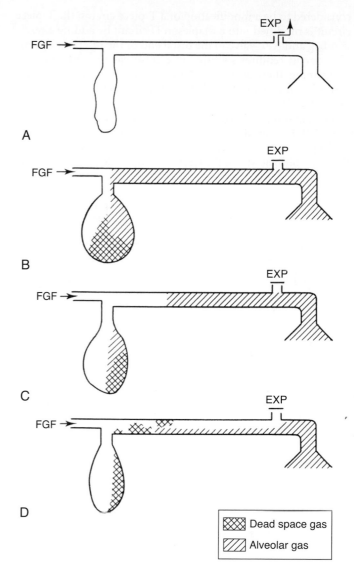

**Fig. 191.3** Mapleson A circuit: Controlled ventilation. **A,** At the end of the inspiratory phase, the reservoir bag is empty. **B,** During expiration, the reservoir bag refills with alveolar gas, fresh gas, and dead-space gas. **C,** The expiratory pause is minimal, and **(D)** the alveolar gas retention in the circuit is quite high. *EXP,* Expiratory valve; *FGF,* fresh-gas flow. (Redrawn from Ward CS. *Anaesthetic Equipment: Physical Principles and Maintenance.* 2nd ed. Bailliere Tindall WB Saunders; 1985:122–126.)

gas in the reservoir tubing immediately before exhalation is dead-space gas because it has not been exchanged within the patient's lung and therefore does not contain alveolar gases. During the expiratory pause, all of the alveolar gases in the reservoir tubing and some of the dead-space gases are pushed by the fresh-gas flow and expelled through the APL valve. However, not all of the dead-space gas is expired before the next cycle. Because of this residual dead-space gas, the amount of fresh gas required to eliminate rebreathing in the Mapleson A circuit during spontaneous ventilation is less than the minute ventilation.

In contrast with spontaneous ventilation, controlled ventilation (hand ventilation) of the Mapleson A circuit empties the reservoir bag at the end of the inspiratory phase (Fig. 191.3). The reservoir bag refills with a mixture of alveolar gases, fresh

gas, and dead-space gases during the expiratory phase. During controlled ventilation, the expiratory pause is minimal, which increases the likelihood of alveolar gas retention in the reservoir tubing and increases the amount of alveolar gases present with the initiation of the next inspiratory phase. Among the Mapleson circuits, the Mapleson A circuit under controlled ventilation is considered to be the least efficient at preventing rebreathing; rebreathing is overcome by increasing fresh-gas flow far exceeding minute ventilation.

## MAPLESON D CIRCUIT

In the Mapleson D circuit, compared with the Mapleson A circuit, the positions of the APL valve and the fresh-gas-flow nipple are reversed; the fresh-gas-flow nipple is located at the patient's end of the circuit, and the APL valve is next to the reservoir bag at the opposite end. The Mapleson D circuit is considered to be a modification of a T-piece circuit; the T-piece circuit is modified into a Mapleson D circuit by adding a reservoir bag and APL valve to the distal end of the reservoir tubing. This circuit requires slightly more fresh-gas flow to eliminate rebreathing than does the Mapleson A circuit. However, for controlled mechanical ventilation, circuit D is the most efficient of the Mapleson circuits.

During spontaneous ventilation with the Mapleson D circuit (Fig. 191.4), the alveolar gases are immediately mixed with fresh-gas flow as the gases pass down the reservoir tubing and fill the reservoir bag. When the reservoir bag is filled with a mixture of alveolar and fresh gases, the mixed gas is vented out the APL valve. The first gas to exit through the APL is the dead-space gas, followed by the mixture of alveolar and fresh gases. During the expiratory pause, fresh-gas flow expels most of the alveolar mixed gas if the minute ventilation is adequate. Therefore to prevent rebreathing, the fresh-gas flow must be twice the minute ventilation, and the expiratory pause has to be sufficiently long to allow all of the alveolar mixed gases to be expelled.

During the expiratory phase of controlled ventilation with the Mapleson D circuit (Fig. 191.5), the fresh-gas flow drives the mixed alveolar gases and dead-space gases out of the APL valve. Furthermore, during the inhalation phase the mixed alveolar gases are pushed and expelled not only by the continuous

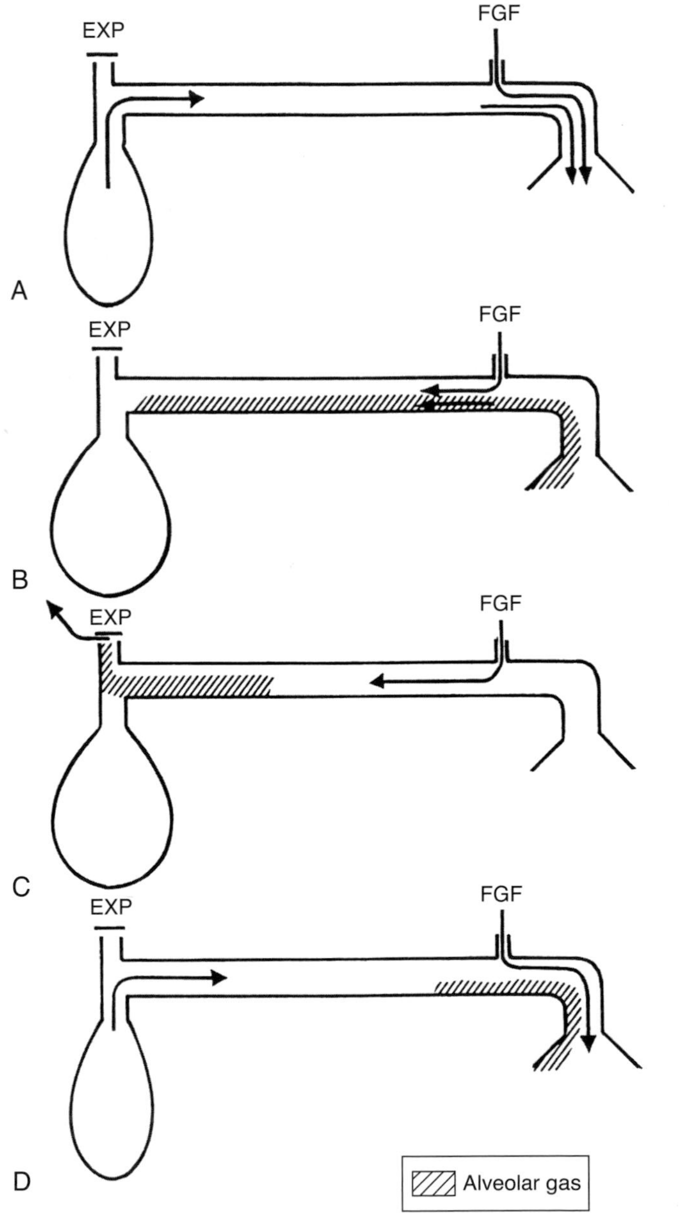

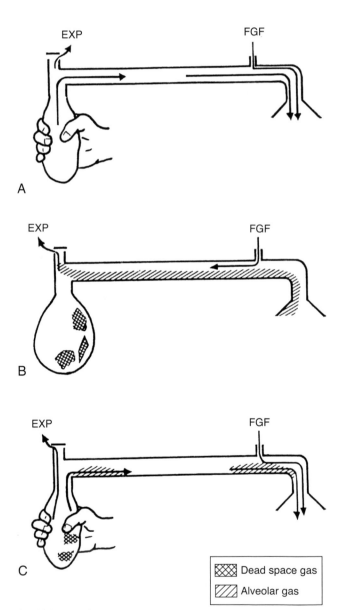

**Fig. 191.4** Mapleson D circuit: Spontaneous ventilation. **A,** The fresh-gas-flow nipple is at the patient's end of the circuit, and the adjustable pressure-limiting valve is at the opposite end with the reservoir bag; therefore **(B)** alveolar and fresh gas mix in the circuit during expiration and **(C)** the alveolar gas is not completely evacuated before **(D)** the next inspiratory phase of spontaneous respiration. *EXP,* Expiratory valve; *FGF,* fresh-gas flow. (Redrawn from Ward CS. *Anaesthetic Equipment: Physical Principles and Maintenance.* 2nd ed. Bailliere Tindall WB Saunders; 1985:122–126.)

**Fig. 191.5** Mapleson D circuit: Controlled ventilation. **A,** During inspiratory phase, the positive pressure (with hand bag-squeeze) will build pressure to expel alveolar mixed gases through adjustable pressure-limiting (APL) valve and the fresh gas flow will also push through APL **(B)** and provide fresh gas to the patient **(C).** *EXP,* Expiratory valve; *FGF,* fresh-gas flow. (Redrawn from Ward CS. *Anaesthetic Equipment: Physical Principles and Maintenance.* 2nd ed. Bailliere Tindall WB Saunders; 1985:122–126.)

fresh-gas flow but also by the positive pressure of controlled ventilation. The amount of fresh-gas flow necessary to minimize rebreathing is greater than the patient's minute ventilation.

The Bain circuit is a modification of the Mapleson D; the two circuits have the same efficiency, but the Bain circuit provides improved humidification of the inspired air and is the most compact of the Mapleson circuits. The position of the reservoir bag, APL valve, and the fresh-gas inflow in these two devices is the same except that the tube carrying fresh gas is an inner coaxial tube within the corrugated tube in the Bain circuit. The inner tube enters the circuit at the reservoir-bag end, and the fresh gas empties at the patient's end of the circuit. The advantages of the Bain circuit over the Mapleson D include (1) less equipment to interfere with the surgical field; (2) less likelihood of kinking the tracheal tube or extubating the patient because the system is lightweight; and (3) the ability to mount the Bain circuit on the anesthesia machine, allowing for expired gases to be scavenged. Gas flows and minute ventilation requirements are similar to those for the Mapleson D circuit.

## Circle System

The circle system is the standard anesthetic circuit on most modern anesthesia machines. Defined by unidirectional valves and a $CO_2$ absorber, the system requires low fresh-gas flow, enabling conservation of heat, humidity, and anesthetic gases. Pediatric circle breathing systems have been developed but are not often used. They are modified to minimize resistance by incorporating narrow-caliber hoses and a smaller $CO_2$ absorber. These pediatric circuits have not been marketed with disposable material, and the adaptation to modern anesthesia is suboptimal.

## Summary

The relevance of the Mapleson circuits, other than the Mapleson D and Bain circuits, is purely academic. However, the relative efficiency of rebreathing prevention and the requirement of fresh-gas flow of these circuits have been described as follows. For spontaneous ventilation, the most efficient to the least efficient is A > DE > CB. During controlled ventilation, the most efficient to the least efficient is DE > BC > A.

Most children are anesthetized with an adult circle breathing system. Infants and neonates who are too small or have sensitive mechanical ventilation requirements need a different class of modern ventilator (e.g., Siemens 300, Dräger Evita). The discussion of the technology behind this class of ventilators is beyond the scope of this chapter. However, these ventilators use technology that can meet the oxygenation and ventilation needs of low-weight infants and neonates and that minimize lung injury more effectively than do the adult anesthesia machines.

## SUGGESTED READINGS

Arnold, P., & Kaufmann, J. (2022). Going around in circles. Is there a continuing need to use the T-piece circuit in the practice of pediatric anesthesia? *Paediatric Anaesthesia, 32*(2), 273–277.

Goenaga-Diaz, E. J., Smith, L. D., Pecorella, S. H., Smith, T. E., Russell, G. B., Johnson, K. N., et al. (2021). A comparison of the breathing apparatus deadspace associated with a supraglottic airway and endotracheal tube using volumetric capnography in young children. *Korean Journal of Anesthesiology, 74*(3), 218–225. doi:10.4097/kja.20518.

Mapleson W. W. (2004). Editorial I: Fifty years after—reflections on 'The elimination of rebreathing in various semi-closed anaesthetic systems'. *British Journal of Anaesthesia, 93*(3), 319–321.

Wenzel, C., Schumann, S., & Spaeth, J. (2018). Pressure-flow characteristics of breathing systems and their components for pediatric and adult patients. *Paediatric Anaesthesia, 28*(1), 37–45. doi:10.1111/pan.13284.

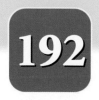

# 192

# Croup Versus Epiglottitis

SARA B. ROBERTSON, MD

Respiratory distress is one of the most common presenting symptoms among pediatric patients in the emergency department and is one of the most common reasons for admission to the intensive care unit (ICU). Both croup (i.e., laryngotracheobronchitis/subglottic inflammation) and acute epiglottitis (supraglottic inflammation) present with evidence of airway obstruction. In 80% of all pediatric patients with stridor, infection is the cause. Of these, 90% are caused by croup, and an increasing minority are cases of epiglottitis. Other causes of respiratory distress include infection (bacterial tracheitis, retropharyngeal abscess, and papilloma), vascular malformations (hemangioma and pulmonary sling), trauma (foreign body and heat injury), and congenital anomalies (subglottic stenosis, vocal cord paralysis, and laryngotracheomalacia)—all of which must also be considered in the differential diagnosis.

Vaccination against *Haemophilus influenzae* type b has resulted in a dramatic reduction (several studies have shown >90% reduction) in the incidence of epiglottitis in children since the late 1980s. The incidence in adults has been less affected, and some authors even report an increasing prevalence in adults of mainly other bacterial infections (e.g., *Staphylococcus*, *Streptococcus*, *Klebsiella*, and *Pseudomonas*).

Because of the possibility of rapid clinical progression to complete obstruction, acute epiglottitis in children requires early and prompt intervention. To provide the appropriate therapeutic interventions, one must be able to differentiate between croup and acute epiglottitis. Table 192.1 compares these two causes of severe stridor.

## Management

### CROUP

The treatment of croup varies according to the severity of the illness. In mild cases, conservative measures (e.g., humidification of air, fever control, hydration) are usually effective. The cause is usually viral, most commonly parainfluenza viruses (types I, II, and III account for 80% of cases), influenza A and B viruses, and respiratory syncytial virus. Additionally, with the recent COVID-19 pandemic, there have been several case reports of croup being caused by SARS-CoV-2 infection. Radiography can be performed to exclude other diagnoses (e.g., a foreign body) and may show the classic "steeple sign" characteristic of croup, though this is neither very sensitive nor specific (Fig. 192.1). In patients who are nontoxic and whose condition is stable, it is increasingly common to perform a flexible laryngoscopy of supraglottic structures to eliminate other diagnoses in the differential diagnosis of croup. In more severe cases, inhaled racemic epinephrine decreases the rate of hospital admission. The inhaled racemic epinephrine solution is prepared according to the child's weight in kilograms—a volume of 2.25% racemic epinephrine is diluted in 2 mL of saline or sterile water (i.e., 0.25 mL of racemic epinephrine for 0–20 kg, 0.5 mL for 20–40 kg, and 0.75 mL for >40 kg). The patient must then be observed for 2 to 3 hours after administration to ensure obstructive symptoms do not return before discharge. Some patients may require more than a single treatment, but if no improvement is seen after more than two inhalation treatments, admission should be considered.

Increasing evidence indicates benefit for steroid use for all cases from mild to severe in terms of alleviation of symptoms, hospital admission, and need for intubation. Dexamethasone, 0.6 mg/kg, can be administered orally, intramuscularly, or parenterally with equal efficacy. The use of helium/oxygen (heliox)

| TABLE 192.1 | Acute Epiglottitis Versus Croup | |
|---|---|---|
| **Clinical Features** | **Acute Epiglottitis** | **Croup** |
| Age (years) | 3–7 | 0.5–5 |
| Family history | No | Yes |
| Prodrome | Usually none ± dysphagia | Usually URI |
| Onset | Abrupt (6–24 h), nonseasonal | Gradual (days), "smoldering," seasonal |
| Clinical course | Rapid, may progress to cardiorespiratory arrest | Usually self-limited |
| **SIGNS AND SYMPTOMS** | | |
| Fever | High (38–40°C) | Low grade |
| Voice | Clear to muffled | Hoarse |
| Dysphagia | Yes | No |
| Dyspnea | Severe | No |
| Inspiratory stridor | Yes | Yes |
| Cough | Usually none | Barking |
| Appearance | Toxic, anxious, sitting upright, leaning forward, mouth open, exaggerated sniffing tripod position | Nontoxic |
| Oral cavity | Pharyngitis with excessive salivation | Minimal pharyngitis |
| Epiglottis | Cherry red, edematous | Normal |
| **RADIOGRAPHIC STUDIES** | | |
| Neck | Enlarged epiglottis ("thumb sign") (Fig. 192.2) | Narrow epiglottis |
| Anteroposterior | Tracheal narrowing | Subglottic narrowing ("steeple sign") (Fig. 192.1) |
| **LABORATORY STUDIES** | | |
| WBC count | Marked elevation with left shift | Variable |
| Etiology | Bacterial: *Haemophilus influenzae* type b, *Staphylococcus*, *Streptococcus*, *Klebsiella*, *Pseudomonas* | Viral: Parainfluenza (types I, II, and III), influenza A and B, RSV, SARS-CoV-2 |

*RSV,* Respiratory syncytial virus; *URI,* upper respiratory infection; *WBC,* white blood cell.

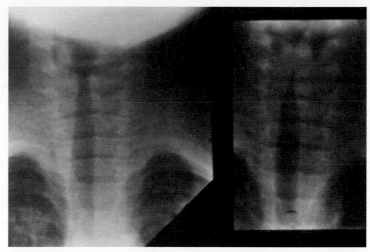

**Fig. 192.1** Anteroposterior neck film demonstrating the "steeple" sign with the characteristic narrowing of the airway. (Used with permission from Hannallah RS, Brown KA, and Verghese ST. Otorhinolaryngologic Procedures. In: Cote CJ, Lerman J, Anderson BJ, eds. *A Practice of Anesthesia for Infants and Children.* 6th ed. Elsevier; 2019:778–781. E-Figure 33-3.)

can be used because the low density of helium attenuates the effects of turbulent flow in the airways. In rare cases (>3%) of croup, humidification, epinephrine, steroids, and heliox are insufficient, and intubation or tracheostomy becomes necessary. An endotracheal tube one size smaller than normal is often appropriate. Antibiotics are indicated only if a secondary bacterial infection develops.

## ACUTE EPIGLOTTITIS

In cases with a more toxic presentation (see Table 192.1) or imminent respiratory collapse, a diagnosis of epiglottitis (supraglottitis) must be suspected. In pediatrics, consider the four "Ds" of epiglottitis (drooling, dysphagia, dysphonia, and dyspnea). The child with acute epiglottitis should be disturbed as little as possible, and no time should be wasted trying to obtain tests (e.g., x-ray) or intravenous (IV) placement. However, if a lateral neck x-ray is obtained, the "thumb" sign is characteristic for the epiglottic edema associated with acute epiglottitis (Fig. 192.2). The child should be transported to the operating room in the sitting position with airway equipment readily available for possible ventilatory support. In severe cases, even attempting to visualize the pharynx can cause acute obstruction. For this reason, the operating room should be set up with all emergency airway equipment readily available: laryngeal mask airways, bougies, fiberoptic bronchoscopes, different blades, and endotracheal tubes in different sizes, as well as a tracheostomy setup. Because of the unpredictable variation in the amount of edema of the epiglottis, and the potential anatomic distortion and difficulty with ventilation, paralytics should be avoided. Inhalational induction and spontaneous breathing should be maintained.

After anesthesia is induced, IV access should be obtained. Laryngoscopy should be performed, and the trachea intubated orally with a tube that is at least a half size smaller than predicted for age. The patient should be admitted to the ICU after the airway is secured for antibiotic administration for several days while the edema resolves. Cases not requiring emergent intubation require intensive observation and readiness in the

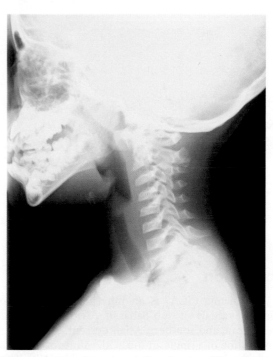

**Fig. 192.2** Soft tissue lateral neck film showing diffuse thickening of the epiglottis, with a thumbprint sign. The aryepiglottic folds are also thickened. (From Eelam A. Adil, Ajman Adil, Rahul K. Shah, Epiglottitis, Clinical Pediatric Emergency Medicine, Vol 16, No 3, Pages 149-153. Figure 2.)

case of deterioration. IV sedation and restraints help prevent accidental extubation. Inspired gases should be humidified, and regular pulmonary toilet should be instituted. Extubation can be considered when pyrexia has subsided and the edema has resolved.

In adults, the course can be more prolonged and less dramatic, but morbidity and mortality remain significant (up to 20%). In contrast to pediatric patients, sore throat and tenderness over the anterior neck are the most common presenting signs. Flexible laryngoscopy provides the diagnosis in 100% of cases. Approximately 70% of children require acute airway intervention, whereas the reported need for adults is closer to 15% to 20%. The presence of stridor, respiratory distress, and rapid onset of symptoms are predictive of the need for airway intervention. Resolution of the symptoms of epiglottitis usually abate within 36 to 48 hours.

Because the cause of epiglottitis is often uncertain, a broad-spectrum cephalosporin such as cefotaxime (200 mcg/kg/day) or ceftriaxone is initiated after blood and epiglottic cultures have been obtained. Alternatively, ampicillin/sulbactam or amoxicillin/clavulanic acid can be used. Levofloxacin or moxifloxacin can be used in patients with a penicillin allergy. The use of corticosteroids has not been shown to be beneficial.

## SUGGESTED READINGS

Al-Qudah, M., Shetty, S., Alomari, M., & Alqdah, M. (2010). Acute adult supraglottitis: Current management and treatment. *Southern Medical Journal*, *103*(8), 800–804.

Chapurin, N., & Gelbard, A. (2019). Epiglottitis. *New England Journal of Medicine*, *381*(9), e15. doi:10.1056/NEJMicm1816761.

Cherry J. D. (2008). Clinical practice. Croup. *New England Journal of Medicine*, *358*(4), 384–391.

Cirilli A. R. (2013). Emergency evaluation and management of the sore throat. *Emergency Medicine Clinics of North America*, *31*(2), 501–515.

Hannallah, R. S., Brown, K. A., & Verghese, S. T. (2019). Otorhinolaryngologic procedures. In C. J. Cote, J. Lerman, & B. J. Anderson (Eds.), *A practice of anesthesia for infants and children* (6th ed., pp. 778–781). Philadelphia: Elsevier.

Smith, D. K., McDermott, A. J., & Sullivan, J. F. (2018). Croup: Diagnosis and management. *American Family Physician*, *97*(9), 575–580.

Sobol, S. E., & Zapata, S. (2008). Epiglottitis and croup. *Otolaryngologic Clinics of North America*, *41*(3), 551–566.

Venn, A. M. R., Schmidt, J. M., & Mullan, P. C. (2021). Pediatric croup with COVID-19. *American Journal of Emergency Medicine*, *43*, 287.e1–287.e3.

# 193

# Sickle Cell Anemia: Anesthetic Implications

MISTY A. RADOSEVICH, MD

## Introduction

Sickle cell anemia (SCA) is an inherited hemoglobinopathy seen in individuals of sub-Saharan Africa, Middle Eastern, Mediterranean, and southern Asian descent. SCA results from the substitution of a single amino acid, valine for glutamic acid, within the beta-globin subunit of hemoglobin (Hb). This molecule is designated Hb S. The amino acid substitution in Hb S results in a defect in the structure of Hb revealing hydrophobic areas of the molecule when deoxygenated. Under certain conditions, these hydrophobic regions may lead to polymerization and precipitation of Hb within the cell, with resultant deformation of the red blood cell (RBC) and the classic sickle-shaped RBC. These sickled, poorly deformable cells lead to intravascular clumping and vessel occlusion, as well as endothelial injury that triggers an inflammatory response involving neutrophils and adhesion molecules (Zhang), as well as interaction with hemostatic factors (platelets, clotting factors). Cell membrane damage and reduced deformability lead to a shortened RBC life span (10–20 days rather than 120 days) as they hemolyze or are removed by the reticuloendothelial system.

The homozygous form of sickle cell anemia (designated Hb SS) results in intra- and extravascular hemolytic anemia and is caused by poor membrane deformability, vasoocclusion that leads to end organ injury under certain physiologic conditions. Repetitive vasoocclusive events and recurrent organ ischemia leads to progressive organ damage (Table 193.1). Manifestations of the disease begin after 3 to 6 months of age as fetal Hb (HbF) concentration wanes and Hb S increases. The heterozygous form of Hb S (sickle cell trait) is mild and typically asymptomatic. Different subtypes including Hb SC and Hb Sβ+, which are compound mutations, may present with severe symptoms with only a single copy of the sickle cell mutation.

## Anesthetic Management

Patients with SCA often require surgery for complications related to their disease, including cholecystectomy (symptomatic gallbladder disease related to pigment stones from chronic hemolysis), orthopedic surgery (avascular necrosis), or splenectomy (splenic sequestration), or for reasons unrelated to their disease (trauma; obstetric; ear, nose, and throat). Perioperative complications are more frequent in SCA patients, especially with increasing age, pregnancy, and preoperative infection (Firth). Overall, 30-day mortality has been estimated at 1.1%.

| TABLE 193.1 | Organ System Effects of Sickle Cell Anemia |
|---|---|
| Hematologic | Chronic hemolytic anemia results in a baseline hemoglobin of 5–9 g/dL. |
| Central nervous system | Vasoocclusion within cerebral vessels may result in ischemic strokes, though hemorrhagic strokes may occur as well. Pain crises are common and related to infarction-mediated pain in bones, hands, and feet. |
| Cardiovascular | Chronic anemia results in a high-output, hyperdynamic state and may result in a cardiomyopathy. Iron overload from frequent transfusions may cause a restrictive cardiomyopathy. Chronic, recurrent vessel occlusion within the pulmonary vasculature may lead to pulmonary hypertension. Cor pulmonale may develop, as well as a sequela of chronic pulmonary insults. Myocardial infarction in the absence of coronary atherosclerosis may also occur. |
| Pulmonary | ACS is a severe complication of SCA involving hypoxemia, cough, chest pain, fever, new pulmonary infiltrate, and respiratory distress. It is likely multifactorial in etiology, including vasoocclusion, infarction and inflammation, infection, and atelectasis. ACS is the leading cause of mortality and hospitalization in SCA and may present in the postoperative period. Recurrent episodes of ACS may lead to pulmonary fibrosis. |
| Renal | Renal failure is a common complication in SCA related to papillary necrosis. Concentrating defects may also be present (isosthenuria). |
| Hepatic | Liver dysfunction and even cirrhosis may develop because of vasoocclusion/infarction, iron overload, or viral hepatitis from frequent transfusions. Cholelithiasis may develop from pigment stones in the setting of chronic hemolysis. |

*ACS*, Acute chest syndrome; *SCA*, sickle cell anemia.

Central to the perioperative care of these patients is avoiding precipitants of erythrocyte sickling, including hypoxia, hypercarbia, acidosis, dehydration, and hypothermia.

## Preoperative

Preoperative management of the patient with SCA should include consultation with a hematologist. History and examination identify high-risk patients; a history of frequent, severe, or recurrent sickle cell crises and evidence of end organ injury are risk factors for perioperative complications. The risk associated with the particular planned procedure is important to consider, as operative risk is associated with postoperative SCA complications (Firth).

Preoperative transfusion management has been evolving. Previously, it was felt that aggressive preoperative transfusion including exchange transfusion to reduce the Hb S concentration to less than 30% was necessary. However, studies have since shown no benefit over conservative transfusion to simply raise the hematocrit to 30% preoperatively. A comparison of preoperative transfusion with no transfusion in 67 patients with SCA (Hb SS type) undergoing low- or medium-risk procedures found a reduced rate of acute chest syndrome (ACS) in those receiving preoperative transfusion to target Hb concentration of 10 g/dL (Transfusion Alternatives Preoperatively in Sickle Cell Disease study, 2013). Though these studies currently inform many clinical decisions, a 2016 Cochrane review including the aforementioned studies rated the level of evidence for the reported outcomes in aggressive versus simple transfusion and in transfusion versus no transfusion to be low to very low because of high risk for bias within the studies.

## Intraoperative

No anesthetic technique is clearly superior to another in the patient with SCA. Pharmacologic alterations may be seen in those with renal or hepatic insufficiency, and dose adjustments may be necessary. Meticulous care to avoid hypovolemia with adequate intravenous fluids and blood products as indicated is necessary. Avoiding hypoventilation, hypercarbia, atelectasis, and targeting oxygen saturation of 100% and partial pressure of

---

### BOX 193.1 INTRAOPERATIVE MANAGEMENT

Supplemental oxygen targeting $PaO_2$ 90% and $SpO_2$ 100%
Hyperoxygenation is not necessary
Ensure adequate ventilation to target normocarbia
Provide adequate fluid resuscitation to avoid hypovolemia and increased blood viscosity
Treat pain aggressively; multimodal analgesia is ideal
Consider regional/neuraxial techniques
Maintain normal acid-base status
Target normothermia, specifically avoiding hypothermia by using forced-air warmers, fluid warmers, and increasing room temperature
Tourniquet use is not strictly contraindicated
Adjust dosing for renal/hepatic function as appropriate
Continue intraoperative management principles into postoperative period

*PaO₂*, Partial pressure of oxygen in arterial blood; *SpO₂*, oxygen saturation.

---

oxygen of at least 90 mm Hg is ideal. Temperature should be monitored and hypothermia avoided. Tourniquets have been used but can increase local hypoxemia, acidosis, and venous stasis favoring erythrocyte sickling (Box 193.1).

## Postoperative

Intraoperative management principles outlined earlier should be continued into the postoperative period. Emphasis should be placed on pulmonary recruitment maneuvers including incentive spirometry and early mobilization. Pain should be treated aggressively, balanced with the need to avoid respiratory depression and hypercarbia. Pain management may be complicated by opioid tolerance often seen in SCA. Postoperative complications in the patient with SCA include painful vasoocclusive events, ACS, stroke, and infection. ACS is a severe complication that may develop 3 days after surgery because of sequestration of sickled cells in the pulmonary vasculature or in the setting of pneumonia, thromboembolism, or fat embolism. It presents similarly to pneumonia, as described previously. Treatment includes correction of hypoxemia, pain control, antibiotics, and transfusion (simple or exchange if severe) (Table 193.2).

| TABLE 193.2 Postoperative Issues and Management | |
| --- | --- |
| **Complication** | **Intervention** |
| Acute chest syndrome | Supplemental oxygen, IS, antibiotics, bronchodilators, transfusion |
| Vasoocclusive events/ pain crises | Aggressive multimodal analgesia, basic SCA cares (oxygen, mobilization, IS, fluid management) |

*IC,* Incentive spirometry; *SCA,* sickle cell anemia.

## SUGGESTED READINGS

Firth, P. G., & Head, C. A. (2004). Sickle cell disease and anesthesia. *Anesthesiology, 101*(3), 766–785.

Howard, J., Malfroy, M., Llewelyn, C., Choo, L., Hodge, R., Johnson, T., et al. (2013). The Transfusion Alternatives Preoperatively in Sickle Cell Disease (TAPS) study: a randomised, controlled, multicentre clinical trial. *Lancet (London, England), 381*(9870), 930–938.

Walker, I., Trompeter, S., Howard, J., Williams, A., Bell, R., Bingham, R., et al. (2021). Guideline on the peri-operative management of patients with sickle cell disease: Guideline from the Association of Anaesthetists. *Anaesthesia, 76*(6), 805–817.

Zhang, D., Xu, C., Manwani, D., & Frenette, P. S. (2016). Neutrophils, platelets, and inflammatory pathways at the nexus of sickle cell disease pathophysiology. *Blood, 127*(7), 801–809.

# 194

# Anesthetic Considerations for the Patient With Down Syndrome

LEAL G. SEGURA, MD

Trisomy 21 (three copies of chromosome 21) accounts for 95% of the cases of Down syndrome (DS), the most common chromosomal abnormality (1:691 live births, according to the Centers for Disease Control and Prevention). The remaining 5% of patients have DS because of mosaicism, Robertsonian translocations, partial trisomy of chromosome 21, isochromosomes, or ring chromosomes. DS is the most common genetic cause of intellectual disability in the United States.

The most significant risk factor for trisomy 21 is maternal age, but more than a century ago it was thought to be "uterine exhaustion." We now know that older mothers have more babies with DS because of the increased frequency of meiotic nondisjunction with increasing maternal age.

Regardless of risk factors, screening recommendations have changed over the last decade. In 2020, the American College of Obstetricians and Gynecologists issued a practice bulletin recommending that all pregnant women be offered screening for DS with ultrasound and serum markers or cell-free DNA, regardless of age or risk for chromosomal abnormality. The practice bulletin recommended that those women with positive screens be offered genetic counseling, comprehensive ultrasound evaluation, and chorionic villus sampling or amniocentesis for definitive diagnosis.

## Clinical Manifestations

Children with DS are often small for age, with multiple characteristic features. Some of these, such as nasal structural abnormalities or decreased right atrial blood flow, are present on ultrasound by 12 weeks' gestation. At birth, hypotonia is common, and characteristic facial features are typical, including oblique palpebral fissures, inner canthal folds, hyperflexible joints, and a single palmar crease. More than half of neonates with DS will have congenital cardiac disease.

## Neurologic Manifestations

Children with DS demonstrate near universal cognitive impairment, and early intervention programs should be instituted soon after birth, with a goal of enhancing development based on each child's needs. For example, receptive language may be a relative strength for a child with DS, versus expressive language, which may be more impaired. Social development may be relatively spared. Although the prevalence of psychiatric disorders is higher in DS than the general population, anesthesiologists should remember that most children with DS do not have behavioral problems.

Anesthesiologists should also be aware of the risk of "diagnostic overshadowing," which occurs when a provider attributes symptoms of a new disorder to the existing, primary diagnosis. For example, a provider may dismiss new behavioral problems in a patient with DS as "just part of the syndrome," rather than the result of new onset medical problems, such as untreated obstructive sleep apnea (OSA), hypothyroidism, or pain.

The incidence of seizures in children with DS is between 5% and 10%, but patients may develop them throughout life. Forty percent of patients with DS may develop infantile spasms or seizures before 1 year, 40% will develop a seizure disorder between 20 and 30 years of age, and some patients develop seizures with advancing age and the onset of dementia. Patients with DS may be at increased risk for stroke, despite fewer typical risk factors, and moyamoya disease, a rare neurovascular lesion, is more prevalent in this population.

## Cardiac Abnormalities

Patients with DS have a high incidence of congenital cardiac abnormalities, the most prevalent of which are atrial and ventricular septal defects. The American Academy of Pediatrics (AAP) recommends an echocardiogram (read by a pediatric cardiologist) in every child with trisomy 21, even if a fetal study was performed in utero and even in babies with DS having otherwise normal cardiovascular examinations. Further, if a child has no echocardiogram for review before surgery, the anesthesiologist should consider delaying the case until a cardiac consultation and echocardiogram can be performed.

Any child with uncorrected or corrected cardiac abnormalities should be considered a candidate for endocarditis prophylaxis, depending on the nature of the surgery and in keeping with American Heart Association guidelines.

Adolescents and older patients with DS should be evaluated annually for newly acquired mitral and aortic valvular disease, and an echocardiogram is indicated in any patient with DS who has cardiovascular symptoms including dyspnea, fatigue, or exercise intolerance, and should be considered for any adult patient with DS without cardiac evaluation since childhood.

## Respiratory Manifestations

Because DS is associated with a high incidence of congenital heart disease, providers may underappreciate the wide spectrum of pulmonary problems experienced by patients with DS. Common pulmonary problems include recurrent bronchitis or pneumonia, OSA, laryngomalacia, tracheobronchomalacia, tracheal bronchus (when a bronchus originates above the carina, more commonly on the right), pulmonary hypertension, subpleural cysts, and subglottic stenosis. Less common abnormalities include complete tracheal rings and interstitial lung disease.

Of these, the AAP recommends discussing specific symptoms of OSA at each well-child visit. The AAP also recommends referral for polysomnography (PSG) in all children with DS by age 4 years because of poor correlation between parental reporting and PSG. If a patient with DS does not have preoperative OSA screening, the anesthesiologist should have a high index of suspicion for an untreated sleep disorder, especially in adults.

## Gastrointestinal Manifestations

Certain surgical malformations of the gastrointestinal (GI) tract are associated with DS (esophageal atresia, duodenal atresia, Hirschsprung disease, and anal atresia) and may present early in the neonatal period. Medical providers who are involved in neonatal resuscitation should be aware that early and massive vomiting may be a sign of GI obstruction because of esophageal or duodenal atresia.

Anesthesia providers may take care of patients with DS as they undergo evaluation of feeding disorders later in childhood as well. Feeding concerns are common in children with DS and may be related to hypotonia, anatomic differences, developmental issues, or celiac disease, which is present in between 7% and 10% of patients with DS. Gastroesophageal reflux is common in infants with DS, and constipation can be a concern across all ages.

## Endocrinologic Manifestations

Patients with DS have an increased prevalence of endocrine disorders, including thyroid disease and diabetes mellitus. Obesity may be more common in older children, adolescents, and adults with DS, and can lead to metabolic syndrome (obesity, hypertension, and diabetes). Despite guidelines recommending annual thyroid screening in patients with DS, yearly testing does not always occur, and thyroid disease may be underdiagnosed.

## Musculoskeletal Abnormalities

Anesthesia providers should be aware that patients with DS are at increased risk of spine abnormalities, including atlantooccipital and atlantoaxial hypermobility, which can lead to cervical or atlantooccipital instability. Although some organizations, such as the Special Olympics and certain schools, require cervical spine screening before participation, the AAP does not recommend routine radiographic evaluation of the cervical spine in asymptomatic children with DS. In fact, radiographic findings may not be consistently visible until 3 years of age because of incomplete bony development and mineralization, and normal films do not guarantee the absence of cervical spine problems.

Anesthesia providers may encounter patients with DS during perioperative visits for other musculoskeletal abnormalities. These include slipped capital femoral epiphysis, patellar instability, and foot deformities. Throughout childhood, nonsurgical interventions such as physical therapy play an important role in the physical development of patients with DS.

## Head and Neck Abnormalities

In addition to cervical spine concerns, patients with DS often have abnormalities of the head and neck that are relevant to the anesthesia provider in the perioperative setting (Box 194.1). In addition, patients with DS may require frequent surgical interventions to address ear, nose, and throat issues. Recurrent otitis media and eustachian tube dysfunction is common secondary to midface hypoplasia, and adenotonsillectomy may be indicated to address OSA. Because children with DS have a higher incidence of post-tonsillectomy respiratory complications, practice guidelines from the Academy of Otolaryngology recommend overnight admission postoperatively.

## Adults With Down Syndrome

Although the prevalence of DS in the pediatric population has been stable for decades, its prevalence in adults in increasing, related to dramatic improvements in life expectancy because of improved medical management over the last 40 years. Thus anesthesiologists should remain familiar not just with progression of childhood disorders but also with independent age-acquired manifestations of DS. These include dementia, acquired valvular heart disease, degenerative cervical spine lesions, obesity, and severe OSA—all more prevalent in DS than the general population. Adults with DS present for all types of surgery and may be more likely to require anesthesia for examinations or minor procedures because of dementia.

## Perioperative Management

### PREOPERATIVE EVALUATION

Patients with DS are frequently encountered by anesthesiologists as they undergo surgical procedures related to numerous comorbidities. Careful perioperative care includes diligent patient education and planning.

Anesthesia providers caring for patients with DS should be particularly attentive to evaluation of the airway, the cardiac system, the pulmonary system, and the cervical spine. The anesthesia provider should ask about symptoms and signs of cord compression, focusing on gait abnormalities, weakness, fatigue, spasticity, or clonus. Even in the absence of abnormal spine films or neurologic symptoms, providers should empirically treat the cervical spine with care, maintaining neutral neck positions during intubation, ventilation, and surgical positioning. If atlantoaxial instability is suspected, any elective procedure should be postponed until orthopedic or neurosurgical evaluation can be performed.

A sedative premedication may or may not be indicated, depending on the individual patient. Optimal agents and routes of administration will depend on the level of patient cooperation and perioperative needs. Preoperative planning should also include discussions with the patient and the patient's primary caregiver regarding postoperative pain control.

## Operative Management

Because of an increased incidence of hip subluxation caused by ligament and tendon laxity, special care should be taken when positioning a patient with DS for any procedure and especially for procedures performed in the lithotomy position.

Surveillance for significant hemodynamic changes with anesthesia is important. Several case reports, series, and retrospective studies describe bradycardia with exposure to inhalation anesthetics. One study reported an incidence of severe bradycardia with inhalation induction as high as 57%, considerably higher than the general population. Such bradycardia may require treatment with anticholinergic agents or epinephrine, if severe. Providers should remember that obtaining rapid intravenous access to administer such drugs may be difficult in patients with DS. Some authors suggest both arterial and peripheral venous cannulation may be more difficult in this population.

Care should be taken in appropriately sizing an endotracheal tube, and providers should remember a high incidence of subglottic narrowing. Again, even in children with normal neck films and no symptoms, intubation should be performed in a neutral position.

## SUGGESTED READINGS

Bull, M. J. (2020). Down syndrome. *New England Journal of Medicine, 382*(24), 2344–2352.

Kraemer, F. W., Stricker, P. A., Gurnaney, H. G., McClung, H., Meador, M. R., Sussman, E., et al. (2010). Bradycardia during induction of anesthesia with sevoflurane in children with Down syndrome. *Anesthesia and Analgesia, 111*(5), 1259–1263.

Malinzak, E. B. (2021). Perioperative care of adults with Down syndrome: A narrative review. *Canadian Journal of Anaesthesia, 68*(10), 1549–1561.

Sulemanji, D. S., Donmez, A., Akpek, E. A., & Alic, Y. (2009). Vascular catheterization is difficult in infants with Down syndrome. *Acta Anaesthesiologica Scandinavica, 53*(1), 98–100.

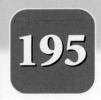

# 195

# Pediatric Neuromuscular Disorders

ASHLEY V. WONG GROSSMAN, MD  |  RANDALL PAUL FLICK, MD, MPH

## Pediatric Neuromuscular Disorders

Pediatric neuromuscular disorders (NMDs) are a diverse group of neurologic and muscular diseases of variable complexity and origin. Perioperative management of these disorders depends on the specific disease pathophysiology and clinical presentation, emphasizing the importance of the preanesthetic medical evaluation. Because the specific NMD or pathophysiology of the NMD is not always known, the anesthetic management of patients with these disorders can be challenging.

NMDs are often associated with other congenital disorders, and it is not uncommon for children with these disorders to present for diagnostic procedures or elective surgery to correct various deformities. The most significant anesthetic concerns to consider when caring for pediatric patients with NMDs are listed in Box 195.1. Several types of NMDs are briefly reviewed here along with their associated perioperative considerations.

## Cerebral Palsy

Cerebral palsy (CP) and static encephalopathy are terms used for a collective group of nonprogressive disorders of movement involving abnormal development or prenatal injury to the brain. Although genetic abnormalities, perinatal anoxia, infection, and trauma have been proposed as etiologic factors in CP, no single cause has been identified. CP has a prevalence of 2 to 4 in 1000 live births, and patients with CP will have a variety of presentations from near normal functional status to complete incapacitation. Clinical manifestations include disorders of posture because of spasticity or hypotonia of lower or upper extremity muscle groups and abnormal speech or vision. Gastroesophageal reflux, behavior problems, intellectual disability, and epilepsy can coexist in some children with CP. The severity of preoperative CP appears to directly correlate with postoperative complications. Factors associated with increased risk of a perioperative adverse event include a high American Society of Anesthesiologists physical status score, history of seizures, upper airway hypotonia, and general surgery.

## Muscular Dystrophy

The muscular dystrophies (MDs) are characterized by progressive degeneration of skeletal muscles. Duchenne MD (DMD) and Becker MD (BMD) are rare (1 per 3000–3500 male newborns), X-linked recessive disorders caused by genetic mutations that result in abnormal dystrophin protein. Symptoms of DMD are more severe than those of BMD; however, both disorders result in myofibril atrophy, necrosis, and fibrosis. In patients with DMD, affected muscles increase in size (pseudohypertrophy) as result of muscle replacement with fat and connective tissue. Muscle weakness may not become evident until the patient is 2 to 5 years of age, but the weakness can rapidly progress such that children with DMD are often wheelchair bound by 8 to 10 years of age and die before 30 years of age.

The preanesthetic medical evaluation of patients with MD should include an assessment of coexisting disease. A thorough review of the cardiac system is important given the increased risk of cardiomyopathy and arrhythmias caused by fibrosis of the cardiac electrical conduction system. Respiratory insufficiency is also common in patients with MD, and the need for postoperative mechanical ventilatory support should be anticipated during the preanesthetic evaluation. Preoperative respiratory optimization and training in the use of noninvasive ventilation and manual or assisted cough techniques can be helpful, especially in patients with preoperative forced vital capacity less than 50% predicted. Patients with MD may also have an increased risk of aspiration secondary to depressed laryngeal reflexes and gastrointestinal hypomobility. Succinylcholine and volatile anesthetics are contraindicated in patients with MD because of the risk of rhabdomyolysis with subsequent hyperkalemic cardiac arrest. In patients with advanced disease, nutritional status should be optimized before surgery to minimize wound infections, and stress-dose steroids should be considered in patients maintained on chronic steroid therapy. Other anesthetic considerations in this high-risk population include known difficult intravenous access, opioid sensitivity, risk of hypothermia secondary to reduced heat production, increased blood loss, and known difficult airways secondary to masseter muscle atrophy, macroglossia, and cervical spine immobility.

---

**BOX 195.1  ANESTHETIC CONSIDERATIONS FOR CHILDREN WITH NEUROMUSCULAR DISORDERS**

- Aspiration risk is increased because of decreased airway reflexes and increased oral secretions
- The use of succinylcholine should be avoided because of the increased risk of rhabdomyolysis and hyperkalemia
- Volatile anesthetics should be avoided in patients with DMD secondary to the risk of rhabdomyolysis and hyperkalemia
- Patients may have increased resistance to the effects of nondepolarizing neuromuscular blocking agents
- MAC may be decreased in patients with NMDs
- Patients with NMDs may have an increased sensitivity to opioids
- Patients with NMDs may have an increased risk of experiencing perioperative blood loss, factor deficiency, or thrombocytopenia
- Patients with NMDs may be more prone to developing hypothermia
- Consider optimizing preoperative respiratory and cardiovascular function, as well as nutrition

*DMD,* Duchenne muscular dystrophy; *MAC,* minimum alveolar concentration; *NMD,* neuromuscular disorders.

---

## Mitochondrial Myopathies

Mitochondrial myopathies are a complex group of disorders with varied presentations characterized by defects in mitochondrial respiratory chain complex function. Clinical manifestations include generalized muscle fatigability, progressive weakness, hypoglycemia, metabolic acidosis, failure to thrive, and stroke. All organ systems can be affected, especially those with high oxygen demands (brain, heart, liver, and kidneys). Mitochondria are the principal source of adenosine triphosphate (ATP), and when patients undergo stress (e.g., surgery), ATP levels may be inadequate to meet the demand; lactate levels are often increased in these patients during periods of physiologic stress. Therefore preoperative fasting should be minimized in these patients. As in children with MD, a thorough preoperative anesthetic medical evaluation is vital to ensuring appropriate perioperative planning, as respiratory compromise, myocardial dysfunction, conduction abnormalities, and dysphagia are also common in these patients.

In addition, it may be prudent to avoid the use of high-dose propofol infusions in pediatric patients with suspected mitochondrial myopathies given the clinical manifestations (metabolic acidosis, rhabdomyolysis, and cardiac impairment) and pathophysiology of both mitochondrial myopathies and propofol infusion syndrome (PRIS) have similarities. Although the myocytotoxic effects of propofol in PRIS have not been entirely elucidated, the mitochondria play an important role.

## Malignant Hyperthermia and Neuromuscular Disorders

Malignant hyperthermia (MH) is a rare, life-threatening disorder manifested by a hypermetabolic state of skeletal muscle often triggered by exposure to halogenated volatile anesthetics and the depolarizing neuromuscular relaxant succinylcholine. Clinically, MH presents nonspecifically with muscle rigidity, acute rhabdomyolysis, fever, hypercarbia, tachycardia, acidosis, hyperkalemia, arrhythmias, and elevated creatine kinase levels. The susceptibility to MH among patients with neuromuscular disorders has been an area of controversy; however, with advances in pharmacogenetics, it is now believed that MH is associated with only a few conditions to date: King-Denborough syndrome, Evans myopathy, central core disease, multiminicore disease, congenital fiber type disproportion, core-rod myopathy, and centronuclear myopathy. Much of the difficulty associated with defining the relationship between MH and MD is related to the phenomenon of acute rhabdomyolysis. Acute rhabdomyolysis leading to hyperkalemic cardiac arrest has been reported to occur in association with many MDs and myopathies and has been understandably confused with MH. Presenting symptoms and signs of acute rhabdomyolysis are very similar to those of MH, and if untreated, both rhabdomyolysis and MH may result in death. Similar to MH, most reported cases of rhabdomyolysis have been associated with the use of succinylcholine; however, several cases have occurred in its absence. Inhalation anesthetic agents have also been implicated, although the mechanism by which this occurs remains, to a large extent, unexplained. For these reasons, it is common to avoid the use of triggering anesthetic agents (succinylcholine and inhalation agents) in patients with MD.

Because both MH and rhabdomyolysis are uncommon, most studies are underpowered to be able to demonstrate the safety of using inhalation anesthetic agents in the setting of suspected myopathy. Studies that include small groups of patients have shown that, in a diverse population of children undergoing muscle biopsy for known or suspected myopathy, the incidence of MH or rhabdomyolysis is extremely uncommon even when succinylcholine or inhalation anesthetic agents have been used. The estimated risk of MH or rhabdomyolysis attributed to the use of these agents is probably less than 1%. Each anesthesia provider must decide based on a patient's clinical situation whether the risk is sufficient to justify the use of an alternative anesthetic agent: propofol (PRIS), etomidate (adrenal suppression), dexmedetomidine (bradycardia and hypotension), ketamine (hallucinations), or a regional technique (feasibility/acceptance/cooperation). Although not currently approved by the U.S. Food and Drug Administration in children, the neuromuscular blockade reversal agent sugammadex has been reported to reverse neuromuscular blockade in these difficult clinical scenarios involving children with neuromuscular disorders when succinylcholine is avoided. Compared with anticholinesterase inhibitors, sugammadex has been shown to have an attractive safety profile with few adverse effects across all pediatric age groups.

## SUGGESTED READINGS

Baum, V. C., & O'Flaherty, J. E. (Eds.). (2007). *Anesthesia for Genetic Metabolic and Dysmorphic Syndromes of Childhood* (2nd ed.). Philadelphia: Lippincott, Williams & Wilkins.

Flick, R. P., Gleich, S. J., Herr, M. M., & Wedel, D. J. (2007). The risk of malignant hyperthermia in children undergoing muscle biopsy for suspected neuromuscular disorder. *Paediatric Anaesthesia, 17*(1), 22–27.

Gaver, R. S., Brenn, B. R., Gartley, A., & Donahue, B. S. (2019). Retrospective analysis of the safety and efficacy of sugammadex versus neostigmine for the reversal of neuromuscular blockade in children. *Anesthesia and Analgesia, 129*(4), 1124–1129.

Racca, F., Mongini, T., Wolfler, A., Vianello, A., Cutrera, R., Del Sorbo, L., et al. (2013). Recommendations for anesthesia and perioperative management of patients with neuromuscular disorders. *Minerva Anestesiologica, 79*(4), 419–433.

Segura, L. G., Lorenz, J. D., Weingarten, T. N., Scavonetto, F., Bojanić, K., Selcen, D., et al. (2013). Anesthesia and Duchenne or Becker muscular dystrophy: Review of 117 anesthetic exposures. *Paediatric Anaesthesia, 23*(9), 855–864.

Shapiro, F., Athiraman, U., Clendenin, D. J., Hoagland, M., & Sethna, N. F. (2016). Anesthetic management of 877 pediatric patients undergoing muscle biopsy for neuromuscular disorders: A 20-year review. *Paediatric Anaesthesia, 26*(7), 710–721.

Tobias, J. D. (2017). Current evidence for the use of sugammadex in children. *Paediatric Anaesthesia, 27*(2), 118–125.

Wass, C. T., Warner, M. E., Worrell, G. A., Castagno, J. A., Howe, M., Kerber, K. A., et al. (2012). Effect of general anesthesia in patients with cerebral palsy at the turn of the new millennium: A population-based study evaluating perioperative outcome and brief overview of anesthetic implications of this coexisting disease. *Journal of Child Neurology, 27*(7), 859–866.

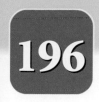

# 196

# Anesthesia for Patients With Myotonic Dystrophy

KELLI C. WATSON, MD, MPH | ARNOLEY S. ABCEJO, MD

## Introduction

Myotonic dystrophy is an autosomal dominant disorder characterized by myotonia—delayed or absent muscle relaxation after voluntary or elicited muscle contraction. Myotonia classically presents with prolonged grip release after a forceful handgrip but can also be stimulated with deep tendon reflex testing or by tapping the thenar eminence. Symptoms classically present in the second or third decade of life as loss of hand coordination and myotonia, with eventual progression to distal muscle weakness and atrophy. Clinical diagnosis is made in the setting of a positive family history with evidence of muscular weakness and clinical myotonia. Confirmative diagnosis is made by genetic testing.

There are two main types of myotonic dystrophy: myotonic dystrophy type 1 (DM1 or Steinert disease) and myotonic dystrophy type 2 (DM2 or proximal myotonic myopathy). DM1 is more common than DM2, presents earlier in life, and is more often associated with significant, more severe multisystem complications. DM1 and DM2 are both caused by a unique trinucleotide repeat sequence that leads to abnormal splicing of various genes, including a chloride channel, cardiac troponin, and insulin receptor (Table 196.1). The trinucleotide repeat sequence lengthens with each subsequent generation, resulting in worsening severity of the disease and its complications within offspring. This genetic phenomenon is known as anticipation.

## Coexisting Organ System Dysfunction

Because of the molecular disease mechanism affecting various genes and downstream proteins, myotonic dystrophy is a complex multisystem disorder. Muscular dysfunction (both smooth and skeletal muscle) results from a dysfunctional adenosine triphosphate system that prevents functional return of calcium to the sarcoplasmic reticulum. The repeat sequence also affects gene splicing of many downstream receptors, placing multiple organ systems at risk for dysfunction. This is particularly true in DM1 (Table 196.2). Because of the potential multiorgan involvement of muscular dystrophy, a thorough preoperative anesthetic evaluation must be completed.

Pulmonary pathophysiology can be both structural and functional. Respiratory muscles, including the diaphragm, chest wall muscles, and bulbar muscles, become progressively weaker, leading to restrictive lung physiology and impaired ventilatory responses to hypoxia and hypercarbia. Weakened oropharyngeal muscles and cough mechanism can predispose these patients to recurrent pulmonary infections and obstructive sleep apnea.

Cardiac involvement is characterized by conduction system abnormalities, supraventricular and ventricular arrhythmias, and, less commonly, myocardial dysfunction and ischemic heart disease. Notably, these conduction abnormalities can be the earliest manifestations of myotonic dystrophy, even before the onset of myotonia or muscle weakness. Because of an increased risk of sudden cardiac death, these patients may undergo pacemaker implantation before development of symptomatic arrhythmias. Other cardiac manifestations of myotonic dystrophy include mitral valve prolapse (up to 20% of affected individuals), cardiomyopathy, and heart failure.

Smooth muscle involvement leads to gastrointestinal hypomotility, which can present as constipation, pseudoobstruction, and increased risk of aspiration. Pregnant women may experience

| TABLE 196.1 | Characteristic Differences Between Myotonic Dystrophy Types 1 and 2 | |
|---|---|---|
| | **Myotonic Dystrophy Type 1** | **Myotonic Dystrophy Type 2** |
| Alternative name | Steinert disease | Proximal myotonic dystrophy |
| Chromosome | 19q13.3 | 3q21 |
| Defect | CTG repeat on DMPK gene | CCTG repeat on ZNF9 gene |
| Prevalence | 2.1–14.3 per 100,000 | Unknown because of variable presentation |
| Age of onset | Birth, childhood, or adult | Adult |
| Pattern of muscle weakness | Distal > proximal | Proximal > distal (mild) |
| Clinical myotonia | Prominent | Less prominent or absent |
| Severity of disease | Moderate to severe (progressive) | Mild |
| Association with coexisting disease | See Table 196.2 | Dilated cardiomyopathy, glucose intolerance, myalgias, sudden cardiac death (rare) |
| Adverse reactions to pharmaceuticals | See Table 196.2 | None (see Suggested Readings) |

| TABLE 196.2 | Complications of Myotonic Dystrophy Type 1 by Organ System | |
|---|---|---|
| **Organ System** | **Comorbidities and Coexisting Diseases** | |
| Central and peripheral nervous system | • Increased sensitivity to sedatives and hypnotics<br>• Decreased ventilatory response to hypercarbia<br>• Presenile cataracts | |
| Musculoskeletal | • Muscular atrophy<br>• Risk for myotonic crises caused by:<br>  • Surgical incision/pain<br>  • Electrocautery<br>  • Muscular twitch monitoring<br>  • Shivering<br>  • Medication administration (see Table 196.3)<br>• Delayed recovery from nondepolarizing neuromuscular blockade | |
| Pulmonary | • Restrictive lung disease<br>• Inspiratory muscle weakness > expiratory muscle weakness<br>• Oropharyngeal muscular weakness leading to obstructive sleep apnea and silent aspiration | |
| Cardiac | • Cardiac conduction abnormalities<br>• Dilated cardiomyopathy<br>• Ischemic heart disease<br>• Mitral valve prolapse | |
| Gastrointestinal | • Gastroesophageal reflux<br>• Delayed gastric emptying<br>• Postoperative ileus<br>• Aspiration risk | |
| Obstetric/reproductive | • Premature and prolonged labor<br>• Uterine atony<br>• Postpartum hemorrhage<br>• Polyhydramnios | |
| Endocrine | • Insulin resistance<br>• Gonadal failure<br>• Testicular and ovarian hypotrophy<br>• Hypothyroidism | |

uterine atony during labor, which increases the risk for prolonged labor, retained placenta, and peripartum hemorrhage.

Endocrine dysfunction presents with pancreatic, adrenal, thyroid, and gonadal insufficiency. Insulin resistance can be common, secondary to impaired insulin receptor function. Patients may also develop presenile cataracts and premature frontal baldness. Central nervous system involvement includes attention disorders, cognitive impairment, and mental retardation. Understanding these multisystem effects of myotonic dystrophy is critical for an anesthesiologist when developing a safe anesthetic plan.

## Anesthetic Considerations

Patients with myotonic dystrophy are at increased risk for perioperative complications, with a rate of 8.0% to 42.9%. Complications are most often pulmonary in nature, including respiratory failure, aspiration, and pneumonia. Respiratory failure is the leading cause of death in these patients, followed by sudden cardiac death secondary to arrhythmia. Risk factors include DM1 genotype, upper abdominal surgery, prolonged surgery duration longer than 1 hour, severe muscular disability,

lack of appropriate reversal after nondepolarizing muscle relaxant administration, and perioperative morphine use. Patients with DM2, on the other hand, have only a 0.6% rate of perioperative complication risk.

## PREANESTHETIC EVALUATION

A detailed evaluation should be performed by the primary care provider and anesthesiologist up to 4 weeks in advance of a planned surgery. Strong consideration should be given to involvement of additional multidisciplinary providers such a cardiologist, pulmonologist, and neurologist. Focus should be given to assessment of neuromuscular weakness, pulmonary function, airway protection capability, and cardiac function. Deconditioning may mask heart failure or stable angina. Cardiac conduction abnormalities do not reliably correspond with neuromuscular weakness and may be present even with mild disease. Typical preoperative workup includes a baseline electrocardiogram, echocardiogram, and pulmonary function tests, as well as pacemaker interrogation if one is present.

## PREMEDICATION

Patients with myotonic dystrophy are highly sensitive to the respiratory depressant effects of sedative medications (Table 196.3). Thus commonly used premedications such as midazolam or opioids should be avoided preoperatively. If medication must be given, ensure appropriate monitoring and airway rescue equipment is available. Preoperative treatment with nonparticulate antacid, $H_2$ blockers, and metoclopramide should be considered to minimize aspiration risk in the setting of gastric hypomotility.

## INDUCTION

These patients often carry multiple risk factors for aspiration including delayed gastric emptying, oropharyngeal muscle

| TABLE 196.3 | Adverse Drug Reactions to Commonly Used Perioperative Medications in Patients With Myotonic Dystrophy Type 1 |
|---|---|
| **Pharmacologic Agent** | **Adverse Drug Reaction** |
| **SEDATIVES** | |
| Propofol* | Prolonged or enhanced sedation<br>Rare association with myotonic crisis |
| Etomidate | Prolonged or enhanced sedation<br>Rare association with myotonic crisis |
| Narcotics, benzodiazepines, barbiturates | Prolonged or enhanced sedation |
| **MUSCLE RELAXANTS** | |
| Succinylcholine | Myotonic crisis and impaired ventilation |
| Nondepolarizing neuromuscular blockers | Prolonged or enhanced muscle weakness |
| **OTHER** | |
| Halothane | Myotonic crisis |
| Neuraxial opioids | Increased sensitivity, high risk of respiratory depression |

*Propofol has been used to terminate myotonic crises.

weakness, and sensitivity to induction agents. Thus modified rapid sequence intubation without neuromuscular blockade is recommended (see later regarding succinylcholine use). Patients' high sensitivity to hypnotic and analgesic agents necessitates careful titration to desired effect. Current literature reports safe use of etomidate and propofol. However, the pain associated with intravenous (IV) administration of these agents has been shown to precipitate myotonic contractions; pretreatment with lidocaine is often useful.

## MAINTENANCE

Volatile anesthetics are safe to use in patients with myotonic dystrophy. Medical literature also reports safe use of propofol and remifentanil infusions for total IV anesthesia.

## NEUROMUSCULAR BLOCKADE

When possible, neuromuscular blockade should be avoided. Despite common misconception, these patients do not have an increased risk of malignant hyperthermia with succinylcholine administration. However, succinylcholine is contraindicated in these patients as it can induce myotonic contractions severe enough to impair ventilation. When neuromuscular blockade is necessary, selection of a short-acting nondepolarizing agent such as rocuronium or cisatracurium is recommended. Of note, neuromuscular blocking agents will not treat myotonic contractions.

Historically, reversal with anticholinesterases was avoided in these patients because of a concern for precipitating myotonic crisis. However, this has been refuted, and current literature suggests that incomplete reversal is associated with much higher risk of adverse perioperative respiratory events. Sugammadex has been used safely in these patients and is recommended for reversal when available. Newer literature suggests that the era of neuromuscular blockade avoidance in patients with myotonic dystrophy may be shifting toward acceptance of safe use of rocuronium and vecuronium with full sugammadex reversal.

## MONITORS

Temperature monitoring is highly recommended, as cold temperatures and shivering can precipitate myotonic contractions.

Neuromuscular blockade should be monitored with peripheral nerve stimulation. However, this electrical stimulation may cause myotonia, which can be mistaken for sustained tetany, falsely suggesting adequate reversal of neuromuscular blockade.

## PAIN MANAGEMENT

Opioid-sparing techniques are favored and have been shown to improve perioperative outcomes and decrease prolonged recovery after anesthesia in patients with myotonic dystrophy. Opioid use is associated with profound respiratory depression and potentially catastrophic postoperative complications. In addition, opioids can exacerbate gastrointestinal hypomotility, leading to increased incidence of pseudoobstruction. Nonsteroidal antiinflammatory drugs and acetaminophen can be safely used for multimodal analgesia.

## REGIONAL ANESTHESIA

Regional anesthesia can be performed safely in patients with myotonic dystrophy and should be considered as an alternative to general anesthesia when feasible. Use of ultrasound guidance for needle placement is preferred over nerve stimulation technique to avoid precipitation of myotonic contractions.

## RECOVERY

Extubation criteria should be strictly followed. Prolonged awakening should be anticipated because of increased sensitivity to sedative and hypnotic agents and impaired response to hypoxia and hypercarbia. Continuous postoperative monitoring including pulse oximetry and electrocardiography is critical in these patients, as they can experience delayed-onset apnea up to 24 hours postoperatively, as well as cardiac arrhythmias. Thus disposition level of care may require observation in a monitored bed setting. Noninvasive ventilation should be used with caution, as these patients are at higher risk for aspiration and iatrogenic stomach insufflation. Use of chest physiotherapy and incentive spirometry is encouraged. Last, postoperative shivering may precipitate myotonic contractions, and preemptive treatment with meperidine may be beneficial.

## SUGGESTED READINGS

Ferschl, M., Moxley, R., Day, J. W., & Gropper, M. (2021). *Practical suggestions for the anesthetic management of a myotonic dystrophy patient.* Retrieved from https://www.myotonic.org/sites/default/files/pages/files/MDF_PracticalSuggestions DM1_Anesthesia2_17_21.pdf. Access date, December 2021.

Mangla, C., Bais, K., & Yarmush, J. (2019). Myotonic dystrophy and anesthetic challenges: A case report and review. *Case Reports in Anesthesiology, 2019,* 4282305.

Teixeira, J., Matias, B., Ferreira, I., Taleço, T., & Duarte, J. S. (2019). Sugammadex is changing the paradigm in neuromuscular blockade in patients with myotonic dystrophy. *Journal of Perioperative Practice, 29*(10), 337–340.

Veyckemans, F., & Scholtes, J. L. (2013). Myotonic dystrophies type 1 and 2: Anesthetic care. *Paediatric Anaesthesia, 23*(9), 794–803.

Weingarten, T. N., Hofer, R. E., Milone, M., & Sprung, J. (2010). Anesthesia and myotonic dystrophy type 2: A case series. *Canadian Journal of Anaesthesia, 57*(3), 248–255.

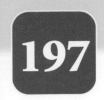

# Regional Anesthesia and Pain Relief in Children

ROBERT J. FRIEDHOFF, MD

Regional anesthesia in the pediatric patient has been undergoing a revival since the early 1990s. This is especially advantageous for the pediatric patient undergoing outpatient surgery. Regional blocks can provide prolonged and predictable postoperative analgesia. Regional techniques are usually performed along with general anesthesia in the pediatric patient. Performance of the block after the induction of anesthesia but before the beginning of surgery will allow general anesthetic agents to be reduced once the block is established and should be considered safe. The clinician should be familiar with the anatomic, physiologic, and pharmacologic differences in the pediatric patient. The use of ultrasound and the advances in technology has allowed faster onset with lower doses of local anesthetic. Hepatic metabolism of local anesthetics is not fully functional until 9 months of age. There is reduced concentration of $\alpha_1$-acid glycoprotein until 1 year of age. Local anesthetic toxicity is rare (approximately 1:10,000) and most often occurs in infants. Lipid resuscitation therapy with 20% intralipid with up to 10 mL/kg should be considered.

Anatomy—Target nerves are smaller, closer to other anatomic structures (vessels), and closer to the skin in pediatric patients. The caudal extent of the dura and spinal cord extends approximately two interspaces lower in an infant than an adult. The epidural fat is more gelatinous, less fibrous in an infant, favoring the spread of local anesthetics and the passage of epidural catheters.

Physiology—Clinically significant decreases in blood pressure secondary to sympathectomy from central neuraxial blockade is rare in children less than 8 years of age.

Cooperation—Essentially all regional techniques with the exception of spinal anesthesia for the high-risk premature infant are performed in a heavily sedated or anesthetized patient. The use of a peripheral nerve stimulator can be very valuable.

Test doses—Use of epinephrine to detect unanticipated intravascular injection in patients under volatile anesthetics is unreliable and controversial.

## Topical Blocks

### EUTECTIC MIXTURE OF LOCAL ANESTHETICS (PRILOCAINE AND LIDOCAINE)

A combination of prilocaine and lidocaine that should be placed on the skin and covered with a Tegaderm dressing at least 45 minutes before an invasive procedure (i.e., needle stick, circumcision).

### LMX

Similar to EMLA. Do not cleanse the skin before applying a thin layer. It works best with the skin's surface oils. Repeat with a thicker layer 10 minutes later. It will take 30 minutes to work.

Iontophoresis of lidocaine requires approximately 10 minutes but requires an apparatus that provides a tingly sensation that can be troublesome to the patient.

### ILIOINGUINAL/ILIOHYPOGASTRIC

Indication: hernia repairs and orchidopexy
Technique: wound edge infiltration before closure or instillation of drug before closure (enough to fill the wound after dissection).
Key: identify the anterior superior iliac spine and place a 23-gauge needle 1 to 2 cm medial and inferior to it. Feel the "pop" through the fascia and fan the local from lateral to medial.
Drug: bupivacaine 0.25% to 0.5% (up to 0.5 mL/kg)

## Transverse Abdominis Plane Block

Indication: for lower abdominal surgeries
Technique: ultrasound guided in-plane approach at the midaxillary line; visualize the external oblique, internal oblique, and transverse abdominus muscles. Inject between the internal oblique and transverse abdominus.
Drug: bupivacaine 0.25% to 0.5% (up to 0.5 mL/kg)

## Rectus Sheath Block

Indication: umbilical or incisional hernia repair
Technique: injection of local under the under the rectus abdominus muscle; visualize the double layer of the transversalis fascia. Two to four injections are needed (bilateral, above and below umbilicus) using an in-plane approach from medial to lateral.
Drug: bupivacaine 0.25% to 0.5% (up to 0.5 mL/kg)

### PENILE

Indication: circumcision, hypospadias repairs
Technique: ring the base of the penis with a superficial wheal of local anesthetic or, while pulling the penis toward the feet, insert a needle 90 degrees just below the symphysis pubis into the shaft of the penis. "Pop" through Buck fascia and inject one half at 11 o'clock and one half at 1 o'clock.

Drug: bupivacaine 0.25% (up to 0.5 mL/kg)
Key: *avoid* epinephrine

## FEMORAL

Indication: quadriceps muscle biopsy, femoral shaft fracture
Technique: remember NAVEL—the nerve is *lateral* to the artery. Just below the inguinal ligament, place an insulated needle attached to a nerve stimulator (patient must not be paralyzed with a muscle relaxant). Set the twitch at 1/s and stimulate at the lowest palpable setting until a twitch is noted in the patella. Alternatively, use an ultrasound-guided approach either in-plane or out of plane.
Drugs: bupivacaine 0.25% or ropivacaine 0.2% (0.2–0.3 ml/kg)

## AXILLARY

Indication: surgery on the arm/hand
Technique: use of the ultrasound to identify the axillary artery and the nerves surrounding it and the musculocutaneous nerve. Alternative is use of nerve stimulator, as in often done in adults (in unparalyzed patient). You can also palpate the axillary artery in the axilla, puncture the skin with a 20-gauge needle, then place a 22-gauge B (blunt) needle through the puncture site, aiming toward the artery until you feel a "pop" through the fascia or "septa" of the axillary sheath. After negative aspiration, inject local anesthetic.
Drugs: bupivacaine 0.25% or ropivacaine 0.2% with epinephrine 1/200,000 (0.2–0.3 mL/kg up to 25 mL)

## CAUDAL

### Single Shot

Indication: surgery below the diaphragm
Technique: with patient in the lateral decubitus position (left lateral for a right-handed anesthesiologist, right lateral for a left-handed anesthesiologist) with the knees flexed up to the belly, palpate and identify with a thumbnail the sacral cornua above the gluteal fold. Using aseptic technique, place a 22- to 23-gauge needle at a 45-degree angle to the skin until a "pop" is felt through the sacrococcygeal ligament. Bring the needle down, parallel to the skin, and advance 1 mm. After negative aspiration for blood and cerebrospinal fluid, inject slowly while observing the electrocardiogram for t-wave changes. Injection of the local should be easy. Any resistance indicates incorrect needle placement.
Drugs: bupivacaine 0.125 to 0.25% or ropivacaine 0.2% depending on patient age and incision location—penile (0.5–0.8 mL/kg), inguinal (1 mL/kg up to 20 mL)

### Continuous

Indication: for prolonged pain relief
Caution: need to maintain clean dressing area in sacral area and access to site (i.e., no spica cast)
Technique: similar to single shot. After identifying the caudal space under sterile technique using either an 18-gauge angiocatheter or Crawford needle, a 20-gauge catheter (with stylet) is advanced to the level of the patient's incision. Dressing with Mastisol is applied.
Drugs: bupivacaine 0.1% with narcotic (hydromorphone 5–10 mcg/mL or fentanyl 2 mcg/mL) at 0.3 mL/kg/h

## POPLITEAL

Indication: unilateral foot and ankle surgery and surgery below the knee
Technique: with patient either supine (leg bent at the knee) or prone using ultrasound guidance, identify the common peroneal and tibial nerve in the popliteal fossa. Moving the transducer cephalad until visualization of the two nerves come together forming the sciatic nerve. Infiltration of the drug at this site with a needle entering laterally, 1 to 3 cm above transducer. This can also be done with a stimulating needle if ultrasound is not available.
Drugs: bupivacaine 0.25 to 0.5% with epinephrine 1:200,000 (0.5 mL/kg up to 25 mL)

## LUMBAR EPIDURAL

Similar to adults. For patients less than 30 kg, a 2-inch, 18-gauge needle can be used.
Drugs: bupivacaine 0.125%–0.25% with epinephrine 1/200,000 (0.5–1.0 mL/kg up to 20 ml)

## SPINAL

Indication: for former premature high risk neonates or infants up to 6 months of age having GU or lower abdominal surgery lasting 30 to 90 minutes
Technique: remember the spinal terminates at L3 in neonates. Try to place the spinal with the patient in the sitting position, upright with the head not flexed. Intranasal dexmedetomidine in preoperative room to sedate. Best to avoid deep sedation, including ketamine to prevent postoperative apnea. Attempt to start the intravenous line in lower extremity after placement of spinal block, and place the blood pressure cuff there as well.
Drugs: tetracaine 1 mg/kg + 10% dextrose

## SUGGESTED READINGS

Cote, C. J., Lerman, J., & Anderson, B. J. (2019). *A practice of anesthesia for infants and children* (3rd ed.). Philadelphia, PA: Elsevier.

Davis, P. J., & Cladis, F. P. (2022). *Smith's anesthesia for infants and children* (10th ed.). Philadelphia, PA: Elsevier.

Gray, A. T. (2013). *Atlas of ultrasound-guided regional anesthesia.* Philadelphia, PA: Elsevier.

Merella, F., Canchi-Murali, N., & Mossetti, V. (2019). General principles of regional anaesthesia in children. *BJA, 10,* 342–348.

Taenzer, A. H., Walker, B. J., Bosenberg, A. T., Martin, L., Suresh, S., Polaner, D. M., et al. (2014). Asleep versus awake: Does it matter? Pediatric regional block complications by patient state: A report from the Pediatric Regional Anesthesia Network. *Regional Anesthesia and Pain Medicine, 39*(4), 279–283.

# SECTION XI

# Pain Medicine

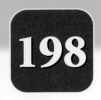

# Perioperative Management of the Opioid-Tolerant Patient

RYAN S. D'SOUZA, MD  |  OLUDARE O. OLATOYE, MD

## Introduction

Adequate postoperative pain management improves patient satisfaction, reduces perioperative morbidity, and allows for adequate postoperative rehabilitation. Presence of preoperative pain is the most significant indicator that the patient will have difficultly controlling postsurgical pain. In the opioid-tolerant patient, providing postoperative pain management can be challenging and often requires a multimodal treatment approach, as well as preoperative evaluation and planning. Opioid tolerance is defined as reduced responsiveness to a dose that was previously providing analgesia and the need for increased dose to achieve a therapeutic effect.

The preoperative setting is ideal for discussing goals of postoperative pain control, establishing expectations for opioid use and tapering, and evaluating preprocedural pain levels. Identifying the patient's current pain severity, chronicity, location along with opioid dose, and duration of use can inform the provider of the patient's risk for difficult-to-control postoperative pain and degree of opioid tolerance. A focused medical history should include evaluation for pertinent comorbidities such as sleep apnea; pulmonary, renal, or liver dysfunction; previous dependence or addiction to opioids, benzodiazepines, or alcohol; and current use of medication for opioid use disorder (MOUD) (use of U.S. Food and Drug Administration (FDA)-approved medications for maintenance treatment of opioid use disorder and to prevent relapse of opioid use), including methadone, buprenorphine, and naltrexone. Preferably, opioid-tolerant patients are introduced to possible regional techniques for pain control in a preoperative visit. Furthermore, addressing fear of postoperative pain has been shown to dramatically improve the patient's experience.

## Postoperative Management

The principles of postoperative analgesia in the chronically opioid-consuming patient include maintenance of multimodal analgesia, continuation of basal opioid requirements, and careful titration of additional opioid therapies and adjuvant agents. In patients able to tolerate oral opioid therapies postoperatively, short-acting oral opioids should be made available as needed but no more frequent than every 3 hours. We recommend refraining from starting or escalating long-acting opioids in the immediate postoperative period. If oral medications are not tolerated, intravenous (IV) administration of opioids via a patient-controlled analgesia device is appropriate for many patients, with plans to transition to oral therapies as soon as possible. Although basal infusions of opioids are not appropriate for most patients, they can be considered for patients with substantial opioid tolerance who are unable to continue their typical oral basal opioid requirements and if appropriate

monitoring is instituted. When preparing for hospital discharge, many patients will require higher opioid doses than what they were receiving preoperatively. In these instances, we recommend that providers work with a pain specialist (or the patient's primary provider for their chronic pain management) to develop a taper plan over 2 to 4 weeks, culminating in return to their preoperative opioid requirements. Further opioid adjustments and prescriptions should be made by the patient's primary pain physician with close outpatient follow-up and monitoring.

## Perioperative Multimodal Analgesia

Multimodal analgesia has become a hallmark of perioperative pain management and is particularly relevant for the opioid-dependent patient.

### ACETAMINOPHEN AND NONSTEROIDAL ANTIINFLAMMATORY DRUGS

Acetaminophen has been shown to decrease perioperative opioid requirements and has no significant renal or hematologic adverse effects when taken at appropriate doses. Hence, preoperative administration of acetaminophen is a logical first step in the management of the patient on chronic opioid therapy and may be continued through the perioperative period, with administration possible via per rectum and IV routes. Nonsteroidal antiinflammatory drugs (NSAIDs) have been studied extensively in the perioperative period and are noted to decrease postoperative pain and opioid requirements. They provide analgesia by inhibiting cyclooxygenase-1 (COX-1) and cyclooxygenase-2 (COX-2), thereby preventing the synthesis of prostaglandins and thromboxanes (selective COX-2 inhibitors will be discussed separately from nonselective NSAIDs). Although caution should be used in patients with renal insufficiency, volume depletion, advanced age, peptic ulcer disease, or coagulopathy, NSAIDs are typically well tolerated. Ketorolac is a particularly potent NSAID that may be administered orally, intravenously, or intramuscularly. Selective COX-2 inhibitors (e.g., celecoxib) have been developed to provide discriminatory inhibition of the enzyme thought to be most responsible for the analgesic, antiinflammatory, and antipyretic effects on nonselective NSAIDs. Notably, this selective inhibition also reduces the risk of gastrointestinal bleeding, though clinical concern has been raised for potential adverse cardiovascular events.

### KETAMINE

Ketamine is an $N$-methyl-$D$-aspartate (NMDA)-receptor antagonist with strong evidence for perioperative analgesia. Specifically, ketamine reduces perioperative opioid tolerance and hyperalgesia, thereby reducing opioid requirements. It is typically administered in subanesthetic doses perioperatively and commonly administered as an infusion at 0.1 to 0.3 mg/kg/h. Although the optimal duration of administration is unclear, we recommend maintenance of a continuous infusion of ketamine in the early postoperative period for opioid-dependent patients after major surgical insults. De-escalation strategies vary and may be down-titrated by 0.1 mg/kg/h every 12 to 24 hours before discontinuation, or simply turned off after short-term use (e.g., 3–5 days). Side effects include hallucinations, dysphoria, and vivid dreams, which some evidence suggests may be attenuated by preemptive administration of low-dose midazolam.

## ANTICONVULSANTS

Gabapentin and pregabalin are calcium channel blockers at the alpha-2-delta subunit, and may be used in the treatment of chronic neuropathic pain. Evidence remains limited. Although some studies have shown that both medications may improve postoperative analgesia and decrease opioid consumption, concerns exist regarding the sedative nature of these medications during the acute postoperative period. The anxiolytic and sedative qualities may increase postoperative somnolence and delay postanesthesia care unit (PACU) discharge. An FDA black box warning has also been issued regarding use of these sedative medications in the perioperative period, which may be associated with severe respiratory complications. As with opioid therapy, home doses should be provided to patients receiving these medications preoperatively. However, patients on these medications chronically may be at increased risk for postoperative respiratory depression, warranting increased monitoring. Appropriate renal dosing is recommended for patients with renal insufficiency.

## ANTIDEPRESSANTS

Serotonin-norepinephrine reuptake inhibitors (SNRIs) and tricyclic antidepressants (TCAs) are commonly used for chronic neuropathic pain. Duloxetine, a medication belonging to the SNRI class, has often been used as an adjunct for treatment of acute postoperative pain, and there is evidence demonstrating reduction of postoperative pain scores and opioid consumption after duloxetine administration. There is insufficient evidence to support the clinical use of TCAs in the acute postoperative setting, likely stemming from its numerous anticholinergic side effects.

## DEXMEDETOMIDINE AND CLONIDINE

Dexmedetomidine is an $\alpha_2$-receptor agonist increasingly used in the perioperative period and intensive care unit (ICU) as a sedative and anxiolytic, with notably less respiratory depression than other sedative agents. Dexmedetomidine has also been shown to decrease postoperative opioid requirements and improve pain scores in multiple unique surgical populations. When administered, most advocates suggest an intraoperative bolus dose of 0.5 mcg/kg followed by a continuous infusion at 0.2 to 1.5 mcg/kg/h, which may be continued postoperatively. Administration of dexmedetomidine often necessitates a closely monitored setting, such as an ICU or progressive care unit. Clonidine, a less selective $\alpha_2$-receptor agonist, may also be

considered in the opioid-dependent patient. Importantly, both medications alleviate symptoms of opioid withdrawal. In addition, both medications may induce hypotension and bradycardia, though only rarely is this life-threatening.

## SODIUM CHANNEL BLOCKER

Perioperative IV lidocaine infusions have regained attention as part of a multimodal analgesia protocol. Although lidocaine's principle mechanism of action as a local anesthetic is through blockade of voltage-gated sodium channels, IV lidocaine also blocks muscarinic receptors and NMDA receptors. At higher concentrations, it may also affect NaV 1.7/1.8 channels, 5-hydroxytryptamine receptors, and voltage-gated calcium channels. Rather than the local anesthetic effect, this multimodal mechanism likely explains lidocaine's ability to have antinociceptive, antihyperalgesic, and antiinflammatory properties. There is evidence that perioperative infusions of IV lidocaine may be associated with decreased postoperative pain, nausea, ileus duration, opioid consumption, and hospital length of stay. Although most trials were performed in patients undergoing abdominal surgeries, evidence also exists for thoracic, cardiac, and prostate surgeries. Although dosing regimens vary, a common protocol is to administer an initial bolus dose of 1 to 1.5 mg/kg of IV lidocaine before induction of general anesthesia, followed by an intraoperative infusion of 0.5 to 1.5 mg/kg/hr. The infusion may be continued at 0.5 to 1.0 mg/kg/hr in the PACU and during the postoperative period in the hospital with adequate monitoring. The analgesic effect of IV lidocaine may exceed the duration of the infusion by over 8.5 hours. Vigilance for local anesthetic systemic toxicity is warranted. This entails not administering IV lidocaine infusions within 4 hours of regional anesthetic blockade. For infusions longer than 12 hours, it is advisable to obtain daily serum lidocaine levels with a goal of 1 to 3 mcg/mL. Higher serum levels have been associated with cardiovascular instability. Furthermore, it is recommended to use the ideal body weight for dose calculations and not to exceed the maximum dose of 120 mg/hr of lidocaine.

Although other sodium channel blockers including phenytoin, carbamazepine, and oxcarbazepine have been used extensively in the chronic pain setting, there is limited evidence of their utility in the acute postoperative period.

## INTERVENTIONAL MODALITIES

### Regional Anesthesia

Regional anesthesia is often considered an ideal technique in those with opioid dependence. Regional anesthesia can be defined by the site of administration (peripheral vs. neuraxial), the duration of administration (single bolus vs. continuous infusion), the clinical context of administration (primary anesthesia vs. perioperative analgesia vs. combined), and the pharmacologic profile of the injectate (local anesthetic vs. opioid vs. combined ± additional adjunct medications). Adjunct medications may include epinephrine, alpha-2-agonists, and neostigmine. Furthermore, in the delivery of epidural analgesia, a fixed continuous infusion or a patient-controlled epidural analgesia mode may be instituted. Numerous studies have shown opioid-sparing effects and improved perioperative pain control after a seemingly endless combination of regional techniques. When possible, regional anesthetic techniques should be initiated before the surgical incision in chronic opioid users for preemptive analgesia.

## LOCAL WOUND INFILTRATION AND TOPICAL ANESTHESIA

Direct wound infiltration with local anesthetic is a simple analgesic technique that may be considered when other regional techniques are not readily applicable or in addition to regional techniques. Topical administration of local anesthetic, most commonly in a 4% or 5% lidocaine patch, is also a simple and widely available analgesic adjunct.

## LIPOSOMAL BUPIVACAINE

Liposomal bupivacaine (Exparel) has gained much traction in recent years, including use in wound infiltration, peripheral regional techniques, and periarticular blocks. Liposomal bupivacaine consists of bupivacaine encapsulated in multivesicular liposomal particles, allowing for slow-release of the drug over a 72-hour time period. It has been approved by the FDA for direct infiltration into the surgical wound. It is increasingly being used intraarticularly and in peripheral regional anesthetic techniques as a substitute for other local anesthetics or in combination with standard bupivacaine. It should not be used near the neuraxis given concerns for prolonged motor and sensory blockade. Of note, liposomal bupivacaine may be administered in the same admixture syringe as standard bupivacaine as long as the milligram dosing of bupivacaine to liposomal bupivacaine does not exceed 1:2. However, liposomal bupivacaine may not be mixed with lidocaine and should not be given in the first 20 minutes after lidocaine administration, as this may cause an immediate release of bupivacaine from the liposomes. Furthermore, lidocaine infusions should not be offered to patients who have received liposomal bupivacaine because of the risk for local anesthetic systemic toxicity.

## Special Situations

### HIGH-DOSE OPIOID THERAPY

For patients taking high-dose opioid therapy, the general principle of treatment is to continue home opioid medications with additional dosing of short-acting oral and/or IV opioids for postoperative needs. Patients with chronic daily use of oral morphine equivalent of 30 mg or greater typically require three to four times the opioid dose needed to adequately control acute pain in their opioid-naïve counterparts. It is imperative, however, to consider incomplete cross-tolerance/dose reduction if a different opioid compared with the patient's home regimen is used for perioperative pain control. Monitoring for respiratory depression with pulse oximetry is prudent while titrating opioids.

### INTRATHECAL DRUG DELIVERY SYSTEM

Intrathecal drug delivery systems are placed for malignant and nonmalignant pain syndromes and for spasticity. These implantable devices include a medication pump reservoir in communication with an intrathecal catheter that delivers a preset daily dose of medication to the cerebrospinal fluid in either via a basal continuous infusion and/or via bolus dosing. Opioid medications are most commonly delivered and can be in combination with adjuvant medications, such as bupivacaine or clonidine. The patient's intrathecal pain medication regimen and daily dose should be profiled after interrogation of the device in the immediate pre- and postoperative periods. Because of the potency of intrathecally delivered opioids, these patients typically have significant opioid tolerance, and postoperative opioid needs can be higher than opioid-naïve patients. Unless prolonged postoperative pain is anticipated, the intrathecal dose is typically held constant and short-acting opioids are added in the perioperative period. Dose modifications should be done with the assistance of a pain specialist.

Intrathecal drug delivery systems are also implanted to deliver intrathecal baclofen in patients with spasticity refractory to medical management. In the perioperative period the intrathecal baclofen is most often held consistent with baseline levels. In situations of disruption or malfunction of the system or catheter, baclofen withdrawal can be life-threatening. Symptoms of baclofen withdrawal include increased spasticity, diffuse pruritis, and altered sensorium. These patients should be carefully monitored (typically in the ICU setting), and aggressive titration of oral baclofen and benzodiazepines is required.

## METHADONE

Methadone may be used for either chronic pain or abstinence maintenance therapy. Outpatient dose of methadone should be continued throughout the perioperative period with vigilance to ensure a dose is not missed. If a patient cannot have oral medications, methadone can be administered intravenously (IV dose = 0.5 oral dose). Because of methadone's long half-life, it is not easily titrated for acute pain. Typically, methadone dose is maintained at preprocedural levels, whereas opioids with a shorter half-life are titrated to effect. Furthermore, down-titration of opioid medication after recovery from surgery is more easily achieved with short half-life opioids compared with methadone and other long-acting opioids.

## PARTIAL AGONIST/ANTAGONIST (SUBOXONE/ BUTRANS/SUBUTEX)

Partial agonist opioid medications such as buprenorphine present specific challenges. Buprenorphine is used for either chronic pain management or opioid cessation treatment. This may be prescribed orally (Subutex) or via a transdermal patch (Butrans). A combination of buprenorphine and naloxone (Suboxone) may be prescribed by an addiction specialist for opioid addiction cessation. Common Suboxone formations provide a 4:1 ratio of buprenorphine to naloxone.

Buprenorphine has a weak analgesic effect because of partial agonist activity along with high affinity for the mu receptor. Historically, it was recommended that before elective surgeries, patients should discontinue buprenorphine 3 to 5 days before the operation to allow for metabolism and elimination of the drug. In addition, in cases of urgent or emergent operations, the medication was discontinued and a multimodal pain treatment initiated. However, more evidence has highlighted that although there is no clear benefit between bridging versus stopping buprenorphine perioperatively, failure to restart it postoperatively introduces concern for relapse of opioid use disorder. Thus recent recommendations have favored continuing buprenorphine in the perioperative period along with a multimodal analgesia protocol. Guidance and approval from the patient's addiction specialist is paramount if the medication has been prescribed for opioid cessation therapy.

## SUGGESTED READINGS

Anderson, T. A., Quaye, A. N. A., Ward, E. N., Wilens, T. E., Hilliard, P. E., & Brummett, C. M. (2017). To stop or not, that is the question: Acute pain management for the patient on chronic buprenorphine. *Anesthesiology, 126*(6), 1180–1186.

Brill, S., Ginosar, Y., & Davidson, E. M. (2006). Perioperative management of chronic pain patients with opioid dependency. *Current Opinion in Anaesthesiology, 19*(3), 325–331.

Carroll, I. R., Angst, M. S., & Clark, J. D. (2004). Management of perioperative pain in patients chronically consuming opioids. *Regional Anesthesia and Pain Medicine, 29*(6), 576–591.

Dunn, L. K., & Durieux, M. E. (2017). Perioperative use of intravenous lidocaine. *Anesthesiology, 126*(4), 729–737.

Kopf, A., Banzhaf, A., & Stein, C. (2005). Perioperative management of the chronic pain patient. *Best Practice & Research Clinical Anaesthesiology, 19*(1), 59–76.

# 199

# Patient-Controlled Analgesia

MARTIN L. DE RUYTER, MD, MS, FASA

Postoperative analgesia is one of the main foci of the convalescing patient. As many as 50% of patients who receive conventional therapy for their postoperative pain do not have adequate analgesia. Additionally, many patients report a high level of dissatisfaction with their pain management. It is recognized that better analgesia is associated with many positives, including earlier mobility, decreased complications, shorter length of stay, and improved patient satisfaction. Thus pain relief has become a top priority for health care facilities. This has been fueled in part by the 2001 Joint Commission statement that pain is the "fifth vital sign" and the U.S. Congress declaring 2001 to 2011 the "Decade of Pain Control and Research." The resulting public benchmarks and financial incentives, all based on patient-reported satisfaction with analgesia, have led to significant changes to the medical professionals' approach to postoperative recovery. Unfortunately, our society today is facing an unanticipated fallout from these changes, namely our current opioid epidemic. Nonetheless, patients should not be denied adequate treatment for their postoperative pain. Improved pain control does lead to overall patient satisfaction with their health care, better quality of life, less frequent progression to chronic pain, more efficient clinical resource management, and reduction of long-term costs both for the individual and society. There are several proposed approaches to achieving better postoperative pain control, with the common theme being multimodal analgesia. This chapter will discuss one modality, patient-controlled analgesia (PCA).

## Evolution and Application of Patient-Controlled Analgesia

PCA enables the patient to self-administer predetermined doses of an analgesic when they deem necessary. In 1968, Sechzer first introduced PCA with intermittent intravenous (IV) doses of opioids delivered "on demand" by the patient, which gave patients the ability to better control their level of analgesia, balanced against their level of sedation and their risks of side effects, namely respiratory depression. In current practice, an infusion pump is programmed to provide a preset dose of an analgesic agent when the patient presses a button on a handheld controller; the "lockout" time—the interval before the next dose can be delivered—is also preset. Although IV PCA with opioids is a widely used modality to treat postoperative pain, it is also commonly used in cancer-related pain and pain associated with nonmalignant conditions (e.g., acute nephrolithiasis and pancreatitis).

Several studies have supported the efficacy of IV PCA over alternative non-PCA based (e.g., intramuscular) analgesic approaches. A 2015 Cochrane review concluded that evidence (moderate to low quality) supports IV PCA, as these patients had lower pain scores, were more satisfied, had higher opioid consumption compared with non-PCA recipients, and, other than a higher incidence of pruritus, both groups were similar in other adverse events. Considering the supporting evidence, the American Pain Society, with input from the American Society of Anesthesiologists, recommends that IV PCA be used for postoperative systemic analgesia when the parenteral route is needed (strong recommendation, moderate-quality evidence).

The concept of PCA has been expanded to include other patient-controlled approaches to analgesia (e.g., patient-controlled epidural analgesia, patient-controlled peripheral nerve catheter analgesia, patient-controlled sublingual opioid analgesia). Unlike IV PCA, patient-controlled epidural analgesia is not limited to infusion of opioids and often includes the coadministration of a local anesthetic agent, whereas patient-controlled peripheral nerve catheter analgesia primarily involves delivery of only local anesthetic agents. A complete discussion of the various types of PCA is beyond the scope of this section; however, key characteristics of an ideal PCA are presented in Box 199.1. This chapter focuses on IV PCA with opioids.

# Intravenous Patient-Controlled Analgesia

## ADVANTAGES

The main advantage of IV PCA with opioids is that it is patient controlled. Traditional intermittent nurse-administered parenteral analgesia, ordered as "scheduled" (e.g., every 6 hours) or "intermittent" (e.g., as needed), is inherently labor intensive and fraught with problems. Typical doses of scheduled analgesic drugs are generalized to most patients rather than individual patient needs and in relatively large doses (often exceeding the minimal effective dose) to achieve a more sustained effect. Further, the time to redosing is often prolonged, resulting in low serum drug concentrations and the recurrence of pain. The as-needed approach is an even less favorable regimen because patients often wait until their pain is significant, thus delaying receipt of their pain medication. With both regimens, patients can experience "peaks" of supratherapeutic analgesia, which can increase the risk of complications (e.g., respiratory depression, nausea, emesis), followed by "valleys" of low serum opioid levels, during which patients experience breakthrough pain. These subtherapeutic levels, with their associated inadequate analgesia, may limit patients' recovery and delay discharge. In comparison, patients with IV PCA have their dose of analgesic agent and lockout interval individualized, and because IV PCA eliminates a second person as a decision maker and facilitator (i.e., the nurse), IV PCA maintains more effective and less variable serum analgesic drug concentrations. Other reported advantages of IV PCA are listed in Box 199.2.

## CHOICE OF OPIOIDS

Morphine, hydromorphone, and fentanyl are commonly administered opioids via IV PCA. Meperidine is largely avoided because of the potential adverse effects (e.g., seizures) associated with its active metabolite, normeperidine, and the recognition of better alternative agents (Table 199.1).

## INITIAL SETUP

When prescribing IV PCA with opioids, the anesthesia provider must select the opioid and set several dosing parameters: the loading dose, demand dose, lockout interval, and maximum dose limit. Other considerations include subsequent bolus doses and continuous infusion. The loading dose administered at the initiation of IV PCA is intended to quickly establish an effective serum concentration of the drug. Satisfactory analgesia is

| TABLE 199.1 | Suggested Dosing Regimens for Opioid-Naïve Patients* Receiving Opioids via Intravenous Patient-Controlled Analgesia | | | | | | |
|---|---|---|---|---|---|---|---|
| Drug | Concentration (mg/mL) | Loading Dose[†], (mg maximum) | Demand Dose (mg) | Lockout Interval (min) | Basal Infusion[‡] (mg/h) | 1-h Limit (mg) | 4-h Limit (mg) |
| Morphine | 1 | 2–4 | 1–2 | 6–10 | 0–1 | 7.5 | 30 |
| Hydromorphone | 0.2 | 0.4 | 0.2–0.4 | 6–10 | 0–0.2 | 1.5 | 6 |
| Fentanyl | 0.01 | 0.02–0.04 | 0.01–0.03 | 6–10 | 0–0.02 | 0.1–0.2 | 0.4–0.8 |

*Older adult patients (>65 years) and patients on chronic opioids may need adjustment of these guidelines.
[†]The loading dose is given as a bolus every 5 min until the patient is comfortable, and then the patient-controlled analgesia is started.
[‡]Most practitioners do not recommend a continuous infusion for most patients.

maintained with subsequent demand doses delivered in a predetermined window or frequency. The loading and demand doses of the drug should be adjusted for the patient's age, comorbid conditions, and concomitant medications. Smaller loading and demand doses of opioids are recommended for older adults, those with pulmonary disease (e.g., chronic obstructive pulmonary disease, obstructive sleep apnea) or tenuous hemodynamic status, or those who are receiving drugs that may act synergistically with opioids (e.g., benzodiazepines). Patients with chronic pain and opioid tolerance will likely need larger demand doses and/or a shorter lockout interval. The maximum dose allowed is usually the cumulative dose allowed at 1 or 4 hours and is a safety measure designed to prevent patients from receiving excessive amounts of opioid. Bolus doses can be administered to a patient by a health care provider if adequate analgesia is not achieved with the initial settings. Most clinicians do not routinely prescribe a continuous or basal infusion of an opioid. Exceptions can be found in challenging situations, such as the patient with opioid dependence who now has acute postsurgical pain superimposed on their chronic pain. An advantage of IV PCA is that the delivery device can be interrogated, and by monitoring the number of patient demands relative to the number of doses delivered, clinicians can tailor and adjust the demand dose and lockout interval to better meet the analgesic needs of the patient. Appropriate strategies to consider when patients have inadequate analgesia include decreasing the lockout interval, increasing the demand dose, adding a basal infusion, or some combination of these parameters.

## ADVERSE EFFECTS AND OUTCOMES

IV PCA with opioids is not without disadvantages, side effects, or adverse outcomes. Box 199.3 lists several recognized disadvantages. With regard to side effects, nausea, vomiting, and pruritus are not uncommon, and excessive somnolence has been

> **BOX 199.3 DISADVANTAGES OF INTRAVENOUSLY ADMINISTERED OPIOIDS VIA PATIENT-CONTROLLED ANALGESIA**
>
> - Patients using patient-controlled analgesia must be mentally alert, physically able to push the button, and able to understand the concept of IV PCA and follow instructions.
> - IV PCA should be used with caution in patients with significant liver, renal, or pulmonary disease.
> - Patients with obstructive sleep apnea are at increased risk of experiencing opioid-induced respiratory depression.
> - Pruritus is more common with IV PCA than with intramuscular administration but less common than with epidural administration.
> - Surrogate (nonpatient, i.e., family members or nursing staff) "pushers" of the button may subject patients to overdosing levels of opioids.
> - Direct costs are increased because of the need for special equipment, setup, and staff training.
>
> *IV PCA,* Intravenously administered patient-controlled analgesia.

observed with cases reports of hypoxia. Unfortunately, much of the observed adverse events are likely secondary to human error (Fig. 199.1). To improve the safety of IV PCA, many hospitals have guidelines that recommend staff members regularly assess and document the patient's pain scores (using a metric such as numeric or visual analog scores), respiratory rate, oxygen saturation via pulse oximetry, state of arousal, and level of sedation. Although it is recognized that oxygen desaturation is a delayed occurrence in the event of respiratory depression, pulse oximetry remains a widely used monitor. Concurrent monitoring of end-tidal carbon dioxide or the use of ventilation acoustic monitors with the hope of earlier detection are becoming more common practice. To address human error, electronic medical record patient verification, pharmacy automation, standard

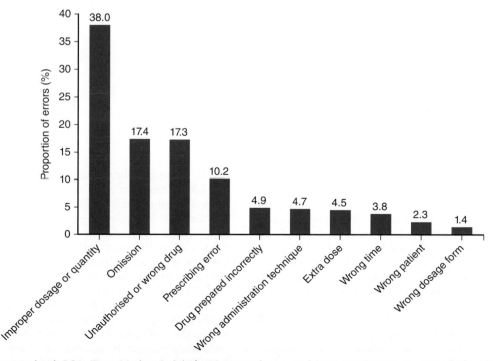

**Fig. 199.1** Errors associated with PCA. (From Morlion B, Schäfer M, Betteridge N, et al. Non-invasive patient-controlled analgesia in the management of acute postoperative pain in the hospital setting. *Curr Med Res Opin.* 2018;34:1179–1186.)

labeling, infusion pump programing protocols, and bedside nursing double-checks are all aimed at making IV PCA a safer modality for analgesic administration.

## Conclusion

In summary, the concept of PCA has been expanded to include not only IV PCA use commonly with opioids but also other nonopioid patient-controlled methods. Although current evidence supports a multimodal approach aiming to limit opioid exposure to patients, opioids delivered through IV PCA will likely continue to have a role particularly for the management of moderate to severe acute postoperative pain. Although PCA is associated with higher startup costs (including devices and training of nursing staff) and requires an engaged patient and a cooperative family, it is cost-effective because its use is associated with improved outcomes and better patient satisfaction.

## SUGGESTED READINGS

Apfelbaum, J., Ashburn, M., & Connis, R. (2012). Practice guidelines for acute pain management in the perioperative setting: An updated report by the American Society of Anesthesiologists Task Force on Acute Pain Management. *Anesthesiology*, 116(2), 248–273.

Chou, R., Gordon, D. B., de Leon-Casasola, O. A., Rosenberg, J. M., Bickler, S., Brennan, T., et al. (2016). Management of postoperative pain: A clinical practice guideline from the American Pain Society, the American Society of Regional Anesthesia and Pain Medicine, and the American Society of Anesthesiologists' Committee on Regional Anesthesia, Executive Committee, and Administrative Council. *Journal of Pain*, 17(2), 131–157.

Gan, T. J., Habib, A. S., Miller, T. E., White, W., & Apfelbaum, J. L. (2014). Incidence, patient satisfaction, and perceptions of post-surgical pain: Results from a US national survey. *Current Medical Research and Opinion*, 30(1), 149–160.

Hicks, R. W., Sikirica, V., Nelson, W., Schein, J. R., & Cousins, D. D. (2008). Medication errors involving patient-controlled analgesia. *American Journal of Health System Pharmacy*, 65(5), 429–440.

McNicol, E. D., Ferguson, M. C., & Hudcova, J. (2015). Patient controlled opioid analgesia versus non-patient controlled opioid analgesia for postoperative pain. *Cochrane Database of Systematic Reviews*, 2015(6), CD003348.

Mitra, S., Carlyle, D., Kodumudi, G., Kodumudi, V., & Vadivelu, N. (2018). New advances in acute postoperative pain management. *Current Pain and Headache Reports*, 22(5), 35.

Morlion, B., Schäfer, M., Betteridge, N., & Kalso, E. (2018). Non-invasive patient-controlled analgesia in the management of acute postoperative pain in the hospital setting. *Current Medical Research and Opinion*, 34(7), 1179–1186.

Schug, S. A., Palmer, G. M., Scott, D. A., Alcock, M., Halliwell, R., & Mott, J. F. (2020). *Acute pain management: Scientific evidence* (5th ed.). Melbourne: ANZCA &FPM.

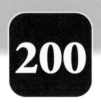

# 200

# Neuraxial Opioids

PAUL E. CARNS, MD

Opioids were first introduced into the central neuraxis in 1979. Since that time, they have been used both epidurally and intrathecally for both acute and chronic pain control and are commonly administered in combination with other neuraxial adjuvant compounds, such as local anesthetics and $\alpha_2$-adrenoreceptor agonists. The clinical benefits of epidural and intrathecal opioids include excellent analgesia in the absence of motor, sensory, and autonomic blockade. This in turn leads to downstream benefits, including earlier ambulation and improved pulmonary function.

The sites of action are the opioid receptors found mainly within layers 4 and 5 of the substantia gelatinosa in the dorsolateral horn of the spinal cord. Activation of these receptors inhibits the release of excitatory nociceptive neurotransmitters within the spinal cord. In addition to producing direct spinal effects, neuraxial-administered opioids may also activate cerebral opioid receptors when cephalad spread of the drug occurs via cerebrospinal fluid (CSF). Some drug is invariably absorbed into the vasculature, leading to systemic effects. The lipid solubility of each opioid, determined by the octanol/water partition coefficient, is the most critical pharmacokinetic property to consider when administering opioid doses near the neuraxis. Molecular weight, dose, and volume of injectate may also play a role in dural transfer (Table 200.1).

Hydrophilic opioids (those with low octanol/water partition coefficients, e.g., morphine) have a high degree of solubility within the CSF, permitting significant cephalad spread. Thoracic analgesia may be accomplished when either epidural or intrathecal doses are administered at the lumbar level. The epidural or intrathecal dose of morphine is significantly less

| TABLE 200.1 | Octanol/Water Partition Coefficients and Molecular Weights of Common Opioids | |
|---|---|---|
| Drug | Octanol/Water Partition Coefficient | Molecular Weight (g/mol) |
| Morphine | 1.4 | 285 |
| Hydromorphone | 2 | 285 |
| Meperidine | 39 | 247 |
| Alfentanil | 145 | 452 |
| Fentanyl citrate | 813 | 528 |
| Sufentanil citrate | 1778 | 578 |

than that required to achieve an equianalgesic effect through intravenous (IV) administration.

When used epidurally, hydrophilic opioids have a slow onset and prolonged duration of action. An initial epidural bolus dose is required, which may be followed by a continuous infusion through an epidural catheter. Because of their slow onset of action, hydrophilic opioids are less suitable for patient-controlled epidural analgesia than are lipophilic opioids. When hydrophilic opioids are used intrathecally, onset of action is more rapid and very low doses are required, resulting in both less systemic toxicity and effective analgesia that lasts for up to 24 hours. The lack of a continuous catheter makes this a cost-effective option and has become an attractive alternative to continuous epidural infusions for enhancing postoperative recovery (e.g., intrathecal opioid used within multimodal, enhanced recovery pathways for colorectal and abdominal, gynecologic, and urologic surgeries).

Lipophilic opioids (those with a high octanol/water partition coefficient, e.g., fentanyl) have a rapid onset and a much shorter duration of action. When used epidurally, these drugs are rapidly taken up by epidural fat and redistributed into the systemic circulation, resulting in poor bioavailability to the spinal cord. In fact, doses of lipophilic opioids needed to achieve equianalgesic effect are nearly identical in the neuraxis compared with IV dosing. Plasma levels attained with equal doses of epidural and IV infusions of fentanyl are also nearly identical, suggesting a significant systemic mode of action. Low CSF solubility permits only a limited amount of cephalad spread, and doses should be placed near the dermatome or dermatomes at which analgesia is desired. For example, lumbar administration of a lipophilic opioid would be a poor choice for thoracic analgesia. Side effects are generally fewer, with a lower incidence of delayed respiratory depression compared with hydrophilic opioid administration. These drugs are ideal for continuous infusions and patient-controlled epidural analgesia.

A biphasic pattern of respiratory depression is seen with epidural doses of hydrophilic opioids. A portion of the initial bolus dose is absorbed systemically, which accounts for an initial phase, and usually occurring within 2 hours of the bolus dose being administered. Remaining drug within the CSF slowly spreads rostrally, producing a second phase as the drug reaches the brainstem, anywhere from 6 to 18 hours later.

This results in direct depression of the respiratory nuclei and chemoreceptors. In contrast, intrathecal doses of hydrophilic opioids produce only a uniphasic pattern of respiratory depression. Effective doses of intrathecally administered hydrophilic opioid are very low compared with the larger epidural doses, thus early respiratory depression is typically not seen. The slow rostral spread of drug deposited directly within the CSF is responsible for the pattern of delayed respiratory depression. Mechanical ventilation and Valsalva maneuvers (coughing/vomiting) that raise intrathoracic pressure may promote rostral spread. Somnolence usually precedes the onset of significant respiratory depression. According to the American Society of Anesthesiologists Task Force on Neuraxial Opioids, patients should be closely monitored for the first 24 hours after a neuraxial dose of a hydrophilic opioid, and this should include pulse oximetry. If an infusion is planned, monitoring is necessary throughout its duration. Naloxone should be readily available for reversal of significant respiratory depression.

Side effects after neuraxial administration of opioids are dose dependent and are generally similar when used either epidurally or intrathecally. They include respiratory depression, somnolence, pruritus, nausea and vomiting, hypotension, and urinary retention. Patients who are elderly, obese, or have obstructive sleep apnea may be at greater risk for respiratory depression. Use of additional sedatives and opioids in all patients should be avoided or used with caution within the first 24 hours after intrathecal opioid administration. Pain management specialist involvement is useful if inadequate pain relief is observed. Hypotension after administration of intrathecal opioids in parturients may result in fetal bradycardia secondary to decreased fetal oxygenation. Generalized pruritus is the most common and least dangerous side effect seen with the use of neuraxial opioids. The mechanism is unclear, but it is not thought to be secondary to histamine release. Postulated mechanisms include the presence of an "itch center" within the CNS, medullary dorsal horn activation and antagonism of inhibitory transmitters, modulation of the serotonergic pathway, and a theory that links pain and pruritus. Treatment includes dilute naloxone infusions, low-dose mixed agonist/antagonist opioids (nalbuphine, 5-HT3 antagonists [ondansetron, granisetron, dolasetron, mirtazapine], gabapentin, propofol, and dopamine D2 antagonists [droperidol, alizapride]). Antihistamines may also be beneficial for the sedation they may provide.

Nausea and vomiting are common complications of neuraxial opioid administration, similar to parenteral opioid use. Reversible causes, such as hypotension, must be initially ruled out and corrected if present. Rostral spread of opioids directly stimulates the medullary vomiting center. Treatment options include the administration of D2 antagonists, phenothiazines (prochlorperazine), 5-HT$_3$ antagonists, dexamethasone, and antihistamines. Phenothiazines may cause significant drowsiness, however, which may hinder evaluation of somnolence secondary to the effects of the opioid itself.

Opioids may reduce the sacral parasympathetic outflow, resulting in urinary retention. Although this may be reversed by direct antagonism with naloxone, the doses of naloxone required are often high and may also result in reversal of analgesia. Placement of an indwelling urinary catheter should be considered.

## SUGGESTED READINGS

Cook, T. M., Counsell, D., Wildsmith, J. A., & Royal College of Anaesthetists Third National Audit Project. (2009). Major complications of central neuraxial block: Report on the Third National Audit Project of the Royal College of Anaesthetists. *British Journal of Anaesthesia, 102*(2), 179–190.

Kumar, K., & Singh, S. I. (2013). Neuraxial opioid-induced pruritus: An update. *Journal of Anaesthesiology, Clinical Pharmacology, 29*(3), 303–307.

Mariano, E. R. (2021). *Management of acute periop-erative pain. Regional Anesthesia and Pain Medicine, 0*, 1–10.

Practice guidelines for the prevention, detection, and management of respiratory depression associated with neuraxial opioid administration: An updated report by the American Society of Anesthesiologists Task Force on Neuraxial Opioids and the American Society of Regional Anesthesia and Pain Medicine. (2016). *Anesthesiology, 124*, 535–552.

Schug, S. A., Saunders, D., Kurowski, I., & Paech, M. J. (2006). Neuraxial drug administration: A review of treatment options for anaesthesia and analgesia. *CNS Drugs, 20*(11), 917–933.

# 201

# Complex Regional Pain Syndrome

ROBALEE L. WANDERMAN, MD | HALENA M. GAZELKA, MD

## Background

Complex regional pain syndrome (CRPS) is a relatively uncommon neuropathic, often chronic pain disorder with reported incidence rates ranging from 5.46 to 26.2 per 100,000 person-years at risk. Morbidity from this syndrome depends on symptom severity and length but can include dependence on pharmacologic interventions, debility from work resulting in lost wages, loss of limb functionality, and overall decreased quality of life. Women are three to four times more likely than men to carry the diagnosis, with the mean age of diagnosis being 47 to 52 years of age. Whites and Asians are the most common ethnic groups diagnosed with this condition. Upper extremity involvement is more common than lower extremity. Fractures, sprains, surgery, and crush injuries are the most common inciting events.

## Definitions

For over a century, CRPS has been described in medical literature, albeit by different nomenclature. CRPS, as defined by the International Association for the Study of Pain (IASP), is a collection of locally appearing painful conditions after a trauma, which chiefly occur distally and exceed in intensity and duration the expected course of the original trauma, often resulting in restricted motor function.

CRPS types I and II—formerly known, respectively, as *reflex sympathetic dystrophy* and *causalgia*—are characterized by varying degrees of hyperalgesia, allodynia, edema, vasomotor and sudomotor instability, trophic changes, and bone rarefaction, with type I encompassing most cases.

In CRPS type I, the initial event, whether spontaneous or a major insult, does not result in an obvious nerve injury. The hallmark of CRPS type I is continuing pain disproportionately more severe than expected given the injury. The pain, dystrophy, and features of autonomic instability progress and affect regions of the extremity not involved in the initial event. Severe cases may involve the entire limb or even the contralateral extremity.

Conversely, CRPS type II results from injury to an identifiable nerve and is characterized by burning pain, allodynia, and hyperpathia. It is distinct from a peripheral mononeuropathy in that the afflicted region often extends beyond the predicted nerve distribution.

CRPS type III does not comply with either of the classical forms and is a distinction that is rarely clinically useful.

## Diagnosis

CRPS is a clinical diagnosis of exclusion; however, some investigations are considered useful and may assist in clarifying the diagnosis. The IASP guidelines (Table 201.1) improve diagnostic specificity (up to 100%) at the expense of sensitivity (as low as 41%), which could potentially lead to overdiagnosis. To improve diagnostic accuracy, it has been suggested the Budapest Criteria (Table 201.2) also be used. In one validation study, the Budapest Criteria resulted in similar sensitivity as the IASP guidelines (99%) but with improved specificity (68%). Because of this improved rigor, the Budapest Criteria are particularly useful for research in CRPS.

The differential diagnosis for CRPS includes but is not limited to small-fiber and diabetic neuropathies, nerve entrapment, degenerative disc disease, thoracic outlet syndrome, cellulitis, vascular insufficiency, thrombophlebitis, lymphedema, angioedema, erythromelalgia, and deep venous thrombosis.

Although CRPS is a clinical diagnosis, several diagnostic studies may provide objective results to assist in the diagnosis of CRPS. Thermometry, the quantitative sudomotor axon reflex

| TABLE 201.1 | International Association for the Study of Pain Criteria for the Diagnosis of Complex Regional Pain Syndrome* | |
| --- | --- | --- |
| **Category** | **Signs and Symptoms** | |
| Sensory | Allodynia<br>Hyperalgesia<br>Hyperesthesia<br>Hypoalgesia | |
| Vasomotor | Livedo reticularis<br>Skin color changes<br>Temperature variability | |
| Sudomotor | Edema<br>Hyperhidrosis<br>Hypohidrosis | |
| Motor | Decreased range of motion<br>Neglect<br>Tremor<br>Weakness | |

*Diagnostic predictability improves when patients report at least one symptom in each category and one sign in two or more categories.

| TABLE 201.2 | Budapest Criteria for the Clinical Diagnosis of Complex Regional Pain Syndrome | |
| --- | --- | --- |
| **Pain** | **Continuing Pain That Is Disproportionate to Inciting Event** | |
| One reported **symptom** in three out of the four categories | Sensory<br>Vasomotor<br>Sudomotor/edema<br>Motor/trophic | |
| One observed **sign** at time of evaluation in two or more categories | Sensory<br>Vasomotor<br>Sudomotor/edema<br>Motor/trophic | |
| Other etiologies | No other unifying diagnosis to explain signs/symptoms | |

| TABLE 201.3 | Studies to Inform Complex Regional Pain Syndrome Diagnosis |
| --- | --- |
| **Evaluation** | **Utility** |
| Sweat test | Useful in the evaluation of small fiber neuropathy<br>Helps document presence/absence of sudomotor dysfunction |
| Thermography | Infrared thermometer measures multiple points on extremities<br>Difference of 1°C is considered significant |
| Quantitative Sudomotor Axon Reflex Test | Measures sweat output to a cholinergic challenge<br>Measure sweat bilaterally and symmetrically |
| Bone densitometry | Decreased bone mineral density and bone mineral content |
| Three-phase bone scan | Increased periarticular activity = increased bone metabolism<br>Sensitivity and specificity of 80% |

| TABLE 201.4 | Stages of Complex Regional Pain Syndrome |
| --- | --- |
| **Stage** | **Presentation** |
| Stage I: Acute/warm | Burning or aching pain increasing with physical contact or emotional stress<br>Edema<br>Unstable temperature and color of limb<br>Increased periarticular uptake on scintigraphy<br>Accelerated hair and nail growth<br>Joint stiffness<br>Muscle spasm |
| Stage II: Dystrophic | Indurated, cool, hyperhidrotic, cyanotic, mottled skin<br>Joint space narrowing<br>Muscle weakness<br>Osteoporotic changes on radiography |
| Stage III: Atrophic/cold | Ankylosis<br>Hair loss<br>Muscle atrophy<br>Tendon contractures<br>Thickening of fascia<br>Thin, shiny skin |

test, thermoregulatory sweat testing, laser Doppler flowmetry, three-phase bone scintigraphy, plain radiographs, and magnetic resonance imaging studies have been shown to be useful in the diagnosis of CRPS (Table 201.3). CRPS types I and II have been thought to progress through several stages, which vary significantly in temporal duration and even sequence, adding yet another challenge to making the diagnosis (Table 201.4). CRPS may resolve spontaneously, but significant disability can persist for years with periods of remission and relapse despite treatment. Cold CRPS appears to prognosticate a worse outcome. Estimated rates of return to original functional status vary from 20% to 40%.

## Etiology

The pathophysiology underlying CRPS remains incompletely understood; however, many theories are currently being entertained. Emerging research points to an element of peripheral sensitization in disease development. Central sensitization or "wind-up" of the dorsal horn neurons, brainstem, or thalamus,

along with remodeling of the primary somatosensory cortex and disinhibition of the motor cortex, appear to play key roles in more severe forms of CRPS. Ischemic rat models support a hypoxic and endothelial dysfunction theory in which hypoxia secondary to vasoconstriction essentially leads to acidosis and increased free radical formation resulting in primary afferent pain. Autonomic nervous system dysfunction holds some credence as an underlying mechanism, as animal models have shown a role for postsynaptic receptors in sensitization. However, sympathetic dysregulation is not an obligatory feature of CRPS. Inflammation might also contribute to the pathophysiology as the early phase of CRPS appears inflammatory, as demonstrated by elevated levels of neuropeptides, and studies have demonstrated injected leukocytes and immunoglobulins travel to the area of CRPS.

Sympathetically mediated pain responding to central or peripheral sympathetic blockade variably contributes to the overall pain experienced by patients. Additional sympathetically independent mediators have been identified. Elevated levels of circulating free radicals, inflammatory cytokines (e.g., interleukin-6 and tumor necrosis factor α), neuropeptides (substance P, bradykinin, neuropeptide Y, and calcitonin G–related protein), and cerebrospinal fluid levels of glutamate have been measured in patients with CRPS. Associations have been demonstrated between disease onset, responsiveness to treatment, features of dystonia, and the presence of human leukocyte antigen class I and II polymorphisms among patients with CRPS, suggesting a possible genetic component to the disease.

## Treatment

The overall goal of CRPS treatment is functional restoration as patients tend to avoid moving the affected limb. Patients should be educated on the neuropathic and centrally mediated nature of CRPS, and how disuse of the painful region can eventually harm the muscle, nerves, and bones if treatment is delayed.

### PHYSICAL AND OCCUPATIONAL THERAPY

Physical and occupational therapy geared toward functional restoration are considered the therapeutic mainstays of treatment. Gentle range-of-motion exercises, bandaging for control of edema, progressive increase in weight-bearing activities, improvement in flexibility and posture, and aerobic conditioning, ergonomics, and resolution of myofascial pain are thought to aid in recovery, although controversy exists regarding the long-term benefit of these interventions. CRPS-specific therapies may include graded motor imagery, mirror therapy, and exposure therapy where desensitization is achieved by subjecting the affected limb to warm and cool contrast baths and to fabrics of varying textures.

### PSYCHIATRIC THERAPY

Depression, anxiety, posttraumatic stress disorder, and kinesophobia often accompany CRPS, and, if present, should be addressed. Recent studies have shown that pain catastrophizing leads to increased opioid use and increased cytokine activity, especially in women, and that emotional distress can lead to increased perception of pain intensity. Psychiatric interventions could theoretically help ameliorate some of these effects; however, data to support these interventions needs development. Therapy focuses on treating underlying psychiatric disease, cognitive behavioral therapy, relaxation techniques, guided imagery, biofeedback, and stress management. Some authors also suggest pain rehabilitation as a possible adjunct to these modalities to optimize pain coping strategies.

### PHARMACOLOGIC THERAPY

In CRPS, the goal of medication management is to facilitate participation in physical and occupational therapy, as discussed earlier. Multimodal analgesia is the mainstay of treatment, and although no "strong" evidence exists for specific therapy, initial medication management typically includes the use of nonsteroidal antiinflammatory drugs, neuropathic agents such as gabapentin or pregabalin, tricyclic antidepressants, and topical lidocaine or capsaicin cream. Bisphosphonates have also been

found beneficial for patients exhibiting abnormal uptake on bone scan. Further, several studies in the orthopedic surgery literature have suggested that vitamin C administered in high doses at the time of fracture or surgical insult may play a role in prevention of CRPS. Not surprisingly, given its usefulness in spasticity, there is also some evidence for the intrathecal administration of γ-aminobutyric acid agonists (baclofen) for symptomatic relief of CRPS-related dystonia.

Additional treatments with less conclusive or even conflicting evidence supporting their use include corticosteroids, parenteral and topical ketamine, opioids, selective norepinephrine/serotonin reuptake inhibitors (or other antidepressants), calcitonin, sildenafil, botulinum toxin injections, cannabinoids for central and neuropathic pain, and intravenously administered lidocaine.

## PROCEDURAL TECHNIQUES

Traditionally, sympathetic blockade techniques such as stellate ganglion and lumbar plexus blocks were long viewed as a gold standard for CRPS treatment, yet there is a paucity of data supporting their therapeutic use. Chemical, thermal, and surgical neurolysis are also used in clinical practice, but controlled studies regarding their long-term utility are also lacking. Contemporary practice limits sympathetic blockade techniques; however, procedures continue to be used to facilitate functional restoration exercises, and sympathetic blockade has been theorized to aid in the prediction of successful treatment with spinal cord stimulation (SCS).

Literature supporting neuromodulation as a treatment modality for CRPS is limited to studies of small samples and mostly limited to case series or retrospective studies. A nonrandomized prospective trial of SCS in patients with CRPS responsive to sympathetic blockade demonstrated significant improvement in pain relief and strength over a mean of 35 months. In another randomized study comparing patients with CRPS treated with physical therapy to patients undergoing physical therapy and SCS, SCS plus physical therapy resulted in decreased pain intensity and improved global perceived effect for up to 2 years after the combination. Yet lasting significant findings were not apparent at the 5-year follow-up, which supports another randomized clinical trial comparing SCS versus physical therapy with no lasting significant findings upon this study's 3-year follow-up.

Dorsal root ganglia (DRG) stimulation has also been used in patients with lower extremity CRPS. Many pain clinics use DRG stimulation as the first-line therapy for neuromodulation in this population. Others reserve this for patients who fail SCS therapy. Some studies show superior symptomatic management with DRG stimulation over SCS therapy.

Although the mechanism of action of SCS remains complex, with a multitude of suggested theories including but not limited to inhibiting sympathetic output, blocking pain transmission, and activation of inhibitory pathways, cost-benefit analyses studying SCS use in patients have shown neuromodulation to be more cost-effective in comparison with conservative and other medical therapies. Limited evidence supports the use of permanent peripheral nerve stimulators in the treatment of CRPS type II. Finally, mirror and motor imagery therapies have been shown in preliminary, randomized crossover studies to significantly decrease pain and improve functionality in all CRPS types.

## SUGGESTED READINGS

Bruehl, S. (2010). An update on the pathophysiology of complex regional pain syndrome. *Anesthesiology, 113*(3), 713–725.

Deer, T. R., Levy, R. M., Kramer, J., Poree, L., Amirdelfan, K., Grigsby, E., et al. (2017). Dorsal root ganglion stimulation yielded higher treatment success rate for complex regional pain syndrome and causalgia at 3 and 12 months: A randomized comparative trial. *Pain, 158*(4), 669–681.

Goebel, A., Barker, C. H., & Turner-Stokes, L. *Complex regional pain syndrome in adults: UK guidelines for diagnosis, referral and management in primary and secondary care.* London: RCP; 2012.

Harden, R. N., Oaklander, A. L., Burton, A. W., Perez, R. S., Richardson, K., Swan, M., et al. (2013). Complex regional pain syndrome: Practical diagnostic and treatment guidelines, 4th edition. *Pain Medicine (Malden, MA), 14*(2), 180–229.

O'Connell, N. E., Wand, B. M., Gibson, W., Carr, D. B., Birklein, F., & Stanton, T. R. (2016). Local anaesthetic sympathetic blockade for complex regional pain syndrome. *Cochrane Database of Systematic Reviews, 7*(7), CD004598.

Poree, L., Krames, E., Pope, J., Deer, T. R., Levy, R., & Schultz, L. (2013). Spinal cord stimulation as treatment for complex regional pain syndrome should be considered earlier than last resort therapy. *Neuromodulation, 16*(2), 125–141.

Sanders, R. A., Moeschler, S. M., Gazelka, H. M., Lamer, T. J., Wang, Z., Qu, W., et al. (2016). Patient outcomes and spinal cord stimulation: A retrospective case series evaluating patient satisfaction, pain scores, and opioid requirements. *Pain Practice, 16*(7), 899–904.

Tran, D. Q., Duong, S., Bertini, P., & Finlayson, R. J. (2010). Treatment of complex regional pain syndrome: A review of the evidence. *Canadian Journal of Anaesthesia, 57*(2), 149–166.

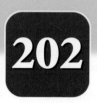

# 202

# Postoperative Headache

JILLIAN MALONEY, MD

Postoperative headache (PH) is one of several bothersome adverse events associated with anesthesia and surgery, along with corneal abrasions, nausea, vomiting, sore throat, back pain, fatigue, and myalgias. These minor adverse events, although rarely prolonged, can delay discharge and contribute to patient suffering and dissatisfaction. This chapter will explore common causes of PH including postdural puncture headache (PDPHA) and postcraniotomy pain, in addition to patient factors associated with PH even when no lumbar puncture or craniotomy was performed.

## Postdural Puncture Headache

Cerebrospinal fluid (CSF) leak that results in headache may be spontaneous or iatrogenic from a dural puncture (lumbar puncture, neuraxial anesthetic) or dural tear (spinal surgery). The International Headache Society (IHS) defines a PDPHA as "headache occurring within 5 days of a lumbar puncture, caused by CSF leakage through the dural puncture. It is usually accompanied by neck stiffness and/or subjective hearing symptoms. The headache remits spontaneously within 2 weeks, or after sealing of the leak with autologous epidural lumbar patch." The headache usually appears within 48 hours but may develop more than 3 days later. Nausea, vomiting, subjective hearing symptoms, and visual disturbances (diplopia, blurred vision, or photophobia) may also occur.

The IHS notes risk factors for PDPHA, including previous PDPHA, female gender, and age range 30 to 50 years. The headache is typically orthostatic (i.e., relieved by lying down), but this is not a reliable diagnostic factor. Evidence of low CSF pressure or leak, as seen on magnetic resonance imaging or other imaging modalities, supports the diagnosis, although neuroimaging is not required unless it is necessary to rule out an alternative diagnosis. The visual symptoms may result from traction on the brain, notably cranial nerve VI (in addition to cranial nerves III and IV). Although traditional teaching held that PDPHA is a result of traction on pain-sensitive meninges, it is more likely that headache results from compensatory venous hypervolemia and dilation of pain-sensitive dural venous sinuses in response to low intracranial CSF volume. Intrathecal air from dural puncture during an air-based epidural loss-of-resistance technique can also cause a headache.

For anesthesiologists, PDPHA is most likely to occur in the setting of obstetric anesthesia. In the postpartum period, headaches are more likely to be tension type and preeclampsia than PDPHA. In a study of 237,437 neuraxial anesthetics, including both spinal and epidural anesthesia, the incidence of PDPHA was 1:144. Approximately 1650 patients had headache, of which 58% required an epidural blood patch (EBP) and 10% required a second blood patch. As mentioned earlier, young females were at highest risk for PDPHA. However, among parturients, increased body mass index may be protective, and cesarean section decreases risk of PDPHA. This may be a result of pushing during delivery increasing the CSF leak and/or size of the dural tear. One study found parturients who had a witnessed dural puncture and who pushed during labor had an increased risk of PDPHA, more days of headache, and were more likely to require an EBP.

## Prevention

Several techniques can be used to reduce the incidence of PDPHA. First, the smallest-gauge pencil-point (vs. cutting or Quincke) needle should be used (Fig. 202.1). A metaanalysis in 2018 by Nath et al. showed the incidence of PDPHA was 11% in the conventional traumatic needle group compared with 4.2% in the atraumatic group. There was no significant difference in the success of lumbar puncture on the first attempt or the mean number of attempts between needle groups. In addition to needle type, the orientation of the spinal needle bevel perpendicular to the long axis of the spinal column can also increase the risk of PDPHA. The literature on prophylactic EBPs is mixed (i.e., injection of ~20 mL of autologous blood at the time of accidental dural puncture with a large-bore Tuohy needle may or may not reduce the incidence of PDPHA). Because a blood patch is not entirely without risk, some providers will wait to see if the patient develops a headache before performing the blood patch, although this requires an additional procedure. Another technique is to leave an intrathecal catheter in place for 24 hours after inadvertent dural puncture. The presence of a catheter may trigger an inflammatory reaction in the dura resulting in sealing the hole. The intrathecal catheter can also be used to provide analgesia or anesthesia, reducing the risk of another dural puncture from a second attempt at epidural catheter placement.

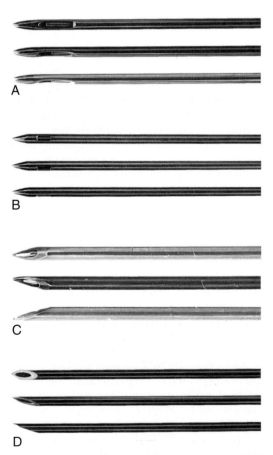

**Fig. 202.1** Frontal, oblique, and lateral views of common spinal needles. (A) Sprotte needle. (B) Whitacre needle. (C) Greene needle. (D) Quincke needle. (From Brown DL. *Regional Anesthesia and Analgesia.* WB Saunders; 1996. Used with permission of Mayo Foundation for Medical Education and Research. All rights reserved.)

## Treatment

Bed rest, hydration, analgesics, abdominal binders, and various medications (including sumatriptan, methylergonovine maleate, hydrocortisone, and gabapentin) have been used to treat PDPHA. Most of the supporting evidence for these therapies is weak, as is the use of caffeine for preventing and treating PDPHA.

Epidural saline infusions may provide short-term benefit. An EBP is used to treat persistent and severe symptoms, although EBPs performed less than 24 hours after dural puncture are associated with a lower success rate. Risks of EBP are low but not negligible; back pain is most common, with rare reports of arachnoiditis occurring after inadvertent intrathecal injection of autologous blood. The mechanism of action of the EBP may be twofold: immediate headache relief results from compression of the intrathecal space by the iatrogenic epidural hematoma, resulting in increased CSF pressure and headache resolution; long-term relief results from sealing of the dural tear.

## Other Postoperative Headaches

Preoperative headache is considered a risk factor for PH. Caffeine withdrawal has been cited as a common cause of PH in surgical patients. Intravenous or oral caffeine has been used successfully in some cases. Inhalation anesthetic agents are associated with PHs. Treatment is symptomatic.

The IHS recognizes acute and persistent postcraniotomy headaches. An acute postcraniotomy headache is defined by the IHS as "a headache of less than 3 months duration caused by craniotomy. In comparison, a persistent postcraniotomy headache is a headache greater than 3 months duration." Headache has been reported in up to 75% of patients undergoing a craniotomy for acoustic neuroma or other cerebellopontine angle tumors, though headache can occur after any craniotomy. Skull-based surgery or other cranial procedures associated with extensive muscle dissection (e.g., suboccipital approach) are higher risk for postoperative pain; craniectomy patients may be more prone to headache than those who have the bone replaced at the end of the procedure (craniotomy or cranioplasty). Surgical cases longer than 4 hours have been associated with a higher incidence of postcraniotomy headache. Neuroma and scar tissue formation may contribute to long-term pain after craniotomy; in the case of craniectomy, muscle tissue may adhere to the dura after surgery and contribute to headache. CSF leak is associated with postdural headache after surgery.

Headaches after craniotomy are often described by patients in ways reminiscent of head trauma headaches. Postcraniotomy headaches may represent a mixture of "site-of-injury" headache at the surgical site plus tension-type headache. Although the pathogenesis of postcraniotomy headache remains unclear, headache caused by head (surgical) trauma may be mediated by meningeal nerves that infiltrate the periosteum via the calvarial sutures. Because there are sensory fibers in the sutures, there may be a good reason to avoid drilling through them during craniotomies.

A pneumocephalus with associated headache can occur after spine operations. Otolaryngologic (e.g., sinus) and ophthalmologic operations have also been complicated by PH.

Hyperperfusion syndrome and associated headache has been described after carotid endarterectomy. Carotid endarterectomy can be associated with headache even in the absence of hyperperfusion, perhaps because of damage to the sympathetic plexus and altered sympathetic tone.

## Patient Characteristics Associated With Postoperative Headache

Several patient characteristics have been put forth as predisposing to PH. These include caffeine and alcohol use, dietary changes perioperatively, and tobacco cessation. Head trauma is an obvious risk factor; in other patients, certain drugs used in the perioperative period may contribute to headache (e.g., 5-hydroxytryptamine receptor antagonists [ondansetron]).

A recent prospective study reported the results of pre- and postoperative patient interviews regarding headache, and risk factors were identified. Overall, 28.3% of patients complained of headache by postoperative day 5. Patients with a history of headache had a 41% incidence of PH, versus those with no headache history who had an incidence of 16%. Independent risk factors included sevoflurane use, hypotension during surgery, female gender, and tobacco use. Among those without a headache history, caffeine but not smoking was associated with PH.

### SUGGESTED READINGS

DelPizzo, K., Luu, T., Fields, K. G., Sideris, A., Dong, N., Edmonds, C., et al. (2020). Risk of postdural puncture headache in adolescents and adults. *Anesthesia and Analgesia, 131*(1), 273–279.

Franz, A. M., Jia, S. Y., Bahnson, H. T., Goel, A., & Habib, A. S. (2017). The effect of second-stage pushing and body mass index on postdural puncture headache. *Journal of Clinical Anesthesia, 37*, 77–81.

Gaiser, R. R. (2017). Postdural puncture headache: An evidence-based approach. *Anesthesiology Clinics, 35*(1), 157–167.

Haldar, R., Kaushal, A., Gupta, D., Srivastava, S., & Singh, P. K. (2015). Pain following craniotomy:

Reassessment of the available options. *BioMed Research International, 2015,* 509164. doi:10.1155/2015/509164.

Headache Classification Committee of the International Headache Society (IHS). (2018). The International Classification of Headache Disorders. *Cephalalgia, 38*(1), 1–211. doi:10.1177/0333102417738202.

Matsota, P. K., Christodoulopoulou, T. C., Batistaki, C. Z., Arvaniti, C. C., Voumvourakis, K. I., & Kostopanagiotou, G. G. (2017). Factors associated with the presence of postoperative headache in elective surgery patients: A prospective single center cohort study. *Journal of Anesthesia, 31*(2), 225–236.

Nath, S., Koziarz, A., Badhiwala, J. H., Alhazzani, W., Jaeschke, R., Sharma, S., et al. (2018). Atraumatic versus conventional lumbar puncture needles: A systematic review and meta-analysis. *Lancet (London, England), 391*(10126), 1197–1204.

Rocha-Filho, P. A. (2015). Post-craniotomy headache: A clinical view with a focus on the persistent form. *Headache, 55*(5), 733–738.

The International Classification of Headache Disorders, 3rd edition (beta version). (2013). *Cephalalgia, 33*(9), 629–808.

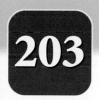

# 203

# Treatment of Cancer-Related Pain

TIM J. LAMER, MD  |  ROSS BARMAN, DO

## Introduction

Pain is exceedingly prevalent among patients with malignancies and is often suboptimally managed. It is estimated that approximately 90% of patients with cancer will experience pain as their disease progresses. One-third of patients experience pain while undergoing active therapy for disease, and more than three-quarters of patients experience pain during the last stages of illness. As survival rates for cancer continue to improve, the prevalence of cancer-free survivors afflicted by chronic pain also increases. Approximately 40% of cancer survivors experience persistent pain as a sequela of their cancer or its treatment. With the use of pharmacologic agents, interventional therapies, and other modalities, effective analgesia can be attained for 70% to 90% of people with cancer.

## Mechanisms of Cancer Pain

Cancer pain generators include direct effects of the neoplasm on surrounding tissues and structures, side effects of treatment, and other causes not related to the malignancy. Mechanistically, cancer pain syndromes can be divided into two major pain categories: nociceptive pain and neuropathic pain. Nociceptive pain results from direct tissue damage and can be further subdivided into somatic and visceral nociceptive pain. Somatic pain may originate from multiple sites—including skin, muscle, joints, connective tissue, and bone—and is mediated by somatic afferent fibers (Aδ and C fibers). Somatic pain is the most common type of cancer pain and is often described based on the location of the tissue involved. Pain from superficial structures such as skin is often described as sharp, throbbing, and well localized, whereas deep tissue pain is often described as dull, aching, and less well localized. Visceral pain originates from solid or hollow organs and is mediated by visceral nociceptive afferent fibers that travel along with visceral sympathetic efferent fibers. This pain is often described as a dull, diffuse pain that is frequently referred in a dermatomal fashion.

Neuropathic pain is involved in approximately 40% of cancer-related pain and may present acutely or as a component of chronic pain. Neuropathic pain occurs when there is damage to or dysfunction of nerves in the peripheral or central nervous system. The pain frequently has dysesthetic (e.g., burning, pricking) or paroxysmal (e.g., stabbing, shooting, electric shock-like) qualities and may be associated with sensory, motor, or autonomic dysfunction. When the pain is coupled with loss of sensory input, it is referred to as *de-afferentation pain* (e.g., phantom limb pain). When dysregulation of the autonomic nervous system plays a major role, the pain is referred to as *sympathetically mediated pain* (e.g., complex regional pain syndrome). Sympathetically mediated pain may occur after a nerve or limb injury; the patient often has diffuse burning pain of the affected extremity associated with allodynia, hyperpathia, sudomotor dysfunction, and signs of impaired vasomotor regulation to the extremity. This pain may be mediated, at least in part, by sympathetic efferent fibers. Compared with nociceptive pain, neuropathic pain is more challenging to effectively treat and is often less responsive to conventional pharmacologic therapy.

One or more of these mechanisms may contribute to a patient's pain and may occur as a result of the primary cancerous lesion, metastatic disease, neural compression, or treatments such as radiation therapy, chemotherapy, or surgery. Pain may also originate from secondary nonmalignant sources (e.g., herniated nucleus pulposus, spinal stenosis, myofascial pain syndrome).

## Medical Therapy

The World Health Organization's three-step analgesic ladder created the foundation of contemporary pain management for patients with cancer. This ladder recommends progressing in a stepwise fashion from nonopioid medications to intermediate- and then high-potency opioids for severe pain, with nonopioid adjuvant medications being used as needed for specific pain types. Although this model initially revolutionized cancer pain management, increasing survival rates and novel interventional therapeutic strategies have necessitated a shift in this linear treatment algorithm. New treatment algorithms use this ladder in a bidirectional fashion allowing clinicians to not only move through the ladder depending on any given disease stage but also skip specific rungs to more quickly address a patient's specific needs. In addition, early application of interventional modalities may be indicated in specific cases to provide optimal pain control, reduce the risk of polypharmacy, and more quickly improve a patient's quality of life. This multimodality approach allows for more aggressive treatment and shorter duration of pain while reducing overall opioid exposure to minimize risk and reduce systemic side effects of oral medications.

## Adjuvant Analgesic Agents

Adjuvant analgesic agents play a major role in treating patients with malignancies (Table 203.1). Most of these medications have a primary indication other than pain but have analgesic

| TABLE 203.1 | Adjuvant Analgesic Agents for the Treatment of Cancer-Related Pain: Major Classes |
|---|---|
| **Drug Class** | **Example(s)** |
| **MULTIPURPOSE ANALGESIC AGENTS** | |
| Antidepressants | |
| Tricyclics | Amitriptyline, desipramine, nortriptyline |
| SSRIs | Citalopram, paroxetine (minimal analgesia activity) |
| SNRIs | Duloxetine, venlafaxine |
| Other agents | Bupropion |
| Corticosteroids | Dexamethasone, prednisone |
| $\alpha_2$-Adrenergic agonists | Clonidine, tizanidine |
| Neuroleptic agents | Olanzapine |
| **ADJUVANTS FOR NEUROPATHIC PAIN** | |
| Anticonvulsants | Carbamazepine, gabapentin, pregabalin, topiramate |
| Local anesthetic agents | Lidocaine, mexiletine |
| NMDA receptor antagonists | Dextromethorphan, ketamine |
| Other agents | Baclofen, cannabinoids, capsaicin, lidocaine, lidocaine/prilocaine, psychostimulants (methylphenidate, modafinil) |
| Topical drugs | Capsaicin, EMLA cream, lidocaine patch or cream |
| **ADJUVANTS FOR BONE PAIN** | |
| Corticosteroids | Dexamethasone, prednisone |
| Calcitonin | |
| Bisphosphonates and monoclonal antibodies | Clodronate, pamidronate, zoledronic acid Denosumab |
| Radiopharmaceuticals | Samarium-153, strontium-89 |
| **ADJUVANTS FOR MUSCULOSKELETAL PAIN** | |
| Muscle relaxants | Carisoprodol, cyclobenzaprine, metaxalone, methocarbamol, orphenadrine |
| Baclofen | |
| Benzodiazepines | Clonazepam, diazepam, lorazepam |
| Tizanidine | |
| **ADJUVANTS FOR PAIN FROM BOWEL OBSTRUCTION** | |
| Anticholinergics | Glycopyrrolate, scopolamine |
| Corticosteroids | Dexamethasone, prednisone |
| Octreotide | |

*EMLA,* Eutectic mixture of local anesthetics (prilocaine and lidocaine); *NMDA,* N-methyl-D-aspartate; *SNRI,* serotonin-norepinephrine reuptake inhibitor; *SSRI,* selective serotonin reuptake inhibitor.

properties as well. The choice of an adjuvant agents is made based on several factors, including the type of pain, pharmacologic characteristics and adverse effects of the drug, interactions with other medications, and patient comorbid conditions (e.g., depression). Adjuvant agents comprise a diverse group of medications and can be broadly classified into multipurpose adjuvant analgesic agents and adjuvants specifically for neuropathic pain, bone pain, musculoskeletal pain, and bowel obstruction.

Multipurpose adjuvant analgesic agents include agents such as tricyclic antidepressants (TCAs), serotonin-norepinephrine reuptake inhibitors (SNRIs), calcium channel blocking agents, corticosteroids, $\alpha_2$-adrenergic agonists, and neuroleptic agents. TCAs are the most common antidepressants used in the treatment of chronic pain conditions; however, their use may be limited by the frequent occurrence of associated adverse effects such as orthostatic hypotension, sedation, cardiotoxicity, and anticholinergic syndrome. The sedating properties of TCAs can sometimes be used to an advantage when a patient's pain is contributing to poor sleep. The SNRI medications venlafaxine and duloxetine have significant analgesic properties and have demonstrated efficacy for both neuropathic pain and musculoskeletal pain. They are less sedating and have a more favorable cardiovascular side effect profile compared with TCAs. Corticosteroids are useful for bone pain, neuropathic pain, headaches secondary to increased intracranial pressure, spinal cord compression, and pain caused by obstruction of a hollow viscus or organ-capsule distention. Corticosteroids may also improve appetite, decrease nausea and malaise, and greatly improve overall quality of life. The $\alpha_2$-adrenergic agonists, such as clonidine and tizanidine, may also be useful in treating selective cancer pain syndromes. Administered in the intrathecal (IT) space, clonidine has been shown to be beneficial in severe, intractable cancer pain. Finally, neuroleptic agents, such as olanzapine, have been found to decrease pain and opioid consumption while improving cognitive functioning and decreasing anxiety.

The gabapentinoids, gabapentin and pregabalin, inhibit neurotransmitter release by binding to the alpha-2-delta subunit of voltage-gated calcium channels. They are considered first-line agents and have demonstrated analgesic efficacy in many neuropathic pain states. Oral and parenterally administered local anesthetic agents also have analgesic properties in patients with neuropathic pain. The *N*-methyl-D-aspartic acid receptor antagonists have been shown to have analgesic effects, with ketamine specifically being found to reduce opioid requirements and reduce cancer pain. Injections of botulinum toxin have been shown to reduce cancer-related pain caused from surgery and radiation.

Bone pain and pathologic fractures are common in patients with cancer. Radiation therapy is commonly used to treat cancer-related bone pain and administered when possible. Adjuvants have been found to be valuable in treating bone pain. These agents include calcitonin, bisphosphonates, and certain radiopharmaceuticals (radionuclides that are absorbed at areas of high bone turnover). Bisphosphonates (e.g., zoledronic acid, pamidronate) and monoclonal antibodies (e.g., denosumab) have been shown to improve pain control and reduce the frequency of pathologic fractures and can be helpful in treating cancer-related hypercalcemia.

If surgical decompression is not feasible in patients with a malignant bowel obstruction, the use of the somatostatin analog octreotide, anticholinergic drugs (hyoscine, glycopyrrolate), and corticosteroids may be beneficial.

Other systemically administered drugs such as baclofen, cannabinoids, benzodiazepines, and psychostimulants have also been used as adjuvant analgesics. Topical lidocaine patches, topical local anesthetic creams, and topical capsaicin may be useful in patients with localized pain syndromes, such as chest pain after mastectomy, radiation-induced dermatitis, postthoracotomy pain, and others.

Not all cancer-related pain can be managed with orally or parenterally administered medications alone. In fact, pharmacologic therapy will not provide adequate pain relief in 10% to 15% of patients with cancer. In these situations interventional therapy is often undertaken.

## Interventional Therapy

Given that the use of the World Health Organization's analgesic ladder does not provide adequate analgesia for all patients with cancer, a revised stepwise approach has been developed that includes the use of interventional techniques (Fig. 203.1).

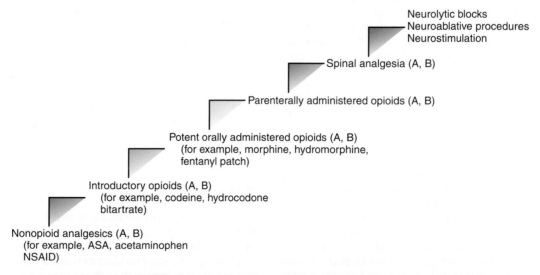

**Fig. 203.1** Revised stepladder approach to the management of cancer pain. *ASA,* Acetylsalicylic acid; *NSAID,* nonsteroidal antiinflammatory drug. (Modified, with permission, from Lamer TJ. Treatment of cancer-related pain: when orally administered medications fail. *Mayo Clinic Proc.* 1994;69:473–480.)

It is now recommended to consider implementing interventional modalities earlier in the treatment plan to provide optimal pain control or to reduce the burden of oral analgesic side effects such as sedation, reduced mental acuity, and constipation.

There are multiple interventional therapies that may provide relief to patients with refractory pain. These therapeutic options include nerve blocks and other injection therapies (e.g., joint and trigger-point injections), neurolytic blocks, epidurally and intrathecally administered analgesia, neuromodulation (e.g., spinal cord stimulation [SCS], dorsal root ganglion [DRG] stimulation), and advanced neurosurgical techniques (e.g., cordotomy, midline myelotomy, rhizotomy).

## NEURAXIALLY ADMINISTERED ANALGESIA

Drug toxicity secondary to opioids and adjuvant medications is a leading cause of treatment failure in the management of cancer-related pain. Patients who experience intractable focal pain or who are intolerant to the effects of systemic opioids are candidates for a neuroaxial analgesic approach. Neuraxial analgesia refers to a temporary or permanently implanted device that delivers an infusion of an analgesic from a drug reservoir to either the epidural or IT space. The benefit of these treatment modalities is that they bypass the blood-brain barrier, reduce the overall amount of medication exposure, and limit toxicities from systemic oral or intravenous therapy. Compared with oral analgesics in patients with intractable cancer-related pain, implantable drug delivery systems are associated with superior reduction in pain scores, decreased fatigue, increased quality of life, and an improved 6-month survival.

Currently, morphine and ziconotide (a selective N-type calcium-channel inhibitor) are the two first-line U.S. Food and Drug Administration (FDA)-approved therapeutic options in IT therapy for chronic pain, which currently includes cancer pain. These medications are recommended for both neuropathic and nociceptive pain. Morphine is an IT agent that has been efficacious for patients who respond to opioid medications. Ziconotide is a preferred IT agent for patients with opioid resistance or have hyperalgesia and who experience intolerable opioid side effects. Ziconotide may also be considered when trying to avoid opioids, such as in in patients with obstructive sleep apnea, underlying lung disease, or in younger patients with a longer life expectancy. Although only morphine and ziconotide are FDA approved, numerous other medications including other opioids (hydromorphone and fentanyl), $\alpha_2$-adrenergic agonists (clonidine), calcium-channel blockers, and local anesthetic agents (e.g., bupivacaine) are commonly used. Other than morphine and ziconotide, these medications are considered as "off-label" when used for neuraxial analgesia. Single agents or a combination of agents may be used, depending on the pain mechanism involved.

Before initiating IT therapy, it is recommended that patients undergo multidisciplinary evaluation for comorbid medical and psychiatric conditions. Evaluation regarding other cancer-related pharmacologic treatments, such as anticoagulation and chemotherapeutic agents, and cancer-related comorbidities, such as immunosuppression, hematologic abnormalities, postradiation scarring, and epidural metastases, should be conducted because these may limit the use of IT therapy.

## NERVE BLOCKS AND ABLATIVE PROCEDURES

Neurolytic nerve blocks and ablative procedures can be effective for treating refractory pain. Neurolytic blocks with phenol, ethanol, radiofrequency ablation, or cryoablation are most appropriate for patients with advanced disease and decreased life expectancy when other, less invasive options have failed to provide adequate relief. Neurolytic celiac plexus block is very effective for pain related to intraabdominal malignancies, particularly pancreatic cancer. Neurolytic blocks targeting the lumbar sympathetic, superior hypogastric plexus, or ganglion impar can be useful for treating pain causes by tumors of the pelvis. Intercostal and paravertebral blocks are valuable for treating chest pain (e.g., rib metastasis, pathologic rib fractures). For carefully selected patients with perineal pain, sacral nerve neurolytic blocks may be beneficial, and trigeminal nerve blocks may be effective for facial pain.

More recently, direct tumor ablative treatments have been demonstrated to be effective for some tumors. Image-guided radiofrequency tumor ablation, cryoablation, and high-intensity focused ultrasound are techniques that use heat, cold, or ultrasound energy to locally destroy pain-producing tumors.

## Neuromodulation

Patients with cancer who have attempted conventional therapy yet continue to suffer from intractable postsurgical or radiation-induced pain, chemotherapy-associated neuropathic pain, or chronic pain may benefit from interventional neuromodulation. Spinal cord stimulation (SCS) usually includes a trial period, which, if successful, is followed by the permanent implantation epidural leads and a pulse generator. Although the benefits of SCS and DRG stimulation have been more extensively studied in the noncancer population, patients with cancer who continue to suffer from refractory pain should be referred to an interventional pain physician to assess their candidacy for neuromodulation or other interventional pain strategies.

## Surgical Procedures

The effectiveness of neuraxial analgesia has significantly reduced the use of destructive neurosurgical procedures to treat cancer pain. In carefully selected patients who have failed less invasive therapies, dorsal root entry zone lesioning, percutaneous cordotomy, or midline myelotomy can be considered.

As with all interventional techniques, these interventions are not without potential complications; therefore the provider must carefully weigh the risks and benefits for each patient (Table 203.2).

## Other Approaches

Therapies other than medications and procedures can be effective for treating cancer-related pain. Relaxation techniques, massage, therapeutic exercise, heat, ice, electrical stimulation, counseling, and other modalities may be valuable. A multidisciplinary or team approach to the management of cancer-related pain, with the participation of oncologists, nurses, psychologists, rehabilitation specialists, palliative care specialists, and pain management specialists, will likely produce the most beneficial treatment program.

| TABLE 203.2 | Potential Complications of Invasive Procedures for the Treatment of Cancer-Related Pain |
| --- | --- |
| **Treatment** | **Potential Adverse Effects** |
| Neurolytic blocks | Sensorimotor impairment<br>Sympathetic or parasympathetic impairment<br>Postural hypotension<br>Bowel or bladder dysfunction<br>Pain recurrence<br>De-afferentation pain<br>Pneumothorax* |
| Spinally administered opioids | Respiratory depression<br>Pruritus<br>Urinary retention<br>Nausea and vomiting<br>Hypogonadism and other endocrinopathies |
| Spinally administered clonidine | Hypotension<br>Sedation |
| Spinally administered local anesthetic agent | Sympathetic blockade[†]<br>Exaggerated spread[‡]<br>Motor block |
| Neurosurgical procedures | Bladder dysfunction<br>Motor weakness<br>De-afferentation pain<br>Respiratory dysfunction[§] |
| Neuraxial catheters | Catheter break or leak<br>Catheter obstruction<br>Infection[‖]<br>CSF leak |
| Spinally administered ziconotide | Psychiatric symptoms[¶]<br>Motor deficits<br>Meningitis<br>Seizures |
| Neuromodulation (e.g., SCS, DRG) | Lead migration<br>Device malfunction (lead fracture, battery failure)<br>Infection[¶]<br>Neurologic injury (CSF leak, epidural hematoma, postdural puncture headache) |

*Celiac plexus.
[†]Hypotension, urinary retention.
[‡]High block.
[§]Cervical cordotomy.
[‖]Cellulitis, epidural abscess, meningitis.
[¶]Hallucinations, new or worsening depression, suicidal ideation.
*CSF*, Cerebrospinal fluid; *DRG*, dorsal root ganglion; *SCS*, spinal cord stimulation.

# SUGGESTED READINGS

Aman, M. M., Mahmoud, A., Deer, T., Sayed, D., Hagedorn, J. M., Brogan, S. E., et al. (2021). The American Society of Pain and Neuroscience (ASPN) best practices and guidelines for the interventional management of cancer-associated pain. *Journal of Pain Research, 14*, 2139–2164. doi:10.2147/JPR.S315585.

Hagedorn, J. M., Pittelkow, T. P., Hunt, C. L., D'Souza, R. S., & Lamer, T. J. (2020). Current perspectives on spinal cord stimulation for the treatment of cancer pain. *Journal of Pain Research, 13*, 3295–3305. doi:10.2147/JPR.S263857.

Lamer, T. J., Deer, T. R., & Hayek, S. M. (2016). Advanced innovations for pain. *Mayo Clinic Proceedings, 91*(2), 246–258. doi:10.1016/j.mayocp.2015.12.001.

Wanderman, R. L., & Hagedorn, J. M. (2021). Intrathecal drug delivery system: A pain management option for refractory cancer-related pain. *Pain Medicine (Malden, MA), 22*(2), 523–526. doi:10.1093/pm/pnaa364.

# Postherpetic Neuralgia

CHRISTINE L. HUNT, DO, MS

## Introduction

The syndrome of postherpetic neuralgia (PHN) is defined as the onset of persistent chronic pain after an attack of acute herpes zoster (AHZ). AHZ is a reactivation of the varicella virus that lies dormant after an episode of infection often preceding AHZ by years known as "chickenpox," which usually occurred during childhood. More than 95% of young adults in North America possess antibodies to the varicella zoster virus, indicating that the virus lies dormant in most of the adult population. When the virus reactivates in the setting of waning immunity, advanced age, illness, or other states of physiologic stress, AHZ may occur. Incidence increases with age, with only 3.4 per 1000 persons at 50 years of age but increasing to 11 per 1000 persons by age 80.

The pain of AHZ typically subsides within 2 to 4 weeks. Approximately 10% of patients with AHZ develop PHN, which is defined as pain in the same dermatomal distribution persisting beyond 3 months after rash onset. The following risk factors increase the likelihood of a patient developing PHN after AHZ: older age (>60 years), greater severity of acute pain during AHZ infection, more extensive or inflammatory rash, infection in the trigeminal distribution, delayed antiviral treatment (more than 72 hours), a prodrome of dermatomal pain before onset of the rash, and patients with immune suppression including cancer, diabetes, immunosuppression, and lymphoproliferative disorders. Patients with these risk factors may have as much as a 50% to 75% risk of having pain that persists for at least 6 months after rash onset. PHN is more common after ophthalmic herpes than after the spinal segment type.

## Description of the Syndrome

The persistence of pain located within a single dermatome from the central dorsal line in a ventral direction after the initial rash of AHZ is the most typical manifestation of the syndrome of PHN. The pain is typically described as constant aching or burning pain, paroxysmal lancinating pain, and/or allodynia, and may be accompanied by pruritus that some patients find quite distressing. The pain is unilateral, most commonly affecting a thoracic dermatome or the ophthalmic division $V_1$ of the trigeminal nerve (cranial nerve V). Lumbar, cervical, and sacral involvement is less common. Occasionally, but rarely, the pain of PHN can occur without a preceding rash.

In PHN, the affected area typically shows changes in the form of pigmentation and scarring where the vesicles of AHZ have healed. Hyperesthesia, hyperpathia, and allodynia may be present. The pain can often be excruciating and intractable, impairing quality of life to the point that the patient may contemplate suicide. The pain of PHN is purely neuropathic.

## Pathophysiology

The varicella zoster virus remains dormant in the dorsal root ganglion (DRG) of the peripheral nerve after initial infection, often occurring in childhood. The cause of its reactivation is not fully understood but could be related to a perturbation in the immune system, an increase in stress, or both. Reactivation leads to replication and propagation of the virus along the nerve associated with the DRG, triggering an inflammatory immune response ultimately leading to cell death of cutaneous cells and sometimes neuronal cells within the central and peripheral nervous system. The dermatomal distribution of the vesicular rash seen in AHZ is related to the transport of the reactivated virus along the sensory nerve fiber to the skin. Damage to peripheral nerves leads to impaired inhibition of pain signals, as well as to descending pathways due to damage to the dorsal horn that leads to central sensitization.

## Treatment

Because of the complex nature of the pathology of PHN, no definitive treatment is available. For this reason, prevention of PHN is vital and consists of recommendations that individuals older than 60 years be vaccinated and, when recurrence is diagnosed, that the AHZ episode be treated early with antiviral medication and steroids.

Often a multimodal analgesic approach is required in cases of moderate to severe PHN. Treatment includes medications (both topical and oral), epidural steroid injections, cognitive behavioral therapy, and advanced interventional therapies, as well as surgical techniques. A balanced combination of conservative modalities has the best potential to achieve the goal of decreasing pain to a level that allows patients a better functional status and improved quality of life (Table 204.1). Referral to a pain rehabilitation center is recommended when the disease is debilitating and when the patient's functional status, emotional status, and quality of life are severely impaired.

### PHARMACOTHERAPY

Topical agents are often considered as initial therapy given their typically low side effect profile and good tolerability in most patients. Topical creams include capsaicin and EMLA (eutectic mixture of local anesthetics) cream, and lidocaine patches are used with success in some patients. Topical capsaicin (8%) transdermal patch is sometimes applied for patients who fail to respond to use of more accessible topical agents. Anticonvulsants including gabapentin or pregabalin are often used as initial therapy for patients with PHN. Care must be taken to adjust the dosage in patients with renal impairment. Other commonly used anticonvulsants include carbamazepine or oxcarbazepine.

| TABLE 204.1 | Treatment Options for Postherpetic Neuralgia | |
| --- | --- | --- |
| **Pharmacotherapy** | **Interventional Therapies (Percutaneous)** | **Surgical Interventions** |
| NSAIDs | Epidural steroid injection | Caudalis DREZ lesioning/stereotactic nucleotomy |
| EMLA cream | Pulsed radiofrequency denervation of DRG | Gamma knife surgery |
| Lidoderm cream and patch | Radiofrequency denervation of intercostal nerves | Motor cortex stimulation |
| Capsaicin cream and patch | SCS | Cordotomy* |
| Gabapentin | PNS | Percutaneous radiofrequency rhizotomy* |
| Pregabalin | Intrathecal drug delivery | Gasserian ganglion stimulation* |
| Amitriptyline | | |
| Nortriptyline | | |
| Duloxetine | | |
| Venlafaxine | | |
| Carbamazepine | | |
| Oxcarbazepine | | |
| Opioid (limited circumstances) | | |

*There is very limited data regarding use of these procedures for treatment of postherpetic neuralgia.
*DREZ*, Dorsal root entry zone lesioning; *DRG*, dorsal root ganglion; *EMLA*, eutectic mixture of local anesthetics; *NSAIDs*, nonsteroidal antiinflammatory drugs; *PNS*, peripheral nerve stimulation; *SCS*, spinal cord stimulation.

Tricyclic antidepressant medications (amitriptyline, nortriptyline) can also be used if initial agents are incompletely effective or poorly tolerated and if patients do not have contraindications such as intolerance to anticholinergic medications or prolonged QT syndrome. Monitoring for anticholinergic side effects is important, particularly in older patients. Other medications commonly employed in the antidepressant class include the serotonin-norepinephrine reuptake inhibitors (e.g., duloxetine, venlafaxine). Like all neuropathic pain, severe cases may require judicious and careful use of medications from more than one class of agent to optimize analgesic effect. Use of multiple medications increases the risk for intolerable side effects and medication interactions, so patients should be closely followed while titrating adjuvant medications.

Because of the risks of tolerance, dependence, addiction, and development of central sensitization, opioid medications are generally discouraged for use in chronic pain syndromes including PHN. Their use may be considered with careful screening for history of substance use disorder and discussion with patients regarding risks, benefits, and goals of care.

## INTERVENTIONAL THERAPIES

Epidural steroid injections performed at the dermatomal level associated with pain from PHN may be considered in patients with persistent and refractory pain symptoms. These are generally performed within 3 months of presentation (after initial infection is resolved), with patients possibly less likely to respond as they approach 1 year after onset of symptoms.

Because transcutaneous electrical nerve stimulation (TENS) has minimal side effects and typically provides at least moderate results, these units should also be tried along with pharmacotherapy.

Emerging interventions for the treatment of PHN have been numerous in the last few years and include pulsed radiofrequency denervation of the intercostal nerve roots/DRG, implanted spinal cord stimulators, and implanted peripheral nerve stimulators (not to be confused with TENS). These should generally be reserved for patients with refractory symptoms not adequately treated with more conservative therapies.

## SURGICAL PROCEDURES

Surgical interventions for the treatment of PHN include dorsal root entry zone (DREZ) lesioning/stereotactic nucleotomy, gamma knife surgery, motor cortex stimulation, and rarely performed surgeries including cordotomy, percutaneous radiofrequency rhizotomy, and Gasserian ganglion stimulation. Results from these procedures in treatment of PHN have variable results and should be considered in select highly refractory cases in consultation with an experienced neurologic surgeon.

## Acknowledgment

The author and editors wish to sincerely thank Salim Michel Ghazi, MD, for his work on a predecessor chapter. [Ghazi SM. Postherpetic neuralgia. In: Trentman TL, ed. *Faust's Anesthesiology Review*. 5th ed. Elsevier; 2020:632–634.]

## SUGGESTED READINGS

Dworkin, R. H., O'Connor, A. B., Kent, J., Mackey, S. C., Raja, S. N., Stacey, B. R., et al. (2013). Interventional management of neuropathic pain: NeuPSIG recommendations. *Pain, 154*(11), 2249–2261.

Ghanavatian, S., Wie, C. S., Low, R. S., Butterfield, R. J., Zhang, N., Dhaliwal, G. S., et al. (2019). Parameters associated with efficacy of epidural steroid injections in the management of postherpetic neuralgia: The Mayo Clinic experience. *Journal of Pain Research, 12*, 1279–1286.

Hadley, G. R., Gayle, J. A., Ripoll, J., Jones, M. R., Argoff, C. E., Kaye, R. J., et al. (2016). Post-herpetic neuralgia: A review. *Current Pain and Headache Reports, 20*(3), 17. [Erratum in: Curr Pain Headache Rep. 20:28, 2016.].

Johnson, R. W., & Rice, A. S. (2014). Clinical practice: Postherpetic neuralgia. *New England Journal of Medicine, 371*(16), 1526–1533.

Liu, B., Yang, Y., Zhang, Z., Wang, H., Fan, B., & Sima, L. (2020). Clinical study of spinal cord stimulation and pulsed radiofrequency for management of herpes zoster-related pain persisting beyond acute phase in elderly patients. *Pain Physician, 23*(3), 263–270.

Mongardi, L., Visani, J., Mantovani, G., Vitali, C., Ricciardi, L., Giordano, F., et al. (2021). Long term results of Dorsal Root Entry Zone (DREZ) lesions for the treatment of intractable pain: A systematic review of the literature on 1242 cases. *Clinical Neurology and Neurosurgery, 210*, 107004.

Texakalidis, P., Tora, M. S., & Boulis, N. M. (2019). Neurosurgeons' armamentarium for the management of refractory postherpetic neuralgia: A systematic literature review. *Stereotactic and Functional Neurosurgery, 97*(1), 55–65.

# Common Interventions for Low Back Pain

BRENDAN J. LANGFORD, MD | MARKUS A. BENDEL, MD

Low back pain (LBP) is a widespread condition affecting greater than 80% of the adult population. Back pain is the third most common reason for an outpatient physician visit. The direct and indirect medical costs related to lost productivity are substantial. In 2016, LBP and neck pain accounted for the largest amount of health care dollars spent on a disorder, totaling $134.5 billion. Back pain can be caused by a multitude of different pathologies (Box 205.1), which is important to consider when formulating a treatment plan ranging from physical therapy to surgical consultation (Box 205.2).

The Centers for Disease Control and Prevention defines acute back pain as back pain lasting less than 4 weeks, subacute as 4 to 12 weeks, and chronic back pain as lasting greater than 12 weeks. Episodes of acute LBP generally respond to conservative measures, with resolution of symptoms within a few weeks. However, patients with persistent pain after a trial of conservative care may be appropriate candidates for percutaneous injection therapy, commonly including facet joint injections, medial branch blocks (MBBs), or sacroiliac joint (SIJ) injections. Historically, this chapter focused on epidural steroid injections for LBP, and although they are still commonly used in clinical practice for radiculitis, there is limited evidence to suggest that they are frontline therapy for LBP. The best intervention must be selected after considering a patient's clinical presentation, physical examination, and advanced imaging findings.

## Facet (Zygapophysial) Joint Injections

Facet joints are diarthrodial joints formed by a superior articular process and inferior articular process that are covered by hyaline cartilage and encapsulated in a synovial-filled capsule. Because of an abundance of nociceptors in this area, stretching or compressing the facet joint can lead to significant LBP. Approximately 15% to 45% of LBP is derived from the facet joints. Patients may have paraspinal tenderness and note that pain is exacerbated with positioning changes. Imaging modalities have low sensitivity for detecting facet joint pain. Facet joint pathology may include osteoarthritis and inflammatory processes. Facet joint injections or MBBs are required to confirm a diagnosis of facetogenic pain.

### BOX 205.1   ETIOLOGIES OF LOW BACK PAIN

Trauma
Myofascial
Malignancy
Osteoarthritis
Discogenic
Sacroiliitis
Inflammatory
Infectious
Stenosis

### BOX 205.2   LOW BACK PAIN INTERVENTIONS

Physical therapy
Medication management
Transcutaneous electrical nerve stimulation
Acupuncture
Osteopathic manipulation
Facet joint injections
Medial branch blocks with subsequent ablation
Sacroiliac joint injections
Epidural steroid injections
Basivertebral nerve ablation
Kyphoplasty/vertebroplasty
Neuromodulation (spinal cord stimulation, dorsal root ganglion stimulation)
Spine surgery

This sterile procedure is performed by pain medicine specialists using fluoroscopy. Steroid and local anesthetic are both injected for diagnostic and therapeutic purposes.

Academic evidence for facet joint injections in treating facetogenic pain has been weak, with studies revealing variable results. Fuchs and colleagues performed a randomized controlled trial (RCT) of hyaluronic acid versus triamcinolone facet joint injections. Both injectates led to reduced visual analog scale scores and functional improvement. Anand and Butt performed a prospective study that revealed 53% of patients who received facet joint injections for lumbar back pain had pain relief (complete or partial) after 8 weeks and 68% of patients had relief (complete or partial) after 6-month follow-up. Celik and colleagues described a randomized study of 80 patients into a control group (diclofenac sodium, thiocolchicoside, and bed rest) versus a treatment group (facet joint injections with prilocaine, bupivacaine, and methylprednisolone). Visual analog scale scores were lower in the treatment group than the control group, but the difference was not statistically significant. However, there was a statistically significant reduction in Oswestry LBP disability questionnaire scores, favoring the treatment group. Finally, Bani and colleagues discussed facet joint injections in 230 patients. At a mean follow-up of 10 months, 18.7% had long-lasting pain relief of either LBP and/or leg pain, whereas 50.4% of patients had no pain relief from the facet joint injections.

## Medial Branch Blocks and Radiofrequency Ablation

The medial branch of the posterior primary ramus innervates the facet joint. These medial branches course along the neck of the superior articular process. MBBs with local anesthetic are intended as a diagnostic block (Fig. 205.1). Two trials are performed: one with short-acting local anesthetic (e.g., lidocaine)

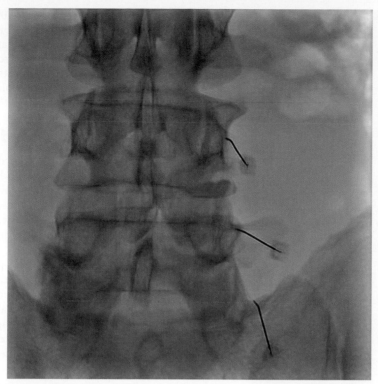

**Fig. 205.1**    Medial branch blocks of the right L3, L4, and L5 medial branch nerves innervating the right L4–L5 and L5–S1 facet joints.

and one with long-acting local (e.g., bupivacaine). Only a small amount of local anesthetic (e.g., 0.5 mL) is used to focus on the intended target and not allow spread to adjacent structures. Two trials are used to increase the specificity of the blocks in diagnosing facetogenic pain and reducing false positive results with single trials. Note that two trials will unfortunately increase the number of false negatives. If appropriate pain reduction is achieved with both trials (at least 50%–80% pain reduction), then therapeutic radiofrequency ablation (RFA) of these medial branches would be offered to the patient. In the therapeutic procedure, a specialized RFA cannula and probe are placed near the medial branch nerve, and an ablative lesion is created at 80°C to 85°C for 90 seconds (Fig. 205.2).

Clinical evidence for RFA of medial branch nerves for treating facetogenic pain is more convincing and promising than the variable evidence seen with facet joint injections. One study by Dreyfuss and colleagues revealed a 90% success rate with RFA when the patients had greater than 80% pain relief for more than 1 to 2 hours with trial 1 (lidocaine) and more than 2 to 3 hours with trial 2 (bupivacaine). Conger and colleagues performed a retrospective chart review and a phone survey to evaluate the efficacy of RFA relieving patients' pain; 56.5% of patients had at least 50% pain reduction at a minimum of 6 months' follow-up.

## Sacroiliac Joint Injections

The SIJ is a diarthrodial joint that connects the pelvis (ilium) with the sacrum. The SIJ has a combination of hyaline cartilage and fibrocartilage. The innervation of the joint is debated but is likely from dorsal rami of lumbar and sacral nerves. The volume of the capsule is less than 2 mL. The SIJ helps transition weight from the spine to the lower extremities. It may be a

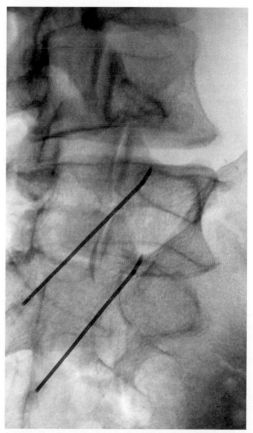

**Fig. 205.2**    An oblique fluoroscopic view of radiofrequency ablation probes denervating the right L5–S1 facet joint.

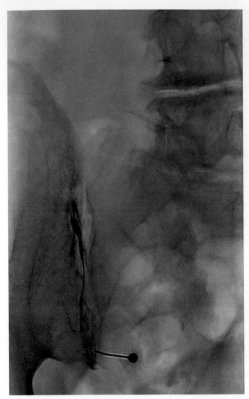

**Fig. 205.3** A left sacroiliac injection with contrast spreading within the joint line.

received saline had at least 50% pain reduction. Jee and colleagues looked at fluoroscopic-guided versus ultrasound-guided SIJ injections, with 55 patients in each group. Fluoroscopic guidance led to a more accurate intraarticular injection (98.2% accuracy vs. 87.3% in the ultrasound group). Mean pain reduction in the fluoroscopic group was 51.3% at 2 weeks and 60.3% at 12 weeks.

## Contraindications and Adverse Effects

Many factors should be considered before proceeding with spine injections, but absolute contraindications are few. Anticoagulation status needs to be thoroughly evaluated as per established guidelines (see Narouze and colleagues in Suggested Readings). Also, active infection should be treated with appropriate antibiotics and resolved before proceeding with an elective percutaneous procedure.

The risks can be divided into procedural adverse events and those related to the administered medications. RFA may cause a local inflammatory response and may also lead to denervation of multifidus muscles. Procedural risks include tissue swelling, back pain, bleeding, nerve damage, and infection. Medication risks from steroids include breakdown of joint cartilage. Fortunately, the mentioned spine injections have proven relatively safe over time.

## Conclusion

Facet joint injections, lumbar RFA, and SIJ injections may be effective in treating LBP in well-selected patients. The best results seem to be in those with significant pain relief from MBBs who proceed to RFA. These interventional spine procedures, when performed by pain medicine specialists, have been shown to be relatively safe procedures with low rates of serious adverse events. Despite the safety associated with these procedures, they should only be performed after a patient has failed conservative management, including but not limited to exercise, physical therapy, and nonopioid medications. There is ongoing debate regarding the efficacy of facet joint injections for facetogenic pain, and these injections may not be covered by insurance companies. Fluoroscopic-guided spine injections continue to be commonly used, and these procedures provide effective pain relief for many patients.

source of low back, buttock, or lower extremity pain. There are no pathognomonic signs or symptoms for SIJ pain. Exam findings that may help suggest SIJ-related pain include positive FABER, compression, Gaenslen's, seated flexion-standing, and tenderness over SIJ. SIJ injections may serve both diagnostic and therapeutic purposes (Fig. 205.3).

The evidence associated with intraarticular SIJ injections for treating LBP is debated. There are studies that have shown promising results. Maugars and colleagues performed an RCT that included 13 injections in 10 patients with sacroiliitis comparing intraarticular saline ($n = 7$) versus steroid ($n = 6$). The study revealed that all patients who received steroid had at least 50% pain reduction at 1 month, whereas only one patient who

## SUGGESTED READINGS

Anand, S., & Butt, M. S. (2007). Patients' response to facet joint injection. *Acta Orthopaedica Belgica, 73*(2), 230–233.

Dieleman, J. L., Cao, J., Chapin, A., Chen, C., Li, Z., Liu, A., et al. (2020). US health care spending by payer and health condition, 1996-2016. *JAMA, 323*(9), 863–884.

Dreyfuss, P., Halbrook, B., Pauza, K., Joshi, A., McLarty, J., & Bogduk, N. (2000). Efficacy and validity of radiofrequency neurotomy for chronic lumbar zygapophysial joint pain. *Spine, 25*(10), 1270–1277.

Forst, S. L., Wheeler, M. T., Fortin, J. D., & Vilensky, J. A. (2006). The sacroiliac joint: Anatomy, physiology and clinical significance. *Pain Physician, 9*(1), 61–67.

Kennedy, D. J., Engel, A., Kreiner, D. S., Nampiaparampil, D., Duszynski, B., & MacVicar, J. (2015). Fluoroscopically guided diagnostic and therapeutic intra-articular sacroiliac joint injections: A systematic review. *Pain Medicine (Malden, MA), 16*(8), 1500–1518.

Narouze, S., Benzon, H. T., Provenzano, D. A., Buvanendran, A., De Andres, J., Deer, T. R., Rauck, R., et al. (2015). Interventional spine and pain procedures in patients on antiplatelet and anticoagulant medications. *Regional Anesthesia and Pain Medicine, 40*, 182–212.

Soto Quijano, D. A., & Otero Loperena, E. (2018). Sacroiliac joint interventions. *Physical Medicine and Rehabilitation Clinics of North America, 29*(1), 171–183.

Staal, J. B., de Bie, R. A., de Vet, H. C., Hildebrandt, J., & Nelemans, P. (2009). Injection therapy for subacute and chronic low back pain: An updated Cochrane review. *Spine, 34*(1), 49–59.

Veizi, E., & Mchaourab, A. (2011). Medial branch blocks and facet joint injections as predictors of successful radiofrequency ablation. *RAPM, 15*, 33–38.

Won, H. S., Yang, M., & Kim, Y. D. (2020). Facet joint injections for management of low back pain: A clinically focused review. *Anesthesia and Pain Medicine, 15*(1), 8–18.

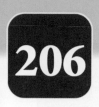

# Stellate Ganglion Block

NICHOLAS CANZANELLO, DO  |  SUSAN MOESCHLER, MD

## Indications

There are numerous indications for a stellate ganglion block, including both chronic pain syndromes and vascular disorders of the upper limb. Chronic pain conditions include chronic regional pain syndromes types I and II, herpes zoster affecting the face and neck, refractory chest pain or angina, and phantom limb pain. Vascular disorders include Raynaud phenomenon, obliterative vascular disease, vasospasm, scleroderma, trauma, embolic phenomenon, and frostbite. Other indications include postembolectomy vasospasm, postreimplantation of a traumatic amputation, undefined arteriopathy, and upper extremity tourniquet-induced hypertension. More recent indications include refractory ventricular arrhythmias, posttraumatic stress disorder, and postmenopausal "hot flashes." Further, stellate ganglion block is also used diagnostically to differentiate sympathetically maintained pain syndromes from sympathetically independent pain syndromes. Relative contraindications include systemic or local infection in the area of the injection, coagulopathy, previous anterior lower cervical surgery, or patient refusal.

## Anatomy

The cervical sympathetic chain is composed of the superior, middle, and inferior cervical ganglia. The inferior cervical ganglion fuses with the first thoracic ganglion to form the cervicothoracic ganglion, also known as the *stellate ganglion*. The stellate ganglion lies anterolateral to the seventh cervical vertebral body at the base of the seventh cervical transverse process.

The peripheral sympathetic nervous system arises from the intermediolateral column of the spinal cord. The efferent preganglionic fibers pass out of the spinal cord via the ventral roots from T1 to L2. The fibers then enter the sympathetic chain through the white rami communicantes. The preganglionic fibers may travel for a variable distance within the sympathetic chain before synapsing in ganglia or exiting the chain to synapse in peripheral ganglia.

The cervical sympathetic chain lies along the anterolateral aspect of the vertebral bodies in a fascial space bounded posteriorly by the prevertebral muscles and in the cervical region anteriorly by the carotid sheath. The nerve fibers in the cervicothoracic chain originate from preganglionic sympathetic fibers from T1 to T6 and visceral afferent fibers from the head, neck, and upper extremity (see Chapter 29, The Sympathetic Nervous System: Anatomy and Receptor Pharmacology). These fibers are distributed to the brain, meninges, eye, ear, glands, skin, and vessels of the head, neck, upper extremity, and some thoracic viscera.

The oval stellate ganglion (0.5–1.5 inches wide) resides in the prevertebral fascial space of the longus colli muscle. It lies anterior to the first rib at the anterior tubercle of C7. The transverse processes of C7 and T1 are posterior to the ganglion. Superior to the ganglion is the C6 vertebrae. The anterior tubercles of the C6 vertebrae are known as the *Chassaignac tubercles*, which are important palpable landmarks separating the carotid artery and the vertebral artery. The medial boundary is the vertebral column, and the scalene muscles form the lateral boundary. The inferior boundary is the pleural dome over the apex of the lung. It is important to note that some thoracic preganglionic sympathetic fibers may bypass the stellate ganglion.

Despite the stellate ganglion's typical location at C7, the block is more commonly performed at the C6 level as the vertebral artery enters the foramina of the transverse process at this level, protecting it from inadvertent needle puncture.

## Technique

Although historically a landmark-based technique, the use of fluoroscopy and ultrasound has been shown to minimize the risk of complications, reduce the amount of medication needed, and improve accuracy in performing this block. Therefore the fluoroscopic- and ultrasound-guided techniques will be highlighted in this chapter. The fluoroscopic-guided technique can be performed in either a straight anterior-posterior approach or a more oblique approach. The patient is positioned supine with their head in neutral position or slightly rotated to the contralateral side. A pillow is placed under the patient's shoulders to promote cervical extension. Arms are adducted at the patient's sides and secured. Because light to moderate sedation is often used to facilitate this block, standard monitors are placed including a blood pressure cuff, pulse oximetry, and electrocardiography leads. Oxygen supplementation via nasal cannula is often also provided. Before the procedure, intravenous access is also obtained. Skin temperature in the upper extremities is monitored pre- and postprocedure.

Fluoroscopy is then used to optimally visualize the C6 superior vertebral endplate and C6 uncinate processes. Next, the c-arm is rotated in an ipsilateral oblique manner to visualize the neural foramina if a lateral-to-medial, oblique approach is desired. After the application of a skin preparation agent, sterile drapes are applied. The skin and subcutaneous tissue is anesthetized with 1% lidocaine using a 25- to 30-gauge 1- to 1.5-inch needle. Using fluoroscopic-guidance and direct palpation of the carotid artery (which may be displaced laterally) to avoid needle entry into the vessel, a 25-gauge 2.5-inch needle with a slight bend at the tip is advanced in a coaxial trajectory under intermittent fluoroscopic guidance until it contacts periosteum between the uncinate process of C6 and the vertebral body. Then the needle is withdrawn approximately 1 to 2 mm so that the tip should be anterior to the longus colli muscle within the prevertebral fascia. Proper needle placement is confirmed with multiple fluoroscopic views including oblique and lateral imaging. After negative aspiration for both blood and cerebral spinal fluid, 2 to 3 mL of contrast are injected through an extension tubing attached to the needle. Dynamic "real-time" fluoroscopy is used with initial contrast injection to rule out intravascular absorption. The contrast should be observed to flow parallel to the spinal column within the prevertebral fascia (Fig. 206.1). Performance of digital subtraction angiography can be considered to further rule out intravascular absorption. When no intravascular uptake of contrast is appreciated, approximately 8 mL of local anesthetic with or without steroid is injected slowly and incrementally with serial negative aspirations and close monitoring for signs of local anesthetic systemic toxicity. This small volume is usually adequate for spread to the first thoracic segment. After the injection, the needle is flushed with an intermediate-acting local anesthetic and withdrawn from the skin. Of note, particulate steroid should be avoided because of the risk of particulate steroid embolization with cases reported to cause neurologic infarction.

More recently, stellate ganglion blocks are being performed under ultrasound guidance or ultrasound guidance in addition to fluoroscopic guidance to improve the success of the block and to decrease vascular complications further. To use ultrasound guidance, an image of the C6 Chassaignac tubercle is obtained along with the corresponding transverse process. Then the probe is moved inferior to identify the C7 transverse process. Identification of unintended targets of the block is important, including the carotid artery, internal jugular vein, esophagus, thyroid, and the longus colli muscle belly. The longus colli muscle will be encapsulated by the prevertebral fascia deep to the carotid sheath. The needle trajectory will be in an oblique, lateral-to-medial approach to the target, which is just 1 to 2 mm superficial to the longus colli muscle within the prevertebral fascia (Fig. 206.2). Postprocedure temperatures are

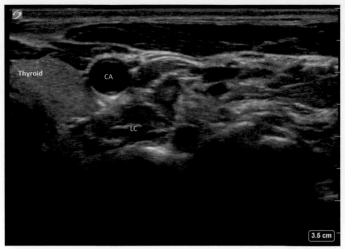

**Fig. 206.2** Ultrasound image of the anatomy for a stellate ganglion block after local anesthetic injection. *CA,* Carotid artery; *LC,* longus colli.

| TABLE 206.1 | Signs of a Successful Stellate Ganglion Block |
| --- | --- |
| Flushing of the conjunctiva and skin |
| Horner syndrome (ptosis, miosis, enophthalmos, anhidrosis) |
| Ipsilateral nasal congestion |
| Temperature increase in the ipsilateral arm and hand |

| TABLE 206.2 | Side Effects and Complications of a Stellate Ganglion Block |
| --- | --- |
| **COMMON SIDE EFFECTS AND COMPLICATIONS**<br>Hematoma<br>Sensation of "a lump in the throat"<br>Temporary hoarseness and dysphagia because of recurrent laryngeal block (a 60% prevalence rate)<br>Unpleasant effects of Horner syndrome |
| **UNCOMMON COMPLICATIONS**<br>Brachial plexus block (rare and often local anesthesia volume dependent)<br>Cardioaccelerator nerve block with hypotension or bradycardia<br>Epidural or subarachnoid block<br>Osteitis of the transverse process or vertebral body<br>Phrenic nerve block<br>Pneumothorax (1% prevalence rate)<br>Puncture of esophagus<br>Puncture of intervertebral disk |
| **POTENTIALLY SEVERE COMPLICATIONS**<br>Intradural injection causing total spinal block<br>Osteomyelitis of the vertebral body or diskitis<br>Vertebral artery injection causing loss of consciousness and seizure<br>Retropharyngeal hematoma |

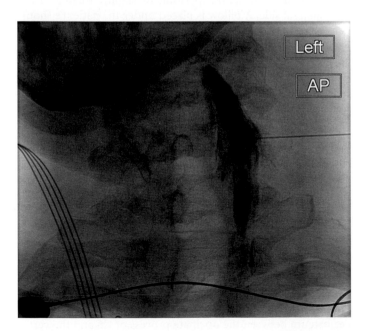

**Fig. 206.1** Oblique fluoroscopic view of needle placement and contrast spread for a stellate ganglion block.

obtained in bilateral upper extremities after the completed injection to confirm the ipsilateral rise in temperature in the blocked upper extremity. Other signs of a successful stellate ganglion block, block complications, and medication side effects are outlined in Tables 206.1 and 206.2, respectively.

## SUGGESTED READINGS

Ganesh, A., Qadri, Y. J., Boortz-Marx, R. L., Al-Khatib, S. M., Harpole, D. H., Jr., Katz, J. N., et al. (2020). Stellate ganglion blockade: An intervention for the management of ventricular arrhythmias. *Current Hypertension Reports, 22*(12), 100.

Goel, V., Patwardhan, A. M., Ibrahim, M., Howe, C. L., Schultz, D. M., & Shankar, H. (2019). Complications associated with stellate ganglion nerve block: A systematic review. *Regional Anesthesia and Pain Medicine, 44,* 669–678.

Narouze, S. (2014). Ultrasound-guided stellate ganglion block: Safety and efficacy. *Current Pain and Headache Reports, 18,* 424.

Raut, M., & Maheshwari, A. (2018). Stellate ganglion block: Important weapon in the anesthesiologists' armamentarium. *Journal of Cardiothoracic and Vascular Anesthesia, 32*(2), e36–e37.

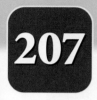

# 207

# Lumbar Sympathetic Blockade

REBECCA A. SANDERS, MD

## Relevant Anatomy

The lumbar sympathetic ganglia are known to control the sympathetic impulses to the lower extremities. These structures may represent either a single fused elongated mass or up to six separate ganglia spanning from the L1 to the L5 vertebrae. As the sympathetic trunk passes into the abdomen, it begins a migration from a position that is more anterior to the vertebral bodies to a true anterolateral position by the midlumbar levels. On the right side, the sympathetic trunk is positioned posterior to the inferior vena cava, and, on the left, it is lateral and slightly posterior to the aorta. Injection techniques that position needles from L2 through L4 have been described. When approaching the ganglion, the best starting point is the area just cephalad to the middle of the body of the L2 or L3 vertebrae. These levels have the highest probability of encountering the ganglion and variation is less, compared with an L4 approach; and moreover, the psoas muscle may terminate at the lower part of the L3 vertebra. This is important, as the psoas muscle is well positioned posterior to the sympathetic chain, thus separating it from the somatic lumbar plexus and leading to fewer complications after injection, compared with approaches to other lumbar levels of the sympathetic chain.

## Indications

The indications for lumbar sympathetic blockade fall into three main categories. First are conditions that result in circulatory insufficiency of the lower extremity including atherosclerotic disease, arterial embolism, thromboangiitis, Raynaud phenomenon, frostbite, and vascular insufficiency after reconstructive vascular operations. Many of these conditions, such as claudication, rest pain, ischemic ulcers, and gangrene, are quite painful. The institution of continuous sympathetic blockade can transiently improve regional blood flow and predict the success of future surgical sympathectomy or neurolytic therapy.

The second category involves pain from nonvascular causes and includes "phantom" or "residual-limb" pain after amputation, postherpetic neuralgia, renal colic, interstitial cystitis, and complex regional pain syndrome. For complex regional pain syndrome, blocks are often performed in succession to improve analgesia and function in conjunction with pharmacologic and physical therapy. A third miscellaneous category includes typically nonpainful conditions such as lower extremity hyperhidrosis. The block is primarily used for diagnostic and predictive purposes before neurolysis or surgical sympathectomy for this category.

## Technique

Patients are placed in the prone position with pillow support to reduce lumbar lordosis. The procedure should be performed by clinicians who are experienced in performing percutaneous procedures. The L2 or L3 vertebral level is chosen (Fig. 207.1). Using an anteroposterior (AP) fluoroscopic image, the endplates of the chosen vertebral level are aligned; an oblique view is used for needle advancement until osseous contact is made and needle is advanced just anterior to the vertebral body, as identified in the lateral image. On AP imaging, the needle is within the shadow of the ipsilateral pedicle's medial border. Contrast agent is used to confirm spread along the ganglia distribution and avoidance of intravascular or neuroaxial uptake. An 8 to 12 mL injectate containing local anesthetic is administered incrementally. Adjuvant medications such as dexamethasone or clonidine may provide additional neuromodulation benefits. Extremity temperature increases between 1°C and 8°C verify blockade.

## Adverse Side Effects

Mild back pain commonly occurs after the procedure because of soft tissue needle passage. This pain usually resolves in a

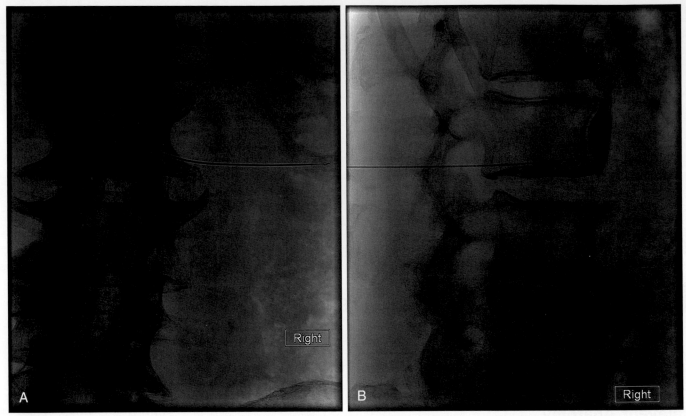

**Fig. 207.1** Needle positioning and contrast spread during right lumbar sympathetic block, performed at L2. **A,** Final needle position in the antero-posterior view, showing needle tip at the medial border of the right L2 pedicle. **B,** Contrast medium injected in the lateral view shows a linear spread along the anterior aspect of L2 vertebral body.

few days with conservative measures including use of ice, rest, acetaminophen, and/or nonsteroidal antiinflammatories. Less commonly, hypotension due to sympathetic blockade can occur; it is typically transient and responds to intravenous fluid administration. Other possible procedural complications include local anesthetic systemic toxicity, neuraxial injection (spinal/epidural), intradiscal injection, and abscess formation. Renal or urethral needle penetration can cause temporary hematuria.

Blockage of the genitofemoral nerve or lumbar plexus within the psoas muscle may occur and can result in numbness of the groin, thigh, or quadriceps after injection of local anesthetic into the psoas fascia. Prolonged weakness and genitofemoral neuralgia can result from injection of any neurolytic agent. This risk has been estimated to be 6% to 16% for neurolytic procedures. Of note, this risk is significantly decreased if the procedure is performed at higher lumbar levels (i.e., L2 vs. L4).

## SUGGESTED READINGS

Awal, S., Madabushi, R., Agarwal, A., & Singla, V. (2016). CRPS: Early lumbar sympathetic block is better compared to other interventions. *Pain Physician, 19*(2), E363.

Gunduz, O. H., & Kenis-Coskun, O. (2017). Ganglion blocks as a treatment of pain: Current perspectives. *Journal of Pain Research, 10*, 2815–2826.

Spiegel, M. A., Hingula, L., Chen, G. H., Legler, A., Puttanniah, V., & Gulati, A. (2020). The use of L2 and L3 lumbar sympathetic blockade for cancer-related pain, an experience and recommendation in the oncologic population. *Pain Medicine (Malden, MA), 21*(1), 176–184.

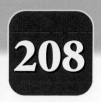

# 208

# Celiac Plexus Block

DAVID P. MARTIN, MD, PhD

## Indications

The celiac plexus provides sensory innervation and sympathetic outflow to most of the upper abdominal viscera. Neurolytic blockade of the celiac plexus is most used to control pain caused by pancreatic cancer, although it can be useful for managing pain related to malignancies of the gastrointestinal tract from the lower esophageal sphincter to the splenic flexure, as well as the liver, spleen, and kidneys. Although potentially long-lasting, neurolytic celiac plexus block is not "permanent" because the nerves in the plexus can regenerate in 3 to 6 months. The block may be repeated in such circumstances, but many patients with pancreatic cancer unfortunately do not outlive this effective duration of neurolytic celiac plexus block. Even after neurolysis, most patients with pancreatic cancer still require oral analgesics after neurolytic celiac plexus block.

Temporary diagnostic blockade of the celiac plexus can be used to differentiate visceral pain from somatic pain. Visceral pain is poorly localized and can be referred to somatic areas. For example, pancreatic pain often presents as epigastric tenderness radiating to the back. Relief of pain after celiac plexus block suggests a visceral origin of the pain. In contrast, pain persisting after celiac plexus block is more likely to be somatic in origin. In addition to its neurolytic and diagnostic uses, celiac plexus injection with a local anesthetic agent and a corticosteroid is sometimes used to treat the pain associated with chronic pancreatitis.

## Anatomy

The celiac plexus is primarily a sympathetic nervous system structure that lies anterior to the aorta near the celiac arterial trunk (Fig. 208.1). Preganglionic sympathetic fibers originate from the nerve roots of T5 to T12 and combine to form the splanchnic nerves. The splanchnic nerves cross the crura of the diaphragm before joining the vagus nerve to form the celiac plexus anterior to the aorta. The location of the plexus varies from the T12 to L2 vertebral levels; approaches to the block are directed at the T12 to L1 level.

Effective visceral pain relief can be achieved by either blocking the splanchnic nerves before they pierce the diaphragm or blocking the nerves and ganglia anterior to the diaphragmatic crura. The splanchnic nerve block (retrocrural) is also termed the *classic celiac plexus block*, as opposed to *true* blockade of the plexus and ganglia (intercrural).

## Procedure

Several approaches to the celiac plexus have been described, including endoscopic, ventral, and dorsal. The endoscopic route is convenient when combined with endoscopic retrograde

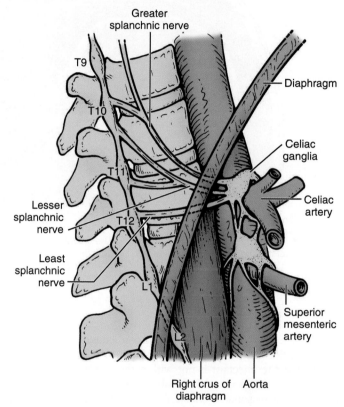

**Fig. 208.1** Anatomy. The celiac ganglion lies anterior to the aorta just superior to the celiac artery. It receives preganglionic fibers from the splanchnic nerves. Visceral analgesia can be achieved by blocking the splanchnic nerves before they pierce the diaphragm or by blocking the plexus and ganglion anterior to the diaphragmatic crura. (Modified from Stanton-Hicks MB. Lumbar sympathetic nerve block and neurolysis. In: Waldman SD, Winnie AP, eds. *Interventional Pain Management.* WB Saunders; 1996:353–359.)

cholangiopancreatography and is done with ultrasound guidance. The ventral approach can be advantageous if tumor obstructs the dorsal route, but it has a higher risk of bowel injury and infection and is therefore often done with guidance from computed tomography. The most common approach used by pain medicine physicians is a retrocrural approach via the dorsal route and is performed with the patient in the prone position with a pillow under the hips. Landmarks are identified and marked on the skin surface, indicating the 12th rib and the thoracolumbar spinous processes. Fluoroscopy is strongly recommended for the posterior approach. Needles are inserted bilaterally under fluoroscopic guidance at a site approximately 7.5 cm lateral to midline at a point 2 cm inferior to the 12th rib. The initial pass is directed to contact the L1 vertebral body at an angle approximately 45 degrees from the sagittal plane (Fig. 208.2). Ideal positioning is anterolateral to the L1 vertebral

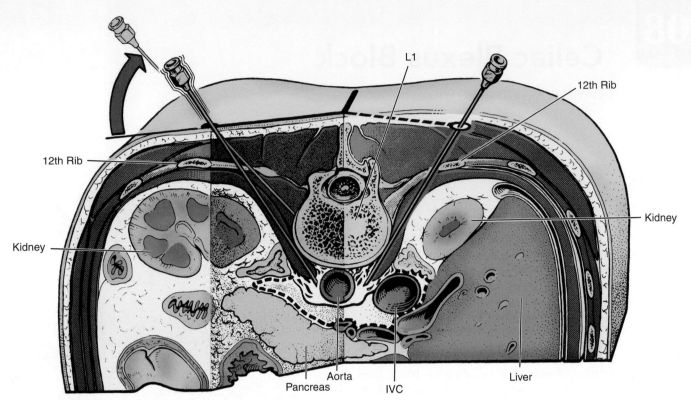

**Fig. 208.2** Performing the celiac plexus block. The needle is inserted approximately 7.5 cm lateral to the midline along a path inferior to the 12th rib. The initial needle path is at a 45-degree angle from the sagittal plane to contact the vertebral body of L1. The needle is then withdrawn and redirected to pass anterolateral to L1. *IVC,* Inferior vena cava. (Modified from Kopacz DJ, Thompson GE. Celiac and hypogastric plexus, intercostal, interpleural, and peripheral neural blockade of the thorax and abdomen. In: Cousins MJ, Bridenbaugh PO, eds. *Neural Blockade in Clinical Anesthesia and Management of Pain.* 3rd ed. Lippincott; 1998:451–485.)

body. Proper drug distribution can be confirmed with the injection of radiocontrast dye under fluoroscopy. It is important to ensure that the injectant is not within the psoas muscle, which could result in blockade of the lumbar plexus. Bupivacaine, 0.25% to 0.5%, is a reasonable choice for the diagnostic nerve block. Typically, 10 to 15 mL is injected on each side. For diagnostic blocks, the procedure ends at this point. At least 15 to 20 minutes must elapse until the effects of blockade can be assessed. In addition to pain relief, motor function should also be tested.

When a neurolytic block is planned, the needles can be left in place during the sensory and motor assessment. If pain is relieved and no motor deficits are observed after injecting local anesthesia, it is reasonable to proceed with neurolysis. For neurolytic procedures, 50% to 100% alcohol is the most used agent. Typically, 10 mL is injected on each side. A small volume of local anesthetic agent can be injected while withdrawing the needles to prevent alcohol from tracking to more superficial tissue.

## Expected Side Effects

The procedure itself can cause local soreness and bruising. These symptoms are usually transient and can be treated conservatively with ice. Psoas muscle spasm is not uncommon after neurolytic celiac plexus block and can be minimized by preventing the escape of neurolytic agent through the needle tract. Psoas muscle spasm often responds well to intravenously or intramuscularly injected nonsteroidal antiinflammatories (e.g., ketorolac).

Interruption of sympathetic innervation to the viscera can blunt normal postural hemodynamic reflexes, resulting in orthostatic hypotension. Patients should be cautioned that they may feel lightheaded upon standing. The sympathectomy can also cause increased gastrointestinal motility and possibly diarrhea for 1 to 2 days. However, the effect of sympatholysis on intestinal motility can be beneficial in counteracting the constipation often caused by concomitant orally administered opioid therapy. Finally, celiac plexus block may mask early presenting symptoms of other intraabdominal diseases, such as cholecystitis and gastric ulceration.

## Adverse Effects

As with any injection, sterile technique should be observed during the performance of celiac plexus block to minimize the risk of infection. Because of the proximity of the celiac plexus to the aorta, vascular injury is possible; hematoma formation, aortic dissection, and distal (lower extremity) ischemia have been reported. Intravascular injection of a local anesthetic agent can cause mental status changes, seizures, and possible hemodynamic collapse.

Unintentional intrathecal or epidural spread may also cause spinal nerve block. The spread of neurolytic agent to unintended nerve or vascular structures introduces the risk of permanent neurologic injury, including paralysis. Therefore careful neurologic evaluation after injection of a local anesthetic is essential before injecting the neurolytic agent. The most common nerve injury after celiac plexus block is genitofemoral neuralgia (pain along the cutaneous regions in the groin and inner thigh). Despite these risks, celiac plexus block is relatively safe when performed by experienced physicians.

In randomized clinical trials, where control groups receive attentive and consistent oral analgesia, celiac plexus block has not been shown to decrease pain or improve quality of life. It is not clear if nerve block offers clinical benefit in circumstances where patients do not receive equivalent ongoing assessment and analgesic optimization. However, of greater concern is more recent evidence suggesting that sympathetic neurolysis may decrease survival in patients with more advanced stages of pancreatic cancer.

## SUGGESTED READINGS

Burton, A. W., Phan, P. C., & Cousins, M. J. (2009). Treatment of cancer pain: Role of neural blockade and neuromodulation. In M. J. Cousins, D. B. Carr, & T. T. Horlocker, & P. O. Bridenbaugh (Eds.), *Neural blockade in clinical anesthesia and pain medicine* (4th ed., pp. 1124–1133). Philadelphia: Lippincott.

Dong, D., Zhao, M., Zhang, J., Huang, M., Wang, Y., Qi, L., et al. (2021). Neurolytic splanchnic nerve block and pain relief, survival, and quality of life in unresectable pancreatic cancer: A randomized controlled trial. *Anesthesiology, 135*(4), 686–698.

Lamer, T. J. (1996). Sympathetic nerve blocks. In D. L. Brown (Ed.). *Regional anesthesia and analgesia* (pp. 357–384). Philadelphia: WB Saunders.

Stanton-Hicks, M. B. (1996). Lumbar sympathetic nerve block and neurolysis. In S. D. Waldman & A. P. Winnie (Eds.), *Interventional pain management* (pp. 353–359). Philadelphia: WB Saunders.

Wong, G. Y., Schroeder, D. R., Carns, P. E., Wilson, J. L., Martin, D. P., Kinney, M. O., et al. (2004). Effect of neurolytic celiac plexus block on pain relief, quality of life, and survival in patients with unresectable pancreatic cancer: A randomized controlled trial. *JAMA, 291*(9), 1092–1099.

# 209

# Neuromodulation Techniques in Pain Medicine

CHRISTOPHER WIE, MD | STEPHEN COVINGTON, DO

## History

Spinal cord stimulation (SCS), also known as *dorsal column stimulation*, was first used in 1967 and approved by the U.S. Food and Drug Administration for the management of chronic pain in 1989; since then, SCS has become an important interventional adjuvant. In the United States common indications for SCS include failed back surgery syndrome (postlaminectomy pain syndrome), complex regional pain syndrome (CRPS), and lumbar radiculopathy. Peripheral nervous system (PNS) stimulation was first tested by Sweet and Wepsic in 1968. The advancement of smaller lead sizes and real-time ultrasound techniques have led to precise treatment of peripheral nerve injuries. These tools are now used on a regular basis by pain physicians to help patients who have failed more conservative therapies.

## Mechanism of Action

Several theories have been postulated regarding the potential mechanism of action behind neuromodulation. In 1965, Melzack and Wall introduced the "gate control" theory. This theory proposes that pulsed energy from neurostimulator electrodes activates large myelinated Aβ fibers that inhibit or "close the gate" to painful peripheral stimuli carried by Aδ and C fibers. In SCS, the electrodes or "leads" are placed in the epidural space so the points of stimulation surround the dermatomes from which the noxious stimuli arise. Ideally, an electrical field is created that stimulates the appropriate spinal cord structures without affecting the nearby nerve roots. In PNS, before lead placement, a diagnostic anesthetic nerve block is performed to ensure the correct nerve is targeted. Leads are placed under real-time ultrasound near the affected nerve. Another potential mechanism of SCS pain relief is the release of neuromodulators (γ-aminobutyric acid, 5-hydroxytryptamine, glycine, and adenosine) in proximity to the dorsal horn of the spinal cord that inhibits afferent spinal cord impulses. Neuropathic pain relief is mediated in part by wide dynamic range neuron suppression in the dorsal horn as well. SCS has also been demonstrated to activate supraspinal nuclei, with an increase in activity of inhibitory descending pathways in the spinal cord.

## Patient Selection

Proper patient selection is a key aspect for success of neuromodulation. As previously stated, the most common indication for neuromodulation is SCS for failed back surgery syndrome and lumbar radiculopathy. Patients must have failed more conservative therapies including over-the-counter pain medications, nonopioid pain medications, and physical therapy, as well as more noninvasive interventional treatments. Patients who are have chronic pain may have comorbid psychosocial factors contributing to their overall pain state. Pain catastrophizing, a tendency to magnify the threat value of a pain stimulus and to feel helpless in the presence of pain, has variable effects on how individuals experience pain. Properly identifying and addressing high levels of pain catastrophizing and/or uncontrolled depression through validated questionnaires before SCS may improve overall outcomes. Because of the high potential for concomitant psychiatric illness in patients with chronic pain, a psychiatric evaluation should be obtained before spinal cord stimulator trial and permanent implantation. In addition, pretrial thoracic magnetic resonance imaging (MRI) is usually warranted to rule out stenosis in the lower thoracic spine where leads are typically placed. The collection of objective measurements (pain improvement percentage, increase in steps walked per day, improved sleep, duration of activity) is highly recommended during the SCS trial as it will decrease the false-positive rates and may reduce the percentage of patients who do not receive adequate relief after permanent implantation.

## Contraindications

Contraindications to SCS are similar to other neuraxial procedures and include active infection, coagulopathies, and continued anticoagulant/antiplatelet therapy. SCS trial and permanent implantation is classified as a high-risk procedure for bleeding complications. Therefore recent international guidelines created by national pain and neuromodulation societies have been published with recommendations that should be followed for any patient on antiplatelet and anticoagulant medications pursuing a neuraxial procedure. Other contraindications include previous spinal surgery at site of needle entry into the epidural space, ongoing litigation, and untreated psychological problems. Although the majority of SCS devices are MRI conditional (pose no known hazards), it is important to discuss the need for future MRI studies with prospective patients, especially in those participating in regular cancer surveillance.

## Types of Spinal Cord Stimulation

Neurostimulation of the spinal cord can be categorized into two main therapies: traditional (low-frequency SCS) and high-frequency SCS (paresthesia free). In traditional SCS, the leads are placed into the epidural space and paresthesia mapping is performed to cover the painful areas. For high-frequency SCS therapy, the trial leads are placed anatomically with coverage of the T9 to T10 intervertebral disc (for low back and lower extremity pain), which is the most common indication for high-frequency therapy. High-frequency neurostimulation is paresthesia-free by using a stimulation frequency of 10 kHz. Neuromodulation companies are constantly searching for novel waveforms, frequencies, and stimulation modes to improve the pain relief in patients. One such new advancement includes the "burst waveform," which can be described as a group of high-frequency, pulsed stimulations separated by pulse-free periods. Research by Sherman and colleagues suggests that this may mimic a pattern similar to our physiologic neuronal firing pattern, leading to improved pain control.

## Types of Peripheral Nerve Stimulation

PNS neuromodulation waveforms mirror SCS therapies as there are both low- and high-frequency options. Burst waveforms have been trialed in few PNS case studies targeting chronic migraine, cluster headaches, and trigeminal neuralgia, though further studies are warranted. A dichotomy exists between temporary externalized and fully implantable devices in the PNS field. Temporary externalized devices such as the SPRINT (SPR Therapeutics) device uses a percutaneous lead placement that is removed after a 60-day trial (Fig. 209.1). Pain relief occurs during stimulation and relief has been shown to be sustained at 12 months in multiple studies. Fully implantable systems include the StimRouter (Bioness Inc.), StimQ (Stimwave Inc.), and Nalu micro-IPG (Nalu Medical). Fully implantable systems may be considered in patients who do not have continued relief once a temporary externalized device is removed.

A recent novel target in the PNS is the dorsal root ganglion (DRG). The DRG is a group of cell bodies that have immediately branched from the spinal cord that are responsible for transmission of sensory input (including nociception) from the PNS to the CNS. When targeting the DRG for stimulation, leads are driven into the epidural space and then directed laterally out the neural foramen to rest adjacent to the DRG. Stimulation of the DRG has dramatically improved treatment of conditions such as CRPS and focal peripheral nerve injuries. Ultimately, the decision to use a temporary externalized, fully implantable device or DRG stimulation relies on the patient's preference for recharging burden, wearing an external pulse transmitter (EPT), and acceptance of a permanently implanted device.

## Procedural Process

The process of SCS involves two phases. The first phase, or trial phase, involves placement of percutaneous leads into the

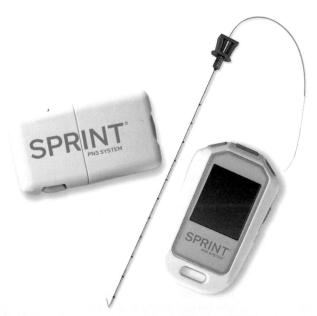

**Fig. 209.1**  Sprint product with lead. (Courtesy SPR Therapeutics.)

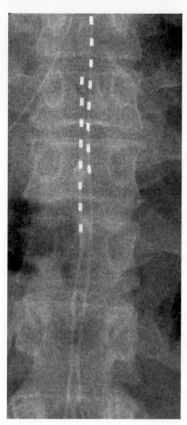

**Fig. 209.2** Fluoroscopic view of cylindrical leads in the epidural space.

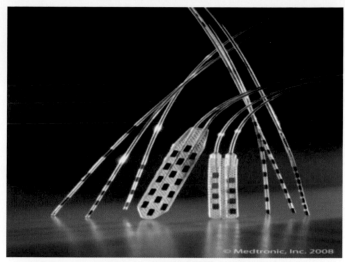

**Fig. 209.3** Variety of leads: cylindrical and paddle. (Courtesy Medtronic, Inc., Minneapolis, MN.)

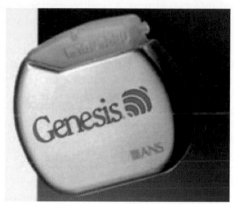

**Fig. 209.4** Implantable pulse generator. (Courtesy Advanced Neuromodulation Systems, Inc./St. Jude Medical, St. Paul, MN.)

epidural space under fluoroscopic guidance. Typically, the T12 to L1 interlaminar space is entered for low back and leg pain, whereas the C7 to T1 epidural space is typically entered for neck and upper extremity pain. Trial stimulation is performed to elicit paresthesia over the painful area for traditional low-frequency neurostimulation. Trial leads are placed anatomically to cover the T9 to T10 intervertebral disc space (Fig. 209.2) for high-frequency neurostimulation. The patient then "test drives" the device for 3 to 10 days by attempting to complete tasks and daily activities that normally cause them pain or discomfort. The trial is considered successful if the patient experiences pain relief of more than 50% improvement in function.

If the first phase is successful, the second phase entails placement of a permanent lead (cylindrical or paddle; Fig. 209.3) in the same location. Cylindrical leads are placed transfascially via 14-gauge epidural needle after the thoracodorsal fascia is exposed. If a paddle lead is required, a midline laminotomy is performed in conjunction with a neurosurgical specialist. The lead is then connected to an implantable pulse generator (IPG) (Fig. 209.4). Criteria for implantation require that (1) the patient failed conservative therapy (e.g., injections, medications, physical therapy); (2) the patient be devoid of major psychiatric conditions; and (3) the patient has completed a successful trial phase.

PNS stimulation typically requires the use of ultrasound for placement of the leads near the targeted peripheral nerve. Common nerves include the greater and lesser occipital nerves for chronic headaches; supraorbital and infraorbital nerves in chronic facial pain; ulnar, median, and radial nerves for posttraumatic-related pain; suprascapular nerve for poststroke shoulder pain; ilioinguinal and genitofemoral nerves for abdominopelvic pain; and the sciatic and common peroneal for lower extremity pain. Some PNS systems can be used to target the medial branches of the lumbar spine for relief from chronic back pain. In this case fluoroscopic guidance is used to place the introducer near the intended targets.

## Outcome Studies

Several studies have reported favorable responses to SCS in patients with either postlaminectomy pain syndrome or CRPS. Kumar and colleagues undertook a prospective multicenter study that included 100 patients with postlaminectomy pain syndrome. Patients were randomly assigned to receive either conventional medical management alone or conventional medical management in combination with SCS. Conventional medical management included any therapy advised by the physician except reoperation, implantation of an intrathecal drug-delivery system, or SCS. At 6 months, the SCS group had a statistically significant reduction in pain, compared with the conventional medical management group (48% vs. 9%, respectively). The SCS group also had improved functionality and improved patient satisfaction. These results were consistent up to the 24-month follow-up visit.

Several studies have analyzed the medical costs of SCS therapy in the setting of postlaminectomy pain syndrome. The consensus remains that, by reducing the demand for medical care, SCS therapy (if effective) pays for itself within 2.1 years.

In 2015, Kapural and colleagues published the SENZA Randomized Controlled Trial with a total of 198 test subjects with both back and leg pain. These patients were randomized equally into traditional SCS therapy versus high-frequency SCS therapy. In total, 171 patients had a successful SCS trial and were implanted with an SCS system. A positive response was defined as having greater than 50% pain relief. At 3 months, 84.5% of implanted high-frequency therapy subjects were responders for back pain and 83.1% for leg pain versus 43.8% and 55.5% for traditional stimulation, respectively.

In 2017, Deer and colleagues aimed to assess the safety and efficacy of DRG stimulation to traditional stimulation. A total of 152 patients with complex regional pain syndrome were randomized into two groups. A positive response was defined as greater than 50% pain relief at end of trial phase and at 3 months postimplant and lack of neurologic deficit. DRG stimulation demonstrated better treatment success (81.2%) than with traditional stimulation (55.7%) and also targeted the paresthesia to the area of pain better than traditional stimulation.

More recent data has revealed successful treatment of postamputation neuropathic pain with PNS stimulation. In 2019, Gilmore and colleagues collected data from 28 patients with lower extremity postamputation pain where half underwent temporary externalized PNS stimulation for 60 days. A significantly greater portion of patients receiving PNS (58%) demonstrated greater than 50% reduction in average postamputation pain than compared with placebo subjects. In addition, 67% of PNS stimulation patients reported greater than 50% reduction in pain interference after 8 weeks of therapy compared with placebo.

A 2021 study (Petersen et al.) suggested that high-frequency SCS in patients with diabetic peripheral neuropathy had an 85% responder rate (pain reduction >50%) at 6 months with improved health-related quality of life.

## Complications

Complications from the use of SCS can occur. Fortunately, severe complications are extremely rare. Complications can include lead migration (15.5%), lead fracture (6.4%), and infection (4.9%). Complications that occur less frequently include pain over implant site, battery failure, unwanted stimulation, and cerebrospinal fluid leak.

## Future Directions

The role of neurostimulation has expanded, and SCS is now being used for various peripheral neuropathies, peripheral vascular diseases, and angina. The introduction of high-frequency neurostimulation has improved the treatment of back pain associated with patients with failed back surgery syndrome. This therapy is now being offered for the treatment of neck and upper extremity pain as well. The "neurorestorative" approach to chronic back pain shows promise, as researchers are now using PNS for chronic low back pain after failing radiofrequency ablation. By targeting the medial branch nerves with peripheral stimulation, Deer and colleagues have reported clinically significant reductions in average pain ($\geq$50%) in 67% of participants after 2 months with 87% improvement in functional outcomes as measured by disability and 80% improvement in pain interference. It is theorized that PNS of the medial branches has a neuromodulatory effect via the gate-control pain theory and normalizes the membrane excitability of neurons in nociceptive pathways, resulting in decreased pain signaling. New technologies such as the ReActiv8 system (Mainstay Medical Limited) has a similar neurorestorative approach by permanent implantation of leads to stimulate the lumbar multifidus to target chronic low back pain. Peripheral vascular disease and angina in patients who are not candidates for surgery are common indications for neurostimulation in Europe, based on the theories that SCS decreases sympathetic outflow, increases regional blood flow, and decreases myocardial oxygen consumption. With advances in technology, there will likely be smaller yet longer-lasting SCS batteries that are all MRI compatible. The technologies and techniques to implement these new therapies continue to grow to help chronic pain patients.

## SUGGESTED READINGS

Cameron, T. (2004). Safety and efficacy of spinal cord stimulation for the treatment of chronic pain: A 20-year literature review. *Journal of Neurosurgery, 100*(3 Suppl Spine), 254–267.

Deer, T. R., Levy, R. M., Kramer, J., Poree, L., Amirdelfan, K., Grigsby, E., et al. (2017). Dorsal root ganglion stimulation yielded higher treatment success rate for complex regional pain syndrome and causalgia at 3 and 12 months: A randomized comparative trial. *Pain, 158*(4), 669–681.

Deer, T. R., Naidu, R., Strand, N., Sparks, D., Abd-Elsayed, A., Kalia, H., et al. (2020). A review of the bioelectronic implications of stimulation of the peripheral nervous system for chronic pain conditions. *Bioelectronic Medicine, 6*, 9.

Kapural, L., Yu, C., Doust, M. W., Gliner, B. E., Vallejo, R., Sitzman, B. T., et al. (2015). Novel 10-kHz high-frequency therapy (HF10 Therapy) is superior to traditional low-frequency spinal cord stimulation for the treatment of chronic back and leg pain: The SENZA-RCT randomized controlled trial. *Anesthesiology, 123*(4), 851–860.

North, R. B., Kidd, D. H., Farrokhi, F., & Piantadosi, S. A. (2005). Spinal cord stimulation versus repeated lumbosacral spine surgery for chronic pain: A randomized, controlled trial. *Neurosurgery, 56*(1), 98–107.

Petersen, E. A., Stauss, T. G., Scowcroft, J. A., Brooks, E. S., White, J. L., Sills, S. M., et al. (2021). Effect of high-frequency (10-kHz) spinal cord stimulation in patients with painful diabetic neuropathy: A randomized clinical trial. *JAMA Neurology, 78*(6), 687–698.

# Critical Care Medicine

# 210

# Hyperbaric Oxygen Therapy

KLAUS D. TORP, MD | ANNA BOVILL SHAPIRO, MD

Hyperbaric oxygen therapy (HBOT) refers to the inhalation of 100% oxygen ($O_2$) in an environment in which the barometric pressure is greater than 1 atmosphere. Note that 1 atmosphere absolute (ATA) is the atmospheric pressure at sea level. For every increase in ambient pressure of 760 mm Hg, or 14.7 psi or 33 feet of seawater (fsw), the pressure increases by 1 ATA. Exposure to increased gas pressures can occur in other situations, such as breathing compressed gas mixtures while diving (scuba) or working in underground tunnels (caisson workers). For HBOT, the pressure in a hyperbaric chamber is typically at least 1.4 ATA.

All gases follow fundamental gas laws:

*Boyle's law:* At a constant temperature, the volume of gas is inversely proportional to the pressure:

$$PV = k$$

where $P$ is absolute pressure, $V$ is volume, and $k$ is a constant, representative of the pressure and volume of the system.

*Dalton's law:* The total pressure of a mixture of gases is equal to the sum of the partial pressures of the component gases.

*Henry's law:* At constant temperature, the amount of gas dissolved in a liquid is directly proportional to the partial pressure of that gas in equilibrium with the liquid.

In clinical medicine, the liquid of interest is blood, and the dissolved gas is $O_2$. The driving pressure of $O_2$ into blood is the partial pressure of $O_2$ in alveoli ($Pao_2$). Note that it is the partial pressure of $O_2$ and not the percentage of $O_2$ that is responsible for its effects (Table 210.1). As the $Pao_2$ increases in arterial blood, the saturation of hemoglobin approaches 100% (at $Pao_2$ ~100 mm Hg). Above that $Pao_2$ level, all additional $O_2$-carrying capacity of blood comes from the oxygen dissolved in the plasma. HBOT can therefore increase $O_2$ content in the face of

severe anemia and also increase $O_2$ delivery in areas of partial obstruction to blood flow. The increased barometric pressure can reduce intravascular air bubbles in patients with decompression sickness or air embolism, improving perfusion and increasing the removal of nitrogen from the blood (Fig. 210.1), in addition to providing an increased gas gradient to help the elimination of nitrogen by breathing 100% $O_2$ under pressure.

The effectiveness of HBOT has been established for several indications, and the basic mechanisms for its effect on the body have been demonstrated. It can be the sole lifesaving therapy in gas embolism, decompression sickness, and severe carbon monoxide poisoning, as well as decrease morbidity and mortality in severe necrotizing infections. With the alarming trend of hyperbaric facilities no longer treating emergencies or critically ill patients, one should be aware of where and how to transfer patients in need of lifesaving HBOT. Table 210.2 lists all the current conditions that are recommended for HBOT by the Undersea and Hyperbaric Medical Society, as well as those that are reimbursed by the Centers for Medicare and Medicaid Services as of December 2017. Before considering any other indications, one should first examine how the basic mechanisms of HBOT (Box 210.1) will affect the underlying pathophysiology of the disease.

## Effects of Hyperbaric Oxygen

### PULMONARY EFFECTS

A high inspired oxygen partial pressure ($Po_2$) is thought to overcome the body's scavenging system for free radicals, resulting in the formation of reactive $O_2$ species, such as superoxides, hydrogen peroxide, and hydroxyl radicals. Although this is beneficial to help certain antibiotics to fight infections, reactive $O_2$

| TABLE 210.1 | Expected Gas Tensions and Arterial Blood Oxygen Content at Various Ambient Pressures in a Normal Individual* | | | | | | |
|---|---|---|---|---|---|---|---|
| Atm | $Fio_2$ | Inspired $Po_2$ (mm Hg) | $PAo_2$ (mm Hg) | $Pao_2$ (mm Hg) | $Cao_2$ | | $Paco_2$ (mm Hg) |
| | | | | | Total | Dissolved | |
| 1 | 0.21 | 150 | 102 | 87 | 18.7 | 0.3 | 40 |
| 1 | 1.0 | 713 | 673 | 572 | 21.2 | 1.7 | 40 |
| 2 | 1.0 | 1473 | 1433 | 1218 | 23.1 | 3.7 | 40 |
| 3 | 1.0 | 2233 | 2193 | 1864 | 25.1 | 5.6 | 40 |
| 6 | 0.21 | 898 | 848 | >750 | 21.8 | 2.3 | 40 |

*Hemoglobin = 14 g/dL.
*Atm,* Atmosphere; *Cao₂,* arterial oxygen content; *Fio₂,* fraction of inspired oxygen; *Paco₂,* partial pressure of carbon dioxide; *MI/DI, ; PAo₂,* partial pressure of oxygen in alveoli; *Pao₂,* arterial partial pressure of oxygen; *Po₂,* inspired oxygen partial pressure.

Modified, with permission, from Moon RE, Camporesi EM. Clinical care in altered environments: at high and low pressure and in space. In: Miller RD, ed.. *Anesthesia.* 8th ed. Churchill Livingstone; 2005:2665–2701.

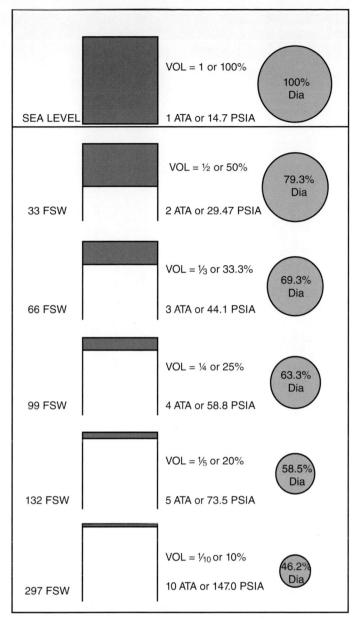

**Fig. 210.1** Gas volume (*Vol*) and bubble size as a function of depth: Boyle's law. *ATA*, Atmosphere(s) absolute pressure; *Dia*, diameter; *FSW*, feet of sea water; *PSIA*, pounds per square inch absolute.

species can cause pulmonary $O_2$ toxicity symptoms, such as retrosternal burning, coughing, and fibrosis, and can lead to a measurable decrease in vital capacity. The pulmonary toxicity is dependent on duration and $Po_2$, and its effect is cumulative. Most HBOT protocols reduce toxicity by introducing air breaks between $O_2$ treatment periods. Pulmonary oxygen toxicity is usually reversible after cessation of treatment.

### CENTRAL NERVOUS SYSTEM EFFECTS

HBOT decreases cerebral blood flow, thereby decreasing intracranial pressure and central nervous system (CNS) edema formation by up to 20%. CNS toxicity manifests when breathing 100% $O_2$ at approximately 3 ATA at rest (or less at exercise). Common signs and symptoms of toxicity include nausea, facial numbness, facial twitching, and unpleasant taste or smell.

Unrecognized CNS toxicity can progress to full tonic/clonic seizures, which will abate on reducing the $Po_2$. Pharmacologic pretreatment can be helpful in patients prone to seizures or who have demonstrated prior HBOT seizures; however, after the HBOT treatment series, no further pharmacologic treatment for HBOT-induced seizures is necessary.

### OPHTHALMOLOGIC EFFECTS

Prolonged HBOT (usually 30–60 treatments) may lead to refraction changes of the lens. This effect is usually reversible, and new vision prescriptions should wait for some time (>6 weeks) after the cessation of HBOT.

### CARDIOVASCULAR EFFECTS

A $Pao_2$ above 1500 mm Hg can increase systemic vascular resistance and peripheral blood pressure, with a resultant reflex bradycardia and a decrease in cardiac output. Flow to the periphery is reduced, leading to a decrease in edema; however, total $O_2$ delivery to tissues is markedly increased. Diffusion of $O_2$ away from the vascular bed into the tissues is greatly enhanced, which is the basis for most of the indications for HBOT. Pulmonary vascular resistance is decreased under hyperbaric conditions.

### EFFECTS ON AIR-CONTAINING CAVITIES

Nasal sinuses, the middle ear, and noncommunicating pulmonary bullae may be affected by the pressure changes in a HBOT chamber. Middle ear barotrauma is the most common problem but highly variable, occurring in 2% to 45% of patients. Nonsurgical therapies such as decongestants and slowing the rate of pressure increase are usually effective, but myringotomy tubes may be needed in those patients who cannot clear their ears. Pulmonary barotrauma is a rare complication that may in some cases require needle or chest tube decompression.

### EFFECTS ON BLOOD SUGAR

In patients with diabetes, HBOT may lead to a drop in blood sugar, which should be monitored before and after each hyperbaric treatment.

## Anesthetic Management in a Hyperbaric Oxygen Therapy Chamber

Providing general anesthesia in a hyperbaric chamber is rare. Potential indications include double-lung lavage and emergent surgical procedures in patients who cannot be brought out of the chamber in a timely manner. The anesthesia provider may, however, be called for airway management or to sedate and provide support for critically ill patients. In monoplace chambers, only the patient is exposed to higher atmospheric pressures in a 100% oxygen environment. All critical care support has to be provided from the outside through electrical, fluid, and ventilator connections across the chamber hull (usually the door). In multiplace chambers, the inside providers are also exposed to changes in ambient pressures but in an air environment. Only the patient is breathing oxygen during most of the treatment time (with the inside provider breathing oxygen during the latter part of the treatment to decrease their risk of

| TABLE 210.2 | Recommended and Reimbursed Indications for Hyperbaric Oxygen Therapy | | |
|---|---|:---:|:---:|
| **Indication** | | **UHMS** | **CMS** |
| Air or gas embolism (1) | | X | X |
| Carbon monoxide poisoning patient meeting certain criteria (1) | | X | X |
| Carbon monoxide poisoning complicated by cyanide poisoning meeting certain criteria (1) | | X | X |
| Clostridial myositis and myonecrosis (gas gangrene) (2) | | X | X |
| Crush injury, compartment syndrome, and other acute traumatic ischemias (2) | | X | X |
| Decompression sickness (1) | | X | X |
| Enhancement of healing in selected problem wounds (2) | | X | |
| Exceptional blood loss (anemia) (2) | | X | |
| Intracranial abscess (2) | | X | |
| Necrotizing soft tissue infections (2) | | X | X |
| Osteomyelitis (refractory) (2) | | X | X |
| Delayed radiation injury (soft tissue and bony necrosis) (2) | | X | X |
| Skin grafts and flaps (compromised) (2) | | X | X |
| Thermal burns (2) | | X | |
| Acute peripheral arterial insufficiency (2) | | X | X |
| Refractory actinomycosis (2) | | | X |
| Diabetic wounds of the lower extremities in patients who meet certain criteria (2) | | | X |
| Idiopathic Sudden Sensorineural Hearing Loss (2) | | X | |
| Central Retinal Artery Occlusion (2) | | X | |

*CMS,* Centers for Medicare and Medicaid Services 20.29 V4, 12/18/2017; *UHMS,* Undersea and Hyperbaric Medical Society 2019; *(1)* primary treatment; *(2)* adjuvant treatment.

---

**BOX 210.1   BASIC MECHANISMS OF HYPERBARIC OXYGEN THERAPY**

Hyperoxygenation
Vasoconstriction
Neovascularization
Increasing pressure and gas gradients (to decrease bubble size and increase off-gassing of bubble content)
Altering cellular functions, such as inhibiting $\beta_2$-integrin molecules on white blood cells or increasing killing power of neutrophils by increasing oxygen radicals

---

decompression sickness). All personnel must be pressure tested and properly trained before entering an HBOT chamber. The induction of anesthesia by inhalation agents depends only the partial pressure of those agents in the brain, not on the concentration that is inhaled. If 1.1 minimum alveolar concentration (MAC) of isoflurane (about 8 mm Hg) produces anesthesia at sea level (1 ATA), then the same effect will be produced by 0.33 MAC of isoflurane at 3 ATA because partial pressure of the drug in the alveoli and brain will still be 8 mm Hg.

However, ambient pressure changes have little effect on the dial settings of variable bypass vaporizers, as the vapor pressure is a physical property of the volatile agent, which then gets diluted by the gas bypassing the vapor chamber, resulting in a similar partial pressure effect on the brain independent of different (clinically) applied ambient pressures.

A vaporizer with a heating element should never be taken into an HBOT chamber because of fire risk. Nitrous oxide has been used successfully in a hyperbaric chamber before but should be avoided because of its increased solubility and the complex changes in pressure and breathing gases in a hyperbaric chamber. Total intravenous anesthesia (TIVA) is preferred over the use of inhalation anesthetic agents in an HBOT chamber because TIVA requires less equipment and eliminates pollution of the HBOT chamber with anesthetic gases. Regional anesthesia is also a very good choice, but the local anesthetic agent should be devoid of any air bubbles when injected.

Increased gas density caused by the increase in atmospheric pressure decreases flow through rotameter flowmeters, leading to falsely high readings under hyperbaric conditions. Gas cylinders should function normally but are usually not found inside an HBOT chamber.

Anesthesia equipment needs to be rated for use in an HBOT chamber because it may not function normally. Cuffs on tracheal tubes and intravenous and bladder catheters should be filled with fluid or carefully monitored during pressure changes. Air-filled cuffs will undergo large volume changes with changes in pressure, as will drip chambers on intravenous lines, which require frequent observation during pressure changes to rapidly identify air and avoid an intravenous air embolus. Mechanical ventilators should be rated for use in an HBOT chamber or, at the least, tested for accuracy and safety under pressure. Petroleum-based lubricants and alcohol must be avoided because they are a fire hazard in an $O_2$-enriched environment.

## HYPERBARIC OXYGEN IN THE TREATMENT OF COVID-19

In the absence of effective pharmacologic intervention for the treatment of hypoxemic respiratory failure secondary to SARS-CoV-2 infection early in the pandemic, HBOT has been used successfully to increase the $PO_2$ and therefore help improve the $PaO_2/FiO_2$ ratio and decrease the need for intubation. Although patients uniformly felt better in the high $Po_2$ environment, particular attention must be paid and a plan established upon reaching ambient pressure resulting in a reduction in $Po_2$ to avoid the effects of sudden hypoxia. Given that HBOT is not readily accessible to all populations, it is unlikely to reach widespread use for hypoxia related to COVID-19 or any future hypoxic respiratory infections in the near future.

## SUGGESTED READINGS

Edmonds, C., Bennett, M., Lippman, J., & Mitchell, S. (Eds). (2020). *Diving and subaquatic medicine.* Boca Raton, FL: CRC Press.

Moon, R. E. (2019). *Hyperbaric oxygen therapy indications* (14th ed.). North Palm Beach, FL: Best Publishing Co.

Moon, R. E., Cherry, A. D., & Camporesi, E. M. (2020). Clinical care in extreme environments: High pressure, immersion, drowning, hypo- and hyperthermia. In M. A. Gropper (Ed.), *Miller's anesthesia* (9th ed., pp. 2337–2366). Philadelphia: Elsevier.

Shinomiya, N., & Asai, Y. (2020). *Hyperbaric oxygen therapy: Molecular mechanisms and clinical applications.* New York: Springer.

# 211

# Perioperative Management of Blood Glucose

BETH L. LADLIE, MD, MPH  |  ALEXANDRA L. ANDERSON, MD  |  MICAH T. LONG, MD

## Introduction

Hyperglycemia is common in hospitalized patients with and without diabetes, especially in the perioperative period. Perioperative physiologic stressors lead to systemic inflammation and a surge in counterregulatory hormones including cortisol, glucagon, catecholamines, and growth hormone. These mediators inhibit insulin release and glucose uptake, creating a state of relative insulin resistance. Critical illness, anesthesia, some medications, altered nutritional intake, and the metabolic stress of surgery result in metabolic dysregulation with glucose mobilization, altered glucose production, and reduced glucose uptake. The net result is hyperglycemia. A growing body of evidence supports the association between dysglycemia (including hyperglycemia, hypoglycemia, and glycemic variability) and adverse outcomes such as surgical site infections, impaired wound healing, and increased length of hospitalization.

Perioperative hyperglycemia is frequent and occurs in approximately 30% of general surgery patients and nearly 80% of those undergoing cardiac surgery. Although absolute hyperglycemia is most frequent in those with diabetes, stress-induced hyperglycemia (SIH) or acute-on-chronic hyperglycemia may be most associated with negative outcomes. Uniquely, of patients with SIH and no prior diagnosis of diabetes, more than half will develop diabetes within a year. Thus managing dysglycemia in the perioperative setting is important to optimize patient outcomes, as well as an opportunity to affect long-term health.

Unfortunately, there is no one set of definitive guidelines for anesthesia clinicians in terms of optimal blood glucose concentrations or management strategy. Perioperative glucose targets were developed as extrapolations of data and recommendations in the critically ill. There, fear of hyperglycemia-induced immune dysfunction and mortality at historical glucose targets (<200 mg/dL) prompted efforts to maintain physiologically normal glucose ranges (80–110 mg/dL). Later work showed that targeting lower glucose goals was associated with hypoglycemia and increased mortality. This is of significant concern as monitoring glucose perioperatively is challenging, and anesthesia may mask symptoms and blunt physiologic response to hypoglycemia. Currently, intermediate blood glucose goals are largely used (130–180 mg/dL), with the goal of preventing concentrations greater than 180 mg/dL by initiating therapy when serum glucose reaches 140 to 150 mg/dL (Table 211.1). Individualization based on changing approaches to glucose monitoring, glycemic management, patient factors, and surgical factors is expected to evolve. Insulin sensitivity, history of hypoglycemia, duration of surgery and recovery, and time to resumption of oral intake should all be

| TABLE 211.1 | Recommendations of Various Professional Societies for Target Plasma Glucose in Hospitalized and Surgical Patients With Diabetes |
| --- | --- |
| American Society of Clinical Endocrinologists | Random glucose <180 mg/dL, fasting glucose <140 mg/dL, <180 mg/dL in intensive care unit |
| American Diabetes Association | Random glucose <180 mg/dL, fasting glucose <140 mg/dL |
| Society for Ambulatory Anesthesiology | Intraoperative glucose <180 mg/dL |
| Society of Critical Care Medicine, *in revision* | Blood glucose most <150 mg/dL, absolutely <180 mg/dL, initiate at ≥150 mg/dL |
| Joint British Diabetes Society/NHS Diabetes | Target blood glucose should be 108–180 mg/dL (acceptable range: 72–216 mg/dL) |
| Australian Diabetes Society | 90–180 mg/dL |
| Center for Disease Control | <200 mg/dL |
| Surviving Sepsis Campaign | <180 mg/dL |
| American College of Surgeons and Surgical Infection Society | 110–150 mg/dL in all patients except <180 mg/dL cardiac surgery patients |

considered when initiating therapy to achieve a defined serum glucose target. For example, it may be reasonable to observe mild hyperglycemia (<250 mg/dL with no signs or symptoms of ketoacidosis or other acute illness) in short outpatient procedures with low risk of physiologic stress when oral intake and home medications are expected to reliably resume shortly thereafter.

## Preoperative Management of Glycemic Control

If a patient is not acutely ill or in need of an emergent life- or limb-saving procedure, further assessment regarding chronic glycemic levels and dysglycemic consequences should be considered. History and physical should look for signs of end organ disease such as cardiovascular disease, renal impairment, neuropathy, or retinopathy. The hemoglobin $A_{1c}$ (Hb $A_{1c}$) reflects the percentage of glycated hemoglobin and can give an estimate of chronic glycemic state. In the preoperative clinic, patients with high HbA$_{1c}$ (>6.5%) and/or a high serum glucose (>140 mg/dL) may be referred to their primary care physician or to an endocrinologist for optimization before elective procedures, noting that there is a lack of data supporting optimal target glucose and HbA$_{1c}$ goals or time frame to achieve them. For patients with diabetes, detailed preoperative medication instructions should be provided and an HbA$_{1c}$ assessed at least 3 to 6 months before surgery. Considerations for the preoperative evaluation of patients with diabetes and medication guidelines are reviewed in the chapter entitled "Anesthesiology for Patients With Diabetes Mellitus."

Hyperglycemia on the day of surgery presents a different dilemma and prompts further investigation. Hyperglycemic emergencies such as diabetic ketoacidosis (DKA) (glucose >250 mg/dL, arterial pH <7.3, serum bicarbonate <18 mEq/L, and anion gap >10) and hyperglycemic hyperosmolar state (HHS) (glucose >600 mg/dL and serum osmolality >320 mOsm/L)

should be ruled out regardless of surgical urgency. In the absence of DKA or HHS, it may be appropriate to proceed with attention to glycemic management and hydration. However, many centers may delay surgery for preoperative blood glucose levels over 200 to 350 mg/dL depending on individual patient considerations, surgical type, surgical urgency, and/or risks. Regardless, plans must be in place for outpatient follow-up to optimize glycemic control, as well as plans to monitor and manage blood glucose perioperatively. A suggested assessment and plan for preoperative hyperglycemia is shown in Fig. 211.1.

It is crucial to note that patients with type 1 diabetes have an absolute insulin deficiency and require a continuous source of insulin. Either a long-acting subcutaneous insulin or an intravenous insulin infusion may be used. Transitioning back to a subcutaneous insulin regimen is important, but dosages may need adjustment as surgery and recovery can transiently influence insulin sensitivity.

Patients with diabetes are increasingly being treated with ambulatory continuous subcutaneous insulin infusions (insulin pumps). Outpatient surgical procedures often allow for continued use of insulin pumps, but longer inpatient stays, pumps that interrupt the surgical field, or circumstances when skin perfusion may be altered (temperature fluctuations or hemodynamic instability) merit conversion to a protocolized intravenous insulin infusion and insulin schedule. It is important to remember that another source of exogenous insulin must be provided. It is also important to consider decreasing basal insulin needs during periods of fasting both for personal subcutaneous pumps and perioperative infusions.

## Intraoperative Management of Glycemic Control

Treatment of hyperglycemia in perioperative patients should proceed with insulin, with the route dictated by patient and procedural context. Frequently reviewed hospital-standardized, validated protocols are mandatory; many are published and/or available online. Protocols must outline blood glucose targets and thresholds for treatment of both hyperglycemia and hypoglycemia, correction-scale insulin, and treatment for hypoglycemia, along with frequency (and modality) of blood glucose checks to monitor glycemic control and avoid hypoglycemia. Both the method of monitoring blood glucose and the means of administering insulin must consider hemodynamic stability, shock states, perfusion, volume status, and duration of surgery. In addition, the pharmacokinetics of various insulin regimens warrant consideration (Table 211.2).

Patients with well-controlled diabetes undergoing shorter, less invasive procedures can be treated with correction-scale subcutaneous fast-acting insulin. The use of long-acting subcutaneous basal insulin with correction-scale insulin can cause hypoglycemia in the setting of prolonged fasting. If long-acting subcutaneous basal insulin is used, it is imperative that protocols for blood glucose monitoring and treatment of hypoglycemia are followed. For longer procedures, critically ill patients, procedures associated with significant physiologic stress, patients with insufficient endogenous insulin, or if administration of subcutaneous insulin is not possible, the use of intravenous insulin infusions should be considered. As mentioned earlier, the use of continuous subcutaneous insulin infusion devices (insulin pumps) during the perioperative period is controversial, but they are generally not advised for longer procedures with high physiologic demand.

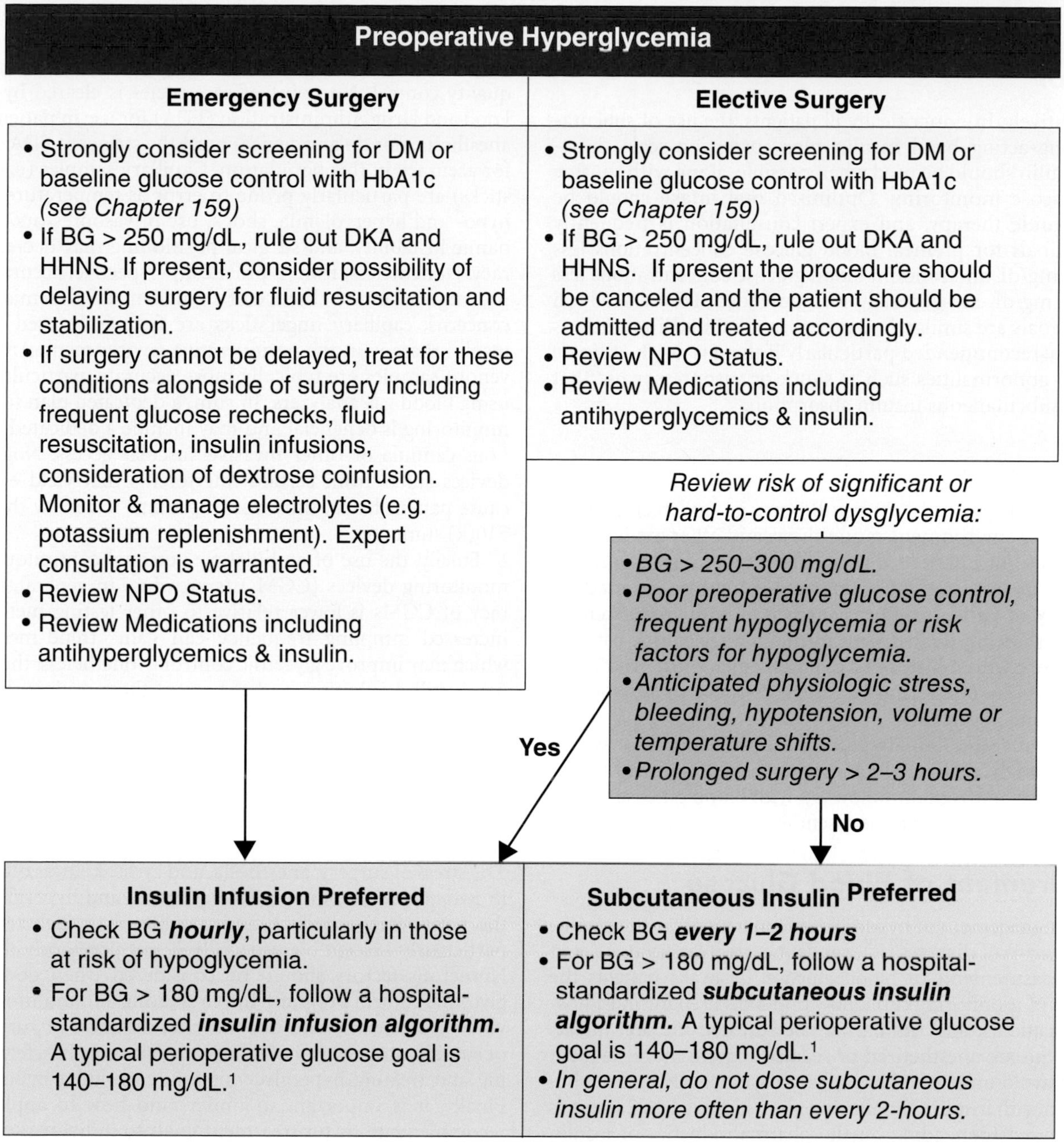

## Preoperative Hyperglycemia

| Emergency Surgery | Elective Surgery |
|---|---|
| • Strongly consider screening for DM or baseline glucose control with HbA1c *(see Chapter 159)*<br>• If BG > 250 mg/dL, rule out DKA and HHNS. If present, consider possibility of delaying surgery for fluid resuscitation and stabilization.<br>• If surgery cannot be delayed, treat for these conditions alongside of surgery including frequent glucose rechecks, fluid resuscitation, insulin infusions, consideration of dextrose coinfusion. Monitor & manage electrolytes (e.g. potassium replenishment). Expert consultation is warranted.<br>• Review NPO Status.<br>• Review Medications including antihyperglycemics & insulin. | • Strongly consider screening for DM or baseline glucose control with HbA1c *(see Chapter 159)*<br>• If BG > 250 mg/dL, rule out DKA and HHNS. If present the procedure should be canceled and the patient should be admitted and treated accordingly.<br>• Review NPO Status.<br>• Review Medications including antihyperglycemics & insulin. |

*Review risk of significant or hard-to-control dysglycemia:*

- *BG > 250–300 mg/dL.*
- *Poor preoperative glucose control, frequent hypoglycemia or risk factors for hypoglycemia.*
- *Anticipated physiologic stress, bleeding, hypotension, volume or temperature shifts.*
- *Prolonged surgery > 2–3 hours.*

**Yes** → **No** ↓

| Insulin Infusion Preferred | Subcutaneous Insulin Preferred |
|---|---|
| • Check BG **hourly**, particularly in those at risk of hypoglycemia.<br>• For BG > 180 mg/dL, follow a hospital-standardized **insulin infusion algorithm.** A typical perioperative glucose goal is 140–180 mg/dL.[1] | • Check BG **every 1–2 hours**<br>• For BG > 180 mg/dL, follow a hospital-standardized **subcutaneous insulin algorithm.** A typical perioperative glucose goal is 140–180 mg/dL.[1]<br>• *In general, do not dose subcutaneous insulin more often than every 2-hours.* |

**Fig. 211.1** Management of preoperative hyperglycemia. Perioperative hyperglycemia warrants comprehensive assessment and consideration of diabetes screening. For severe elevations, diabetic ketoacidosis *(DKA)* and hyperglycemic hyperosmolar nonketoic syndrome *(HHNS)* should be ruled out and, if present and possible, surgery should be rescheduled. Insulin algorithms should be followed per local guidelines with frequent reassessments of glucose, particularly in those at risk of hypoglycemia. *BG*, Blood glucose; *DM*, diabetes mellitus; *HbA1c*, hemoglobin $A_{1c}$; *NPO*, nothing by mouth. [1]Some centers initiate therapy at plasma glucose above 160 mg/dL if the plasma glucose is rising, to prevent hyperglycemia.

**TABLE 211.2  Examples of Insulin Used for Correction and Maintenance of Glycemic Control**

| Intravenous Insulin | Examples | Onset | Peak | Duration |
|---|---|---|---|---|
| Rapid-acting | Insulin | 15 min | 15–30 min | 2–6 hours |
| **Subcutaneous Insulin (Correction)** | | | | |
| Rapid-acting | Aspart Lispro | 5–15 min | 30–120 min | 3–5 hours |
| Short-acting | Regular | 30 min | 2–4 hours | 5–8 hours |
| *Subcutaneous Insulin (Basal)* | | | | |
| Intermediate-acting | Insulin NPH | 2–4 hours | 4–10 hours | 10–18 hours |
| Long-acting | Detemir | 1–3 hours | 6–8 hours | 18–20 hours |
| | Glargine | 2–4 hours | No peak | 20–24 hours |

*NPH*, Neutral protamine Hagedorn.

# Postoperative Management of Glycemic Control

Postoperatively, in noncritically ill patients, the use of subcutaneous long-acting basal insulin plus correction-scale short-acting insulin should be used when possible, along with routine blood glucose monitoring. Optimized oral intake should be used to guide therapy, and expert consultation is frequently helpful. Goals for premeal blood glucose concentrations less than 140 mg/dL and random blood glucose concentrations less than 180 mg/dL are generally recommended. For critically ill patients, goals are similar, however parenteral insulin infusions are usually recommended particularly if there is a risk of tissue perfusion abnormalities such as shock or vasopressor use that can alter subcutaneous insulin absorption.

## HYPOGLYCEMIA

Hypoglycemia (glucose <70 mg/dL) may go undetected in the perioperative environment as anesthesia and other medications can mask and/or interfere with normal physiologic response. A high index of suspicion for hypoglycemia must be maintained, particularly in patients who have received antihyperglycemics and in those being treated with insulin. Other at-risk patients include those with a history of hypoglycemia, those who graze through the day (vs. eating larger meals), and those who are insensate to hypoglycemia.

For patients who develop glucose below 70 mg/dL or symptomatic hypoglycemia, rapid administration of 25 to 50 mL of 50% dextrose and vigilant follow-up with blood glucose checks at 5- to 15-minute intervals is essential.

## Measurement of Blood Glucose

The safe management of hyperglycemia in patients with or without a diagnosis of diabetes is dependent on regular, accurate, and precise measurements of blood glucose. In awake patients the frequency of monitoring can follow protocols used for most hospitalized patients, and timing may be adjusted for oral intake. Patients who are anesthetized or sedated require more frequent testing to avoid undetected hypoglycemia, especially in those being treated with insulin. Monitoring glucose every 1 to 2 hours is recommended (depending on the pharmacokinetics of insulin used), with increased frequency for intravenous insulin infusions or increased sensitivity to the effects of insulin.

Point-of-care glucose testing with glucose meters is used for convenience and rapid results, though it requires training and quality control. No point-of-care meter is cleared by the U.S. Food and Drug Administration (FDA) for use in patients under anesthesia, nor do any devices meet the stringent FDA guidance for accuracy in this population. Capillary samples (e.g., fingersticks) are particularly prone to error as temperature changes, hypo- and hypervolemia, shock, use of vasopressors, hemodynamic instability, and surgical positioning may decrease accuracy. Nonetheless, from a practical perspective, accuracy is improving and in the absence of significant dysglycemia or other concerns, capillary fingersticks are frequently used to titrate insulin therapy in the perioperative environment. Arterial and venous samples are typically more accurate, particularly when using blood gas analyzers. In sum, a dedicated plan for glucose monitoring is beneficial and may include a dedicated distal venous cannula or other invasive vascular access. Note that all devices suffer from certain interferents that yield errors and cause patient harm; thus it is important to review the device's 510(k) summary.

Finally, the use of ambulatory personal continuous glucose monitoring devices (CGMs) is growing. In general, the accuracy of CGMs is lower relative to other testing methods, but increased sampling frequency can gain "trend-monitoring," which may improve glycemic control. Nonetheless, the technology is still developing, and at present these devices should not be used perioperatively to guide insulin therapy. Likewise, newer closed-loop artificial pancreas device systems integrating a CGM and insulin pump should not be used perioperatively.

## Summary

The stress of surgery, anesthesia, and critical illness often results in patients developing insulin resistance and hyperglycemia in the perioperative period, and patients with diabetes may be particularly susceptible especially if not previously diagnosed. Numerous factors should be considered when developing a glycemic control program and in treating and monitoring individual patients. Insulin dependence, duration of surgery, type of surgery, and severity of illness all play a role in safely preventing and treating hyperglycemia while avoiding hypoglycemia. Finally, it is important to understand how to apply various recommendations for treatment goals to individual patients to achieve safe management of diabetes and hyperglycemia in the perioperative period.

## SUGGESTED READINGS

Berríos-Torres, S. I., Umscheid, C. A., Bratzler, D. W., Leas, B., Stone, E. C., Kelz, R. R., et al. (2017). Centers for disease control and prevention guideline for the prevention of surgical site infection, 2017. *JAMA Surgery, 152*(8), 784–791.

Duggan, E., & Chen, Y. (2019). Glycemic management in the operating room: Screening, monitoring, oral hypoglycemics, and insulin therapy. *Current Diabetes Reports, 19*(11), 134.

Duggan, E. W., Carlson, K., & Umpierrez, G. E. (2017). Perioperative hyperglycemia management: An update. *Anesthesiology, 126*(3), 547–560.

Duggan, E. W., Klopman, M. A., Berry, A. J., & Umpierrez, G. (2016). The emory university perioperative algorithm for the management of hyperglycemia and diabetes in non-cardiac surgery patients. *Current Diabetes Reports, 16*(3), 34.

Joshi, G. P., Chung, F., Vann, M. A., Ahmad, S., Gan, T. J., Goulson, D. T., et al. (2010). Society for Ambulatory Anesthesia consensus statement on perioperative blood glucose management in diabetic patients undergoing ambulatory surgery. *Anesthesia and Analgesia, 111*(6), 1378–1387.

Long, M. T., Anderson, A. L., & Curry, T. B. (2022). What is new in perioperative dysglycemia? *Intensive Care Medicine, 48*(9), 1230–1233.

Long, M. T., & Coursin, D. B. (2020). The perils of perioperative dysglycemia. *International Anesthesiology Clinics, 58*(1), 21–26.

Marathe, P. H., Gao, H. X., & Close, K. L. (2017). American Diabetes Association standards of medical care in diabetes 2017. *Journal of Diabetes, 9*(4), 320–324.

Peters, A. L., Ahmann, A. J., Battelino, T., Evert, A., Hirsch, I. B., Murad, M. H., et al. (2016). Diabetes technology-continuous subcutaneous insulin infusion therapy and continuous glucose monitoring in adults: An Endocrine Society clinical practice guideline. *Journal of Clinical Endocrinology and Metabolism, 101*(11), 3922–3937.

Simha, V., & Shah, P. (2019). Perioperative glucose control in patients with diabetes undergoing elective surgery. *JAMA, 321*(4), 399–400.

Sreedharan, R., & Abdelmalak, B. (2018). Diabetes mellitus: Preoperative concerns and evaluation. *Anesthesiology Clinics, 36*(4), 581–597.

Underwood, P., Askari, R., Hurwitz, S., Chamarthi, B., & Garg, R. (2014). Preoperative A1C and clinical outcomes in patients with diabetes undergoing major noncardiac surgical procedures. *Diabetes Care, 37*(3), 611–616.

# 212

# Acute Respiratory Distress Syndrome

RICHARD K. PATCH III, MD   |   MEGAN N. MANENTO, MD

## Introduction

Acute respiratory distress syndrome (ARDS) is an inflammatory lung condition with associated noncardiogenic pulmonary edema and impairment of gas exchange resulting in acute hypoxic respiratory failure. It is a major cause of respiratory failure in patients in the intensive care unit (ICU). Patients in the perioperative setting who undergo major surgical procedures are at risk of developing ARDS, particularly in those who aspirate. The incidence of ARDS in the United States is estimated at almost 200,000 adult patients per year. The incidence is decreasing due to lung protective ventilation, more conservative use of blood products, and a reduction in nosocomial infections. Mortality from ARDS is estimated to range from 26% to 58%, and in-hospital mortality remains high at 46.1% for those with severe ARDS.

## Pathophysiology

The histopathologic feature of ARDS is diffuse alveolar damage with lung capillary endothelial cell injury. The histopathologic features develop over time, and ARDS is divided into two phases: the early exudative phase and the late fibroproliferative phase. An alteration in the relationship between the alveolar epithelium and the capillary endothelium occurs during the exudative phase. This allows an influx of protein-rich edema fluid into the alveoli. Neutrophils are recruited to the lungs, and cytokines such as tumor necrosis factor (TNF) and interleukin (IL)-1, IL-6, and IL-8 are among the inflammatory mediators involved. Injury to type II alveolar cells results in disruption of epithelial fluid transport, impairs removal of alveolar fluid, and alters surfactant production. The damage to the alveolar epithelial cells impairs resorption of the fluid from the alveolar space, enhancing parenchymal injury. During the late fibroproliferative phase, increasing numbers of fibroblasts and myofibroblasts enter the alveolar walls leading to deposition of collagens and other components of the extracellular matrix. The end result is impaired gas exchange, decreased lung compliance, and pulmonary hypertension.

## Etiology

ARDS typically results from a direct insult to the lung, such as aspiration of gastric contents. Pneumonia (either community acquired, pandemic related such as H1N1 or COVID-19, or nosocomial) is likely the most common cause, though sepsis is a close second. Direct injury may also be related to pulmonary contusion, fat embolus, inhalation or drowning injury, or transfusion of blood products. ARDS also occurs as part of a systemic illness such as acute pancreatitis, although not every case has an identifiable etiology (Table 212.1).

| TABLE 212.1 | Etiologies of Acute Respiratory Distress Syndrome | |
| --- | --- | --- |
| **Pulmonary** | | **Extrapulmonary** |
| Pneumonia (community acquired, nosocomial, pandemic-related) | | Sepsis |
| Gastric aspiration/aspiration pneumonitis | | Shock states |
| Inhalation injury (e.g., inhaled crack cocaine) | | Pancreatitis |
| Near drowning | | Trauma (e.g., long bone fractures, fat embolism) |
| Lung contusion | | Massive transfusion |
| Amniotic fluid embolism | | Burns and smoke inhalation |
| Hematopoietic stem cell transplantation | | Postcardiopulmonary bypass |
| Drug overdose (e.g., aspirin) | | Primary graft failure in lung transplantation |
| Medication induced (chemotherapeutic agents, radiation, amiodarone) | | |

## Clinical Presentation

Clinical manifestations of ARDS can evolve rapidly or a have a subacute course of up to 72 hours. Respiratory distress with worsening dyspnea, tachypnea, and diffuse rales on lung auscultation, accessory muscle use, diaphoresis, and overall increased work of breathing are common. Arterial blood gas analysis shows an elevated alveolar-arterial $O_2$ gradient with severe hypoxemia, consistent with right-to-left shunt physiology. Respiratory alkalosis may be present in early ARDS; however, respiratory acidosis usually develops later in the course of the condition.

## Diagnosis

The diagnosis of ARDS is made clinically, as it is a clinical syndrome. In 2012, the Berlin Definition of ARDS (Table 212.2) replaced the American-European Consensus Conference's definition published in 1994. The term "acute lung injury" was eliminated and pulmonary capillary wedge pressure was removed as a diagnostic criteria. A moderate to severe oxygen impairment must be present as defined by the ratio of arterial oxygen tension to fraction of inspired oxygen ($Pao_2/Fio_2$). To diagnose ARDS, all of the following criteria are required.
- Acute respiratory symptoms that start within 7 days of a precipitating event or new or worsening symptoms during the past week.
- Bilateral opacities consistent with pulmonary edema on chest radiography or CT scan.

| TABLE 212.2 | The Berlin Criteria for Acute Respiratory Distress Syndrome | |
|---|---|
| Timing | Acute process < 7 days from presentation |
| Chest imaging | Bilateral opacities consistent with pulmonary edema |
| Origin of edema | Respiratory failure not fully explained by cardiac failure or fluid overload |
| **SEVERITY** | |
| Mild ARDS | P/F ratio > 200 mm Hg, but ≤ 300 mm Hg on ventilator settings that include a PEEP or CPAP ≥ 5 cm $H_2O$ |
| Moderate ARDS | P/F ratio > 100 mm Hg, but ≤ 200 mm Hg on ventilator settings that include a PEEP ≥ 5 cm $H_2O$ |
| Severe ARDS | P/F ratio ≤ 100 mm Hg on ventilator settings that include a PEEP ≥ 5 cm $H_2O$ |

*ARDS,* Acute respiratory distress syndrome; *CPAP,* continuous positive airway pressure; *PEEP,* positive end-expiratory pressure; *P/F ratio,* arterial $pO_2$ divided by $FiO_2$

- Respiratory failure that cannot be fully explained by cardiac failure or fluid overload, and an objective evaluation (e.g., echocardiography) is required to exclude hydrostatic pulmonary edema.

## Management

Lung protective mechanical ventilation is the foundation of ARDS management. This is achieved by maintaining appropriate arterial oxygenation and protecting the injured lung from ventilator-associated lung injury (VALI). Limiting alveolar overdistention, trauma from repetitive opening and closing of the alveoli, and the further release of inflammatory cytokines will protect against further injury.

### LOW TIDAL VOLUME VENTILATION

The ARDSNet lower tidal volume trial (ARMA) proved that use of low tidal volume ventilation (LTVV) of 6 mL/kg of predicted body weight and a plateau pressure (Pplat) of 30 cm $H_2O$ or less compared with 12 mL/kg and Pplat of 50 cm $H_2O$ or less decreased mortality. The decrease was secondary to minimizing lung overdistention and VALI. Predicted body weight is based on patient height and sex. LTVV has become a standard of care in the management of patients with ARDS in the ICU. Although volume-control ventilation was used in the ARDSNet low tidal volume study, pressure-control ventilation (which may provide superior oxygenation because of its flow pattern) can be used instead, providing tidal volumes are limited.

### PERMISSIVE HYPERCAPNIA

In permissive hypercapnia, the $Paco_2$ is allowed to increase, even to the point of acidemia, to maintain a LTVV strategy. Over time, the respiratory acidosis will be compensated for by renal retention of bicarbonate to bring the pH back toward normal.

### OPEN LUNG VENTILATION

Open lung ventilation refers to the strategy of combining LTVV with enough positive end-expiratory pressure (PEEP) to maximize alveolar recruitment and allow ventilation above the lower inflection point. As a result, alveolar overdistention is decreased and more alveoli remain open throughout the respiratory cycle. Typically PEEP and $Fio_2$ are titrated in concert using incremental increases in both to achieve the aforementioned oxygenation goal. Levels of PEEP can range from 12 to 24 mm Hg. Recruitment maneuvers are the application of high levels of positive airway pressure (e.g., 40 cm $H_2O$) to open collapsed alveoli. Adverse effects include hypotension and desaturation; however, these are self-limited.

### DRIVING PRESSURE

Driving pressure ($\Delta P$) is an important variable that allows optimization of mechanical ventilation in patients with moderate to severe ARDS. It is calculated by subtracting Pplat from the applied PEEP ($\Delta P = Pplat - PEEP$). Retrospective analysis revealed that increased driving pressure, even with LTVV and an open lung strategy, was associated with an increased risk of death. A goal $\Delta P$ of less than 15 cm $H_2O$ is associated with improved outcomes.

### FLUID MANAGEMENT

Conservative fluid management even in patients who are not volume overloaded is beneficial. Once the period of active resuscitation is over, diuretics should be used to decreased extravascular lung water. Both ventilator-free days and ICU-free days increased without worsening nonpulmonary organ failure in patients who received conservative fluid management.

### NEUROMUSCULAR BLOCKADE

Patients with ARDS who underwent neuromuscular blockade within 48 hours of initiating mechanical ventilation saw a mortality benefit. Treatment with cisatracurium had a higher 90-day survival, more ventilator-free days, and less barotrauma. ICU-acquired weakness did not increase in the group receiving paralytics. Moreover, neuromuscular blockade eliminates ventilator asynchrony and reduces chest wall elastance.

### GLUCOCORTICOIDS

No definitive role for glucocorticoid use in ARDS has been established. Low-dose steroids during the early phase, as defined by within 72 hours of presentation, showed a reduction in duration of mechanical ventilation, ICU length of stay, and ICU mortality. Caveats to these results include small and unbalanced treatment groups. Evaluation of corticosteroids in the late fibroproliferative stage did not show an outcome benefit.

### ESOPHAGEAL PRESSURE MONITORING

Transpulmonary pressure ($P_{tp}$) is equal to the airway pressure minus the pleural pressure. Pleural pressure can be estimated using an esophageal balloon, and thus a patient-specific, optimal level of PEEP can be determined. PEEP titration with a goal of achieving a $P_{tp}$ between 0 and 10 mm Hg was compared with the PEEP titration algorithm outlined in the ARMA trial. Patients with PEEP levels guided by esophageal monitoring had higher total levels and better P/F ratios, arterial $pO_2$ ("P") from the ABG divided by the $FiO_2$ ("F"). However, there was no difference in ICU-free or ventilator-free days.

## TRACHEAL GAS INSUFFLATION

Permissive hypercapnia is generally well tolerated, although in some patients control of the hypercapnia is limited due to the presence of a large physiologic dead space. A point is reached where increasing respiratory rate to increase minute ventilation without a coinciding increase in tidal volume will not change the ratio of dead space ventilation to alveolar ventilation. As such, the $Pco_2$ continues to increase and the patient can develop acidosis. Tracheal gas insufflation involves the continuous flow of fresh $O_2$ (usually ~6 L/min) through a small tube placed through or alongside the tracheal tube and exiting above the carina. The gas washes out $CO_2$ and is an adjunct to the $CO_2$ removal provided by mechanical ventilation.

## Refractory Hypoxemia

Refractory hypoxemia does not have an official definition. Essentially, it is continued hypoxemia with a $Pao_2/Fio_2$ less than 100 mm Hg, Pplat 30 mm Hg or greater, and an oxygenation index greater than 30 [($Fio_2 \times$ mean airway pressure $\times$ 100)/ $Pao_2$] despite LTVV and an optimal level of PEEP.

### PRONE POSITION VENTILATION

Placement of a patient in the prone position increases end-expiratory lung volume, improves ventilation-perfusion matching, and causes regional changes in ventilation associated with alterations in chest wall mechanics. Oxygenation is improved. However, the improvement may or may not be sustained when the patient is returned to the supine position. Prone position ventilation had an absolute mortality risk reduction of 17% and a relative risk reduction of 50%. Contraindication to prone positioning include but are not limited to increased intracranial pressure, spinal instability, pregnancy, active bleeding including hemorrhagic shock or massive hemoptysis, unstable fractures, and recent tracheal surgery or sternotomy.

### VENOVENOUS EXTRACORPOREAL MEMBRANE OXYGENATION

In 2009, the multicenter, Conventional ventilator support versus Extracorporeal membrane oxygenation for Severe Acute Respiratory failure (CESAR) trial showed increased survival in the patient group referred to the extracorporeal membrane oxygenation (ECMO) center compared with conventional management. It is important to note that not all patients who were referred to the center received ECMO. Some received conventional management due to the fact that they did not receive it at the outside facility.

The EOLIA trial, published in 2018, compared the use of early ECMO to conventional LTVV. The LTVV control group could crossover and receive late ECMO as a rescue therapy for refractory hypoxemia. The study was stopped early with a primary end point of 60-day mortality. The results were not statistically significant but were in favor of early ECMO with a 35% mortality in the ECMO group compared with 46% mortality in the conventional group.

## Alternative Management Strategies

Alternative modes of ventilation such as airway pressure release ventilation and bilevel ventilation have been used as a rescue strategy in patients with refractory hypoxemia. Neither improved mortality. High-frequency oscillatory ventilation (HFOV) uses an oscillating pump to deliver a small tidal volume (1–4 mL/kg) at a frequency of 3 to 15 Hz. By delivering small tidal volumes, the mode maintains constant lung recruitment and prevents lung injury from overdistention. Unfortunately, patients receiving HFOV had an increased mortality compared with those with LTVV and high PEEP. Inhaled nitric oxide (iNO) dilates the pulmonary vasculature by stimulating guanylate cyclase resulting in increased cyclic GMP, smooth muscle relaxation, and increased oxygenation. A metaanalysis revealed iNO had no effect on mortality, and additional studies have suggested increased renal impairment. Prostacyclin $E_1$ is another pulmonary vasodilator that improves oxygenation, but the efficacy in ARDS is not known.

## Post-ARDS Outcomes

Survivors of ARDS may have significant short-term to medium-term disability. The morbidity among survivors is extensive with neurocognitive dysfunction, physical disabilities, and psychiatric illnesses such as depression, anxiety, posttraumatic stress disorder, and post–intensive care syndrome (PICS). Additionally, some patients may require a tracheostomy and a prolonged period of ventilator weaning. In the long term, lung function usually returns to near normal, but mild abnormalities on pulmonary function tests may persist.

## SUGGESTED READINGS

Amato, M. B., Meade, M. O., Slutsky, A. S., Brochard, L., Costa, E. L., Schoenfeld, D. A., et al. (2015). Driving pressure and survival in the acute respiratory distress syndrome. *New England Journal of Medicine, 372*(8), 747–755.

Beitler, J. R., Thompson, B. T., Baron, R. M., Bastarache, J. A., Denlinger, L. C., Esserman, L., et al. (2022). Advancing precision medicine for acute respiratory distress syndrome. *Lancet Respiratory Medicine, 10*(1), 107–120.

Combes, A., Hajage, D., Capellier, G., Demoule, A., Lavoué, S., Guervilly, C., et al. (2018). Extracorporeal membrane oxygenation for severe acute respiratory distress syndrome. *New England Journal of Medicine, 378*(21), 1965–1975.

Mega, C., Cavalli, I., Ranieri, V. M., & Tonetti, T. (2022). Protective ventilation in patients with acute respiratory distress syndrome related to COVID-19: Always, sometimes or never? *Current Opinion in Critical Care, 28*(1), 51–56.

Ranieri, V. M., Rubenfeld, G. D., Thompson, B. T., Ferguson, N. D., Caldwell, E., Fan, E., et al. (2012). Acute respiratory distress syndrome: The Berlin Definition. *JAMA, 307*(23), 2526–2533.

Singh, A. R., Kumar, R., & Sinha, A. (2022). Understanding COVID-19 acute respiratory distress syndrome. *Annals of the American Thoracic Society, 19*(1), 150.

Siuba, M. T., Sadana, D., Gadre, S., Bruckman, D., & Duggal, A. (2022). Acute respiratory distress syndrome readmissions: A nationwide cross-sectional analysis of epidemiology and costs of care. *PLoS One, 17*(1), e0263000.

Thompson, B. T., Chambers, R. C., & Liu, K. D. (2017). Acute respiratory distress syndrome. *New England Journal of Medicine, 377*(6), 562–572.

Young, D., Lamb, S. E., Shah, S., MacKenzie, I., Tunnicliffe, W., Lall, R., et al. (2013). High-frequency oscillation for acute respiratory distress syndrome. *New England Journal of Medicine, 368*(9), 806–813.

# Pulmonary Hypertension

BARRY A. HARRISON, MBBS, FRACP, FANZCA   |   WESLEY L. ALLEN, MD

## Introduction

Pulmonary hypertension (PH) is an abnormal increase in mean pulmonary artery pressure (mPAP). At rest, the normal mPAP is $14 \pm 3.3$ mm Hg (upper limit, 20 mm Hg) and increases with exercise. A sustained elevation of mPAP to more than 25 mm Hg at rest, as measured by right heart catheterization, or to more than 30 mm Hg with exercise, is diagnostic of PH.

## Pathophysiology

There are multiple etiologies of PH; however, they are divided into five general classifications (Table 213.1). Pulmonary arterial hypertension (PAH) constitutes Group 1, which in the past was known as primary PH. Vasoconstriction of the pulmonary arterioles and thickening of the pulmonary artery (PA) vessel wall through remodeling and inflammation leads to plexiform lesions and thrombosis in situ. With disease progression, vascular elasticity is reduced along with the pulmonary vasculature total cross-sectional area. In combination with an imbalance of endogenous pulmonary vasodilator and vasoconstrictor regulation, pulmonary vascular resistance (PVR) increases, leading to increased right ventricular afterload. The right ventricle (RV) hypertrophies in response to maintain RV-PA coupling, but with disease progression, the RV becomes uncoupled and fails because of its inability to match output to rising afterloads.

## Clinical Features

All groups of PH have progressive dyspnea initially with exercise progressing to dyspnea at rest. Box 213.1 illustrates the classification of clinical severity of PH. In PAH, other symptoms include fatigability, cough, syncope, dizziness, and signs of venous congestion (lower extremity edema, hepatic congestion, abdominal distension). The incidence is higher in women than men, and peak occurrence is the 20- to 40-year age group. Because of the nonspecific nature of symptoms, roughly >20% of patients have symptomatic PAH more than 2 years before diagnosis. With progression of PH, the RV dilates and fails, indicating severe disease. Previously, when there was no effective treatment available, death usually ensued within 3 years.

## Diagnosis

Physical examination may be unremarkable, but can include elevated jugular venous pressure (JVP), an increased or widened splitting of P2 (pulmonary component) of the second heart sound, right-sided S3 or S4 with increased venous volumes (JVP), and/or low blood pressure with increased resting heart rate. The electrocardiograph may demonstrate peaked P

| TABLE 213.1 | Updated Classification of Pulmonary Hypertension |
|---|---|

1. PAH
  1.1 Idiopathic PAH
  1.2 Heritable PAH
    1.2.1 BMPR2
    1.2.2 *ALK–1, ENG, SMAD9, CAV1, KCNK3*
    1.2.3 Unknown
  1.3 Drug and toxin induced
  1.4 Associated with:
    1.4.1 Connective tissue disease
    1.4.2 HIV infection
    1.4.3 Portal hypertension
    1.4.4 Congenital heart diseases
    1.4.5 Schistosomiasis
1'. Pulmonary venoocclusive disease and/or pulmonary capillary hemangiomatosis
1''. PPHN

2. PH due to left-sided heart disease
  2.1 LV systolic dysfunction
  2.2 LV diastolic dysfunction
  2.3 Valvular disease
  2.4 Congenital/acquired left heart inflow/outflow tract obstruction and congenital cardiomyopathies

3. PH due to lung diseases and/or hypoxia
  3.1 COPD
  3.2 Interstitial lung disease
  3.3 Other pulmonary diseases with mixed restrictive and obstructive pattern
  3.4 Sleep-disordered breathing
  3.5 Alveolar hypoventilation disorders
  3.6 Chronic exposure to high altitude
  3.7 Developmental lung diseases

4. CTEPH

5. PH with unclear multifactorial mechanisms
  5.1 Hematologic disorders: chronic hemolytic anemia, myeloproliferative disorders, splenectomy
  5.2 Systemic disorders: sarcoidosis, pulmonary histiocytosis, lymphangioleiomyomatosis
  5.3 Metabolic disorders: glycogen storage disease, Gaucher disease, thyroid disorders
  5.4 Others: tumoral obstruction, fibrosing mediastinitis, chronic renal failure, segmental PH

*BMPR*, Bone morphogenic protein receptor type II; *CAV1*, caveolin-1; *COPD*, chronic obstructive pulmonary disease; *CTEPH*, chronic thromboembolic pulmonary hypertension; *ENG*, endoglin; *HIV*, human immunodeficiency virus; *LV*, left ventricular; *PAH*, pulmonary arterial hypertension; *PH*, pulmonary hypertension; *PPHN*, persistent pulmonary hypertension of the newborn.

From Simonneau G, Gatzoulis MA, Adatia I, et al. Updated clinical classification of pulmonary hypertension. *JACC*. 2013;62:D34–D41.

waves and right ventricular hypertrophy. The chest x-ray may only demonstrate enlarged pulmonary arteries and right ventricular enlargement. Pulmonary function tests may be normal with the exception of a decrease in the carbon monoxide diffusing capacity. The initial screening test is a transthoracic echocardiogram, which may demonstrate increased right ventricular systolic pressure and any associated cardiac conditions. However, right-sided cardiac catheterization is performed to confirm the diagnosis of PH by measuring the pulmonary artery pressure (PAP), the PA occlusion pressure (PAOP), and cardiac output, allowing calculation of the PVR:

$$PVR = \frac{(mPAP - PAOP)}{CO}$$

Increased pulmonary pressure due to left heart disease results in an increase in PAOP that eventually progresses to an increase in PAP. Thus these patients have a lower PVR (<3 Wood units, where 1 Wood unit = 80 dyn · sec$^{-1}$ · cm$^{-5}$) because both pulmonary arterial pressure and pulmonary venous pressure are elevated. However, in PAH, pulmonary pressure elevation is predominately on the arterial (precapillary) side of the pulmonary circulation (PAOP normal), resulting in increased PVR (>3 Wood units).

## Treatment of Pulmonary Hypertension

Treatment of PH is dependent on its etiology and severity, and there are four broad categories for therapeutic options.

1. Treat underlying comorbid disease
   In PH secondary to lung disease, it is important to treat the lung disease. Most important is to administer oxygen either nocturnally or continuously to correct any hypoxemia.
2. Pulmonary vasodilators
   Pulmonary vasodilators are used to counteract the vasoconstriction, smooth muscle cell and endothelial cell proliferation, and prothrombotic state present in PAH. They include the following:
   a. Calcium channel blockers: Calcium channel blockers are relatively inexpensive and, with the exception of verapamil (the use of which is associated with too much negative inotropy), can be used if the patient responds with at least a 10% decrease in mPAP.
   b. Prostacyclin analogs: Studies have demonstrated an association between PAH and decreased endogenous prostacyclin synthase, an enzyme involved in the synthesis of prostacyclin, a potent endogenous pulmonary vasodilator. Several prostacyclin analogs are

therefore used to treat PAH. Epoprostenol (prostacyclin) is given by continuous intravenous (IV) infusion, whereas iloprost (a prostacyclin analog) is delivered by an aerosol route.
   c. Phosphodiesterase inhibitors: Phosphodiesterase inhibitors, especially sildenafil, have a role in the treatment of PAH by inhibiting the breakdown of cyclic guanosine monophosphate, which, in turn, leads to relaxation in smooth muscle cells within the vascular intima, resulting in vasodilation.
   d. Endothelin receptor antagonists are a newer class of drugs that block endothelin receptors, decreasing the vasoconstrictive and vascular remodeling effects of endothelin-1. Bosentan, an oral preparation, increases exercise capacity and delays disease progression but, unfortunately, is hepatotoxic and teratogenic and causes anemia.
3. Surgery
   Cardiac surgery to correct the left-sided cardiac lesions precipitating the PHT is important. Also, at the time, treating any moderate to severe tricuspid regurgitation is of benefit. PA thromboembolectomy or balloon angioplasty may be necessary in the treatment of chronic thromboembolism disease.
4. Lung transplantation
   Before the use of pulmonary vasodilators, lung transplantation was considered lifesaving surgery. However, it is now only considered for combined heart-lung transplantation, this transplant is undertaken extremely rarely.

## Anesthetic Management of the Patient With Pulmonary Arterial Hypertension

Increased awareness, improved diagnosis, and effective treatment have resulted in early death becoming uncommon. Thus the prevalence of PH patients undergoing surgery for unrelated conditions has increased. Because of their PH, these patients have significant perioperative morbidity and mortality rates; one study found a perioperative mortality rate of 7%.

General or regional anesthesia has been used with success; however, the following principles of anesthesia care for the patient with PH need to be followed:

1. Avoid exacerbation of the pulmonary arterial pressure by preventing hypoxemia, acidosis, hypercarbia, hypothermia, and pain.
2. Maintain right ventricular function by optimizing fluid balance and avoiding hypotension. Goals for these patients then include maintaining normal sinus rhythm, with a heart rate of approximately 80 to 90 beats/min to optimize cardiac output. Right ventricular function is sensitive to both intravascular volume depletion and excess; therefore fluids should be administered slowly and in small volumes, with a goal of maintaining a central venous pressure of 12 mm Hg or less.
3. Patients with PAH have elevated sympathetic activation that inversely correlates with RV function. As RV function declines, rapid or significant alterations in the sympathetic tone can have deleterious effects on the hemodynamics and RV performance. Preinduction inotropic support has been described in patients with chronic thromboembolic pulmonary hypertension and RV dysfunction with success to supplement the sympathetic depression seen with induction of anesthesia.

## Preoperative

Clinically, severity of dyspnea is associated with severity of PH. Syncope is a harbinger of poor outcome and symptoms and signs of right-sided heart failure. A right atrial pressure of more than 20 mm Hg, pericardial effusion, and a cardiac output of less than 2 L · min$^{-1}$ · m$^{-2}$ have each been associated with adverse perioperative outcomes. Appropriate review of specialty consultations is important to understand the severity of the patient's condition; if such a consultation has not been recent or there has been deterioration in the patient's condition, then additional consultation is valuable. All PAH medications should be continued throughout the perioperative period, especially any of the prostacyclin analogs, because abrupt discontinuation can result in severe rebound in PH.

## Intraoperative

### MONITORING

Basic standard monitoring is applied; however, pulse oximetry and end-tidal carbon dioxide hold particular importance. The use of invasive arterial pressure monitoring allows prompt treatment of hypotension. If the operation is long, associated with large fluid shifts, risk of hemorrhage is high, and hemodynamic lability is present, then consideration of use of central venous catheter, PA catheter, and or transesophageal echocardiography is warranted.

### GENERAL ANESTHESIA

IV induction agents (e.g., propofol) should be carefully titrated to avoid precipitous decreases in systemic arterial pressure and myocardial depression. Etomidate may cause less hemodynamic instability, as it has little effect on the sympathetic tone. Ketamine shown to be safe despite increasing mPAP, as it does not alter PVR or the ratio of PVR to systemic vascular resistance (SVR). Inhaled induction with volatile anesthetic also has been used effectively. Nitrous oxide should be avoided because of its pulmonary vasoconstrictive properties. Although sympathomimetic agents act on the systemic circulation, they may also increase mPAP and thus need to be administered in incremental doses. Histamine-releasing medications should be avoided. Vasopressin is an ideal drug of choice for treatment of low SVR as it does not alter PVR. Norepinephrine is a safe alternative in that it may increase PVR but will not affect RV ejection fraction (EF) because of its $\beta_1$ component. Phenylephrine should be used with extreme caution, especially in end-stage PH, as it increases the PVR to a greater extent than SVR and reduces RV EF. If a supraglottic airway is selected, the combination of respiratory depressant drugs and spontaneous ventilation may cause a deleterious shift of the $CO_2$ response curve to the right, resulting in hypercapnia and hypoxia and exacerbation of PAH. The use of mechanical ventilation is neither indicated nor contraindicated. Conversely, the use of controlled ventilation with high tidal volumes and peak airway pressures increases mean airway pressure, thereby increasing PVR; however, extremely low tidal volumes will also increase PVR. High peak end-expiratory pressures ($>10$ cm $H_2O$) will also increase PVR. Thus the effects of both spontaneous and controlled ventilation require close monitoring.

### REGIONAL TECHNIQUES

Neuraxial anesthesia may be indicated, especially for procedures below the level of the umbilicus, but it must be borne in mind that prostacyclin analogs have an inhibitory effect on platelet aggregation. Neuraxial anesthesia and analgesia can result in significant systemic vasodilation, which can result in decreased coronary artery perfusion pressure to the RV and decreased preload to the RV.

### MONITORED ANESTHESIA CARE

Sedation techniques can also be used, especially in conjunction with local anesthesia techniques. However, deep sedation techniques may lead to hypercarbia and hypoxemia.

## Postoperative

The patient with PAH needs intense monitoring in the immediate recovery and hospitalization. Supplemental $O_2$ should be administered to all patients with PAH in the postoperative period and monitored with pulse oximetry. Effective analgesia is important; however, opioids must be carefully titrated, if used at all, to minimize the potential for hypercapnia. Treatment of pain with multimodal analgesia, nonopioid medications, and regional techniques is preferred.

## Conclusion

The prognosis of PAH patients has improved markedly since the late 20th century. When these patients present for elective operations, the anesthesia provider must understand the complex pathophysiology and etiology of the PH, be familiar with the multiple drugs the patient may be taking, develop an anesthetic plan that minimizes the chances of increasing PVR, avoid significant alterations to the sympathetic tone, and be prepared to intervene if the patient develops acute right-sided heart failure (Box 213.2).

## BOX 213.2   MANAGEMENT OF ACUTE INCREASE PULMONARY HYPERTENSION AND DECOMPENSATION OF RIGHT VENTRICLE FUNCTION

I. Decrease PH and PVR
   a. Correct—hypoxemia, acidosis, hypothermia
   b. Induce hypocapnia—if lung mechanics allow
   c. Decrease oxygen consumption—increase anesthesia depth and analgesia and use neuromuscular blockers
II. Maintain hemodynamics
   a. Maintain systolic arterial pressure >90 mm Hg and/or 40 mm Hg > PAP
      i. Use phenylephrine, norepinephrine, vasopressin
   b. Maintain normal sinus rhythm and rate 80–90 beats/min
   c. Minimize CVP: <12 mm Hg
      i. Limit intravascular fluid, cautious use of diuretics
   d. Maintain cardiac index >2.2 L/min/m²
III. Pulmonary vasodilator
   a. Inhaled pulmonary artery vasodilators
      i. Nitric oxide (gas) up to 30 ppm—continuous administration usually via a ventilator
      ii. Inhaled prostacyclin (liquid)—continuous or intermittent administration via a nebulizer, preferably an electronic nebulizer

IV. Increase right ventricular function
   a. Pharmacology
      i. Intravascular inodilators—milrinone (load 50 µg/kg, infuse 0.25–0.75 µg/kg/min)
      ii. Dobutamine (2–5 µg · kg⁻¹ · min⁻¹)—will increase right ventricular contractility and decrease mPAP
      iii. Systemic hypotension may result, requiring the use of vasopressors
   b. Mechanical devices
      i. An intraaortic balloon pump may be of benefit by augmenting myocardium perfusion, improving function of both ventricles
      ii. A right ventricular assist device may be of benefit, especially if the patient's right ventricular failure has been exacerbated by left ventricular failure, or vice versa

*CVP*, Central venous pressure; *mPAP*, mean pulmonary arterial pressure; *PAP*, pulmonary arterial pressure; *PH*, pulmonary hypertension; *PVR*, pulmonary vascular resistance.

## SUGGESTED READINGS

Gelzinis, T. A. (2022). Pulmonary hypertension in 2021: Part I–definition, classification, pathophysiology, and presentation. *Journal of Cardiothoracic and Vascular Anesthesia, 36*(6), 1552–1564.

Hirani, N., Brunner, N. W., Kapasi, A., Chandy, G., Rudski, L., Paterson, I., et al. (2020). Canadian Cardiovascular Society/Canadian Thoracic Society Position Statement on Pulmonary Hypertension. *Canadian Journal of Cardiology, 36*(7), 977–992.

Kim, B., Satya, K., & Berkowitz, R. (2019). *Critical care medicine: Principles of diagnosis and management in the adult* (p. 690–703.e5). New Jersey: Elsevier.

Maron, B. A., & Leopold, J. A. (2015). Emerging concepts in the molecular basis of pulmonary arterial hypertension: Part II: Neurohormonal signaling contributes to the pulmonary vascular and right ventricular pathophenotype of pulmonary arterial hypertension. *Circulation, 131*(23), 2079–2091.

Pritts, C. D., & Pearl, R. G. (2010). Anesthesia for patients with pulmonary hypertension. *Current Opinion in Anaesthesiology, 23*(3), 411–416.

Ramakrishna, G., Sprung, J., Ravi, B. S., Chandrasekaran, K., & McGoon, M. D. (2005). Impact of pulmonary hypertension on the outcomes of noncardiac surgery: Predictors of perioperative morbidity and mortality. *Journal of the American College of Cardiology, 45*(10), 1691–1699.

Strumpher, J., & Jacobsohn, E. (2011). Pulmonary hypertension and right ventricular dysfunction: Physiology and perioperative management. *Journal of Cardiothoracic and Vascular Anesthesia, 25*(4), 687–704.

Teo, Y. W., & Greenhalgh, D. L. (2010). Update on anaesthetic approach to pulmonary hypertension. *European Journal of Anaesthesiology, 27*(4), 317–323.

# Management of Stroke

NYCOLE K. JOSEPH, MD  |  SHERRI A. BRAKSICK, MD

## Initial Evaluation of Acute Stroke Patients

### ISCHEMIC STROKE

Ischemic strokes make up about 87% of all strokes and occur when a large intracranial artery (e.g., middle cerebral artery, basilar artery) or small perforating intracranial artery is occluded, causing ischemia to downstream brain tissue. There are multiple possible causes of ischemic stroke (Box 214.1).

The area of irreversible cellular death is termed the *infarct core* and is no longer salvageable. In contrast, ischemic (but not infarcted) brain tissue that is potentially salvageable is termed the *penumbra*. Brain tissue in the penumbra will progress to infarct in a time-dependent fashion unless blood flow is reestablished acutely. Adequate hemodynamic management and avoiding drops in blood pressure (BP) are important to optimize collateral blood flow and help maintain viability of the penumbra. BP targets should be individualized based on the patient's history of chronic hypertension and baseline BP, location of vessel occlusion, degree of collaterals, and acute stroke treatment(s) provided (e.g., intravenous [IV] thrombolytics and/or endovascular thrombectomy [EVT]).

IV thrombolysis with recombinant tissue plasminogen activator (rtPA) or tenecteplase (TNK) is indicated in ischemic stroke patients who meet criteria within 4.5 hours after symptom onset. In patients who are candidates for IV thrombolysis, BP should be lowered safely to 180/105 mm Hg or less before administering these medications and maintained at that goal for the first 24 hours after treatment. A short half-life antihypertensive should be administered under continuous hemodynamic monitoring to allow careful dose titration. Continuous infusions (e.g., nicardipine, clevidipine) may be necessary to avoid rebound hypertensive episodes. Orolingual angioedema is a rare but potentially serious complication of rtPA, especially in patients who are on angiotensin-converting enzyme inhibitors. When severe, this can result in airway compromise. Treatment includes dexamethasone (10 mg IV) and diphenhydramine (50 mg IV).

Careful clinical assessment and patient selection for reperfusion therapy is imperative to optimize functional neurologic outcomes and avoid secondary brain injury. The neurology team should be consulted to determine the appropriate imaging and treatment course in stroke patients. Noncontrast head computed tomography (CT) scan is the primary imaging tool used to rule out hemorrhage and identify features of an evolving ischemic stroke. CT angiography of the head and neck visualizes the extracranial and intracranial blood vessels supplying the brain to evaluate for a large vessel occlusion. Advanced imaging such as CT perfusion provides a snapshot of blood flow to identify infarcted core and salvageable penumbra (Fig. 214.1).

EVT with a stent retriever or catheter aspiration device is the standard of care for acute ischemic stroke patients with a large vessel occlusion who present (1) within 6 hours of symptom onset or (2) within 6 to 24 hours of symptom onset when specific criteria are met. In cases of cervical internal carotid artery occlusions, angioplasty and/or carotid artery stenting may be done acutely. Conscious sedation (CS) is often considered an ideal compromise for mechanical thrombectomy to facilitate patient cooperation, comfort, and procedural speed. In three single-center randomized clinical trials of patients with ischemic stroke undergoing EVT, general anesthesia (GA) was not found to be superior compared with CS. However, a recent study showed that GA during EVT was associated with a lower rate of favorable outcomes compared with CS, and GA was associated with lower rates of favorable outcomes and a higher rate of death compared with local anesthesia. The decision to proceed with CS or GA is often decided after discussion between anesthesia and the proceduralist.

The ideal BP goals during and after EVT are not well defined and need further investigation. For example, in select patients with a proximal artery occlusion, permissive hypertension is recommended and it is reasonable to support with IV fluid and vasopressors, if needed. After successful recanalization, the BP target should be lowered, as studies have found that increased mean systolic BP levels in the first 24 hours after EVT are associated with higher odds of symptomatic intracranial hemorrhage, early neurologic deterioration, and worse functional outcomes.

### HEMORRHAGIC STROKE

Hemorrhagic strokes result from a ruptured intracranial vessel. Spontaneous intracerebral hemorrhage (ICH) may occur in deep locations (basal ganglia, pons, or cerebellum) and are often due to hypertension. The remaining ICHs occur more superficially and are termed *lobar hematomas*, which are often due to cerebral amyloid angiopathy or hypertension. However, many of these patients require additional evaluation to ensure no underlying vascular malformation or tumor as a source of the hemorrhage. The ICH score is used as a mortality risk predictor in patients with a spontaneous ICH. Components of this score

---

**BOX 214.1  CAUSES OF ISCHEMIC STROKE**

Cardioembolic (e.g., atrial fibrillation, aortic thromboembolism)
Large artery atherosclerosis to distal artery (e.g., carotid artery atheroembolism)
Small vessel occlusion (e.g., lacunar)
Other mechanism (e.g., vasculitis, vasculopathy, dissection, hypercoagulable states)
Cryptogenic (stroke of undetermined cause)

---

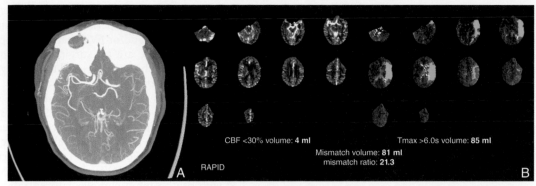

**Fig. 214.1** A 75-year-old patient who presented with right hemiparesis and aphasia, consistent with left middle cerebral artery (MCA) territory ischemia. **A,** Computed tomography angiography demonstrates a left MCA occlusion. **B,** The perfusion map demonstrates a small core infarct (*purple*) with a large surrounding penumbra (*green*).

include hemorrhage location, hemorrhage volume, presence of intraventricular blood, patient age, and admission GCS score.

Compared with ischemic strokes (except massive ischemic stroke with cerebral edema), hemorrhagic stroke is more commonly associated with increased intracranial pressure (ICP), progressive mass effect with compression of adjacent normal brain tissue, and cerebral edema. Increased ICP is proportionate to the volume of blood introduced into the closed intracranial vault (i.e., Monro-Kellie doctrine), and this blood may further increase ICP by obstructing cerebrospinal fluid pathways (obstructive hydrocephalus) or the arachnoid granulations, preventing absorption of cerebrospinal fluid (communicating hydrocephalus). Regardless of the mechanism, increased ICP can compromise global cerebral perfusion pressure (CPP) [CPP = mean arterial pressure (MAP) − ICP] and induce brain ischemia. BP is more tightly regulated in patients with spontaneous ICH, generally with a target of 140 mm Hg or less systolic. Overall, a 20% reduction in MAP is generally well tolerated in acute hypertensive states. When the ICP is being measured, a standard goal for CPP is 50 to 70 mm Hg to ensure adequate cerebral perfusion.

It should be noted that localized mass effect and brain compression may cause irreversible brain injury before the measured ICP increases. For this reason, patients should be carefully monitored, and if neurologic deterioration is found to be due to local edema, aggressive management of cerebral edema should be initiated.

Subarachnoid hemorrhage typically occurs from a ruptured cerebral aneurysm around the circle of Willis, which will require endovascular coiling or surgical clipping to secure the aneurysm. These patients often have prolonged ICU stays to monitor for late complications, including cerebral salt wasting, hydrocephalus, and vasospasm. Trauma may result in small, superficial subarachnoid hemorrhage and does not require specific intervention.

Other causes of intracranial bleeding include epidural hematoma, subdural hematoma, and intraventricular hematomas, which may occur spontaneously, as a consequence of trauma or from a vascular anomaly.

## Anesthetic Management

### PREOPERATIVE EVALUATION

Perioperative risks depend on the comorbidities of cerebrovascular disease and in patients who have had a stroke, it is important

| TABLE 214.1 | Perioperative Cardiovascular Risks of Surgery | |
|---|---|---|
| **Surgery** | | **Stroke Risk (%)** |
| General surgery | | 0.2 |
| General surgery with or without carotid bruit | | 0.5 |
| General surgery after prior stroke | | 2.9 |
| General surgery with carotid stenosis and bruit or prior symptoms | | 3.6 |
| CABG retrospective studies | | 1.4 |
| CABG prospective studies | | 2.0 |
| CABG surgery after prior stroke or TIA | | 8.5 |
| CABG surgery + valve surgery | | 4.2–13.0 |
| CABG surgery + unilateral >50% carotid stenosis | | 3.0 |
| CABG surgery + bilateral >50% carotid stenosis | | 5.0 |
| CABG surgery + carotid occlusion | | 7.0 |
| Surgery with symptomatic vertebrobasilar stenosis | | 6.0 |

*CABG,* Coronary artery bypass graft; *TIA,* transient ischemic attack.
With permissions from Blacker D, Flemming KD, Link MJ, Brown RD Jr. The preoperative cerebrovascular consultation: common cerebrovascular questions before general or cardiac surgery. *Mayo Clin Proc.* 2004;79:223–229.

to perform and document a baseline neurologic examination. If feasible, patients with a recent stroke should have elective operations postponed to enable the care team to elucidate the cause of the stroke and to initiate therapy, as well as to allow recovery of cerebral blood flow (CBF) autoregulation. It is important for the anesthesia provider to know the patient's preoperative baseline systemic BP, given that chronic hypertension shifts the autoregulation curve to the right, thereby necessitating higher MAP to maintain CBF. Patients with known carotid artery disease are more susceptible to large drops in BP and the perioperative stroke risk is higher in patients with high-grade carotid artery stenosis (70%–99% by ultrasound) and high-grade extracranial/intracranial vessel stenosis or occlusion (Table 214.1).

### INTRAOPERATIVE MONITORING

When a patient is undergoing GA, new-onset neurologic deficits are impossible to recognize until the patient emerges from anesthesia. Therefore to detect ischemia as early as possible, neuromonitoring techniques (e.g., evoked potentials, electromyography, electroencephalography, frontal near-infrared spectroscopy, transcranial Doppler) may be used. Discovery of intraoperative ischemia by neuromonitoring should lead to immediate action to reverse the deficit (e.g., correcting surgical clamping of a carotid artery, increasing MAP, optimizing $O_2$ carrying capacity). The use of inhaled anesthetic agents can lead to reduced CBF in patients with impaired vascular reserve, which can be due to any of the following: large vessel extracranial or intracranial artery stenosis or occlusion, lack of a complete circle of Willis, impaired vascular autoregulation from ischemia, or chronic hypertension with right-shifted autoregulation.

## POSTOPERATIVE MANAGEMENT

The differential diagnosis of postoperative neurologic symptoms include a new cerebrovascular accident, reappearance of previously resolved neurologic deficits from a prior stroke on emerging from anesthesia (often termed "recrudescence"), hypoglycemia, hypotension, seizure with subsequent Todd's paralysis, complicated migraine, hypertensive encephalopathy, and conversion disorder. Differential awakening is a phenomenon that occurs in patients with preexisting impaired vascular reserve of the brain or spinal cord who undergo GA, and in whom focal neurologic deficits are unmasked. These symptoms are transient and typically resolve within 30 minutes in the postoperative period. One possible mechanism is that the pharmacologic effect of GA may linger in the areas affected by prior insult and escape more slowly compared with healthy brain areas. It has also been proposed that previously injured areas might be more sensitive to anesthetic agents or that secondary pathways develop after an insult and might function only in a completely awake state.

Patients with new neurologic deficits postoperatively should receive an emergency neurology consultation while the anesthesia team assesses the patient's $O_2$ carrying capacity (e.g., serum hemoglobin concentration, arterial blood gas analysis), obtains other serologic tests (e.g., glucose, coagulation studies, electrolytes, troponin), and arranges for an immediate noncontrast cerebral CT scan to evaluate for evolving ischemia or hemorrhagic stroke. In patients experiencing an ischemic stroke event, thrombolytic therapy and/or EVT may be appropriate considerations assuming there are no surgical contraindications. The surgical team should be involved in all thrombolytic decisions in the postoperative setting.

In patients given IV thrombolysis, all other antithrombotic agents should be avoided for the first 24 hours. Patients who have intracranial hemorrhage who were therapeutically anticoagulated should have rapid anticoagulation reversal to prevent hematoma expansion. For patients taking warfarin, the international normalized ratio (INR) should be corrected (e.g., INR <1.5) with prothrombin complex concentrate (PCC) or fresh frozen plasma (FFP) in addition to IV vitamin K (10 mg, slow infusion over 30 minutes). The choice between PCC and FFP is largely determined by product availability and patient factors. PCC can increase the risk of subsequent thrombosis, whereas FFP requires a much higher volume to achieve adequate anticoagulation reversal. For patients on direct-acting oral anticoagulants (DOACs), PCC or the specific reversal agent andexanet alfa may be used. Dabigatran can be reversed with idarucizumab or removed with dialysis.

The use of continuous cardiac monitoring or telemetry is advised because of the risk of cardiac arrhythmias and electrocardiographic abnormalities that may occur. Hypotonic fluids should be avoided because of a "leaky" blood-brain barrier and the attendant risks of worsening cerebral edema. In patients with increased ICP who require intubation, coughing, performing the Valsalva maneuver, and excessive straining should be avoided. For management of increased ICP, inducing mild hyperventilation and hypocapnia ($Paco_2$ 30–35 mm Hg) may be used temporarily until definitive neurosurgical intervention (e.g., surgical decompression or placement of an external ventricular drain) or administration of osmotic agents can take place. Generally, hyperventilation should not be continued for prolonged periods because of the risk of cerebral vasoconstriction-related ischemia. A core body temperature of 38.5°C or higher should be treated with antipyretic medications and cooling techniques if needed, to avoid temperature-mediated exacerbations of neurologic injury.

## SUGGESTED READINGS

Cappellari, M., Pracucci, G., Forlivesi, S., Saia, V., Nappini, S., Nencini, P., et al. (2020). General anesthesia versus conscious sedation and local anesthesia during thrombectomy for acute ischemic stroke. *Stroke, 51*(7), 2036–2044.

Connolly, E. S., Jr., Rabinstein, A. A., Carhuapoma, J. R., Derdeyn, C. P., Dion, J., Higashida, R. T., et al. (2012). Guidelines for the management of aneurysmal subarachnoid hemorrhage: A guideline for healthcare professionals from the American Heart Association/American Stroke Association. *Stroke, 43*(6), 1711–1737. doi:10.1161/STR.0b013e3182587839.

Hemphill, J. C., III, Greenberg, S. M., Anderson, C. S., Becker, K., Bendok, B. R., Cushman, M., et al. (2015). Guidelines for the management of spontaneous intracerebral hemorrhage: A guideline for healthcare professionals from the American Heart Association/American Stroke Association. *Stroke, 46*(7), 2032–2060. doi:10.1161/STR.0000000000000069.

Katsanos, A. H., Malhotra, K., Ahmed, N., Seitidis, G., Mistry, E. A., Mavridis, D., et al. (2022). Blood pressure after endovascular thrombectomy and outcomes in patients with acute ischemic stroke: An individual patient data meta-analysis. *Neurology, 98*(3), e291–e301. doi:10.1212/WNL.0000000000013049.

Powers, W. J., Derdeyn, C. P., Biller, J., Coffey, C. S., Hoh, B. L., Jauch, E. C., et al. (2015). 2015 American Heart Association/American Stroke Association focused update of the 2013 guidelines for the early management of patients with acute ischemic stroke regarding endovascular treatment: A guideline for healthcare professionals from the American Heart Association/American Stroke Association. *Stroke, 46*(10), 3020–3035. doi:10.1161/STR.0000000000000074.

Wang, A., & Abramowicz, A. E. (2017). Role of anesthesia in endovascular stroke therapy. *Current Opinion in Anaesthesiology, 30*(5), 563–569. doi:10.1097/ACO.0000000000000507.

Zhang, Y., Jia, L., Fang, F., Ma, L., Cai, B., & Faramand, A. (2019). General anesthesia versus conscious sedation for intracranial mechanical thrombectomy: A systematic review and meta-analysis of randomized clinical trials. *Journal of the American Heart Association, 8*(12), e011754.

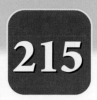

# 215

# Acute Kidney Injury

PATRICK O. MCCONVILLE, MD, FASA  |  ROBERT M. CRAFT, MD

## Incidence, Signs, and Symptoms

Affecting approximately 5% to 10% of all hospitalized patients and up to 50% of critical care patients, acute kidney injury is subcategorized into subclinical and functional categories. Although subclinical acute kidney injury does not result in symptoms commonly associated with acute kidney failure, patient sequelae include increased hospital length of stay and a doubling of mortality. Functional acute kidney injury is manifested in symptoms from failure to eliminate nitrogenous waste products including nausea, confusion, anorexia, asterixis, pericarditis, and pruritus. Systemic edema and dysrhythmias may result from a loss in fluid and electrolyte homeostasis. Additionally, inflammation triggered from acute kidney injury can result in multiple organ system effects. Cardiac and pulmonary dysfunction such as shortness of breath, central nervous system (CNS) symptoms of altered consciousness, and hepatic inflammation resulting in fatigue may all manifest from acute kidney injury.

## Risk Factors

Risk factors for acute kidney injury include patient factors such as chronic kidney disease, diabetes, cardiovascular disease, hypertension, advanced age, and obesity. Autoimmune disorders such as systemic lupus erythematosus, scleroderma, and polyarteritis likewise can result in acute kidney injury. Conditions that reduce renal perfusion such as hypovolemia, sepsis, bleeding, and congestive heart failure increase the incidence of acute kidney injury. Medications including contrast dye, nonsteroidal antiinflammatory drugs, and antibiotics can result in nephrotoxicity. Major surgical cases that results in bleeding, volume shifts, or direct injury increases the risk of acute renal failure and include cardiac, vascular, and trauma surgery.

## Laboratory Analysis

Although timely recognition of acute kidney injury is paramount to prevention of further damage, most signs of clinical manifestations are not apparent until such damage is advanced. Commonly used serum laboratory analysis such as rising blood urea nitrogen or creatinine are delayed, resulting in hours or even days of insult before diagnosis, which limits the ability of clinicians to mitigate sequelae. Research has focused on biomarker identification that are sufficiently sensitive and specific to allow for intervention and treatment before long-term damage occurs. Biomarkers including neutrophil gelatinase-associated lipocalin and kidney injury molecule-1 are molecules released in early renal ischemia that show potential as early identifiers of injury. Continued challenges exist, however, including a lack of sensitivity and availability of point-of-care devices. Tissue inhibitor of metalloproteinases-2

and insulin-like growth factor binding protein-7 likewise continue undergoing investigation as predictive markers of acute kidney injury with encouraging results. Although identification of accurate and timely biomarkers for acute kidney injury appears promising, demonstrating improvements in clinical outcomes remains a challenge to investigators.

## Causes and Treatment

Traditional categories of acute kidney injuries, though conceptually clear, oversimplify the processes that cause perioperative renal disease. The kidneys are autoregulated with the ability to increase or decrease glomerular afferent and efferent flow in response to the hormones prostaglandin and the renin-angiotensin-aldosterone systems. Such autoregulation allows for maintenance of fluid volume both within the glomerulus and in the vascular system as a whole. Disruptions in these processes through low-flow input states, disease or injury of the renal structures themselves from inflammation, or outflow obstructions of various causes can result in a complex interconnected injury to the kidney. Prolonged hypoxic injury to the renal tubules or the glomeruli can then result in collagen deposition and fibrosis resulting in irreversibility of function for these individual nephrons. Rapid recognition of the sources contributing to ischemia of various portions of the nephron and prompt removal of the offending source is the most important treatment to prevent long-term injury.

## Management

Rapid identification of acute kidney injury and prompt treatment are key to limiting damage and further morbidity. Fluid or blood administration and vasoactive medications may support renal perfusion. Treatment of infections with appropriate antibiotics or systemic inflammation with corticosteroids may be needed. Removal of nephrotoxic medications or intravenous hydration before contrast administration may be indicated. In other cases, surgery to remove sources of systemic infection or mechanical obstruction may limit further morbidity. Supportive therapy including dialysis should be instituted in some cases.

## Complications

Although acute kidney injury that results in organ dysfunction directly impairs the ability to maintain normovolemia, electrolyte homeostasis, and acid-base balance, the number of other organ systems affected should be recognized. Kidney injury causes systemic release of cytokines and other inflammatory mediators that affect every major organ system. Increased vascular permeability in the CNS can cause confusion and encephalopathy. Inflammatory hepatic effects can reduce metabolic function of the liver and result in prolonged effects of various medications commonly administered in hospitalized patients. Fluid overload and accumulation of urea can result in cardiac failure in some patients resulting in significant morbidity and mortality. Immune impairment from a reduction in cytokine clearance likewise can cause increases in nosocomial infections.

## SUGGESTED READINGS

Gumbert, S. D., Kork, F., Jackson, M. L., Vanga, N., Ghebremichael, S. J., Wang, C. Y., et al. (2020). Perioperative acute kidney injury. *Anesthesiology*, *132*(1), 180–204.

Haase-Fielitz, A., Bellomo, R., Devarajan, P., Story, D., Matalanis, G., Dragun, D., et al. (2009). Novel and conventional serum biomarkers predicting acute kidney injury in adult cardiac surgery—a prospective cohort study. *Critical Care Medicine*, *37*(2), 553–560.

Huo, W., Zhang, K., Nie, Z., Li, Q., & Jin, F. (2010). Kidney injury molecule-1 (KIM-1): A novel kidney-specific injury molecule playing potential double-edged functions in kidney injury. *Transplantation Reviews (Orlando, FL)*, *24*(3), 143–146.

Jia, H. M., Huang, L. F., Zheng, Y., & Li, W. X. (2017). Prognostic value of cell cycle arrest biomarkers in patients at high risk for acute kidney injury: A systematic review and meta-analysis. *Nephrology (Carlton, Vic.)*, *22*(11), 831–837.

Kashani, K., Al-Khafaji, A., Ardiles, T., Artigas, A., Bagshaw, S. M., Bell, M., et al. (2013). Discovery and validation of cell cycle arrest biomarkers in human acute kidney injury. *Critical Care (London, England)*, *17*(1), R25.

Kork, F., Balzer, F., Spies, C. D., Wernecke, K. D., Ginde, A. A., Jankowski, J., et al. (2015). Minor postoperative increases of creatinine are associated with higher mortality and longer hospital

length of stay in surgical patients. *Anesthesiology*, *123*(6), 1301–1311.

Koyner, J. L., Shaw, A. D., Chawla, L. S., Hoste, E. A., Bihorac, A., Kashani, K., et al. (2015). Tissue inhibitor metalloproteinase-2 (TIMP-2). IGF-binding protein-7 levels are associated with adverse long-term outcomes in patients with AKI. *Journal of the American Society of Nephrology*, *26*(7), 1747–1754.

McIlroy, D. R., Wagener, G., & Lee, H. T. (2010). Biomarkers of acute kidney injury: An evolving domain. *Anesthesiology*, *112*(4), 998–1004.

# 216

# Sepsis and Septic Shock

ONUR DEMIRCI, MD

Sepsis is a complex syndrome involving a host response to an infection. This response in some cases can be exaggerated by endogenous factors and can cause a gamut of tissue damage. The resulting dysfunctions can involve every organ system. Sepsis is the leading cause of death in critically ill patients. In the United States sepsis occurs in 750,000 people every year and results in over 200,000 mortalities. The financial burden of sepsis on the U.S. health system is more than $20 billion per year, which corresponds to over 5% of yearly hospital costs. The incidence of sepsis is increasing, and it is especially common in the elderly. Sepsis is also commonly seen in the perioperative period and is a frequent cause of admission to the surgical intensive care unit.

In 1991, the American College of Chest Physicians and the Society of Critical Care Medicine published consensus-derived definitions of systemic inflammatory response syndrome (SIRS) (Table 216.1), sepsis, and organ failure. In 2001, a list of signs and laboratory findings that should prompt a clinician to consider sepsis in the differential diagnosis was proposed. In addition to tachypnea, tachycardia, and alterations in temperature and white blood cell count, these findings include chills, poor capillary refill, decreased skin perfusion, thrombocytopenia,

| TABLE 216.1 | Systemic Inflammatory Response Syndrome Criteria Based on 1991 Consensus Definitions |
|---|---|
| Two or more of the following:<br>• Temperature >38°C or <36°C<br>• Heart rate >90 beats/min<br>• Respiratory rate >20 breaths/min or Paco$_2$ <32 mm Hg<br>• WBC count >12 × 10$^9$/L or <4 × 10$^9$/L or >10% immature band forms | |

*WBC*, White blood cell.

hypoglycemia, oliguria, alteration in mental status, and skin mottling. After 14 years, a similar task force proposed updated definitions for sepsis and septic shock (Table 216.2). Along with the revised 2015 definitions, this group also acknowledged some weaknesses of the commonly used criteria such as SIRS and severe sepsis, and introduced a bedside clinical score termed qSOFA (quick sepsis-related organ failure assessment) to predict sepsis-related in-hospital mortality (Table 216.3). Because the clinician can now more accurately determine the

| TABLE 216.2 | Third International Consensus Definitions for Sepsis and Septic Shock |
|---|---|
| **Term** | **Definition** |
| Sepsis | Life-threatening organ dysfunction caused by a dysregulated host response to infection.<br>• Clinically: Suspected or documented infection and an acute increase of ≥2 SOFA points. |
| Septic shock | Subset of sepsis in which underlying circulatory and cellular/metabolic abnormalities are profound enough to substantially increase mortality.<br>• Clinically: Sepsis with persistent hypotension requiring vasopressors to maintain MAP 65 mm Hg and having a serum lactate level >2 mmol/L despite adequate volume resuscitation. |

*MAP,* Mean arterial pressure; *SOFA,* sepsis-related organ failure assessment.

| TABLE 216.3 | Quick Sepsis-Related Organ Failure Assessment Score |
|---|---|
| Respiratory rate >22 breaths/min | |
| Altered mentation | |
| Systolic blood pressure <100 mm Hg | |

A patient who meets two out of three qSOFA criteria incurs an overall mortality risk of approximately 10% in a general hospital population with presumed infection. This risk increases to >25% with 3 positive qSOFA criteria.
*qSOFA,* Quick sepsis-related organ failure assessment.

severity of a septic patient's condition using qSOFA, severe sepsis as a term was abandoned.

Since its introduction in the 1991 guidelines, the term *SIRS* has been seen as a precursor to sepsis, and SIRS criteria has been used widely as a screening tool. However, SIRS can occur in the absence of infection and may be secondary to surgical insult, trauma, or inflammatory conditions, such as pancreatitis. Also, although the qSOFA scoring system was initially developed to predict poor outcome, it has become the de facto screening tool since the 2015 SEPSIS-3 definitions. However, since then a plethora of evidence surfaced against its use as a suitable screening tool. Studies have shown that qSOFA is more specific but less sensitive than having two of four SIRS criteria in early sepsis recognition. Updated management guidelines published in 2021 by the Society of Critical Care Medicine (SCCM) and European Society of Intensive Care Medicine (ESICM) acknowledged qSOFA's limitations as a screening tool and recommended against using this scoring system, compared with other commonly used screening tools such as SIRS, National Early Warning Score (NEWS) or Modified Early Warning Score (MEWS) as a single screening tool. Advances in machine learning are already showing superior recognition of hospital acquired sepsis compared with the previously mentioned screening tools and might soon replace them as well.

Sepsis is the result of a complex interaction among the patient's immune, inflammatory, and coagulation systems and an infecting organism. At the site of injury or infection, a local inflammatory response is antagonized by a local antiinflammatory response (Fig. 216.1). Such proinflammatory and antiinflammatory responses often become systemic. Both excessive and inadequate host immune responses can lead to progression of

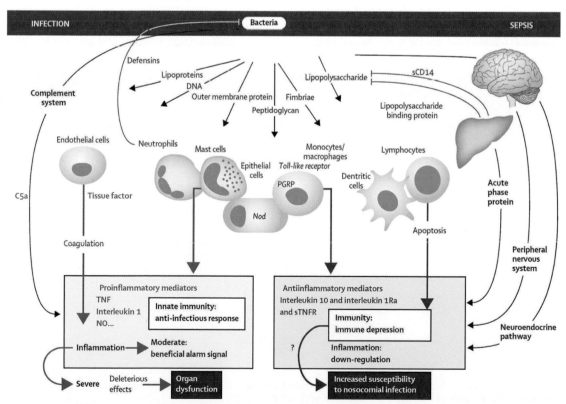

**Fig. 216.1** Mechanisms of disease after bacterial infection. *Barred lines* indicate inhibition; *lines with arrows,* activation or consequences. *C5a,* Complement component 5a; *NO,* nitric oxide; *Nod,* nucleotide-binding oligomerization domain; *PGRP,* peptidoglycan recognition proteins; *sCD14,* soluble CD14; *sTNFR,* soluble tumor necrosis factor (TNF) receptor. (From Annane D, Bellissant E, Cavaillon JM. Septic shock. *Lancet.* 2005;365:63–78.)

disease and organ dysfunction. Further, a highly pathogenic infectious agent may cause organ dysfunction even in the presence of a competent immune system. Neutrophils play a key role in the development of sepsis. An initial toxic stimulus (e.g., bacterial endotoxin) leads to production of proinflammatory cytokines, such as interleukin 1 and tumor necrosis factor. Migration of neutrophils to vascular endothelium subsequently occurs, with concomitant activation of clotting and generation of secondary inflammatory mediators.

Organ system failure as a result of sepsis tends to follow a predictable course, independent of the inciting insult, unless the process is halted by therapeutic interventions. Intravascular volume depletion and vasodilation initially lead to hypotension. The acute respiratory distress syndrome (ARDS) may also occur relatively early. Subsequently, acute kidney injury, ileus, mental status changes, and hepatic dysfunction may occur. As the process continues, direct myocardial depression and bone marrow suppression may develop. The task force consensus also recommended ways of assessing the severity of the organ dysfunction is the use of the SOFA score (Table 216.4). This scoring system can accurately predict the mortality of a septic patient in the ICU based on the degree of dysfunction of six organ systems (respiratory, coagulation, liver, cardiovascular, central nervous, and renal).

Common sites of infection, in descending order of frequency, include the lung, the abdominopelvic region, urinary tract, and soft tissue. In 20% to 30% of patients, a definite site of infection is not identified, and blood cultures may be positive only 30% of the time.

Sepsis is associated with a vasodilated state; intravascular volume depletion results from "third spacing." The classic picture shows a hyperdynamic, high cardiac output state with a low systemic vascular resistance. However, this hemodynamic pattern may be absent in the early stages before adequate volume resuscitation has taken place or when sepsis-associated myocardial depression leads to a decrease in stroke volume.

Septic shock is a medical emergency requiring prompt intervention. Guidelines for management have been developed by a multinational, multidisciplinary collaboration of experts as part of an education initiative known as the Surviving Sepsis Campaign, the latest iteration in 2016. Many institutions have incorporated these therapies into "sepsis bundles" to promote best practice. Suggested algorithms for investigating potential sepsis and managing patients with sepsis are provided in Fig. 216.2. Elements of sepsis management include initial resuscitation, diagnosis, antibiotic therapy, source control, and supportive therapy.

## Initial Resuscitation

Fluid resuscitation and identification of the infection with surgical site control, if possible, are hallmarks of treatment. Large-volume intravenous (IV) fluid resuscitation is often required to reverse organ hypoperfusion. Current guidelines recommend at least 30 mL/kg of IV-balanced crystalloid fluid be given within the first 3 hours. Side effects of normal saline such as hyperchloremic metabolic acidosis have been recognized for a long time. The SMART trial published in 2018 showed lower 30-day mortality in patient receiving saline versus balanced fluids and as such, normal saline should not be used in sepsis resuscitation. In adults, the deficit is often more than 6 L, and further crystalloids and colloids may be administered, preferably according to a protocol. Although the hallmark multicenter SAFE (Saline vs. Albumin Fluid Evaluation) study failed to show a benefit of colloid (albumin) over crystalloid (saline) in most patient populations, more recent studies showed some mortality reduction with albumin administration, especially in the septic shock patients. Therefore the 2021 Surviving Sepsis Guidelines suggest using albumin in addition to balanced crystalloids for initial resuscitation and subsequent intravascular volume replacement in patients with sepsis and septic shock. Use of hydroxyethyl starches and gelatins for fluid resuscitation

| TABLE 216.4 | Sequential (Sepsis-Related) Organ Failure Assessment Score | | | | |
|---|---|---|---|---|---|
| | **SCORE** | | | | |
| **System** | **0** | **1** | **2** | **3** | **4** |
| **Respiration** Pao$_2$/Fio$_2$ (mm Hg) | ≥400 | <400 | <300 | <200 with respiratory support | <100 with respiratory support |
| **Coagulation** Platelets ($10^3$/μL) | ≥150 | <150 | <100 | <50 | <20 |
| **Liver** Bilirubin (mg/dL) | <1.2 | 1.2–1.9 | 2.0–5.9 | 6.0–11.9 | >12.0 |
| **Cardiovascular** | MAP ≥70 | MAP <70 | Dopamine <5 mcg/kg/min or dobutamine (any dose) | Dopamine 5.1–15 mcg/kg/min or epinephrine ≤0.1 mcg/kg/min or norepinephrine ≤0.1 mcg/kg/min | Dopamine >15 mcg/kg/min or epinephrine >0.1 mcg/kg/min or norepinephrine >0.1 mcg/kg/min |
| **Central nervous system** Glasgow Coma Scale | 15 | 13–14 | 10–12 | 6–9 | <6 |
| **Renal** Creatinine (mg/dL) Urine output (mL/day) | <1.2 | 1.2–1.9 | 2.0–3.4 | 3.5–4.9 <500 | >5.0 <200 |

Record worst score every 24 hours. An increase in SOFA score of 1 from baseline in 72 hours after ICU admission is associated with 23% mortality. Similarly, an increase in SOFA score of 2 or more is associated with 42% mortality.

*Fio$_2$,* Fraction of inspired oxygen; *ICU,* intensive care unit; *MAP,* mean arterial pressure; *Pao$_2$,* partial pressure of oxygen; *SOFA,* sepsis-related organ failure assessment.

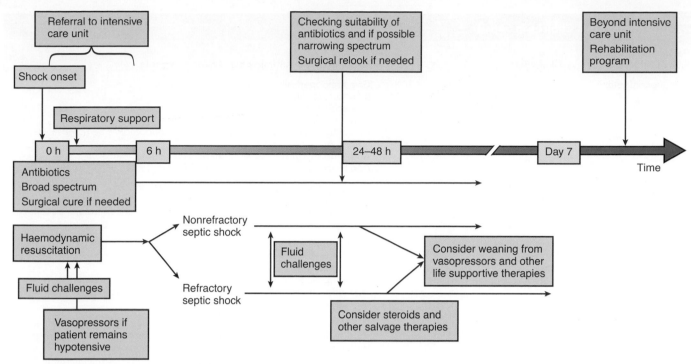

**Fig. 216.2** Principles of the treatment of septic shock. *Pink boxes* refer to interventions; *brackets,* timing of interventions. (Modified from Annane D, Bellissant E, Cavaillon JM. Septic shock. *Lancet.* 2005;365:63–78.)

in sepsis is not recommended due to safety concerns. Arterial and central venous catheters for measuring central venous pressure and venous oximetry are often placed to guide resuscitation. "Early goal-directed" resuscitation has been demonstrated to improve outcomes in septic shock, and since its publication, this has become the usual care. The 2021 Surviving Sepsis Guidelines recommend using dynamic measures such as capillary refill time, leg raising combined with cardiac output measurement, and fluid challenges to increase stroke volume or decrease pulse pressure to guide fluid resuscitation, rather than static measures such as central venous pressure and systolic blood pressure.

Based on Transfusion Requirements In Septic Shock (TRISS) and Protocol-Based Care for Early Septic Shock (ProCESS) trials, red blood cell transfusion for a hemoglobin goal of greater than 10 g/dL is no longer recommended in the absence of certain circumstances, such as myocardial ischemia, severe hypoxemia, or acute hemorrhage. Compared with the current recommendation of restrictive transfusion goal of hemoglobin 7 g/dL, both studies failed to show improved mortality with the previously recommended higher transfusion goal.

Although nonspecific, trending serum lactate, C-reactive protein, and procalcitonin concentrations may be useful in determining resuscitation success.

## Diagnosis

Appropriate cultures should be obtained before antimicrobial therapy is initiated, assuming that performance of such cultures does not significantly delay antibiotic administration. Two sets of blood cultures should be drawn in addition to appropriate cultures of other potential sites of infection. Imaging studies should be performed expeditiously, weighing

the risk of transport, if required, against the potential benefit of the study.

## Antimicrobial Therapy and Source Control

In patients with possible septic shock or a high likelihood of sepsis, empiric combination antibiotic therapy using at least two antibiotics of different antimicrobial classes directed against likely pathogens should be intravenously administered within the first hour of diagnosis. Antimicrobial agents that effectively penetrate into the presumed site of infection should be chosen. The initial therapy should cover a wide spectrum of pathogens, with subsequent daily reassessment based on culture data and clinical response. Given the high incidence of methicillin-resistant *Staphylococcus aureus* (MRSA) in Western countries, in patients with high risk of MRSA, empiric antimicrobials with MRSA coverage should be chosen. Also, based on risk of fungal infection (e.g., immunosuppression, gastrointestinal tract perforation), antifungal coverage should be considered. Antimicrobial options are presented in Table 216.5. Identification of an anatomic site of infection should prompt consideration of intervention to control the source (e.g., drainage of empyema or intraabdominal abscess, debridement of infected necrotic tissue, removal of an infected device).

## Vasopressors and Inotropes

After adequate volume resuscitation, mean arterial pressure should be maintained at a minimum of 65 mm Hg, though preexisting comorbid conditions (e.g., long-standing hypertension) may alter this pressure goal. Surviving Sepsis Campaign recommendations for hemodynamic support are provided in

| TABLE 216.5 | Antimicrobial Choices in Sepsis | |
|---|---|---|
| **Patient Population/ Site of Infection** | **Likely Pathogen** | **Recommended Antimicrobial Agent or Agents** |
| Immunocompetent | Gram-positive Gram-negative | Give ureidopenicillins + one of the following: β-Lactamase inhibitors Carbapenems Third- and fourth-generation cephalosporins Add antipseudomonal fluoroquinolone if *Pseudomonas aeruginosa* is a likely pathogen. Add vancomycin or linezolid if there is concern for MRSA. Add linezolid if there is concern for VRE. |
| Immunocompromised | Gram-positive Gram-negative Fungal | Treat as for an immunocompetent patient, with inclusion of vancomycin or linezolid and antipseudomonal agent. Add antifungal (amphotericin B, caspofungin, or voriconazole) if patient is at high risk for fungal infection. |
| Intravascular catheter-related infections | Gram-positive Gram-negative Fungal | Provide broad-spectrum antimicrobial coverage. In settings with a significant MRSA prevalence, vancomycin should be administered. Add antipseudomonal agent in immunocompromised patients. Add intravenously administered amphotericin B or fluconazole if fungemia is suspected. |
| VAP, HCAP, HAP* | *Streptococcus pneumoniae, Haemophilus influenzae,* MSSA, enteric gram-negative bacilli | In the absence of risk factors that necessitate use of broad-spectrum antibiotics, fluoroquinolone, ampicillin/sulbactam, or ceftriaxone can be given. With recognized risk factors, use antipseudomonal cephalosporin (cefepime, ceftazidime), antipseudomonal carbapenem (imipenem, meropenem), or piperacillin/tazobactam and antipseudomonal fluoroquinolone (ciprofloxacin, levofloxacin) or aminoglycoside. Add vancomycin or linezolid if there is concern for MRSA. Add macrolide or fluoroquinolone if there is concern for *Legionella pneumophila.* |
| Severe community-acquired pneumonia | Typical organisms (*S. pneumoniae, H. influenzae, Staphylococcus aureus*) and atypical organisms (*Mycoplasma pneumoniae, Chlamydia pneumoniae, L. pneumophila*) | Give third-generation cephalosporin and intravenously administered macrolide or nonpseudomonal fluoroquinolone. Give antipseudomonal fluoroquinolone if *P. aeruginosa* is a likely pathogen. |
| Fungal infections | *Candida* spp., *Aspergillus* | Caspofungin, amphotericin B, voriconazole, itraconazole, or fluconazole may be chosen depending on individual patient and organism factors. |

*Certain patients (e.g., those with recent antibiotic therapy, prolonged hospitalization, or immunosuppression or on dialysis) require broad-spectrum antibiotics targeting gram-positive, gram-negative, and atypical organisms, such as *Legionella pneumophila* and MRSA.
*HAP,* Hospital-acquired pneumonia; *HCAP,* health care–associated pneumonia; *MRSA,* methicillin-resistant *Staphylococcus aureus;* *MSSA,* methicillin-sensitive *Staphylococcus aureus; VAP,* ventilator-associated pneumonia; *VRE,* vancomycin-resistant *Enterococcus.*

Box 216.1. Norepinephrine is recommended as the first-choice vasopressor in septic shock. Vasopressin followed by epinephrine may be added when the patient is poorly responsive to the initial choice. Phenylephrine is devoid of β-adrenergic effects and is not recommended as a first-line agent because it is likely to decrease stroke volume. Also, high-dose vasopressin (>0.03 units/min) and phenylephrine should be avoided due to concerns for splanchnic ischemia. Angiotensin II, which works as a vasoconstrictor through the activation of the renin-angiotensin system, has shown physiologic effectiveness in achieving mean arterial pressure goals. However, because of the lack of good-quality evidence, it should not be considered as a first-line agent but might have some usefulness as adjunctive therapy. Based on evidence, short-term administration of vasopressors (<6 hours) via a peripheral route is safe, especially if the access site is distal to the antecubital fossa, and therefore vasopressor administration should not be delayed until central venous access can be obtained. When myocardial dysfunction is suggested by elevated cardiac filling pressures and low cardiac output, additional dobutamine or epinephrine as monotherapy should be administered to attain a normal (though not *supra*normal) cardiac index.

## Corticosteroids

Relative adrenal insufficiency may be a feature of the "endocrinopathy of critical illness." Based on multiple large randomized controlled trials published since 2016 and their metaanalysis, 2021 Surviving Sepsis Guidelines now recommend administration of IV steroids such as 200 mg/day hydrocortisone in divided doses for adults with septic shock who require vasopressors. Systemic corticosteroids have been found to accelerate resolution of shock and increase vasopressor days. However, one should always consider the risk of increased muscle weakness with prolonged steroid administration and taper them off as soon as feasible. Patients who have documented adrenal insufficiency or who are likely to have suppression of the hypothalamic–pituitary–adrenal axis because of long-term steroid use should also receive supplemental IV hydrocortisone during episodes of critical illness.

## Recombinant Human-Activated Protein C

With its antiinflammatory, antithrombotic, and profibrinolytic activities, recombinant human activated protein C (rhAPC)

## BOX 216.1 SURVIVING SEPSIS CAMPAIGN 2021 RECOMMENDATIONS FOR HEMODYNAMIC THERAPY

Balanced crystalloids instead of normal saline should be the initial resuscitation fluid in severe sepsis and septic shock.

Albumin should be added when substantial amounts of crystalloids are required. Hydroxyethyl starches and gelatins are not recommended.

A fluid bolus of 30 mL/kg should be administered in hypoperfusion states with presumed hypovolemia. Fluid challenges should be repeated based on response (change in pulse pressure, stroke volume variation, arterial pressure, heart rate).

Resuscitation should be guided to normalize lactate in patients with elevated lactate levels as a marker of tissue hypoperfusion.

RBC transfusion should only occur when hemoglobin concentration decreases to <7.0 g/dL in adults in the absence of certain circumstances such as myocardial ischemia.

Vasopressor therapy should target a MAP of 65 mm Hg.

Vasopressor therapy should not be delayed to obtain central venous access; peripheral administration of pressors is safe for a limited time.

Norepinephrine is the first-choice vasopressor. Vasopressin followed by epinephrine should be added when an additional agent is needed to maintain MAP.

Dopamine should be used only in highly selected cases. Avoid in patients at risk for arrythmias.

Dobutamine should be added or therapy should be switched to Epinephrine if myocardial dysfunction with signs of hypoperfusion is present despite adequate intravascular volume and MAP.

*MAP,* Mean arterial pressure; *RBC,* red blood cell.

---

was the first drug to target the mechanism of sepsis that appeared to offer a survival benefit. Initial iterations of the Surviving Sepsis Guidelines recommended its careful use in select patient groups; however, further trials such as PROWESS-SHOCK failed to show any effectiveness of rhAPC in septic shock. As more studies were conducted, other safety concerns were demonstrated, and the manufacturer withdrew the product from the market in October 2011.

## Vitamin C

Although the use of IV vitamin C as the last line of therapy in pressor refractory septic shock has become commonplace since the publication of a single-center trial in 2017, further metaanalysis was unable to show an association between vitamin C and reduced mortality. Also, in patients with impaired kidney function, which is common in patients with septic shock, there is an increased risk of oxalate nephropathy and associated renal failure with use of high-dose vitamin C. Therefore the 2021 Surviving Sepsis Guidelines recommend against using IV vitamin C.

## Supportive Therapy

Multiple supportive therapies are often required for patients with sepsis. Noninvasive or invasive mechanical ventilation may be needed for patients with ARDS. When required, sedation should be guided by protocols that target predetermined end points (e.g., sedation scales), with daily interruption or lightening of sedation with awakening and retitration of sedative agents. Neuromuscular blocking agents should be avoided, if possible, to decrease the likelihood of the development of critical illness polyneuromyopathy, although a short (≤48-hour) course of neuromuscular blocking agents is recommended for patients with ARDS and sepsis. Glycemic control in critically ill patients has been the subject of considerable debate, with evolution of target values over the past decade. The NICE-SUGAR (Normoglycemia in Intensive Care Evaluation and Survival Using Glucose Algorithm Regulation) study from 2009 has greatly influenced the Surviving Sepsis Guidelines in this regard. A use of a protocol-based approach is recommended, commencing with intravenously administered insulin when two consecutive blood glucose levels are greater than 180 mg/dL and targeting an upper blood glucose level of 180 mg/dL or less. Stricter blood glucose control (levels of ≤110 mg/dL), as suggested by van der Berghe and colleagues in the Leuven study in 2001, is no longer recommended.

Renal failure is common in patients with septic shock, and renal replacement therapy should be initiated as appropriate. Continuous renal replacement therapy and intermittent hemodialysis are equivalent in patients with severe sepsis and acute renal failure, but continuous techniques may facilitate management of fluid balance in hemodynamically unstable patients.

In addition to the aforementioned therapies, other proven practices (e.g., deep venous thrombosis and stress ulcer prophylaxis, optimal nutrition support) should be used in patients with sepsis.

Unfortunately, septic shock has a mortality rate between 25% and 50%, which is directly related to the number of organ failures. An important aspect of management is communication of likely outcomes to family members or health care surrogates and, when appropriate, consideration for limitation of support.

## SUGGESTED READINGS

Evans, L., Rhodes, A., Alhazzani, W., Antonelli, M., Coopersmith, C. M., French, C., et al. (2021). Surviving sepsis campaign: International guidelines for management of sepsis and septic shock 2021. *Intensive Care Medicine, 47*(11), 1181–1247.

Finfer, S., Bellomo, R., Boyce, N., French, J., Myburgh, J., Norton, R., et al. (2004). A comparison of albumin and saline for fluid resuscitation in the intensive care unit. *New England Journal of Medicine, 350*(22), 2247–2256.

Finfer, S., Chittock, D. R., Su, S. Y., Blair, D., Foster, D., Dhingra, V., et al. (2009). Intensive versus conventional glucose control in critically ill patients. *New England Journal of Medicine, 360*(13), 1283–1297.

Holst, L. B., Haase, N., Wetterslev, J., Wernerman, J., Guttormsen, A. B., Karlsson, S., et al. (2014). Lower versus higher hemoglobin threshold for transfusion in septic shock (TRISS). *New England Journal of Medicine, 371*(15), 1381–1391.

Rivers, E., Nguyen, B., Havstad, S., Ressler, J., Muzzin, A., Knoblich, B., et al. (2001). Early goal-directed therapy in the treatment of severe sepsis and septic shock. *New England Journal of Medicine, 345*(19), 1368–1377.

Russell J. A. (2006). Management of sepsis. *New England Journal of Medicine, 355*(16), 1699–1713.

Semler, M. W., Self, W. H., Wanderer, J. P., Ehrenfeld, J. M., Wang, L., Byrne, D. W., et al. (2018). Balanced crystalloids versus saline in critically ill adults. *New England Journal of Medicine, 378*(9), 829–839.

Singer, M., Deutschman, C. S., Seymour, C. W., Shankar-Hari, M., Annane, D., Bauer, M., et al. (2016). The third international consensus definitions for scpsis and septic shock (Sepsis-3). *JAMA, 315*(8), 801–810.

Sprung, C. L., Annane, D., Keh, D., Moreno, R., Singer, M., Freivogel, K., et al. (2008). The CORTICUS study group: Hydrocortisone therapy for patients with septic shock. *New England Journal of Medicine, 358*(2), 111–124.

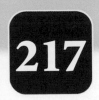

# 217 Anesthesia for Burn-Injured Patients

CHRISTOPHER V. MAANI, MD | PETER A. DESOCIO, DO, MBA, CPE, FASA

## Acute Injury

The first 24 to 48 hours after burn injury is the resuscitation phase. Patients suffering from major burns in excess of 20% to 40% total body surface area (TBSA) often require resuscitation with significant volumes of intravenous fluids (IVF) to maintain intravascular volume and urine output. Although there are several formulas that may guide acute burn resuscitation, hourly IVF goals are best titrated to maintain urine output between 0.5 and 1.0 mL/kg/h. Overresuscitation should be avoided, as it is associated with increased edema and complications such as extremity compartment syndrome, intraabdominal hypertension, respiratory insult, and circulatory overload. During this acute phase, burn patients may require escharotomy and/or fasciotomy to preserve blood flow to extremities and to improve ventilation. Less commonly, a decompressive laparotomy may be required to treat abdominal hypertension. Nonburn injuries, such as those seen in polytrauma patients, may dictate other operative procedures during this early resuscitation phase. During the resuscitation phase, the goal is maintaining organ perfusion as demonstrated by urine output or other goal-directed therapy (e.g., central venous pressure, arterial line, or transesophageal [TEE] or transthoracic [TTE] echocardiograms), rather than volume loading to perceived intravascular euvolemia with little or no objective evidence.

Anesthesiologists may be called on for airway management during this period. For patients with burns as their only injury, less than 40% TBSA burns usually do not require intubation; however, greater than 60% TBSA almost always require intubation. Patients with inhalation injury are at increased risk of intubation regardless of the size of their burn. Generally, intubation should be performed earlier rather than later. The decision to intubate burn patients in the acute setting requires considerable deliberation and clinical judgment. Serial airway exams are required as subtle physical exam clues, such as changes in the quality and character of a patient's voice, may tip the decision. Succinylcholine (SCh) is thought to be safe in the first 48 hours after burn injury. If intubation is delayed until the patient is in respiratory distress, the time remaining before complete ventilatory arrest may be short. Larger endotracheal tubes (ETTs) are preferred because of the frequent need for bronchoscopy and the increased likelihood of plug/clot production associated with mucus, blood, epithelial sloughing, and friable mucosal linings compromised by soot and edema. In emergent situations and especially when there is concern for supraglottic edema making placement of a larger ETT difficult, clinicians may understandably elect to initially secure the airway with a smaller tube. The smaller ETT may then be changed to a larger tube under controlled circumstances.

## Excision and Grafting

Full-thickness burns, unless very small (e.g., <3%–5%), are commonly managed with excision and grafting (E&G).

Partial-thickness burns may also require E&G, or they may be treated nonoperatively depending on depth, size, location, and patient comorbidities. Burn dressings and wound care agents (e.g., Manuka honey, silver-impregnated wound dressings) are in constant development and should be carefully examined for potential anesthetic implications. Silver sulfadiazine (Silvadene) and mafenide acetate (Sulfamylon) are the most used topical salves. For instance, mafenide acetate has been associated with hyperchloremic metabolic acidosis, which may not resolve until the offending agent is withdrawn. Excision of burned skin and placement of dermal grafts (either skin grafts or dermal substitutes) remain the primary objective of burn surgery. Modern-day practice defines excision within 48 hours of injury as early. There is some controversy over the optimal timing for initial surgery, but many burn centers will conduct the first operation within a few days, or even hours, after thermal injury. However, there is no optimal timing for all patients. Likewise, the aggressiveness and extent of initial E&G surgeries is often debated. Some surgeons will restrict the scope of each operation to 20% TBSA excision, 2 L of estimated blood loss, or even 2 hours of operative time. Other surgeons prefer to remove as much, if not all, of the burn as possible on the first procedure.

Excision technique may be either tangential (shaved until unburned tissue is exposed) or fascial (en bloc removal down to the fascial layer, usually by using electrocautery). Tangential excision often produces a better functional and cosmetic result. However, fascial excision is widely considered to be faster and require decreased transfusion owing to less blood loss. Whatever surgical technique the surgeon elects, there is often significant intraoperative blood loss, which may vary from 123 to 387 mL for each 1% TBSA excised. Several factors affect the volume of intraoperative blood loss (Table 217.1). Less blood loss is associated with fascial excisions, fresh burns, more centrally located burns, and tourniquet use on limb burns. Greater degrees of blood loss are typically seen with older burns, infected burns, extremity burns, and comorbidities such as cirrhosis or other coagulopathies. The use of intraoperative sterile tourniquets, medical hemostatic agents (e.g., recombinant-activated Factor VII [rFVIIa], desmopressin, antifibrinolytics such as tranexamic acid), hemostatic sprays such as fibrin glue, thrombin spray, and other topical hemostatic agents may reduce blood loss.

| TABLE 217.1 | Factors Related to Blood Loss in Patients With Burns | |
|---|---|---|
| | **Blood Loss** | |
| **Factor** | **Decreases** | **Increases** |
| Excision technique | Fascial | Tangential |
| Age of burns | Fresh | Older |
| Location of burns | Torso | Hands, feet, or shoulders |

Harvesting of the skin graft may also produce considerable blood loss. This is especially evident when the scalp is harvested. Infiltration of epinephrine solution in the area to be harvested can reduce blood loss and transfusion requirements. Pitkin solution is lactated Ringer solution with 1 to 2 mg of epinephrine per liter. Other combinations of vasoconstrictors in crystalloid solutions are also available and may be equally effective. Postoperatively, most patients report that the donor site (site of graft harvest) is much more painful than the excision site (site of the excised burn injury). Donor harvest sites should be prioritized preoperatively for either neuraxial or peripheral nerve block selection. Of note, most patients are treated with a chemoprophylactic deep venous thrombosis regimen, which should be considered if regional anesthesia techniques are planned.

## Operating Room Setup

For large TBSA burns (i.e., >20%), the room should be heated to greater than 90°F if possible. The patient's entire body may be completely exposed, limiting the utility of both overbody and underbody forced air warming blankets. A rapid infusion system capable of warming and infusing blood at 100 to 200 mL/min should be available for major excisions. Blood should be crossmatched, with 2 to 6 units of red blood cells (RBCs) immediately available. For large excisions with multiple surgeons excising simultaneously, 10 to 20 units of RBCs may be needed within the first 2 to 3 hours. Platelets and plasma may also be required for larger excisions even if the patient's preoperative baseline demonstrates a normal coagulation profile.

## Preoperative Phase

In addition to the standard preoperative evaluation, there are several additional clinical considerations that warrant extra attention in burn patients.

### INTRAVASCULAR ACCESS AND MONITORS

Large-bore peripheral IV is sufficient for most cases less than 20% TBSA; however, a central line often may be required for resuscitations of greater than 20% TBSA burns, especially when vasoactive support is required. A sheath introducer type central line is only needed for the largest TBSA cases. An arterial line can be very useful for larger excisions, both for hemodynamic monitoring ability and the need for serial lab draws. An arterial line may also be indicated if the surgical plan leaves no suitable site for application of a noninvasive blood pressure cuff. Placement of all lines must be made with attention to and coordination with the surgical plan. Catheters are prepped into the surgical field when necessary. Even peripheral IV catheters may be routinely secured with sutures and/or staples, as burn creams or prep solutions can render adhesive tape useless.

### AIRWAY

Patients with burn cream on their faces may pose challenges for mask ventilation due to difficulty obtaining adequate seal. A standard hand towel may be used to give additional traction on the face, and early adoption of two-hand masking techniques should be considered. Tracheostomy management may become an issue when the patient is no longer ventilator dependent, but

removing the tracheostomy tube may make future airway management challenging. Patients may develop problematic burn scar contractures or scarring that limits mouth opening and/or neck extension. Decisions regarding the tracheostomy must be individualized and made as a team.

For patients who will be/remain intubated, the ETT may best be secured with cloth ties (focused on avoidance of venous congestion or vascular compromise); suturing to a tooth is another viable option. Nasal intubation with cloth ties around or through the nasal septum is also quite effective. If suture or umbilical tape is used to tie the oral ETT in place, it is again important to minimize injury related to constriction/tightness of the ties or further swelling of the head and neck.

### PULMONARY

Burn patients routinely have higher than normal minute ventilation. High ventilator pressures and $Fio_2$ requirements combined with nonreassuring arterial blood gas trends indicate respiratory insult and potential difficulty oxygenating or ventilating in the operating room (OR). This is especially concerning if the prone position is planned. The combination of marginal lung performance, clot production, and position changes can result in rapid deterioration and inability to oxygenate and ventilate. Very ill patients may need to remain on an intensive care unit (ICU) ventilator rather than using the anesthesia machine. In this case the anesthetic plan will require total IV anesthetic (TIVA) as most ICU ventilators are not compatible with anesthetic volatile gases. Patients with high ventilator pressures and high inspired oxygen levels may desaturate very rapidly when disconnected even briefly from their ventilator.

### CIRCULATION

Patients who survive their initial injury and shock have essentially passed a physiological stress test. Of note, large burns often result in a rise of serum troponin levels, even in patients who do not have cardiac disease. Burn patients are typically hyperdynamic and may remain so for weeks or months after their injury. Heart rates of 110 to 120 bpm in adults are typical, even in the absence of notable pain. If a patient is hypotensive early in their resuscitation (burn shock), inadequate preload is the common culprit. Later in their course, afterload is more often the cause of hypotension; however, both preload and afterload may be simultaneously compromised.

### NEUROLOGIC

The primary neurologic issue is pain control and sedation. Burn patients often require larger doses of narcotic or sedative drugs and yet remain surprisingly awake. Serial assessments of the patient's level of consciousness and drug doses can facilitate titration of analgosedatives needed to optimize perioperative care.

### NUTRITION

Fasting times should be minimized whenever possible and safe, especially for daily burn dressing changes and wound care. For patients with feeding tubes beyond the pylorus, feeds may be continued until transport to the OR, with controversy whether to stop them at all. The clinical rationale for holding tube feeds in the OR is that these patients frequently are treated with vasoactive medications during and after surgery. This may result in compromised splanchnic circulation and may predispose them to an increased risk for mesenteric ischemia.

## Intra- and Postoperative Phases

Consideration should be given to induction and intubation on the patient's bed if movement (transfer to the OR bed) may be especially painful or harmful for the patient. Monitor placement may be limited by injuries and dressings. Traditional adhesive electrocardiogram (ECG) leads may not adhere well to burn patients but may be stapled in place after induction. Exhaled $CO_2$ monitoring is essential in burn patients. It is a reliable indicator of adequate ventilation and a rough guide to cardiac output. It may be the "perfusion monitor" that is most readily available, most reliable, and least likely to fail in these patients. Alternatively, the most sensitive monitor for guiding intraoperative resuscitation may be real-time echocardiography. At present time, there is insufficient evidence to demonstrate improved patient outcomes, but future studies may demonstrate significant utility of TEE and TTE as a diagnostic tools for perioperative care of burn patients.

Creativity may be needed in placing a pulse oximeter. Other than fingers and toes, the ears, nose, lips, forehead, and hard palate are some of the other common sites that may be successful. Less common sites for oxygen saturation trend monitoring include intrarectal and periscrotal placement when necessary. Core temperature monitoring is typically used because burn patients are more prone to hypothermia. Inability to maintain a temperature of 96.8°F warrants maximum effort to warm the patient and may necessitate aborting the remainder of surgical plans for the day. Indwelling urinary catheters should be used to monitor strict urine output for most cases.

Induction of anesthesia usually involves muscle relaxant drugs. SCh is widely recognized as being contraindicated in burn patients after 48 hours postinjury. SCh is considered safe for the first 24 to 48 hours after a burn; however, some studies suggest this safe period may extend out to 4 to 6 days. Beyond that period and for up to several years after healing, SCh may cause a dramatic and potentially fatal hyperkalemia (hyperkalemic cardiac arrest). Nondepolarizing muscle relaxants are used in burn patients with the understanding that larger and more frequent dosing is required. The exception to that rule is mivacurium, which lasts as long or longer in burned patients as nonburned patients. The introduction of sugammadex for rapid reversal of paralysis from nondepolarizers (especially during rapid sequence intubations) remains the most notable change in current induction considerations. Aside from intubation, muscle relaxants are generally not required during burn surgery.

Burn patients may be resistant or tolerant to opiates. Tachyphylaxis is especially notable when patients are given large doses for several days, but they generally respond normally to the usual induction agents. Another drug response that is altered in burn patients is catecholamines and vasomotor tone. Burn patients often require larger doses of phenylephrine and other vasopressors.

Potent inhalation agents supplemented with opiates work well for most patients. If an IV anesthetic is chosen, propofol (with or without ketamine) supplemented by opiates also works well. For patients with a large or ongoing blood loss, myocardial depression may be compounded by propofol, necessitating that propofol infusions be decreased to very low rates even in well-resuscitated patients. Ketamine has been a traditional choice in burn patients and works well either as a supplement to other IV agents or as the main anesthetic agent. Emergence delirium is seldom an issue in critically ill ICU patients who often remain intubated after surgery and are generally maintained on sedatives for days afterward. Despite its reputation, long-term untoward psychological sequelae have not been documented with ketamine. The addition of dexmedetomidine, either as a bolus or a continuous infusion, may also complement the anesthetic provision of care.

Blood loss during the excision portion may be dramatic, with 1 to 2 L of blood loss in a short period of time. As a general rule, if the patient is hypotensive during intraoperative hemorrhage, initiate RBC transfusion while investigating the cause, especially if they are not responding well to IV fluid challenges and phenylephrine. Choice of crystalloid and/or colloid will vary. At many burn centers, the principle IV fluid is Plasma-Lyte or lactated Ringer solution. Plasma-Lyte is not as acidic as normal saline and is compatible with blood products coadministration. Although some emerging studies suggest avoidance of hydroxyethyl starches (HES) in burn and septic patients (because of the higher risk of renal injury and mortality), there is no clear consensus to contraindicate HES in burn surgery. The need for non-RBC products varies considerably from case to case. Component-based transfusion practices are driven by laboratory values, clinically observed bleeding, and the judgment of the staff involved. Cases involving large blood loss have used rFVIIa occasionally, but at present there is insufficient data to warrant routine use. Base deficit, lactate, and hematocrit guide resuscitative fluid and volume. It is not uncommon to require vasoactive medications to maintain adequate blood pressure and anesthetic tolerance after surgery has begun. Decreased vasomotor tone may be due to the release of bacteria and inflammatory mediators or other burn factors during excision of the wound. Care must be taken to ensure that anemia or lack of preload is not the cause of hypotension before relying on vasopressors to maintain blood pressure.

If severe blood loss outpaces resuscitation during surgery, it may be necessary to have surgeons temporarily cease surgery while the resuscitation catches up. Holding pressure to stop bleeding from excision/harvest sites can be very effective. Epinephrine-soaked lap pads are employed to assist in hemostasis. Barring direct intravascular uptake, patients tend not to show a significant response to epinephrine. Patients may receive several milligrams of subcutaneous epinephrine from Pitkin solution without significant change of heart rate or blood pressure. Despite a long history of use in burn patients, halothane anesthesia may not be desirable in the face of additional epinephrine use because of the risk of ventricular arrhythmias. Thus ongoing research continues to investigate the safety of halothane anesthesia in burn surgery. Of note, halothane is no longer commercially available in the United States, but it remains a viable anesthetic option in certain austere environments such as military deployments and developing nations. For large burn E&G cases, the patient may receive several liters of Pitkin solution, which will be mobilized over the next 24 hours along with IV crystalloids. This volume and the potential for third spacing during fluid equilibration must be taken into account when considering extubation after surgery.

After skin grafts are placed, they may be covered with negative pressure dressings or conventional gauze dressings. At this point, nearing the end of the surgery, protecting the graft from shearing is very important. Smooth emergence and adequate analgesia will help prevent patient movement or combativeness that may shear the grafts. Patients with negative pressure dressings in place should be reconnected to suction without delay.

In the absence of regional anesthesia techniques, patients may require larger analgesic doses to achieve adequate analgesia. Pain control usually requires treatment with opiates. Ketamine infusions may be considered. Meperidine is not used because of the potential for toxic metabolites to accumulate. Methadone has also been used successfully, sometimes when other opiates have failed; although inherent QT prolongation risks warrant serial ECG monitoring.

## Outfield Procedures

Burn patients often require wound care procedures performed in a shower room or hydro-tank. Pain control for removing large adherent dressings or for blunt wound debridement can be challenging. Some patients cannot tolerate their care without more profound acute pain control, inspiring quick onset and short-duration benzodiazepines and opioid analgesic regimens for procedural pain control. Complementary regional anesthesia techniques are also gaining favor. Choosing an anesthetic plan that is familiar and comfortable for the anesthesia provider is probably more important than any particular drug selection. If propofol alone is chosen but inadequate, small doses of ketamine can be added, typically 10 to 20 mg at a time with up to 1 mg/kg cumulative dosing. A newer therapeutic option is dexmedetomidine, the alpha-adrenergic agonist. Typical infusion rates for procedural sedation are 0.2 to 1.4 mcg/kg/h, with or without a loading dose of 1 to 2 mcg/kg. These cases are routinely performed without the need for positive pressure ventilation or supplemental oxygen. When monitoring capability is limited, pulse oximetry and ventilation monitors are emphasized. Exhaled $CO_2$ monitoring can be very reassuring when available. Additional monitors may be considered based on individual patient and procedure issues.

## Electrical Injuries

Electrical injuries are similar to thermal injuries with a few distinctions. There may be extensive underlying tissue destruction beyond the obvious contact point, especially with high-voltage injury. Muscle destruction is common with electrical injury, and monitoring potassium, creatine kinase levels and blood urea nitrogen/creatinine are mandatory for electrical injuries. Patients with electrical injuries are usually monitored in an ICU for 24 hours even with small burns to observe for cardiac arrhythmias. Malignant cardiac arrhythmias are rare. Patients with electrical injury commonly have a superimposed thermal burn injury if the electrical current has ignited their clothing.

## Nonthermal Skin Diseases

Any injury or disease that causes a significant loss of skin may be suitable for admission and treatment in a burn unit. One of the most common disorders is toxic epidermal necrolysis syndrome (TENS). TENS has a reported 30% to 50% mortality. The disease causes a partial-thickness skin injury that may also involve the mucosal membranes. This disease does not usually require skin grafting, but the anesthesiologist may be involved for airway issues. The important thing to consider with TENS is that mucous membranes may slough and collapse into the airway, and manipulation of these friable mucous membranes during airway management may result in significant bleeding. Direct laryngoscopy in a TENS patient may result in bleeding sufficient to totally obscure the view of the airway. The first attempt at laryngoscopy may provide the only good view, and fiberoptic bronchoscopy may be difficult or impossible afterward. TENS patients may also produce mucoepithelioid plugs that can acutely completely obstruct ETT lumens.

## Conclusion

Providing anesthesia service to burn patients requires detailed knowledge of and deliberate preparation for some specific issues. With proper planning and close coordination alongside the rest of the burn care team, these cases can be performed smoothly and safely. Burn patients often return to the OR multiple times over the course of weeks to years. This provides an opportunity for continuity that anesthesiologists seldom get with other patients, as well as the satisfaction of seeing patients progress from critically ill to recovered and functional.

## SUGGESTED READINGS

Bittner, E. A., Shank, E., Woodson, L., & Martyn, J. A. (2015). Acute and perioperative care of the burn-injured patient. *Anesthesiology, 122*(2), 448–464.

Guilabert, P., Usúa, G., Martín, N., Abarca, L., Barret, J. P., & Colomina, M. J. (2016). Fluid resuscitation management in patients with burns: Update. *British Journal of Anaesthesia, 117*(3), 284–296.

Romanowski, K. S., Carson, J., Pape, K., Bernal, E., Sharar, S., Wiechman, S., et al. (2020). American Burn Association guidelines on the management of acute pain in the adult burn patient: A review of the literature, a compilation of expert opinion, and next steps. *Journal of Burn Care & Research, 41*(6), 1129–1151.

Sheckter, C. C., Stewart, B. T., Barnes, C., Walters, A., Bhalla, P. I., & Pham, T. N. (2021). Techniques and strategies for regional anesthesia in acute burn care: A narrative review. *Burns & Trauma, 9,* tkab015.

Wolf, S. E., Kauvar, D. S., Wade, C. E., Cancio, L. C., Renz, E. P., Horvath, E. E., et al. (2006). Comparison between civilian burns and combat burns from Operation Iraqi Freedom and Operation Enduring Freedom. *Annals of Surgery, 243*(6), 786–795.

# SECTION XIII

# Risk Management

# Medical Ethics

ELLEN C. MELTZER, MD, MSc   |   TIMOTHY J. INGALL, MB BS, PhD

Medical ethics is a fundamental part of medical practice and serves to provide a framework for systematically approaching ethical problems that arise in clinical care. Medical ethics has been an integral part of the practice of medicine for ages. Perhaps the most famous code of ethics is the Oath of Hippocrates, which includes many of the principles that still guide the modern-day physician. As modern medical practice has evolved, many ethical dilemmas have become manifest because of advances in technology. This has forced a rapid evolution in medical ethics from the relatively simplistic codes that have guided the "virtuous" physician for centuries to a clinical practice that can be applied at the bedside. Accordingly, medical ethics is now a fundamental part of clinical care and serves to provide a framework for systematically approaching ethical problems that arise in clinic care. This chapter offers a brief review of the principles of medical ethics and explores ethical issues relevant to anesthesia providers.

## Principles of Medical Ethics

The principles of autonomy, beneficence, nonmaleficence, and justice, expounded on at length by Beauchamp and Childress, are cornerstones of current ethical writings.

### AUTONOMY

Autonomy is derived from the Greek root words *autos* (self) and *nomos* (rule, governance, or law). Autonomy is a key component of contemporary Western medical ethics and is evident through such practices as informed consent and informed refusal, whereby capacitated patients have the right to make their own medical decisions. The courts and medical ethicists have long agreed that patients with the capacity to understand the consequences of their actions have the right to accept or reject medical care, including "life-saving" care.

### BENEFICENCE

Beneficence is an obligation to help others further their important and legitimate interests. This requires the removal of harm as well as the provision of benefit, often expressed clinically through a consideration of proportionality. Proportionality is a consideration of the benefits and burdens of a proposed intervention. In general, efforts are made to maximize benefit while minimizing potential harm or burden.

### NONMALEFICENCE

Nonmaleficence is an obligation not to inflict harm on others. It is clearly associated with the maxim *primum non nocere:* "above all, do no harm." The Hippocratic Oath addresses the

duty to promote nonmaleficence and beneficence with the statement, "I will use treatment to help the sick according to my ability and judgment, but I will never use it to injure or wrong them."

### JUSTICE

Justice in medical ethics considers fair and equitable distribution of medical resources. Advocating for an individual patient is but one example of justice in clinical care; this principle extends far beyond the bedside to larger, systemic societal issues that affect medical care. With the COVID-19 pandemic, justice became a fundamental, guiding principle in determining how best to proceed when presented with a shortage of clinical resources.

One should be cognizant that approaching an ethical challenge through the lens of any one of these principles may lead to a dramatically different, and yet equally "ethical," solution. Accordingly, rather than simply relying on principles to determine a best course of action, a systematic process for approaching clinical ethics cases is advised.

## A Method of Resolving Ethical Challenges in Clinical Care

As proposed by Jonsen and colleagues, and outlined only briefly here, an ethically challenging situation can be approached in much the same way as any clinical concern. Anesthesiologists faced with an ethical challenge should consider requesting an ethics consultation to assist with this process. The familiar chief complaint, history of the present illness, past medical history, and review of systems are obtained. In addition, contextual and historical features are considered. Ethical features of a clinical case include (1) medical indications, including the patient's diagnosis if known, current clinical recommendations for evaluation and management, and likely prognosis or outcomes depending on the pursued course of action; (2) patient preferences, including the patient's current expressed wishes, as well as their historical approach to medical care and medical decision-making; (3) quality-of-life consideration from the perspective of the patient; and (4) the contextual features surrounding the case, such as social, economic, legal, and administrative features. Systematically examining this information often serves to reveal an initial course of action. Follow-up and revision to the ethical plan of care, as needed, are advised.

## When Patients Lack Capacity

Adult patients generally make decisions for themselves, unless they lack capacity or defer decision-making to another person. When adult patients lack capacity, clinical teams will turn to advance directives and appointed medical powers of attorney, also called health care agents, for assistance with medical decisions. Reflecting growing societal interest and concern brought about by court decisions in so-called right-to-die cases, such as that of Nancy Cruzan, Congress enacted the Patient Self-Determination Act in 1991 to increase the use of advance directives. Advance directives include durable powers of attorney for health care and living wills. Durable powers of attorney for health care, also called health care proxy documents, serve to appoint a person (often a spouse, adult child, relative, or close friend) to make medical decisions should a patient lack capacity. Living wills are mechanisms for patients to provide specific directives for medical care, in advance, to be used if they ever lack capacity. In the absence of an appointed decision-maker, living wills have limitations, as their terms can be hard to define and interpret. Furthermore, one's preferences for medical care might understandably change over the various stages of an illness, but the living will might not be updated to reflect and communicate these new wishes. Thus patients are always advised to appoint an agent, preferably someone who has knowledge of the patient's wishes and preference for medical care, who can work with the medical team and help make decisions.

If a patient lacks capacity and does not have a designated agent, then clinical teams must identify a surrogate, or alternate decision-maker. States vary with respect to establishing a priority order for surrogate decision-makers, and anesthesiologists should be aware of local governance. There is an ethical approach for working with surrogate decision-makers. In general, surrogate decision-makers are ethically obligated to promote an incapacitated patient's autonomy by making medical decisions based on the patient's own previously expressed capacitated preferences for medical care, whether documented in an advance directive, written in the medical record, or known from prior personal conversations about this sensitive topic. If there are no specific prior, expressed wishes, then substituted judgment is used, whereby surrogates are asked to make decisions based on their knowledge of the patient and what the patient would likely decide. In the absence of knowledge regarding patients' wishes or preferences, the best-interest standard should be employed, and surrogates should be counseled to make decisions that are in a patient's best interest. For children (<18 years of age), as well as for adults who have never been capacitated, decision-making can be more complicated. Again, decisions should be made that are in the best interest of the patient and should maximize benefit while minimizing harm. In general, parents may not refuse potentially life-saving interventions on behalf of their minor children, unless a terminal diagnosis and poor prognosis argue in favor of a palliative approach to care. It is advised that anesthesiologists faced with ethical challenges related to the care of minors consult their hospital ethicist for additional assistance and guidance.

## Patient Refusal of Blood Products

Anesthesiologists often question how to proceed when a patient refuses potentially life-saving blood products, which many Jehovah's Witnesses prefer to forgo. The American Society of Anesthesiologists (ASA) has developed Guidelines for the Anesthesia Care of Patients with Do-Not-Resuscitate Orders or Other Directives that Limit Treatment that can inform practice. An adult patient of sound mind (i.e., capacitated) legally has the right to refuse blood products even if this could cause significant morbidity or mortality. Parents or guardians, however, do not have the legal right to refuse potentially life-saving blood products on behalf of their minor children. *Prince v. Commonwealth of Massachusetts,* 321 U.S. 158 (1944), was a Supreme Court case that served to establish that parents do not have the absolute right to refuse medical care on behalf of their children based on religious objections, particularly if the refusal could result in harm to the minor child. Difficulties can arise when an older adolescent Jehovah's Witness (<18 years of age) is faced with the prospect of needing blood products and expresses a refusal. Anesthesiologists are advised to seek ethical and legal guidance to ensure appropriate management of the minor adolescent patient should this conflict arise. It must be noted that not all Jehovah's Witnesses approach decisions regarding blood products uniformly. It is imperative that all patients be given the opportunity to speak confidentially with their health care providers about the risks and benefits of blood products, to have all their questions answered, and to be empowered to decide privately, autonomously, and free from coercion whether to accept or refuse blood products. When it comes to operating in the context of a refusal of blood products, anesthesiologists similarly have agency. Anesthesiologists who feel that the risks of surgery in this context outweigh the potential for benefit should discuss their concerns with the surgical team and consider an ethics consultation.

## Do Not Resuscitate in the Operating Room

Ethical questions arise when a patient who has a Do Not Resuscitate (DNR) designation is planning for surgery. How does one proceed? Should the DNR be continued, or should it be automatically rescinded for the perioperative period? The American College of Surgeons recommends a policy of "required reconsideration," through which the DNR designation is discussed with the patient, or their surrogate decision-maker, as a part of the informed consent process. This should include a discussion about the risks and benefits of surgery and anesthesia. As anesthesiologists and surgeons generally prefer to have consent to provide resuscitation to treat *reversible* causes of cardiopulmonary arrest that can develop in the perioperative period, it is imperative that the entire clinical team be aware of the patient's preferences in advance and that any conflict be addressed. In situations in which honoring patient autonomy would create an ethical conflict for the treating anesthesiologist, consideration should be given for consulting ethics and potential transfer of the patient to another physician. The ASA provides additional guidance for the ethical care of patients with DNR orders or other directives that limit treatment.

## Conclusion

Anesthesiologists face many ethical challenges in clinical care, by virtue of their scope of practice extending far beyond the operating room to virtually every setting in clinical care, including the intensive care unit, obstetrics and gynecology, pediatrics, and pain management.

Anesthesiologists are uniquely positioned to identify ethical challenges that exist or may be at risk for developing. Ethics consultation can support these efforts and provide a systematic approach and help all involved parties, patients, family members, and the clinical team determine an appropriate course of action.

## SUGGESTED READINGS

American College of Surgeons. (2014). Statement on advance directives by patients: "Do not resuscitate" in the operating room. *Bulletin of the American College of Surgeons*, 99(1), 42–43.

American Society of Anesthesiologists. (2018). *Ethical guidelines for the anesthesia care of patients with do-not-resuscitate orders or other directives that limit treatment*. Retrieved from Ethical-guidelines-for-the-anesthesia-care-of-patients. pdf. Accessed November 18, 2021.

Ivascu, N. S., & Meltzer, E. C. (2018). Teacher and trustee: Examining the ethics of experiential learning in transesophageal echocardiography education. *Anesthesia and Analgesia*, 126(3), 1077–1080.

Jonsen, A., Siegler, M., & Winslad, W. (2006). *Clinical ethics: A practical approach to ethical decisions in clinical medicine* (6th ed.). New York: McGraw-Hill.

Mason, C. L., & Tran, C. K. (2015). Caring for the Jehovah's witness parturient. *Anesthesia and Analgesia*, 121(6), 1564–1569.

Meltzer, E. C., Shi, Z., Suppes, A., Hersh, J. E., Orlander, J. D., Calhoun, A. W., et al. (2017). Improving communication with surrogate decision-makers: A pilot initiative. *Journal of Graduate Medical Education*, 9(4), 461–466.

Swetz, K. M., Burkle, C. M., Berge, K. H., & Lanier, W. L. (2014). Ten common questions (and their answers) on medical futility. *Mayo Clinic Proceedings*, 89(7), 943–959.

Waisel D. (2007). Physician participation in capital punishment. *Mayo Clinic Proceedings*, 82(9), 1073–1082.

West, J. M. (2014). Ethical issues in the care of Jehovah's Witnesses. *Current Opinion in Anaesthesiology*, 27(2), 170–176.

Woolley, S. (2005). Children of Jehovah's Witnesses and adolescent Jehovah's Witnesses: What are their rights? *Archives of Disease in Childhood*, 90(7), 715–719. doi:10.1136/adc.2004.067843.

# 219

# Medicolegal Principles: Informed Consent

## J. ROBERT SONNE, JD, BA

Informed consent is the process of providing sufficient information to the patient or surrogate decision-maker to allow that patient or surrogate decision-maker to fully participate in respective decisions regarding medical care. This process includes securing authorization from the patient or surrogate decision-maker for any proposed surgical or significant diagnostic treatment or procedure.

Along with the moral and ethical obligations that are involved in obtaining informed consent, there are also associated legal requirements. Various state, federal, and accreditation (e.g., The Joint Commission) statutes, regulations, and guidelines govern and address the legal parameters of the informed-consent process. In addition to general process requirements, legal proscriptions often dictate specific informed-consent provisions for certain treatment or diagnostic procedures (e.g., HIV/AIDS testing). Investigation into specific state and federal law on informed consent is encouraged.

In situations in which patients have filed lawsuits, central questions often arise as to whether the anesthesia provider acted within the limits of the patient's consent and whether the patient was given sufficient information to adequately consent to the proposed treatment or diagnostic procedure. Such lawsuits are generally brought under negligence or battery theories.

## The Informed-Consent Process

Informed consent for anesthesia often occurs when the patient and anesthesia provider meet moments before the surgical procedure is scheduled to begin. For anesthesia providers, the informed-consent process should occur before administration of preprocedure sedation and generally should include a discussion of the elements outlined in Box 219.1. It is largely impractical to discuss all associated risks related to a specific anesthesia treatment or procedure. Thus in determining what relevant risks to discuss, the physician should consider covering those procedure or treatment risks that are most common and most severe. In defining how much information a physician should disclose, there are two dominant standards. The "professional" standard holds that the anesthesia provider must disclose information that other anesthesia providers possessing the same skills and practicing in the same or similar community would disclose in a similar situation. The "materiality" standard considers what a reasonable patient would have considered important in making a decision.

---

**BOX 219.1 ELEMENTS TO BE DISCUSSED BY THE PATIENT AND ANESTHESIA PROVIDER DURING THE PREOPERATIVE VISIT**

The patient's diagnosis
The nature and purpose of the proposed anesthesia treatment or procedure
The relevant risks and benefits of the proposed anesthesia treatment or procedure
The relevant risks and benefits of reasonable alternatives (including no treatment) to the proposed anesthesia treatment or procedure

During the informed-consent discussion, the anesthesia provider is encouraged to ask patients if they have questions or other concerns about the proposed treatment or procedure. Good communication is often an effective deterrent against future patient complaints and legal claims. During this process, the patient also is generally asked to review and sign a written informed-consent form before the proposed surgical or significant diagnostic treatment or procedure. Whether a signed written informed-consent form is warranted may vary based on applicable state, federal, and accreditation statutes, regulations, or guidelines (e.g., see Center for Medicaid Services Conditions of Participation guidelines). Informed-consent forms generally list the specific procedure or treatment to be performed and may include specific risks, complications, or alternatives. Such forms also may include language indicating that not all discussed risks, complications, or alternatives are expressly listed in the form. Overall, the informed-consent form serves as valuable evidence that the informed process occurred and that the patient consented to the recommended treatment or procedure.

As noted previously, good documentation is effective in preventing and defending complaints and legal claims. Consequently, anesthesia providers are additionally encouraged to timely dictate or otherwise enter a note into the medical record (independent of the signed informed-consent form) that substantiates that the informed-consent discussion occurred. In preparing this note, the anesthesia provider should consider listing the most significant discussed risks and alternatives and should expressly note the patient's consent and election to proceed.

## Obtaining Informed Consent When Treating the Incompetent or Minor Patient

If the patient is unable to make their own health care decisions or is a minor (underage), an appropriate surrogate decision-maker most likely needs to be consulted to make decisions and consent to the patient's care and treatment.

If the patient is an incompetent adult, informed consent is generally obtained from the patient's legal guardian or health care power of attorney. If the patient does not have either a legal guardian or a health care power of attorney, state laws often provide a priority list of surrogate decision-makers. These state statutes usually provide highest priority to spouses and then proceed to other family members (e.g., adult children, parents, siblings, grandchildren) and individuals (e.g., domestic partners, close friends). If no surrogate decision-maker is available or willing to provide informed consent, some state statutes allow attending physicians to make and consent to health care decisions. This form of consent, however, is typically only permitted after additional approval is obtained from a hospital ethics committee or a second physician.

If the patient is a minor, informed consent is usually obtained from the patient's parents or legal guardian, with assent obtained from the minor, if possible. In certain circumstances, however, a minor may consent without approval from a parent or legal guardian. For example, some states may allow a minor to independently consent to their own care if the minor is emancipated, married, in the U.S. military service, or homeless. In addition, states may allow a minor to independently consent to care related to sexually transmitted diseases, substance abuse treatment, HIV testing, contraception, abortion, or sexual assault. Anesthesia providers are encouraged to review applicable state law for consent exceptions for minors.

## Obtaining Informed Consent in Emergent Circumstances

If the anesthesia provider determines that an emergency exists, informed consent is not required to undertake surgical or significant procedures that are necessary to treat or diagnose the patient's emergent condition. When informed consent is not obtained because the circumstances are emergent, the physician should document the circumstances that support the emergency.

## SUGGESTED READING

Paterick, T. J., Carson, G. V., Allen, M. C., & Paterick, T. E. (2008). Medical informed consent: General considerations for physicians. *Mayo Clinic Proceedings, 83*(3), 313–319.

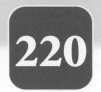

# 220

# Medicolegal Principles: Medical Negligence

J. ROBERT SONNE, JD, BA

A medical negligence or malpractice lawsuit is a civil action commenced by a patient or an authorized representative of the patient seeking monetary damages for injuries claimed to have resulted from negligent treatment. Medical negligence is the most common threat of liability faced by physicians in the United States.

## Elements of Malpractice Actions

A patient is entitled to recover monetary compensation from a physician if the patient can prove that the physician's conduct was below the standard of care and that the conduct caused the patient's injury. It is not enough that the patient suffered a complication or was injured as a result of medical care. The patient must show that the medical care provided by the physician was below the standard of care.

To prevail in a lawsuit, the patient has the burden of proving that a deviation from the standard of care occurred and that the injury was directly caused by that deviation. In most cases, a preponderance of the evidence must support the allegations, and proof must be to a "reasonable degree of medical certainty." To prove deviation from the standard of care, it must be shown that an anesthesiologist failed to use that amount of care and skill commonly exercised by other anesthesiologists with similar training and experience under the same circumstances. Physicians should not be found negligent if they elect to pursue one of several recognized courses of treatment, provided that a respectable number of physicians accept the course of treatment. In addition, reasonable medical judgment, even if in error, should not be considered negligence.

Most often, expert testimony establishes the applicable standard of care. A physician sued for medical malpractice has the right to a jury trial. Because jurors are usually unable to independently evaluate whether medical care is appropriate, physicians and experts explain the medical issues to assist the jury in reaching a conclusion. The expert witness generally has credentials and experience like those of the physician on trial and testifies as to whether the physician acted in accordance with the accepted standards of care. The stringency of the rules on expert qualifications varies by state.

The standard of care may also be established by a variety of other means, including medical treatises or guidelines written by professional organizations, policies of the hospital in which care was provided, and recommendations of drug and device manufacturers. Out-of-court statements by physicians (such as statements to the patient or other colleagues) or documents may constitute admissions against interest and may also be introduced as evidence of a deviation from the standard of care.

If a deviation from the standard of care can be proved, some type of injury must also be proved. Generally, at least some physical injury is necessary. Damages may be awarded to compensate for lost income, past or future medical expenses, and other, less tangible elements of an injury, such as pain and suffering and embarrassment.

Finally, a patient must prove that the physician's deviation from the standard of care proximately caused injury and that the injury was not caused by an underlying disease process. A physician's negligent conduct may be a legal cause of harm if it is a substantial factor in bringing about the injury.

## Types of Claims Against Anesthesia Personnel

The Anesthesia Quality Institute's Closed Claims Program provides important information about the types of claims against anesthesia personnel. The Program, initiated in 1984 as the Closed Claims Project, collects information from insurance companies about closed claims related to events leading to anesthesia-related injury. Numerous references have been published from the data about specific types of anesthetic injuries and resultant malpractice claims, giving a broad-based rather than an anecdotal picture. In general, the types of injuries that result in malpractice claims against anesthesia personnel include dental injury, nerve injury, and death or brain injury caused by either respiratory or cardiac events.

## Lack of Informed Consent

Courts have long recognized that patients have a right to consent to medical treatment. (For more information on informed consent, see Chapter 219, Medicolegal Principles: Informed Consent.) A patient may allege that no consent was given for a procedure and may seek damages for battery. More often, however, patients allege lack of informed consent or negligent nondisclosure. A physician has a legal obligation to advise the patient of certain risks and benefits associated with medical care, as well as available alternatives. Liability may be based on whether the physician failed to disclose a risk that should have been disclosed and whether that risk occurred.

## The Process

Medical malpractice lawsuits are formally commenced by filing or service of a summons and complaint. Notification of the claim may occur before formal commencement of a lawsuit and may come in the form of a letter or formal notice. Both individuals and corporations may be named as defendants. The lawsuit must be commenced within the statute of limitations, a time period that varies by state. If the lawsuit continues, pretrial discovery occurs in the form of either depositions or written documentation. A relatively small percentage of cases are tried; most are either settled or dismissed. If a trial occurs, a jury is generally charged with determining the facts, and the presiding judge is responsible for determining the applicable law.

## Managing Legal Risk

Practicing within accepted standards is the best defense against malpractice liability. Good communication among health care providers and with the patient is critical. Documentation is an essential part of a risk management strategy and should be comprehensive, accurate, objective, and timely. Inadvertent admissions against interest should be avoided. The most common forms of admissions against interest are self-criticism or criticism of colleagues after an adverse outcome and speculation about the cause of an event before all the facts are known. Guidelines and policies should be realistic and written to allow for emergencies and physician discretion.

## SUGGESTED READINGS

Anesthesia Quality Institute. *Closed claims project.* Retrieved from https://www.aqihq.org/ACCMain.aspx. Accessed March 17, 2022.

Cheney, F. W., Posner, K. L., Lee, L. A., Caplan, R. A., & Domino, K. B. (2006). Trends in anesthesia-related death and brain damage: A closed claims analysis. *Anesthesiology, 105*(6), 1081–1086.

Choctaw, W. (2008). *Avoiding medical malpractice: A physician's guide to the law.* New York: Springer.

Sandnes, D. L., Stephens, L. S., & Posner, K. L. (2008). Liability associated with medication errors in anesthesia: A closed claims analysis. *Anesthesiology, 109,* A770.

# 221

# Anesthesia Quality Registries

PATRICK J. MCCORMICK, MD, MEng  |  KATHERINE WOCHOS, MPPA, CAE (past)

## Genesis of Anesthesia Quality Registries

An anesthesia quality registry is an organized system that collects observations in a secure, uniform, structured manner to improve understanding of patient outcomes after anesthesia care. Registries are the primary method by which anesthesiologists can move from anecdote to data and demonstrate their value to patients undergoing surgery or other procedures that require anesthesia.

Initial efforts to identify patterns in adverse anesthetic outcomes focused on critical incidents. A critical incident is a significant occurrence that leads to a desirable or undesirable outcome. Critical incident reporting is a mainstay of industries that put people at risk, such as aviation, railroads, and nuclear power. In 1978, Cooper and colleagues published the results of critical incident analysis applied to anesthesia, finding that the major cause of these incidents was human error (Cooper, Newbower, Long, & McPeek, 1978). Since then, multiple anesthesia incident registries have been founded in different countries. Some registries, such as the Australia/New Zealand anesthetic incident reporting system, started on paper and have since transitioned to internet-based entry.

The intent is for all incidents to be reported, not just ones that lead to a disastrous outcome. The Agency for Healthcare Research and Quality has developed a set of Common Formats for Event Reporting, which can be used for incidents, near misses, or unsafe conditions. An incident is one that reaches the patient; a near miss does not reach the patient; and an unsafe condition is one that increases the likelihood of an incident. For each incident, the reporter is asked to determine the level of harm from no harm to death, and the duration of harm. The common formats also provide a structured method to collect information about who was involved, where the incident occurred, and what contributing factors were at play. Contributing factors include everything from equipment problems to communication difficulty to production pressure.

Another type of registry is the clinical quality registry (CQR). A CQR is designed to provide feedback to health care providers about the quality of care that is delivered. This type of registry includes data about all patient encounters that may be included in the denominator of one or more quality measures. The breadth of data collected allows a CQR to generate compliance rates with process measures and outcome measures.

The American Society of Anesthesiologists (ASA) has made quality measurement a core part of the organization's mission. In October 2008, the ASA created a related organization to facilitate practice-level quality measurement called the Anesthesia Quality Institute (AQI). The remainder of this chapter will explore the quality registries maintained by the AQI.

## The Anesthesia Closed Claims Program

One of the first comprehensive anesthesia incident registries was the Anesthesia Closed Claims Program. The Closed Claims Project was started in 1985 by the ASA in collaboration with malpractice insurance providers to identify common themes in closed malpractice claims against anesthesiologists. After almost 40 years of practice-changing findings, it is apparent that the benefits of this registry will continue. The Project is now referred to as the Closed Claims Program and has been moved to the AQI.

The Closed Claims database is curated by specially trained board-certified anesthesiologists who review selected records at participating medical liability insurance companies. The primary limitation of the database is that malpractice claims constitute only a tiny fraction of all patient injuries due to negligence, estimated at 3% to 4%.

The database is a rich source of uncommon adverse outcomes that has contributed to major changes in anesthesia practice. As of December 2021, the Program has 11,773 claims. Fig. 221.1 shows the breakdown of case types. The majority are surgical (72%), followed by obstetric (12%), chronic pain

(11%), and acute pain (4%). Fig. 221.2 shows the complications documented in the claims. Death resulted in 3485 claims, and severe brain damage in 1141.

In 1990, the project published findings that respiratory adverse events accounted for the majority of death or brain damage claims in the 1970s and 1980s. This finding, along with the increased availability of advanced monitors, led the ASA to adopt pulse oximetry as a standard intraoperative monitor. In 2011, the ASA adopted capnography as a standard monitor for monitored anesthesia care.

Another area where the Closed Claims Project drove improvement is operating room (OR) fires. The Emergency Care Research Institute estimated that OR fires occurred 600 times a year in 2009, but now that number has been reduced to 90 to 100 times a year. Closed Claims research found that 90% of fire claims were due to electrocautery, and most cases involved monitored anesthesia care for upper chest, neck, and head procedures.

Despite advances in technology and training, the number of closed claims where the patient suffers death or brain damage remains above 25%. Situational awareness (SA) errors are a contributor to these incidents. An SA error is defined as a failure to perceive data, integrate that data, or project future trends. A study of cases from a German critical incident reporting system found that 81.5% involved an SA error. A 2017 Closed Claims analysis by the same author found that SA errors contributed to death or brain damage in 74% of those claims.

Communication is another anesthesiologist responsibility where failures are known to be associated with critical incidents. In a 2021 Closed Claims study using claims from 2004, communication failure was a contributor to injury in 43% of claims. Failure in content (inaccurate or insufficient information transmitted) were responsible for 60% of failures.

The Closed Claims project generates new studies every year covering many areas of anesthetic practice, some of which have changed the standard of care.

## Anesthesia Incident Reporting System

In 2011, the AQI introduced an anesthesiology-specific registry for critical incidents open to any practitioner in the United

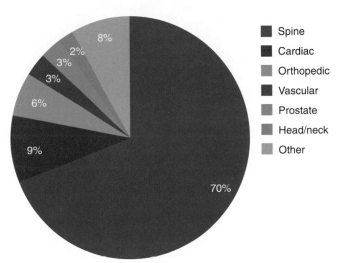

**Fig. 221.1**  Types of claims in the Closed Claims database.

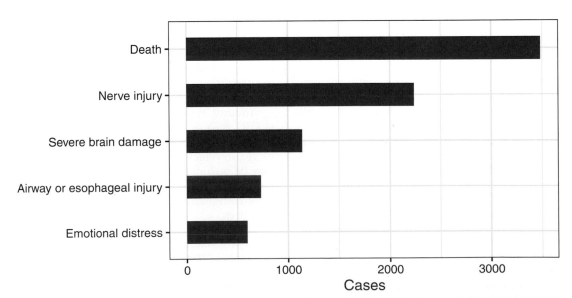

**Fig. 221.2**  Complications documented in the Closed Claims database. Note that a single case may have multiple complications.

States. This registry is known as the Anesthesia Incident Reporting System (AIRS). Because AQI is a federally listed Patient Safety Organization (PSO), the submitted reports are protected by federal law from legal discovery. This federal protection, along with an option to report anonymously, removes major barriers that have prevented anesthesiologists from reporting alarming incidents at their institutions.

Cases submitted to AIRS are reviewed by a steering committee within AQI that publishes monthly case reports in the ASA newsletter. By the end of 2021, the AIRS steering committee had published 123 case reports. Topics include specific problems of respiration and circulation, the role of different cognitive biases in poor decision-making, and environmental factors leading to unsafe anesthesia.

Safe Table forums are another way that the AIRS steering committee uses the reported incidents to help anesthesiologists. A Safe Table forum is a protected space for anesthesiologists to discuss cases from AIRS and from their own institutions. The Patient Safety Act protects these discussions from legal discovery or disclosure because at a Safe Table, all anesthesiologists are PSO participants. The AIRS committee has led Safe Table forums at several national meetings starting in 2018. The Safe Table discussions fill the gap between simply reading a case report and learning one-on-one how others have addressed specific risks in their own institutions.

The goal of critical incident registries such as AIRS is not to determine the prevalence of these incidents, which requires a known denominator. Instead, the registry is used to illuminate unsafe practices for all anesthesiologists so that the quality of everyone's practice is improved.

## National Anesthesia Clinical Outcomes Registry

The AQI's National Anesthesia Clinical Outcomes Registry (NACOR) contains data starting from 2010 onward. The current scope of NACOR includes deidentified anesthesia case data and patient outcomes from participating practices. By including all cases and not just those relating to critical incidents, NACOR aims to determine the incidence of rare events. Any U.S. anesthesiology practice can participate. An electronic dashboard displaying practice-specific summary data is available for free to anesthesiologist members of the ASA and at a nominal cost to nonmember anesthesiologists. There are higher-paid tiers of NACOR participation that include benchmarking of single-practice data against national averages. NACOR supports the AQI's role as a Qualified Clinical Data Registry that facilitates the compliance of anesthesiologists with the Centers for Medicare and Medicaid Services Quality Payment Program.

NACOR data arrives electronically from practices. The minimal data set includes the data usually sent for billing: patient zip code, age, sex, ASA physical status, Common Procedural Terminology codes describing the anesthetic and the procedure, procedural dates and times, and National Provider Identifiers for the anesthesiology staff involved. NACOR also accepts status flags regarding adverse outcomes as defined in the NACOR Data Definitions. These outcomes include hemodynamic instability, cardiac ischemia or arrest, respiratory complications, postoperative nausea and vomiting, anaphylaxis, and other uncommon adverse events. Practices using Anesthesia Information Management System software can also include complete vital signs, medication doses, event times, and other rich data.

As of the end of 2021, NACOR contains over 88 million cases performed by over 50,000 clinicians. Of the practices currently contributing data, 42% have 1 to 25 clinicians, 35% have 26 to 75, 20% have 76 to 250, and 3% have over 250 clinicians. The high proportion of small practices makes NACOR unlike other registries that primarily collect data from large health care enterprises.

Research based on NACOR has used its national scope to make conclusions about U.S. anesthesia care. A study by Whitlock and colleagues of mortality in cases from 2010 through 2014 found a crude mortality rate of 33 per 100,000 and an association with case start time after 4:00 pm (adjusted odds ratio 1.64; 95% confidence interval 1.22–2.21) (Whitlock, Feiner, & Chen, 2015). A study of non–operating room anesthesia (NORA) by Nagrebetsky and colleagues reported that the proportion of NORA cases increased from 28.3% in 2010 to 35.9% in 2014 (Nagrebetsky, Gabriel, Dutton, & Urman, 2017). Also, there was a statistically significant increase in ASA physical status from year to year. A study by Andreae and colleagues of NACOR practices reporting antiemetic prophylaxis and insurance coverage data found an association between low socioeconomic status and antiemetic prophylaxis with ondansetron and dexamethasone (Andreae, Gabry, Goodrich, White, & Hall, 2018).

Several studies on regional anesthesia provided some answers to questions as to how often regional anesthesia is being offered for common procedures. Gabriel and colleagues found the overall prevalence of peripheral nerve blocks (PNBs) to be only 3.3% of all possible cases (Gabriel & Ilfeld, 2018). Shoulder arthroscopies and anterior cruciate ligament construction had the highest rate of PNB at 41% and 32%, respectively. Also, the PNB rate increased during the study period of 2010 to 2015. A study by Lam and colleagues found that PNB use for mastectomy rose to 13% in 2018 and that PNB use for mastectomy was associated with procedures after 2014, female sex, facility region, and use of tissue expanders (Lam et al., 2021).

Use of NACOR for outcomes research has been limited by the lack of consistent and standardized reporting of patient outcomes within 30 days. Many anesthesia practices simply do not know if patients, especially outpatients, have sequelae such as postdischarge nausea and vomiting. Even practices that conduct patient outreach with surveys report poor completion rates. To enhance reporting of more immediate outcomes such as postoperative reintubation, cardiac ischemia, or stroke, NACOR developed a set of data definitions to standardize these outcomes. However, it is not clear how many practices are adhering to these definitions, as there is limited auditing of submitted data. Some practices limit their reporting scope to that required by the federal government for annual quality reporting.

## Future of Anesthesia Quality Registries

This chapter examines some of the larger anesthesia registries available in the United States. Data is also available from health care industry sources that do not focus on anesthesia but that do contain some information about anesthesia type and patient outcomes. The current effort is to change the question from "Should we contribute data to a registry?" to "Which registry should we contribute to?" Practices need quality registry data to inform themselves and the institutions they serve about how the anesthetic care provided compares to other practices nationally.

## SUGGESTED READINGS

Andreae, M. H., Gabry, J. S., Goodrich, B., White, R. S., & Hall, C. (2018). Antiemetic prophylaxis as a marker of health care disparities in the national anesthesia clinical outcomes registry. *Anesthesia and Analgesia, 126*(2), 588–599. doi:10.1213/ANE.0000000000002582.

Anesthesia Quality Institute. (2021). *Anesthesia incident reporting system case reports.* Retrieved from https://www.aqihq.org/casereportsandcommittee.aspx. Accessed December 12, 2021.

Cooper, J. B., Newbower, R. S., Long, C. D., & McPeek, B. (1978). Preventable anesthesia mishaps: A study of human factors. *Anesthesiology, 49*(6), 399–406. doi:10.1097/00000542-197812000-00004.

Dutton, R. P. (2015). Large databases in anaesthesiology. *Current Opinion in Anaesthesiology, 28*(6), 697–702. doi:10.1097/ACO.0000000000000243.

Douglas, R. N., Stephens, L. S., Posner, K. L., Davies, J. M., Mincer, S. L., Burden, A. R., et al. (2021). Communication failures contributing to patient injury in anaesthesia malpractice claims. *British Journal of Anaesthesia, 127*(3), 470–478. doi:10.1016/j.bja.2021.05.030.

Gabriel, R. A., & Ilfeld, B. M. (2018). Use of regional anesthesia for outpatient surgery within the United States: A prevalence study using a nationwide database. *Anesthesia and Analgesia, 126*(6), 2078–2084. doi:10.1213/ANE.0000000000002503.

Glance, L. G., Dutton, R. P., Feng, C., Li, Y., Lustik, S. J., & Dick, A. W. (2018). Variability in case durations for common surgical procedures. *Anesthesia and Analgesia, 126*(6), 2017–2024. doi:10.1213/ANE.0000000000002882.

Gliklich, R. E., Leavy, M. B., & Dreyer, N. A. (Eds.). (2020, September). *Registries for Evaluating Patient Outcomes: A User's Guide* (4th ed.). (Prepared by L&M Policy Research, LLC, under Contract No. 290-2014-00004-C with partners OM1 and IQVIA) AHRQ Publication No. 19(20)- EHC020. Rockville, MD: Agency for Healthcare Research and Quality. Posted final reports are located on the Effective Health Care Program search page. Retrieved from https://doi.org/10.23970/AHRQEPCREGISTRIES4.

Lam, S., Qu, H., Hannum, M., Tan, K. S., Afonso, A., Tokita, H. K., & McCormick, P. J. (2021). Trends in peripheral nerve block usage in mastectomy and lumpectomy: Analysis of a national database from 2010 to 2018. *Anesthesia and Analgesia, 133*(1), 32–40. doi:10.1213/ANE.0000000000005368.

Nagrebetsky, A., Gabriel, R. A., Dutton, R. P., & Urman, R. D. (2017). Growth of nonoperating room anesthesia care in the United States: A contemporary trends analysis. *Anesthesia and Analgesia, 124*(4), 1261–1267. doi:10.1213/ANE.0000000000001734.

Schulz, C. M., Burden, A., Posner, K. L., Mincer, S. L., Steadman, R., Wagner, K. J., et al. (2017). Frequency and type of situational awareness errors contributing to death and brain damage: A closed claims analysis. *Anesthesiology, 127*(2), 326–337. doi:10.1097/ALN.0000000000001661.

Whitlock, E. L., Feiner, J. R., & Chen, L. L. (2015). Perioperative mortality, 2010 to 2014: A retrospective cohort study using the National Anesthesia Clinical Outcomes Registry. *Anesthesiology, 123*(6), 1312–1321. doi:10.1097/ALN.0000000000000882.

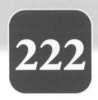

# 222

# Depth of Anesthesia

RISA L. WOLK, MD  |  DANIEL J. COLE, MD  |  KAREN B. DOMINO, MD, MPH

A fundamental component of general anesthesia is unconsciousness. Patients consenting to general anesthesia do so with the expectation that they will not see, hear, feel, or remember intraoperative events. However, studies show that a large percentage of patients who undergo general anesthesia report preoperative fears of awareness or recall. In the past, conventional monitoring of anesthetic depth (i.e., risk for awareness) has included rudimentary signs such as patient movement, autonomic changes, and subjective clinical instinct. Considerable effort has been devoted to establishing a monitor that will reliably determine a patient's depth of anesthesia. Several different methods have been evaluated, yet none is 100% effective. At present, there are at least three inherent obstacles in the development of a "foolproof" monitor of anesthetic depth and the ability of that monitor to prevent intraoperative awareness. The first is that we have an incomplete understanding of the mechanism of general anesthesia. The second is that general anesthesia occurs on a continuum without a quantitative dimension, and the third is that there is considerable interpatient and interanesthetic variability. Attempting to translate a conscious or unconscious state into a quantitative number can, at best, be limited to the practice of probability (Fig. 222.1). Finally, the sensitivity and specificity of measured cortical electrical activity may not be related to a general anesthesia–induced biochemical event within subcortical structures.

## Incidence and Experience of Intraoperative Awareness

The incidence of awareness is greater than most practitioners believe because the incidence is best estimated by formally interviewing patients postoperatively. Patients may not voluntarily report awareness if they were not disturbed by it. In addition, memory for awareness may be delayed. A minority of cases are identified in the immediate postanesthetic period. Although the data are variable and controversial in prospective studies in which a structured interview has been used, it was found that intraoperative awareness occurs with surprising frequency. A prospective evaluation of awareness in nearly 12,000 patients undergoing general anesthesia conducted in Sweden by Sandin and colleagues revealed an incidence of awareness of 0.18% in cases in which neuromuscular blocking agents were used and

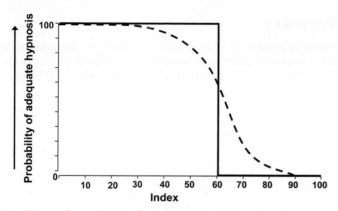

**Fig. 222.1** The probability of adequate hypnosis based upon brain function monitoring index. The *solid line* is the ideal probability curve with 100% sensitivity and specificity. The *dashed line* is a more realistic expectation of monitoring in which a progressive decrease of the monitored index value correlates with increased probability of adequate hypnosis.

0.10% in the absence of such agents. A similar incidence has been observed in tertiary care centers in the United States, with a higher proportion among patients with coexisting morbidity. Studies showing a lower incidence have relied upon quality improvement data rather than the structured interview. Davidson and colleagues report the incidence of awareness is higher in children (0.5%–1%), but psychological sequelae are fewer. Patients experiencing intraoperative awareness report auditory perception of voices or noises, as well as the sensation of loss of mobility or weakness. They may also report feelings of helplessness, anxiety, panic, or impending death. Postoperative sequelae include sleep problems, fear of future anesthetics, daytime anxiety, and posttraumatic stress disorder.

## Risk Factors for Intraoperative Awareness

The most common causes of intraoperative awareness include light anesthesia, increased anesthetic requirement, or malfunction

or misuse of the anesthetic delivery system (Table 222.1). Light anesthesia may be necessary for physiologic stability in hypovolemic patients, in those with limited cardiovascular reserve, or for patients undergoing trauma surgery. Patients with an American Society of Anesthesiologists physical class of 3 or greater who undergo emergency surgery or cesarean section or who have a history of intraoperative awareness have a higher likelihood of experiencing awareness. Neuromuscular blockade prevents the most common sign of light anesthesia, patient movement. An inadequately anesthetized nonparalyzed patient usually moves first, as lower anesthetic concentrations are needed to prevent awareness than to render immobility. Some patients, such as those using alcohol, opiates, amphetamines, and cocaine, may require an increase in anesthetic dose. In addition, equipment problems with the vaporizer or intravenous infusion devices may lead to awareness, although these are less common causes of awareness, especially with use of end-tidal anesthetic gas analysis.

## Prevention of Awareness

Suggestions for the prevention of awareness include premedicating the patient with an amnesic agent, giving adequate doses of induction agents, avoiding muscle paralysis unless necessary, and administering at least a 0.7 minimum alveolar concentration (MAC) of an inhalation agent with monitoring of end-tidal levels to ensure delivery of adequate levels of inhalation anesthetic gases. Importantly, hypertension and tachycardia do not reliably predict awareness.

### BRAIN FUNCTION MONITORING

In general, devices that monitor brain electrical activity for the purpose of assessing depth of anesthesia record electroencephalographic (EEG) activity. Some process spontaneous EEG and electromyographic activity, and others measure evoked responses to auditory stimuli. Most of the research concerning depth of anesthesia and all of the research concerning awareness have been performed on the Bispectral Index (BIS, Covidien, a subsidiary of Medtronic, Minneapolis, MN) monitor.

| TABLE 222.1 | Causes of Awareness | | |
|---|---|---|---|
| **Anesthesia Delivery Problems** | | | |
| Vaporizer malfunction | Medication error | TIVA administration problems | |
| **Increased Anesthetic Requirements** | | | |
| Heavy alcohol use | Chronic benzodiazepine or opioid use | Chronic cocaine use | |
| Prior history of awareness | Genetic factors | | |
| **Light Anesthesia: Patient Factors** | | | |
| ASA 4–5 | Children, teens, young adults | Severe cardiopulmonary disease | |
| Hemodynamic instability | | | |
| **Light Anesthesia: Surgical Factors** | | | |
| Emergency surgery | After hours procedures | Cardiac, cesarean section, trauma, ophthalmic surgery | |
| ICU admission | | | |
| **Light Anesthesia: Anesthetic Factors** | | | |
| Neuromuscular blockade | Nitrous oxide | Low-dose volatile agents | |
| TIVA | Difficult intubation | | |

*ASA,* American Society of Anesthesiologists; *ICU,* intensive care unit; *TIVA,* total intravenous anesthesia.

The BIS uses a proprietary algorithm to convert a single channel of frontal EEG activity into an index of hypnotic level, ranging from 100 (awake) to 0 (isoelectric EEG). Specific ranges (40–60) reflect a low probability of consciousness during general anesthesia. A number of other events (cerebral ischemia or hypoperfusion), other drugs (neuromuscular blocking agents or ephedrine), or conditions (elderly with low-amplitude EEG) may affect BIS level.

Several randomized controlled trials have investigated the effect of BIS-guided anesthesia on the incidence of awareness. Most studies were performed on patients with high risk for intraoperative awareness (e.g., high-risk cardiac surgery, impaired cardiovascular status, trauma surgery, cesarean section, and patients with chronic benzodiazepine or opioid use, heavy alcohol intake, or prior history of awareness). Myles and colleagues compared BIS-guided anesthesia (BIS 40–60) to routine care. Intraoperative awareness occurred in two patients (0.17%) when BIS monitors were used to guide anesthesia and in 11 patients (0.91%) managed by routine clinical practice ($P <$ 0.02). Two subsequent studies compared the incidence of awareness with BIS-guided anesthesia to end-tidal gas-guided anesthesia (0.7%–1.3% age-adjusted MAC). These studies found no difference in awareness between the two monitoring modalities. A Cochrane systematic review by Punjasawadwong concluded that BIS-guided anesthesia is superior to routine care, especially in patients receiving total intravenous anesthesia and in patients at high risk for awareness. This review, as well as a recent metaanalysis by Gao and colleagues, found that BIS does not decrease the incidence of awareness in patients receiving inhalational anesthetics but does reduce risk for patients undergoing intravenous anesthesia. Sedline (Masimo Corporation, Irvine, CA) is a similar brain function monitor that has not been formally studied for prevention of awareness but is plausibly similarly effective.

## Summary

Depth of anesthesia is an important factor in the anesthetic management of patients. When considering depth of anesthesia as it relates to the risk of intraoperative awareness, the following points are key:

- The incidence of intraoperative awareness is 1 to 2 per 1000 inhalation anesthetic procedures, and the incidence is higher with light anesthesia and in children.
- The potential exists for serious psychological or medicolegal sequelae to occur.
- Ensuring the functionality of equipment to be used to deliver general anesthesia is paramount in the prevention of intraoperative awareness.
- The clinician may consider administering an amnestic agent as a premedicant in patients who are at risk for developing intraoperative awareness or as a treatment when patients are lightly anesthetized.
- Readministering hypnotic agents may be suitable in clinical situations that place patients at increased risk for developing intraoperative awareness (e.g., difficult airway).
- Hemodynamic measures are unreliable predictors of inadequate anesthesia.
- No monitor has proved to be 100% sensitive and specific for detecting awareness.
- The end-tidal anesthetic gas concentration should be monitored.
- Consider administering at least a 0.7 MAC of an inhalation anesthetic agent.
- Neuromuscular blocking agents will mask an important indicator of inadequate anesthesia: movement.
- Consider monitoring brain function as an adjunct to other available indicators of anesthetic depth, particularly with total intravenous anesthesia.

## SUGGESTED READINGS

American Society of Anesthesiologists Task Force on Intraoperative Awareness. (2006). Practice advisory for intraoperative awareness and brain function monitoring: A report by the American society of anesthesiologists task force on intraoperative awareness. *Anesthesiology*, 104(4), 847–864.

Avidan, M. S., Jacobsohn, E., Glick, D., Burnside, B. A., Zhang, L., Villafranca, A., et al. (2011). Prevention of intraoperative awareness in a high-risk surgical population. *New England Journal of Medicine*, 365(7), 591–600.

Avidan, M. S., Zhang, L., Burnside, B. A., Finkel, K. J., Searleman, A. C., Selvidge, J. A., et al. (2008).

Anesthesia awareness and the bispectral index. *New England Journal of Medicine*, 358(11), 1097–1108.

Davidson, A. J., Huang, G. H., Czarnecki, C., Gibson, M. A., Stewart, S. A., Jamsen, K., et al. (2005). Awareness during anesthesia in children: A prospective cohort study. *Anesthesia and Analgesia*, 100(3), 653–661.

Gao, W. W., He, Y. H., Liu, L., Yuan, Q., Wang, Y. F., & Zhao, B. (2018). BIS Monitoring on intraoperative awareness: A meta-analysis. *Current Medical Science*, 38(2), 349–353.

Myles, P. S., Leslie, K., McNeil, J., Forbes, A., & Chan, M. T. (2004). Bispectral index monitoring

to prevent awareness during anaesthesia: The B-Aware randomised controlled trial. *Lancet (London, England)*, 363(9423), 1757–1763.

Punjasawadwong, Y., Phongchiewboon, A., & Bunchungmongkol, N. (2014). Bispectral index for improving anaesthetic delivery and postoperative recovery. *Cochrane Database of Systematic Reviews*, 2014(6), CD003843. John Wiley & Sons, Ltd. Retrieved from https://www.cochranelibrary.com/cdsr/doi/10.1002/14651858.CD003843.pub3/epdf/full. Accessed November 1, 2018.

# Patient Safety and Quality Improvement

KARL A. POTERACK, MD

Although patient safety and quality improvement (QI) have been areas of focus in health care for some time, they became priorities after the Institute of Medicine's report "To Err is Human" in 1999, which highlighted the morbidity and mortality associated with iatrogenic injury in hospitals. Chief executive officers of Fortune 500 companies and third-party payers found the report to be in keeping with their thoughts on the health care industry: reimbursement for health care was increasing at double-digit rates every year, but outcomes were no better, and days of work lost because of illness were not decreasing. Accordingly, over the last several years, QI and the safety of patients in health care institutions has become an area of emphasis.

## Quality Improvement

QI has its roots in engineering and manufacturing, where systems theory and statistical process control were combined with general management methods to produce a formal approach to the analysis and improvement of performance. QI is variously defined as the reduction of variability in products and processes and as an organized process that assesses and evaluates health services to improve practice or quality of care. International Standards Organization standard 9000 to 2015 defines quality as "the degree to which a set of inherent characteristics of an object fulfils requirements." The Institute of Medicine (IOM) defines health care quality as "the degree to which health care services for individuals and populations increase the likelihood of desired health outcomes and are consistent with current professional knowledge." The IOM further established six aims, or domains, of health care quality: safe, effective, patient-centered, timely, efficient, and equitable. W. Edwards Deming defined quality as "meeting customer requirements at a price they are willing to pay." Peter Drucker wrote that quality is not what the supplier (health care organization) puts in; it is what the user (patient or payer) gets out of it.

QI programs in health care are guided by requirements of regulatory bodies, such as state governments, the Center for Medicare and Medicaid Services, and deeming entities such as The Joint Commission (TJC). Unfortunately, many clinicians view QI programs as being driven solely by mandates of these external regulatory groups, which results in the whole system being perceived as "red tape" and "overhead" that add cost but no real value. Such an approach can easily become a self-fulfilling prophecy by consuming resources through the production of unread reports and paperwork, thus diverting resources that could be devoted to actually increasing quality.

Different elements of a QI program may focus on the structure, process, and outcome of health care delivery programs. Structure refers to the conditions under which care is provided (e.g., personnel, facilities, how they are organized). *Process* is defined by the National Quality Forum (NQF) as "the activities that constitute health care, usually carried out by professional personnel, but also including other contributions to care, particularly by patients and their families." *Outcome* refers to any changes in the patient's health after the care was performed or "the health and well-being of the patient and the associated costs of care" per the NQF. QI programs, therefore, address all areas of hospital operations.

There is nomenclature around various types of events that can be confusing and varies according to the source. The NQF defines a *patient safety event* as "a process or act of omission or commission that resulted in hazardous health care conditions and/or unintended harm to the patient." A patient safety event can be, but is not necessarily, the result of a defective system or process design, a system breakdown, equipment failure, or human error. Common types of patient safety events include *sentinel events*, *adverse events*, *no-harm events*, *close calls* (aka "near misses"), and *hazardous conditions*.

TJC defines a *sentinel event* as "a patient safety event that results in death, permanent harm or severe temporary intervention harm." Because the occurrence of a sentinel event may indicate a systems problem, TJC requires all sentinel events to undergo root-cause analysis. In this analysis, the stakeholders who were involved in the care of the affected patient at the hospital in which the sentinel event occurred analyze the events to identify flaws in the system.

An *adverse event* is a patient safety event that results in unintended harm to the patient by an act of commission or omission rather than by the underlying disease or condition of the patient. A *no-harm event* is a patient safety event that reaches the patient but does not cause harm. A *close call* (or "near miss" or "good catch") is a patient safety event or a situation that did not produce patient harm but only because of intervening factors, such as patient health or timely intervention. A *hazardous* (or "unsafe") *condition* is a circumstance (other than a patient's own disease process or condition) that increases the probability of an adverse event. A *medical error* is a type of adverse event that is preventable with the current state of medical knowledge.

Continuous QI views patient care as a complex system in which undesired results occur because of either a random event or a system problem. The default assumption is that errors are systems based until proven otherwise. System problems should be controllable through changing the system. These systems problems ("opportunities for improvement") are identified on an ongoing basis, and strategies are implemented to prevent their occurrence.

Identifying these opportunities for improvement may occur in one of several ways. A common method of identification, mandated by regulatory bodies and with a long history of use in medicine, is to focus on undesirable outcomes—the mortality and morbidity method. In contrast with the shame, blame, and scapegoating of many traditional mortality and morbidity processes, continuous QI focuses not on finding fault with a particular individuals' acts or omissions but rather on identification of the system causes of undesirable outcomes. A second way of identifying areas of improvement is the "suggestion box method": giving the opportunity to those involved in the process to identify problems and suggest solutions. This method may range from planned gatherings at various intervals to specifically gather input to a very informal open-door policy that fosters and encourages input from those on the front line. A third category is through the systematic measurement of predefined indicators of quality, such as wait times, turnover times, materials waste, and rates of adverse outcomes.

Once specific opportunities for improvement are identified, their status is measured. The process of care leading to these problems is analyzed. There are multiple formal QI tools applicable to these situations, such as fishbone charts, five whys, and the Plan-Do-Study-Act cycle. A complete discussion of these is beyond the scope of this review; a more complete discussion can be found in the Suggested Readings section. Several key points apply to all of these tools: (1) all individuals with responsibilities for the different areas involved in the actual process (the stakeholders) need to be involved in the analysis; (2) the analysis must be as detailed as possible; (3) the temptation to jump to conclusions must be resisted ("if only the residents would correctly fill out the paperwork, we wouldn't have a problem"); and (4) the goal is to change the system, *not* "reeducate the users" to facilitate the desired outcome.

If change is identified that should lead to improvement, it is implemented. A key part of implementation is identifying process owners who have responsibility for assessing and monitoring the success of the new process. After an appropriate time period, the status is measured again to determine whether improvement actually occurred. Attention may then be directed to continuing to improve this process or turning to a different process to target for improvement.

## Medication Errors, Assessment, and Prevention

A common focus of QI programs is the prevention of medication errors. The U.S. National Coordinating Council for Medication Error Reporting and Prevention defines a *medication error* as "any preventable event that may cause or lead to inappropriate medication use or patient harm while the medication is in the control of the health care professional, patient, or consumer. Such events may be related to professional practice, health care products, procedures, and systems, including prescribing, order communication, product labeling, packaging, and nomenclature, compounding, dispensing, distribution, administration, education, monitoring, and use." An *adverse drug event* refers to any incident in which the use of a medication (drug or biologic) at any dose, a medical device, or a special nutritional product (e.g., dietary supplement, infant formula, medical food) may have resulted in an adverse outcome in a patient. This includes both errors in the medication use process ("medication error") and adverse outcomes from the proper administration of the drug ("adverse drug reaction"). An *adverse drug reaction* is defined more formally by the World Health Organization as "a response to a drug which is noxious and unintended, and which occurs at doses normally used in man for the prophylaxis, diagnosis, or therapy of disease, or for the modifications of physiologic function." The aforementioned IOM report identified medication errors as the most common type of error in health care and attributed several thousand deaths to medication-related events.

Numerous organizations have published recommendations for the prevention of medication errors, including, for example, the Agency for Health Care Research and Quality, the Institute for Health Care Improvement, the Institute for Safe Medication Practices, TJC, and the NQF. These recommendations include implementing computerized provider order entry, using barcoding technology at the point of care, ensuring availability of pharmaceutical decision support, having a central pharmacist supply high-risk intravenously administered medications and pharmacy-based admixture systems, standardizing prescription writing and prescription rules, and eliminating certain abbreviations and dose expressions.

## Programs to Improve Outcome

QI efforts that are focused on the operating room, in which anesthesiologists are very involved, have included, as a few examples, efforts to decrease medication errors, surgical wound infections, and bloodstream infections and to reduce the complications with central venous catheter placement. Multiple groups, including the Centers for Disease Control and Prevention and the American Society of Anesthesiologists, have promulgated clinical practice guidelines for the placement of central venous catheters. These programs are not static. As part of the QI initiative, the processes are monitored; compliance with the recommendations, systems' problems in implementing the recommendations, and the outcomes themselves must be monitored and assessed, and changes to the recommendations must be implemented when necessary.

## Disclosure of Errors to Patients

Although not a part of the QI process, one of the areas that has come under increased scrutiny in the last several years concerns how and what to reveal to patients and their family member when errors are discovered. Fear of malpractice action has traditionally made physicians hesitant to disclose medical errors to patients. However, regulatory bodies now encourage, and in some cases state law may require, the disclosure of "serious unanticipated outcomes" to patients. Such disclosure is frequently not protected from admissibility in a legal action. Surveys suggest that most patients want disclosure of errors, an explanation of how the error occurred and how the effects of the error will be minimized, and what actions will be taken to prevent the error from occurring to other patients. Most hospitals and medical staffs, with input from their legal departments, have developed guidelines on how errors and adverse events are disclosed to patients and their families.

## SUGGESTED READINGS

Dekker, S. (2014). *Field guide to understanding human error*. Surrey, England: Ashgate Publishing.

Fondahn, E., DeFer, T. M., & Lane, M. (2018). *Washington manual of patient safety and quality improvement*. Philadelphia: Wolters Kluwer Health.

Institute of Medicine. (2006). *Preventing medication errors: Quality chasm series*. Retrieved from https://psnet.ahrq.gov/resources/resource/4053. Accessed December 16, 2021.

NQF Definitions. *NQF Patient safety terms and definitions*. Retrieved from https://www.qualityforum.org/Topics/Safety_Definitions.aspx. Accessed December 16, 2021.

*The 7 basic quality tools for process improvement*. Retrieved from http://asq.org/learn-about-quality/seven-basic-quality-tools/overview/overview.html. Accessed December 16, 2021.

The Joint Commission. *Sentinel event*. Retrieved from https://www.jointcommission.org/resources/patient-safety-topics/sentinel-event/. Accessed December 16, 2021.

Institute of Medicine (US) Committee on Quality of Health Care in America, Kohn, L. T., Corrigan, J. M., & Donaldson, M. S. (Eds.). (1999). *To err is human: Building a safer health system*. Washington (DC): National Academies Press. Retrieved from https://

nap.nationalacademies.org/resource/9728/To-Err-is-Human-1999—report-brief.pdf. Accessed December 16, 2021.

World Health Organization (2016). *Medication errors: Technical series on safer primary care*. Retrieved from http://apps.who.int/iris/bitstream/10665/252274/1/9789241511643-eng.pdf. Accessed December 16, 2021.

# 224

# Perioperative Pulmonary Aspiration

MEGAN HAMRE BLACKBURNE, MD

Pulmonary aspiration is defined as the inhalation of oropharyngeal or gastric contents into the lower respiratory tract. The physiologic mechanisms that prevent regurgitation and aspiration under normal circumstances include the lower esophageal sphincter, the upper esophageal sphincter, and the laryngeal reflexes. The most common risk factors for perioperative pulmonary aspiration are emergency surgery and gastrointestinal obstruction. Trauma, depressed level of consciousness, history of neurologic disease, and age greater than 60 years are also associated with increased risk for aspiration. Altered physiologic states such as obesity, pregnancy, diabetes mellitus, gastrointestinal motility dysfunction, and reflux disease are associated with prolonged gastric emptying and increased risk for aspiration, as are patients receiving enteral tube feeding. Additionally, patients may be at increased risk of pulmonary aspiration due to retention of gastric contents secondary to pain or inadequate fasting. Of those patients who do aspirate, patients with American Society of Anesthesiologists (ASA) physical classification status 3 or greater are at greatest risk for severe pulmonary morbidity or death after the aspiration event. In a 2021 closed claims analysis by Warner and colleagues, death occurred in 57% of pulmonary aspiration claims and severe permanent injury in another 16% of claims.

## Importance of Pulmonary Aspiration

Pulmonary aspiration is the single most common cause of death among airway management complications. Two large studies have documented the frequency of perioperative pulmonary aspiration during anesthesia. In 1993 Warner and colleagues reported an overall incidence of one aspiration event in 3216 anesthetics from 215,488 general anesthetics performed from 1985 to 1991 at Mayo Clinic. The difference in incidence between the two studies may be attributed to stricter definition of pulmonary aspiration by Warner and colleagues.

Accurate diagnosis of aspiration is difficult unless the event is witnessed and gastric contents are noted in the tracheobronchial tree. Among those patients who have a witnessed aspiration, mortality rate is 5%. Depending on condition and composition of the aspirates, three different complications may result from pulmonary aspiration. These include acid-associated aspiration pneumonitis, bacterial infection, and particle-associated aspiration. Pulmonary aspiration associated with aspiration pneumonitis accounts for 10% to 30% of all deaths associated with anesthesia. This is the most important risk factor in the development of acute respiratory distress syndrome, which is associated with a 30% to 40% mortality rate.

Based on the information in Table 224.1, the expected mortality resulting from perioperative pulmonary aspiration in the United States would be approximately 200 deaths annually. However, aspiration of gastric contents may also lead to serious morbidity, with approximately 25% of patients who aspirate requiring critical care support.

Over the last two decades there has been a notable increase in surgical procedures performed on the elderly population. These patients are much more likely to have preexisting

| TABLE 224.1 | **Risk of Aspiration-Associated Pulmonary Complications and Death After General Anesthesia by American Society of Anesthesiologists Physical Status Classification** | | |
|---|---|---|---|
| | | **FREQUENCY** | |
| **ASA Physical Status Classification** | **Pulmonary Complications*** | **Deaths†** | |
| I | 1/39,865 (1:39,865) | 0 | |
| II | 2/87,471 (1:43,735) | 0 | |
| III | 7/78,714 (1:11,245) | 1/78,714 (1:78,714) | |
| IV and V | 3/9438 (1:3146) | 2/9438 (1:4719) | |
| Total | 13/215,488 (1:16,576) | 3/215,488 (1:71,829) | |

*Pulmonary complications include acute respiratory distress syndrome, pneumonitis, and pneumonia (with or without positive viral or bacterial identification).
†Death from aspiration-associated pulmonary complications within 6 months of aspiration.
*ASA*, American Society of Anesthesiologists.
From Warner MA, Warner ME, Weber JG. Clinical significance of pulmonary aspiration during the perioperative period. *Anesthesiology.* 1993;78:56–62.

| TABLE 224.2 | **Summary of 1999 American Society of Anesthesiologists Task Force Pharmacologic Recommendations to Reduce the Risk of Pulmonary Aspiration*** |
|---|---|
| **Drug Type and Common Examples** | **Recommendation** |
| **GASTROINTESTINAL STIMULANTS** Metoclopramide | No routine use |
| **GASTRIC ACID SECRETION BLOCKERS** Cimetidine | No routine use |
| Famotidine | No routine use |
| Lansoprazole | No routine use |
| Omeprazole | No routine use |
| Ranitidine | No routine use |
| **ANTACIDS** Sodium citrate | No routine use |
| Sodium bicarbonate | No routine use |
| Magnesium trisilicate | No routine use |
| **ANTIEMETIC AGENTS** Droperidol | No routine use |
| Ondansetron | No routine use |
| **ANTICHOLINERGIC AGENTS** Atropine | No use |
| Scopolamine | No use |
| Glycopyrrolate | No use |
| Combinations of the medications above | No routine use |

*A 2017 update of these guidelines states that, in patients who have no apparent risk of pulmonary aspiration, the routine preoperative use of gastrointestinal stimulants, antacids, gastric acid blockers, antiemetics, anticholinergics, or combinations thereof is not recommended.
*ASA*, American Society of Anesthesiologists.

comorbidities and to experience regurgitation and/or aspiration in the perioperative period. Obesity also contributes to increased risk of pulmonary aspiration. The mechanism is likely multifactorial due to increased intraabdominal pressure, high residual gastric volume, delayed gastric emptying, and increased incidence of gastroesophageal reflux disease.

## Pulmonary Aspiration in Children

The incidence of aspiration in the pediatric population is similar to that observed in the adult population; however, children tend to have fewer pulmonary complications and a lower mortality rate resulting from aspiration. Their outcomes after aspiration are generally better, and their recoveries seem to be faster. The children at highest risk for aspiration include those undergoing emergency procedures and those younger than 1 year.

## Use of Medications and Preoperative Fasting

Pharmacologic aspiration prophylaxis consists of several classes of medications, including antacids, histamine-2 receptor antagonists, proton pump inhibitors, anticholinergic agents, antiemetics and gastrointestinal stimulants. Antacids rapidly neutralize the acidic pH of the stomach contents but also increase gastric volume whereas H2-receptor antagonists and proton pump inhibitors inhibit secretion of acid and reduce volume and acidity of the stomach contents. Medications that block gastric acid secretion may be preoperatively administered to patients at increased risk of pulmonary aspiration. However, no data suggest that the use of any of these medications decreases the risk of pulmonary aspiration. Per the ASA 2017 guidelines, routine use of these medications is not recommended in patients who have no apparent increased risk for pulmonary aspiration. The recommendations of the ASA for medications and fasting are given in Tables 224.2 and 224.3, respectively.

## Occurrence of Aspiration in the Perioperative Period

Numerous studies have indicated that a significant number of aspiration events occur during tracheal intubation and extubation. In a 2021 closed claims analysis, Warner and colleagues noted that aspiration occurred during induction or airway manipulation in 60% of claims and during emergence or extubation in 7% of claims. Inadequate depth of anesthesia, inadequate muscle relaxation, and difficult intubation are risk factors for aspiration events during induction and laryngoscopy, whereas weakness and nonresponsiveness are risks for aspiration during extubation. There is insufficient information on the effectiveness of laryngeal mask airways to prevent aspiration, but there are case reports of aspiration associated with their use in both high-risk and low-risk patients. Placement of a cuffed endotracheal tube allows for isolation of the airway from the gastrointestinal tract; however, aspiration has been documented to occur perioperatively and in the intensive care unit (ICU) setting in the presence of both endotracheal and tracheostomy tubes.

| TABLE 224.3 | Summary of 2017 Updated American Society of Anesthesiologists Committee on Standards and Practice Parameters' Recommendations on Preoperative Fasting and the Use of Pharmacologic Agents to Reduce the Risk of Pulmonary Aspiration* | |
|---|---|---|
| **Ingested Material** | **Minimum Fasting Period (h)[†]** | |
| Clear liquids[‡] | 2 | |
| Breast milk | 4 | |
| Infant formula | 6 | |
| Nonhuman milk[§] | 6 | |
| Light meal[¶] | 6 | |

*These recommendations apply to healthy patients who are undergoing elective procedures. They are not intended for women in labor. Following the guidelines does not guarantee complete gastric emptying.
[†]The recommended fasting periods apply to all ages.
[‡]Examples of clear liquids are water, fruit juices without pulp, carbonated beverages, clear tea, and black coffee.
[§]Because nonhuman milk is similar to solids in gastric emptying time, the amount ingested must be considered in determining an appropriate fasting period.
[¶]A light meal typically consists of toast and clear liquids. Meals that include fried or fatty foods or meat may prolong gastric emptying time and require additional fasting time (e.g., ≥8 h). Both the amount and type of foods ingested must be considered when determining an appropriate fasting period.

# Management of Perioperative Pulmonary Aspiration

The most important step in minimizing aspiration events is perioperative optimization. Preoperative assessment and identification of patients with risk factors for pulmonary aspiration allow the anesthesiologist to ensure preoperative fasting, appropriate anesthetic technique, and administration of medications to minimize perioperative risk. Preoperative ultrasound examination of the gastric antrum may also be performed to assess a patient's aspiration risk. When measured with the patient in a semirecumbent position, the appearance of any fluid or solid contents in the antrum corresponds to significant gastric content volume.

Supportive care remains the cornerstone of management of perioperative pulmonary aspiration and may range from observation and respiratory support to management of sepsis and severe lung injury. If aspiration occurs during induction or tracheal intubation, the patient should be placed in a head-down position to minimize the amount of pulmonary contamination. The airway should be cleared of debris with suctioning followed by securing the airway with an endotracheal tube. Once the airway is established, the patient should receive further suctioning of the tracheobronchial tree. Bronchoscopy may be useful to check for residual particulate matter and remove any obstructing debris. Lavage with saline is not recommended because it may increase the spread of aspirate and has not been associated with improved outcomes. Further actions are guided by subsequent clinical findings. In general, prophylactic treatment with antibiotics and/or steroids is not recommended, as both of these measures are ineffective in decreasing the incidence of aspiration pneumonia and lung inflammation.

After confirming the diagnosis of pulmonary aspiration, the decision to proceed with surgery must be discussed between the surgical and anesthesiology teams. Items to consider include the urgency of the procedure, the extent of aspiration and resulting clinical status, and the patient's comorbid conditions. Postoperative disposition and need for ICU monitoring depends on the clinical manifestation of the aspiration event.

# Conclusion

Pulmonary aspiration is an infrequent event in healthy surgical patients, with low associated morbidity and mortality. However, because many aspiration events are unwitnessed, the reported incidence and complication rates may be falsely low. Risk factors include emergency surgery, gastrointestinal obstruction, trauma, depressed level of consciousness, age greater than 60 years, and comorbid conditions such as pregnancy, diabetes mellitus, neurologic disease, gastrointestinal motility dysfunction, and reflux disease. Approximately 25% of patients who aspirate in the perioperative period develop significant pulmonary complications. The overall mortality rate is 5% in the adult population, whereas children rarely experience severe complications or death as a result of aspiration. The routine use of preoperative medications to reduce the risk of pulmonary aspiration is not recommended. Ultrasound examination of the gastric antrum may be performed to assess aspiration risk and formulate an appropriate anesthetic plan. Preoperative assessment and identification of risk factors followed by selection of appropriate anesthetic techniques is critical in avoiding perioperative aspiration.

## SUGGESTED READINGS

American Society of Anesthesiologists Committee. (2017). Practice guidelines for preoperative fasting and the use of pharmacologic agents to reduce the risk of pulmonary aspiration: Application to healthy patients undergoing elective procedures: An updated report by the American Society of Anesthesiologists Task Force on Preoperative Fasting and the Use of Pharmacologic Agents to Reduce the Risk of Pulmonary Aspiration. *Anesthesiology, 126*(3), 376–393.

Bouvet, L., Desgranges, F. P., Aubergy, C., Boselli, E., Dupont, G., Allaouchiche, B., et al. (2017). Prevalence and factors predictive of full stomach in elective and emergency surgical patients: A prospective cohort study. *British Journal of Anaesthesia, 118*(3), 372–379.

Kalinowski, C. P., & Kirsch, J. R. (2004). Strategies for prophylaxis and treatment for aspiration. *Best Practice & Research Clinical Anaesthesiology, 18*(4), 719–737.

Warner, M. A. (2000). Is pulmonary aspiration still an important problem in anesthesia? *Current Opinion in Anaesthesiology, 13*(2), 215–218.

Warner, M. A., Meyerhoff, K. L., Warner, M. E., Posner, K. L., Stephens, L., & Domino, K. B. (2021). Pulmonary aspiration of gastric contents: A closed claims analysis. *Anesthesiology, 135*(2), 284–291.

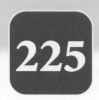

# Eye and Dental Complications

ANDREW GORLIN, MD

## Eye Injury

Anesthesia-related eye injuries are relatively uncommon, but anesthesia providers focus a great deal of attention on avoiding injury to the eye because the eye is one of the major sense organs. An analysis of eye injury claims against anesthesiologists published in 1992 as part of the American Society of Anesthesiologists (ASA) Closed Claims Project found that 3% of all claims in the database were for eye injury. The frequency of payment for eye injury claims was significantly higher than that for claims not related to eye injuries (70% vs. 56%); however, the median cost of eye injury claims was significantly less than that for other claims ($24,000 vs. $95,000).

### CORNEAL INJURY

The most often reported eye complications after general anesthesia are corneal abrasion and corneal exposure, both of which are very painful and blur vision. An abrasion is caused by trauma, with complete loss of corneal epithelium, whereas corneal exposure is caused by damage to (but not loss of) the corneal epithelium due to exposure and secondary loss of tear film protection, which is necessary for protecting the integrity of corneal epithelium. Most injuries are thought to be secondary to lagophthalmos, an incomplete closure of the eyelid, with an abrasion being the result of direct trauma to the cornea from facemasks, surgical drapes, fingers, or other foreign objects that inadvertently contact the cornea. Laparoscopic and robotic surgery is also associated with an increased risk (4- and 6.5-fold, respectively) of corneal injury, possibly because of increased corneal edema from the steep Trendelenburg position or the increased duration of these procedures compared with open surgery.

The prevalence of corneal injuries varies depending on the methods used to detect them, but the incidence—as defined by clinical symptoms in patients whose eyes were taped closed during a surgical procedure—ranges from 0.05% to 0.15%. A specific cause of injury can be determined in only approximately 20% of the cases. Because the mechanisms of corneal injury are poorly understood, it is difficult to formulate preventive strategies that will completely eliminate the risk of injury. However, a review of the literature reveals several recurring themes. The pulse oximeter probe should be placed on patients' fourth or fifth finger because patients are less likely to rub their eyes with these fingers. Patients' eyes should be taped closed immediately after induction of anesthesia (do not wait until after intubation). Studies show that if patients' eyes are taped closed, no extra protection is achieved by using eye ointment unless the surgical procedure is prolonged or if patients are placed in other than the supine position. Even when patients' eyes are taped shut, the anesthesia provider must use caution to prevent foreign objects from coming into contact with the

patients' eyes during intubation (e.g., stethoscope draped around the clinician's neck, identification badge clipped to the chest pocket, a loose watchband or bracelet). The patient should be checked periodically, particularly after repositioning, to ensure that movement, moisture, or tears have not loosened or repositioned the tape.

In patients with proptosis, in patients undergoing head and neck procedures, for procedures performed with the patient prone or in the lateral position, and for procedures that are going to last for more than 90 minutes, the use of ointment on the eyes in addition to taping should be considered. Ointment provides good protection if there is concern that the eyelid tape may come off, but patients who have ointment on their eyes may have some blurred vision at the end of the procedure. The use of petroleum-based ointment is recommended for longer procedures, but because it is flammable, petroleum-based ointment should not be used if electrocautery or electrosurgery is used around the patient's head and neck. Methylcellulose ointment is also an option; because it dissipates more quickly than petroleum-based ointment, it can be used for shorter procedures, and its use is associated with less blurring of vision postoperatively compared with petroleum-based products. Finally, practitioners need to be well educated about the risks and prevention of corneal injuries and provided feedback about their own clinical performance. One study demonstrated that being cared for by an inexperienced provider (in this case, a student nurse anesthetist) was an independent risk factor for developing a corneal injury. In this same study, a department-wide educational and practice feedback protocol was introduced, which resulted in a significant decrease (1.51–0.79 per 1000) in the incidence of corneal injuries.

Corneal injury should be suspected postoperatively if the patient has pain, photophobia, blurred vision, or the sensation of having a foreign body in the eye. All but the most serious injuries can be managed conservatively. Ophthalmic antibiotic ointment should be administered to the eye, and the patient should be reassured that the injury will resolve within 24 to 48 hours without permanent sequelae. An eye patch can be taped in place, but because it is so often done incorrectly, the use of an eye patch is associated with additional problems.

### POSTOPERATIVE VISUAL LOSS

Postoperative visual loss (POVL) is a rare but devastating complication seen most commonly after spine, cardiac, and head and neck surgical procedures (Fig. 225.1). During the 1990s, the incidence of POVL seemed to be increasing, so in 1999, the ASA Committee on Professional Liability established the ASA POVL Registry to tabulate data on POVL after nonocular operations. Seven years later, a review of the registry identified 93 cases of POVL associated with spine operations; most were caused by

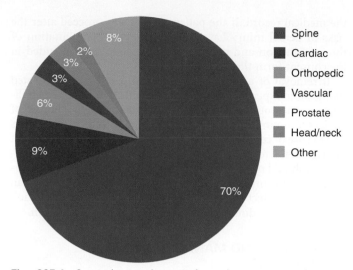

**Fig. 225.1** Surgical procedures performed in 175 cases from the American Society of Anesthesiologists Postoperative Visual Loss Registry database.

ischemic optic neuropathy (ION), either anterior or posterior, and not by compression of the globe. Only 10 of the patients had a central retinal artery occlusion, whereas the remainder had ION. Patients with ION, compared with those without ION, were relatively healthy, were more likely to have an associated blood loss of 1000 mL or greater, or were more likely to have had an anesthetic duration of 6 hours or longer; such conditions were found in 96% of the patients.

More recently, the ASA released a Practice Advisory for POVL associated with spine operations. The recommendations are based on observational studies; because the incidence of POVL is so low, prospective randomized studies would be impossible to perform. Among the factors that might increase the incidence of POVL are preexisting vascular disease (e.g., hypertension, diabetes, peripheral vascular disease, coronary artery disease), obesity, tobacco use, and anemia. As reported previously, the advisory commented that POVL is more likely to occur during prolonged procedures (>6.5 hours), during procedures in which substantial blood loss occurs, and during prolonged procedures combined with substantial blood loss.

## REDUCING THE RISK OF POSTOPERATIVE VISUAL LOSS

Of more importance to clinicians were the recommendations of the panel on the intraoperative management of patients as to what might be done to decrease the likelihood of POVL. The panel recommended that special attention be given to the management of blood pressure, intraoperative fluids, and anemia; the use of vasopressors; patient positioning; and staging of surgical procedures.

### Blood Pressure Management

Many preoperative factors—including the presence of chronic hypertension, cardiac dysfunction, and renal and vascular disease—need to be taken into account in terms of intraoperative blood pressure goals and management for patients undergoing prolonged spine operations in the prone position. In addition, many intraoperative factors must also be taken into account—such as the amount of fluid administered, rate of blood loss, degree of hypotension, and requirement for vasopressors to maintain blood pressure—when making decisions regarding intraoperative blood pressure goals. The use of deliberate hypotension is not contraindicated for these patients but should be determined on a case-by-case basis.

**Management of Intraoperative Fluids.** Monitoring of central venous pressure in patients at high risk of developing POVL should be considered, with administration of both crystalloids and colloids to maintain central venous pressure in patients who have significant blood loss.

**Management of Anemia.** Hemoglobin levels should be monitored periodically during surgery in at-risk patients if sustained or significant blood loss occurs. A hemoglobin target that would eliminate the possibility of POVL has not been established.

**Use of Vasopressors.** Because there have been no controlled trials evaluating the use of α-adrenergic agonists to maintain blood pressure in patients at risk for developing POVL, the decision to use α-adrenergic agonists should be made on a case-by-case basis.

**Patient Positioning.** Other than recognizing that the risk of POVL is increased in patients undergoing procedures in the prone position, the only other recommendation of the ASA task force was to avoid direct pressure on the ophthalmic globe and to periodically check to ensure that nothing impinges or presses on the eye during the surgical procedure.

### Recognizing and Treating Postoperative Visual Loss

As soon as at-risk patients are alert after surgery, their visual acuity should be assessed. If they have any evidence of having experienced visual loss, an ophthalmologist should be consulted immediately and asked to examine the patient to document the degree of impairment and to advise as to possible cause. Hemoglobin values, $O_2$ saturation, and hemodynamics should be optimized, and consideration should be given to ordering a magnetic resonance imaging study to rule out intracranial causes of POVL. There is no evidence to support the administration of diuretics, corticosteroids, anticoagulants, antiplatelet drugs, or drugs that decrease intraocular pressure.

## Dental Injury

Damage to the oropharynx is one of the most common, if not the most common, iatrogenic injuries that patients experience while under general anesthesia, occurring in up to 5% of general anesthetics. Injury to the hypopharynx (sore throat) is the most common; in one survey, injury occurred in 45% of patients. One-fifth of oral injuries (1% of all general anesthetics) are the result of trauma to teeth, usually to the upper incisors in patients older than 50 years. Surprisingly few of these injuries to the teeth require dental or oral surgical intervention, and yet dental injury is the most frequent cause of complaints and litigation against anesthesia providers.

Fractures of tooth enamel or of crowns account for approximately 40% of cases of dental injury, loosening or frank avulsion of teeth occurs in another 40% of reported cases (in one-fourth of those, or 10% of the time, a tooth or teeth are found to be missing), and the remaining 20% of cases are due to damage to veneers, dental restorations, prosthetic crowns, and fixed partial dentures.

## ETIOLOGY

### Patient Factors

Children aged 5 to 12 years (who have a mixture of primary and permanent teeth) and adults with carious teeth, gum disease, protruding or loose upper incisors, and difficult airways are at highest risk of experiencing dental injury.

### Anesthetic Factors

Dental injury occurs most commonly during induction and emergence from anesthesia. Patients with difficult airways, as mentioned previously, are as much as 20 times more likely to be injured during tracheal intubation compared with patients without a difficult airway. The anesthesia provider's skill is also a factor; less experienced providers are more likely to inflict dental injury, as evidenced by one study in which these providers were more likely to contact the laryngoscope with the left upper incisor during intubation. During emergence (or during induction of anesthesia if the depth of anesthesia is not sufficient or if the patient is not adequately relaxed), patients commonly bite, which can generate considerable force concentrated on the incisors and on an oropharyngeal airway, if an oropharyngeal airway is used as a bite block.

## PREVENTION

A thorough preoperative evaluation and examination of the oropharynx should be performed, not only to document whether the patient has a difficult airway but also to identify those patients with loose or carious teeth. In patients with poor dentition, consideration should be given to postponing the procedure if time permits to allow patients to see their dentists before the planned surgical procedure to attend to the dental problem (Fig. 225.2). Because two-thirds of injuries in one review were due to preexisting conditions (e.g., caries, prostheses, loose or damaged teeth, a single isolated tooth, or functional limitations), the anesthesia provider should document these in the medical record. If the patient requests to proceed after the risks of dental injury have been explained, documentation of the examination and of the counseling should be included in the consent form that the patient signs.

If removal of a partial denture or bridge leaves an isolated tooth, some experts advise that the benefits of leaving the appliance in place outweigh the benefit of removing it. The use of devices to optimize intubation in patients with difficult airways and the use of certain dental guards can decrease the incidence of damage to the teeth but do not eliminate the potential for damage and should not be relied on exclusively. Clearly, in these situations, it is incumbent on the anesthesia provider to have a plan for how to protect the airway during induction and intubation and to minimize direct contact with and trauma to the teeth.

## TREATMENT AND MANAGEMENT OF DENTAL INJURY

Despite our best efforts, injury to teeth can and will occur. Anesthesia departments should have a protocol in place to guide the management and care of dental injuries (Fig. 225.3). This protocol should include, at a minimum, the following items:

- Any missing teeth or fragments must be found. If the teeth or fragments are not identified, the patient should have a chest radiograph and an abdominal radiograph, if necessary, to identify fragments that may have been aspirated or swallowed.
- In children, the loss of a primary tooth does not require treatment. However, if a permanent tooth is avulsed, it should be stored in cool, sterile saline until placed back in the socket from which it came.
- Once the patient has recovered from anesthesia, she or he should be offered an explanation. A plan for postoperative care should be documented in the patient's medical record. If indicated, an oral surgical consultation should be obtained while the patient is still in the postanesthesia care unit, or, if treatment is not urgent, arrangements should be made, with a written plan given to the patient, for the patient to see his or her personal dentist.

---

**Identify patient factors that increase the risk of dental injury**

- Primary teeth
- Loose tooth
- Cavities
- Gum disease
- Mallampati score > 2
- Limited mouth opening
- Partial bridge
- Age > 50 y

**Perform a preoperative examination**

- Obtain history
- Examine the airway and teeth
- Thoroughly explain findings/risks of proceeding to patient
- Document results

**Develop the anesthetic plan**

- Assess or plan for removable bridges or partial dentures
- Provide adequate depth of anesthesia and relaxation before instrumentation
- Use a bite block between solid molars in high-risk patients
- Ensure additional safeguards for patients with difficult airways and poor dentition

**Refer high-risk patients to a dentist or oral surgeon**

**Fig. 225.2** Strategies for decreasing the incidence of intraoperative dental injury.

---

**Avulsed tooth**

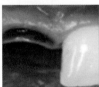

- Act quickly.
- Do not touch the root surfaces.
- Place the tooth in sterile saline.
- Assess whether the tooth can be replaced.
- Consult with a dentist.
- If dentist agrees to see the patient in follow-up, place the tooth back into the socket and hold for several minutes.

**Subluxated or chipped tooth**

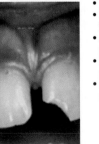

- Find missing teeth, tooth, or fragments.
- Perform imaging studies if unable to account for all fragments.
- Apologize and explain to patient in the presence of her or his responsible companion.
- Document findings and explanation in the medical record.
- Provide the patient with a written follow-up plan.

**Fig. 225.3** Managing avulsed or subluxated or chipped tooth. Avulsed teeth that are more likely to be able to be replaced include permanent teeth in patients with otherwise good dental health and no evidence of being immunocompromised.

## SUGGESTED READINGS

American Society of Anesthesiologists Task Force on Perioperative Visual Loss. (2012). Practice advisory for perioperative visual loss associated with spine surgery: An updated report by the American Society of Anesthesiologists Task Force on Perioperative Visual Loss. *Anesthesiology, 116*(2), 274–285.

Christensen, R. E., Baekgaard, J. S., & Rasmussen, L. S. (2019). Dental injuries in relation to general anaesthesia: A retrospective study. *Acta Anaesthesiologica Scandinavica, 63*(8), 993–1000.

Contractor, S., & Hardman, J. G. (2006). Injury during anaesthesia. *Continuing Education in Anaesthesia Critical Care Pain, 6*, 67–70.

Gaudio, R. M., Barbieri, S., Feltracco, P., Tiano, L., Galligioni, H., Uberti, M., et al. (2011). Traumatic dental injuries during anaesthesia. Part II: Medicolegal evaluation and liability. *Dental Traumatology, 27*(1), 40–45.

Lee, L. A. (2000). Postoperative visual loss data gathered and analyzed. *ASA Newsletter, 64*, 25–27.

Lee, L. A. (2003). ASA postoperative visual loss registry: Preliminary analysis of factors associated with spine operations. *ASA Newsletter, 67*, 7–8.

Lee, L. A., Roth, S., Posner, K. L., Cheney, F. W., Caplan, R. A., Newman, N. J., et al. (2006). The American Society of Anesthesiologists Postoperative Visual Loss Registry: Analysis of 93 spine surgery cases with postoperative visual loss. *Anesthesiology, 105*(4), 652–868.

Lin, J. C., French, D. D., Margo, C. E., & Greenberg, P. B. (2022). Epidemiology of postoperative visual loss for non-ocular surgery in a cohort of inpatients. *Eye (London, England), 36*(6), 1323–1325. doi:10.1038/s41433-021-01791-9.

Windsor, J., & Lockie, J. (2008). Anaesthesia and dental trauma. *Anaesthesia Intensive Care, 9*, 355–357.

# 226

# Intraoperative Patient Positioning and Positioning Complications

RYAN CHADHA, MD   |   REBECCA L. JOHNSON, MD

## Commonly Used Positions

The basic patient positions for surgery are supine, prone, and lateral, with the head down (Trendelenburg position) (Fig. 226.1), or with the head up (reverse Trendelenburg). Most other positions are variations on these. Lithotomy (supine) with the legs elevated and flexed (Fig. 226.2), jackknife (prone and flexed), lateral decubitus (Fig. 226.3), beach chair, and sitting are other commonly used positions.

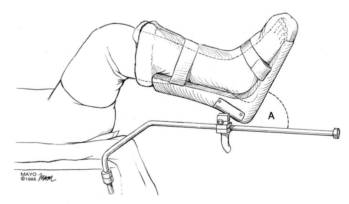

Correct position – Lower leg weight distributed to foot of stirrup by increasing angle A of stirrup to support bar.

**Fig. 226.2**   Correct lower limb positioning in a patient in the lithotomy position. The weight of the lower leg can be distributed to the foot of the stirrup by increasing angle A between the stirrup and the support bar. (By permission of Mayo Foundation for Medical Research and Education. All rights reserved.)

## Recommendations for Correct Positioning

### UPPER EXTREMITY POSITIONING

When patients are in the prone position, one or both arms are placed on arm boards in the "surrender" position. In some cases, the arms are tucked beneath the arched frame; in others,

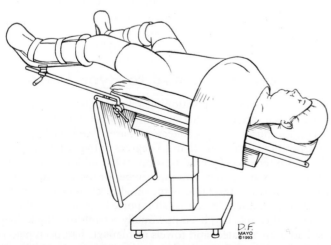

**Fig. 226.1**   The Trendelenburg position. (Used with permission of Mayo Foundation for Medical Education and Research, all rights reserved.)

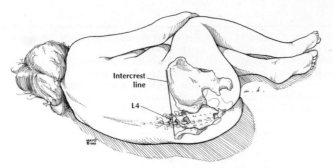

both arms are placed at the patient's sides. Risks to the arms, regardless of the surgical positioning, include pressure on or stretching of the brachial plexus and pressure on the ulnar nerve. It is usually prudent to place the arms in a neutral position within the patient's limits of awake ranges of motion. This may require that during the procedure, arms be tucked at their sides, as many patients have changes in somatosensory-evoked potentials when their arms are abducted. The brachial plexus can often be palpated at the axilla, and the shoulder can be maneuvered so as to ensure that the plexus is not under tension or pressure. For the lateral position, the use of an axillary (chest) roll is important to protect the brachial plexus (Fig. 226.4). Abduction of a shoulder to greater than 90 degrees potentially stretches the plexus (Fig. 226.5). It is prudent to avoid abduction greater than 90 degrees of any joint, and the cervical spine should be in a neutral position, especially for extended periods of time.

### LOWER EXTREMITY POSITIONING

The anterior iliac crest must be well padded to avoid pressure injury on the lateral femoral cutaneous nerve with subsequent paresthesias of the lateral thigh. If the patient's legs are large, the

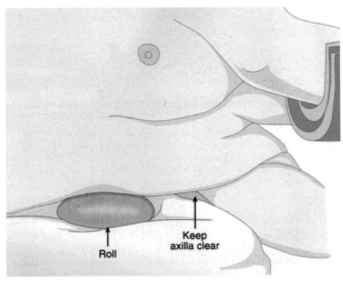

knees must be padded or even suspended to prevent pressure blisters between the legs. In older adult patients, care must be taken to avoid overflexing the hips, which can cause sciatic nerve stretch.

## Complications Resulting From Incorrect Positioning

### PRESSURE INJURIES

Evidence suggests that intraoperative positioning problems are often multifactorial and may not be preventable, despite our best efforts. Pressure injuries are common; these include tape "burns," skin blisters from prolonged pressure on surfaces, and evidence of skin breakdown from contact with the edge of positioning devices. Fortunately, point pressure injuries are usually shallow enough to heal without an ulcer. However, prolonged pressure on any soft tissue may reduce local blood flow and result in ischemia. Bony prominences such as on the occiput, elbows, and heels are vulnerable and should be padded. The greatest care must be taken around the patient's face and head. Although the skin of the face is vascular and heals well, an ischemic area at a fold in the facial tissue can lead to poor healing and scarring. Particular care must be taken with taping of the eyes and securing the endotracheal tube. Additionally, pressure alopecia (or hair loss due to ischemia) can result in the occipital region of the head with the combination of prolonged pressure, hypotension, and hypothermia.

### NERVE INJURY

Among the most serious complications of poor positioning are central and peripheral nerve injuries. Anesthetized patients lose the ability to respond to painful stimuli. Postoperative neuropathy is mostly associated with stretch and compression. However, patient-specific factors (e.g., sex, extremes of body weight, age, multiple comorbidities) and perioperative inflammatory responses such as use of anesthesia drugs and blood transfusion have also been shown to be contributors. Understanding these risk factors for central and peripheral nerve injury may provide anesthesiologists with future research themes and targets for prevention. Recent research suggests that perioperative inflammatory responses are present in patients who have prolonged postoperative neuropathies. A neurologic consultation should be considered, as potential exists for therapeutic interventions (e.g., immunomodulation and high-dose steroids) that may reduce both severity and duration of symptoms.

## Complications Related to Hyperlordosis

Among the most severe positioning-related injuries, spinal cord ischemia is a rare event that occurs when patients undergoing pelvic procedures (e.g., prostatectomy) are placed in a hyperlordotic position, with more than 15 degrees of hyperflexion at the L2 to L3 interspace. Operating room (OR) tables made in the United States are designed to limit hyperlordosis in supine patients, even when the table is maximally retroflexed with the kidney rest elevated. In almost all reported cases of spinal cord ischemia, the table had been maximally retroflexed, the kidney rest had been elevated, and towels or blankets had been placed under the patient's lower back to promote further anterior or forward tilt of the pelvis (to improve the surgeon's vision of

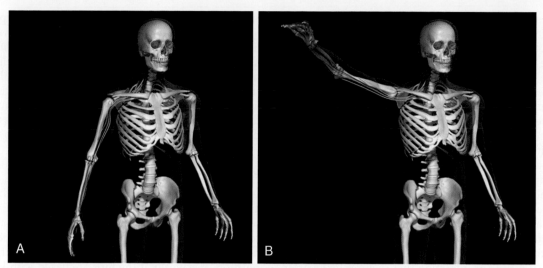

**Fig. 226.5 A,** The neurovascular bundle to the upper extremity passes on the flexion side of the shoulder joint when the arm is at the side or abducted less than 90 degrees. **B,** Abduction of the arm beyond 90 degrees transitions the neurovascular bundle to where it now lies on the extension side of the shoulder joint. Progressive abduction greater than 90 degrees increases stretch on the nerves at the shoulder joint. (By permission of Mayo Foundation for Medical Research and Education. All rights reserved.)

deep pelvic structures). In general, anesthesia providers should not allow placement of materials under the patient's lower back for this purpose.

## Complications of Upper Extremity Positioning

Surgical procedures involving the shoulder, elbow, wrist, and hand require positioning that has been associated with postoperative neurologic injury including brachial plexopathies. By far the most common brachial plexopathies involve the ulnar, median, and radial nerves.

Ulnar neuropathy, the most common of all positioning-related injuries, illustrates pathologic stretch and compression effects. Stretch of any nerve by more than 5% of resting length

may restrict arterial flow to the nerve and/or venule drainage away from nervous tissue, leading to direct and indirect ischemic insults, respectively. Prolonged elbow flexion of more than 90 degrees increases intrinsic pressure on the nerve and may be an etiologic factor, as is prolonged extrinsic pressure. The ulnar nerve passes behind the medial epicondyle and then runs under the aponeurosis that holds together the two muscle bodies of the flexor carpi ulnaris. The proximal edge of this aponeurosis is sufficiently thick, especially in men, to be separately named the cubital tunnel retinaculum. This retinaculum stretches from the medial epicondyle to the olecranon. Flexion of the elbow stretches the retinaculum and generates high pressure on the nerve as it passes underneath the retinaculum (Fig. 226.6).

Approximately 40% of sensory-only ulnar neuropathies resolve within 5 days; 80% resolve within 6 months. In contrast,

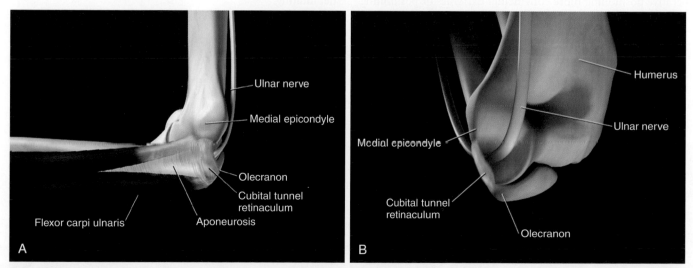

**Fig. 226.6 A,** The ulnar nerve of the right arm passes distally behind the medial epicondyle and underneath the aponeurosis that holds the two heads of the *flexor carpi ulnaris* together. The proximal edge of the aponeurosis is sufficiently thick in 80% of men and 20% of women to be distinct anatomically from the remainder of the tissue. It is commonly called the *cubital tunnel retinaculum.* **B,** Viewed from behind, the ulnar nerve is intrinsically compressed by the *cubital tunnel retinaculum* when the elbow is progressively flexed beyond 90 degrees and the distance between the olecranon and the medial epicondyle increases. (By permission of Mayo Foundation for Medical Research and Education. All rights reserved.)

few combined sensorimotor ulnar neuropathies resolve within 5 days; only 20% resolve within 6 months, and most result in permanent motor dysfunction and pain. The motor fibers in the ulnar nerve are primarily located in the middle of the nerve. Injury to these fibers is likely associated with more significant ischemia or pressure insult to all ulnar nerve fibers.

Thoracic outlet syndrome, a group of conditions that develop when the blood vessels or nerves in the thoracic outlet become compressed, provides another example of positioning upper extremity neuropathy. Perioperatively, thoracic outlet obstruction occurs when patients with this syndrome are positioned prone or lateral. In almost all reported cases, the shoulder had been abducted more than 90 degrees. In that position, the vasculature to the upper extremity is compressed either between the clavicle and rib cage or between the two heads of the sternocleidomastoid muscle, leading to ischemia. When ischemia is prolonged, the results range from minor disability to severe tissue ischemia or infarction that requires forequarter amputation. A simple preoperative question such as "Can you use your arms to work above your head for more than a minute?" may elicit a history of thoracic outlet obstruction.

## Complications of Lower Extremity Positioning

In comparison with upper extremity injuries, lower extremity peripheral neuropathies are less frequently seen in the perioperative period. Common lumbosacral neuropathies associated with abdominal and pelvic surgery involve the sciatic, obturator, femoral, and lateral femoral cutaneous nerves. Like postoperative injuries that occur after upper extremity surgery, the mechanism for neurologic injury after lower extremity, abdomen, and pelvic surgery is not clear and may be multifactorial with patient, anesthesia, and surgical factors influencing occurrences. However, the evidence to implicate intraoperative positioning may be stronger for postoperative lower extremity neuropathies compared with upper extremity complications. Lower extremity neuropathies are reported earlier than upper extremity neuropathies, with symptoms noted within hours of surgery, making the link to operative positioning more convincing. Extremes of positioning

and external compression of the legs against supports has led to intraoperative nerve injuries and compartment syndromes. Warner and colleagues discovered that the risk of motor neuropathy increased nearly 100-fold for each hour spent in lithotomy position. It is recommended that surgeons and anesthesiologists restrict total time in the lithotomy position. Reducing duration in lithotomy position is important in those with multiple risk factors including patients with body mass index less than 20 kg/m$^2$, diabetes, peripheral vascular disease, and tobacco use.

### SCIATIC NERVE INJURY

Injuries to the proximal and distal portions of the sciatic nerve are rare (0.2%–0.3% after vaginal surgeries). The proximal sciatic and common fibular (peroneal) nerves are fixed at the sciatic notch and the neck of the fibula, respectively. These nerves are susceptible to excessive stretch during lithotomy position, specifically if the hips are flexed with knees extended or even if hips and knees are bent with excessive external rotation of the thigh at the hip. Intraoperative injuries have been reduced when lithotomy positioning has been adjusted to moderate hip flexion and abduction of the thighs with near neural hip rotation. The common fibular nerve, after separating from the tibial nerve in the thigh, takes a superficial course across the head of the fibula before descending down the leg. This nerve is most susceptible to compression injury.

### OBTURATOR NEUROPATHY

Hip abduction of more than 30 degrees results in strain on the obturator nerve. The nerve passes through the pelvis and out the obturator foramen. With hip abduction, the superior and lateral rim of the foramen serves as a fulcrum (Fig. 226.7). The nerve stretches along its length and is also compressed at this fulcrum point. Thus excessive hip abduction should be avoided whenever possible. With obturator neuropathy, motor dysfunction is common, and approximately 50% of patients who have motor dysfunction in the perioperative period will continue to have it 2 years later. The dysfunction is not painful, but it can be debilitating.

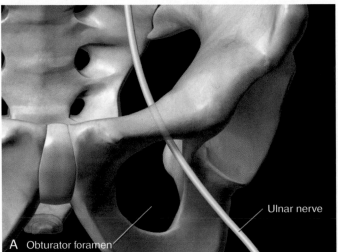 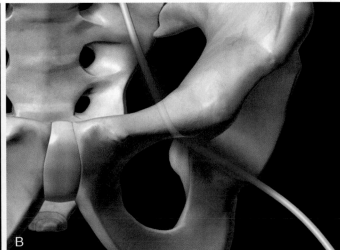

A   Obturator foramen

Ulnar nerve

B

**Fig. 226.7    A,** The obturator nerve passes through the pelvis and exits out the superior and lateral corner of the obturator foramen as it continues distally down the inner thigh. **B,** Abduction of the hip stretches the obturator nerve and can provoke ischemia, especially at the exit point of the obturator foramen. The point serves as a fulcrum for the nerve during hip abduction.

## FEMORAL AND LATERAL FEMORAL CUTANEOUS NEUROPATHY

One-third of the fibers of the common femoral and lateral femoral cutaneous nerves pass through the inguinal ligament as the fibers pass into the thigh (Fig. 226.8). Prolonged hip flexion will result in lateral displacement of the anterior superior iliac spine and increased stretch of the inguinal ligament. Branches of these nerves can become ischemic, resulting in sensory loss of the anterolateral thigh. The lateral femoral cutaneous nerve carries only sensory fibers, so no motor disability occurs when this nerve is injured. However, patients with this perioperative neuropathy can have disabling pain and dysesthesias of the lateral thigh (meralgia paresthetica). Approximately 40% of these patients have dysesthesias that can last for more than a year. Femoral neuropathies, although rare, have been reported in patients undergoing urologic, gynecologic, transplant, general, and colorectal surgery and can result in significant disability.

## Complications of Steep Trendelenburg Position

As surgeons gain experience with new technologies (e.g., robotics for use in pelvic procedures), they often request that the patient be placed in a steep Trendelenburg position (Fig. 226.9). Venous engorgement of the face can be impressive, sometimes resulting in marked conjunctival edema. Airway edema can also result, although this is rarely clinically significant. Pulmonary compliance is reduced when the contents of the abdomen press on the diaphragm, like in the steep Trendelenburg position, with variable effects depending on patient-specific factors. Reduced pulmonary compliance appears to be a transient problem that can be corrected by returning the patient to the supine position. It is reasonable to assume that these patients may have an increase in interstitial lung water that could impair diffusion. An unexplained decrease in $O_2$ saturation is not uncommon in patients experiencing reduced pulmonary compliance. Applying positive-pressure ventilation when the patient resumes the supine position should correct this phenomenon.

There are also reports of patients sliding off the OR table and of extremity compartment syndromes with the weight of the patient pressing against arm straps, with the straps occluding venous return. Although intracranial pressure also increases, it rarely results in a negative outcome.

## Complications Related to the Sitting Position

The sitting position also has associated risks but also many unique benefits that benefit surgical exposure. The primary risks are of venous air embolism and cerebral ischemia. When intra-arterial cannulas are placed to measure blood pressure when the patient is in the sitting position, placing the transducer at the level of the external auditory meatus is considered the gold standard to measure cerebral perfusion pressure.

## Complications Related to Head Positioning

For many operations involving the cranial nerve or ear, nose, or throat, the patient's head is turned to the side. Degenerative disease of the cerebral vertebrae or vascular impingement may limit the degree to which the patient's head can be turned. Only rarely will such a patient have somatosensory-evoked potentials monitored to detect spinal cord compromise. The best way to determine the degree of cervical movement that the patient can tolerate is to place the patient in the desired position while awake and check the range of motion carefully before inducing anesthesia. The head should not be flexed to the point where there are less than two fingerbreadths of space between the bone of the chin and the sternal notch, as quadriplegia may result (Fig. 226.10). Age should be considered when positioning the patient with the head turned, flexed, or extended. The cervical and vascular degeneration that contribute to problems can begin in middle age and are nearly always present by the seventh decade of life.

Some have suggested that prolonged prone cases should be performed with the patient's head pinned to reduce the risk of postoperative vision loss (POVL). Because POVL occurs

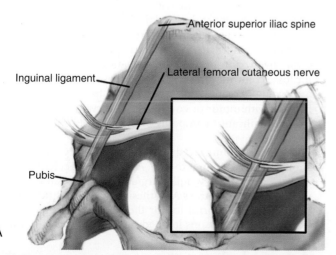
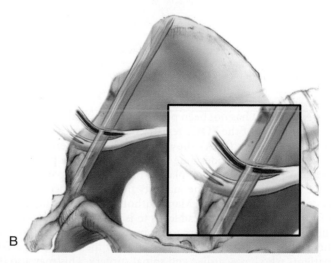

**Fig. 226.8 A,** Approximately one-third of the lateral femoral cutaneous nerve fibers penetrate the inguinal ligament as the nerve passes out of the pelvis and distally into the lateral thigh. **B,** Hip flexion, especially when greater than 90 degrees, leads to stretch of the inguinal ligament as the ilium is displaced laterally. This stretch causes the intraligament pressure to increase and compresses the nerve fibers as they pass through the ligament. (By permission of Mayo Foundation for Medical Research and Education. All rights reserved.)

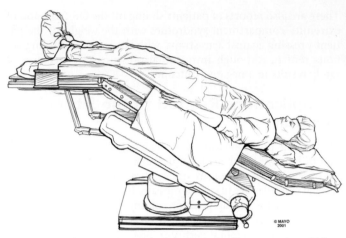

**Fig. 226.9** The steep Trendelenburg position. (By permission of Mayo Foundation for Medical Research and Education. All rights reserved.)

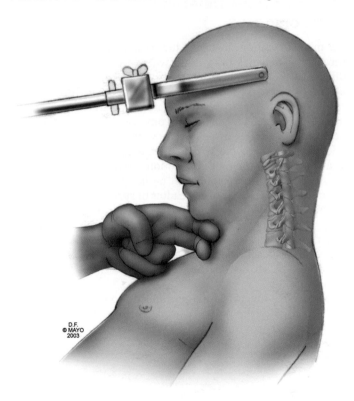

**Fig. 226.10** Two-finger technique for preventing cervical compression, and therefore quadriplegia, during anesthesia. (By permission of Mayo Foundation for Medical Research and Education. All rights reserved.)

infrequently, it has not been possible to specifically identify the cause. Review of the POVL registry of the American Society of Anesthesiologists (ASA) shows that 67% of patients who develop POVL have undergone spine surgery in the prone position, so positioning likely plays a role. In those patients who have developed POVL, the majority had spine procedures that lasted between 5 and 9 h. Many authorities assume that edema of the retina and optic head leads to ischemia. POVL occurs in all age groups but appears to be more common in older patients; however, this may be a reflection of the number of older patients who have cardiac and spinal surgery. This may also be due to peripheral vascular disease in older patients. Atherosclerosis, along with hypotension and anemia, may play an important role in the development of POVL.

## Practical Considerations for Preventing Positioning-Related Injury

*Use padding to distribute compressive forces and position joints to avoid excessive stretch.* Do not exceed comfortable awake range of motions of any joint. Tailor the positioning to avoid discomfort, strain, pull, or compression (recognizing variation among individuals). Although few studies have been conducted to demonstrate that padding has any impact on the frequency or severity of perioperative neuropathies, it makes sense to distribute point pressure. The use of padding has been viewed favorably as a positive marker of vigilant care by jurors in several medicolegal cases.

*Avoid bilateral tucked arm positioning.* Tucking of one or both arms has been associated with persistent ulnar neuropathy. Hence it will be important for the perioperative team to discuss the potential for modifying arm positioning. Avoid tucking of both arms or tucking an arm with preexisting neuropathy, especially in patients with multiple risk factors for development of perioperative ulnar neuropathy (e.g., male sex, higher body mass index, history of cancer, or when cases are expected to run longer).

*Act to prevent vision loss.* Maintaining the head at or above the level of the heart to reduce venous congestion, avoiding pressure on the eyes, using colloids along with crystalloids for volume replacement, and splitting long operations into stages in high-risk patients has been advocated by the ASA Task Force on Perioperative Visual Loss. More controversial are intraoperative practices of transfusion to maintain upper range of normal hemoglobin levels and chemical methods to maintain normotension during operations.

*Limit the length of the operation.* With soft tissue injury, visual loss, and peripheral and neuraxial neuropathies more likely occurring with prolonged cases times, limiting surgical duration or consider staging procedures that require an operating time greater than 5 h to reduce risk.

## What to Do When Injury Occurs

If your patient develops a peripheral neuropathy and the neural loss is only sensory, it is reasonable to follow the patient's condition daily for up to 5 days. Many sensory deficits in the immediate postoperative period will resolve during this time. If the deficit persists longer than 5 days, it is likely that the neuropathy will have an extended impact. It is appropriate if the sensory deficit lasts longer than 5 days to request that a neurologist become involved to provide an evaluation and long-term care. If the loss is only motor or combined sensory and motor, it would be prudent to request that a neurologist become involved earlier. Patients with motor or combined sensory and motor loss likely have a significant neuropathy and will need prolonged postoperative care.

Positioning injuries should be reported. Confidential and anonymous reporting to the Anesthesia Incident Reporting System (https://www.aqihq.org/airs), a repository of cases maintained by the ASA's Anesthesia Quality Institute, is important. There is opportunity for the case to be reviewed by colleagues with the lessons learned, aggregated, and disseminated.

## Acknowledgment

The authors wish to acknowledge the contributions of Drs. Cucchiara and Warner to previous editions of this chapter.

## SUGGESTED READINGS

American Society of Anesthesiologists Task Force on Perioperative Visual Loss. (2012). Practice advisory for perioperative visual loss associated with spine surgery: An updated report by the American Society of Anesthesiologists Task Force on Perioperative Visual Loss. *Anesthesiology, 116*(2), 274–285.

Pulos, B. P., Johnson, R. L., Laughlin, R. S., Njathi-Ori, C. W., Kor, T. M., Schroeder, D. R., et al. (2021).

Perioperative ulnar neuropathy: A contemporary estimate of incidence and risk factors. *Anesthesia and Analgesia, 132*(5), 1429–1437.

Staff, N. P., Engelstad, J., Klein, C. J., Amrami, K. K., Spinner, R. J., Dyck, P. J., et al. (2010). Postsurgical inflammatory neuropathy. *Brain, 133*(10), 2866–2880.

Warner, M. E., & Johnson, R. L. (2017). Patient positioning and potential injuries. In P. G. Barash (Ed.), *Clinical anesthesia* (8th ed., pp. 809–825). Philadelphia: Wolters Kluwer Health/Lippincott Williams & Wilkins.

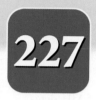

# 227

# Malignant Hyperthermia

KLAUS D. TORP, MD  |  SHER-LU PAI, MD

## Introduction

Malignant hyperthermia (MH) is a serious and potentially life-threatening hypermetabolic skeletal muscle disorder that can be triggered in response to all volatile anesthetics, as well as succinylcholine, in MH-susceptible (MHS) individuals, whereas all other anesthetics appear to be safe. Prior to the introduction of intravenous dantrolene, MH episodes had a very high mortality. Present management requires an understanding of MH genetics along with early recognition of clinical signs and treatment strategies. Referral for genetic counseling is helpful in identifying susceptible family members when a causative mutation for MH is found. MH is known to be linked with central core and minicore myopathies. Recent reports also suggest a possible link with other muscle abnormalities, including exercise-induced rhabdomyolysis.

## History

In 1960, Denborough and Lovell reported the first case of anesthesia-induced hypermetabolism in a patient with a familial history of multiple anesthetic deaths during ether administration. The patient, a young man with a lower extremity fracture, survived a halothane-induced MH episode with symptomatic treatment in this predantrolene era. The strong familial history rendered this a particularly clear description of a genetically linked condition. Little further attention was paid to this condition until 1969, when Kalow and Britt described a metabolic error of skeletal muscle metabolism in patients from Wausau, Wisconsin, who had recovered from MH episodes. This finding formed the scientific basis for modern diagnostic contracture testing. In 1975, Harrison reported the efficacy of dantrolene in treating porcine MH, a treatment that has

lowered the mortality rate associated with this rare condition from as high as 80% to less than 10%.

## Incidence and Mortality

The incidence of MH is variably reported as ranging from 1:4500 to 1:60,000 general anesthetics (geographic variation is related to the gene prevalence); however, genetic predisposition has been reported with much higher frequency at 1:2000 to 1:3000, which suggests incomplete penetrance. Approximately 50% of MH-susceptible individuals have had at least one previous triggering anesthetic without developing MH symptoms. MH is rare in infants, and incidence decreases after age 50 years, with the highest prevalence of clinical symptoms in males. The reasons for these variations are not understood.

MH has been clearly associated with central core disease (CCD). MH-like symptoms have been associated with other neuromuscular disorders, such as Duchenne's muscular dystrophy; nontriggering anesthesia is recommended for these patients. Association with other conditions such as myotonia, sudden infant death syndrome, serotonin syndrome, and neuroleptic malignant syndrome (NMS) is controversial and unlikely. More recently, exercise-induced muscle disorders (rhabdomyolysis), hyperthermia, and death have been linked to genetic markers associated with MH.

## Genetics of Malignant Hyperthermia

MH has an autosomal dominant pattern of inheritance with clinical heterogeneity and variable expression. The rate of spontaneous mutation is unknown but is probably less than 10%. A single gene mutation responsible for MH was identified in the affected swine model involving the ryanodine receptor gene. The ryanodine receptor is a protein that controls the calcium release channel in the skeletal muscle sarcoplasmic reticulum, a site shown to be defective in MH-susceptible swine. Unfortunately, human MH is far more complicated genetically. The ryanodine gene (RYR1) (MHS1 locus) encodes the type 1 ryanodine receptor. Mutations in this gene can be identified in 70% to 80% of MHS and CCD patients, and more than 180 mutations (over one-half of these mutations are found in a few families) have been identified. The other known MH gene is the CACNA1S (MHS5 locus), which encodes the subunit of the dihydropyridine (DHP) receptor L-type calcium channel. Mutations in this gene account for only about 1% of all MHS; two mutations have been identified. There are three additional mapped loci without identified genes: MHS2, MHS4, and MHS6. Another much less common gene locus is STAC 3 on chromosome 12, which encodes a protein ligand between RYR1 and DHP.

Patient selection for genetic testing is very important. In a patient with a positive caffeine-halothane muscle biopsy or very strong family history of unequivocal MH, complete sequence analysis of RYR1 coding gives 70% to 80% detection. In the case of a multigenerational family (two or more) with unequivocal MH in at least 10 members, linkage analysis for all MHS loci can be performed and new sites can be detected. However, screening of a single individual with a new diagnosis of clinical MH against the MH genes will be negative in up to 50% of cases. In addition, the CACNA1S and RYR1 genes are naturally highly variant, and only a very small subset has been characterized as a causative mutation. Thus a single preoperative genetic screening test in humans is unlikely in the near future.

## Clinical Presentation

Onset of clinical signs can be acute and fulminant or delayed. MH can occur at any time during the anesthetic and has been reported to occur as late as 24 h postoperatively.

Trismus (masseter muscle rigidity [MMR]) after inhalation induction and succinylcholine is associated with an approximately 50% incidence of MH diagnosed by contracture testing. MMR is often not associated with signs of a fulminant MH episode; however, patients must be closely observed for evidence of rigidity, hypermetabolism, and rhabdomyolysis. Minor symptoms, such as unusual muscle cramping after MMR in the recovery room in the absence of any other symptoms, has led to genetically confirmed diagnosis of MH.

**Clinical signs and symptoms** reflect the state of highly increased metabolism. The onset of hyperthermia may be delayed, but a recent review of MH cases suggests that in many cases, trending temperature increases may be an early indication of hypermetabolism (Table 227.1). Therefore the earliest

| TABLE 227.2 | Differential Diagnosis of Hypermetabolic Conditions During Surgery |
|---|---|
| Malignant hyperthermia | |
| Neurolept malignant syndrome | |
| Pheochromocytoma | |
| Thyrotoxicosis | |
| Serotonin syndrome | |
| Recreational drug abuse | |
| Iatrogenic overheating | |
| Sepsis | |
| Baclofen withdrawal | |
| Brain injury | |
| Light anesthesia | |
| Exhausted soda lime or hypoventilation | |
| Excessive carbon dioxide during laparoscopic surgery | |

signs of MH include increased end-tidal $CO_2$ levels, sinus tachycardia, hyperthermia, and tachypnea (in an unparalyzed patient). Although it is important to begin treatment for MH (e.g., administering dantrolene) as soon as possible, one should at least consider other potential diagnoses of highly increased metabolism and temperature during surgery, especially if the patient does not react to treatment (Table 227.2).

**Supportive laboratory tests** for confirmation of MH diagnosis include:
- Elevated end-tidal $CO_2$
- Elevated temperature
- Muscular abnormalities
- Blood gas analysis: mixed venous, arterial, or venous samples will show a metabolic acidosis. Recent data show that respiratory acidosis alone is the most common presentation with metabolic acidosis present in only one-third of cases
- Elevated serum creatine phosphokinase (CK): draw every 6 h for 24 h
- Myoglobin in serum and urine
- Increased serum $K^+$, $Ca^{2+}$, lactate

**Triggers** include:
- All potent volatile anesthetics
- Succinylcholine

**Safe anesthetic agents** include nitrous oxide, etomidate, ketamine, propofol, benzodiazepines, all narcotics, all local anesthetics, all barbiturates, and all nondepolarizing muscle relaxants. Agents used for reversal of muscle relaxants are also safe.

**Mechanism.** Exposure to triggering anesthetics causes decreased control of intracellular calcium, resulting in excessive release of free unbound ionized $Ca^{2+}$ from storage sites. The calcium pumps attempt to restore homeostasis, which results in increased adenosine triphosphate utilization, increased aerobic and anaerobic metabolism, and a runaway hypermetabolic state. Rigidity occurs when unbound myofibrillar $Ca^{2+}$ approaches the contractile threshold, when it cannot be removed due to overwhelmed calcium pumps.

**Treatment.** Discontinue triggers immediately and hyperventilate with high-flow (>10 L) 100% oxygen. Place activated charcoal filters on both inspiratory and expiratory limbs and replace in 1 h as per manufacturer guidelines. They are very effective in quickly reducing the concentration of volatile anesthetics. Although replacing the breathing circuit and soda lime may further help decrease the volatile anesthetic reservoir, this should not distract from other important tasks during the crisis.

| TABLE 227.1 | Clinical Signs of Malignant Hyperthermia | |
|---|---|---|
| **Increased Temperature** | **Increased Sympathetic Activity** | |
| Tachypnea | Tachycardia | |
| Rhabdomyolysis | Dysrhythmias | |
| Metabolic/respiratory acidosis | Sweating | |
| Rigidity (75% humans) | Hypertension/hypotension | |
| Widened QRS complex | Peaked T-waves | |

When MH is suspected, dantrolene should be given early in a dosage of 2.5 mg/kg (ideal body weight) intravenously (IV), repeated every 5 min until symptoms start to resolve. Often this can be accomplished with doses up to 10 mg/kg; however, higher doses (up to 30 mg/kg) have been reported. The newer dantrolene formulation (e.g., Ryanodex) is more concentrated (250 mg/5 mL) as opposed to the traditional vials (20 mg/60 mL) and much easier to reconstitute, which may free up personnel to help with other tasks during the crisis. After successful treatment, dantrolene is continued at 1 mg/kg IV every 4 to 6 h for 24 to 48 h to prevent recrudescence of symptoms, which can occur in up to 25% of patients. In case of recrudescence this dose may need to be increased. Calcium channel blockers should not be given in the presence of dantrolene because myocardial depression has been demonstrated in swine. Treatment efficacy is monitored with arterial blood gases, serum CK, and vital signs. Dantrolene has unpleasant side effects (nausea, malaise, muscle weakness) but is generally well tolerated and has minimal toxicity in IV doses for MH treatment.

**Symptomatic treatment** includes, as appropriate:

- Cooling (caution: avoid hypothermia; stop cooling at core temperature of 38°C)
- Antiarrhythmics (avoid calcium channel blockers)
- Management of hyperkalemia with insulin and glucose
- Diuretics: mannitol, furosemide (rarely needed because of mannitol in the traditional dantrolene, but only contains small amounts in the new concentrated Ryanodex)
- Sodium bicarbonate
- Cases of successful venovenous and venoarterial extracorporeal membrane oxygenation have been reported in patients who are refractory to standard therapy

The use of printed checklists (one example can be found at https://emergencymanual.stanford.edu/) can be very helpful to manage an MH crisis. A newly developed app endorsed by the European MH group and the Malignant Hyperthermia Association of the United States (MHAUS) (http://www.girard.li/MHApp/MHApp_/MHApp.html) is also available. Both resources are free to download.

## Anesthesia for Malignant Hyperthermia-Susceptible Patients

Pretreatment with dantrolene is not recommended. Only nontriggering anesthetic agents should be used. Prepare the machine by removing vaporizers (if possible), and replace breathing circuits and soda lime. Previous recommendations suggested that flushing with high-flow air or oxygen (10 L/min) for 10 min would be adequate; however, newer machines have been shown to require flushing up to 70 min to reach the recommended volatile agent level of less than 5 ppm. In addition, if flows are then decreased, there is a rebound of volatile concentration. Using high flows (>10 L/min), adding activated charcoal filters to each limb of the breathing circuit, or using autoclaved internal breathing system components minimizes the risk of residual machine contamination. Trying to schedule MHS patients as the first case of the day makes turnover time much more efficient and allows for longer observation of the patient in the postanesthesia care unit. A minimum observation period of 2 h has been recommended.

Monitoring should include all standard monitors with an emphasis on end-tidal $CO_2$, oxygen saturation, and core temperature (skin monitors may not reflect core changes). A recent review reported that mortality is many times higher when core temperature was not monitored. Arterial and central venous pressures should be monitored only if indicated by the surgical procedure or the patient's medical condition.

## Evaluation of Susceptibility

Patients are referred for evaluation for a number of reasons:

- Unexplained intraoperative death in family members
- History of adverse anesthetic event (e.g., trismus)
- History of known MH in a family member
- Idiopathic elevated CK levels
- History of exertional rhabdomyolysis
- Associated myopathies (e.g., CCD, multiminicore disease, King-Denborough syndrome)

A serum CK level is often obtained in patients suspected of being susceptible to MH. This value is elevated in approximately 70% of affected individuals but may be inconsistent.

Standardized muscle biopsy contracture testing is the only reliable diagnostic test for MH, and it is extremely sensitive. Muscle is tested with caffeine and halothane in separate testing vessels, and contracture responses are measured. Because this test requires live muscle, it can only be performed in specialized testing centers. A list of these centers can be found at https://www.MHAUS.org, along with a list of current genetic testing centers in the United States. Patients who may benefit from referral for genetic testing include:

1. Patients who have a positive muscle biopsy contracture test
2. Patients who have had an unequivocal MH episode
3. Family members of patients who have a known mutation
4. Family members of patients who have had a mutation identified in a research center

MHAUS (https://www.MHAUS.org) is a lay organization with a medical MH-expert advisory group that provides support for patients and physicians. It publishes books, pamphlets, and a quarterly newsletter at nominal cost, sponsors the website (https://MHAUS.org), and manages a 24-hour hotline (1–800-MHHYPER) to provide assistance to physicians managing MH-susceptible patients or treating acute MH episodes.

## Dantrolene Availability and Patient Safety

Consensus guidelines issued by various anesthesia professional societies and MHAUS state that dantrolene must be available at anesthetizing locations where MH-triggering agents are routinely administered. However, recommendation controversies exist on the requirement of dantrolene availability in office-based anesthesia where succinylcholine is stocked for the sole purpose of treating life-threatening airway emergencies. Office-based surgery facilities are generally categorized into three classes based on the type of anesthesia administered: in class A facilities, local or topical anesthesia is administered; in class B facilities, sedation medication and regional anesthesia are administered; and in class C facilities, general anesthesia is administered.

The Society for Ambulatory Anesthesia proposes that in class B ambulatory facilities, where patients exclusively received oral or intravenous medications for sedation without volatile anesthetics, dantrolene should not be required as no known MH triggers are routinely used. Although uncommon, airway emergencies may lead to significant morbidity and mortality when not effectively managed. Succinylcholine's rapid onset, short duration, and compatibility with intramuscular administration have made it a crucial medication for emergency airway rescues. Because of the substantial cost of maintaining a stock of dantrolene, some have argued that a class B facility should not be required to keep dantrolene even though it has a stock of succinylcholine for rare event of airway emergencies, so long as it ensures a preexisting agreement with a close health care center that has dantrolene. Alternatively, some class B facilities have replaced succinylcholine with rocuronium and sugammadex, planning to administer high-dose sugammadex for rocuronium reversal to facilitate the return of spontaneous ventilation in patients during "cannot intubate and cannot ventilate" situations.

## Acknowledgment

The authors wish to thank Denise J. Wedel, MD for her contributions to previous editions of this chapter.

## SUGGESTED READINGS

Brislin, R. P., & Theroux, M. C. (2013). Core myopathies and malignant hyperthermia susceptibility: A review. *Paediatric Anaesthesia, 23*(9), 834–841.

Huh, H., Jung, J. S., Park, S. J., Park, M. K., Lim, C. H., & Yoon, S. Z. (2017). Successful early application of extracorporeal membrane oxygenation to support cardiopulmonary resuscitation for a patient suffering from severe malignant hyperthermia and cardiac arrest: A case report. *Korean Journal of Anesthesiology, 70*(3), 345–349.

Larach, M. G., Brandom, B. W., Allen, G. C., Gronert, G. A., & Lehman, E. B. (2014). Malignant hyperthermia deaths related to inadequate temperature monitoring, 2007-2012: A report from the North American Malignant Hyperthermia Registry of the Malignant Hyperthermia Association of the United States. *Anesthesia and Analgesia, 119*(6), 1359–1366.

Larach, M. G., Gronert, G. A., Allen, G. C., Brandom, B. W., & Lehman, E. B. (2010). Clinical presentation, treatment, and complications of malignant hyperthermia in North America from 1987 to 2006. *Anesthesia and Analgesia, 110*(2), 498–507.

Larach, M. G., Klumpner, T. T., Brandom, B. W., Vaughn, M. T., Belani, K. G., Herlich, A., et al. (2019). Succinylcholine use and dantrolene availability for malignant hyperthermia treatment: Database analyses and systematic review. *Anesthesiology, 130*(1), 41–54.

Litman, R. S., Smith, V. I., Larach, M. G., Mayes, L., Shukry, M., Theroux, M. C., et al. (2019). Consensus statement of the malignant hyperthermia association of the United States on unresolved clinical questions concerning the management of patients with malignant hyperthermia. *Anesthesia and Analgesia, 128*(4), 652–659.

Riazi, S., Kraeva, N., & Hopkins, P. M. (2018). Malignant hyperthermia in the post-genomics era: New perspectives on an old concept. *Anesthesiology, 128*(1), 168–180.

Skerritt, C., & Carton, E. (2019). Veno-venous extracorporeal membrane oxygenation in the management of malignant hyperthermia. *British Journal of Anaesthesia, 122*(6), e82–e83.

# 228 Anaphylactic and Anaphylactoid Reactions in Anesthesia

CARMELINA GURRIERI, MD

Severe intraoperative allergic reactions are associated with substantial morbidity and mortality, with anesthesia-related mortality estimated to be as high as 6%. The reported rate of intraoperative anaphylactic reactions ranges from 1:10,000 to 1:20,000. The primary risk factor for intraoperative anaphylaxis is a history of a reaction during surgery. Other risk factors include female sex and atopic disorders (e.g., asthma, eczema, hay fever).

## Pathophysiology

Anaphylaxis is a potential lethal multisystem syndrome resulting from the sudden release of mast cell and basophil derived vasoactive mediators including histamine, serum protease (e.g., tryptase), proteoglycans, prostaglandins, and leukotrienes into the circulation. Two mechanisms are implicated: immunoglobulin (Ig)E-mediated (anaphylactic) reactions, which account for approximately 60% of cases; and non–IgE-mediated (anaphylactoid) reactions.

## Clinical Features

Then clinical presentation of allergic reactions in the perioperative period can be variable but typically present as sudden changes in cardiovascular and/or respiratory parameters. Clinical manifestations may include:

- Cardiovascular instability, which ranges from hypotension to cardiac arrest and collapse.

- Tachycardia occurs in the majority of cases, but bradycardia can develop.
- Bronchospasm, which presents as increased peak pressure, upsloping pattern in the end-tidal carbon dioxide waveform, decrease in end-tidal carbon dioxide, and decrease in arterial oxygen saturation.
- Laryngeal edema, which can manifest as difficult intubation and/or postextubation stridor.
- Skin symptoms such as erythema, flushing, and urticaria can present, but may be difficult to recognize if the skin is draped or covered.

## Causative Agents

### NEUROMUSCULAR BLOCKING AGENTS

Neuromuscular blocking agents (NMBAs) are the most common causative agents of anaphylactic reactions in many European countries and Australia, with the majority to succinylcholine and rocuronium. Cross-sensitivity among the neuromuscular blockers is approximately 60% to 70%, with pairs found between pancuronium and vecuronium, succinylcholine and gallamine, and cis-atracurium and atracurium. NMBAs can cause anaphylaxis through both IgE-mediated and non–IgE-mediated reactions. The IgE recognition site for the neuromuscular blockers is their substituted ammonium ions and molecular environment. Given their ammonium structures, possible sensitization to neuromuscular blockers can occur with exposure to environmental factors containing tertiary and quaternary ammonium groups including many over-the-counter drugs, cosmetics, disinfectants, and food products. Pholcodine, an opioid antitussive widely available in several European countries and Australia, can produce high levels of antibodies, which may react with NMBAs. This drug is now believed to be the primary culprit for the high rates of anaphylactic reactions to NMBAs in countries where pholcodine was available. Anaphylactic reactions toward NMBAs have dramatically decreased in Norway after the withdrawal of pholcodine. Other countries (e.g., Sweden, Australia) where pholcodine remains available have not had similar reductions of NMBA reactions. Pholcodine has never been available in the United States, which accounts for the low rate of reactions to NMBAs in North America.

### ANTIBIOTICS

Antibiotics are reported to be the most common culprits of perioperative anaphylactic reactions in the United States and Spain, accounting for up to 55% of the cases. β-Lactam antibiotics (penicillins and cephalosporins) are the most frequent agents reported with cefazolin being the most common, followed by vancomycin (which causes reactions secondary to histamine release) and quinolones. Cross-reactivity between penicillins and first generation cephalosporins may approach 10%.

### CHLORHEXIDINE

Allergic reactions to chlorhexidine are considered rare, although a Danish study found chlorhexidine triggered 19% of perioperative allergic reactions. Initial reports of these reactions were often type IV delayed hypersensitivity reactions quite difficult to diagnose. Subsequently, immediate type I hypersensitivity reactions (ranging from widespread urticaria to anaphylactic shock) have been reported to chlorhexidine via topical skin application, ophthalmic wash solution, chlorhexidine bath, coated central venous catheter, and urethral gels. The exact mechanism of sensitization to chlorhexidine is not entirely clear, although, in many cases, it requires contact with mucous membranes or direct penetration into the bloodstream.

### LATEX

Latex allergy was one of the most common cause of perioperative anaphylaxis in the 1990s in the setting of increased production of latex-containing gloves to meet the demand of hospital hygiene practices during the HIV epidemic. However, over the past few decades the rate of allergic reactions to latex has substantially decreased in response to institutional initiatives to limit the use of latex products. High-risk group populations include health care workers, patient undergoing multiple surgical procedures (e.g., patients with spina bifida), and patients with allergies to mango, kiwi, and/or bananas.

### OTHER SUBSTANCES

- Hypnotic agents. Most of the cases were attributed to barbiturates, which were reported to account for up to 38% of perioperative allergic reactions, but this rate has reduced to approximately 2% because of widespread adoption of propofol. Propofol is suspended in an emulsion that contains soybean oil, egg lecithin, and glycerol. True allergic reactions to propofol are likely to be secondary to the two isopropyl groups. Concerns have been raised about the safety of propofol in patients with allergies to egg, soy, and peanut. However, soybean and egg allergies are typically triggered by proteins contained in these foods, not the fatty components (i.e., oils, lecithin). Because of this, many consider propofol safe in these patients.
- Opioids. The reported rate of allergic reactions to opioids is 1 in 100,000 to 200,000 anesthetics. Morphine, meperidine, and codeine are well known to cause direct degranulation of dermal mast cells, resulting in release of histamine and other mediators without, however, the involvement of opioid-specific IgE antibodies. This can lead to flushing and urticaria, which can mimic an allergic reaction. Rarely, true IgE-mediated allergic reactions have occurred with the use of fentanyl and sufentanil. Diagnosis of opioid-related anaphylactic reaction relies mostly on a detailed clinical history focused on the timing of the administration to the reaction, as well as the exclusion of other etiologies. Skin testing, in fact, could be precluded by the histamine release mechanism mentioned earlier.
- Local anesthetics. Local anesthetics are classified as either ester or amide compounds. Esters are associated with a higher incidence of allergic reactions because of a p-aminobenzoic acid (PABA) metabolite. However, preservative compounds (methylparaben) used in the preparation of amide-type agents are metabolized to PABA and can cause allergic reactions to amide local anesthetic solutions.
- Sugammadex. Sugammadex is a reversal agent for neuromuscular agents approved in the United States in 2015. First reports of allergic reaction to sugammadex were described in Japan with an incidence of 1 in 2500 anesthetics. Reactions usually occur late in surgery because of its use as a reversal agent. The mechanism of the sensitivity to sugammadex is not well known yet, although it seems to

be correlated to the cyclodextrin, which is also found in food additives and cosmetics. There have been reports also of sensitivity reactions to sugammadex-rocuronium complex. Interestingly, in these cases, testing to rocuronium and sugammadex individually may be negative.

- Dyes. Dyes are becoming more recognized as perioperative culprits for anaphylactic reactions. The most used are patent blue dye and methylene blue. Although very rare, there are few reports of cross-reactivity between methylene blue and patent blue.
- Protamine. Protamine can cause hypersensitivity reactions that have been classified in three subtypes: type I, related to histamine release; type II or IgE mediated; and type III related to thromboxane A2 (TXA2) release. Reactions occur in less than 1% of cases but are a widely recognized phenomenon. Reactions can be seen with higher doses, rapid administration, or repeated doses. Patient factors associated with increased risk include previous protamine exposure (especially for type II reaction), use of protamine-containing drugs (e.g., neutral protamine hagedorn insulin or neutral protamine hagedorn insulin (NPH), protamine zinc insulin or protamin zinc insulin (PZI), and certain β-blockers), previous vasectomy (because sperm contains protamine, which is then released into the systemic circulation), and food allergies to fish. Also, severe left ventricular dysfunction or abnormal preoperative pulmonary hemodynamics may be risk factors.
- Colloid volume expanders. Allergic reactions can occur to colloid volume expanders, with gelatins and dextrans having the highest risk and hetastarch the least. They may cause both IgE-mediated and non–IgE-mediated allergic reactions. Usually allergic reactions to volume expanders are rare, with a reported rate of less than 1% of cases in some European studies. Even more rare are allergic reactions to albumin.

## Diagnosis

Diagnosis of allergic reactions is based upon clinical history, skin testing (skin prick test and intradermal testing), and serum tryptase levels. Tryptase is a serine protease indicative of mast cell degranulation. An acute elevation of tryptase serum level suggests anaphylaxis, but normal levels do not exclude an anaphylactic reaction. Anaphylactic reactions may generate higher tryptase levels than anaphylactoid reactions, but this is not consistent. Serum tryptase level should be obtained shortly after the reaction (15 minutes to 3 hours), as serum tryptase has approximately a 2-hour half-life. A second tryptase measurement should be obtained 24 hours later, as a normalized second level supports the diagnosis, whereas a persistently elevated level suggests another process that can mimic anaphylaxis (e.g., mastocytosis). Patients should be referred to an allergist for skin testing to determine the causative factor. Meticulous records regarding the temporal relationship between the timing of medications administration and symptom onset is crucial. Reactions occurring within 30 minutes of induction are more likely related to antibiotics, NMBAs, or hypnotic agents, whereas later reactions suggest reactions to latex, sugammadex, blood products, protamine, and colloid volume expanders.

## Treatment

The aim of treatment is to support the cardiopulmonary system to prevent serious morbidity and death. General management of a patient with suspected allergic reaction can be summarized in the follow steps:

1. Call immediately for additional help and notify the surgical team.
2. Discontinue any potential allergens.
3. Prepare a code cart and epinephrine.
4. If patient is in cardiac arrest, begin advanced cardiac life support.
5. Increase fraction of inspired oxygen fraction of inspired oxygen ($FiO_2$) to 100%.
6. Secure or establish the airway.
7. Cardiovascular support: administer intravenous (IV) fluids bolus (patient may require liters of fluids). Administer epinephrine in escalating doses every 2 minutes. Start at 10 to 100 mcg IV and increase dose every 2 minutes until clinical improvement is noticed.
8. Adjuvant therapies: albuterol (4–8 puffs); H1 antagonist (e.g., diphenhydramine 25–50 mg IV) and H2 antagonist (e.g., ranitidine 50 mg IV); steroids (e.g., methylprednisolone 125 mg IV or hydrocortisone 100 mg IV).
9. Vasopressin or norepinephrine may be considered for refractory hypotension.
10. When patient is more stable, obtain serial serum tryptase levels and refer the patient for postoperative allergy testing.

## SUGGESTED READINGS

Florvaag, E., & Johansson, S. G. (2009). The pholcodine story. *Immunology and Allergy Clinics of North America, 29*(3), 419–427.

Fujita, A., Kitayama, M., & Hirota, K. (2007). Anaphylactoid shock in a patient following 5% human serum albumin infusion during off-pump coronary artery bypass grafting. *Journal of Anesthesia, 21*(3), 396–398.

Gurrieri, C., Weingarten, T. N., Martin, D. P., Babovic, N., Narr, B. J., Sprung, J., & Volcheck, G. W. (2011). Allergic reactions during anesthesia at a large United States referral center. *Anesthesia and Analgesia, 113*(5), 1202–1212.

Mertes, P. M., Alla, F., Tréchot, P., Auroy, Y., Jougla, E., & Groupe d'Etudes des Réactions Anaphylactoïdes Peranesthésiques. (2011). Anaphylaxis during anesthesia in France: An 8-year national survey. *Journal of Allergy and Clinical Immunology, 128*(2), 366–373.

Min, K. C., Woo, T., Assaid, C., McCrea, J., Gurner, D. M., Sisk, C. M., et al. (2018). Incidence of hypersensitivity and anaphylaxis with sugammadex. *Journal of Clinical Anesthesia, 47*, 67–73.

Nybo, M., & Madsen, J. S. (2008). Serious anaphylactic reactions due to protamine sulfate: A systematic literature review. *Basic Clinical Pharmacology & Toxicology, 103*(2), 192–196.

Takazawa, T., Mitsuhata, H., & Mertes, P. M. (2016). Sugammadex and rocuronium-induced anaphylaxis. *Journal of Anesthesia, 30*(2), 290–297.

Volcheck, G. W., & Hepner, D. L. (2019). Identification and management of perioperative anaphylaxis. *Journal of Allergy and Clinical Immunology in Practice, 7*(7), 2134–2142.

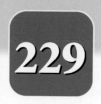

# Central Line Safety

JEFFREY T. MUELLER, MD

## Introduction

The insertion and use of central lines are an integral component of anesthesiology practice. This chapter will briefly review essential safety steps for the insertion, maintenance, and removal of centrally inserted central lines (also referred to as central venous catheters [CVCs]). This discussion does not include peripherally inserted central catheters. Complete education and training for the insertion and use of central lines should include hands-on learning in simulation and clinical environments. It is also recommended that anesthesiologists be familiar with the more comprehensive content of the American Society of Anesthesiologists' (ASA) *Practice Guidelines for Central Venous Access 2020,* the American Society of Echocardiography and Society of Cardiovascular Anesthesiologists' *Guidelines for Performing Ultrasound Guided Vascular Cannulation,* and the Society of Health Care Epidemiology and Infectious Disease Society of America's (SHEA-IDSA) *Strategies to Prevent Central Line–Associated Bloodstream Infections in Acute Care Hospitals; 2014 Update.*

## Indications

The indications for insertion of CVCs include establishment of high-reliability or long-term venous access, administration of medications unsuitable for peripheral venous administration, monitoring central venous pressure, insertion of pulmonary artery catheters, cardiac pacing, temporary hemodialysis, blood sampling, and the contingency ability to aspirate venous air in situations presenting a high risk of venous air embolism. The important first step in central line safety is to ensure that the benefits of central line placement and usage outweigh the risks.

## Complications

The risks of specific mechanical and infectious complications related to central venous access vary with the site of insertion, such as increased risk of pneumothorax with subclavian vein insertions and carotid injury with internal jugular vein insertions. The overall risks include injury to any surrounding structure, including arterial injury, airway compromise, pneumothorax, hemothorax, and cardiac tamponade. Venous thrombosis and unintended guidewire retention are additional mechanical complications. Infectious complications include both infection at the insertion site and central line–associated bloodstream infections resulting from central line–related seeding of pathogens. Finally, misinterpretation of central venous pressure measurements leading to ineffective or harmful therapeutic intervention is an additional complication of central venous catheter utilization.

## Insertion Procedure

Site selection is determined by several factors including indication, urgency, comorbidities, patient anatomy, planned catheter duration, infectious risks, and coagulation status. The inserting physician must balance these factors to select the optimal site for a given patient. Anatomic considerations influence the relative risks of certain mechanical complications, such as increased risk of pneumothorax with subclavian insertion or carotid injury with internal jugular insertion. Determination of the relative infection risks of different access sites is controversial. Current guidance recommends avoiding the femoral vein in obese adult patients in nonurgent situations.

Other site selection factors include neck immobilization, pulmonary impairment, clinical setting, and the physician's specific skill and experience. Generally, the internal jugular vein offers intraoperative access to the catheter site for most surgical situations, good access to the right side of the heart, and a lower incidence of pneumothorax; the subclavian vein may offer a lower incidence of infection and increased patient comfort; and the femoral vein removes the risk of pneumothorax or carotid injury but presents increased risks of thrombosis and infection in adult patients.

## Insertion Procedure Safety Steps

The ASA *Practice Guidelines for Central Venous Access* should be consulted for complete evidence-based recommendations. Selected insertion safety steps include use of a checklist, the participation of an assistant, use of a supply cart and insertion kits that contain all necessary components for insertion, placing the patient in head-down (Trendelenburg) position for chest or neck insertion sites, use of static (prepuncture) ultrasound before site skin preparation to verify presence of an acceptable vein, and use of real-time (during puncture) ultrasound guidance for internal jugular insertions and possibly selected subclavian and femoral insertions. Additional infection prevention steps should include hand hygiene before gloving, maximal sterile barrier precautions (cap, mask, sterile gown, sterile gloves, large sterile drape), and skin preparation with chlorhexidine alcohol-based antiseptic unless it is specifically contraindicated.

It is important to recognize that although use of real-time ultrasound guidance reduces the incidence of mechanical complications such as carotid artery injury during internal jugular vein insertion, it does not eliminate complications. An ultrasound imaging error, such as misinterpretation due to reverberation artifacts, or unidentified through-and-through puncture of the vein into an underlying carotid artery, can lead to erroneous arterial cannulation in spite of ultrasound guidance. It is therefore important to properly use a venous verification test after the vessel is punctured under ultrasound guidance but before vessel dilation and placement of the large bore catheter. Possible venous verification tests include manometry as described by Fabian and Jesudian, pressure transduction through a small-bore catheter, or imaging of the intravessel guidewire before dilation (the latter if the proceduralist possesses the necessary expertise in the respective imaging modality). The ASA *Practice Guidelines for Central Venous Access* statement "Blood color or absence of pulsatile flow should not be relied upon for confirming that the thin-walled needle resides in the vein" further emphasizes the importance of objectively confirming venous access before dilation.

## Safe Central Line Use, Maintenance, and Removal

SHEA-IDSA recommendations include 5-sec disinfection of catheter hubs, connectors, and injection ports with alcoholic chlorhexidine, povidone–iodine, or 70% alcohol before accessing catheters. This includes operating room usage. In addition to safe insertion, anesthesiologists engaged in central line insertion should also ensure that the subsequent maintenance and removal of the catheter occurs in a clinical environment providing high-quality and safe care based on authoritative guidance. This includes the daily assessment of ongoing need for the catheter and daily inspection of the catheter insertion site by qualified clinical staff.

The removal of central lines exposes patients to very significant risks including venous air embolism and bleeding. Central line removal therefore also includes important safety steps such as ensuring that an existing peripheral or other venous catheter is in place; assessing coagulation status, including review of any available related laboratory results; monitoring of patient vital signs throughout the removal procedure; ensuring availability of the equipment and supplies necessary to oxygenate and ventilate the patient; positioning the patient head down (Trendelenburg) for removal of internal jugular and subclavian catheters and head up with legs extended for removal of femoral catheters; and cleansing of the site with alcoholic chlorhexidine. During the act of removal, spontaneously ventilating patients should perform a Valsalva maneuver and be asked to "continue to bear down until the line is removed." Steady pressure should be applied to the site with a gauze pad as the catheter is removed and a sterile air-occlusive dressing immediately applied; this recommendation does not apply to patients receiving positive-pressure mechanical ventilation. The patient's vital signs and neurologic status should be monitored and bed rest maintained for a predetermined interval after catheter removal.

## SUGGESTED READINGS

American Society of Anesthesiologists Task Force on Central Venous Access, Rupp, S. M., Apfelbaum, J. L., Blitt, C., Caplan, R. A., Connis, R. T., et al. (2020). Practice guidelines for central venous access 2020: An updated report by the American Society of Anesthesiologists task force on central venous access. *Anesthesiology, 132,* 8–43.

Ezaru, C. S., Mangione, M. P., Oravitz, T. M., Ibinson, J. W., & Bjerke, R. J. (2009). Eliminating arterial injury during central venous catheterization using manometry. *Anesthesia and Analgesia, 109*(1), 130–134.

Fabian, J. A., & Jesudian, M. C. (1985). A simple method for improving the safety of percutaneous cannulation of the internal jugular vein. *Anesthesia and Analgesia, 64*(10), 1032–1033.

Keegan, M. T., & Mueller, J. T. (2012). Removal of central venous catheters. *Anesthesiology, 117*(4), 917–919.

Marschall, J., Mermel, L. A., Fakih, M., Hadaway, L., Kallen, A., O'Grady, N. P., et al. (2014). Strategies to prevent central line-associated bloodstream infections in acute care hospitals: 2014 update. *Infection Control and Hospital Epidemiology, 35*(7), 753–771.

Parienti, J. J., Mongardon, N., Mégarbane, B., Mira, J. P., Kalfon, P., Gros, A., et al. (2015). Intravascular complications of central venous catheterization by insertion site. *New England Journal of Medicine, 373*(13), 1220–1229.

Troianos, C. A., Hartman, G. S., Glas, K. E., Skubas, N. J., Eberhardt, R. T., Walker, J. D., et al. (2012). Special articles: Guidelines for performing ultrasound guided vascular cannulation: Recommendations of the American Society of Echocardiography and the Society of Cardiovascular Anesthesiologists. *Anesthesia and Analgesia, 114*(1), 46–72.

Vannucci, A., Jeffcoat, A., Ifune, C., Salinas, C., Duncan, J. R., & Wall, M. (2013). Special article: Retained guidewires after intraoperative placement of central venous catheters. *Anesthesia and Analgesia, 117*(1), 102–108.

# SECTION XIV

# Practice Management

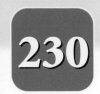

# American Society of Anesthesiologists Evidence-Based Practice Parameters

KAREN B. DOMINO, MD, MPH  |  MARK GRANT, MD, PhD

The American Society of Anesthesiologists' (ASA) practice parameters provide guidance to anesthesiologists to improve their decision-making and promote beneficial patient outcomes. The ASA has three types of practice parameters: practice standards, practice guidelines, and practice advisories. Practice parameters are developed under the direction of the ASA Committee on Practice Parameters, with final approval by the ASA House of Delegates. The ASA began publishing practice guidelines and advisories in 1993 with the publication of the difficult airway and pulmonary artery catheterization guidelines. Fourteen guidelines and eight advisories have been published, with over 25 updates. In 2021, the Web of Science reported almost 12,000 citations to the ASA practice guidelines and advisories. Over the years, practice parameters have improved the quality of patient care, decreased patient harm, reduced unnecessary variation of care, and provided medicolegal benefits to anesthesiologists and many other health care providers.

## Practice Parameters and Their Influence on Clinical Practice

### PRACTICE STANDARDS

Practice standards are generally accepted principles of anesthetic patient management that provide rules or minimal requirements for clinical anesthesia practice. Practice standards may be modified only under unusual circumstances, extreme emergencies, or lack of availability of equipment. The ASA has three practice standards, one aimed at each phase of anesthesia care: preoperative, intraoperative, and postoperative care (https://www.asahq. org/standards-and-guidelines). The "Basic Standards for Preanesthesia Care" dictate requirements for medical record review, history and focused physical examination, ordering and reviewing of appropriate tests and consultations, ordering appropriate preoperative medications, obtaining anesthesia care consent, and documentation of these requirements in the medical record. The "Standards for Basic Anesthetic Monitoring" set the requirement for qualified anesthesia personnel to be present in the room throughout the conduct of all general and regional anesthetics and monitored anesthesia care. This practice standard also specifies the continual evaluation of patient's oxygenation, ventilation, circulation, and temperature during anesthesia care. Finally, the "Standards for Postanesthesia Care" dictate care requirements in the postanesthesia care unit (PACU), transport from the procedural area to the PACU by a member of the anesthesia care team, handoff of care to a PACU nurse, PACU nursing care, and physician discharge of a patient from the PACU.

### PRACTICE GUIDELINES AND PRACTICE ADVISORIES

In contrast to practice standards that are requirements for minimally acceptable anesthesia practice, practice guidelines and practice advisories provide recommendations and guidance for care of patients undergoing anesthetic care. Variance in care from the recommendations of practice guidelines and advisories is acceptable, based upon the clinical judgment of the responsible anesthesiologist.

Practice guidelines and practice advisories are evidence-based documents developed by a rigorous process. The systematic review follows a standardized approach to the collection, assessment, analysis, and reporting of the relevant scientific literature and allows for public comment. The ASA development of practice guidelines and advisories adheres to the standards for trustworthy guidelines, including transparency and strict disclosure and management of potential conflicts of interest (Graham et al., 2011). Although practice guidelines and advisories employ similar approaches and methodologies, the evidence base supporting practice guidelines is stronger in quantity, quality, and consistency compared with practice advisories. Practice guidelines provide recommended patient management strategies to optimize care and improve outcomes. Examples of recent practice guidelines include the Practice Guideline for Central Venous Access (Apfelbaum et al., 2020b) and the Difficult Airway Practice Guideline (Apfelbaum et al., 2022).

In contrast, practice advisories assist anesthesiologists in decision-making when there is insufficient published evidence. Examples of recent informative ASA practice advisories include the prevention of Perioperative Visual Loss Associated with Spine Surgery (Apfelbaum et al., 2019) and the Perioperative Management of Patients with Cardiac Implantable Electronic Devices (Apfelbaum et al., 2020). Unfortunately, in these areas of perioperative care, the evidence quality is poor or lacking. However, the care of these patients is complex, and the advisories represent the best available evidence-based clinical advice. Therefore the practice advisories summarize the scientific evidence and provide suggestions for perioperative care.

A recent systematic review of the evidence supporting North American and European Perioperative Care Guidelines for Anesthesiologists between 2010 and 2020 found that half of the 2,280 recommendations in anesthesiology clinical practice guidelines were based on a low level of evidence (Laserna et al., 2021). Fewer than one in six recommendations were based upon the highest quality of evidence: randomized controlled trials or meta-analyses of multiple randomized controlled trials. Sadly, the proportion of perioperative recommendations supported by a high quality of evidence did not increase between 2010 and 2020. Therefore improving the number, diversity, and quality of randomized studies in anesthesiology and perioperative care is the path to improve the quality of evidence (Neuman and Apfelbaum, 2021). The finding of low quality of evidence driving the guideline recommendations is concerning as the consensus-based recommendations of the expert panel members may lead to harmful recommendations (Yao et al., 2021).

As the judgments and interpretations of the evidence and the formation of recommendations are made by the task force members, individual anesthesiologists must decide for themselves whether there are important differences in their own clinical and patient setting compared with those considered by the task force (Brignardello-Petersen et al., 2021).

## Practice Guideline and Practice Advisory Methodology

The ASA practice guideline and advisory methodology uses comprehensive systematic literature reviews, well-formulated clinical questions, explicit study inclusion and exclusion criteria, risk of bias assessments, assigning importance to outcomes and their value to patients, strength of evidence evaluation to summarize findings, and developing recommendations for clinical care. Fig. 230.1 summarizes the essential steps in the development of practice guidelines and practice advisories.

### CLINICAL QUESTIONS

The first step in the systematic review process is to define the clinical questions for the review. Clinical questions are formulated into PICOTS (population, interventions, comparators, outcomes, timing, and setting) for the systematic review (Counsell, 1997). Well-formulated questions facilitate and guide the systematic review and evidence synthesis. The questions, PICOTS, and evidence availability determine the types of studies and study designs that are included in a systematic review. Randomized controlled trials provide the strongest evidence, and if present, other study designs are often excluded in the assessment of treatment efficacy. Evidence from nonrandomized and retrospective designs is commonly used to assess harms and adverse safety events because of the often-rare occurrence of adverse events.

### OUTCOMES

Outcomes are ranked according to their importance for decision-making. Patients care most about health outcomes rather than intermediate outcomes (e.g., intraoperative hypotension, laboratory test results). Evidence is considered direct when an intervention leads to a health outcome and indirect when it leads to an intermediate outcome. The assessment of outcome importance also incorporates patient preferences and values.

## SYNTHESIS AND ASSESSMENT OF STRENGTH OF EVIDENCE

Data are abstracted from published research and then synthesized using quantitative and qualitative approaches, summarized in tables, and include meta-analyses when appropriate. Interpretation of a meta-analysis assesses the methods used to combine study results, statistical heterogeneity, small study effects, and potential publication bias. The strength of the evidence is evaluated using tools to assess whether study results are believable and internally valid (i.e., risk of bias). The strength of evidence is evaluated with two frameworks: evidence hierarchy and certainty of evidence. The evidence hierarchy approach ranks studies according to design with randomized controlled trials and meta-analyses providing the most convincing evidence. The certainty of evidence model incorporates the study design hierarchy but defines the strength of evidence in terms of confidence that the range of effects reflect some "true effect" now and in the future. Older ASA practice guidelines and advisories were evaluated by study design hierarchy, but current practice guidelines and advisories are evaluated by both methods.

## DEVELOPING RECOMMENDATIONS FOR CLINICAL CARE

A panel (task force) of experts, methodologists, and, in most cases, a patient representative evaluates the evidence and develops recommendations. Task force members consider the effect of the interventions on benefits and harms, which are weighed according to how each is valued. The task force then formulates recommendations and describes the strength of each recommendation. Conflicts of interest for task force members are disclosed and managed, with the chair/cochairs and more than half of the task force free of relevant conflicts of interest. Drafts of practice guidelines and advisories are circulated for public comment and revised. After approval by the House of Delegates, practice parameters are available on the ASA's website. Practice guidelines and practice advisories are also published in the ASA's journal, *Anesthesiology*.

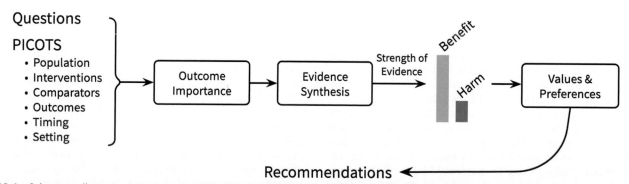

**Fig. 230.1** Schematic illustrating an overview for development of American Society of Anesthesiologists practice guidelines and advisories, including questions and PICOTS (population, interventions, comparators, outcomes, timing, and setting) that drive the systematic review; outcome importance; evidence synthesis; incorporating values and preferences; and recommendations for care.

## Discussion

In 2023, the ASA continues to provide practice parameters as a service to its members and other health care practitioners. Other professional societies may collaborate with the ASA to develop these documents for use by practitioners in their specialties. For instance, the American Association of Oral and Maxillofacial Surgeons, the American College of Radiology, the American Society of Dentist Anesthesiologists, and the Society of Interventional Radiology collaborated with the ASA on the 2018 Moderate Procedural Sedation Guideline.

### SUGGESTED READINGS

Apfelbaum, J. L., Hagberg, C. A., Connis, R. T., Abdelmalak, B. B., Agarkar, M., Dutton, R. P., et al. (2022). 2022 American Society of Anesthesiologists practice guidelines for management of the difficult airway. *Anesthesiology, 136*(1), 31–81.

Apfelbaum, J. L., Roth, S., & Rubin, D., Connis R. T., Agarkar, M., Arnold, P. M., et al. (2019). Practice advisory for perioperative visual loss associated with spine surgery 2019: An updated report by the American Society of Anesthesiologists Task Force on Perioperative Visual Loss, the North American Neuro-Ophthalmology Society, and the Society for Neuroscience in Anesthesiology and Critical Care. *Anesthesiology, 130*(1), 12–30.

Apfelbaum, J. L., Schulman, P. M., Mahajan, A., Connis, R. T., & Agarkar, M. (2020a). Practice advisory for the perioperative management of patients with cardiac implantable electronic devices: Pacemakers and implantable cardioverter-defibrillators 2020. *Anesthesiology, 132*, 225–252.

Apfelbaum, J. L., Rupp, S. M., Tung, A., Connis, R. T., Domino, K. B., Grant, M. D., et al. (2020b). Practice guidelines for central venous access 2020. An updated report by the American Society of Anesthesiologists Task Force on Central Venous Access. *Anesthesiology, 132*, 8–43.

Brignardello-Petersen, R., Carrasco-Labra, A., & Guyatt, G. H. (2021). How to interpret and use a clinical practice guideline or recommendation: Users' guides to the medical literature. *JAMA, 326*(15), 1516–1523.

Counsell, C. (1997). Formulating questions and locating primary studies for inclusion in systematic reviews. *Annals of Internal Medicine, 127*(5), 380–387.

Graham, R., Mancher, M., Miller Wolman, D., Greenfield, S., & Steinberg, E. (2011). *Clinical practice guidelines we can trust*. Washington DC: The National Academies Press.

Laserna, A., Rubinger, D. A., Barahona-Correa, J. E., Wright, N., Williams, M. R., Wyrobek, J. A., et al. (2021). Levels of evidence supporting the North American and European perioperative care guidelines for anesthesiologists between 2010 and 2020: A systematic review. *Anesthesiology, 135*(1), 31–56.

Neuman, M. D., & Apfelbaum, J. L. (2021). Clinical practice guidelines in anesthesiology: Adjusting our expectations. *Anesthesiology, 135*(1), 9–11.

Yao, L., Ahmed, M. M., Guyatt, G. H., Yan, P., Hui, X., Wang, Q., et al. (2021). Discordant and inappropriate discordant recommendations in consensus and evidence based guidelines: Empirical analysis. *BMJ (Clinical Research), 375*, e066045.

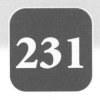

# 231

# Value-Based Payment Models

JONATHAN GAL, MD, MBA, MS, FASA  |  SHARON K. MERRICK, MS, CCS-P  |
VANESSA SALCEDO, MPH

## The Medicare Access and CHIP Reauthorization Act of 2015

### BACKGROUND AND TIMELINE

The Resource-Based Relative Value System (RBRVS), described in Chapter 242, dramatically changed the way most physicians are paid for their services. Its fundamental premise was to determine payments based on the resources required without regard to specialty or location. In RBRVS, resources are the value of physician work, practice expenses, and liability costs. With ongoing refinements, RBRVS has been reasonably successful in meeting these objectives. Health policy experts recognized that implementing RBRVS would possibly lead to an increased volume or intensity of services, as that would be the only way to increase income for clinicians in a fixed-rate system. Since RBRVS was implemented, Congress has attempted to constrain spending growth for what it considered to be unnecessary services. The first effort implemented in the early 1990s was called the Medicare Volume Performance Standard (MVPS), touted at the time to be a viable alternative to legislatively mandated spending targets. The MVPS received much criticism from organized medicine, including aggressive lobbying for its replacement, because growth targets were so low as to virtually guarantee cuts in payments.

In 1997, Congress passed the Balanced Budget Act, which included a new way to control Medicare physician spending through a formula called the Sustainable Growth Rate (SGR). The SGR was a replacement for MVPS, first applied in 1998. This formula limited growth in spending to overall economic growth, with adjustments for health care cost inflation and introduction of new technologies and services. Robust economic growth in the late 1990s led to positive payment updates; however, health care expenditures began to far outpace economic growth during most of the next decade. As a result, the SGR formula began requiring cuts in payments to clinicians. This solution to the MVPS became an entirely new problem. Congress faced strong political lobbying from organized medicine to avoid these cuts. Fearing the political impact of reduced access for Medicare beneficiaries, Congress repeatedly voted to *delay* implementing SGR cuts—with the exception of a single instance; however, these delays led to an ever-worsening SGR debt that would need to be paid at some point. By the early 2010s, the accrued SGR debt would have resulted in a 25% cut in the Medicare conversion factor to balance the books, something that members of Congress widely recognized as being politically toxic.

Concurrently with the growth in the SGR debt, a proposed better way to control health care expenses and improve health care quality gained traction among policy experts. This approach would pay for the *value* of care received rather than only for the *volume* of services rendered. Value, in this context, was broadly defined as quality divided by cost. This meant that cost-adjusted outcomes for patients would drive payments to the health care provider community. Beginning with legislation passed during the great recession, the Medicare program has slowly, and in a piecemeal fashion, experimented with several ways to financially reward clinicians successfully pursuing improvements in value. Medicare's Physician Quality Reporting System (PQRS), meaningful use (MU) of electronic health records, and the value-based payment modifier (VM) programs separately provided incentives and penalties for clinician performance for several years. These early value-based programs were not well coordinated, and the administrative burdens of participating were significant. Medicare has also experimented with major payment redesign, known as alternative payment models (APMs). Examples include bundled payments for episodes of care, such as total joint replacements or bariatric surgery, accountable care organizations (ACOs), patient-centered medical homes, and more. These APMs can take on upside risk by sharing in any savings resulting from reduced health care costs, downside financial risk resulting in paying the insurer back should costs of care rise, or both, known as two-sided risk. In each arrangement, shared savings or penalties are weighted based on participant performance demonstrated through satisfactory quality health outcomes.

In 2015, Congress addressed the need to fix the SGR problem by mandating a transition to value-based care through legislation known as the Medicare Access and CHIP Reauthorization Act (MACRA). This bill passed by overwhelming majorities in both houses of Congress. MACRA wiped out the SGR debt, replacing it with a system mandating transition to value-driven care. The legislation included sections that unified the various experiments in quality improvement and cost containment into a single structure.

After Congress passed legislation, the executive branch of government created regulations to implement the new law. For MACRA, the Centers for Medicare and Medicaid Services (CMS) published their first round of regulations in 2016. They called the value-based part of MACRA the Quality Payment Program (QPP). The first year that *payments* to clinicians reflected bonuses or penalties under MACRA was in 2019, based on performance that occurred by eligible clinicians in 2017. There is a 2-year gap between performance and payment adjustments. Clinicians collect data on QPP measures during the performance year, submit them to CMS the next year to be scored and adjudicated, then receive bonus payments based on those performance scores in the following year. For example, throughout 2018 eligible clinicians collected data of their required metrics and reported them in 2019 to CMS for review and validation to determine each clinician's payment update for 2020.

CMS provides annual updates to these regulations to address any problems encountered and further refine the program as it evolves. With more than 50% of total Medicare payments to physicians and other clinicians tied to quality and cost, CMS continues to push for increasing the percentage toward 100% quickly. As part of this push, CMS has made some value-based payment models mandatory.

The QPP has two payment pathways: the Merit-based Incentive Payment System (MIPS) track and the Advanced APM track (Fig. 231.1). These will be described in the following sections. The QPP applies only to Medicare Part B (physician and other clinician professional) services, although APMs can affect

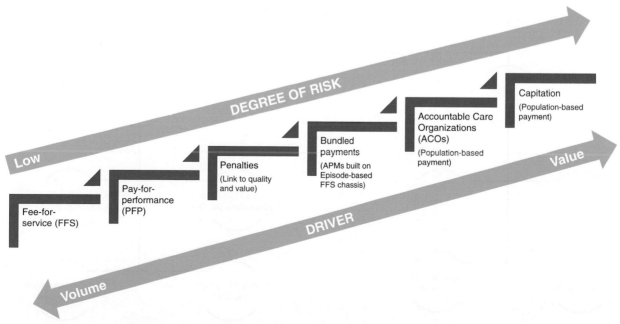

**Fig. 231.1** Payment models and their degree of risk and what drives them.

payments to hospitals and other nonclinician providers through risk-sharing arrangements.

## MERIT-BASED INCENTIVE PAYMENT SYSTEM

The MIPS pathway takes the existing RBRVS fee-for-service (FFS) system and attaches value-based components to modify payment. The old PQRS, MU, and VM programs received new names: Quality, Advancing Care Initiative (ACI), and Cost. In addition, a new category to encourage improving care was added. This component is called Improvement Activities (IA), and it rewards individual clinicians' participation in practice improvement activities (Fig. 231.2). The requirements for the existing programs have been simplified and aligned to eliminate conflicts between program elements and to reduce reporting burdens.

Each MIPS component receives a percentage weight and has specified performance criteria. Each clinician or practice group receives a score based on their success in meeting these performance criteria. The sum of the scores multiplied by the weights results in an overall performance score for a given *performance year*. The Medicare program then determines relative performance for clinicians and groups to provide bonuses or penalties. As previously mentioned, these payment adjustments lead to modification of the conversion factor for the clinician 2 years later. For example, performance in 2017 affects payments in 2019.

Incentives and penalties gradually increase over time, starting at up to +/– 4% in 2019 and increasing to as much as +/– 9% by the early 2020s. These incentives and penalties are budget neutral, meaning that cuts to poor performers will pay for incentives to good performers. Congress additionally allocated $500 million a year that CMS may use to reward outstanding performance. This additional pool is not subject to budget neutrality. However, if the vast majority of clinicians avoid penalties, as was observed in the first three MIPS performance years, the funds for bonuses are smaller and therefore the maximum bonuses received were all observed to be under 2%.

CMS considered the first performance year as a transitional year and relaxed a number of the program requirements to ease the transition for clinicians and to minimize downside financial risk. The MACRA law provided some leeway to slow the phase-in during the first few years of the program. CMS exercised this option by not including cost of care in the MIPS performance calculation and only requiring limited reporting of other components in that first year of the QPP. That relaxation in requirements reduced both the upside and downside financial risk for participants. Regulations since the creation of the QPP have continued at a slow pace with introduction of new innovations in payment. However, these new innovations in payment are intended to incrementally create greater financial risk and reward for those in MIPS.

One such example, is the MIPS Value Pathways (MVPs), a subset of measures and activities, established through rulemaking, that can be used to meet MIPS reporting requirements. The MVPs framework attempts to align and connect measures and activities across the Quality, Cost, Promoting Interoperability, and Improvement Activities performance categories of MIPS for different specialties or conditions. Rather than multiple specialties reporting MIPS measures in siloes while caring for the same patient, through MVPs those clinicians coordinate those measures and report them in a patient-centered manner. In addition, the MVPs framework incorporates a foundation that leverages Promoting Interoperability measures and a set of administrative claims–based quality measures that focus on population health, public health priorities, and reduced reporting. CMS

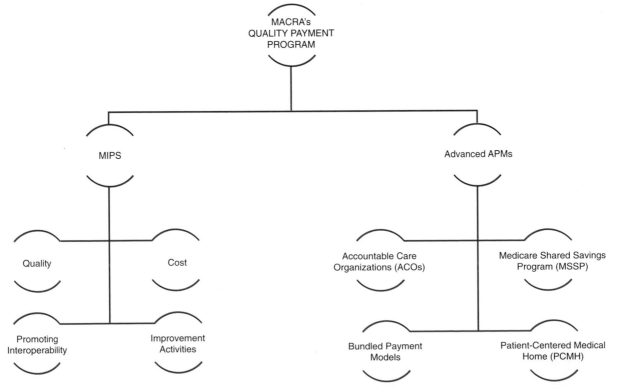

**Fig. 231.2** The Medicare Access and CHIP Reauthorization Act Quality Payment Program's payment models.

believes this combination of administrative claims–based measures and specialty/condition specific measures will streamline MIPS reporting, reduce complexity and burden, and improve measurement. CMS issued a call for MVP candidates in 2020, and seven MVPs were selected and announced in 2021 for implementation in 2023. The American Society of Anesthesiologists' (ASA) proposed MVP was one of the MVPs selected. CMS referred to it as the Patient Safety and Support of Positive Experiences with Anesthesia MVP. Additionally, the ASA's Perioperative Surgical Home (PSH) Care Coordination Improvement Activity (IA_CC_15) was changed from a medium-weight to a high-weight activity, reflecting the increased significance of the measure and its relevance on patient outcomes.

## ADVANCED ALTERNATIVE PAYMENT MODELS

APMs are slowly replacing traditional FFS health care with new, integrated approaches that typically involve financial risk for participating clinicians and health care organizations. APMs often take one of two common approaches. They either integrate systems of care to improve overall health of a population of patients or seek to improve care delivered during an acute episode surrounding a patient's illness or need for a procedure. Within the QPP there are also two pathways for APMs depending on their risk: MIPS-APMs are those that take only upside risk, whereas Advanced-APMs take on both upside and downside risk. Examples of population health approaches include ACOs and medical homes. Their goals are to care for a population of patients over an extended period of time by providing evidence-informed preventative care, encouraging wellness, managing chronic conditions to limit disease progression, and assuring effective coordination of care when multiple clinicians become involved in treating a patient. ACOs have the highest level of risk and reward, as pictured in Fig. 231.1 and can be either physician-led (large multispecialty practices) or formed by a hospital-physician partnership. ACOs have significantly grown in the last 20 years, and some have successfully achieved cost savings. Data from the American Medical Association's Physician Practice Benchmark Survey demonstrated that in 2020, 55% of physicians reported participation in at least one type of ACO (up 11 percentage points from 2016).

Episode-based approaches include bundled payments for common surgical conditions for time-limited but costly medical treatments. As an example, Medicare's first episode-based model, the Comprehensive Care for Joint Replacement (CJR) program, provides a fixed and discounted target payment amount for Medicare FFS total joint replacements, including hospital fees, professional services fees, and acute postdischarge care fees. If total cost of care is less than this target price and quality metrics are met, Medicare shares the savings with those who provided care. If costs are greater than targeted, the providers are on the hook for at least some of the excess spending. Initially, hospitals bore the financial risk for CJR; however, CMS expanded the risk/reward calculation to include other members of the care team, most notably the physicians and other clinicians providing care. Another acute episode example is the Oncology Care Model, a program that focuses on reducing costs and improving quality and care coordination for Medicare patients undergoing chemotherapy. Medicare offers care coordination payments to help improve care while also offering shared savings payments if certain cost containment goals are met. Once again, this assumes that quality targets are met or exceeded.

MACRA's Advanced-APM pathway allows physicians and certain other clinicians to participate in qualifying programs and potentially avoid being subject to MIPS requirements. Successfully meeting Advanced APM requirements results in annual fixed 5% bonuses to the Medicare RBRVS conversion factor from 2019 until the mid-2020s; furthermore, beginning in the late 2020s, the APM pathway participants will garner larger annual updates in the conversion factor than seen for MIPS participants. One of the requirements for successful participation is to meet a specified threshold, recently 35%, of Medicare beneficiaries receiving care through the APM. The threshold considers both participation and payment rates. If unsuccessful in meeting these thresholds, APM clinicians will have to participate in MIPS; however, their participation in an Advanced APM gives the clinicians a significant amount of credit toward reaching MIPS bonus targets. These clinicians also have reduced reporting requirements in MIPS. The volume and payment thresholds noted above will increase over time.

By creating these bonus payments and higher conversion factor updates for the Advanced-APM pathway, Congress deliberately created incentives to encourage clinicians to move away from FFS and into risk-bearing, value-based care delivery. Whether or not the APM meets its performance targets, APM clinicians reporting through MIPS have an easier pathway for receiving financial incentive payments than those at the individual clinician level. A recent review of publicly published CMS data for MIPS performance by providers demonstrated that anesthesia provider performance in the first 2 years of MIPS was strong with most receiving bonus payments. There was also an observed shift in reporting for anesthesia providers from individuals to groups or APMs between the first and second year. In 2020 per the American Medical Association's Survey, 67% of physicians were in practices that received at least some payment through APMs (up 9 percentage points from 2012). About 70% of practice revenue still comes from FFS, although there was a shift away from complete reliance on FFS. The COVID-19 pandemic demonstrated that sole reliance on FFS is not financially sound when elective health care significantly decreases. Early evidence in 2021 suggested that medical practices with revenue based on capitation or other value-based designs fared better than those only in FFS arrangements.

## Anesthesia Considerations

Much of the focus in the value-based care movement has been on improving population health status, including effectively managing chronic disease conditions, assuring preventative measures take place, and controlling costs. Population health APMs have to meet overall expenditure and quality targets; therefore compensation arrangements for clinicians in APMs typically include significant incentives for meeting quality and cost goals at the individual patient level that are believed to affect the entire population. More money being available to reward value means less is available to reward volume.

Although anesthesiologists can play an important role in both managing chronic disease and encouraging health improvement during an acute procedural episode, calculating the value of these efforts in a population health APM such as an ACO is very difficult. For this reason, anesthesiologists may face downward pressure on incomes as they may receive payments only for the procedures they perform and not for chronic disease management or population health improvement. This would put anesthesiologists at a financial disadvantage compared with most ACO participants.

As mentioned previously, another APM approach targets cost and quality for brief episodes of care. The anesthesiologist plays an important role in patient assessment, risk stratification, disease optimization, pain management, and care coordination for a surgical episode. Measuring and rewarding these contributions in acute procedural episodes like those for total joint replacements, spine surgery, and cardiac bypass procedures are pathways by which anesthesiologists can fully participate in an APM. Anesthesiologists play a key role toward cost-saving through care coordination because of their involvement as gatekeepers in resource-intensive procedural services.

Recognizing the need for anesthesiologists to measurably provide value-based care, the ASA supported the development of the PSH—a care model that facilitates improved, cost-effective care during a procedural episode. Conceptually, the PSH fosters patient-centeredness, care coordination, standardization of care, attention to resource use, and aggressive management of clinical outcomes to continually improve the delivery of major procedural care. ASA has hosted learning collaboratives and educational conferences and offered consultative services to assist its members in implementing the PSH. ASA has also worked with surgical specialties to identify areas of collaboration. Although the PSH is not an APM, it provides a pathway to APM success.

Most physicians, whether anesthesiologists or not, continue to be MIPS participants. As described in the MIPS section, clinicians who have a sufficient volume of Medicare cases must report quality metrics, improvement activities, and advancing care information performance. This can be managed either through group or individual reporting. In the general quality measure set, the specialty of anesthesiology only had nine measures applicable in the first performance year. Some measures did not apply to all anesthesiologists, such as the one assessing use of beta-blockers before isolated coronary artery bypass surgery. All but one of these current measures evaluate processes of care (did the clinician accomplish the desired steps at the correct time for the appropriate patient). An example process measure is using a checklist at time of transfer to postanesthesia care unit care. The only current clinical outcome measure in the current set evaluates whether the patient achieved normothermia around the end of anesthesia.

Specialty-specific registries, like those sponsored by ASA, the American College of Surgeons, and the Society of Thoracic Surgeons, have contributed to improved quality of care over many years. MIPS allows for reporting quality and other requirements for Medicare patients through registries. Qualified Clinical Data Registries (QCDRs) are more recent innovations to help simplify meaningful quality reporting to Medicare and other payers. QCDRs provide the anesthesiologist or anesthetist with greater flexibility for MIPS participation, because the QCDR can develop specialty specific measures without going through the cumbersome approval process for standard CMS measures. The Anesthesia Quality Institute, created by ASA to promote quality improvement in the specialty, offers a QCDR to ASA members and others. It is known as the National Anesthesia Clinical Outcomes Registry. A number of university-affiliated practices participate in the Anesthesiology Performance Improvement and Reporting Exchange QCDR, an outgrowth of a research registry housed at the University of Michigan. This research program is called the Multicenter Perioperative Outcomes Group. Other QCDRs are available as well. In addition to quality reporting, QCDRs may also serve as a clearinghouse for all MIPS requirements, including reporting ACI measures and IA on behalf of those participating. Important advantages of using a QCDR include simplification of reporting MIPS requirements, benchmarking against peers, tracking all patients (not just those in Medicare), potential for use of actual physiologic data from electronic health records in assessing outcomes, and readily available, clinically important, and actionable data for quality improvement initiatives.

The QPP is the most significant change in decades in how Medicare pays clinicians. A fundamental operating principle is to control costs while maintaining quality, and often includes a transfer of financial risk to clinicians. Commercial payers are implementing similar changes in payment with a focus on high quality and decreased costs in their contracts with clinicians, as these payers, not surprisingly, also seek to transfer financial risk to others. The synopsis of the QPP in this chapter is only a brief introduction to a continuously evolving and complex payment system. Anesthesiologists, certified registered nurse anesthetists, and certified anesthesiologist assistants who care for Medicare patients will need to closely follow the QPP's implementation, working with their practice managers to assure compliance and maximize performance.

MACRA repealed the SGR formula that had long been used to determine conversion factors within the Medicare Physician Fee Schedule. MACRA introduced the QPP that includes both the MIPS and APM pathways. The QPP is having a marked effect on both how care is delivered and paid. Anesthesiologists need some understanding of both QPP and basic coding and billing in order to meaningfully participate in value-based payment arrangements that recognize and reward anesthesiologists' contributions.

## SUGGESTED READINGS

A foundational article that explains all health care payment methods including fee-for-service and the implications for anesthesiologists, Gal, J. S., Vaidyanathan, M., & Morewood, G. (2021). Anesthesiology payment methods: US perspective. *International Anesthesia Clinics*, 59, 37–46. doi:10.1097/AIA.0000000000000334.

Gal, J. S., Morewood, G. H., Mueller, J. T., Popovich, M. T., Caridi, J. M., & Neifert, S. N. (2022). Anesthesia provider performance in the first two years of merit-based incentive payment system: Shifts in reporting and predictors of receiving bonus payments. *Journal of Clinical Anesthesia*, 76, 110582. doi:10.1016/j.jclinane.2021.110582.

The American Medical Association. (2021). *Policy research perspectives: Payment and delivery in 2020: Fee-for-Service revenue remains stable while participation shifts in accountable care organizations during the pandemic.* Chicago: The American Medical Association.

The American Society of Anesthesiologists (ASA). *Hosts information on the QPP that is particularly relevant to anesthesiologists, including specialized educational modules and tools available to members.* Retrieved from https://www.asahq.org/macra. Accessed December 9, 2021.

The ASA's Perioperative Surgical Home service delivery model helps leverage the expertise of anesthesiologists in improving procedural care episodes and when implemented have helped organizations meet cost and quality targets in CJR, BPCI, and ACOs. Retrieved from https://www.asahq.org/psh. Accessed December 9, 2021.

The ASA sponsors the Anesthesia Quality Institute (AQI). *Access AQI's Qualified Clinical Data Registry (QCDR).* Retrieved from https://www.aqihq.org/introduction-to-nacor.aspx. Accessed December 9, 2021.

The Medicare program's Quality Payment Program (QPP). Retrieved from https://qpp.cms.gov. Accessed December 9, 2021. This site has extensive, official information about MIPS, MIPS Value Pathways, APMs, and all requirements.

# Perioperative Surgical Home

CHRIS STEEL, MD | ROSEANNE M. FISCHOFF, MPP

## What Is the Perioperative Surgical Home Model?

The Perioperative Surgical Home (PSH) model is a physician-led, patient-centric, team-based system of coordinated care that guides patients through the entire surgical experience, from the decision to undergo a surgery/procedure to discharge and beyond. This is achieved through shared decision-making and seamless continuity of care for surgical and other procedural patients. The goal of the PSH model is to achieve the "quadruple aim": provide cost-effective, high-quality perioperative care and exceptional patient experiences while reducing provider burnout. Fig. 232.1 is a visual representation that describes the PSH model.

## Why Was the Perioperative Surgical Home Model Created?

The PSH model was designed to reduce the overall cost and improve the quality and experience of perioperative care in the United States. The PSH team must reengineer the entire perioperative process to:
- Coordinate care and transition planning
- Focus on early patient engagement with preoptimization of their condition
- Eliminate unnecessary testing
- Improve intraoperative efficiency
- Enable early patient mobility postprocedure
- Reduce complications

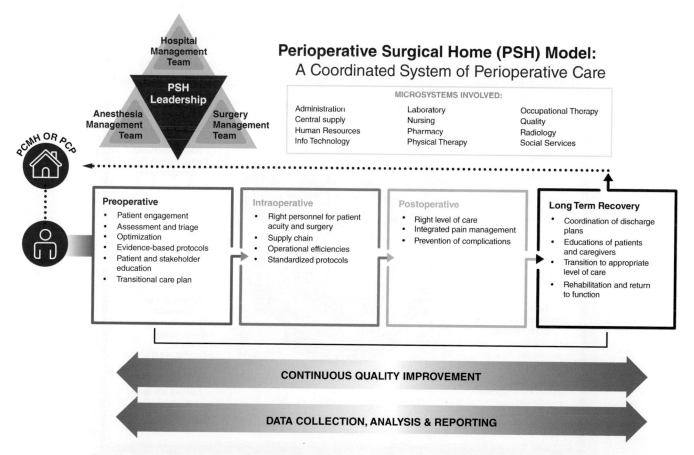

**Fig. 232.1** Overview of the Perioperative Surgical Home (PSH) model. *PCMH,* Patient-centered medical home; *PCP,* primary care physician. (Image from the American Society of Anesthesiologists PSH website with permission.)

- Improve clinical outcomes
- Decrease the total cost of care
- Enhance the patient's perception of the entire surgical experience
- Reduce the administrative burden on individual providers to reduce burnout

## What Are the Components and Principles of the Perioperative Surgical Home Model?

In 2021, a workgroup was assembled with representatives from the American Hospital Administration, the American Academy of Orthopaedic Surgeons, the American Society of Anesthesiologists, and the National Health Council. This group was charged with developing a PSH Implementation Guide. This guide was developed "to accelerate the widespread adoption of the PSH principles, which focus on optimizing outcomes and experiences for patients undergoing a procedural or a surgical episode of care".[1] The workgroup was asked to reflect on their experiences with implementing a PSH model at their institutions and for the first time define the model's core principles and components. Fig. 232.2 is an infographic detailing these principles and components.

## Who Are the Stakeholders in the Perioperative Surgical Home Model?

Collaborating with team-based care members is a critical component of the PSH initiative. Because the model is based on coordinated care, it is essential that all members of the care team work together to determine the best clinical protocols for how to treat their patients. With this in mind, the most successful PSH pilots have the following stakeholders as a part of the PSH care team:

- Administrative champion(s)
- Anesthesiology champion(s)
- Surgeon champion(s)
- Appropriate physician specialties including primary care, physiatrists, emergency, etc.
- Nurses
- Information technology champion(s)
- Project management champion(s)
- Many other clinicians, including care managers, physical therapists, pharmacists, etc.

## How Is the Perioperative Surgical Home Implemented?

The PSH team must include key stakeholders in the perioperative continuum. This team must employ team leadership skills, establish a performance improvement methodology, and understand how to assist with project management. But most importantly, the leaders of the PSH team must have strong competencies in change management. To develop this skill, Dr. John P. Kotter offers eight steps for implementing change: generate urgency, build a team, create change vision and strategy, achieve buy-in, empower others, celebrate short-term wins, be relentless, and anchor change in the culture.

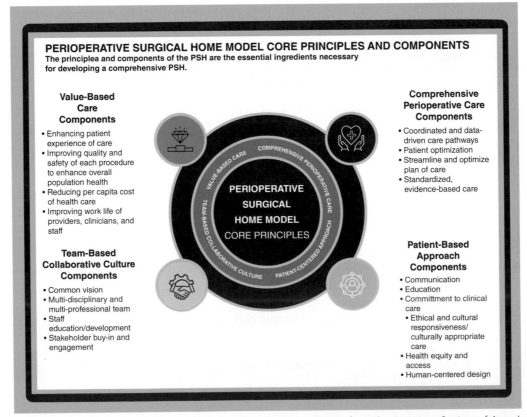

**Fig. 232.2** Perioperative Surgical Home model core principles and components. (Image from the American Society of Anesthesiologists PSH Implementation Guide with permission.)

# What Organizational Capabilities Are Associated With a Successful Perioperative Surgical Home Pilot?

In addition to having the right team in place, a successful PSH pilot will require a variety of organizational capabilities, including:
- Ability to collect and analyze data to assess performance
- Ability to gather support and resources from beyond the immediate project team
- Ability to implement evidence-based clinical protocols and pathways
- Ability to monitor compliance with evidence-based protocols and pathways
- Access to financial decision support and expertise
- Access to performance improvement support and expertise
- Familiarity with clinical registries (e.g., American Joint Replacement Registry, National Surgical Quality Improvement Program, National Anesthesia Clinical Outcomes Registry, Society of Thoracic Surgeons National Database)
- Eventual access to claims data through Centers for Medicare and Medicaid Services, commercial, Accountable Care Organization, hospital programs facilitator conveners, or third-party vendors

# What Types of Institutions Are Piloting the Perioperative Surgical Home Model?

One of the benefits of the PSH model is that it is incredibly flexible. Because its tenets are based on coordinated care in the surgical suite and beyond, any type of institution that is delivering surgical care can implement a PSH pilot. This notion is supported by the publications from various types of institutions that have successfully launched a PSH pilot such as:
- Mayo Clinic—a large integrated care system
- Lee Health—a community-based hospital system
- Jamaica Hospital Medical Center—a community-based hospital system
- Ohio State University—an academic medical center

To review these publications, visit www.asahq.org/psh or see the "Suggested Readings" section of this chapter.

# What Are Some of the Outcomes of the Perioperative Surgical Home Pilots?

Although the results of individual PSH pilot programs vary by institution, depending on variables such as service line chosen and key areas of focus, institutions that have launched PSH pilots have reported success in enhancing clinical quality, controlling costs, and/or improving patient experiences as a result of their PSH initiatives. Some examples of these outcomes include:
- Decreases in lengths of stay
- Decreases in direct costs or increases in cost savings
- Decreases in readmission rates
- Decrease in surgical complications and/or decrease in surgical site infection
- Increase in discharge to home or home health care
- Increase in patient satisfaction scores
- Decrease in same day surgical case cancellations
- Improved operating room efficiency
- Decreases in total oral morphine

# What Are Examples of Institutions That Have Implemented a PSH Pilot?

One example of an institution that has implemented a PSH pilot is Bellin Health Partners. In 2021, Bellin Health Partners in northeast Wisconsin reported that through their PSH programs they were able to see decreases in length of stay, readmission rates, skilled nursing facility use, and same day cancellations. Fig. 232.3 compares outcomes between their PSH patients and their non-PSH patients.

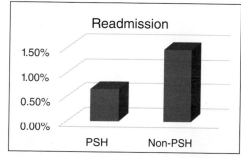

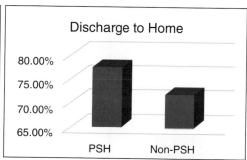

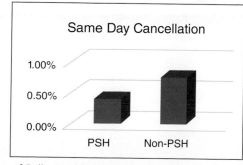

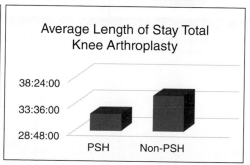

**Fig. 232.3** Examples of Bellin Health Partners' PSH patient outcomes as compared with non-PSH patient outcomes. (Image from the American Society of Anesthesiologists Monitor with permission.)

Dr. Saied Assef, president of Bellin Health Partners, states: "We feel that the collective efforts of specialists involved in the implementation of PSH has provided a significant contribution to Bellin Health Partners' success in accountable care, such as the achievement of the highest quality and lowest per capita cost in the pioneer and next-generation accountable care outcomes during three of the 6 years of participation in these programs".[2]

Another example of an institution that has implemented a PSH pilot is the Kettering Health Network in Southwest Ohio. The Kettering PSH program officially started in July 2018 in their colorectal service line. The outcomes of this pilot included a 45% reduction in length of stay, a 25% reduction in complication rates, a 20% increase in patient satisfaction scores, and improved pain control with less opioid usage. Fig. 232.4 compares outcomes between their PSH patients and their non-PSH patients.

Because of the success of the Kettering PSH program, less than 2 years later, six additional service lines were added to their PSH portfolio, including hernia, gynecology-oncology surgeries, spinal fusions, total joints, and major urology/urology-gynecology surgeries.

COVID-19 presented significant challenges for the Kettering team. However, because of the PSH framework that they had already in place, the perioperative care team was able to quickly streamline a process for COVID-19 testing preoperatively. In addition, they were able to address concerns in the postoperative and discharge process and meet with their primary care colleagues to build a road map for both the clinicians and the patients, including optimization resources to enhance population health strategies before a surgical intervention was determined. Because of these efforts and many more, at the end of 2020, the Kettering team, through great teamwork, was able to add four additional service lines to their PSH portfolio.

## Conclusion

Developing a PSH model in your community will more closely align perioperative care with the transition to value-based payments and population health medicine. Anesthesiologists should learn the skills involved in team leadership, performance improvement, and project management to serve in PSH leadership roles together with the other specialist champions.

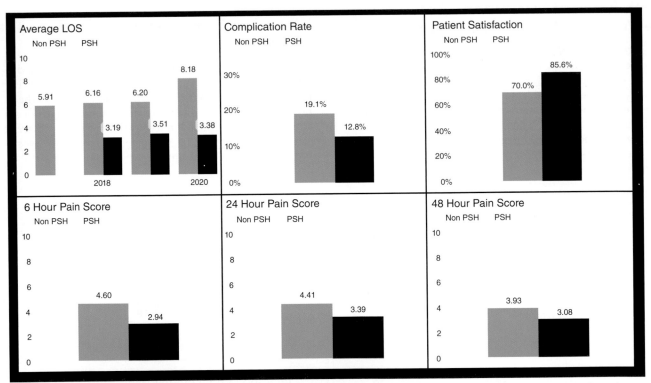

**Fig. 232.4** Examples of Kettering Health Network's PSH patient outcomes as compared with non-PSH patient outcomes. (Image from the American Society of Anesthesiologists Monitor with permission.)

## REFERENCES

1. Steel, C., Brouhard, D., Duggan, K., et al. (2021). *Perioperative Surgical Home Implementation Guide 2021.* Schaumburg, IL: American Society of Anesthesiologists. Retrieved from https://education. asahq.org/course/view.php?id=4095. Accessed December 8, 2021.

2. Assef, S., Suplinski, C., Ames, A. R., & Brouhard, D. M. (2021). Bellin Health Partners standardizes surgical process with perioperative surgical home and Kettering Health Network PSH proves resilient through a pandemic. *ASA Monitor, 85*(1), 6–7. doi:10.1097/01.ASM.0000725816.59371.e4.

## SUGGESTED READINGS

American Society of Anesthesiologists. (2020). *PSH Learning collaborative roadmap to success.* Retrieved from https://www.asahq.org/about-asa/-/media/55 a81760da5c421985cb72c952ebb4e5.ashx.

Cline, K. M., Clement, V., Rock-Klotz, J., Kash, B. A., Steel, C., & Miller, T. R. (2020). Improving the cost, quality, and safety of perioperative care: A systematic review of the literature on implementation of the perioperative surgical home. *Journal of Clinical Anesthesia, 63,* 109760. doi:10.1016/j.jclinane.2020.109760.

Glantz, G. (2021). Mayo clinic sees tangible gains from project OASIS practice optimization. *ASA Monitor, 85*(11), 36–37. doi:10.1097/01.ASM.0000798568. 59898.

Holt, C. (2021). ASA Model helps Florida's Lee health optimize perioperative surgical care. *ASA Monitor, 85*(11), 40–41. doi:10.1097/01.ASM.0000798584. 48931.01.

Humeidan, M., Harter, R., Blackburn, J., Koons, C., & Slatton, T. (2020). The Ohio State University reduced total oral morphine equivalents through perioperative surgical home and Pikeville Medical Center reduces postoperative opioid consumption in total knee arthroplasty patients. *ASA Monitor, 84*(12), 23. doi:10.1097/01.ASM.0000724044.86844.19.

Kotter, J. P., & Rathgeber, H. (2005). *Our iceberg is melting: Changing and succeeding Uuder any conditions.* New York: St. Martin's Press.

Mesarch, J., Rubin, J., Adler, A., Snyder, E., & Koch, M. (2020, November). *How a West Texas hospital used a PSH to improve outcomes and cut costs.* Downers Grove, IL: Healthcare Financial Management Association. https://www.hfma.org/cost-effectiveness-of-health/financial-sustainability/how-a-west-texas-hospital-used-a-psh-to-improve-outcomes-and-cut/.

Tumolo, J. (2020). Jamaica hospital medical center sees benefits with perioperative surgical home model. *ASA Monitor, 84*(11), 44. doi:10.1097/01. ASM.0000722196.92474.39.

Vetter, T. R., & Bader, A. M. (2020). *Continued evolution of perioperative medicine: Realizing its full potential.* Anesthesia and Analgesia, 130(4), 804–807.

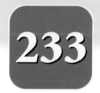

# 233

# Licensure, Credentialing, and Privileging

JEFFREY T. MUELLER, MD | MATTHEW THOMAS POPOVICH, PhD

Health care organizations such as hospitals, health plans, and provider networks must be certain that individuals who provide health care services for their respective organizations are fully qualified, competent, and able to perform those services. This process includes not only evaluating an applicant's licensure and reviewing credentials but also granting specific clinical privileges to that physician. The determination of both qualifications and competency is essential if a health care organization is to provide safe competent care while avoiding lawsuits, bad publicity, and financial loss.

Licensure is the process whereby a government board or agency reviews a physician's education, training, background, and any ethical concerns and, if the standards are adequately met, thereafter grants the physician the right to provide health care services within its jurisdiction. The government views licensure as its primary mechanism of protecting the public from substandard care. The requirements for licensure vary from state to state and sometimes include specific education requirements. Additionally, some states require supplemental competency testing if the physician is several years past formal medical training, received their medical training outside the United States, or is not board certified.

Credentialing is the process of assessing and verifying the qualifications to obtain appointment to a medical staff or to be approved as a provider in a health plan or health care network. Although many of the requirements for credentialing are similar to those for licensure, each health care organization determines its own criteria and processes. The health care organization may therefore set standards and expectations for quality, safety, and other performance measures that go beyond licensure standards.

Privileging is the process of evaluating the training, experience, and current competency of an individual to perform specific medical services as a part of a medical staff. Privileges are detailed and specific, and providers may only offer medical services in those areas in which they hold privileges. For most requested privileges, the designated individuals within the health care organization will review the provider's education and training, past clinical performance, malpractice history, and the number of cases performed. An organization's decision to limit a physician's privileges can be grounds for legal action by the applicant or require the organization to submit a report to the applicable state or federal regulatory agency and, therefore, must be done with great care and consistency. Today, most health care organizations also employ a process of ongoing concurrent review after the granting of privileges to ensure that competency is maintained.

Anesthesia services are typically overseen by a director of anesthesia services or similar position within hospitals and other facilities. In the Centers for Medicare and Medicaid Services Hospital Conditions of Participation, medical staff bylaws "must include criteria for determining the anesthesia service privileges to be granted to an individual practitioner and a procedure for applying the criteria to individuals requesting privileges for any type of anesthesia services." Ambulatory surgery center conditions of participation describe similar arrangements, including those related to who may supervise another practitioner administering anesthesia. Anesthesia leadership, including the director of anesthesia services, often works with hospital and facility leadership to determine the criteria used for granting such privileges.

## How Health Care Organizations Credential and Privilege Physicians

The specific processes for credentialing and privileging are delineated in a combination of the health care organization's medical staff bylaws, rules and regulations, and policies and procedures. For legal and regulatory reasons, it is essential that the processes are clearly outlined and precisely followed. Otherwise, the health care organization may have a limited ability to correct or dismiss providers for inadequate performance.

In most health care organizations, the data collection involved with credentialing and privileging is performed by individuals specifically designated by the organization. These individuals may function solely as credentialing/privileging personnel, or this function may be part of the broader services provided by medical staff services. After the collection of data, a credentialing or personnel committee or designee reviews the data and makes recommendations to the governing body. In acute care hospitals, the medical executive committee is responsible for forwarding recommendations to the governing body of the health care organization, which is ultimately responsible for the decisions concerning staff membership and clinical privileges.

The information used in licensure, credentialing, and privileging comes from a variety of sources. To decrease the risk that an individual will submit falsified documents for review, licensing boards and health care organizations check information through a process known as primary source verification. This means that verification of an applicant's education, training, experience, work history, board certification, licensure, malpractice history, and legal background check must be obtained directly from the originating source. Although this process can be time-consuming, much of the information is now available on secure Internet sites.

At times, questions, concerns, or issues (i.e., "red flags," such as incomplete or inconsistent information found on the application form) confront those who are reviewing an application. Among the red flags that cause the greatest concern for reviewers are:

- Conflicting information between the information provided on the application and the information received in the verification process.
- Unexplained gaps in time. Organizations may determine what time period is considered an acceptable time gap between transitions (e.g., a time gap between training programs or when relocating). Unexplained or extended time gaps are considered red flags and require additional information.
- Frequent moves from location to location or practice to practice. This situation not only can make competency evaluation for privileging difficult but may also suggest problems in other areas, such as poor interpersonal skills, health problems, issues with a state licensing board or agency, or excessive malpractice claims.
- Negative references or reference requests that are not returned. References can be a powerful source of information, but because applicants have a tendency to select individuals who will give a positive review, a negative response is particularly important.
- Unanswered questions on the application. Although an omission may be a simple error, it can also signal an effort by the applicant to hide something.
- A large number of liability suits. Recently, the number of lawsuits associated with a provider has become linked to their ability to communicate with patients, as well as competency.

## License Renewal, Reappointment, and Continuation of Clinical Privileges

No longer is it acceptable for licensing bodies or health care organizations to simply "rubber-stamp" a health care physician's request for licensure renewal, reappointment to a health care organization, or continuation of clinical privileges. Regulators and medical staff leaders expect the renewal process to be every bit as rigorous and perhaps more evidence based than was the initial licensure, appointment, or privileging process. This rigor is supplemented by the data that can be collected on a provider during the previous practice period. Not only can the information collected during initial licensure, appointment, and privileging be reassessed, but new information may now be available. This information may include:

- Quality and safety information, including compliance with practice guidelines
- Complication and infection rate data
- Compliance with policies and procedures
- Patient satisfaction (e.g., number of patient complaints)
- Continuing medical education hours
- Maintenance of board certification
- Peer references
- Malpractice history
- Current competency
- Utilization management

Gathering this information can be a complex and sometimes difficult task, but it is necessary if a health care organization is to make the reappraisal process meaningful in terms of patient protection and institution liability.

Perhaps of greatest importance during this reassessment is the ability to more reliably assess providers' competency to continue to provide the services specified in their initial privileging. This competency is usually assessed through a review of cases performed, success and complication rates, and an assessment of competency by peers or the individual's department chair. To demonstrate an individual's competency, most health care organizations have established criteria, which may include the number and type of procedures performed. When possible, objective data should be used in this evaluation process, because any limitation of privileging may greatly affect the applicant provider's ability to continue their practice of medicine.

## Delegated Credentialing

Delegated credentialing is the process used when a health care organization outsources or delegates the credentialing responsibility to an outside vendor or credentialing verification organization (CVO) or another health care organization. Often this involves a health insurer or health care network delegating the credentialing to a participating provider group within the health plan or network. The participating provider group or CVO, rather than the health insurer, performs the credentialing process. This process assumes that the participating provider group or CVO is capable of performing the credentialing process and meets the standards set by the delegating organization. Not only does this arrangement obviate the need for the outsourcing organization to perform the detailed work already being done by the provider group or CVO, but it also means less work for the practitioners who would otherwise be burdened with additional, often duplicative, paperwork.

If health care organizations that delegate credentialing are serious about protecting their patients and decreasing their own liability, they must include oversight of the provider group or CVO. The health care organization that delegates credentialing must set standards for the delegated credentialing process that includes a periodic audit of the credentials files and policies and procedures of the provider group or CVO. Review of quality, safety, patient satisfaction or complaints, liability, and other specific data should be included. Only those outsourced provider groups or CVOs that meet these standards are allowed to continue with delegated credentialing status. In most circumstances, the final decision about whether a provider is credentialed by a delegating health care organization rests not with the outsourced group or CVO but with the health care organization itself.

## SUGGESTED READINGS

Centers for Medicare and Medicaid Services (CMS). *Strategic plan.* Retrieved from https://www.cms.gov/. Accessed September 17, 2021.

NCQA. *Credentials verification organization certification.* Retrieved from https://www.ncqa.org/ programs/health-plans/credentials-verification-organization-cvo/. Accessed September 17, 2021.

National Association Medical Staff Services (NAMSS). Retrieved from http://www.namss.org/. Accessed September 17, 2021.

Utilization Review Accreditation Commission (URAC). *Credentials verification organization accreditation.* Retrieved from https://www.urac.org/accreditation-cert/credentials-verification-organization-accreditation/. Accessed September 17, 2021.

# 234

# Board Certification and Maintenance of Certification

KATHRYN S. HANDLOGTEN, MD

Although participation in the American Board of Anesthesiology (ABA) certification process is voluntary, achieving and maintaining certification are increasingly important to secure and maintain medical licensure and hospital privileges. Board certification and maintenance of certification are often requirements for membership in a private group practice or an academic anesthesiology department. Therefore achieving and maintaining certification are important goals for practicing anesthesiologists.

## Primary Certification Examination Process

The ABA, a member board of the American Board of Medical Specialties (ABMS), has established threshold criteria, training, and education requirements, as well as acquisition of the knowledge and skills that anesthesiologists require so that the ABA can certify (and recertify) an anesthesiologist as meeting these criteria. Certification by an ABMS member board, such as the ABA, has been shown to correlate with medical school evaluations and grades, the duration and type of residency training, and faculty assessment of procedural skills. Interestingly, personal characteristics such as trait anxiety (the tendency to respond to a wide range of situations as dangerous or threatening) and the ability to maintain focused attention (vigilance) and process information quickly are also associated with clinical competence. However, certification by an ABMS member board is recognition of competence that is more widely accepted by the public.

Because physicians' knowledge and skill sets may erode over time, and because medical technology and science continue to advance, ABMS member boards have largely evolved from life-time certification to time-limited certification. In general, certification of anesthesiologists correlates with better patient outcomes. A retrospective cohort study demonstrated that physician anesthesiologists who fail the Structured Oral Examination (SOE) have a higher incidence of having disciplinary action taken against them by their state medical board compared with those who pass the exam on the first attempt. In this study, failing the written examination did not have a similar impact if the candidate successfully passed the oral examination. Additional studies comparing pass rates and construct validation between the written examinations, oral examinations, and Objective Structured Clinical Examinations (OSCEs) confirm that differing exam formats test different components of clinician aptitude and are important for assessing overall competency.

## Continuum of Education in Anesthesiology

The ABA Continuum of Education in Anesthesiology consists of 4 years of full-time training after a medical or osteopathic degree has been conferred. This continuum includes 1 year of clinical base year training (CBY) and 3 years of training in clinical anesthesiology (CA; CA-1, CA-2, and CA-3 years). The CBY must be completed in a transitional year or primary specialty training program that is accredited by the Accreditation Council for Graduate Medical Education (ACGME) or the American Osteopathic Association. Training outside the United States and its territories must be conducted in a program affiliated with a medical school that is approved by the Liaison Committee on Medical Education.

The 3-year clinical anesthesia curriculum includes basic anesthesia training, subspecialty anesthesia training, and advanced anesthesia training during which residents provide care for progressively more complex patients and progressively more difficult procedures. Basic anesthesia training focuses on fundamental aspects of anesthesia. Subspecialty anesthesia training is focused on the subdisciplines of anesthesiology, such as obstetric anesthesia, pediatric anesthesia, cardiothoracic anesthesia, neuroanesthesia, anesthesia for outpatient surgery, the postanesthesia care unit, perioperative evaluation, regional anesthesia, critical care medicine, and pain medicine. Advanced anesthesia training occurs in the CA-3 year. Training in the CA-3 year is distinctly different from that obtained during the CA-1 and CA-2 years and is characterized by increasing independence to prepare residents for the unsupervised practice of anesthesiology after residency completion. Additional details about the specific requirements for completion of the Continuum of Education in Anesthesiology are available in the ABA Booklet of Information accessible on the ABA website.

Clinical anesthesia training (CA-1 through CA-3 years) must be conducted in no more than two ACGME-accredited programs with at least 3 months of uninterrupted training in each. The 6-month period of clinical anesthesia training in any one program must end with receipt of a satisfactory Certificate of Clinical Competence for this training to receive credit toward requirements to complete the Continuum. Part-time training is assessed on an individual basis by the ABA Credentials Committee and must be approved prospectively. The absence from training policy for anesthesia residency was revised in July 2019. Previously, the total absence from training could not exceed 60 working days during the CA-1 through CA-3 years. Since the revision of this policy in 2019, the ABA will consider requests for up to an additional 40 days away from training after a formal request is placed for serious medical illness, parental, or family leave. Absences beyond this limit require extension of total training time based on the duration of the absence. After a prolonged absence from training (>6 months), the ABA Credentials Committee will determine the number of months of training after the absence that are required.

## ABA Staged Examinations

Physicians who successfully complete the requirements for residency training in an ACGME-accredited anesthesiology residency program may qualify to enter the examination process for primary certification by the ABA if they meet the threshold requirements for primary certification in anesthesiology (Box 234.1).

Trainees beginning the CBY in 2012 or later are required to complete three stages of ABA examinations (previously referred to as Part 1 and Part 2 exams). The ABA Basic examination is administered after successful completion of 18 months of clinical training, including 12 months of CBY and 6 months of the CA-1 year. It is administered twice per year, with most candidates completing the examination near the end of the CA-1 year. The ABA Advanced examination is administered after successful completion of the Basic examination. Candidates can register for the Advanced examination after 30 months of residency training. The Advanced examination is typically administered in July after completion of the CA-3 year. The ABA Applied examination, which consists of an SOE and OSCE, may be taken after successful completion of the Basic and Advanced written examinations. The Applied examination components are administered at the ABA assessment center in Raleigh, North Carolina. During the COVID-19 pandemic, the ABA held select Applied examinations in a virtual format because of local and national travel restrictions.

Candidates completing residency training after January 1, 2012 must complete all certification requirements within 7 years of the last day of the year in which residency training was completed.

## Maintenance of Certification

Maintenance of Certification in Anesthesiology (MOCA) is required for ongoing certification of anesthesiologists who achieved primary certification in anesthesiology during or after 2000. The MOCA process is completed in 10-year cycles intended to assure the public of a diplomate's continuing

---

**BOX 234.1  THRESHOLD REQUIREMENTS FOR PRIMARY CERTIFICATION IN ANESTHESIOLOGY**

A permanent, unconditional, unrestricted, and unexpired medical license to practice medicine or osteopathy in one or more states or jurisdictions of the United States or province of Canada

Completion of the requirements of the Continuum of Education in anesthesiology

An ABA Certificate of Clinical Competence with an overall satisfactory rating covering the final 6-month period of clinical anesthesia training in each anesthesiology residency program on file with the ABA

Documentation of professional standing that is satisfactory to the ABA capability to perform independently the entire scope of anesthesiology practice without restriction, or with reasonable accommodation

Successful completion of Basic, Advanced, and Applied exams

*ABA, American Board of Anesthesiology.*

| Part | Requirement(s) |
|------|----------------|

**TABLE 234.1 Maintenance of Certification in Anesthesiology Requirements**

| Part | Requirement(s) |
|------|----------------|
| 1 | **Professionalism and Professional Standing (PPS)** <br> Continual assessment of professional standing through maintenance of valid medical licensure |
| 2 | **Lifelong Learning and Self-Assessment (LLS)** <br> Current knowledge through CME and other forms of learning 250 CME credits <br> 250 must be category 1 <br> Limited to ≤60 per year <br> Some CME activity must be completed in at least 5 years of each 10-year cycle (125 credits by end of year 5). <br> ≥20 must be category 1 patient safety CME <br> *Beginning in 2016, self-assessment CMEs are no longer required. |
| 3 | **Assessment of Knowledge, Judgment, and Skills (KJS)** <br> Diplomates must complete 30 MOCA Minute pilot questions per calendar quarter (120 per year by 11:59 p.m. EST on December 31). |
| 4 | **Improvements in Medical Practice (IMP)** <br> Beginning in 2016, simulation is an optional Part 4 activity. The ABA has developed a point system for Part 4. Diplomates must earn 25 points per 5-year period for a total of 50 points during the 10-year MOCA cycle. |

*ABA*, American Board of Anesthesiology; *CME*, continuing medical education; *MOCA*, Maintenance of Certification in Anesthesiology.

**BOX 234.2 REQUIREMENTS FOR SUBSPECIALTY CERTIFICATION STATUS AS A DIPLOMATE OF THE ABA**

Fulfillment of the licensure requirement for certification
Fulfillment of the specialty training requirements as determined by the ABA
Satisfactory completion of the subspecialty certification examination requirements as determined by the ABA
Professional standing satisfactory to the ABA
Capability of performing independently the entire scope of subspecialty practice without or with reasonable accommodations
For subspecialty certification in sleep medicine and pediatric anesthesiology, enrollment in the MOCA process

*ABA*, American Board of Anesthesiology; *MOCA*, Maintenance of Certification in Anesthesiology.

competence in the practice of anesthesiology. A certificate is valid until December 31 of the 10th year after certification. MOCA requirements are divided into four parts: professional standing; lifelong learning and self-assessment; assessment of knowledge, judgment, and skills; and improvements in medical practice. MOCA requirements are summarized in Table 234.1.

## Maintenance of Certification in Anesthesiology 2.0

In January 2016, the ABA launched MOCA 2.0. This is a web-based learning platform designed to facilitate achievement of MOCA requirements. A primary aspect of MOCA 2.0 is the MOCA Minute. This is a pilot of an online learning tool that allows candidates to participate in multiple-choice questions to fulfill the MOCA Part 3 requirement (see Table 234.1). MOCA Minute questions are multiple-choice questions with a single best answer, like those presented on previous MOCA and subspecialty

recertification exams. The board will use this tool to make judgments about diplomates who fall below a minimum standard.

## Subspecialty Certification

The ABA also offers subspecialty certification in critical care medicine, pain medicine, hospice and palliative care medicine, sleep medicine, neurocritical care, and pediatric anesthesiology (Box 234.2). The ABMS has also approved subspecialty certification for adult cardiac anesthesiology through the ABA as early as 2023. Subspecialty recertification is offered through successful completion of ongoing examinations via MOCA Minute multiple-choice specialty and subspecialty questions. Importantly, ABA diplomates who choose to maintain both primary certification in anesthesiology and subspecialty certification will benefit from one set of program requirements for all parts of MOCA 2.0.

## Summary

Board certification and MOCA are critical achievements that can affect medical licensure, maintenance of licensure, hospital privileges, and employment. The requirements for certification and MOCA are detailed, numerous, and dynamic as they adapt to changing advancements and needs in our specialty. This chapter provides an overview of current primary certification, subspecialty certification, and MOCA requirements. However, it is important for candidates and diplomates to periodically review current requirements on the ABA website to be aware of the most current requirements.

## SUGGESTED READINGS

Brennan, T. A., Horwitz, R. I., Duffy, F. D., Cassel, C. K., Goode, L. D., & Lipner, R. S. (2004). The role of physician specialty board certification status in the quality movement. *JAMA, 292*(9), 1038–1043.

Reich, D. L., Uysal, S., Bodian, C. A., Gabriele, S., Hibbard, M., Gordon, W., et al. (1999). The relationship of cognitive, personality, and academic measures to anesthesiology resident clinical performance. *Anesthesia and Analgesia, 88*(5), 1092–1100.

Rose, S. H., & Burkle, C. M. American Board of Anesthesiology Clinical Competence Committee. (2006). Accreditation council for graduate medical education competencies and the American Board of Anesthesiology Clinical Competence

Committee: A comparison. *Anesthesia and Analgesia, 102*(1), 212–216.

The American Board of Anesthesiology. *What we do: Training information.* Retrieved from: https://www.theaba.org/what%20we%20do.html#training%20info. Accessed November 8, 2021.

The American Board of Anesthesiology. *What we do: Policies.* Retrieved from https://www.theaba.org/what%20we%20do.html#POLICIES. Accessed November 8, 2021.

Wang, T., Sun, H., Zhou, Y., Chen, D., Harman, A. E., Isaak, R. S., et al. (2021). Construct validation of the American Board of Anesthesiology's APPLIED examination for initial certification. *Anesthesia and Analgesia, 133*(1), 226–232.

Warner, D. O., Lien, C. A., Wang, T., Zhou, Y., Isaak, R. S., Peterson-Layne, C., et al. (2020). First-year results of the American board of anesthesiology's objective structured clinical examination for initial certification. *Anesthesia and Analgesia, 131*(5), 1412–1418.

Zhou, Y., Sun, H., Culley, D. J., Young, A., Harman, A. E., & Warner, D. O. (2017). Effectiveness of written and oral specialty certification examinations to predict actions against the medical licenses of anesthesiologists. *Anesthesiology, 126*(6), 1171–1179.

# Professional Liability Insurance

BRIAN J. THOMAS, JD

Medical professional liability insurance is provided by third-party liability insurance companies and is purchased by an insured to protect against potential tort liability, a civil wrong, to others. When a civil wrong occurs, it creates liability against the wrongdoer (tortfeasor) in favor of the injured party. The civil wrong in a medical malpractice case typically involves an alleged breach of the standard of care by a physician or other health care provider in the form of a negligent act or omission that substantially leads to the patient's injury or death. The physician–patient relationship gives rise to the "duty" owed by the physician to the patient. A patient can recover money from a physician if the patient can prove that the physician's conduct fell below the accepted standard of care and caused the patient's injury or death. Most physicians purchase medical professional liability insurance to defend and pay claims resulting from medical malpractice lawsuits.

## Scope of Coverage—What Is Covered?

The purpose of medical professional liability insurance is to protect the insured physician's personal assets from the risk of paying the costs to defend a lawsuit and the risk of having to pay any settlement or judgment to the plaintiff as a result of a lawsuit. Most medical professional liability insurance policies cover both risks: contractually obligating the insurance company to pay the cost of defending lawsuits and to indemnify the insured for settlements and judgments. Medical professional liability insurance generally provides coverage for a physician's legal liability for "injury" that results from professional services provided or that should have been provided by the physician. "Injury" might include bodily injury or death and intangible injury such as pain, mental suffering, and loss of consortium (conjugal fellowship of husband and wife including not only material services but also such intangibles as society, guidance, companionship, and sexual relations). "Injury" might also include purely economic losses, such as lost past and future wages, past and future medical expenses, and funeral expenses, if the loss derives from an act or omission of a professional nature. The protection provided by medical professional liability insurance varies and is typically defined by a policy's "scope of coverage" provision.

## Exclusions—What Is Not Covered?

Medical professional liability insurance policies generally contain exclusionary language expressly limiting coverage in specifically defined situations. Although the exclusionary language varies among different policies, most medical professional liability policies routinely exclude coverage for specific situations (Box 235.1).

> **BOX 235.1 TYPICAL EXCLUSIONS BY MEDICAL PROFESSIONAL LIABILITY INSURANCE POLICIES**
>
> Any intentional, willful, wanton, fraudulent, or malicious acts or omissions
> Liability arising from substance abuse
> Liability arising from the alteration, falsification, or destruction of medical records with fraudulent intent
> Liability assumed under a written or oral contract or agreement
> Punitive or exemplary damages
> The performance of administrative duties as a medical director on behalf of a hospital, health care facility, or insurance entity

## Limits of Liability—How Much Is Covered?

A medical professional liability insurance policy limits the amount of damages the insurance company will pay under the policy. Most medical professional liability insurance policies contain a "per claim" limit and an aggregate limit. The per claim limit is the maximum amount of damages the insurance company will pay for each claim. The aggregate limit is the total amount of damages the insurance company will pay for all claims within a specified period—typically 1 year. Physicians may purchase different limits of liability coverage, generally ranging from $200,000 to $1 million per claim and with an annual aggregate that is typically three times the per claim limit. The amount of professional liability coverage purchased depends on the individual physician's needs. Additionally, some states and health care facilities may require physicians to carry a minimum amount of professional liability coverage.

In addition to the limits of liability, most medical professional liability insurance policies provide coverage for the costs of defending a covered claim. The costs of defending a medical negligence lawsuit usually include attorney fees, expert fees, deposition fees, textbooks, and trial exhibits. The costs of defending a medical negligence lawsuit are most often provided in addition to the limits of liability to indemnify the insured for any settlement or judgment. However, under some policies, the limits of liability are reduced by defense expenditures, also known as a "wasting" liability policy.

## Duties of the Insurance Company and the Insured

The professional liability insurance contract (also known as the policy) defines the rights, responsibilities, and duties of the insurance company and insured. Generally, the professional liability contract gives the insurance company the right to investigate any claim or lawsuit, the duty to defend the insured against the claim or suit, the right to control the defense—including selecting defense counsel—and the right to settle covered claims. The professional liability contract requires the insured to notify the insurance company promptly of any claim or lawsuit and cooperate with the insurance company's investigation and defense of any claim or lawsuit against the insured.

## Consent-to-Settle Clauses

The relationship between a physician and their medical professional liability insurance company is also defined by the extent to which the physician can influence the settlement of claims. Some medical professional liability insurance policies contain consent-to-settle clauses that require the insurance company to obtain the insured physician's permission before settling a claim. Because many physicians view an out-of-court settlement as an admission of guilt or feel strongly that their care and treatment were appropriate, a consent-to-settle clause might be an essential policy provision for those physicians. Some insurance policies do not include consent-to-settle clauses and allow the insurance company the right to settle claims—even those without merit—without the insured physician's consent. Some states prohibit consent-to-settle clauses by law, regulation, or public policy.

## Coverage Forms

Medical professional liability insurance was traditionally written on an occurrence form. Coverage is triggered when the injury that precipitates a claim for damages occurs during the policy period. Because many claims are not recognized, reported, or filed until years after the alleged negligent act occurred, insurance companies have difficulty calculating how much premium should be collected today to cover claims that might not be reported for years.

Many medical professional liability insurance companies now use a claims-made form instead of the occurrence form to address this problem. Under a claims-made form, coverage is triggered when the claim is asserted. The term *claims-made* refers to the notification that an injured third party is seeking redress from the insured. Typically, coverage is triggered when a physician receives a demand for money from an injured patient or receives a notice or summons from the patient's legal representative and, in turn, gives notice to the insurance company. The policy definition of claims-made frequently allows coverage to be triggered by precautionary reporting of adverse outcomes or incident reports to the insurance company within the policy period regardless of third-party involvement. Such forms are referred to as *modified* claims-made.

Another feature of claims-made policies is the extended reporting period, which, in return for additional premium, guarantees the insured an extended period in which claims may be reported if the policy is canceled or not renewed. The extended reporting period—also known as *tail coverage*—applies only to claims made after the policy expires or is canceled and arising from events that occur after the date the policy was issued and before the policy expired. These provisions and their costs vary substantially among insurance companies.

Prior acts insurance coverage – also referred to as *nose coverage* – provides coverage for claims for negligent acts or omissions that occurred during a period in which the physician was insured under a previous claims-made policy. To avoid gaps in coverage when changing insurance companies, physicians must purchase prior acts coverage for any incidents that might arise unless they purchased tail coverage from their previous insurance company. Understanding the coverage form and the ease of moving coverage from one form to another are important considerations.

## SUGGESTED READINGS

American College of Physicians. (2021). *Medical malpractice insurance.* Retrieved from https://www. acponline.org/about-acp/about-internal-medicine/ career-paths/residency-career-counseling/resident-career-counseling-guidance-and-tips/medical-malpractice-insurance. Accessed January, 2022.

Medical Professional Liability Association. *MPL insurance – a practitioner's primer.* 2019 ed. Retrieved from https://www.mplassociation.org/store/detail.aspx?id=P19PRIMER&WebsiteKey=d190c161-263f-44b3-bcce-a9540a8281c4.

National Association of Insurance Commissioners. (2021). *Medical malpractice insurance.* Retrieved from https://content.naic.org/cipr_topics/topic_medical_malpractice_insurance.htm. Accessed January, 2022.

# Anesthesia Information Management Systems

PATRICK J. GUFFEY, MD, MHA  |  KARL A. POTERACK, MD

An anesthesia information management system (AIMS) is the perioperative component of an electronic health record (EHR). AIMS serve to document the anesthesia care during a perioperative episode or when anesthesia is provided in a nonoperative remote area. This system collects data automatically from the anesthesia machines, physiologic monitors, and other electronic medical devices. AIMS also allow the anesthesiologist to document case events, care provided, and medications given. These data are then stored, organized, and displayed in both real time and retrospectively. An AIMS may also provide documentation of preoperative evaluation and postoperative care, information for billing and coding, clinical decision support, scheduling, resource and equipment management, and quality improvement functions. A well-designed and -implemented AIMS can minimize manual clinical documentation, facilitate increased situational awareness and attention to critical tasks, and provide access to higher-resolution data and information than was possible in a paper record environment. However, an AIMS that is inadequately implemented or optimized can increase clerical burden and provider frustration, detract attention from patient care, and even propagate errors in the medical record.

The very first "automated anesthesia charts" appeared in the early 1980s. Given that a single anesthetic can create millions of bits of information and that in a paper system up to 40% of an anesthesia provider's time is spent as a scribe, computer automation was seen as a natural way to create a higher-quality record with less manual input. Early systems were almost exclusively "homebuilt," stand-alone designs that did not benefit from standardization or integration with other systems. Currently, vendors provide AIMS products with wide variations in functionality from fully integrated systems into leading EHRs to stand-alone products that run on a tablet with no interfaces to the EHR.

## Architecture and Configuration

An AIMS can be a stand-alone system or can be integrated within a larger EHR. Even in stand-alone systems, there are typically some types of interfaces providing data to other clinical systems, at the minimum scheduling and basic patient demographics. In integrated environments, data moves seamlessly and instantly in a bidirectional fashion. In some circumstances, it may no longer be appropriate to call an integrated system an AIMS versus a group of tools specialized to anesthesia documentation within the EHR. Examples of other clinical systems receiving data from an AIMS include a computerized physician order entry system, medication administration record (MAR), surgical scheduling, supply management, quality improvement, and coding and billing software.

A proper AIMS requires high-reliability hardware, software, and networks. In contrast to many other parts of an EHR or other electronic clinical systems, there is a greater need for "real-time" access to data. Vital sign data is typically recorded, at a minimum, every minute and is documented in an unvalidated fashion, meaning the anesthesiologist does not manually validate the information and it is automatically recorded versus almost all other areas of the EHR, where a nurse or provider must declare the data to be accurate. Additionally, the spatial and temporal constraints of the perioperative environment provide special challenges with regard to human factors, engineering, and user interface technologies. These have been shown to be extremely important for the successful design, deployment, and, perhaps most important, user acceptance of any AIMS installation. An AIMS presents all the attendant requirements of a mission critical system. Dedicated support from the organization's information technology department is essential. Expertise in device integration methodology is of particular importance. Some organizations are beginning the process of interfacing medication pump data with the AIMS/EHR, and more operative equipment will move in this direction in the coming years.

## Prevalence and Utilization

The Health Information Technology for Economic and Clinical Health (HiTECH) Act in 2009 (part of the American Recovery and Reinvestment Act) provided approximately $27 billion over a 10-year period to facilitate the transformation to EHRs of all types, including AIMS. Due in large part to this financial incentive, the prevalence of these records has greatly increased since then. With regard to AIMS prevalence specifically, a 2011 survey of American Society of Anesthesiologists members suggested that 24% of respondents were using an AIMS, although methodologic difficulties with this study make it difficult to translate this to data about practice locations per se. A 2014 survey of academic anesthesiology departments (with a 100% response rate) reported that 67% of academic anesthesiology departments were using an AIMS, with an additional 8% planning to have one installed within 12 months. This survey estimated that 85% of programs would be using an AIMS by the 2018 to 2020 timeframe. Given the foregoing, it is likely that at some point around that 2018 to 2020 timeframe, more than 50% of anesthetics provided in the United States were charted in an electronic system, and that number has likely grown some since then.

Whether an AIMS is "homegrown" or vended, stand-alone or integrated, the degree of data integration with other systems, such as hospital EHRs, operating room management systems (e.g., surgical scheduling, patient tracking, supply management), and other operational systems (e.g., pharmacy, blood banking, physician orders, accounting, billing, quality reporting, preanesthesia evaluations, barcode-enabled drug and blood product administration and charting, drug conflict checking, and user-accessible databases for outcomes research and quality reporting) is variable. However, evolving requirements created by pay-for-performance, quality, and safety initiatives and other administrative expectations are increasing the demand for integration and advanced AIMS. Although these developments have created a demand for these functions, there can be significant downsides if these capabilities are poorly integrated with EMRs and hospital-wide information systems.

A new requirement in 2021 was the implementation of the 21st Century Cures Act. Phase 1 required that whenever technically feasible, and without causing harm, much of the data in the EHR must be electronically released to patients in real time. At this time, pre- and postanesthetic notes, procedure notes, laboratory results, and other consultations must be released directly to the patient. Phase 2 is planned for implementation in 2022 and will require most data in the EHR, including vital signs, medication administration, and all clinical documentation, to be released. Releasing this information to the patient (or their proxies) in real time is a new era in medical transparency and is sure to evolve over the coming years.

## Benefits/Disadvantages

The most obvious benefit of an AIMS is the elimination of manual charting on a paper anesthesia record, which not only reduces the need for human input but also provides real-time display of more accurate, higher-resolution, clinically relevant information. In fact, first-generation systems provided little more than the convenience of automatic charting and a legible record. As AIMS technology has progressed, additional benefits have been realized. A well-designed AIMS can add value to an anesthesia practice and the associated facility that is not attainable with paper anesthesia records. Benefits in quality improvement, safety, cost management, revenue capture, and medical liability have all been demonstrated. However, deploying any new and evolving technology introduces risks, and many of these risks and pitfalls have also been noted in the literature. Institutions without the necessary financial and technical resources or the full commitment of senior leadership should consider AIMS implementation carefully. Making an informed decision includes consulting the literature and specialty organizations for guidelines, policies, technical recommendations, and best practices.

One item that deserves discussion is patient identification and associated safety checks. AIMS systems integrated with EHRs are able to display patient photos, reducing errors surrounding documenting on the wrong patient, and making the electronic time-out process more reliable.

Although an increasing array of benefits have been attributed to AIMS technologies, the question of whether these systems broadly and consistently produce a positive financial return remains hotly debated. One significant confounding factor regarding return-on-investment discussions is determining who receives the benefit and who pays the cost. Although both anesthesia groups and facilities may realize significant benefit from an AIMS, the acquisition and support costs are frequently provided by the health system, or business owner for free-standing surgery centers. For the limited number of organizations that have deployed an AIMS, survey findings show that return-on-investment expectations have "generally been met," with specific benefits attributed to improved clinical documentation, data collection for clinical research, enhancement of quality improvement programs, and improved regulatory compliance.

## Summary

In its most basic stand-alone form, an AIMS provides the essential function of collecting intraoperative anesthesia data and automating some documentation workflows. An advanced AIMS interfaces with other systems and provides various information management functions. These capabilities can directly facilitate improvements in billing, regulatory compliance, quality improvement, safety, and research. A fully integrated AIMS can facilitate improved and more efficient care far beyond the operating room. Generally, health care lags behind other industries in the utilization of integrated information technology. However, AIMS implementation and use should continue to increase significantly as the technology matures and its value becomes increasingly demonstrated and understood.

## SUGGESTED READINGS

Poterack, K. A., & Ramakrishna, H. (2015). Converting data into information and knowledge: The promise and the reality of electronic medical records. *Annals of Cardiac Anaesthesia, 18*(3), 290–292.

Raymer, K. (2011). The anesthetic record: How content and design influence function in anesthetic practice and beyond. *Journal of Anesthesia and Clinical Research, 4*, 1–7.

Simpao, A. F., & Rehman, M. A. (2018). Anesthesia information management systems. *Anesthesia and Analgesia, 127*(1), 90–94. doi:10.1213/ANE.0000000000002545.

Stol, I. S., Ehrenfeld, J. M., & Epstein, R. H. (2014). Technology diffusion of anesthesia information management systems into academic anesthesia departments in the United States. *Anesthesia and Analgesia, 118*(3), 644–650.

Stonemetz, J. (2009). *Anesthesia informatics.* London: Springer Verlag.

Stonemetz, J., & Dutton, R. (2014). 2014 Anesthesia information management systems (AIMS) market update. *ASA Newsletter, 78*(10), 38–40.

Thomas, J. J., Yaster, M., & Guffey, P. (2020). The use of patient digital facial images to confirm patient identity in a children's hospital's anesthesia information management system. *Joint Commission Journal on Quality and Patient Safety, 46*(2), 118–121. doi:10.1016/j.jcjq.2019.10.007.

Trentman, T. L., Mueller, J. T., Ruskin, K. J., Noble, B. N., & Doyle, C. A. (2011). Adoption of anesthesia information management systems by US anesthesiologists. *Journal of Clinical Monitoring and Computing, 25*(2), 129–135.

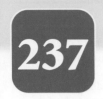
# Medical Coding and Payment Systems

SHARON K. MERRICK, MS, CCS-P  |  JEFFREY T. MUELLER, MD

Coding, billing, and payment are important elements of every medical practice. Failure to understand coding and payment systems can harm the cash flow and viability of an anesthesia practice. Contracts with payers, in addition to a complex web of laws and regulations, govern correct coding. Compliance with these rules, laws, and contractual terms protects against allegations of fraudulent or abusive practices and the potentially severe legal consequences that may occur. In this chapter, we will provide a top-down review, starting with coding and billing issues that are relevant to all medical specialties, and then drill down to those that are unique to anesthesia. It is important to note that emerging value-based and alternative payment models are often built upon the coding systems described in this chapter; see Chapter 231, Value-Based Payment Models, for an overview of the Quality Payment Program (QPP) within the Medicare Access and CHIP Reauthorization Act of 2015 (MACRA).

## Medical Diagnosis and Procedure Codes

Medical codes provide a convenient shorthand way to tell payers and others what you did and why you did it. The Health Insurance Portability and Accountability Act of 1996 standardized the code sets to be used on claims submitted to Medicare, Medicaid, and most third-party payers. CPT (current procedural terminology) codes describe professional services. The American Medical Association (AMA) owns and maintains this code set. Professional medical services include patient visits with a physician or other qualified health care professional; diagnostic and therapeutic procedures, including major and minor operations; anesthesia care; certain diagnostic tests; and many other categories.

Some procedures or services are not part of CPT but are included in the Healthcare Common Procedural Coding System (HCPCS). HCPCS codes also describe drugs, supplies, and durable medical equipment. The HCPCS code set is maintained through the joint efforts of the Centers for Medicare and Medicaid Services (CMS), the Health Insurance Association of America, and the Blue Cross and Blue Shield Association (BCBSA).

Physicians use ICD-10-CM codes to explain the reason or reasons behind the need for a medical service. ICD stands for International Classification of Diseases, and CM means that the code set has been clinically modified to be relevant for use in the United States. The World Health Organization created and maintains the ICD, and the U.S. government, through the National Center for Health Statistics and CMS, maintains ICD-10-CM, including instructions for proper use. ICD-10-CM codes are occasionally referred to informally as "diagnosis" codes. The ICD-10 code set also includes ICD-10-PCS, where PCS stands for procedural coding system. ICD-10-PCS is used only by hospitals to describe and report services and procedures. Physicians and other qualified health care professionals do not use ICD-10-PCS; they report services and procedures with CPT or HCPCS codes.

### Code Sets Used by Physicians and Other Qualified Health Care Professionals

| | |
|---|---|
| CPT | Codes and modifiers to report services and procedures |
| HCPCS | Codes and modifiers to report services and procedures and to submit claims for separately reportable drugs, supplies, and durable medical equipment |
| ICD-10-CM | Codes that describe the patient's condition or diagnosis |

## Current Procedural Terminology Code Development and Valuation Process

CPT codes describe a medical service; payment systems link these codes to a defined value. This section will describe the method in which CPT codes are created and the most common systems of payment important to anesthesia professionals.

When a specialty society, payer, industry, individual, or any interested stakeholder identifies a need for a new procedure code, that individual or group submits a formal proposal to the AMA, which has established a well-defined process that must be followed. Representatives from all specialties seated in the AMA House of Delegates have the opportunity to review all proposals and offer comments or suggestions. The members of the CPT Editorial Panel make decisions on acceptance, rejection, final wording, and guidelines for use. The 2023 Panel consists of 21 members, including its chair and cochair. The AMA Board of Trustees selects most members from a pool of physicians nominated by the participating specialty societies. Additional members represent nonphysician health care professionals nominated by the AMA Healthcare Professionals Advisory Committee (HCPAC). The remaining members are representatives from CMS, America's Health Insurance Plans, the American Hospital Association, and the BCBSA.

In 1992, the U.S. government introduced a payment system for the Medicare program to value medical procedures based on the resources used, rather than using the local usual and customary fee. Each service paid under this resource-based relative value system (RBRVS) scale has associated relative value units (RVUs) to account for work, practice expense, and professional liability insurance. Long before the introduction of RBRVS, the American Society of Anesthesiologists (ASA) developed a relative value system for anesthesia services. This system uses a different scale in which each anesthesia code has an associated base unit value assigned, recognizing the complexity of the case. Time units calculated by the exact minutes reported on a claim reflect the time taken to perform the anesthetic service, and modifier units reflect patient condition, emergency status, and several other situations that impact anesthesia care. Medicare uses a modification of the ASA system to pay for anesthesia care in the RBRVS. At this time, nearly all payers use the anesthesia payment system, and over 75% use RBRVS. This method of assigning a relative value to each specific service holds its importance under MACRA's QPP. These values, as published each year in the Medicare Physician Fee Schedule, are the baseline for the positive or negative QPP adjustments that are applied to Medicare Part B payments.

Once the CPT Editorial Panel approves a new code or revises an existing code, the next step is to assign or update the value of the code in the RBRVS. In the early 1990s, the AMA and many medical specialty societies jointly created a committee to provide comments to CMS on the value of services covered by this new system. This AMA/Specialty Society Relative Value Scale Update Committee, known as the RUC, has played a very important role in the ongoing refinement of the RBRVS over the ensuing years. The composition of the RUC includes representatives from the AMA, the CPT Editorial Panel, the American Osteopathic Association, HCPAC, and permanent and rotating seats for specialty societies. Representatives from CMS attend the meetings as well. For new and revised codes, specialty societies conduct surveys of physicians who are knowledgeable about the service under review, comparing the work associated with this service with that of a service with an established and accepted valuation. Specialty societies analyze the data and present the results, along with their recommendations as to the value of the service, to the RUC. The specialty societies also submit information on clinical staff, equipment, and supply expenses associated with the service that CMS uses in creating practice expense relative values. The RUC reviews all the materials and listens to the specialty societies' arguments. The RUC then forwards its own recommendations to CMS. These recommendations require a two-thirds vote to approve, helping ensure that the RUC's submissions reflect the consensus opinion of organized medicine. It is important to note that CMS makes the ultimate decision on the value to be assigned to a service. For codes reviewed for the 2022 fee schedule, CMS accepted approximately 77% of the RUC's work value recommendations. Revaluation of a service via the RUC survey process can also be triggered if the service is identified by the RUC or CMS as being potentially misvalued.

## Anesthesia Coding

Anesthesia services are described by CPT codes 00100 through 01999. This section of CPT is subdivided into body regions. For example, anesthesia for procedures on the upper arm and elbow is grouped into codes 01710 to 01782. Codes 01810 to 01860 are used to report anesthesia for procedures on the forearm, wrist, and hand. When coding for anesthesia care, modifiers are used to provide additional information about the patient, provide additional information about the circumstances in which the care was provided, or both. The former is accomplished via a physical status (PS) modifier and the latter with a qualifying circumstance code. The ASA PS assessment, which ranges from 1 for healthy patients through 5 for moribund patients and 6 for an organ donor, has corresponding modifiers (P1 to P6). Depending on the payer, these modifiers can yield higher payments. Information to assist anesthesiologists in making the clinically based PS assignment is available from ASA at https://www.asahq.org/standards-and-guidelines/asa-physical-status-classification-system.

Medicare does not recognize additional units for PS or qualifying circumstances, but many private payers will do so. This should be clearly addressed in contracts with private payers.

A number of practice models exist for delivering anesthesia care in the United States. Sometimes anesthesiologists work alone. Sometimes resident physicians or nonphysician anesthesia clinicians (certified anesthesiologist assistants or certified registered nurse anesthetists [CRNAs]) work with an anesthesiologist on the anesthesia care team; sometimes the nonphysician anesthetist may work under the supervision of a surgeon or, depending on state law, independently. Medicare and some private payers have specific payment rules that affect payment, depending on the mode of anesthesia practice. Medicare has created certain payment modifiers to report these various circumstances, which many private payers use as well.

ASA publishes two very important resources to aid practices in coding for the anesthesia services they provide. The Relative Value Guide (RVG) provides a basic overview of anesthesia coding, along with a list of all the anesthesia CPT codes with the associated base unit value. The CROSSWALK offers assistance in selecting the exact code that best describes the anesthesia service provided, based on the surgical service or services performed. All the coding resources cited in this chapter (CPT, HCPCS, ICD-10-CM, RVG, and CROSSWALK) are reviewed and updated each year. For this reason, use of outdated editions is penny wise and dollar foolish, because it will eventually lead to incorrect codes being submitted, may be seen as fraudulent or abusive practice, and could lead to civil or criminal prosecution.

## Payment Methodology Illustrations—Anesthesia

The following formula is used to determine payment for an anesthesia service:

$$\text{Allowed amount} = (\text{Base units} + \text{Time units} + \text{Modifying factors}) \times \text{Conversion factor}$$

where the allowed amount is the total payment for the service received from the insurer and the patient.

The base unit is a measure of the work involved in providing the anesthesia care. The higher the base unit value, the more complex the care. The work covered by the base unit value includes all of the typical preanesthesia and postanesthesia work and excludes only the time spent directly delivering anesthesia and any modifying factors.

Anesthesia time according to the ASA RVG, is determined as follows: "Anesthesia time is defined as the period during which an anesthesia practitioner is present with the patient. It starts when the anesthesia practitioner begins to prepare the patient for anesthesia services in the operating room or in an equivalent area and ends when the anesthesia practitioner is no longer furnishing anesthesia services to the patient, that is, when the patient is safely placed under postoperative care." Anesthesia time is reported in actual minutes, and the payer will convert that to time units based on the specifics agreed to by contract. Medicare uses a 15-minute unit and will calculate the number of time units out to one decimal place. Commercial payers often use 15-minute units, but this should be verified because other intervals may be used.

The modifying factor is a modifier based on the PS or qualifying circumstance code. The *conversion factor* is the number of dollars paid per unit.

Medicare has specific payment rules that apply when an anesthesiologist medically directs anesthesia care or is involved in teaching of residents. Separate Medicare teaching rules also apply to teaching of CRNA students. Some commercial and other governmental payers have adopted Medicare teaching rules in whole or in part. Because of the complexity of the rules and variability in implementation by payer, we will not discuss these scenarios in this chapter.

## ILLUSTRATION 1

A physician anesthesiologist provided anesthesia care for a patient undergoing a cholecystectomy. Anesthesia time was 57 minutes, and the patient had severe systemic disease, classifying him as a P3, worth one unit. According to the group's contract with the patient's insurer, the conversion factor is $85 per unit and time is calculated using a 15-minute unit out to one decimal place. Per the ASA CROSSWALK, the proper anesthesia code associated with a cholecystectomy is 00790. Code 00790 has seven base units. Assuming the payer uses a 15-minute time unit, calculation is as follows:

$$\text{Allowed amount} = (\text{Base units} + \text{Time units}$$
$$+ \text{Modifying factors}) \times \text{Conversion factor}$$
$$= (7 + 3.8 + 1) \times \$85$$
$$= \$1003.00$$

## ILLUSTRATION 2

The anesthesiologist provided anesthesia care for a female patient undergoing drainage of a deep periurethral abscess. In this instance the CROSSWALK offers two potential anesthesia codes. The primary selection is code 00920—Anesthesia for procedures on male genitalia (including open urethral procedures); not otherwise specified. The alternate code is code 00942—Anesthesia for vaginal procedures (including biopsy of labia, vagina, cervix, or endometrium); colpotomy, vaginectomy, colporrhaphy, and open urethral procedures. The patient's sex directs you to select the alternate offering. The RVG tells you that code 00942 has four base units. The anesthesia time is 46 minutes and there are no modifying factors. The contracted conversion factor is $75 per unit and time units are calculated to a whole unit:

$$\text{Allowed amount} = (\text{Base units} + \text{Time units}$$
$$+ \text{Modifying factors}) \times \text{Conversion factor}$$
$$= (4 + 3 + 0) \times \$75$$
$$= \$525.00$$

Medicare payments adjust to account for economic differences based on geography. Each Medicare billing area applies slightly different adjustments to the national anesthesia conversion factor, which was $21.56 in 2021. For example, the 2021 Medicare anesthesia conversion factor ranged from $29.88 in Alaska to $20.24 in Nebraska.

## Payment Methodology Illustrations—Resource-Based Relative Value System

A different formula is used to determine payment for nonanesthesia services. Medicare and many private payers use the RBRVS. Under RBRVS, RVUs are assigned to the work, practice expense, and professional liability insurance components of each service.

These RVUs are added together, and the resulting sum is multiplied by a conversion factor. The formula is as follows:

$$\text{Allowed amount} = (\text{Work RVU} + \text{PE RVU} + \text{PLI RVU})$$
$$\times \text{Conversion factor}$$

where PE refers to practice expense and PLI to professional liability insurance.

## ILLUSTRATION 3

A physician anesthesiologist provides anesthesia care for a patient, and the patient requires placement of an arterial line to provide a more detailed level of monitoring. We will use the 2021 Medicare RBRVS conversion factor of $34.8931 per unit. Placement of an arterial line is reported with CPT code 36620. The RVUs assigned to this code in 2021 are shown in Table 237.1.

Multiplying the total RVUs by the conversion factor results in an allowed amount of $45.01.

The RBRVS method accounts for geographic differences by making adjustments to the RVUs assigned to each component (work, PE, and PLI) of each service, leaving the conversion factor constant across the country.

A physician's Medicare participation status is another determinant of their Medicare payment. The details of Medicare participation are beyond the scope of this chapter, and the reader is referred to the AMA's Guide on Medicare Participation.

## Conclusion

Anesthesiologists perform some services for Medicare patients, which are paid by the anesthesia methodology, and other services that are paid under the RBRVS method. Commercial payers might use these same methods. As such, anesthesiologists must understand both systems. Terms of payment are also increasingly determined or modified by value-based or alternative payment models (see Chapter 231, Value Based Payment Models). Anesthesiologists should also have a broad-based understanding of the overall CPT coding system because the anesthesia codes they report depend on the more than 6000 diagnostic and therapeutic CPT-described services that may require anesthesia care. Finally, anesthesiologists must understand how to code for line placement, image guidance, pain procedures, transesophageal echocardiography, critical care, inpatient and outpatient evaluation and management visits, and other services unrelated to anesthesia care and may be separately reported.

| TABLE 237.1 | RBRVS Relative Value Units for Arterial Line Placement | | | |
|---|---|---|---|---|
| Code | Descriptor | 2021 Work RVU | 2021 Facility PE RVU | 2021 PLI RVU | Total 2021 RVUs |
| 36620 | Arterial catheterization or cannulation for sampling, monitoring, or transfusion (separate procedure); percutaneous | 1.00 | 0.20 | 0.09 | 1.29 |

PE, Practice expense, PLI, professional liability insurance; RVU, relative value unit.

## SUGGESTED READINGS

AMA. *Medicare participation guide.* Retrieved from https://www.ama-assn.org/system/files/2019-05/know-options-medicare-participation-guide.pdf. Accessed September 8, 2021.

AMA/Specialty Society. *RVS Update Committee.* Retrieved from https://www.ama-assn.org/about/rvs-update-committee-ruc. Accessed October 28, 2021.

AMA. *CPT (Current Procedural Terminology).* Retrieved from https://www.ama-assn.org/about/cpt-editorial-panel. Accessed September 8, 2021.

Healthcare Common Procedures Coding System (HCPCS). *HCPCS general information.* Retrieved from https://www.cms.gov/Medicare/Coding/MedHCPCSGenInfo/index.html. Accessed October 28, 2021.

CMS. *ICD-10-CM.* Retrieved from https://www.cms.gov/Medicare/Coding/ICD10/index.html. Accessed October 28, 2018.

# 238

# Chemical Dependence in Anesthesia Personnel

RICARDO VERDINER, MD

The past two decades has seen an explosion in the consumption and abuse of controlled substances by the general population. Overdose deaths have increased 200% since 2000. A potential contributor to this trend was the changes in the 1990s in government policies toward regulation of prescription opiates along with changing sentiment of the medical community. Opioid manufacturers were influential in shifting pain management strategies. The campaigns to view pain as a fifth vital sign led to increases in the number of opioid prescriptions. Pain relief and opioid addiction were disassociated from the minds of the prescribers, as well as the recipients of opioids. The belief was simply that addiction risk was minimal in the presence of pain; to restrict opioids was to allow the patient to undergo undue suffering. Since then, regulations and policies have tightened in an attempt to counter the epidemic. However, the increasing trend toward substance abuse still persists within the general population. This will likely result in higher percentages of the workforce requiring treatment or having had treatment for substance abuse. This trend will no doubt be reflected in future students entering medical school and, by extension, future residents in the specialty of anesthesiology. Thus it is imperative that the stakeholders within the subspecialty assume the responsibility of taking a proactive approach to mitigating the risks that substance abuse and addiction have on the practice of anesthesiology. The aim of this chapter is to identify the risk factors for substance use disorder (SUD), discuss prevention, recognize the signs of addiction, discuss intervention, and acknowledge the risk of relapse despite treatment.

The potency, addictive potential, and accessibility of mind-altering substances within the operating room setting were always viewed as contributors to the increased prevalence of substance abuse among anesthesia providers. Studies have suggested that risk factors besides accessibility and pharmacology may also exist. An analysis of anesthesiology residents in the United States by Warner in 2015 suggested that males were much more likely to develop SUD than females. Despite comparable scores in the clinical base year, the study also showed individuals with SUD had lower in-training exam scores by the second year of training in comparison to their cohorts. Other studies suggested a history of psychiatric disorders, younger age of trainees, family history of substance abuse, and repetitive exposure to microscopic amounts of anesthetic drugs in the operating room may contribute to the increased prevalence and recurrence of SUD in anesthesia care providers. These risk factors have translated into a rising incidence of SUD of 2.87 per 1000 resident years during the period of 2003 to 2009 in Warner's study. The outcomes of that increased incidence include failure to complete residency, failure to become board certified or achieve subspecialty certification, increased risk of loss or restriction of medical licensure, and increased risk of death. In a survey by Booth and colleagues, 7% to 18% of substance abuse by physicians had the presenting symptom of death or near fatal overdose.

Given these consequences, the desire to reduce substance abuse through prevention has taken many forms. Education of trainees on the hazards of SUD and the appropriate handling of controlled substances have been a staple of training programs for decades. Many pharmacy departments routinely audit controlled substance transactions and assay wasted drugs to verify consistency with the anesthetic records. Any deviation or unusual administration pattern flags the pharmacy of potential substance abuse or drug diversion by anesthesia care providers. Some anesthesiology departments have implemented random drug screenings as both a layer of surveillance and deterrent to substance abuse. However, this approach has been met with some resistance, and national consensus has yet to be established.

Though preventive measures have their merits, identification of signs of substance abuse in many cases has been lifesaving. Workplace performance has historically been a late sign of SUD. Addiction focuses the individual's attention on securing a drug source. In most cases the anesthesia care provider's job has been their access to the drug and therefore not likely to be placed in jeopardy through lapsed assignments, tardiness, or absences. Instead, changes in behavior like mood swings, increased episodes of irritability, and withdrawal from loved ones and leisure activity have been earlier signs. Dramatic increases in the amounts of medications administered or wasted have also been a potential sign of SUD.

When abuse is suspected, the importance has been placed on intervention versus waiting until evidence of addiction or drug diversion was secured "beyond a reasonable doubt." The risk of death or severe brain injury from substance abuse increases the longer intervention is delayed. Waiting for certainty has been viewed as too great a cost. Instead, an approach should be undertaken that *does not* include a one-on-one with the suspect. Confronting the person one-on-one may result in them reacting impulsively or attempting suicide. A collective and coordinated intervention should include representation from the employee health department, the wellness department, and/or an addiction specialist. The individual should be escorted from the work environment to the employee health clinic or emergency department where immediate drug testing would be performed. Once confirmed, the individual should be transferred to an addiction facility that specializes in treatment of health care professionals to avoid self-harm or an unexpected response.

Controversy does exist on whether addicted physicians should return to anesthesiology after treatment. A study by Warner estimated a 43% risk of at least one relapse by 30 years from the initial episode. This rate has remained consistent for 40 years. In that study 13% of those who did relapse died as a direct result of substance abuse. Not surprisingly, the risk for relapse somewhat parallels the risk for SUD. In a study by Domino a 13-fold increase in relapse risk was seen when a family history of SUD, history of psychiatric disorder, and history of opioid addiction were simultaneously present. Greater rates of recovery from addiction were found when there was late onset of addiction (addicts older than 30 vs. teenage addiction), random urine testing, employment jeopardy, 12-step recovery groups, and long-term treatment with inpatient/outpatient 5-year components.

Substance abuse remains an occupational hazard in the field of anesthesiology. Despite decades of education and hospital-mandated protocols on the handling of controlled substances, the rates of SUD have demonstrated an increasing trend. New methods of clinical practice surveillance and screening for those considered at high risk for substance abuse may one day be necessary. Treatment of substance abuse alone, particularly opioid abuse, have not demonstrated sufficient success in those who return to practice anesthesiology. The high rate of relapse and death provide enough evidence to warrant further modification of treatment and prevention tactics. When considering whether an anesthesiologist, anesthesiologist assistant, or nurse anesthetist should return to practice, the present data suggests engagement in long-term treatment, abstinence from all mind-altering substances, random urine testing, and 12-step recovery groups should be mandatory.

## SUGGESTED READINGS

Berge, K. H., Seppala, M. D., & Schipper, A. M. (2009). Chemical dependency and the physician. *Mayo Clinic Proceedings, 84*(7), 625–631.

Booth, J. V., Grossman, D., Moore, J., Lineberger, C., Reynolds, J. D., Reves, J. G., et al. (2002). Substance abuse among physicians: A survey of academic anesthesiology programs. *Anesthesia and Analgesia, 95*(4), 1024–1030. table of contents.

Bryson, E. O., & Hamza, H. (2011). The drug seeking anesthesia care provider. *International Anesthesiology Clinics, 49*(1), 157–171.

Bryson, E. O. (2018). The opioid epidemic and the current prevalence of substance use disorder in anesthesiologists. *Current Opinion in Anaesthesiology, 31*(3), 388–392.

Domino, K. B., Hornbein, T. F., Polissar, N. L., Renner, G., Johnson, J., Alberti, S., et al. (2005). Risk factors for relapse in health care professionals with substance use disorders. *JAMA, 293*(12), 1453–1460.

DuPont, R. L., McLellan, A. T., White, W. L., Merlo, L. J., & Gold, M. S. (2009). Setting the standard for recovery: Physicians' health programs. *Journal of Substance Abuse Treatment, 36*(2), 159–171.

Gold, M. S., Melker, R. J., Dennis, D. M., Morey, T. E., Bajpai, L. K., Pomm, R., et al. (2006). Fentanyl abuse and dependence: Further evidence for second hand exposure hypothesis. *Journal of Addictive Diseases, 25*(1), 15–21.

Long, M. W., Cassidy, B. A., Sucher, M., & Stoehr, J. D. (2006). Prevention of relapse in the recovery of

Arizona health care providers. *Journal of Addictive Diseases, 25*(1), 65–72.

Ostling, P. S., Davidson, K. S., Anyama, B. O., Helander, E. M., Wyche, M. Q., & Kaye, A. D. (2018). America's opioid epidemic: A comprehensive review and look into the rising crisis. *Current Pain and Headache Reports, 22*(5), 32.

Samuelson, S. T., & Bryson, E. O. (2017). The impaired anesthesiologist: What you should know about substance abuse. *Canadian Journal of Anaesthesia, 64*(2), 219–235.

Warner, D. O., Berge, K., Sun, H., Harman, A., Hanson, A., & Schroeder, D. R. (2015). Risk and outcomes of substance use disorder among anesthesiology residents: A matched cohort analysis. *Anesthesiology, 123*(4), 929–936.

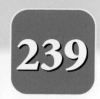

# 239

# Sustainability in Anesthesiology and the Operating Room

ANDREW MURRAY, MBChB

Climate change has been noted to be a significant health risk by the Lancet Commission on Climate change. It has also been estimated by the World Health Organization to cause 250,000 excess deaths per year. For perspective, this is similar to the number of deaths ascribed to medical errors in "To Err Is Human." As health care providers, we are on the front lines of dealing with the increases in health risk while being, as anesthesia providers, significant contributors to the problem of environmental contamination with anesthetic gas and solid waste.

Along with this concern, the degradation of the natural environment needs to be mentioned as well. Health care as an industry has been identified as a significant contributor to climate change, with some estimates stating that the contribution to greenhouse gas (GHG) emissions is between 4.6% and 10% of the national greenhouse gas production in the United States and Canada. Furthermore, the impact of the health care industry also takes the form of excess resource utilization and production of nonrecyclable waste that contributes to landfill operations.

More pointedly, we will discuss the areas that anesthesiologists and certified registered nurse anesthetists can directly influence by adjusting their practice.

## Inhaled Anesthetic Gases

Although historically, the risk of anesthetic gases has centered on the exposure of the provider to these gases, more recent emphasis on their effects on the atmosphere and climate change has started to change provider awareness. Anesthetic gases, though they contribute a small amount to waste, are very potent greenhouse gases. Their impact as measured by global warming potential for 100 years ($GWP_{100}$) is the projected greenhouse gas effect when related to carbon dioxide ($CO_2$), with $CO_2$ forming the base value of 1.

To provide perspective, the US contribution of inhaled anesthetic gases to the atmosphere is estimated to be equivalent to the $CO_2$ emissions of one coal-fired powerplant or one million cars per year. Another example quoted is that a car traveling for 210 hours from northern Norway to Cape Town, South Africa, will emit an amount similar to a 7-hour anesthetic with 2 L/m fresh gas flow (FGF) and desflurane (DES) at 1 minimum alveolar concentration (MAC) with 66% $N_2O$.

Anesthetic gases implicated are the hydrofluorocarbons sevoflurane (SEV), halothane (HAL), DES, and isoflurane (ISO), as well as nitrous oxide ($N_2O$). ISO and HAL contain bromine and chlorine that deplete the ozone layer, thus also limiting the protective effect of the ozone layer on ultraviolet radiation. SEV and DES, though not containing bromine or chlorine, still function as greenhouse gases by absorbing outbound infrared radiation, thus limiting nocturnal cooling.

Although volatile anesthetic gases are a small absolute amount compared with $CO_2$ emissions, their effect is relatively

| TABLE 239.1 | Greenhouse Gas Effect of Anesthetic Gases Relative to Carbon Dioxide | |
|---|---|---|
| **Gas** | **$GWP_{100}$** | |
| $CO_2$ | 1 | |
| ISO | 510 | |
| SEV | 130 | |
| DES | 2540 | |
| $N_2O$ | 298 | |

*$CO_2$*, Carbon dioxide; *DES*, desflurane; *$GWP_{100}$*, global warming potential for 100 years; *ISO*, isoflurane; *$N_2O$*, nitrous oxide; *SEV*, sevoflurane.

| TABLE 239.2 | Lifetime of Gases |
|---|---|
| **Compound** | **Lifetime in Atmosphere (years)** |
| $N_2O$ | 114 |
| DES | 14 |
| HAL | 4 |
| ISO | 3.2 |
| SEV | 1.1 |

*DES*, Desflurane; *HAL*, halothane; *ISO*, isoflurane; *$N_2O$*, nitrous oxide; *SEV*, sevoflurane.

outsized because of their significantly increased effect compared with $CO_2$, as well as their long half-lives. Most of these gases are exhausted via the waste anesthesia gas (WAG) system with little or no metabolism in the patient. The GHG effect of each gas relative to $CO_2$ can be seen in Table 239.1. The lifetime of the gases can be seen in Table 239.2.

Limiting the use of the worst offenders can have a profound effect. Simply eliminating the availability of DES unless requested has been shown to decrease the amount used by 25%. This can also have a financial benefit, as DES is the most expensive volatile anesthetic and has been reported to make up to 83% to 86% of volatile costs.

Nitrous oxide when combined with SEV/oxygen ($O_2$) was found to increase emissions intensity by 900% compared with SEV/$O_2$/air. It is recommended to use $N_2O$ only where there is a clear clinical benefit. Consideration can also be given to use of regional and/or local anesthetic techniques in locations where $N_2O$ is used heavily, such as dental offices or labor and delivery suites.

The method in which the anesthesia provider chooses to use a volatile anesthetic can impact its environmental effect especially when looking at FGF chosen to deliver the anesthetic (Table 239.3).

**775**

| TABLE 239.3 | Effectiveness of Fresh Gas Flow on Environmental Impact of an Anesthetic | | | |
|---|---|---|---|---|
| 1 MAC Inhaled Agent at FGF | Atmospheric Lifetime | $GWP_{100}$ | Equivalent Miles Driven per Hour of Anesthetic | |
| SEV 2% @ 2L | 1.1 | 130 | 8 | |
| ISO 1.2% @ 2L | 3.2 | 510 | 18 | |
| ISO 1.2%@ 1L | | | 9 | |
| DES 6% @ 2L | 14 | 2540 | 400 | |
| DES 6% @ 1L | | | 200 | |
| 60% $NO_2$ @ 1L | 114 | 298 | 61 | |

DES, Desflurane; FGF, fresh gas flow; $GWP_{100}$, global warming potential for 100 years; ISO, isoflurane; MAC, minimum alveolar concentration; $N_2O$, nitrous oxide; SEV, sevoflurane.

## Intravenous Anesthetic Agents

Intravenous anesthetic agents (IVAA) have the benefit that they are not exhaled by the patient in significant quantities; however, they present challenges of their own. They produce glass, needle, and plastic waste, as well as the risk of accumulation in the environment. Many of these agents are excreted unchanged from the patient and are not captured or eliminated by the wastewater management systems. They have been implicated in alteration of endocrine and neurologic systems, and some have carcinogenic or teratogenic effects

## Mitigation Efforts for Environmental Effects of Anesthetic Agents

When evaluating the effect of anesthetic gases, one must take into account how they are used. Higher FGF, MAC, and the atmospheric persistence of the agent in question must be weighed. Increased FGF will lead to greater use and thus greater atmospheric venting. The higher an agent's MAC, the greater amount of the agent must be used to obtain the desired anesthetic effect. The higher atmospheric persistence of the DES and $N_2O$ makes both agents less desirable. Some will propose the use of $N_2O$ to lessen the amount of volatile gas being used, but this ignores the higher flows needed, as well as the inherent detrimental effects of $N_2O$.

A relatively simple mitigation strategy for limiting the effects of these agents is to either eliminate DES or limit it to special request only. If it is to be used, it should be used without $N_2O$ and with ultralow flow technique. $N_2O$ should only be considered if there is a clear clinical benefit to be gained by the patient.

Lowering FGF is not always a solution because of the concern, in the case of SEV, of reactive compounds being created by reaction with the $CO_2$ absorber, specifically compound A. This compound is nephrotoxic and is produced when SEV interacts with traditional $CO_2$ absorbers. This can be mitigated with the adoption of calcium hydroxide and lithium hydroxide absorbers. In the setting of traditional sodium chloride and potassium chloride absorbers, the use of lower gas flows for 2 hours has been found to have low risk of Compound A production.

Another strategy is to shut off FGF when disconnecting the patient from the breathing circuit (e.g., during intubation) instead of shutting off the volatile only. This technique eliminates the venting of the residual volatile agent in the circuit into the room.

Ensuring that the ventilatory system is devoid of any leaks will also minimize inadvertent contamination of the environment.

Sequestration systems exist that serve to capture the volatile anesthetic as it is vented from the machine while allowing for the near-complete capture of all volatile anesthetic agents in a canister. Exploration is ongoing about whether these agents can be reclaimed, purified, and then reused for clinical use. These systems need to be attached to the anesthetic machine and will be collected for further processing either on-site or remotely by a third-party vendor. However, this may incur a fee for the health care institution in the form of a charge by the vendor. One hurdle for the employment of this system is that in the United States, the U.S. Food and Drug Administration (FDA) has not approved the resale and/or reuse of captured volatile anesthetic agents. One potential benefit of a recapture and reuse system is that it may remove the need for a WAG system from the design of operating rooms. Although still theoretical, a clear benefit would be reduction in construction costs by the elimination of the need for a WAG system.

Propofol is not degraded in the environment and has been shown to have toxic effects on aquatic animals. In addition to this, propofol accounts for 45% of drug waste by volume. Because of the concern for infection risk, single-use vials are used, but if care is not taken in selecting an appropriate size container, significant waste may occur. Because of the lack of environmental degradation, the only feasible way to eliminate propofol is through incineration, which is typically energy intensive.

All things considered, switching from inhaled anesthetics to IVAA results in a net environmental benefit in favor of the intravenous (IV) anesthetic, which includes accounting for the increased plastic and glass waste.

## Reusable, Reprocessed, or Disposable

There has been a noticeable move toward the use of single-use devices (SUD) driven somewhat by unit cost and fear of infection. Unfortunately, this has led to an increase in the amount of waste being generated in the operating room. This includes disposable drapes, gowns, instruments, and, more specifically to anesthesia, the advent of disposable laryngoscopes, handles, and even bronchoscopes.

SUD are designated as such by the manufacturer, not the FDA, leaving the opportunity for reprocessing equipment for multiple uses when cleaned, tested, and packaged by a medical reprocessing company. This concept has been applied to surgical instrumentation and can also be applied to airway management equipment like videolaryngoscope handles.

Other devices can be made of materials that allow for sterilization and high-level disinfection. An example is the silicone supraglottic airway, which can be cleaned and reused safely as many as 40 times (manufacturer-recommended reuse). This has the effect of lessening waste produced (packaging), and a cost savings might also be achieved, thus benefiting the health system and allowing the purchase of other much-needed services.

It must be recognized that this cannot be applied to all devices. A complete life cycle analysis (LCA) should be used to determine whether disposable or reusable equipment is more beneficial for both the environment and the institution. LCAs have shown that a 50% GHG reduction is possible in laparoscopic surgery using reusable instruments. Likewise, limited-use reusable SGAs have a carbon footprint of almost half of that of SUDs. Although disposable devices may be viewed as cheaper to acquire, an LCA showed the cumulative annual excess cost of disposable laryngoscopes was approximately $500,000 for handles and $200,000 for blades. The above examples point to the cost benefits of reusable devices, but an opposing example exists where an LCA looking at central cannulation devices concluded that disposable devices had a less deleterious environmental impact than reusable devices.

## Solid Waste

A commonly used estimate is that each surgical procedure produces an equivalent amount of solid waste as a family of four does in a week. Eighty percent of the solid waste from a procedure is generated even before the patient enters the room, thus presenting an opportunity to limit the amount of "clean" waste in the form of more recyclable packaging. Manufacturers should be rethinking the way items come packaged to limit the number of individually wrapped items and instead having systems (e.g., IV tubing sets) preconfigured and assembled in a single package of recyclable plastic.

An active recycling program at a hospital can seek to capture as much recyclable plastic and paper waste as possible. This will necessitate education of staff about what is suitable to recycle while also providing receptacles to facilitate this activity. Also required is enough staffing support from the environmental services department, as well as support from a recycling vendor.

## Putting It Into Practice

Traditionally the three Rs have been employed: reduce, reuse, and recycle. One author has suggested that two more Rs be added: rethink and research.

Reduction would incorporate finding ways to limit individual packaging for multiple small pieces of equipment that could be bundled in a single container. In addition, working with equipment vendors to remove unnecessary items in a container can help eliminate excess waste. Only opening what one needs for a procedure can further enhance this effort.

Reuse of items previously deemed SUD by the manufacturer can be achieved in some situations where it is deemed safe for the patient and economical for the institution. This can also be achieved by adopting reusable drapes, gowns, and surgical equipment.

Recycling should be promoted and encouraged at every opportunity, but this does take a significant amount of education, as well as possible staffing and infrastructure management to maximize this opportunity.

Rethink should encourage us all to consider the way we carry out our daily tasks and actively search for opportunities to improve our environmental impact in ways that are favorable for patient safety and potential cost savings.

Researching which actions help providers practice in a more environmentally responsible way can limit waste. Investigating how providers respond to messaging is important. Messaging may take the form of "nudges" designed to help the provider as they make decisions throughout their day. This can be delivered by a high-tech method, such as prompts in the electronic health record, or a low-tech method, such as simple signs placed on machines to encourage lower flows or gas choices.

Eliminating choice may also serve to achieve this if it is done in a responsible manner that does not frustrate the provider. Examples of this might be restricting the use of DES or the size of propofol vials available to eliminate waste

## Summary

As anesthesia providers, we are able to significantly influence the impact of the operating room on both patient and environmental well-being. This can be achieved by responsible anesthetic choices and limiting excess waste generation. However, our greatest impact comes from interaction with hospital and operating room decision makers to change practices to minimize waste. Shared goals include curbing institutional costs while maximizing patient, societal, and environmental benefits of the dollars spent. The cost savings may be a powerful incentive for health care institutions to make these needed changes.

## SUGGESTED READINGS

Choi, B. J. J., & Chen, C. L. (2022). The triple bottom line and stabilization wedges: A framework for perioperative sustainability. *Anesthesia and Analgesia, 134*(3), 475–485.

ASA. (2017). *Greening the operating room and perioperative Arena: Environmental sustainability for anesthesia practice*. American Society of Anesthesiologists. Retrieved from https://www.asahq.org/about-asa/governance-and-committees/asa-committees/environmental-sustainability/greening-the-operating-room. Accessed April 28, 2022.

Muret, J., & Kelway, C. Members of the SFAR's Sustainability Group French Society of Anaesthesia & Intensive Care. (2019). Why should anaesthesiologists and intensivists care about climate change? *Anaesthesia Critical Care & Pain Medicine, 38*(6), 565–567.

Petre, M. A., Bahrey, L., Levine, M., van Rensburg, A., Crawford, M., & Matava, C. T. (2020). Anesthesia environmental sustainability programs: A survey of Canadian department chiefs and residency program directors. *Canadian Journal of Anaesthesia, 67*(9), 1190–1200.

Petre, M. A., & Malherbe, S. (2020). Environmentally sustainable perioperative medicine: Simple strategies for anesthetic practice. *Canadian Journal of Anaesthesia, 67*(8), 1044–1063.

Van Norman, G. A., & Jackson, S. (2020). The anesthesiologist and global climate change: An ethical obligation to act. *Current Opinion in Anaesthesiology, 33*(4), 577–583.

Page numbers followed by "*f*" indicate figures, "*t*" indicate tables, and "*b*" indicate boxes.